Greenberg's

TEXT-ATLAS OF EMERGENCY MEDICINE

ASSOCIATE EDITORS

Robert G. Hendrickson, MD
Assistant Professor
Department of Emergency Medicine
Oregon Health and Science University
Medical Toxicologist
Oregon Poison Center
Portland, Oregon

Mark Silverberg, MD
Assistant Professor
Department of Emergency Medicine
SUNY Downstate Medical Center
Director of Senior Medical Student Education
Department of Emergency Medicine
Kings County Hospital Center
Brooklyn, NY

ASSISTANT EDITORS

Colleen J. Campbell, MD
Associate Clinical Professor
Department of Emergency Medicine
University of California, San Diego
San Diego, CA

Anthony P. Morocco, MD
EMS Medical Director
Guam Department of Public Health and Social Services
Mangilao, Guam
Attending Physician, Medical Toxicologist
Department of Emergency Medicine
Guam Memorial Hospital
Oka, Tamuning, Guam

Christy Ann Salvaggio, MD
Assistant Professor
Department of Emergency Medicine
Director of Pediatric Emergency Medicine
Drexel University College of Medicine
Pediatric Emergency Medicine Attending
St. Christopher's Hospital for Children
Philadelphia, PA

Matthew T. Spencer, MD
Assistant Professor
Department of Emergency Medicine
University of Rochester School of Medicine and Dentistry
Associate Residency Director
Department of Emergency Medicine
Strong Memorial Hospital
Rochester, NY

Greenberg's TEXT-ATLAS OF EMERGENCY MEDICINE

EDITOR-IN-CHIEF

Michael I. Greenberg, MD, MPH

Professor of Emergency Medicine
Department of Emergency Medicine
Drexel University College of Medicine
Professor of Public Health
Drexel University School of Public Health
Clinical Professor of Emergency Medicine
Department of Emergency Medicine
Temple University School of Medicine
Philadelphia, PA

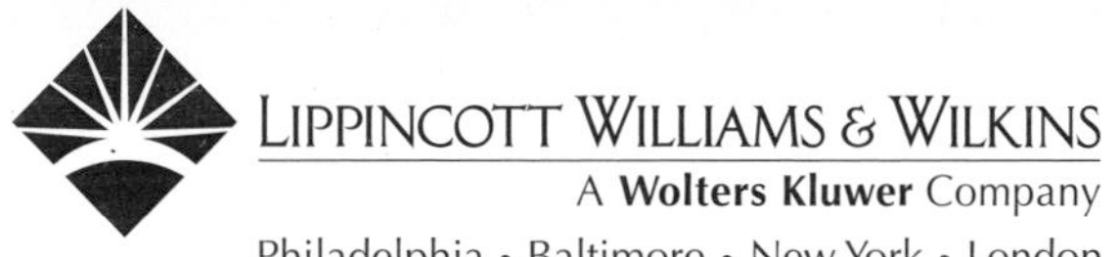
LIPPINCOTT WILLIAMS & WILKINS
A Wolters Kluwer Company
Philadelphia • Baltimore • New York • London
Buenos Aires • Hong Kong • Sydney • Tokyo

Acquisitions Editor: Anne Sydor
Developmental Editor: Kerry Barrett
Production Editor: Bridgett Dougherty
Manufacturing Manager: Benjamin Rivera
Marketing Manager: Adam Glazer
Cover Designer: Bill Donnelly
Compositor: Graphic World Publishing Services
Printer: Quebecor World Kingsport

530 Walnut Street
Philadelphia, PA 19106 USA
LWW.com

Printed in the USA

Library of Congress Cataloging in Publication

Greenberg's text-atlas of emergency medicine / editor-in-chief, Michael I. Greenberg ; associate editors, Robert G. Hendrickson, Mark Silverberg ; assistant editors, Colleen Campbell . . . [et al.].
p. ; cm.
Includes bibliographical references and index.
ISBN 0-7817-4586-1
1. Emergency medicine. 2. Emergency medicine--Atlases. I. Title: Text-atlas of emergency medicine. II. Greenberg, Michael I.
[DNLM: 1. Emergencies--Atlases. 2. Wounds and Injuries--Atlases. 3. Emergency Medicine--methods--Atlases. WB 17 G798 2005]
RC86.7.G745 2005
616.0295--dc22

2004048553

Care has been taken to confirm the accuracy of the information presented and to describe generally accepted practices. However, the authors and publisher are not responsible for errors or omissions or for any consequences from application of the information in this book and make no warranty, expressed or implied, with respect to the currency, completeness, or accuracy of the contents of the publication. Application of this information in a particular situation remains the professional responsibility of the practitioner.

The authors and publisher have exerted every effort to ensure that drug selection and dosage set forth in this text are in accordance with current recommendations and practice at the time of publication. However, in view of ongoing research, changes in government regulations, and the constant flow of information relating to drug therapy and drug reactions, the reader is urged to check the package insert for each drug for any change in indications and dosage and for added warnings and precautions. This is particularly important when the recommended agent is a new or infrequently employed drug.

Some drugs and medical devices presented in this publication have Food and Drug Administration (FDA) clearance for limited use in restricted research settings. It is the responsibility of the health care provider to ascertain the FDA status of each drug or device planned for use in their clinical practice.

10 9 8 7 6 5 4 3 2 1

This work is dedicated to Annette Toni Marie Gara and Jeffrey Scott McCabe, whose love changed my life for the better in ways that words simply cannot adequately express.

It is also dedicated to the memory of two people who I think about each and every day and whose incredible lives have helped me define my own: my daughter, Alexandra Jane Greenberg and my father, Alex Ellis Greenberg.

Michael I. Greenberg, MD, MPH
Wayne, Pennsylvania, July, 2004

To my wife, Jen, for her support, her energy, and her incredible ability to melt away the stresses of a long day at work with her smile. To all of the students, residents, and colleagues whose unending interest in emergency medicine are the source of my professional inspiration and motivation. And thank you to our patients who allow us to photograph their ailments for the benefit of others.

Robert G. Hendrickson, MD
Portland, Oregon, July, 2004

I dedicate this book to the physicians and colleagues who profoundly influenced my academic career, especially Dr. Rich Sinert, Dr. Lewis Kohl and my Department Chair, Dr. Michael Lucchesi. In addition, I dedicate this work to all the Emergency Medicine residents at Kings County Hospital who contributed written topics to this atlas and who searched tirelessly to find many of the images, x-rays, CTs and ultrasounds included in this atlas.

Mark Silverberg, MD, MMB, FACEP
Brooklyn, New York, July 2004

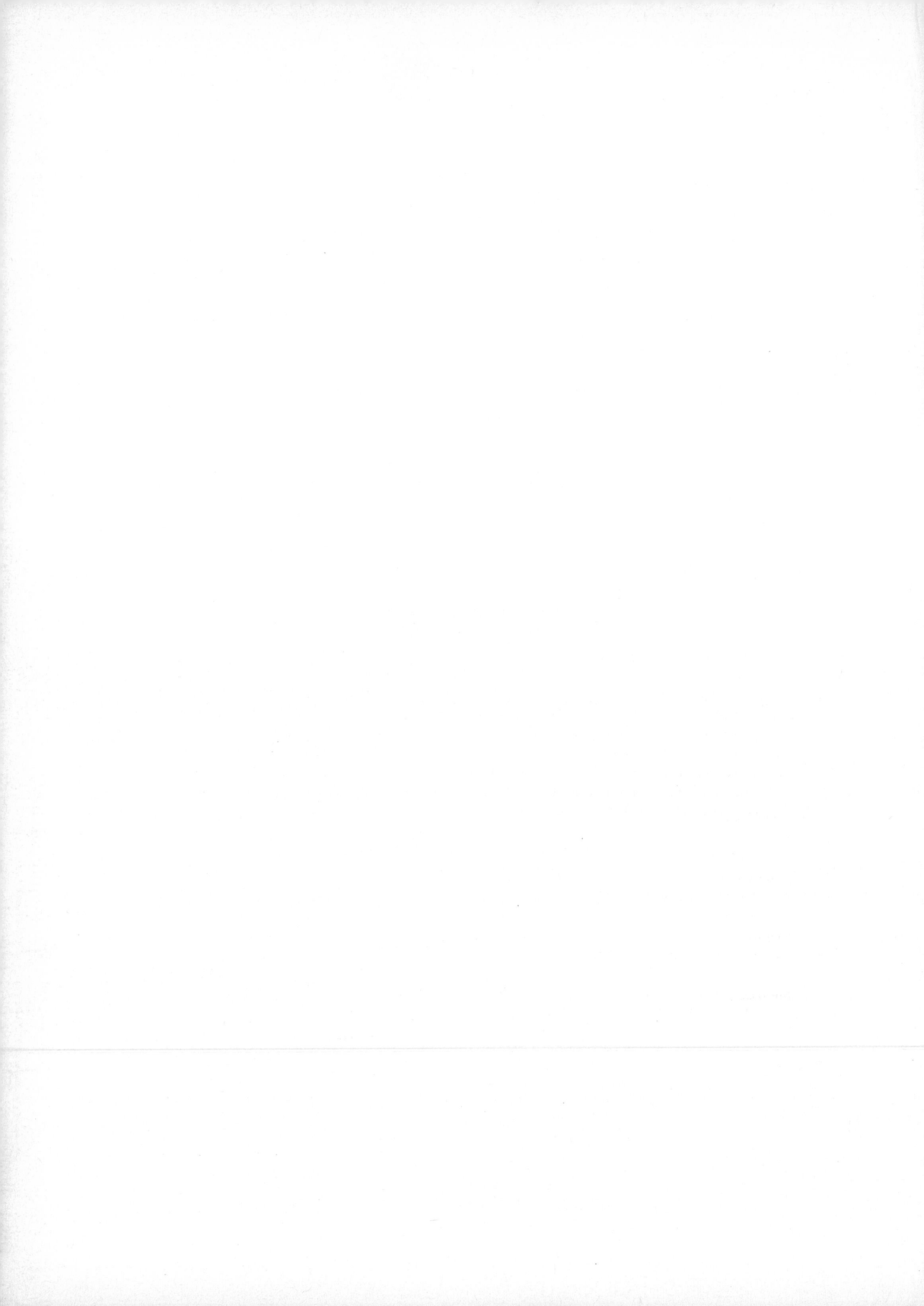

CONTENTS

SECTION V.
SPECIAL ISSUES, 927

FOREWORD

"Hearing a hundred times is not as good as seeing once."

-Ancient Japanese proverb

Drawings found on the walls of caves are the earliest record of human communication. Whether pictorial communication developed before language and whether we use pictures or words for thinking are subjects of on going debate. Regardless of the answers, the spoken and written word has been the dominant form of human communication for thousands of years, with literacy considered an essential skill in modern society. In recent years, however, images have assumed an increasing role in communication, particularly for enduring records (in medicine as well as history) and in education, entertainment, influence peddling (advertising), and journalism (news). Advances in visual imaging technology are partly responsible for this trend.

The popular adage "One picture is worth a thousand words" is attributed to Fred R. Barnard, who proposed the advantages of advertising with pictures and used similar phrases in two advertisements in a trade journal called *Printers' Ink* in the 1920s. Since then, this concept has been espoused by publicists and journalists as the most efficient way of communicating a message. That images can convey an idea or emotion more effectively than words has long been the unspoken mantra of painters and the appeal of visual art. We now know that some individuals are predominantly visual rather than auditory learners and that images improve comprehension of the written word for all. When information is presented as a combination of words and pictures (compared to when it is simply read or heard), learning is enhanced. Without words, however, the meaning of a picture is subject to misinterpretation and its educational value is greatly diminished.

While vision is an essential diagnostic tool in all specialties of medicine, with the exception of dermatology, pathology, and radiology, images in medical textbooks are few and far between and frequently consist of line drawings, sketches, or poorly reproduced black and white photographs. Part of the reason for this is that color images are expensive to reproduce and images add to the size and cost of a textbook, both of which can affect textbook sales and viability.

As the name suggests, *Greenberg's Text-Atlas of Emergency Medicine* combines written text with a collection of images and covers a wide variety of conditions encountered in the emergency department. The text is succinct, up-to-date, clinically-oriented, and includes supporting references. Pictures of anatomic findings, toxic exposures, electrocardiographs, radiographs, and other diagnostic tests, along with figures and tables, are used to illustrate and complement the prose. Color photographs abound and are vividly reproduced.

The liberal use of high-quality visual aids distinguishes *Greenberg's Text-Atlas of Emergency Medicine* from other emergency medicine textbooks and is the recipe for an optimal educational experience. By limiting the text to essential clinical information and focusing on conditions whose diagnosis is enhanced by images, *Greenberg's Text-Atlas of Emergency Medicine* offers a great bedside and learning tool at an affordable price.

Christopher H. Linden, MD
Professor
Department of Emergency Medicine
Division of Medical Toxicology
University of Massachusetts Medical School
Worcester, Massachusetts

ACKNOWLEDGMENTS

We would like to acknowledge the un-ending hard work and dedication of all the Associate Editors and Assistant Editors whose names appear on the cover of this *Atlas*. Without them the *Atlas* certainly would not have come to fruition. Their skill and expertise is unmatched. Special thanks go to all the photo and text contributors as well. Many people allowed us to use their "one of a kind" images which have gone a long way to making this *Atlas* unique. We would like to extend special recognition to the emergency medicine residents who authored topics in this work. For many of these residents, it was their first foray into the world of medical writing and they are to be commended on an excellent job. Hopefully it will not be their last contribution to the literature in the specialty of emergency medicine.

We would like to recognize the hard work and dedication of the entire team at Lippincott, Williams and Wilkins (LWW). Our publisher, Anne Sydor, provided insight into the publication process and guided us through some very difficult seas during the course of this project. Mr. Charley Mitchell of LWW was also a valuable asset in the organization of the book and was extremely helpful in bringing the project to a successful completion. We would also like to acknowledge Ms. Kerry Barrett of LWW whose patience and professionalism were very much appreciated. Without the excellent help of the LWW professionals, the making of this book would have been immeasurably more difficult.

We would also like to thank and acknowledge the following who contributed high-quality images and text that we were, unfortunately, unable to publish. Thank you for your hard work and dedication to the project:

Laurel Berge, MD
Robert Cloutier, MD
Pegeen Eslami, MD
Jason D. Hanley, MD
Robyn R. Heister, MD
William Perhoples, MD
Carlos Sanchez, MD
David Wright, MD
Kabir Yadav, MD

Finally, we would like to acknowledge Ms. Kate Buchert whose organizational and copy editing skills kept the project on track. Kate's input was extraordinarily valuable and without her help the book simply would not have been possible.

Michael I. Greenberg, MD, MPH
Robert G. Hendrickson, MD
Mark Silverberg, MD

CONTRIBUTING AUTHORS

Eric Adar, MD
Assistant Professor of Emergency Medicine
Department of Emergency Medicine
SUNY Downstate Medical Center
Brooklyn, NY
Attending Physician
Department of Emergency Medicine
Staten Island University Hospital
Staten Island, NY

Allon Amitai, MD
Resident
Department of Emergency Medicine
SUNY Downstate Medical Center
Kings County Hospital Center
Brooklyn, NY

Mohamed K. Badawy, MD
Senior Instructor
Departments of Emergency Medicine and Pediatrics
University of Rochester
Attending Physician
Department of Emergency Medicine
Strong Memorial Hospital
Rochester, NY

Heatherlee Bailey, MD
Assistant Professor
Associate Program Director
Department of Emergency Medicine
Drexel University College of Medicine
Medical College of Pennsylvania Hospital
Philadelphia, PA

Ellen S. Bass, MD, MPH
Clinical Instructor
Department of Emergency Medicine
University of Rochester
Clinical Faculty
Department of Emergency Medicine
Strong Memorial Hospital
Rochester, NY

Craig Bates, MD
Attending Physician
Department of Emergency Medicine
MetroHealth Medical Center
Senior Clinical Instructor of Emergency Medicine
Case Western Reserve University School of Medicine
Cleveland, OH

Jason R. Bell, MD
Resident Physician
Department of Emergency Medicine
Temple University School of Medicine
Philadelphia, PA

Taura A.D. Blyth, MD, MPH
Clinical Instructor
Department of Emergency Medicine
University of Rochester Medical Center
Strong Memorial Hospital
Rochester, NY

Stephen C. Boos, MD
Clinical Associate Professor of Pediatrics
University of Medicine & Dentistry of New Jersey
School of Osteopathic Medicine
Stratford, NJ

Reid Brackin, MD
Resident
Department of Emergency Medicine
Harbor-UCLA Medical Center
Los Angeles, CA

Colleen J. Campbell, MD
Associate Clinical Professor
Department of Emergency Medicine
University of California, San Diego
San Diego, CA

Mamie Caton, MD
Clinical Assistant Instructor
Department of Emergency Medicine
SUNY Downstate Medical Center
Brooklyn, NY

Cara Marie Cenera
Medical Student (MS III)
Drexel University College of Medicine
Philadelphia, PA

Kimberly J. Center, MD
Associate Director, Clinical Affairs, Vaccines
Global Medical Affairs
Wyeth Pharmaceuticals
Collegeville, PA

Arthur S. Chang, MD
Resident Physician
Department of Emergency Medicine
Drexel University College of Medicine
MCP-Hahnemann University Hospital
Philadelphia, PA

Robert Chisholm, MD
Resident
Department of Emergency Medicine
Oregon Health and Science University
Portland, OR

Edgar Collazo, MD
Clinical Attending
Department of Emergency Medicine
Section of General Pediatrics
St. Christopher's Hospital for Children
Philadelphia, PA

Gregory P. Conners, MD, MPH, MBA
Associate Professor of Emergency Medicine and Pediatrics
Vice Chair for Academic Affairs
University of Rochester
Acting Chief of Pediatric Emergency Medicine
Strong Memorial Hospital/Golisano Children's Hospital at Strong
Rochester, NY

Richard T. Cook, Jr., MD, MPH
Associate Professor
Departments of Emergency Medicine and Pediatrics
Drexel University College of Medicine
Director of Research and Performance Improvement
Department of Emergency Medicine
St. Christopher's Hospital for Children
Philadelphia, PA

John Curtis, MD
Fellow in Medical Toxicology
Department of Emergency Medicine
Drexel University College of Medicine
Philadelphia, PA
Attending Physician
Department of Emergency Medicine
MCP-Hahnemann University Hospital
Philadelphia, PA

Brandt Arran Delhamer, MD
Resident
Department of Emergency Medicine
University of Texas-Houston Health Science Center
Houston, TX

Ian deSouza, MD
Assistant Professor
Department of Emergency Medicine
SUNY Downstate/Kings County Hospital
Brooklyn, NY

Polly Dole, MD
Attending Physician
Department of Emergency Medicine
Inova Fairfax Hospital
Fairfax, VA

Christopher I. Doty, MD
Assistant Professor
Department of Emergency Medicine
SUNY Downstate Medical Center
Kings County Hospital Center
Brooklyn, NY

Katherine A. Douglass, MD
Resident Physician
Department of Emergency Medicine
Drexel University College of Medicine
Philadelphia, PA

Swapan Dubey, MD
Assistant Professor of Emergency Medicine
Assistant Medical Director - Memorial Hermann EC
The University of Texas-Houston Medical School
Houston, TX

Melissa A. Eirich, MD
Associate Professor of Clinical Emergency Medicine
University of Rochester
Strong Memorial Hospital
Rochester, NY

Judith M. Eisenberg, MD
Instructor
Department of Emergency Medicine
Drexel University College of Medicine
Philadelphia, PA

David R. Fintak, MD
Resident Physician
Wills Eye Hospital
Philadelphia, PA

David Flores, RN
Department of Emergency Medicine
University of California, San Diego School of Medicine
San Diego, CA

Lori D. Frasier, MD
Associate Professor
Department of Pediatrics
University of Utah School of Medicine
Salt Lake City, UT

Lisa Freeman, MD
Clinical Assistant Professor
Department of Emergency Medicine
University of Texas-Houston School of Medicine
Houston, TX

Mary Anne Fuchs, MD
Assistant Clinical Professor
University of California, San Diego School of Medicine
San Diego, CA

Steven C. Gabaeff, MD
Attending Physician
Department of Emergency Medicine
Long Beach Veterans Affairs Hospital
Long Beach, CA

Madelyn Garcia, MD
Fellow, Pediatric Emergency Medicine
Department of Emergency Medicine
University of Rochester
Golisano Children's Hospital
Rochester, NY

Bryan Gargano, MD
Resident
Department of Emergency Medicine
University of Rochester
Strong Memorial Hospital
Rochester, NY

Marco G. Garza, MD
Assistant Professor
Department of Emergency Medicine
University of Texas Medical School at Houston
Houston, TX

Wendymarie Gejer, MD
Resident
Department of Emergency Medicine
Drexel University College of Medicine
Philadelphia, PA

Evan Geller, MD
Assistant Professor
Department of Radiologic Sciences
Drexel University College of Medicine
Chief of Musculoskeletal Imaging
Department of Diagnostic Radiology
St. Christopher's Hospital for Children
Philadelphia, PA

Angelo P. Giardino, MD, PhD
Associate Professor & Associate Chair
Department of Pediatrics
Drexel University College of Medicine
Vice President, Clinical Affairs
St. Christopher's Hospital for Children
Philadelphia, PA

Jonathan Glauser, MD
Assistant Clinical Professor
Department of Emergency Medicine
Case Western Reserve University
Attending Staff
Department of Emergency Medicine
Cleveland Clinic Foundation
Cleveland, OH

Matthew Goldman, MD
Clinical Assistant Instructor
Department of Emergency Medicine
Kings County Hospital Center
Brooklyn, NY

Andrew Gorlin, MD
Clinical Instructor
Department of Emergency Medicine
SUNY Downstate Medical Center
Resident
Department of Emergency Medicine
Kings County Hospital Center
Brooklyn, NY

Nicholas Ryan Gorton, MD
Emergency Physician
New Orleans, LA

Michael I. Greenberg, MD, MPH
Professor of Emergency Medicine
Department of Emergency Medicine
Drexel University College of Medicine
Professor of Public Health
Drexel University School of Public Health
Clinical Professor of Emergency Medicine
Department of Emergency Medicine
Temple University School of Medicine
Philadelphia, PA

James T. Guille, MD
Assistant Professor
Department of Orthopaedic Surgery
Thomas Jefferson University
Philadelphia, PA
Co-Director, Spine and Scoliosis Service
Alfred I. duPont Hospital for Children
Wilmington, DE

In-Hei Hahn, MD
Assistant Professor
Department of Clinical Medicine
Columbia University College of Physicians and Surgeons
New York, NY
Associate Attending, Assistant Director of Research
Department of Emergency Medicine
St. Luke's - Roosevelt Hospital Center
New York, NY

Barry Hahn, MD
Assistant Professor
Department of Emergency Medicine
Staten Island University Hospital
Staten Island, NY

Maria L. Halluska-Handy, MD
Director of Medical Student Education
Clinical Assistant Professor
Attending Physician
Department of Emergency Medicine
Albert Einstein Medical Center
Philadelphia, PA

Derek Halvorson, MD
Resident
Department of Emergency Medicine
Oregon Health and Science University
Portland, OR

Richard J. Hamilton, MD
Associate Professor of Emergency Medicine
Program Director, Emergency Medicine
Department of Emergency Medicine
Drexel University College of Medicine
Philadelphia, PA

Madhu D. Hardasmalani, MD
Attending Physician
St. Joseph's Regional Medical Center
Paterson, NJ

Marc A. Hare, MD
Assistant Clinical Professor of Medicine
Department of Emergency Medicine
University of California, San Diego
San Diego, CA
Medical Director
Center for Wound Healing
Paradise Valley Hospital
National City, CA

Rachel Haroz, MD
Toxicology Fellow
Department of Emergency Medicine
Drexel University College of Medicine
Attending Physician
Department of Emergency Medicine
Medical College of Pennsylvania
Philadelphia, PA

Jennifer Harris, MD
Department of Emergency Medicine
Drexel University College of Medicine
MCP-Hahnemann University Hospital
Philadelphia, PA

Anita Lynn Haynes, MD

Jennifer Railo Hendrickson, MD
Staff Physician
Department of Obstetrics and Gynecology
Tuality Community Hospital
Hillsboro, OR

Robert G. Hendrickson, MD
Assistant Professor
Department of Emergency Medicine
Oregon Health and Science University
Portland, OR
Medical Toxicologist
Oregon Poison Center
Portland, OR

Treve M. Henwood, DO, MMS
Resident Physician
Department of Emergency Medicine
Case Western University
Cleveland Clinic Foundation/MetroHealth Medical Center
Cleveland, OH

Oren Hirsch, MD
Assistant Professor
Department of Emergency Medicine
SUNY Downstate Medical Center
Brooklyn, NY

Leo E. Ho, MD
Assistant Professor
Department of Pediatrics
Drexel University College of Medicine
Director, Urgent Care & Atttending Physician
Department of Emergency Medicine
St. Christopher's Hospital for Children
Philadelphia, PA

Michael H. Horowitz, MD
Resident
Department of Emergency Medicine
Drexel University College of Medicine
MCP-Hahnemann University Hospital
Philadelphia, PA

Joseph A. Iocono, MD
Assistant Professor of Pediatric Surgery
Associate Director, Minimally Invasive Surgery Center
University of Kentucky Chandler Medical Center
Lexington, KY

Yanick A. Isaac, MD
Clinical Assistant Instructor
Department of Emergency Medicine
SUNY Downstate Medical Center
Brooklyn, NY
PGY 4
Department of Emergency Medicine
Kings County Hospital Center
Brooklyn, NY

Paul Ishimine, MD
Assistant Clinical Professor
Departments of Medicine and Pediatrics
University of California, San Diego School of Medicine
San Diego, CA
Attending Physician
Department of Emergency Medicine
UCSD Medical Center
Division of Pediatric Emergency Medicine
Children's Hospital and Health Center
San Diego, CA

Jay S. Itzkowitz, MD
Resident
Department of Emergency Medicine
SUNY Downstate Medical Center
Kings County Hospital Center
Brooklyn, NY

Charles Felzen Johnson, MD
Professor
Department of Pediatrics
Ohio State University College of Medicine and Public Health
Columbus, OH

Kelly Johnson-Arbor, MD
Resident Physician
Department of Emergency Medicine
University of Rochester School of Medicine
Rochester, NY

Raffi Kapitanyan, MD
Clinical Assistant Instructor
Department of Emergency Medicine
Kings County Hospital Center
Brooklyn, NY

Douglas A. Katz, MD
Assistant Professor of Pediatrics and Surgery
Surgical Director of ECMO
Director of Minimally Invasive Center
Director of Surgical Education
St. Christopher's Hospital for Children
Philadelphia, PA

Christopher Keane, MD
Residency Program in Emergency Medicine at MetroHealth Medical Center and the Cleveland Clinic
Cleveland, OH

Boris Khodorkovsky, MD
Clinical Assistant Instructor
Department of Emergency Medicine
SUNY Downstate Medical Center
Brooklyn, NY
Resident
Department of Emergency Medicine
Kings County Hospital Center
Brooklyn, NY

George S. Kim, MD
Staff Physician
Department of Emergency Medicine
Elkhart General Hospital
Elkhart, IN

Samuel Kim, MD
Resident
Department of Emergency Medicine
Oregon Health and Science University
Portland, OR

Edward H. Kim, MD
Resident Physician
Department of Emergency Medicine
University of Rochester School of Medicine and Dentistry
Rochester, NY

Jennifer P. Kiss, MD
Emergency Medicine Physician
Department of Emergency Medicine
Tri-City Medical Center
Oceanside, CA

Jason Kitchen, MD
Resident Physician
Drexel University School of Medicine
Philadelphia, PA

Michele Puszkarczuk Lambert, MD
Clinical Instructor
Department of Pediatrics
Drexel College of Medicine
Chief Resident
Department of Pediatrics
St. Christopher's Hospital for Children
Philadelphia, PA

Jennifer Larson, MD
Resident
Oregon Health and Science University
Portland, OR

Karen J. Lefrak, MD
Resident
Department of Emergency Medicine
Drexel University College of Medicine
MCP-Hahnemann University Hospital
Philadelphia, PA

George Ting Lin, MD
Resident
Department of Emergency Medicine
University of Rochester
Strong Memorial Hospital
Rochester, NY

Kevin Y. Lin, MD

Andrew S. Liteplo, MD
Clinical Assistant Instructor
Department of Emergency Medicine
SUNY Downstate Medical Center
Brooklyn, NY

Brenda L. Liu, MD
Resident
Department of Emergency Medicine
Drexel University College of Medicine
Philadelphia, PA

Timothy E. Lum, MD
Resident
Department of Emergency Medicine
University of Rochester
Strong Memorial Hospital
Rochester, NY

James M. Madsen, MD, MPH, COL, MC-FS, USA
Assistant Professor
Department of Preventive Medicine and Biometrics
Uniformed Services University of the Health Sciences (USUHS)
Bethesda, MD
Scientific Advisor
Chemical Casualty Care Division
U.S. Army Medical Research Institute of Chemical Defense (USAMRICD)
Aberdeen Proving Ground-Edgewood Area (APG-EA), MD

Danielle M. Mailloux, MD
Resident
Department of Emergency Medicine
SUNY Downstate Medical Center
Kings County Hospital Center
Brooklyn, NY

Anthony S. Mazzeo, MD
Resident Physician
Department of Emergency Medicine
Drexel University College of Medicine
MCP-Hahnemann University Hospital
Philadelphia, PA

Maria DiGiorgio McColgan, MD
Assistant Professor
Department of Emergency Medicine
Drexel University College of Medicine
Urgent Care Physician
Department of Emergency Medicine
St. Christopher's Hospital for Children
Philadelphia, PA

R. Zachary McDonald, MD
Department of Emergency Medicine
University of California, San Diego School of Medicine
San Diego, CA

Todd McGrath, MD
Resident
Department of Emergency Medicine
Drexel University College of Medicine
Philadelphia, PA

Sharon McGregor, MD
Clinical Assistant Professor
Department of Emergency Medicine
St. Christopher's Hospital for Children
Philadelphia, PA

Erica S. McKernan, MD
Resident Physician
Department of Emergency Medicine
Temple University Hospital
Philadelphia, PA

Tanisha Medlock, MD
Resident Physician
Department of Emergency Medicine
SUNY Downstate Medical Center
Brooklyn, NY

William J. Meurer, MD
Resident Physician
Department of Emergency Medicine
Case Western Reserve University
Cleveland, OH

Bjorn Miller, MD
Attending Physician
Department of Emergency Medicine
St. Joseph's Hospital
Savannah, GA

Cherie Mininger, DO
Assistant Professor
Department of Emergency Medicine
Temple University School of Medicine
Philadelphia, PA

Rakesh D. Mistry, MD
Fellow, Section of Pediatric Emergency Medicine
Children's Hospital of Wisconsin
Clinical Instructor
Department of Pediatrics
Medical College of Wisconsin
Milwaukee, WI

Steven D. Moonblatt, MD
Resident Physician
Department of Emergency Medicine
Temple University School of Medicine
Philadelphia, PA

Anthony P. Morocco, MD
EMS Medical Director
Guam Department of Public Health and Social Services
Mangilao, Guam
Attending Physician, Medical Toxicologist
Department of Emergency Medicine
Guam Memorial Hospital
Oka, Tamuning, Guam

Mark Mossey, MD
Resident Physician
Department of Emergency Medicine
Case Western University
Cleveland Clinic Foundation/MetroHealth Medical Center
Cleveland, OH

Arun Nagdev, MD
Resident Physician
Department of Emergency Medicine
SUNY Downstate Medical Center
Kings County Hospital Center
Brooklyn, NY

James A. Nelson, MD
Department of Emergency Medicine
University of California, San Diego School of Medicine
San Diego, CA

Dziwe W. Ntaba, MD, MPH
Resident Physician
Drexel University College of Medicine
Philadelphia, PA

Lorenzo Paladino, MD
Assistant Professor
Department of Emergency Medicine
SUNY Downstate Medical Center
Attending Physician
Department of Emergency Medicine
Kings County Hospital
Brooklyn, NY

Sharad A. Pandit, MD
Consultant Physician
Department of Emergency Medicine
Royal Adelaide Hospital
Adelaide, Australia

Dante A. Pappano, MD
Clinical Instructor
Department of Emergency Medicine
University of Rochester
Strong Memorial Hospital
Rochester, NY

Aman K. Parikh, MD
Resident Physician
Department of Emergency Medicine
Drexel University College of Medicine
Philadelphia, PA

Sarah Jane Paris, MD
Resident
Department of Emergency Medicine
University of Rochester
Strong Memorial Hospital
Rochester, NY

Alexander S. Paxson, MD
Resident
Department of Emergency Medicine
University of Washington/Madigan Army Medical Center
Seattle, WA

Catherine Elise Pelletier, MD
Resident Physician
Department of Emergency Medicine
Drexel University College of Medicine
Philadelphia, PA

Michelle C. Peters, MD
Attending Physician
Department of Emergency Medicine
BayCare Clinic Emergency Physicians
Green Bay, WI

Matthew A. Pius, MD
Assistant Professor
Department of Emergency Medicine
SUNY Downstate Medical Center
Brooklyn, NY
Department of Emergency Medicine
Staten Island University Hospital
Staten Island, NY

Paul Prator
Medical Student
University of Texas-Houston Health Science Center
Houston, TX

John R. Queen, MD
Attending Physician
Department of Emergency Medicine
Cleveland Clinic Foundation
Attending Physician
Department of Emergency Medicine
MetroHealth Medical Center
Cleveland, OH

Shalini Ramasunder, MD
Resident Physician
Department of Orthopaedics
Drexel University College of Medicine
Philadelphia, PA

Tara M. Randis, MD
Clinical Fellow in Neonatology
Columbia University
Children's Hospital of New York
New York-Presbyterian Hospital
New York, NY

Laura J. Rendano, MD, MBA
Resident
Department of Emergency Medicine
Strong Memorial Hospital
Rochester, NY

Kyung E. Rhee, MD
Attending Physician
St. Christopher's Hospital for Children
Philadelphia, PA

Benjamin Roemer, MD
Resident Physician
Department of Emergency Medicine
Drexel University College of Medicine
Philadelphia, PA

Gail S. Rudnitsky, MD
Associate Professor
Department of Emergency Medicine
Drexel University College of Medicine
Director, Department of Pediatric Emergency Medicine
St. Christopher's Hospital for Children
Philadelphia, PA

Christopher J. Russo, MD
Assistant Professor
Department of Pediatric Emergency Medicine
Drexel University College of Medicine
Attending Physician
Department of Pediatric Emergency Medicine
St. Christopher's Hospital for Children
Philadelphia, PA

Christy Ann Salvaggio, MD
Assistant Professor
Department of Emergency Medicine
Director of Pediatric Emergency Medicine
Drexel University College of Medicine
Pediatric Emergency Medicine Attending
St. Christopher's Hospital for Children
Philadelphia, PA

John P. Salvo, MD
Assistant Director, Sports Medicine
Cooper Bone & Joint Institute
Voorhees, NJ
Cooper University Hospital
Camden, NJ

Gregory W. Schneider, MD
Attending Physician
Department of Emergency Medicine
Albert Einstein Medical Center
Philadelphia, PA

Harneet Sethi, MD
Attending Physician
Department of Emergency Medicine
Benedectine Hospital
Kingston, NY

Sachin J. Shah, MD
Assistant Professor
Department of Emergency Medicine
Temple University School of Medicine
Assistant Clinical Director
Department of Emergency Medicine
Temple University Hospital
Philadelphia, PA

Lekha Shah, MD
Clinical Assistant Professor
Department of Emergency Medicine
SUNY Downstate Medical Center
Kings County Hospital Center
Brooklyn, NY

Mark Silverberg, MD, MMB
Assistant Professor
Department of Emergency Medicine
SUNY Downstate Medical Center
Brooklyn, NY
Director of Senior Medical Student Education
Department of Emergency Medicine
Kings County Hospital Center
Brooklyn, NY

Christian M. Sloane, MD
Assistant Clinical Professor
Department of Emergency Medicine
University of California, San Diego
UCSD Medical Center
San Diego, CA

Matthew T. Spencer, MD
Assistant Professor
Department of Emergency Medicine
University of Rochester School of Medicine and Dentistry
Rochester, NY
Associate Residency Director
Department of Emergency Medicine
Strong Memorial Hospital
Rochester, NY

Laura A. Spivak, MD
Toxicology Fellow
Department of Emergency Medicine
Drexel University College of Medicine
Attending Physician
Department of Emergency Medicine
Medical College of Pennsylvania
Philadelphia, PA

Adriana Klucar Stoudt, DO
Clinical Instructor of Pediatrics
University School of Medicine
Pediatric Emergency Medicine Attending
Childrens Hospitals and Clinics
Minneapolis, MN

Marisa F. Stumpf, MD
Resident
Department of Emergency Medicine
Beth Israel Deaconess Medical Center
Boston, MA

Mark Su, MD
Assistant Professor
Department of Emergency Medicine
SUNY Downstate Medical Center
Assistant Residency Director/Director of Medical Toxicology
Department of Emergency Medicine
Kings County Hospital Center
Brooklyn, NY

Jason Sundseth, MD
Resident
Department of Emergency Medicine
Oregon Health and Science University
Portland, OR

Cameron Symonds, DO
Chief Resident Physician
Department of Emergency Medicine
Case Western University
Cleveland Clinic Foundation/MetroHealth Medical Center
Cleveland, OH

E. Douglas Thompson, Jr., MD
Assistant Professor
Department of Pediatrics/Section of General Pediatrics
Drexel University College of Medicine
Director, Pediatric Generalist Service
St. Christopher's Hospital for Children
Philadelphia, PA

Roger D. Tillotson, MD
Clinical Assistant Instructor
Department of Emergency Medicine
SUNY Downstate Medical Center
Kings County Hospital Center
Brooklyn, NY

Carolyn Trend, MD
Assistant Professor of Pediatrics
St. Christopher's Hospital for Children
Philadelphia, PA

Renee M. Turchi, MD, MPH
Robert Wood Johnson Clinical Scholars Program
Johns Hopkins University School of Medicine
Baltimore, MD

Jacob W. Ufberg, MD
Assistant Professor
Department of Emergency Medicine
Temple University School of Medicine
Philadelphia, PA

Tyler F. Vadeboncoeur, MD
Resident
Department of Emergency Medicine
University of California, San Diego School of Medicine
San Diego, CA

Carla C. Valentine, MD
Department of Emergency Medicine
University of California, San Diego School of Medicine
San Diego, CA

Louisette Vega, MD
Resident Physician
Department of Emergency Medicine
Temple University School of Medicine
Philadelphia, PA

Gary M. Vilke, MD
Associate Professor of Clinical Medicine
Department of Emergency Medicine
University of California, San Diego
Medical Director
Emergency Medicine Services
San Diego County Health and Human Services
San Diego, CA

Jesse Walck, MD
Associate Professor
Department of Emergency Medicine and Pediatrics
St. Christopher's Hospital for Children
Philadelphia, PA

David A. Wald, DO
Assistant Professor of Emergency Medicine
Director of Undergraduate Medical Education
Department of Emergency Medicine
Temple University School of Medicine
Philadelphia, PA

Mark L. Waltzman, MD
Assistant Professor
Department of Pediatrics, Harvard Medical School
Division of Emergency Medicine and Travel & Geographic Medicine
Children's Hospital Boston
Boston, MA

Matt Warner, MD

Grant Wei, MD
Resident Physician
Department of Emergency Medicine
Drexel University College of Medicine
MCP-Hahnemann University Hospital
Philadelphia, PA

Ralph Weiche, MD
Resident
Department of Emergency Medicine
Oregon Health and Science University
Portland, OR

Moshe Weizberg, MD
Chief Resident
Department of Emergency Medicine
SUNY Downstate Medical Center
Kings County Hospital Center
Brooklyn, NY

Jennifer Wiler, MD, MBA
Resident
Department of Emergency Medicine
Drexel University College of Medicine
Philadelphia, PA

Sigrid Wolfram, MD
Assistant Professor
Assistant Residency Director
Department of Emergency Medicine
SUNY Downstate Medical Center
Kings County Hospital Center
Brooklyn, NY

Phillip Woodward, DO
Private Practice
The Woodlands
Spring, TX

Gerald Wydro, MD
Assistant Professor
Department of Emergency Medicine
Temple University School of Medicine
Philadelphia, PA

Lalena Yarris, MD
Resident
Department of Emergency Medicine
Oregon Health and Science University
Portland, OR

IMAGE CONTRIBUTORS

Eric Adar, MD
Assistant Professor of Emergency Medicine
Department of Emergency Medicine
SUNY Downstate Medical Center
Brooklyn, NY
Attending Physician
Department of Emergency Medicine
Staten Island University Hospital
Staten Island, NY

Alfredo Aguirre, DDS, MS
Director, Advanced Oral and Maxillofacial Pathology Professor
Department of Oral Diagnostic Sciences School of Dental Medicine
SUNY at Buffalo
Buffalo, NY

Ryan Baer, MD
Department of Emergency Medicine
University of Rochester
Strong Memorial Hospital
Rochester, NY

William Banner, Jr., MD, PhD
Clinical Professor of Pediatrics
University of Oklahoma-Tulsa
Tulsa, OK
Medical Director
Children's Hospital at Saint Francis
Saint Francis Hospital
Tulsa, OK

José Biller, MD
Professor
Department of Neurology
Loyola University Medical Center
Maywood, IL

Richard F. Bishop, MD
Education Chairman and Past President
Oregon Mycological Society
Portland, OR

H.C. "Skip" Bittenbender, PhD
Extension Specialist for Coffee, Kava and Cacao
Tropical Plant and Soil Sciences
CTAHR/ University of Hawaii
Honolulu, HI
CTAHR's Farmer's Bookshelf
www.CTAHR.Hawaii.edu/fb/

Jorge G. Burneo, MD, MSPH
Clinical Instructor
Department of Neurology
University of Alabama at Birmingham
Birmingham, AL

Jeffrey P. Callen, MD
Professor of Medicine (Dermatology)
University of Louisville
Louisville, Kentucky

Colleen J. Campbell, MD
Associate Clinical Professor
Department of Emergency Medicine
University of California, San Diego
San Diego, CA

Leslie (Toby) Carroll, MD
Assistant Professor
Department of Emergency Medicine
Temple University School of Medicine
Philadelphia, PA

Charles A. Catanese, MD
Clinical Assistant Professor
Department of Pathology
SUNY Downstate Medical Center
Brooklyn, NY

Mamie Caton, MD
Clinical Assistant Instructor
Department of Emergency Medicine
SUNY Downstate Medical Center
Brooklyn, NY

Kimberly J. Center, MD
Associate Director, Clinical Affairs, Vaccines
Global Medical Affairs
Wyeth Pharmaceuticals
Collegeville, PA

Sam N. Chawla, MD
Department of Urology
Temple University School of Medicine
Philadelphia, PA

Jerrica Chen, MD
Clinical Assistant Instructor (Resident)
SUNY Downstate Medical Center
Kings County Hospital Center
Brooklyn, NY

Robert Chisolm, MD
Resident
Oregon Health and Science University
Portland, OR

Kristin Curtis, MD
Clinical Assistant Instructor
Department of Emergency Medicine
SUNY Downstate Medical Center
Kings County Hospital Center
Brooklyn, NY

Nicole DeIorio, MD
Assistant Professor
Department of Emergency Medicine
Oregon Health and Science University
Portland, OR

Shoma Desai, MD
Resident Physician
SUNY Downstate Medical Center
Kings County Hospital Center
Brooklyn, NY

Christopher I. Doty, MD
Assistant Professor
Department of Emergency Medicine
SUNY Downstate Medical Center
Kings County Hospital Center
Brooklyn, NY

David Effron, MD
Assistant Professor of Surgery
Case Western Reserve University
Cleveland, OH

Judith M. Eisenberg, MD
Instructor
Department of Emergency Medicine
Drexel University College of Medicine
Philadelphia, PA

Glenn B. Everett, BS
Special Agent/Forensic Scientist
Tennessee Bureau of Investigation Crime Laboratory
Nashville, TN
Tennessee Technological University
Cookeville, TN

Richard L. Fischer, MD
Associate Professor
Department of Obstetrics and Gynecology
University of Medicine and Dentistry of New Jersey-Robert Wood Johnson Medical School at Camden
Co-Division Head, Division of Maternal-Fetal Medicine
Cooper University Hospital
Camden, NJ

John P. Fojtik, MD
Assistant Professor
Department of Emergency Medicine
Drexel University College of Medicine
Attending Physician
Department of Emergency Medicine
MCP-Hahnemann University Hospital
Philadelphia, PA

Anthony R. Forestine, MD
Assistant Professor
Department of Emergency Medicine
Mount Sinai Medical Center/Jersey City Medical Center
Jersey City, NJ

Abbas Foroutan, MD
Associate Professor
Department of Physiology
Shaheed Beheshti University of Medical Sciences
Chief, Distance Learning Network Center
Shohada Hospital
Tehran, Iran

Don Fortin, MD
Assistant Professor
Department of Surgery
Division of Plastic Surgery
University of Missouri-Kansas City School of Medicine/Truman Medical Center
Kansas City, MO

Madelyn Garcia, MD
Fellow, Pediatric Emergency Medicine
Department of Emergency Medicine
University of Rochester
Golisano Children's Hospital
Rochester, NY

Evan Geller, MD
Assistant Professor
Department of Radiologic Sciences
Drexel University College of Medicine
Chief of Musculoskeletal Imaging
Department of Diagnostic Radiology
St. Christopher's Hospital for Children
Philadelphia, PA

Michael I. Greenberg, MD, MPH
Professor of Emergency Medicine
Department of Emergency Medicine
Drexel University College of Medicine
Professor of Public Health
Drexel University School of Public Health
Clinical Professor of Emergency Medicine
Department of Emergency Medicine
Temple University School of Medicine
Philadelphia, PA

James T. Guille, MD
Assistant Professor
Department of Orthopaedic Surgery
Thomas Jefferson University
Philadelphia, PA
Co-Director, Spine and Scoliosis Service
Alfred I. duPont Hospital for Children
Wilmington, DE

Barry Hahn, MD
Assistant Professor
Department of Emergency Medicine
Staten Island University Hospital
Staten Island, NY

Richard J. Hamilton, MD
Associate Professor of Emergency Medicine
Program Director, Emergency Medicine
Department of Emergency Medicine
Drexel University College of Medicine
Philadelphia, PA

Rachel Haroz, MD
Toxicology Fellow
Department of Emergency Medicine
Drexel University College of Medicine
Attending Physician
Department of Emergency Medicine
Medical College of Pennsylvania
Philadelphia, PA

Barry Hendler, DDS, MD
Associate Professor/Clinician Educator
Department of Oral and Maxillofacial Surgery
University of Pennsylvania School of Dental Medicine
Philadelphia, PA

Robert G. Hendrickson, MD
Assistant Professor
Department of Emergency Medicine
Oregon Health and Science University
Portland, OR
Medical Toxicologist
Oregon Poison Center
Portland, OR

B. Zane Horowitz, MD, FACMT
Medical Director
Oregon Poison Center
Oregon Health and Sciences University
Portland, OR
Professor
Department of Emergency Medicine
Oregon Health and Sciences University
Portland, OR

William Hughes, MD

Gregory S. Hunt, MD
Department of Emergency Medicine
University of Rochester School of Medicine and Dentistry
Rochester, NY

David Iacobelli, MD
Clinical Assistant Professor
Wayne State University
Detroit, MI

Joseph A. Iocono
Assistant Professor of Pediatric Surgery
Associate Director
Minimally Invasive Surgery Center
University of Kentucky Chandler Medical Center
Lexington, KY

Rafi Israeli, MD
Clinical Assistant Instructor
SUNY Downstate Medical Center
Kings County Hospital Center
Brooklyn, NY

Jay S. Itzkowitz, MD
Resident
Department of Emergency Medicine
SUNY Downstate Medical Center
Kings County Hospital Center
Brooklyn, NY

Paul C. Johnston, MD
Resident Physician
Department of Surgery
UCSF Medical Center
San Francisco, CA

Gregory A. Juhl, MD
Department of Emergency Medicine
University of Rochester School of Medicine and Dentistry
Strong Memorial Hospital
Rochester, NY

Raffi Kapitanyan, MD
Clinical Assistant Instructor
Department of Emergency Medicine
Kings County Hospital Center
Brooklyn, NY

Lewis J. Kaplan, MD
Associate Professor and Director, Emergency General Surgery
Department of Surgery
Division of Trauma, Surgical Critical Care, and Surgical Emergencies
Yale University School of Medicine
New Haven, CT

Boris Khodorkovsky, MD
Resident, Emergency Medicine
SUNY Downstate Medical Center
Kings County Hospital Center
Brooklyn, NY

Edward C. Klatt, MD
Professor and Academic Administrator
Department of Biomedical Sciences
Florida State University College of Medicine
Tallahassee, FL

Mridul Kumar, MD
Clinical Assistant Instructor
SUNY Downstate Medical Center
Kings County Hospital Center
Brooklyn, NY

Alexander D. Lapidus, MD
Resident Physician
Department of Emergency Medicine
Oregon Health and Science University
Portland, OR
Attending Physician
Department of Emergency Medicine
Mid-Columbia Medical Center
The Dalles, OR

CW Leung, MD
Department of Paediatrics and Adolescent Medicine
Princess Margaret Hospital
Lai Chi Kok, Kowloon
Hong Kong

George Ting Lin, MD
Resident
Department of Emergency Medicine
University of Rochester
Strong Memorial Hospital
Rochester, NY

Andrew S. Liteplo, MD
Clinical Assistant Instructor
Department of Emergency Medicine
SUNY Downstate Medical Center
Brooklyn, NY

Yiju Teresa Liu, MD
Assistant Clinical Instructor
Department of Emergency Medicine
SUNY Downstate Medical Center
Brooklyn, NY

Michael Lucchesi, MD
Associate Professor and Chairman
Department of Emergency Medicine
SUNY Downstate Medical Center
University Hospital of Brooklyn and Kings County Hospital Center
Brooklyn, NY

Timothy Lum, MD
Resident Physician
Department of Emergency Medicine
University of Rochester
Strong Memorial Hospital
Rochester, NY

Thorsten Lundsgaarde, MD
Clinical Instructor
University of Washington School of Medicine
Department of Family Medicine
Family Medicine of Southwest Washington
Vancouver, WA

Jamarcy McDaniel, MD
Clinical Assistant Instructor
Department of Emergency Medicine
SUNY Downstate Medical Center
Kings County Hospital Center
Brooklyn, NY

Todd McGrath, MD
Resident
Department of Emergency Medicine
Drexel University College of Medicine
Philadelphia, PA

John McManus, MD
Adjunct Assistant Professor
Department of Emergency Medicine
Oregon Health and Science University
Portland, OR

Phillip S. Mead, MD
Assistant Professor
Department of Emergency Medicine
Drexel University College of Medicine
Philadelphia, PA

Seth Mehr, MD
Resident Physician
Department of Emergency Medicine
Oregon Health and Science University
Portland, OR

Raymond Moreno, MD
Assistant Residency Director
Department of Emergency Medicine
Oregon Health and Science University
Portland, OR

Brent W. Morgan, MD
Assistant Professor
Department of Emergency Medicine
Emory University
Director, Medical Toxicology Fellowship
Georgia Poison Center
Atlanta, GA

Anthony P. Morocco, MD
EMS Medical Director
Guam Department of Public Health and Social Services
Mangilao, Guam
Attending Physician, Medical Toxicologist
Department of Emergency Medicine
Guam Memorial Hospital
Oka, Tamuning, Guam

Rahul Nath, MD
Assistant Professor
Department of Surgery
Division of Plastic Surgery
Baylor College of Medicine
Houston, Texas

Jaimee O'Connor, MD
Department of Emergency Medicine
SUNY Downstate Medical Center
Brooklyn, NY
Department of Emergency Medicine
Staten Island University Hospital
Staten Island, NY

Olufunmilayo Ogundele, MD
Clinical Assistant Instructor
SUNY Downstate Medical Center
Kings County Hospital Center
Brooklyn, NY

Lorenzo Paladino, MD
Assistant Professor
Department of Emergency Medicine
SUNY Downstate Medical Center
Brooklyn, NY
Attending Physician
Department of Emergency Medicine
Kings County Hospital Center
Brooklyn, NY

Sarah Jane Paris, MD
Resident
Department of Emergency Medicine
University of Rochester
Strong Memorial Hospital
Rochester, NY

Scott Phillips, MD
Associate Clinical Professor
Departments of Medicine and Surgery
University of Colorado Health Sciences Center
Denver, CO

Elzbieta Pilat, MD
Clinical Assistant Instructor
SUNY Downstate Medical Center
Kings County Hospital Center
Brooklyn, NY

Anthony Polimeni, DMD
Huntington Bay, NY

Robert H. Poppenga, DVM, PhD
Professor
Department of Pathobiology
School of Veterinary Medicine
University of Pennsylvania
Philadelphia, PA
Chief, Toxicology Laboratory
New Bolton Center
School of Veterinary Medicine
University of Pennsylvania
Kennett Square, PA

Kevin Reinhard, MD
Resident Physician
Department of Emergency Medicine
University of Rochester
Strong Memorial Hospital
Rochester, NY

Claritza L. Rios, MD
Clinical Assistant Instructor
SUNY Downstate Medical Center
Kings County Hospital
Brooklyn, NY

James R. Roberts, MD
Professor and Vice Chair
Department of Emergency Medicine
Drexel University College of Medicine
Director, Division of Medical Toxicology
Hospital of the Medical College of Pennsylvania and Hahnemann University Hospital
Chair
Department of Emergency Medicine
Director, Division of Medical Toxicology
Fitzgerald Mercy Hospital and Mercy Hospital of Philadelphia
Mercy Catholic Medical Center
Philadelphia, PA

Judy Roger, MD
Mycological Services
Gladstone, OR

Eric Rueckmann, MD
Resident Physician
Department of Emergency Medicine
University of Rochester
Strong Memorial Hospital
Rochester, NY

Daniel E. Rusyniak, MD
Assistant Professor
Departments of Emergency Medicine and Pharmacology and Toxicology
Indiana University School of Medicine
Indianapolis, IN

Alfredo Sabbaj, MD
Assistant Professor of Emergency Medicine
Oregon Health and Sciences University
Portland, OR

Donald Sallee, MD
Commander, US Navy
Naval Medical Center
San Diego, CA

Christy Ann Salvaggio, MD
Assistant Professor
Department of Emergency Medicine
Director of Pediatric Emergency Medicine
Drexel University College of Medicine
Pediatric Emergency Medicine Attending
St. Christopher's Hospital for Children
Philadelphia, PA

Wayne Satz, MD
Assistant Professor
Department of Emergency Medicine
Temple University School of Medicine
Philadelphia, PA

Gregory Schneider, MD
Attending Physician
Department of Emergency Medicine
Albert Einstein Medical Center
Philadelphia, PA

William S. Schroder, MD
Associate Professor and Chief
Section of Vascular Surgery
University of Missouri-Kansas City School of Medicine/Truman Medical Center
Kansas City, MO

Gregory Schutt, MD
Resident
Department of Emergency Medicine
Oregon Health Science University
Portland, OR

Michael D. Schwartz, MD
Fellow in Medical Toxicology
ATSDR/Centers for Disease Control/Georgia Poison Center
Atlanta, GA

Sandra R. Scott, MD
Assistant Professor
Division of Emergency Medicine
Department of Surgery
University of Medicine and Dentistry of New Jersey
Newark, NJ

Lekha Shah, MD
Clinical Assistant Professor
Department of Emergency Medicine
SUNY Downstate Medical Center
Kings County Hospital Center
Brooklyn, NY

Binita R. Shah, MD
Professor of Emergency Medicine and Pediatrics
SUNY Downstate Medical Center
Director, Pediatric Emergency Medicine
Kings County Hospital Center
Brooklyn, NY

Sanjay Shetty, MD
Department of Emergency Medicine
University of South Florida
Tampa General Hospital
Tampa, FL

Tor Shwayder, MD
Director, Pediatric Dermatology
Henry Ford Hospital
Detroit, MI

Mark Silverberg, MD, MMB
Assistant Professor
Department of Emergency Medicine
SUNY Downstate Medical Center
Brooklyn, NY
Director of Senior Medical Student Education
Department of Emergency Medicine
Kings County Hospital Center
Brooklyn, NY

Susan Smolinske, PharmD, DABAT
Managing Director
Children's Hospital of Michigan Regional Poison Control Center
Associate Professor
College of Medicine, Department of Pediatrics
Wayne State University
Detroit, MI

Samara Soghoian, MD
Clinical Assistant Instructor
SUNY Downstate Medical Center
Kings County Hospital Center
Brooklyn, NY

Matthew T. Spencer, MD
Assistant Professor
Department of Emergency Medicine
University of Rochester School of Medicine and Dentistry
Rochester, NY
Associate Residency Director
Department of Emergency Medicine
Strong Memorial Hospital
Rochester, NY

Laura A. Spivak, MD
Toxicology Fellow
Department of Emergency Medicine
Drexel University College of Medicine
Attending Physician
Department of Emergency Medicine
Medical College of Pennsylvania
Philadelphia, PA

Michael Stein, PA
Department of Emergency Medicine
Kings County Hospital Center
Brooklyn, NY

Lowan Stewart, MD
Resident
Department of Emergency Medicine
Oregon Health and Science University
Portland, OR

Eustacia (Jo) Su, MD
Assistant Professor
Department of Emergency Medicine
Oregon Health and Science University
Portland, OR

Mark Su, MD
Assistant Professor
Department of Emergency Medicine
SUNY Downstate Medical Center
Assistant Residency Director/Director of Medical Toxicology
Department of Emergency Medicine
SUNY Downstate Medical Center/Kings County Hospital Center
Brooklyn, NY

Bronson E. Terry, MD
Resident Physician
Department of Pediatrics
Oregon Health and Science University
Doernbecher Children's Hospital
Portland, OR

Roger D. Tillotson, MD
Clinical Assistant Instructor
Department of Emergency Medicine
SUNY Downstate Medical Center
Brooklyn, NY

Kristina M. Vogel, MD
Attending Physician
Obstetrics and Gynecology
United States Naval Hospital
Guam

David K. Wagner, MD
Professor and Chair
Department of Emergency Medicine
Drexel University College of Medicine
Philadelphia, PA

Ron M. Walls, MD
Chairman, Department of Emergency Medicine
Brigham and Women's Hospital
Associate Professor of Medicine
Harvard Medical School
Boston, MA

Ralph Weiche, MD
Resident
Oregon Health and Science University
Portland, OR

Michael S. Weingarten, MD
Chief, Department of Vascular Surgery
Professor of Surgery
Drexel University College of Medicine
Hahnemann University Hospital
Philadelphia, PA

Moshe Weizberg, MD
Chief Resident
Department of Emergency Medicine
SUNY Downstate Medical Center
Kings County Hospital Center
Brooklyn, NY

Scott C. Wickless, DO
Department of Dermatology
Oakwood Health System/Oakwood Southshore Medical Center
Dearborn, MI

Robert Yin
Marine Photographer
La Jolla, CA

SECTION I

ABCs

1

Airway, Breathing, Circulation

1-1

Normal Airway

Arun Nagdev

Anatomically, the upper airway begins at the nares and continues to the proximal aspect of the trachea.

Clinical Presentation

Patients with an intact and patent upper airway should show no difficulty in breathing.

Pathophysiology

Functions of the upper airway include acting as a conduit for oxygenation and ventilation, phonation, and prevention of gastric aspiration.[1] Impediment of flow in the upper airway can result in stridor, agitation, hypoxia, or complete loss of upper airway sounds and flow.[1] Obstruction of air flow can occur at any location along the upper airway, commonly including oropharyngeal obstruction secondary to decreased tone of the genioglossus muscle, posterior nasopharyngeal obstruction by hypertrophied lymphoid tissue, and hypopharyngeal obstruction due to inflammatory epiglottitis.[1,2]

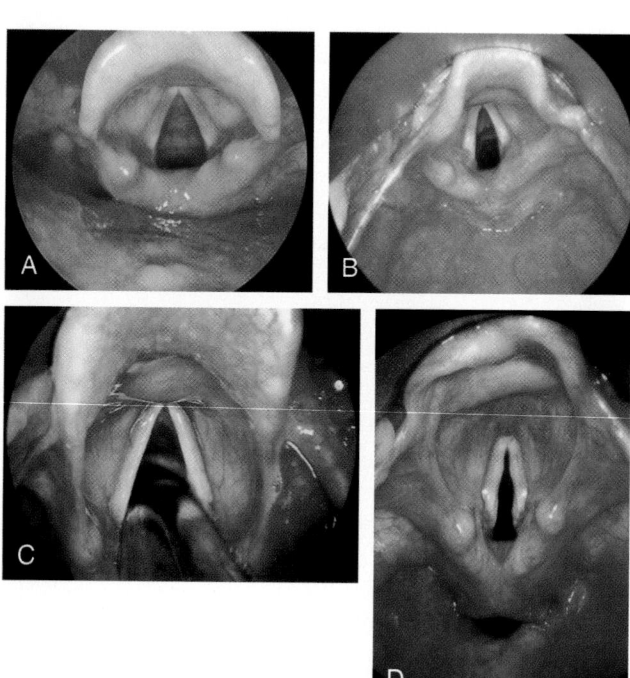

FIGURE 1–1 **A:** Preintubation view of adult airway. **B:** Preintubation view of pediatric airway. **C:** Endotracheal tube passed through vocal cords. **D:** Laryngoscopic view of larynx and hypopharynx. (From Benjamin et al., with permission.)

Diagnosis

Clinicians must be able to detect alterations in normal upper airway anatomy or function clinically. Ancillary testing, such as lateral soft tissue neck radiographs or direct or fiberoptic laryngoscopy, may aid in determining alterations in airway anatomy.

Clinical Complications

Patients who are unable to maintain a normal airway can develop pulmonary aspiration, sepsis, hypoxia, and eventually death if airway alteration is allowed to progress uncorrected.

Management

Ensuring a functioning upper airway is critical in all patients. If compromise of the upper airway has occurred, measures ranging from repositioning of the patient to nasal trumpet placement to orotracheal intubation must be attempted.[1-3]

REFERENCES

1. Issacs RS, Sykes JM. Anatomy and physiology of the upper airway. *Anesthesiol Clin North Am* 2002;20:733–745.
2. Morris IR. Functional anatomy of the upper airway. *Emerg Med Clin North Am* 1988;6:639–669.
3. Behringer EC. Approaches to managing the upper airway. *Anesthesiol Clin North Am* 2002;20:813–832.

Difficult Airway

Arun Nagdev

Difficult intubation is defined as inability to place an endotracheal tube (ET) after three attempts or after 10 minutes via conventional laryngoscopy.[1] Difficulty in mask ventilation is defined as an inability to maintain oxygen saturation greater than 90% using 100% facemask ventilation.[1]

Clinical Presentation

Between 1% and 2% of intubations in the emergency department (ED) become "difficult airways."[2] Facial or neck trauma, oral swelling, morbid obesity, and abnormal facies are common causes of the difficult airway.[3]

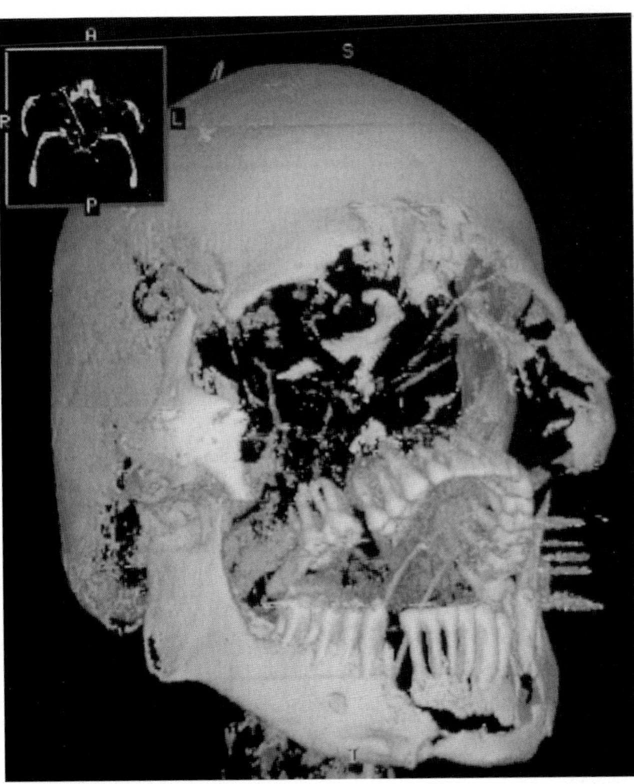

FIGURE 1–2 Facial computed tomogram of a patient with a difficult airway. (Courtesy of Ralph Weiche, MD.)

Pathophysiology

No single factor has been shown to predict a difficult airway. The modified Mallampati score, based on glottic exposure along with mouth opening, jaw size, and thyromental distance, may help predict the difficult airway.[1,3]

Diagnosis

Although many factors can alert the physician that intubation will be difficult, it is not until the procedure is actually started and difficulty is encountered that the diagnosis is realized.

Clinical Complications

Laryngoscopic trauma and hypoxia are the most common complications of the difficult airway. The laryngoscope can cause tooth or mouth injuries or laryngeal fractures. Hypoxia can be caused by esophageal tube placement, prolonged laryngoscopy, or aspiration of secretions.[1-3]

Management

The operator must be experienced in alternative airway techniques in the event of a failed intubation. These "rescue techniques" include the laryngeal mask airway (LMA) and the newer intubating laryngeal mask airway (ILMA), fiberoptic-guided nasal intubation, the Combitube, and the lighted stylet.[1-3]

REFERENCES

1. Orebaugh SL. Difficult airway management in the emergency department. *J Emerg Med* 2002;22:31–48.
2. Levitan RM, Kush S, Hollander JE. Devices for difficult airway management in academic emergency departments: results of a national survey. *Ann Emerg Med* 1999;33:694–698.
3. Butler KH, Clyne B. Management of the difficult airway: alternative airway techniques and adjuncts. *Emerg Med Clin North Am* 2003;21:259–289.

ACE Inhibitor-Associated Angioedema

Arun Nagdev

Angioedema involves extravasation of fluid into the interstitial tissues secondary to the action of inflammatory mediators leading to leakage of the capillary beds.[1]

Clinical Presentation

Patients have acute swelling, usually in the head and neck region and frequently involving the mouth, tongue, pharynx, and larynx.[1] In severe cases involving the upper airway, stridor may be present.

Pathophysiology

The primary therapeutic objective of the use of angiotensin-converting enzyme (ACE) inhibitors is to decrease blood pressure (BP) by preventing the conversion of angiotensin I to angiotensin II, a potent vasoconstrictor. However, ACE inhibitors also cause bradykinin to accumulate, which leads to increased capillary permeability. This results in the formation of interstitial edema within certain tissues. Unlike edema due to increased vascular pressures, the swelling caused by angioedema is usually rapid in onset, asymmetric in distribution, nonpitting, and not confined to dependent areas. ACE inhibitors have been implicated as the cause in 0.1% to 7.9% of angioedema cases.[2] ACE inhibitor–associated angioedema is hypothesized to be caused by a bradykinin-dependent increase in vascular permeability.[1]

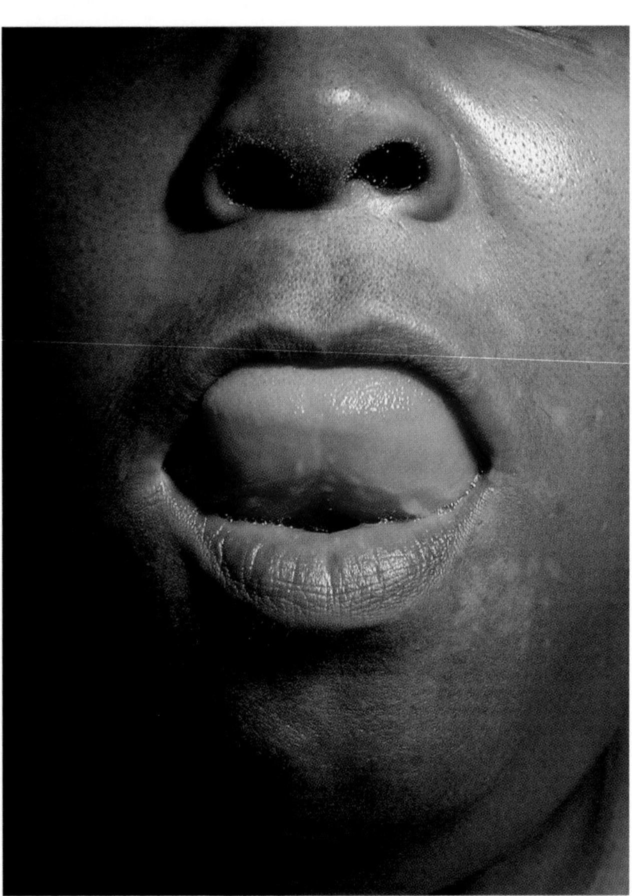

FIGURE 1–3 Swollen tongue caused by angiotensin-converting enzyme (ACE) inhibitor–associated angioedema. (Courtesy of Robert Hendrickson, MD.)

Diagnosis

Angioedema is a clinical diagnosis. If the patient presents with the characteristic swelling of the mouth, lips, tongue, or pharynx and is also taking an ACE inhibitor, the diagnosis should be highly suspected.[2]

Clinical Complication

Airway compromise secondary to swelling of the tongue, uvula, soft palate, and larynx is a common and potentially life-threatening complication of ACE inhibitor–associated angioedema.[2]

Management

Patients with impending airway compromise require the immediate establishment of a definitive airway. Those with less severe findings need early medical management with intravenous (IV) antihistamines, steroids, and subcutaneous epinephrine.[2] After discontinuation of the ACE inhibitor and administration of the appropriate medications, most cases of ACE inhibitor–induced angioedema resolve within 12 to 48 hours.[2] However, this angioedema can proceed rapidly to life-threatening airway closure and must be treated as a serious emergency.

REFERENCES

1. Israili ZH, Hall WD. Cough and angioneurotic edema associated with angiotensin-converting enzyme inhibitor therapy: a review of the literature and pathophysiology. *Ann Intern Med* 1992;117: 234–242.
2. Vleeming W, van Amsterdam JG, Stricker BH, de Wildt DJ. ACE inhibitor-induced angioedema: incidence, prevention and management. *Drug Saf* 1998;18:171–188.

Ludwig's Angina

Arun Nagdev

Ludwig's angina is cellulitis originating in the submandibular space of the mouth.[1]

Clinical Presentation

Symptoms include sore throat, dysphonia, dysphagia, submandibular swelling, and halitosis.

Pathophysiology

Extraction or infection of teeth allows oral flora to enter the submandibular space.[1] Organisms isolated from these infections include *Streptococcus* and *Staphylococcus* species in addition to anaerobes. Edema and abscess formation in the tissues below the tongue result in swelling and encroachment on the airway, eventually leading to respiratory compromise.[1]

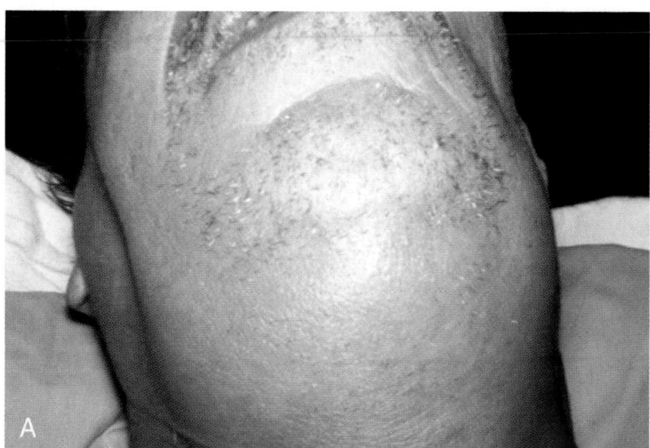

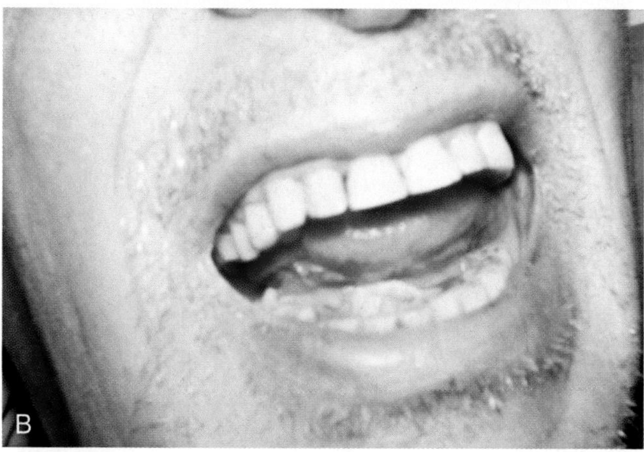

FIGURE 1–4 **A:** Note induration with submandibular redness and swelling. **B:** Note elevation of tongue secondary to swelling of floor of the mouth. (Courtesy of Barry Hendler, DDS, MD.)

Diagnosis

Patients are often febrile and dehydrated from decreased oral intake. Locally, the floor of the mouth appears "full" or swollen, and the tongue may be elevated. The submandibular region is usually tender. The floor of the mouth may appear even with the level of the teeth and may be tense to tongue blade application. In patients with no signs of airway compromise, soft tissue films of the neck may demonstrate widening or gas within soft tissue spaces. Trismus and drooling may be seen.[1]

Clinical Complications

Ludwig's angina can spread through the fascial planes of the oral cavity into the neck and chest. This can lead to retropharyngeal and mediastinal infections in addition to pericardial and pleural effusions.[2] If the involved tissues continue to expand, complete airway occlusion and death may result.

Management

Airway management is a clear priority. Fiberoptic-guided nasotracheal intubation is the preferred method for obtaining a definitive airway, because soft tissue swelling makes laryngoscopic intubation difficult.[2] Stable patients should be kept sitting upright in a comfortable position with intubation equipment at bedside. Antibiotics—penicillin G with metronidazole, ampicillin-sulbactam, or, in penicillin-allergic patients, clindamycin—must be started in the emergency department.[2] Corticosteroid therapy is controversial.[3]

REFERENCES

1. Moreland LW, Corey J, McKenzie R. Ludwig's angina: report of a case and review of the literature. *Arch Intern Med* 1988;148: 461–466.
2. Spitalnic S, Sucov A. Ludwig's Angina: a case report and review. *J Emerg Med* 1995;13:499–503.
3. Freund B, Timon C. Ludwig's angina: a place for steroid therapy in its management? *Oral Health* 1992;82:23–25.

Epiglottitis

Matthew Spencer

Clinical Presentation

Patients typically present with complaints of fever, sore throat, odynophagia, shortness of breath, and a hoarse or muffled voice.[1–3] On examination, there is often an associated pharyngitis, anterior neck tenderness, lymphadenopathy, drooling, or stridor.[1–3] Patients in severe distress may be sitting upright and leaning forward with the mouth open and the jaw thrust forward in what is commonly referred to as the "tripod position."[1,3] There is some variation in presentation between adult and pediatric patients. Adults present most commonly with complaints of sore throat, odynophagia, and anterior neck tenderness, whereas children usually have difficulty breathing, stridor, and a hoarse or muffled voice.[1]

Epiglottitis was previously considered a disease of children, but with the widespread use of the *Haemophilus influenzae* type b (Hib) vaccine, it is now seen more often in adults, at a ratio of 0.4 to 1.[2] It has an incidence of 0.97 to 1.8 per 100,000 in the adult population and peaks between 35 and 47 years of age.[1,2] Epiglottitis is most commonly seen in children between the ages of 7 months and 16 years, with the peak at 2 to 6 years of age.[3] The mortality rate is currently less than 1% in children and 6% to 7% in adults.[2]

Pathophysiology

Epiglottitis is caused by local inflammation and swelling of the epiglottis, aryepiglottic folds, and adjacent soft tissue.[3] Usually the swelling and inflammation are the result of an infection, although in most cases a single organism cannot be identified.[1,2] The organisms most commonly identified are Hib and β-hemolytic streptococci.[1,2]

Diagnosis

The diagnosis should be suspected in all patients who have relatively acute onset of a severe sore throat with fever and odynophagia. The diagnosis is confirmed by direct or fiberoptic laryngoscopy, which is considered the gold standard but should be performed in a controlled environment by a practitioner who is experienced with advanced airway control techniques.[1] In the emergency department, fiberoptic laryngoscopy is considered to be a safe procedure in adults but not in children.[2] Pediatric patients with suspected epiglottitis who have moderate to severe symptoms should go immediately to the operating room for simultaneous airway control and diagnosis confirmation.[3] Mildly symptomatic pediatric patients may have portable soft tissue neck radiographs taken to help establish the diagnosis but should not leave the direct observation of the emergency physician.[3] Lateral soft tissue neck films may show swelling of the

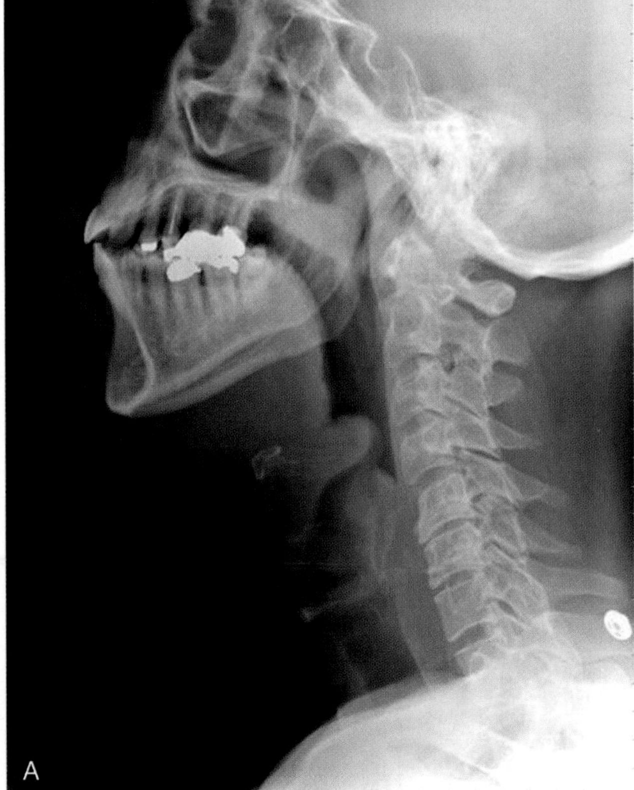

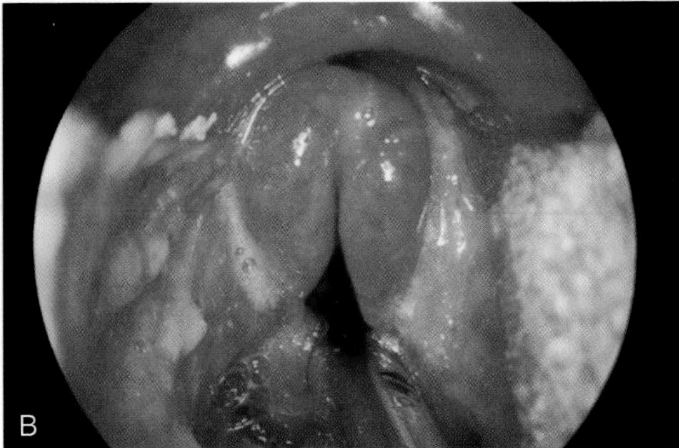

FIGURE 1–5 **A:** Soft tissue radiograph showing a swollen epiglottis (thumbprint sign). (Courtesy of Ryan Baer, MD.) **B:** Cherry-red epiglottis with partial obstruction, shown before intubation. (From Benjamin et al., with permission.)

epiglottitis as evidenced by a "thumbprint sign," swelling of the arytenoids and aryepiglottic folds, a narrowed airway, or prevertebral soft tissue swelling. All of these signs have low sensitivity and specificity except for a decrease in the vallecular airspace (the "vallecular sign").[1,2] Computed tomography (CT) is useful only if the epiglottitis cannot be visualized by laryngoscopy or an abscess is suspected.[1]

Clinical Complications

The most common and most serious complication is complete airway obstruction leading to respiratory compromise and possibly death.[1,2] Bacteremia may lead to the development of sepsis and multiorgan system failure despite antibiotic use.

Management

Airway control is paramount. Only one third of patients require intubation, but practitioners should be prepared for emergency airway management at all times. Many recommend prophylactic intubation.[1] In adult patients, intubation with rapid-sequence induction is recommended, but the physician should be prepared for possible emergency cricothyrotomy.[2] Children should be placed in a quiet, nonstimulating environment and allowed to assume whatever position they find most comfortable.[3] It may be prudent in some cases to allow the parents to be present to comfort the child. Airway management comes before all other procedures in pediatric patients and optimally should be performed in the operating room with the use of inhalation anesthesia.[2,3] All patients should receive empiric antibiotic therapy that covers Hib and β-hemolytic streptococci; current first-line agents are second- or third-generation cephalosporins such as cefotaxime, ceftizoxime, ceftriaxone, or ceftazidime.[1-3] Humidified oxygen and IV fluids should also be administered; steroids and racemic epinephrine remain controversial.[1,2]

REFERENCES

1. Sack JL, Brock CD. Identifying acute epiglottitis in adults. *Postgrad Med* 2002;112:81–86.
2. Carey MJ. Epiglottitis in adults. *Am J Emerg Med* 1996;14:421–424.
3. Bank DE, Krug SE. New approaches to upper airway disease. *Emerg Med Clin North Am* 1995;13:473–487.

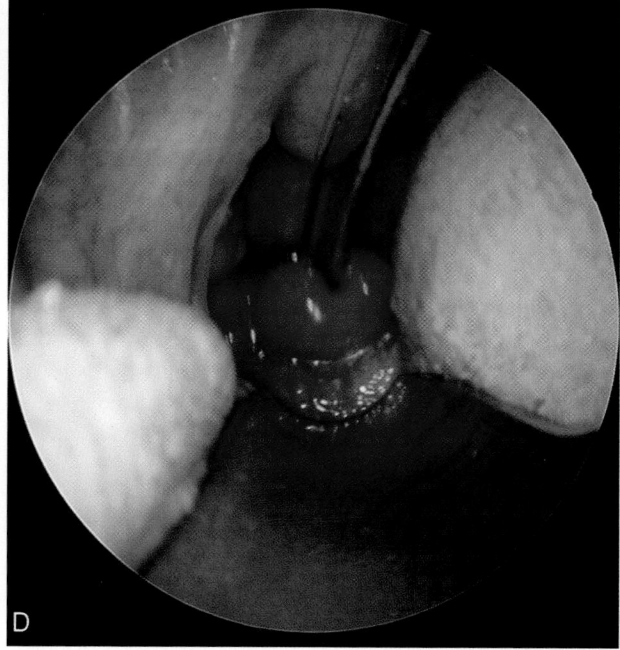

FIGURE 1–5, cont'd C: Child assuming typical body position seen in epiglottitis. (From Fleisher, Baskin, and Ludwig, with permission.) **D:** Cherry-red epiglottis after intubation. (From Fleisher, Baskin, and Ludwig, with permission.)

Orofacial Trauma

Danielle Mailloux

Clinical Presentation

Patients present after injuries that are isolated to the head and face or are part of a more extensive multiple trauma setting. Facial injuries may range from minor abrasions to severe injuries such as gunshot wounds and crush injuries. The presentation of airway compromise in these cases ranges from complete apnea to partial airway obstruction with strider due to debris or foreign matter in the airway. Patients may present with endotracheal tubes that have been incorrectly inserted in the field or that have become dislodged in transit.

Pathophysiology

Facial injuries may be caused by blunt or penetrating trauma. In either case, such injuries require special consideration because of the potential for airway compromise as well as the social and psychological impact that disfiguring injuries of the face can create.[1] Complex facial fractures may occur, teeth may be avulsed or broken, and the sensory organs such as the eyes or ears may be damaged.

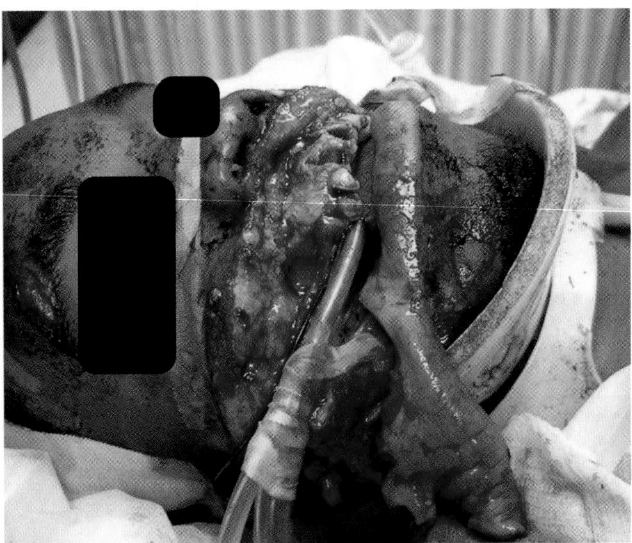

FIGURE 1–6 Severe orofacial trauma. (Courtesy of Mark Silverberg, MD.)

Diagnosis

Diagnosis is based on the history and physical examination. Radiologic studies may be needed to confirm specific injuries.

Clinical Complications

Complications include extensive skin loss, cosmetically deforming injuries, airway compromise due to tissue destruction or foreign materials (e.g., fractured teeth, blood) in the airway, infection, sepsis, and death.

Management

Emergency management of facial trauma should follow advanced trauma life support (ATLS) protocols, addressing airway, breathing, and circulation first and then promptly moving on to alleviating pain and caring for local injuries.[1] Orofacial fractures often require consultation with ear, nose, and throat (ENT) specialists, oral surgeons, ophthalmologists, or plastic surgeons. Empiric antibiotic administration should be considered for intraoral or sinus fractures, contaminated wounds, and injuries involving extensive amounts of devitalized tissue. Tooth fractures with pulp exposure need immediate dental care to prevent necrosis of the neurovascular bundle.[2] Most patients with serious facial injuries need admission for airway management, parenteral antibiotic therapy, and surgical repair.[1,2]

REFERENCES

1. Laskin DM, Best AM. Current trends in the treatment of maxillofacial injuries in the United States. *J Oral Maxillofac Surg* 2000;58:207–215.
2. Flores MT, Andreasen JO, Bakland LK. Guidelines for the evaluation and management of traumatic dental injuries. *Dent Traumatol* 2001;17:193–198.

Laryngeal Trauma

Karen Lefrak

Clinical Presentation

Signs and symptoms of laryngeal trauma include hoarseness, laryngeal pain, dyspnea, dysphagia, cough, hemoptysis, stridor, tenderness or deformity of the larynx, subcutaneous emphysema, and aphonia.[1] Bleeding, expanding hematomas, bruits, and loss of pulses may be associated with vascular injury.

Pathophysiology

Laryngeal trauma is uncommon (1 in 30,000 emergency department visits), and in most of the severe cases the patient dies before arriving at a hospital.[1-3] Blunt trauma causes compression of the larynx on the anterior cervical bodies with tearing of the cartilage and mucosa. Pediatric injuries differ in that the larynx is more protected by the mandible and the cartilaginous skeleton is more flexible in the pediatric age group.[1-3]

Diagnosis

The history of the trauma (e.g., motor vehicle accident, sports injury, personal assault including strangulation) should help the physician make the diagnosis; a good physical examination is necessary to delineate the seriousness of the injury. Airway problems in a patient with signs of trauma should raise suspicion for laryngeal trauma and must be addressed immediately. Flexible fiberoptic nasopharyngolaryngoscopy is the examination of choice. In stable patients, computed tomography (CT) can be useful for determining the extent of the injury.[2]

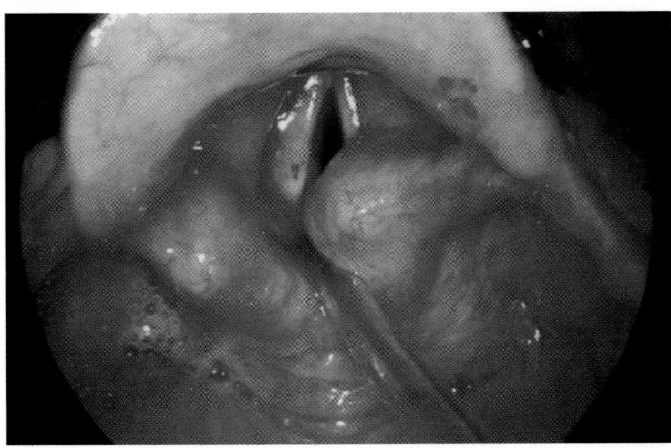

FIGURE 1–7 Laryngeal trauma: dislocated arytenoids. (From Benjamin et al., with permission.)

Clinical Complications

A patient with laryngeal trauma may have a difficult airway and require a surgical airway.[1] Iatrogenic damage to the larynx can occur during intubation, especially if the stylette extends beyond the length of the endotracheal tube. The small size of the pediatric airway and the potential for large amounts of soft tissue swelling make early treatment essential in this population.[1-3]

Management

Maintaining a patent airway is the hallmark of treatment. Some patients require immediate tracheostomy and open exploration in the operating room. Ear, nose, and throat (ENT) and surgical specialists should be consulted to evaluate the patient as early as possible. Patients with laryngeal trauma should be admitted for airway observation and examination by laryngoscopy.[1-3]

REFERENCES

1. Kleinsasser NH, Priemer FG, Schulze W, Kleinsasser OF. External trauma to the larynx: classification, diagnosis, therapy. *Eur Arch Otorhinolaryngol* 2000;257:439–444.
2. O'Mara W, Hebert AF. External laryngeal trauma. *J La State Med Soc* 2000;152:218–222.
3. Verghese ST, Hannallah RS. Pediatric otolaryngologic emergencies. *Anesthesiol Clin North Am* 2001;19:237–256.

Subglottic Stenosis

Barry Hahn

Clinical Presentation

Mild cases of subglottic stenosis in children may manifest as repeated episodes of coughing and may erroneously be given the diagnosis of recurrent croup. Adults with mild congenital stenosis are usually asymptomatic and are often diagnosed after a difficult intubation or while undergoing endoscopy for another purpose. Patients with acquired disease may become symptomatic a few days to years after the initial injury.[2] These symptoms can include dyspnea, stridor, hoarseness, cough, recurrent pneumonitis, and cyanosis.[2]

Pathophysiology

Subglottic stenosis is a congenital or acquired narrowing of the region that extends from the lower surface of the true vocal cords to the lower surface of the cricoid cartilage.[1,2] Congenital stenosis may be diagnosed only in patients with no history of intubation or laryngeal trauma; it is thought to be secondary to failure of the laryngeal lumen to recanalize properly during embryogenesis.[2] Most acquired cases results from laryngoscope injury or pressure necrosis with subsequent scarring.[2] Duration of intubation is a primary factor in the development of laryngeal stenosis.[1,2] Less common causes of scar formation and stenosis are foreign body, infection, inflammation, and chemical irritation.[1,2]

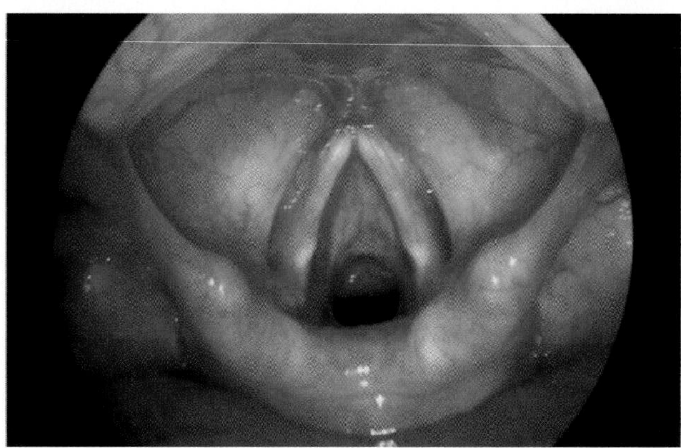

FIGURE 1–8 Subglottic stenosis secondary to Wegener's granulomatosus. (From Benjamin et al., with permission.)

Diagnosis

The diagnosis should be suggested based on the clinical history, but radiographic studies such as plain films, barium esophagram, airway fluoroscopy, magnetic resonance imaging (MRI), and computed tomography (CT) may be helpful adjuncts.[1,2] Plain films are more useful in children and can help exclude other causes of stridor (e.g., foreign bodies). However, the gold standard for diagnosis is still direct laryngoscopy and tracheobronchoscopy.[2]

Clinical Complications

Complications include airway obstruction, respiratory failure, increased risk of respiratory infections, preoperative and postoperative risks of surgical repair, and problems secondary to tracheostomy. Complications of pediatric stenosis also include feeding difficulties.[1]

Management

Most children outgrow congenital stenosis and require only expectant care.[1] Curative surgical procedures include anterior laryngotracheal decompression (cricoid split) and laryngotracheal reconstruction with cartilage grafting.[2] Tracheostomy is a last resort and should be avoided if possible.[2] The use of corticosteroids to prevent airway stenosis is controversial.[1,2] 5-Fluorouracil (5-FU) and mitomycin-C have been suggested to reduced scar formation in the endoscopic treatment of subglottic stenosis.[1,2]

REFERENCES

1. Loh KS, Irish JC. Traumatic complications of intubation and other airway management procedures. *Anesthesiol Clin North Am* 2002; 20:953–969.
2. Lorenz RR. Adult laryngotracheal stenosis: etiology and surgical management. *Curr Opin Otolaryngol Head Neck Surg* 2003;11: 467–472.

Airway Mass

Allon Amitai

Clinical Presentation

Patients with an airway mass may present with snoring or persistent nasal congestion or with dyspnea, stridor, or hemoptysis.[1] Intrathoracic airway masses can cause loss of lung function or postobstructive pneumonia.[2] Some airway masses go unrecognized until airway intervention or radiography is performed for unrelated reasons.

Pathophysiology

Nasal or vocal cord polyps, laryngeal papillomatosis, epiglottitis, granulomata, cysts, tumors, abscesses, and hematomas may all encroach on the upper or lower airway.[1] Mediastinal masses of various kinds (e.g., carcinoma) may obstruct the trachea and bronchi.[2] These processes can be exacerbated by inflammation and edema and result in an acute compromise of a narrowed airway.

Diagnosis

The diagnosis can be made by direct visualization of the mass if it is in a region where this is possible. Direct or fiberoptic laryngoscopy, bronchoscopy, plain radiography, computed tomography (CT), or magnetic resonance imaging (MRI) may assist in visualization of lesions in various locations in the respiratory tract.

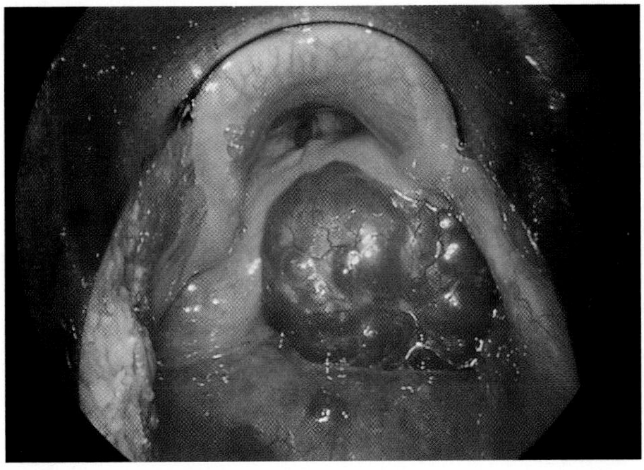

FIGURE 1–9 Severe airway obstruction due to hemangioma. (From Benjamin et al., with permission.)

Clinical Complications

Complications include total airway obstruction and rupture of abscess or hematoma into the airway leading to hypoxemia, aspiration, or respiratory arrest. Tumors and infections may spread to contiguous structures, the mediastinum, or surrounding neck tissue planes and may compromise adjacent neurovascular structures.[1]

Management

Airway assistance techniques, such as raising the head of the bed and extending the atlanto-occipital joint, may be attempted. Adjuncts such as a nasopharyngeal airway may be useful. Oxygen should be administered by facemask. If airway edema is suspected, nebulized racemic epinephrine and corticosteroids may be helpful in some cases.[1] The presence of complete obstruction or an unstable airway necessitates immediate intubation or the establishment of a surgical airway. Because abscess rupture can occur during laryngoscopy, Ludwig's angina or a retropharyngeal abscess may be best managed by establishment of a surgical airway in the operating room. Airway compression from anterior mediastinal masses may be relieved by placing the patient in a lateral decubitus position. If the cause is infection, immediate empiric antibiotic coverage should be instituted. All patients with threatened or impending airway obstruction should be admitted to a monitored setting and should never be left unattended.

REFERENCES

1. Doyle DJ, Arellano R. Upper airway diseases and airway management: a synopsis. *Anesthesiol Clin North Am* 2002;20:767–787.
2. Wood DE. Management of malignant tracheobronchial obstruction. *Surg Clin North Am* 2002;82:621–642.

Cricothyroidotomy

Moshe Weizberg

Indications

Cricothyroidotomy is indicated in cases of failed or unattainable orotracheal intubation.[1,2] Other indications include upper airway obstruction, laryngeal edema, and facial trauma or burns that render orotracheal intubation impossible or contraindicated.[1,2]

Contraindications

Absolute contraindications include the ability to easily perform orotracheal intubation, transection of the trachea with retraction of the distal end, and fractured larynx.[1] Relative contraindications include age younger than 10 years, coagulopathy, and massive neck edema. Relative contraindications may be disregarded in an emergency situation in which airway control is imperative.[1,2]

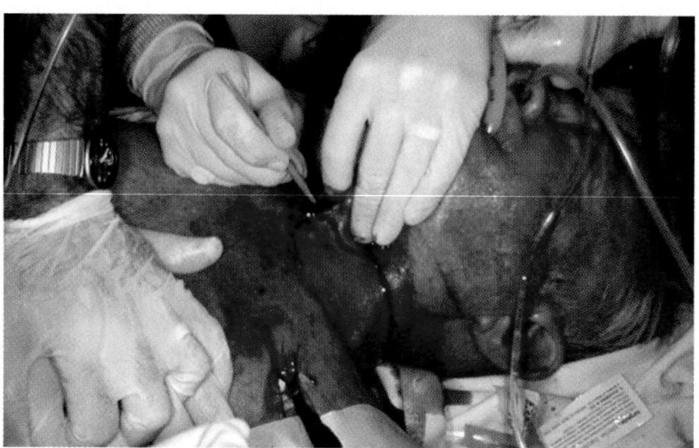

FIGURE 1–10 Emergency cricothyrotomy. (© 2004, Ron M. Walls, MD, used with permission.)

Technique

The neck is prepared and draped in the usual sterile fashion and hyperextended, provided the cervical spine is stable. The landmarks are identified, starting superiorly with the thyroid cartilage and moving inferiorly to the cricothyroid membrane and cricoid cartilage. If the landmarks are distorted, the little finger may be placed in the suprasternal notch. The ring, middle, and index fingers are then placed adjacent to the little finger; the index finger should be resting on the cricothyroid membrane.[1] The larynx is immobilized with the nondominant hand, and a vertical midline incision is made starting at the inferior edge of the thyroid cartilage and extending to the superior border of the cricoid cartilage. Next, a blunt dissection is performed down to the shiny cricothyroid membrane. A transverse incision is then made in the membrane. If available, a tracheal hook is used to apply gentle traction to the thyroid cartilage in a cephalad direction. The incision is dilated to allow passage of a definitive airway, such as a tracheostomy or endotracheal tube. The cuff of the tube is inflated, and a bag-valve device is attached to ventilate the patient. Proper tube placement is confirmed, and the tube is secured in place.[1,2]

Management

Complications include subglottic stenosis, bleeding (sometimes due to laceration of a thyroid vessel), improper tube placement, and infection, as well as transient hoarseness and voice changes.[1]

REFERENCES

1. Walls RM. Cricothyroidotomy. *Emerg Med Clin of North Am* 1988;6:725–736.
2. Hamilton PH, Kang JJ. Emergency airway management. *Mt Sinai J Med* 1997;64:292–301.

Transtracheal Jet Ventilation

Mark Silverberg

Indications

Transtracheal jet ventilation (TJV) is indicated for failed endotracheal intubation or upper airway obstruction.[1,2]

Contraindications

Contraindications to TJV include the ability to easily perform intubation, transection of the trachea with retraction of the distal end, and fractured larynx.

Clinical Complications

The overall complication rate is reported to be approximately 30%.[1,2] Occasionally, TJV fails because of a misplaced catheter, distorted landmarks, or a kinked catheter. The most common complication of TJV is subcutaneous emphysema (7% to 10%).[1,2] Other complications include pneumothorax, pneumomediastinum (2% to 4%), bleeding, hemoptysis, and esophageal injury.

Technique

If time permits, the neck is prepared and draped in sterile fashion. In emergency situations, it is considered reasonable to pour povidone-iodine on the neck. The head is hyperextended, provided that the cervical spine is stable and relevant landmarks have been identified. The index finger is placed on the laryngeal prominence and then slid inferiorly until it "drops off" onto the cricothyroid membrane. If the landmarks are distorted, the little finger may placed in the suprasternal notch. The ring, middle, and index fingers are then placed adjacent to the little finger; the index finger should come to rest on the cricothyroid membrane.

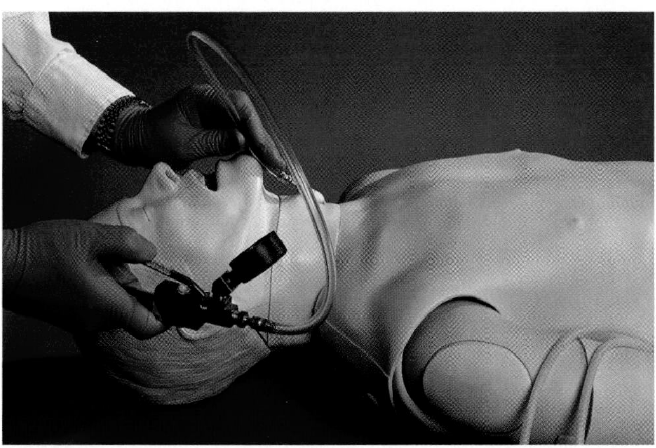

FIGURE 1–11 Proper catheter placement caudally through the cricothyroid membrane with oxygen insufflation using a high-pressure (30 to 60 psi) oxygen source and pushbutton release valve. (© 2004, Ron M. Walls, MD and STRATUS Center for Medical Simulation, Bringham and Women's Hospital, used with permission.)

A 3-mL syringe is attached to a 12- to 14-gauge Angiocath at least 2 cm long. Special 6F transtracheal catheters are available. The larynx is immobilized with the nondominant hand, and the needle is inserted in the midline into the inferior aspect of the cricothyroid membrane. This is done in a caudad direction, at an angle of 45 degrees to the skin. Air should freely return into the syringe when the cricothyroid membrane is punctured. Some practitioners recommend the use of a saline-filled syringe, with the development of bubbles in the syringe confirming intratracheal placement. The syringe and needle are removed, and the catheter is connected to a high-pressure oxygen source and secured in place. Tubing must be connected directly to an oxygen source, without a regulator. A pressure of 50 psi is required for adequate oxygenation. Attachment of a bag-valve device to the catheter does not provide effective ventilation. Equal breath sounds should be confirmed and a chest radiograph obtained. TJV is effective for 20 to 30 minutes, at which time it must be converted to a definitive airway.[1,2]

REFERENCES

1. Patel RG. Percutaneous transtracheal jet ventilation: a safe, quick, and temporary way to provide oxygenation and ventilation when conventional methods are unsuccessful. *Chest* 1999;116:1689–1694.
2. Benumof JL, Scheller MS. The importance of transtracheal jet ventilation in the management of the difficult airway. *Anesthesiology* 1989;71:769–778.

Retrograde Intubation

Moshe Weizberg

Indications

Indications for retrograde intubation include failed or difficult orotracheal intubation, cervical spine injury, and facial or laryngeal distortion.[1,2]

Contraindications

Absolute contraindications to retrograde intubation are inability to open the mouth and easily performed orotracheal intubation.[1] Relative contraindications include systemic coagulopathy and infection on the skin overlying the cricothyroid membrane.[1]

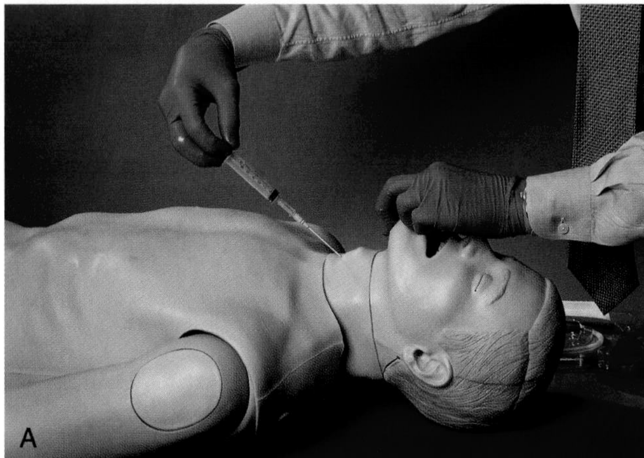

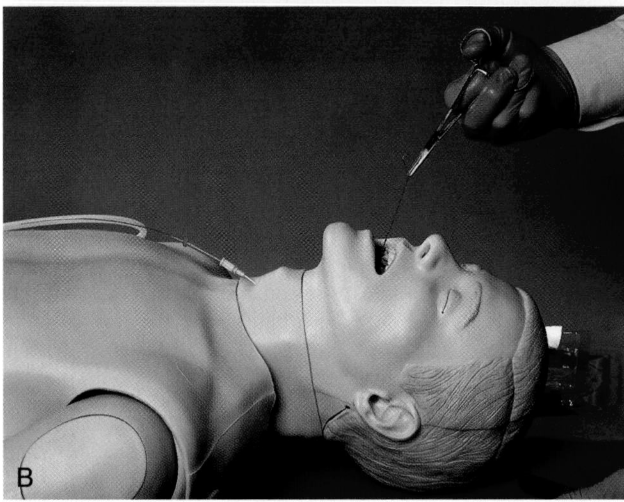

FIGURE 1–12 **A:** Introducer needle is inserted cranially through the cricothyroid membrane. **B:** Long guidewire is introduced through the catheter and retrieved from the pharynx with a hemostat. (© 2004, Ron M. Walls, MD and STRATUS Center for Medical Simulation, Bringham and Women's Hospital, used with permission.)

Technique

The neck is prepared and draped and anatomic landmarks are identified, including the thyroid cartilage, cricothyroid membrane, and cricoid cartilage. The larynx is stabilized with the nondominant hand, and a 16-gauge Angiocath or an epidural needle attached to a syringe is used to puncture the skin. The needle is then angled 30 to 40 degrees cephalad, and a puncture is made through the cricothyroid membrane. Air should be aspirated freely on entering the trachea. The syringe is then removed, and a guidewire from a central line kit is passed into the oropharynx. Magill forceps may be employed to bring the end of the guidewire out of the mouth. The needle or catheter is then removed from the wire, and the guidewire is clamped at the skin, outside the neck. The other end is inserted into the side hole (Murphy eye) of the endotracheal tube and threaded out the proximal end. The endotracheal tube is slowly advanced over the guidewire until resistance is met. If the tube has successfully passed through the vocal cords, slight tension should be felt on the distal guidewire. Light pressure is then exerted on the tube, the clamp is released, and the guidewire is pulled out the proximal end of the tube. The endotracheal tube is then advanced to its proper depth, and placement is confirmed in the usual fashion.[1,2]

Management

Complications include hemorrhage, vocal cord injury, and subcutaneous emphysema.[1] Misplacement of the endotracheal tube into the esophagus can also occur. Puncture of the cricothyroid membrane has been associated with laryngospasm and soft tissue neck infections.[1]

REFERENCES

1. McNamara RM. Retrograde intubation of the trachea. *Ann Emerg Med* 1987;16:680–682.
2. Heller EM, Schneider K, Saven B. Percutaneous retrograde intubation. *Laryngoscope* 1989;99:554–555.

Fiberoptic Intubation

Tanisha Medlock

Fiberoptic intubation is an aid to tracheal intubation in which a flexible fiberoptic rhinolaryngoscope is used to pass an endotracheal tube (ET) into the trachea.[1,2]

Indications

Fiberoptic intubation is used to provide a definitive airway in a patient with a difficult airway. It is a useful adjunct to intubation for patients in whom respiratory depression and paralysis are undesirable. This awake technique can benefit patients with cervical spine or facial injuries, oropharyngeal masses, edema, and other laryngeal pathology that would make direct laryngoscopy difficult or impossible.[2]

Contraindications

Difficulty arises if large amounts of secretions or blood are present. The fiberoptic rhinolaryngoscope has limited suction, which may result in poor visualization and intubation failure. Operator inexperience may also be considered a relative contraindication for this procedure in critically ill patients.[1]

Technique

Two approaches may be employed: the nasotracheal route and orotracheal route. The nasotracheal method is the preferred style, because it is easier to aim the laryngoscope at the glottis with this approach. A vasoconstrictor and a topical anesthetic should be applied to the nasal passage and posterior pharynx. The lubricated ET is placed over the laryngoscope, which is inserted into the most patent nostril. The laryngoscope is then advanced toward the larynx and through the vocal cords. Once this has occurred, the ET can be advanced over the laryngoscope and into final position.[1,2]

Management

Difficulty visualizing the anatomy has been noted. Adequate suction throughout the procedure is important to sufficiently identify the laryngeal anatomy. Visualization can be improved by attaching an oxygen source to the suction channel and insufflating to blow secretions and debris out of view.[1] In the trachea, the ET may be difficult to advance. To solve this problem, the ET may be withdrawn, rotated 90 degrees, and readvanced.[1] Nasopharyngeal trauma and epistaxis are also common complications.

REFERENCES

1. Butler KH, Clyne B. Management of the difficult airway: alternative airway techniques and adjuncts. *Emerg Med Clin North Am* 2003;21:259–289.
2. Rodricks MB, Deutschman CS. Emergent airway management: indications and methods in the face of confounding conditions. *Crit Care Clin* 2000;16:389–409.

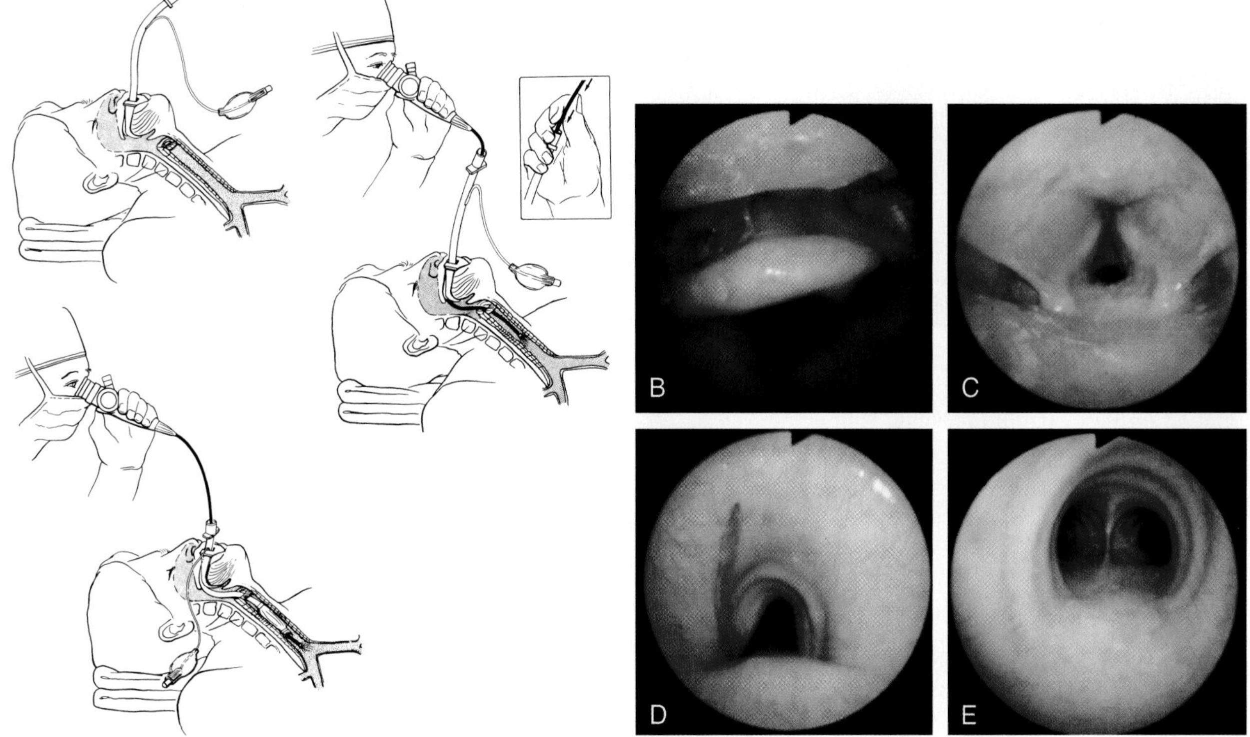

FIGURE 1–13 **A:** Technique for fiberoptic intubation. **B:** Tip of fiberscope in oropharynx. **C:** Tip of fiberscope passed beneath the tip of the epiglottis; glottis is in view. **D:** Tip of fiberscope passed just beyond vocal cords. **E:** Tip of fiberscope in lower trachea; carina is in view. (From Ovassapian et al., with permission.)

Tracheal Foreign Body

Steven Moonblatt

Clinical Presentation

The acute presentation of an airway obstruction caused by a tracheal foreign body (TFB) includes an initial brief period of choking, gagging, or wheezing. This may be associated with hoarseness, cyanosis, aphonia, or dysphonia. In children, up to 50% of acute aspirations are unwitnessed.[1] If the foreign body passes into the trachea, these symptoms resolve and cough, inspiratory stridor, wheezing, tachypnea, suprasternal retractions, and diminished breath sounds may be noted.

Pathophysiology

Eighty-five percent of all foreign body aspirations occur in children younger than 15 years of age, and most occur in children 1 to 3 three years old.[2] Food products are frequently aspirated, with peanuts being the most common source for TFB in children. In adults, there is a propensity for objects to lodge on the right side. In children, reported ranges are 30% to 40% on the left, 40% to 70% on the right, and 10% to 20% in the laryngotracheal area.[2]

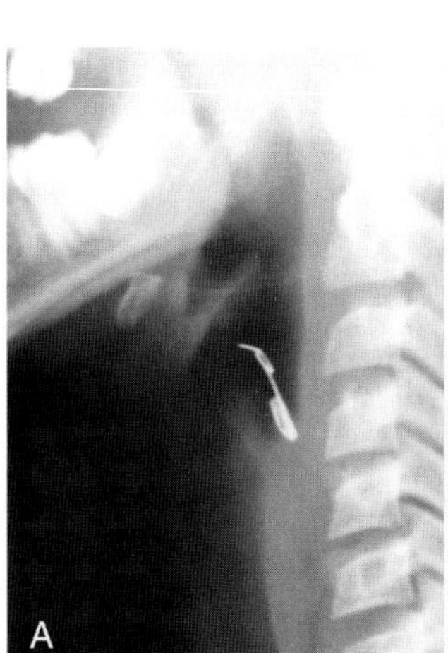

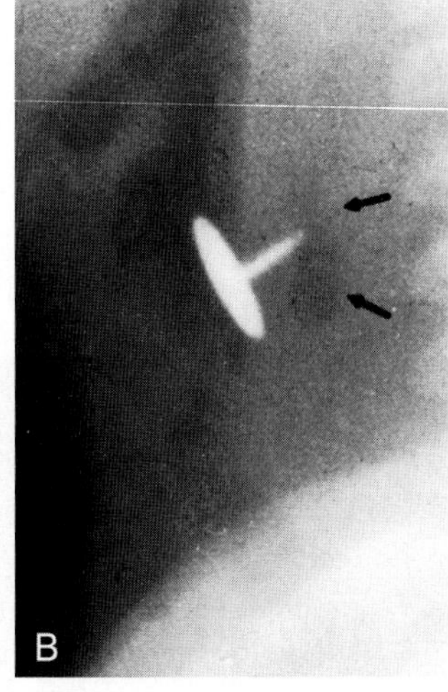

FIGURE 1–14 Tracheal foreign bodies: **(A)** Open safety pin in hypopharynx; **(B)** thumbtack in hypopharynx with retropharyngeal air *(arrows)*. (From Swischuk, with permission.)

Diagnosis

Routine diagnostic imaging should include anteroposterior and lateral chest radiographs (inspiratory and expiratory). Most foreign bodies are radiolucent, but radiographs are useful for detecting indirect signs of TFB, including air trapping, obstructive emphysema, and mediastinal shift. Left and right lateral decubitus films may be helpful. The dependent lung should deflate unless it is obstructed by a foreign body. Up to 50% of patients with TFB have normal radiographs. The gold standard for the identification and localization of an airway foreign body is bronchoscopy.[1,3]

Clinical Complications

The most common complication of a foreign body is pulmonary infection. Other complications include pneumothorax, fistula formation, perforation, atelectasis, and stricture.[3]

Management

Complete occlusion of the airway manifests as the inability to make sounds or exchange air. For an infant younger than 1 year of age, back slaps and chest thrusts with the infant in a head-down position should be done immediately. For children older than 1 year and for adults, abdominal thrusts should be performed according to American Heart Association guidelines. If the patient is able to cough, speak, or cry, no immediate measures need to be undertaken.[3] Pulmonary and surgery services should be consulted. The procedure of choice to retrieve a foreign body is bronchoscopy. Some TFBs cannot be removed by bronchoscopy, and open thoracotomy is required.[2,3]

REFERENCES

1. Friedman EM. Tracheobronchial foreign bodies. *Otolaryngol Clin North Am* 2000;33:179–185.
2. Rafanan AL, Mehta AC. Adult airway foreign body removal: what's new? *Clin Chest Med* 2001;22:319–330.
3. Rovin JD, Rodgers BM. Pediatric foreign body aspiration. *Pediatr Rev* 2000;21:86–90.

Laryngospasm

Tanisha Medlock

Clinical Presentation

Laryngospasm may occur during induction of anesthesia or conscious sedation, or it may be induced by gastroesophageal reflux (GER), aspiration of stomach contents, or inhaled irritants.[1,3] Breathing becomes difficult, and patients complain of dyspnea while coughing and gasping to breathe against a closed glottis. Spasm is more common in the pediatric patient population, especially in children with GER, upper respiratory tract infection, asthma, or exposure to smoke.[1,2]

Pathophysiology

Laryngospasm is essentially an exaggeration of the protective glottic closure reflex in response to irritants such as gases, food, vomit, blood, or foreign bodies.[2,3] This reflexive closure of the glottis can persist after the initial irritation ceases. During laryngospasm, the epiglottic body, false cords, and extrinsic muscles of the larynx prohibit the movement of air through the larynx.[3] No vocalization is possible, and the vocal cords usually cannot be visualized. As hypoxia and hypercarbia develop, the superior laryngeal nerve is inhibited and the laryngospasm usually resolves.[2,3]

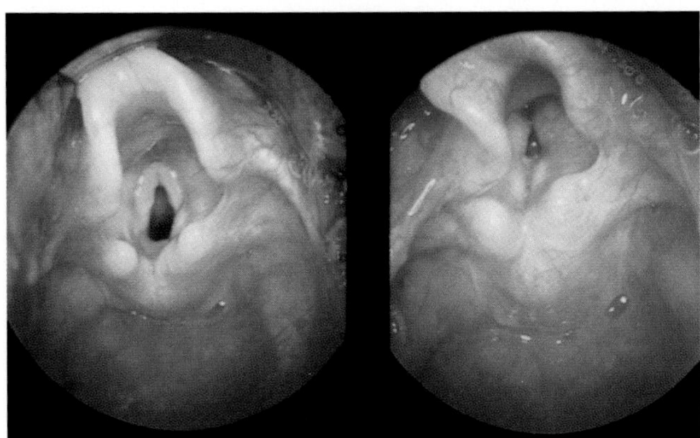

FIGURE 1–15 Laryngeal spasm. Normal larynx *(left)* during spontaneous respiration and (right) with temporary laryngospasm. (From Benjamin et al., with permission.)

Diagnosis

This is a clinical diagnosis that should be suspected in a patient who is desaturating or gasping for air during induction.[3] The diagnosis can be confirmed by direct laryngoscopy or fiberoptic endoscopy. The vocal cords, if visible, should appear totally adducted.

Clinical Complications

Complications include hypoxia, hypercarbia, postobstructive pulmonary edema, and cardiopulmonary arrest.[1,2]

Management

Laryngospasm is classically associated with induction, and it may be relieved by deeper anesthesia. Topical lidocaine may play a role in preventing such occurrences. Some authors recommend tracheal anesthesia with an injection of lidocaine through the cricothyroid membrane.[3] If hypoxia does not resolve with supplemental oxygen, positive-pressure ventilation should be started. If the spasm persists, muscle relaxants may be useful.[3]

REFERENCES

1. Orenstein SR. An overview of reflux-associated disorders in infants: apnea, laryngospasm, and aspiration. *Am J Med* 2001;111[Suppl 8A]:60S–63S.
2. Green SM, Rothrock SG, Lynch EL, et al. Intramuscular ketamine for pediatric sedation in the emergency department: safety profile in 1,022 cases. *Ann Emerg Med* 1998;31:688–697.
3. Davis DP, Hamilton RS, Webster TH. Reversal of midazolam-induced laryngospasm with flumazenil. *Ann Emerg Med* 1998;32: 263–265.

Flail Chest

Erica McKernan

Flail chest occurs when three or more ribs are fractured in more than two areas, resulting in chest wall instability and subsequent paradoxic chest wall motion.[1]

Clinical Presentation

Patients present complaining of chest pain and dyspnea after direct trauma to the chest.

Pathophysiology

Because significant traumatic forces are required to cause flail chest, intrathoracic or intraabdominal injuries (or both) are also usually present. The incidences of concomitant contusion and pneumothorax are 50% and 77%, respectively.[1] Free-floating rib segments reduce the stability of the chest wall, resulting in increased work of breathing. The associated hypoxemia is secondary to the underlying pulmonary contusion and splinting and hypoventilation from pain.[2]

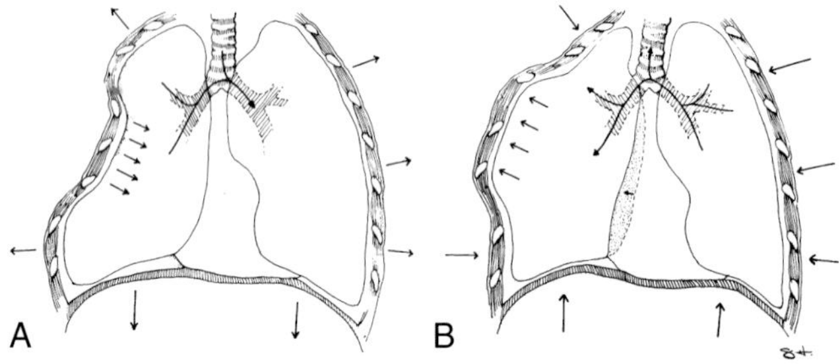

FIGURE 1–16 Paradoxic movement of the unstable "flail" segment of the chest wall during inspiration **(A)** and expiration **(B)**. (From Schwartz et al., with permission.)

Diagnosis

The diagnosis of flail chest is clinical and radiographic. On examination, paradoxic inward motion of the involved chest wall during inspiration and outward motion during expiration may be seen. Computed tomography (CT) of the chest is considered the gold standard for detection of flail chest.[3]

Clinical Complications

Hypoxemia, atelectasis, and pneumonia may complicate flail chest. The mortality rate ranges from 10% to 50% because of the severity of the underlying injuries.[2]

Management

Treatment depends on the severity of the underlying lung injury and pulmonary dysfunction. Selective intubation decreases morbidity and mortality.[1] Noninvasive management, including incentive spirometry, adequate analgesia, chest physiotherapy, and continuous positive airway pressure, reduce the incidence of pulmonary infections, length of stay in the intensive care unit, duration of hospitalization, and mortality.[2] Intubation and mechanical ventilation may be necessary for the patient with severe pulmonary failure. Shock, closed head injury, requirement for surgery, respiratory failure or distress, and airway obstruction are cited in multiple studies as criteria for mechanical ventilation.[1]

REFERENCES

1. Ullman EA, Donley LP, Brady WJ. Pulmonary trauma: emergency department evaluation and management. *Emerg Med Clin North Am* 2003;21:291–313.
2. Domino KB. Pulmonary function and dysfunction in the traumatized patient. *Anesthesiol Clin North Am* 1996;14:59–84.
3. Greenberg MD, Rosen CL. Evaluation of the patient with blunt chest trauma: an evidence-based approach. *Emerg Med Clin North Am* 1999;17:41–62.

Escharotomy

Steven Moonblatt

Clinical Presentation

Burns that require escharotomy may involve the extremities, chest, neck, or penis and are usually full thickness and circumferential. Burns to the chest and upper abdomen may compromise respirations as a result of decreased chest wall compliance.[1]

Pathophysiology

Full-thickness burns result in loss of the ability of the skin to stretch. Edema develops both from fluid resuscitation and directly from thermal injury. As edema increases, circumferentially burned skin becomes a constricting tourniquet. Venous and lymphatic return is impaired. Perfusion through vessels and nerve function may become compromised.

Diagnosis

If an obvious full-thickness, circumferential burn is present, an escharotomy should be preformed on an emergency basis. In the extremities, pulses should be evaluated by Doppler ultrasonography, capillary refill assessed, and a sensory examination performed. These examinations should be done hourly; any abnormality found is an indication for escharotomy. If the skin feels tense or unyielding, an escharotomy is needed. Loss of a pulse is a late finding, and ischemic muscle damage can occur even with discernible Doppler pulses.[2,3]

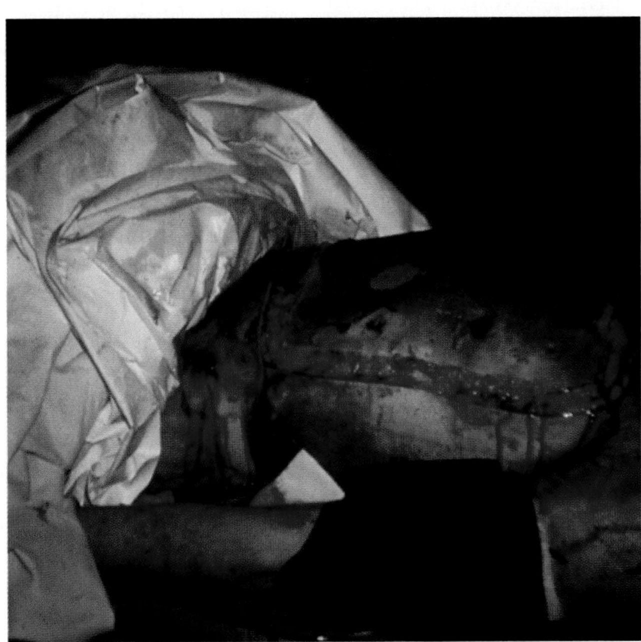

FIGURE 1–17 Severe body burns with chest escharotomy. (Courtesy of Michael Greenberg, MD.)

Clinical Complications

Complications include bleeding, infection, and injury to underlying structures.[1]

Management

Escharotomies are often bedside procedures. The incision is made into the subcutaneous fat; IV sedation may be necessary. For torso escharotomies, axial incisions are made along the anterior axillary line bilaterally and then connected across the midline.[1] For the upper extremity, the escharotomy is made along the medical (ulnar) and lateral (radial) aspects of the arm, extending the full extent of the full-thickness burn and just into the unburned or partial-thickness burn areas. The elbow and wrist should be crossed if needed, and forearm incisions may be extended into the thenar and hypothenar eminences. The hand is incised with dorsal incisions, usually three incisions placed between the metacarpal bones. Incisions in the digits are done in the midlateral line on the radial and ulnar sides.[3] Escharotomy of the lower extremity is similar to that of the upper extremity. Silver sulfadiazine or a similar agent should be applied to the area. Transfer to a burn center should be considered.

REFERENCES

1. Sheridan RL. Burns. *Crit Care Med* 2002;30[11 Suppl]:S500–S514.
2. Brown RL, Greenhalgh DG, Kagan RJ, Warden GD. The adequacy of limb escharotomies-fasciotomies after referral to a major burn center. *J Trauma* 1994;37:916–920.
3. Wong L, Spence RJ. Escharotomy and fasciotomy of the burned upper extremity. *Hand Clin* 2000;16:165–174.

Emergency Department Thoracotomy

Jennifer Kiss

Clinical Presentation

Emergency department thoracotomy (EDT) is best applied to patients with penetrating thoracic injuries who arrive promptly after injury. Witnessed signs of life just before the thoracotomy is performed, including pupillary response, spontaneous ventilation, carotid pulse, extremity movement, and cardiac electrical activity, justify EDT in most cases. EDT after blunt trauma has low survival and poor neurologic outcomes. These guidelines apply to the pediatric as well as the adult population.[1]

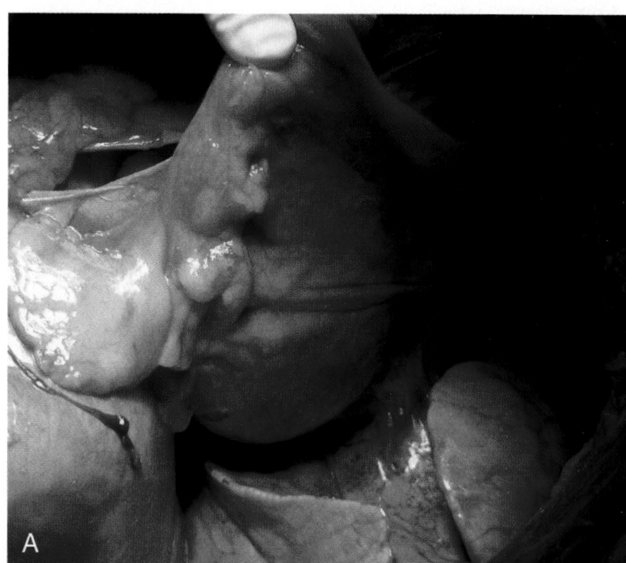

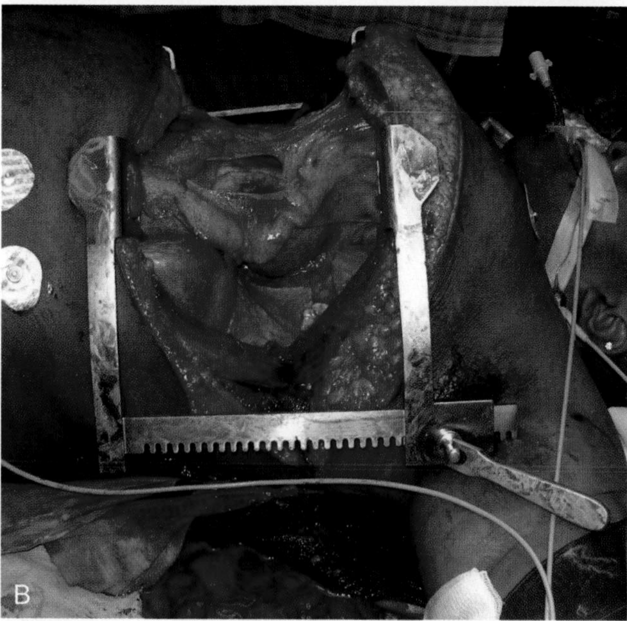

FIGURE 1–18 **A:** Thoracotomy, showing the phrenic nerve running down the pericardium. **B:** Clam shell with double rib spreaders shown from the left. (Courtesy of Mark Silverberg, MD.)

Epidemiology

EDT is associated with a low survival rate (8%).[1–3] When stratified by mechanism, the survival rate for EDTs performed for penetrating thoracic injuries is 11%, that for blunt trauma is less than 2%, and that for penetrating cardiac injury is highest, at 31%.[1]

Diagnosis

Cardiac penetrating injury has a higher survival rate than noncardiac penetrating injury, but EDT may be necessary to discern the specific injury site.[1] Pericardial tamponade is the most common reversible injury caused by penetrating thoracic trauma. Focused abdominal sonography for trauma (FAST) may facilitate the identification of tamponade before thoracotomy.[2]

Clinical Complications

Long-term neurologic impairment is a major complication of thoracotomy. Up to 15% of EDT survivors have neurologic impairment.[1]

Management

Because pericardial tamponade is a reversible injury, the initial objective on opening the chest is rapid pericardotomy and control of cardiac hemorrhage, followed by control of other sources of hemorrhage.[2] Cross-clamping of the descending aorta is the secondary goal to increase perfusion of the heart and brain as well as possibly decreasing distal hemorrhage. Direct cardiac massage and control of air embolism can also be achieved.[3]

REFERENCES

1. Working Group, Ad Hoc Subcommittee on Outcomes, American College of Surgeons, Committee on Trauma. Practice management guidelines for emergency department thoracotomy. *J Am Coll Surg* 2001;193:303–309.
2. Grove CA, Lemmon G, Anderson G, McCarthy M. Emergency thoracotomy: appropriate use in the resuscitation of trauma patients. *Am Surg* 2002;68:313–317.
3. Rhee PM, Acosta J, Bridgeman A, Wang D, Jordan M, Rich N. Survival after emergency department thoracotomy: review of published data from the past 25 years. *J Am Coll Surg* 2000;190: 288–298.

Cardiogenic Shock

Mark Silverberg

Clinical Presentation

Cardiogenic shock is usually secondary to acute myocardial infarction (AMI), and patients often present with typical cardiac complaints. On physical examination, hypotension with evidence of poor tissue perfusion is indicative of the shock state. Electrocardiographic (ECG) findings can include ST elevations or depressions.[1]

Pathophysiology

The most common cause of cardiogenic shock is massive AMI, although smaller infarctions in patients with previously compromised left ventricular function can also precipitate shock.[1] Other possible causes are acute mitral regurgitation and rupture of the interventricular septum or ventricle free wall.[1] The anterior region is the most common infarction zone associated with cardiogenic shock, but right-sided infarctions can also manifest similarly. Less likely causes include myocarditis, end-stage cardiomyopathy, myocardial contusion, and hypertrophic obstructive cardiomyopathy.[1] Shock with a delayed onset may result from infarct extension, reocclusion of a previously patent coronary vessel, or decompensation of myocardial function in the noninfarct zone due to metabolic derangements.[1]

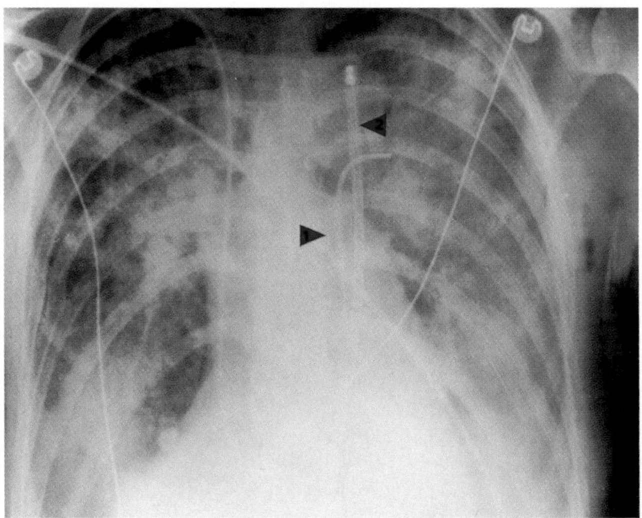

FIGURE 1–19 Radiograph of patient with myocardial infarction and cardiogenic shock, showing a normal-sized heart and bilateral pulmonary alveolar edema. *Arrow 1,* Swan-Ganz catheter; *Arrow 2,* intra-aortic balloon catheter. (From Kassner EG. *Atlas of radiologic imaging.* New York: Gower, 1989.)

Diagnosis

Hemodynamic criteria include sustained hypotension with a systolic blood pressure (BP) of less than 90 mm Hg for 30 minutes or longer, a reduced cardiac index (less than 2.2 L/min/m^2), and an elevated wedge pressure (greater than 15 mm Hg).[1] Clinical clues include signs of poor tissue perfusion such as oliguria, clouded sensorium, and cool, mottled extremities. Other causes of shock (e.g., hypovolemia, sepsis) must be ruled out.[1]

Clinical Complications

If cardiogenic shock is not addressed and reversed rapidly, it usually progresses to refractory hypotension and, eventually, death.[1]

Management

Treatment centers on therapy for the AMI, including aspirin, nitrates, β-blockers, and reperfusion therapy. Fluid resuscitation is important unless there is frank pulmonary edema. The resuscitation should be guided by invasive monitoring, with central venous and arterial access and bladder catheterization. Pain and anxiety may be alleviated with morphine. Cardiovascular support with inotropic agents may be attempted, using dobutamine for a systolic BP greater than 80 mm Hg or dopamine for lower values.[1] Endotracheal intubation should be considered if the patient is hypoxic despite supplemental oxygen, or to reduce the work of breathing in anticipation of cardiac catheterization.[1] Electrolyte abnormalities such as hypokalemia and hypomagnesemia must be addressed, because they may predispose to ventricular arrhythmias. Thrombolytic therapy to open obstructed vessels has been studied, but poor results were reported for patients in cardiogenic shock.[1] Other adjuncts that may raise BP until the patient can be revascularized with percutaneous transluminal coronary angioplasty (PTCA) or coronary artery bypass grafting (CABG) include insertion of an intraaortic balloon pump or a left ventricular assist device.[1]

REFERENCES

1. Hollenberg SM. Cardiogenic shock. *Crit Care Clin* 2001;17:391–410.

Anaphylactic Shock

Boris Khodorkovsky

Clinical Presentation

Patients present after exposure to an offending antigen. Manifestation of allergic reactions can occur within seconds to hours and can vary from local inflammation and itching to multisystem organ failure.[1]

Pathophysiology

Anaphylactic shock results after the exposure of an antigen to the immune system produces mast cell degranulation and mediator release. Mast cell activation can occur either by immunoglobulin E (IgE)–mediated (anaphylactic) or non-IgE-mediated (anaphylactoid) pathways. Triggers of anaphylactic shock include insect stings or bites, medications, and foods; anaphylaxis can also be idiopathic. Inflammatory mediators include histamine, leukotrienes, tryptase, and prostaglandins. When released, they cause increased mucus secretion, increased bronchial smooth muscle tone, airway edema, decreased vascular tone, and capillary leakage. The constellation of these mechanisms leads to respiratory compromise and cardiovascular collapse.[2]

Diagnosis

The diagnosis of anaphylactic shock is clinical and should be considered in any patient with history of allergen exposure and physical signs suggestive of anaphylaxis. Presenting symptoms may include wheezing (26%), pruritus, urticaria, weakness, dizziness, syncope (3%), nausea, vomiting, and diarrhea. Physical examination may reveal tachypnea, tachycardia, hypotension, stridor, angioedema (15%), and urticaria (98%).[2,3]

Clinical Complications

Complications include possible future recurrence and death.

Management

Securing a patent airway is the first priority. Endotracheal intubation may be difficult due to angioedema and laryngeal spasm. Consequently, cricothyroidotomy or transtracheal jet insufflation equipment should be readily available. Subcutaneous epinephrine (1:1,000), 0.3 to 0.5 mg, is indicated for patients with airway symp-

TABLE 1-20 Symptoms and Signs of Anaphylaxis

Reaction	Symptom	Sign
Urticaria	Itching	Raised wheals diffusely, wandering, evanescent
Angioedema	Nonpruritic tingling	Swelling of lips, eyes, hands, uvula, tongue
Laryngeal edema	Hoarseness	Inspiratory stridor
	Dysphagia	Intercostal and clavicular retractions
	Lump in throat	Cyanosis
	Airway obstruction	
	Sudden death	
Bronchospasm	Cough	Wheezing
	Dyspnea	Tachypnea
	Chest tightness	Retractions
Hypotension	Dizziness	Hypotension (mild to severe)
	Syncope	Tachycardia
	Confusion	Oliguria
Rhinitis	Nasal congestion	Mucosal edema
	Itching and fluid	
Conjunctivitis	Tearing	Lid edema, injection, chemosis
	Itching	
Gastroenteritis	Cramping	Normal examination
	Diarrhea	
	Vomiting	

Signs and symptoms of anaphylaxis. (From Harwood-Nuss, with permission.)

toms or unstable vital signs. IV epinephrine (1:10,000), 0.3 to 0.5 mg, may be given in cases of severe shock. Administration of high-flow oxygen with β-agonists via nebulizer may help relieve difficulty in breathing. Hypotension should be treated with crystalloid IV fluids. Pressor agents such as dopamine or epinephrine and invasive monitoring can be instituted in refractory cases. All patients with anaphylactic shock should receive antihistamines (H_1 and H_2 antagonists) and corticosteroids. Further exposure to the offending antigen should be prevented. Patients with profound shock on presentation require admission to an intensive care monitoring setting. Consultation with an allergist for desensitization therapy may be appropriate.[3]

REFERENCES

1. The diagnosis and management of anaphylaxis. Joint Task Force on Practice Parameters. *J Allergy Clin Immunol* 1998;101(6 Pt 2): S465–S528.
2. Weiler JM. Anaphylaxis in the general population: a frequent and occasionally fatal disorder that is underrecognized. *J Allergy Clin Immunol* 1999;104(2 Pt 1):271–273.
3. Lin RY, Curry A, Pesola GR, et al. Improved outcomes in patients with acute allergic syndromes who are treated with combined H_1 and H_2 antagonists. *Ann Emerg Med* 2000;36:462–468.

Hypovolemic/Hemorrhagic Shock

Boris Khodorkovsky

Hypovolemic shock is defined as decreased tissue perfusion and oxygenation with circulatory collapse caused by acute loss of the intravascular volume secondary to various medical or surgical conditions.

Clinical Presentation

Patients with hemorrhagic shock present with a history of recent trauma, recent surgery, or a bleeding disorder. Physical examination findings may include hypotension, tachycardia, depressed mental status, low urine output, and obvious signs of trauma or hemorrhage. Acute blood loss from injuries to the thorax, abdomen, pelvis, or lower extremities can produce the state of shock. Patients may present with respiratory distress, decreased breath sounds, and dullness to percussion, indicating injury in the thorax; abdominal distention, diffuse tenderness, and peritonitis in abdominal injury; and flank ecchymosis in pelvic injury. The initial hematocrit, although unlikely to reflect the degree of blood loss, is useful as a baseline. An arterial blood gas/shock panel may reveal a decrease in base deficit and an increase in lactate values, reflecting lactic acidosis caused by hypoperfusion. Individual response to acute blood loss is varied and is influenced by many factors, including the patient's age, state of health, and medications.[1]

Pathophysiology

Hemorrhagic shock results from inadequate tissue perfusion and oxygenation secondary to acute blood loss. The most common cause is trauma; surgery, gastrointestinal bleeding, and childbirth are less frequent causes. Physiologic compensation to hemorrhage includes vasoconstriction and augmentation of cardiac output through tachycardia. At a later stage of the shock, hypotension ensues secondary to decreased circulatory blood volume. On the cellular level, the tissue hypoperfusion results in an inadequate supply of oxygen to the cells, leading to anaerobic metabolism and production of lactate. The decrease in base deficit and rise in lactate typically precede the physical signs of shock.[1]

Diagnosis

Hemorrhagic shock is possible in any patient with hemorrhage, unstable vital signs, and evidence of hypoperfusion. Shock can be defined by the ATLS classification, which takes into account physical signs only:

- Type I (<15% blood loss)—normal pulse, BP, and pulse pressure
- Type II (15%–30% blood loss)—tachycardia, normal BP, decreased pulse pressure
- Type III (30%–40% blood loss)—tachycardia, hypotension, decreased pulse pressure
- Type IV (40% blood loss)—tachycardia, hypotension, decreased pulse pressure

Diagnosis of the cause of hemorrhagic shock may require laboratory testing, focused abdominal sonography for trauma (FAST) examination, diagnostic peritoneal lavage, computed tomography (CT), and plain radiography.

Clinical Complications

Complications include acute renal failure, acute respiratory distress syndrome, disseminated intravascular coagulation, multisystem organ failure, sepsis, and death.

Management

In hemorrhagic shock, to ensure adequate tissue perfusion and oxygenation, decreased IV volume and oxygen demand must be addressed. Patients should receive supplemental oxygen; venous access and urine output monitoring should be established. Hypotension in these patients must be treated with crystalloid IV fluids and administration of blood products. The site of acute blood loss must be determined, and early control of hemorrhage must be instituted. The success of resuscitation is indicated by clinical and laboratory parameters. Appropriate consultations are warranted to guide further management. Patients in hemorrhagic shock must be admitted to a monitored setting.[1]

REFERENCES

1. Baron BJ, Scalea TM. Acute blood loss. *Emerg Med Clin North Am* 1996;14:35–55.

TABLE 1–21 Classification of Hypovolemic Shock

Parameter	Class 1	Class 2	Class 3	Class 4
Blood loss (mL)	<1000	1000–1500	1500–2000	>2000
Blood loss (%)	<15	15–30	30–40	>40
Systolic blood pressure	Normal	Normal	Reduced	Markedly reduced
Diastolic blood pressure	Normal	Elevated	Reduced	Markedly reduced
Heart rate	≤100	>100	>120	>140
Capillary refill	Normal	May be delayed	Usually delayed	Delayed
Urinary output (mL/hr)	>30	20–30	5–20	0–5
Mental status	Normal	Agitated	Confused	Obtunded

Adapted from American College of Surgeons Committee on Trauma. *Advanced trauma life support for doctors: student course manual.* 6th ed. Chicago: American College of Surgeons, 1997.

Neurogenic Shock

Boris Khodorkovsky

Neurogenic shock is defined as autonomic dysfunction, secondary to spinal cord injury, that results in hypotension and bradycardia.[1]

Clinical Presentation

Patients with neurogenic shock present after either blunt or penetrating trauma to the spinal cord.[1]

Pathophysiology

Neurogenic shock results from injury to the spinal cord that leads to disruption of the sympathetic autonomic outflow. These signals originate in the lateral gray horns of the central cord between the T1 and L2 levels. The consequences of decreased adrenergic tone are inability to properly increase the inotropic work of the heart and poor constriction of the peripheral vasculature in response to excitational stimulation. The unopposed vagal tone produces hypotension and bradycardia. The peripheral vasodilation results in the skin's being warm and flush. Hypothermia may result from the absence of autonomic regulatory vasoconstriction of blood redistribution to the body's core. The higher the level of the cord injury, the more severe the neurogenic shock, because more body mass is cut off from its sympathetic regulation. Neurogenic shock usually does not develop if the injury is below the level of T6.[1,2]

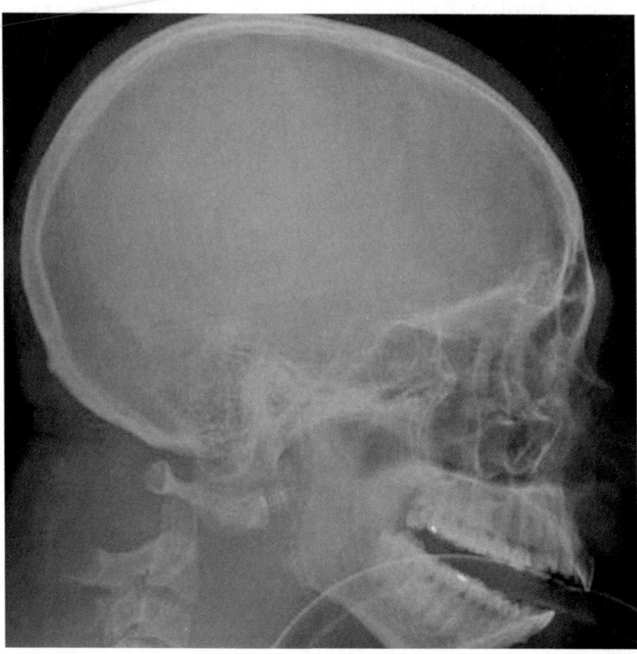

FIGURE 1–22 C1/C2 dislocation with spinal cord injury resulting in neurogenic shock. (Courtesy of Mark Silverberg, MD.)

Diagnosis

Neurogenic shock should be suspected in any patient with a spinal cord injury and cardiovascular collapse. Multiple factors, such as the mechanism of injury, the history, and the physical examination including vital signs, help to confirm the diagnosis of neurogenic shock. Hemorrhagic shock, a more common cause of hypotension in trauma patients, must be excluded. In patients with traumatic spinal cord injury, shock may be caused by blood loss, autonomic dysfunction, or both. Physical examination findings include hypotension, bradycardia (90%), and warm, dry skin, as well as signs of the initial trauma that caused the cord injury.[1,2]

Management

Hypotension in patients with neurogenic shock should initially be treated with crystalloid IV fluids. Pressor agents such as dopamine and dobutamine and invasive monitoring can be instituted if the response to IV fluids is suboptimal. Bradycardia should be treated with atropine, but pacing can be employed in refractory cases. Hypothermia should be treated by the usual conventional methods. Corticosteroid administration is a routine aspect of the treatment of traumatic spinal cord injuries. Emergency neurologic and neurosurgical evaluations are warranted in all cases.[2]

REFERENCES

1. Proctor MR. Spinal cord injury. *Crit Care Med* 2002;30[11 Suppl]: S489–S499.
2. Gerndt SJ, Rodriguez JL, Pawlik JW, et al. Consequences of high-dose steroid therapy for acute spinal cord injury. *J Trauma* 1997;42:279–284.

Interosseous Access

Jennifer Wiler

Interosseous access (IOA) may be used for the administration of crystalloids, colloids, medications, or blood products, as well as diagnostic interventions. It should be considered in all children 6 years of age or younger if peripheral lines are unsuccessful (after two attempts). IOA should be attempted before a central line or venous cutdown, because there is a high incidence of thrombosis with common femoral venous access.[1,2] IOA should be discontinued as soon as other venous access is obtained.

Technique

The preferred insertion location for IOA is the flat anteromedial medial surface of the proximal tibia, at a point 1 cm (about one fingerbreadth) medial and 1 cm inferior to the tibial tubercle, to avoid damaging the growth plate. Other sites include the distal femur, the iliac crest, and the distal tibia near the lateral and medial malleoli. The area of insertion should be cleansed with an appropriate solution and sterilely draped. For a traditional tibial placement, the leg should be supported at a 30- to 45-degree angle (a towel roll or IV bag can be helpful as a support). A bone marrow aspiration needle is inserted, with the bevel facing the patient's feet, at a 90-degree angle. After passage through the cortex, there is a decrease of resistance; the needle is then directed 45 to 60 degrees away from the epiphyseal plate. The needle is advanced with the use of a gentle twisting or boring motion.[1–3]

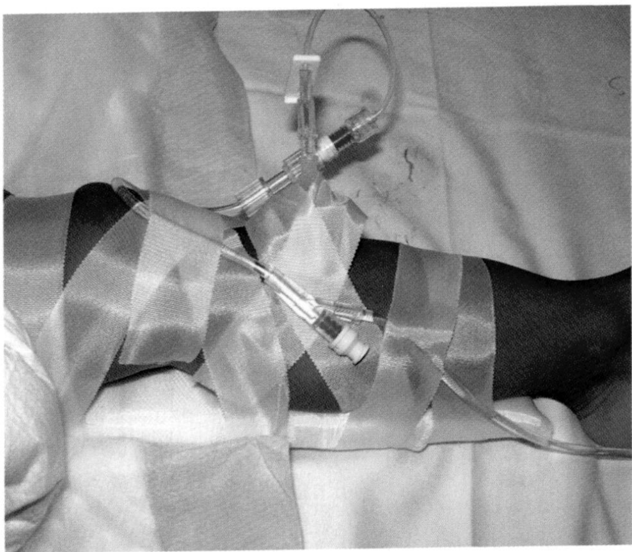

FIGURE 1–23 Anterior tibial intraosseous access. (Courtesy of Mark Silverberg, MD.)

To confirm appropriate placement, the needle should stand erect without support, marrow should be aspirated, and fluid should easily be infused without evidence of subcutaneous infiltration. The needle can then be attached to large-caliber IV tubing and the infusion begun. Antibiotic ointment should be applied around the needle base and covered with sterile dressing, and the needle and tubing should be properly secured.[1,2]

Clinical Complications

Osteomyelitis, through and through bone penetration, tibial fracture, growth plate damage, subcutaneous or subperiosteal infiltration, compartment syndrome, hematoma, and pressure necrosis of the skin may complicate IOA.[1-3]

REFERENCES

1. American Heart Association. Vascular access. In: Chameides L, Hazinski MF, eds. *Pediatric advanced life support.* Dallas: AHA, 1997:5–1.
2. Pediatric vascular access. In: American College of Surgeons Committee on Trauma. *Advanced trauma life support for doctors: student course manual.* 6th ed. Chicago: American College of Surgeons, 1997.
3. Schoenfeld PS, Baker MD. Management of cardiopulmonary and trauma resuscitation in the pediatric emergency department. *Pediatrics* 1993;91:726–729.

Pericardiocentesis

Jennifer Wiler

Indications

Pericardial fluid can accumulate for a variety of reasons, including cardiac trauma or chamber rupture, pericarditis, uremia, malignancy, acquired immunodeficiency syndrome (AIDS), and hypothyroidism. In the emergency department, a prime indication for pericardiocentesis is hemodynamic instability from a pericardial effusion that is refractory to resuscitation techniques. Because the pericardium is a fibrinous sac, minimal amounts of blood or fluid can cause restriction to inflow. Removal of only 15 to 20 mL of fluid may result in hemodynamic improvement.[1]

Technique

The patient is best placed in a semi-upright position, if possible, to facilitate dependent fluid pooling. Time permitting, the subxyphoid and xyphoid areas should be cleansed, and topical and local anesthetic agents may be infiltrated. Vital signs and electrocardiographic (ECG) findings should be monitored throughout the procedure.

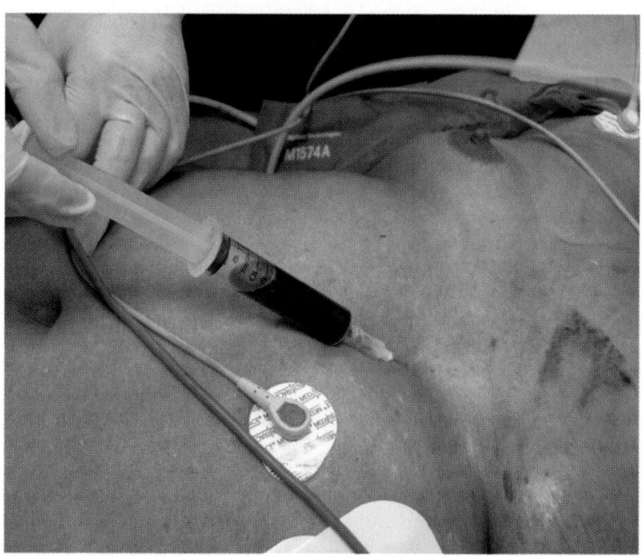

FIGURE 1–24 Emergency pericardiocentesis. (Courtesy of Mark Silverberg, MD.)

A needle over a needle catheter, with an empty syringe and three-way valve, is inserted 1 to 2 cm inferior to the left xiphochondral junction at a 45-degree angle to the skin. The needle is advanced toward the left scapula with constant aspiration traction on the syringe until fluid or blood appears. Attention to the ECG is necessary, because acute myocardial injury caused by the needle may result in changes in ST or QRS complex morphologies. Increased T-wave voltages or premature ventricular contractions may be appreciated as the needle touches the epicardium.[1] If this occurs, the needle should be withdrawn until the ECG returns to baseline. The drainage catheter is left in place until definitive management is available.[1,2]

Because blind techniques are associated with complications and up to 6% mortality, ultrasonography is used to guide needle placement in nonemergency procedures.[2] With echocardiographic guidance, a 3.5- to 5.0-MHz probe is held in the subcostal position while the needle is placed in the left chest wall where the deepest pocket of pericardial fluid is closest to the skin surface.

Clinical Complications

Complications include needle advancement through the pericardium with aspiration of ventricular blood, coronary artery or vein or myocardial laceration, pneumopericardium, arrhythmia induction, damage to local heart structures, pneumothorax, and laceration of the esophagus or peritoneum with subsequent infection. Recurrence of pericardial fluid accumulation is a common occurrence.

REFERENCES

1. Pediatric vascular access. In: American College of Surgeons Committee on Trauma. *Advanced trauma life support for doctors: student course manual.* 6th ed. Chicago: American College of Surgeons, 1997.
2. Tsang TS, Freeman WK, Sinak LJ, Seward JB. Echocardiographically guided pericardiocentesis: evolution and state-of-the-art technique. *Mayo Clin Proc* 1998;73:647–652.

SECTION II

EMERGENCY MEDICAL SERVICES

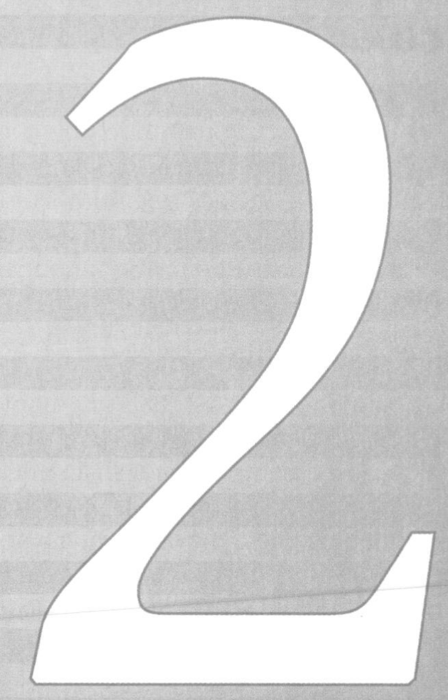

Emergency Medical Services and Pre-Hospital Care

2-1

Vehicular Rollover

Gerald Wydro

Of the five types of vehicle collisions—head-on, T-bone, rear-ended, rotational impact, and rollover—rollover has the greatest mechanistic potential for passenger injuries, which are directly proportional to the amount of force required to overturn the vehicle.

Clinical Presentation

The most common rollover is the "side rollover," which is common in accidents involving sport utility vehicles. It is usually caused by a T-bone collision or when a vehicle strikes a curb, has a blowout, or comes in contact with uneven topography. The second type of rollover involves an end-over-end mechanism by which the vehicle flips bumper-over-bumper. Passenger ejection is common in all rollovers.[1]

Pathophysiology

Three distinct collisions occur during a motor vehicle collision. The first collision occurs when the vehicle strikes an object. The second collision occurs when the body of the patient strikes the interior of the vehicle or is thrown from the vehicle. The third collision occurs when the organs of the patient strike surfaces within the body.[1] Kinetic energy is directly responsible for all second and third collision injuries. The amount of kinetic energy is proportional to the severity of injuries that occur during the accident. Most second collision injuries are easily identified through a good physical examination. They can manifest as soft tissue damage, from simple contusions to major lacerations and avulsions or as musculoskeletal injuries, from closed or open fractures to gross dislocations. Third collision injuries typically are not visible on external examination. Examples include lacerated liver or spleen, other gastrointestinal injuries, brain injuries, and closed chest trauma.

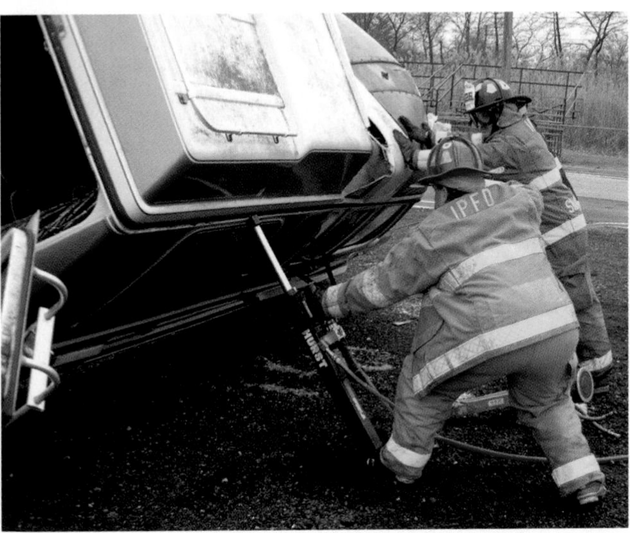

FIGURE 2–1 Ram used to right a rolled-over vehicle. (Courtesy of Mark Silverberg, MD.)

Clinical Complications

Vehicles that have come to rest on their roof or side present obstacles to responders. These vehicles tend to shift, especially with live loads (e.g., patients moving around inside the vehicle). Any vehicle that is on its side or roof is considered to be extremely unstable and should not be entered until it is stabilized. Procedures such as manual cervical spine immobilization and airway control may be complicated by patient positioning.

Management

Scene safety for all responders and patients is the first priority. All vehicles that are unstable must be stabilized before access is gained. All potential passengers must be accounted for. A basic rule of thumb is that the number of passengers to be ruled out is the number the vehicle can legally hold.

REFERENCES

1. Limmer D, O'Keefe M, Grant HD, Murray RH, Bergeron JD. Scene size-up. *Emergency care.* 9th ed. New Jersey: Prentice-Hall, 2001.

Significant Mechanism of Injury

Allon Amitai

Clinical Presentation

Prehospital systems and emergency departments define significant mechanisms of injury (SMOI) as those traumatic events that carry a substantial risk that a patient will have sustained a major injury in an incident.[1,2] The 1999 advanced trauma life support (ATLS) field triage protocol recommended "consideration of transport to a trauma center with trauma team activation" for any of the following: ejection from an automobile, a death occurring in the same passenger compartment, extrication time exceeding 20 minutes, falls greater than 20 feet, rollover motor vehicle crash, auto crash speed greater than 40 mph, auto deformity greater than 20 inches, intrusion into the passenger compartment greater than 12 inches, auto-pedestrian or auto-bicycle injury with speed greater than 5 mph, pedestrian struck or run over, and motorcycle crash with speed greater than 20 mph or with rider separated from motorcycle.[1,2] Other significant mechanisms include penetrating injuries to the head, neck, torso, and proximal extremities and major burns.[1,2]

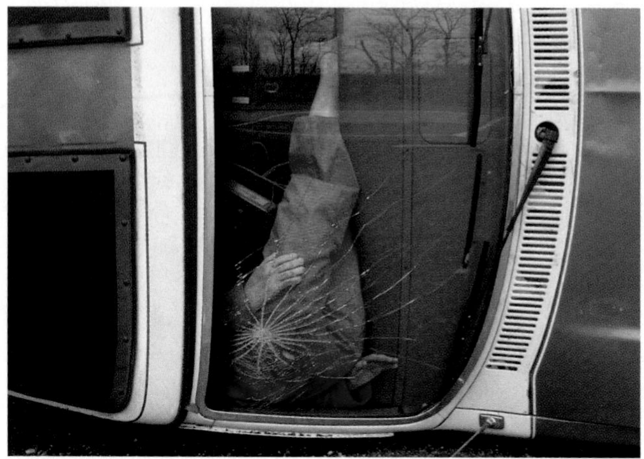

FIGURE 2–2 Significant mechanism of injury: starred windshield. (Courtesy of Mark Silverberg, MD.)

Pathophysiology

Patients with traumatic injuries may initially have normal vital signs that progressively decompensate. Reliance on these physiologic parameters without consideration of the mechanism of injury has been implicated as a cause of undertriage.[1] Informally, the term SMOI can denote any mechanism of injury that involves sufficient energy transfer, focused narrowly enough, or in a rapid enough time interval so that major trauma is likely to have been inflicted.[1,2]

Clinical Complications

Health care providers define SMOIs in order to identify patients who are likely to have sustained a serious, possibly life- or limb-threatening, wound. If such injuries are not identified and addressed, any form of morbidity or even mortality can result.

Management

The ATLS protocols should be adhered to as with any major traumatic injury. Institutional policy may differ from hospital to hospital concerning trauma team activation. Although many patients with SMOIs eventually have insignificant sequelae, a full trauma workup and admission to an intensive care setting or to the operating room is prudent and should be undertaken based on the mechanism of injury alone.[1,2]

REFERENCES

1. Lowe DK, Oh GR, Neely KW, Peterson CG. Evaluation of injury mechanism as a criterion in trauma triage. *Am J Surg* 1986;152: 6–10.
2. Bond RJ, Kortbeek B, Preshaw RM. Field trauma triage: combining mechanism of injury with the prehospital index for an improved trauma triage tool. *J Trauma* 1997;43:283–287.

2–3

Hazardous Materials Placards

Michael Greenberg

Hazardous materials (HAZMAT) placards are required whenever hazardous materials cargo is shipped by truck or other carrier anywhere within the United States. The regulations regarding HAZMAT placards are published in Title 49 of the U.S. Code of Federal Regulations (49CFR), also known as the Federal Motor Carriers Safety Regulations (FMCSR). Canada and Mexico have similar regulations requiring placarding.[1,2] UN/NA numbers (four-digit numbers) are located on bulk placards and refer to specific chemicals or groups of chemicals and are assigned by the United Nations or by the U.S. Department of Transportation, or both. The meaning of these numbers can be found in the *North American Emergency Response Guidebook* (ERG), which is produced by the U.S. Department of Transportation, Transport Canada, and the Secretariat of Transport and Communications (Mexico).[1]

Emergency physicians should be familiar with HAZMAT placards, and a copy of the ERG should be available in all emergency departments and carried in all emergency response vehicles.

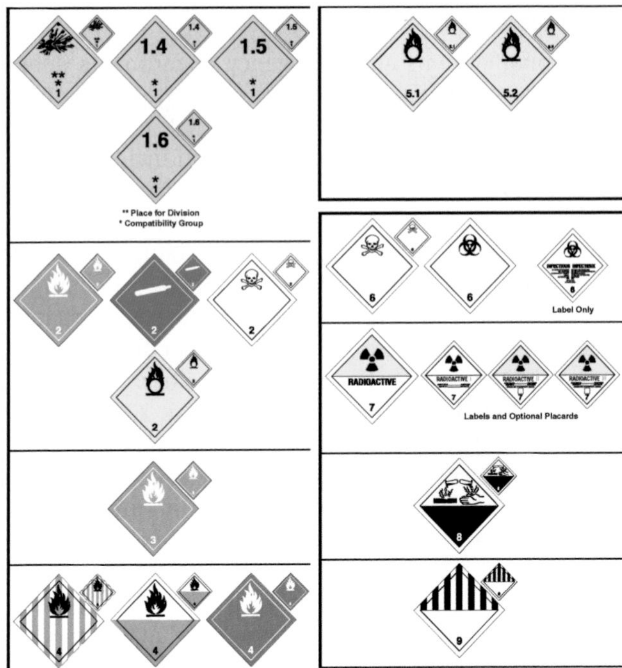

FIGURE 2–3 Hazardous materials placards and labels. Class One—Explosives: 1.1, mass explosion hazard; 1.2, fragment projection hazards; 1.3, fire hazard with minor blast hazard, minor projection hazard, but not mass explosion hazard; 1.4, no significant hazard—explosion effects confined to package; 1.5, insensitive substance with mass explosion hazard; 1.6, extremely insensitive substance with no mass explosion hazard (e.g., blasting agents). Class Two—Gases: 2.1, flammable gas (e.g., propane); 2.2, nonflammable, nontoxic gas (e.g., nitrogen); 2.3, toxic gas (e.g., sulfur dioxide); 2.4, oxygen and oxidizing gases. Class Three—Flammable Liquids: 3.1, flammable liquids with closed-cup flash point not greater than 60.5°C (e.g., gasoline, kerosene). Class Four—Flammable Solids: 4.1, solid that is readily combustible; 4.2, solid liable to spontaneous combustion; 4.3, solid that on contact with water emits flammable gases or becomes spontaneously combustible. Class Five—Oxidizing Substances and Organic Peroxides: 5.1, substances that contribute to combustion of other material by yielding oxygen (e.g., ammonium nitrate); 5.2, organic oxidizing compounds. Class Six—Toxic or Infectious Substances: 6.1, solid that is toxic through inhalation, skin contact, or ingestion; 6.2, microorganisms that are infectious or believed to be infectious to humans. Class 7—Radioactive Materials: categories I, II, and III (lowest to highest in radiation). Class Eight—Corrosives: a substance that causes destruction of skin or corrodes steel or nonclad aluminum (e.g., sodium hydroxide). Class 9—Miscellaneous Products, Substances, or Organisms: hazardous substances that do not meet the criteria of classes 1 through 8. (From Dart, with permission.)

REFERENCES

1. Code of Federal Regulations, 49CFR 173. United States Department of Transportation.
2. *2000 North American emergency response guide book.* U.S. Department of Transportation, Transport Canada, Secretariat of Transport & Communications, 2000.

Vehicular Extrication

Michael Greenberg

Extrication is the process of removal of a victim from a vehicle after a motor vehicle crash; to some extent, it is an indicator of the severity of the crash event, as well as the degree of vehicular internal and external damage. As many as 19% of crashes involve fatalities and require extrications. Extrication time—the time it takes to actually remove the victim from the vehicle, is a critical factor in fatal crash events. The estimated maximum speed immediately before the crash is higher in extrication incidents, and the incidence of brain injuries and lower extremity injuries is higher.[1–3]

Indications

Victims trapped inside or under vehicles may require extrication. Victims with underlying medical problems that interfere with exiting the vehicle also require extrication. The medical management of trapped victims begins before extrication and may proceed during extrication maneuvers. This may include airway control, neck and extremity stabilization, initiation of intravenous fluid therapy and treatment of life-threatening injuries (e.g., exsanguinating hemorrhage, tension pneumothorax) and other injuries.

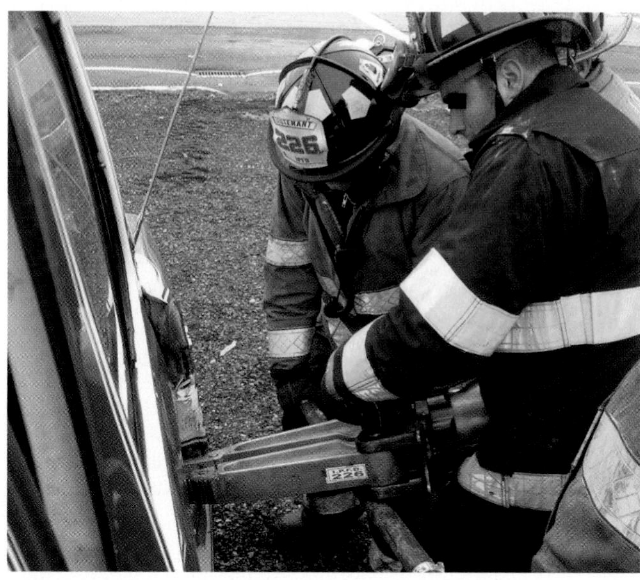

FIGURE 2–4 Jaws of life used to "pop open" a door to extricate a patient. (Courtesy of Mark Silverberg, MD.)

Contraindications

Extrication may need to be delayed if undue risk to the lives of rescuers is evident. Examples include active gunfire in the immediate area, conflagration of the vehicle, contamination of the immediate area with certain chemicals, a high potential or probability for electrocution, and other immediate life threats to rescuers.

Technique

During extrication, victims are at risk for sustaining additional injuries, especially neurologic injuries. The risk is increased if rescuers are not practiced or knowledgeable regarding proper extrication techniques. Rescuers themselves are also at risk for injury during the extrication process. Specific techniques for extrication are beyond the scope of this discussion.

Clinical Complications

Some studies have shown no correlation between extrication time (duration) and mortality.[3] The deployment of previously undeployed airbags during extrication can severely injure rescuers as well as victims.[4]

REFERENCES

1. Siegel JH, Mason-Gonzalez S, Dischinger PC, et al. Causes and costs of injuries in multiple trauma patients requiring extrication from motor vehicle crashes. *J Trauma* 1993;35:920–931.
2. Wilmink AB, Samra GS, Watson LM, Wilson AW. Vehicle entrapment and pre-hospital trauma care. *Injury* 1996;27:21–25.
3. Sanson G, Di Bartolomeo S, Nardi G, et al. Road traffic accidents with vehicular entrapment: incidence of major injuries and need for advanced life support. *Eur J Emerg Med* 1999;6:285–291.
4. Research note http://www.nhtsa.dot.gov/people/injury/ems/disconne.htm

Immobilization

Mark Silverberg

Spinal immobilization can be accomplished with a combination of devices, including hard cervical collars, scoop-stretchers, rigid backboards, and a variety of commercially available neck immobilization devices that attach to the backboard. Additionally, foam blocks, towels, intravenous fluid bags, and sandbags have been used to augment standard equipment and improve immobilization.[2] The patient can then be secured in place within these devices using various straps and tape.[1]

Indications

Patients who sustain major trauma must be presumed to have a spinal cord injury until proven otherwise and therefore must be immobilized.[1,2] Any patient with signs of a neurologic injury (e.g., numbness, paresthesias, weakness, incontinence) should also be immobilized. In addition, any patient complaining of neck pain should undergo spinal immobilization.[2]

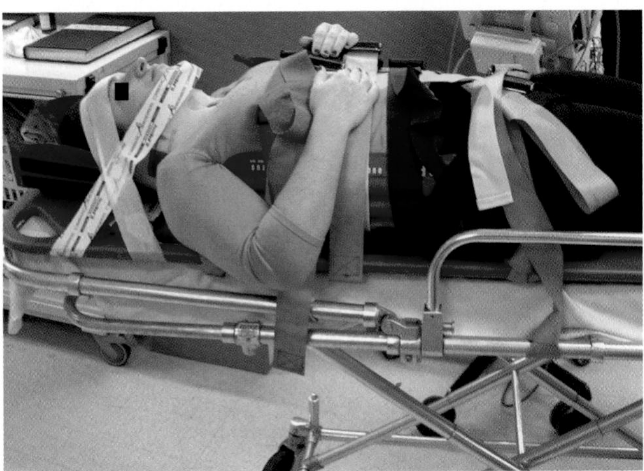

FIGURE 2–5 Immobilization on long board. (Courtesy of Mark Silverberg, MD.)

Contraindications

There are no absolute contraindications to immobilizing a trauma patient. However, airway management should be secured by manual immobilization before mechanical immobilization is performed. Full spinal immobilization may not be possible in confined spaces where a backboard does not fit, but a rigid cervical collar should always be applied.[1]

Technique

The patient should be lying supine with the neck straight and anatomically neutral. A rigid cervical collar should be gently placed on the neck when it is in a neutral position.[1] Then, while the head is held in line with the spine, the patient should be "log-rolled" to one side so that the board can be slid under the patient. Once that is accomplished, the patient can be rolled back supine onto the board, and sandbags or head supports can be fixed in place to prevent neck rotation. The rest of the body is then secured in place with straps and tape to prevent loss of in-line stabilization.[1,2]

Clinical Complications

If immobilization is done incorrectly or not at all, the patient may be placed at risk for severe neurologic sequelae. Additionally, if left on the board for a prolonged period, the patient may develop back pain, muscular spasm, or even pressure ulcers in the regions of maximal board contact, such as occiput, sacrum, and heels.[2]

REFERENCES

1. De Lorenzo RA, Olson JE, Boska M, et al. Optimal positioning for cervical immobilization. *Ann Emerg Med* 1996;28:301–308.
2. Podolsky S, Baraff LJ, Simon RR, Hoffman JR, Larmon B, Ablon W. Efficacy of cervical spine immobilization methods. *J Trauma* 1983;23:461–465.

Pneumatic Antishock Garment

Mark Silverberg

Description

The pneumatic antishock garment (PASG), also known as military antishock trousers (MAST), is an inflatable "pair of pants" that can be applied to trauma patients. It has three compartments that can be inflated separately: one for each leg and one for the pelvis and lower abdomen. It functions as a noninvasive means to increase blood pressure by increasing peripheral vascular resistance.[1] The PASG can also provide a tamponade effect to bleeding wounds under the inflated device.[1] Because the garment becomes semirigid when inflated, it can splint fractures.[1]

Indications

In 1984, the American College of Surgeons' Committee on Trauma made the PASG a standard of care for trauma patients with signs or symptoms of shock and a systolic blood pressure lower than 100 mm Hg, and for any trauma patient with a systolic blood pressure lower than 80 mm Hg.[1] However, subsequent investigations found that the PASG did not increase survival in these patients. In fact, the trend, although not statistically significant, was toward worse outcomes, and for this reason the device has fallen out of favor.[1] Currently, the only indication for EMS personnel to use the PASG is as a splinting device for pelvic fractures.[1]

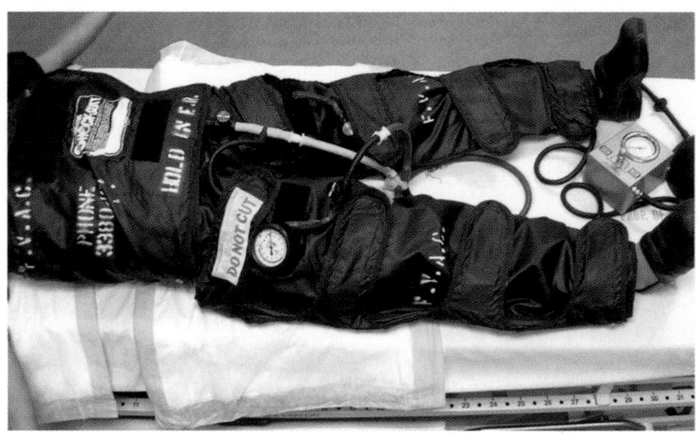

FIGURE 2–6 Pneumatic Antishock Garment (PASG). (Courtesy of Jamarcy McDaniel, MD.)

Contraindications

Although the PASG was used for all hypotensive trauma patients in the past, those with penetrating thoracoabdominal injuries were found to have a statistically significant increase in mortality.[1] Therefore, the PASG has become contraindicated in this patient population. This effect may have been related to the extra time spent in the field applying the PASG, which delayed definitive surgical intervention.[1]

Technique

The PASG should be applied to the lower body of the trauma patient using the Velcro fasteners. The compartments are then blown up sequentially, with the legs first and then the pelvis. When the device is deflated, the reverse order is followed—pelvis first and then each leg.

Clinical Complications

The PASG has been reported to be associated with the development of compartmental syndrome in both the abdomen and the lower extremities. It may also lead to hypotension when it is deflated. Therefore, a pump should be on hand to re-inflate the device should this occur. Researchers also believe that the PASG hinders diaphragm excursion and can cause respiratory difficulty even in uninjured test subjects. Autonomic disturbances such as emesis, urination, or defecation have been recorded with PASG application.[1]

REFERENCES

1. Pepe PE, Eckstein M. Reappraising the prehospital care of the patient with major trauma. *Emerg Med Clin North Am* 1998;16:1–15.

SECTION III

MEDICAL AND SURGICAL EMERGENCIES

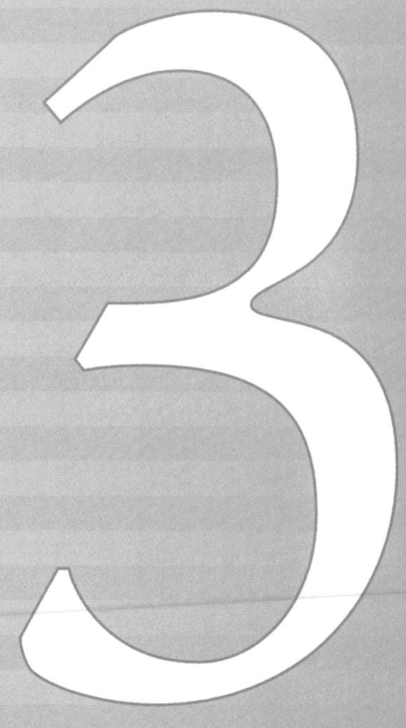

Neurologic

3–1

Intracranial Hemorrhage

Allon Amitai

Clinical Presentation

Patients with intracranial hemorrhage (ICH) typically present with headache, nausea, and vomiting, with or without focal neurologic deficits. Onset of ICH is gradual in comparison to ischemic infarct or subarachnoid hemorrhage (SAH). Altered level of consciousness may arise from increased intracranial pressure (ICP), direct damage to the reticular activating system, or herniation.[1]

Pathophysiology

Most ICHs occur spontaneously, secondary to long-standing hypertension.[1] Age, hematoma volume, presenting Glasgow Coma Scale (GCS) score, and presence of intraventricular blood are the most important prognostic variables.[2] Common locations for ICH are the basal ganglia, external capsule, cerebellum, and brainstem secondary to rupture of perforating arteries. However, hemorrhages in the posterior fossa carry a substantially worse prognosis than supratentorial bleeds and often require surgical decompression.[1] Identified risk factors include anticoagulation, thrombolysis, antiplatelet therapy, African-American race, end-stage renal disease, hypocholesterolemia, vasculitis, amyloidosis, diabetes mellitus, and abuse of alcohol, tobacco, heroin, or sympathomimetics.[1] Structural disorders such as arteriovenous malformation, intracranial aneurysm, and neoplasia are frequently encountered in younger patients. ICH may also develop from hemorrhagic conversion of ischemic stroke or from trauma.

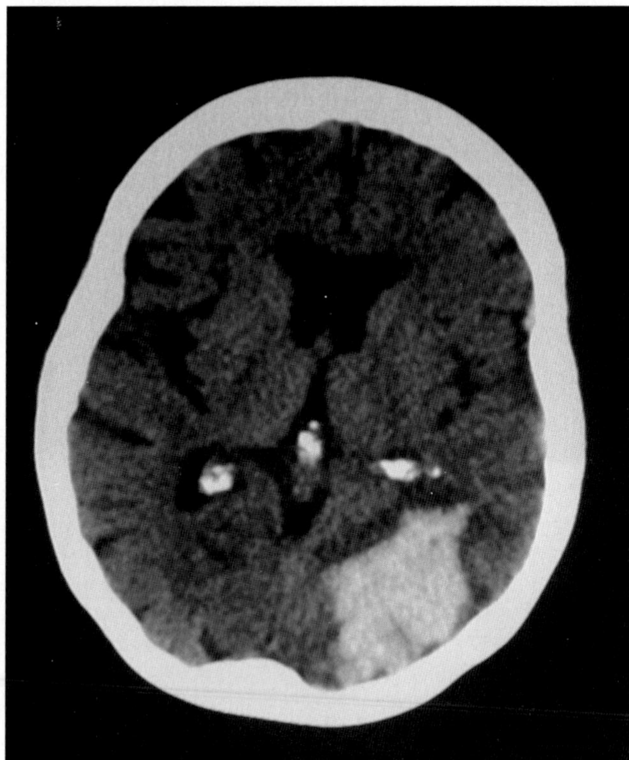

FIGURE 3–1 Computed tomogram showing intracerebral hemorrhage. (Courtesy of Robert Hendrickson, MD.)

Diagnosis

Noncontrast computed tomography (CT) detects most clinically significant acute ICHs and differentiates ICH from ischemic infarct. CT can also indicate the need for interventions such as ventriculostomy placement or surgical decompression.[1]

Clinical Complications

Complications include herniation, obstructive hydrocephalus, seizures, disequilibrium of centrally regulated homeostasis, syndrome of inappropriate secretion of antidiuretic hormone (SIADH), and aspiration. Between 30% and 50% of patients presenting with ICH die within 1 month, and, by 6 months, only 20% will be functioning independently.[1]

Management

Patients who are unable to protect their airway and those with rapidly progressing neurologic deficits should be intubated. Blood pressure should be reduced to a mean arterial pressure (MAP) of 130 mm Hg to maintain cerebral perfusion while reducing the risk of extension of bleeding. Hyperglycemia should be treated. Antiseizure prophylaxis is indicated only if there is clinical evidence of seizure. Midline shift and mass effect may be partly alleviated by administration of mannitol, diuretics, and corticosteroids; elevation of the head of the bed; and hyperventilation to a carbon dioxide tension (P_{CO_2}) of 35 mm Hg. Angiography or magnetic resonance imaging (MRI) is indicated in younger patients who are likely to have surgically treatable structural pathology. Urgent neurosurgical consultation and admission to an intensive care unit (ICU) are usually indicated.[1,2]

REFERENCES

1. Panagos PD, Jauch EC, Broderick JP. Intracerebral hemorrhage. *Emerg Med Clin North Am* 2002;20:631–655.
2. Dubinsky I, Penello D. Can specific patient variables be used to predict outcome of intracranial hemorrhage? *Am J Emerg Med* 2002;20:26–29.

Subarachnoid Hemorrhage

Cherie Mininger

Clinical Presentation

Patients with nontraumatic subarachnoid hemorrhage (SAH) present with the "worst headache of their life," the so-called thunder-clap headache with sudden onset, usually during exertion.[1,2] Patients may exhibit a depressed level of consciousness, transient loss of consciousness, nausea, vomiting, nuchal rigidity, and focal neurologic signs.[1,2] They may also provide history of prior severe headache, known as a warning or "sentinel" headache.[2]

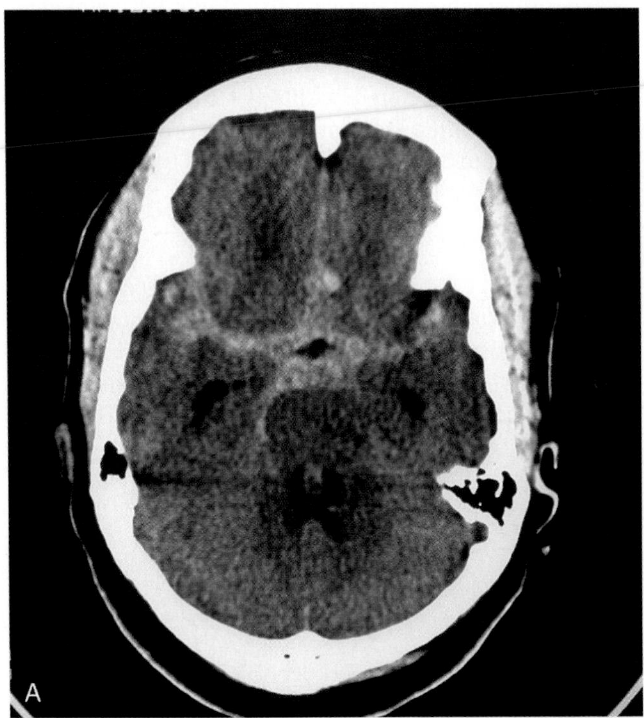

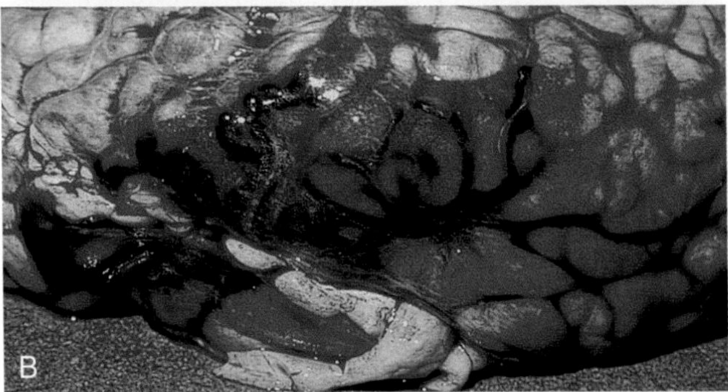

FIGURE 3–2 **A:** Computed tomogram showing subarachnoid hemorrhage. (Courtesy of Robert Hendrickson, MD.) **B:** Postmortem specimen showing massive subarachnoid hemorrhage. (From Reece, with permission.)

Diagnosis

Diagnosis is made by computed tomography (CT) in 93% of patients, if the scan is done within 24 hours after headache onset.[2] Patients with a normal CT scan and a high index of suspicion for SAH should have a lumbar puncture performed. The cerebrospinal fluid (CSF) should be evaluated for both erythrocytes and xanthochromia. There is no set number of red blood cells needed in the CSF to exclude SAH.[1] Xanthochromia is considered to be the most important CSF finding supporting the diagnosis.[2]

Pathophysiology

Bleeding into the subarachnoid space may be traumatic or nontraumatic. Traumatic injury is the most common cause of SAH.[1,2] Of the nontraumatic cases, 80% are caused by ruptured aneurysms.[1,2]

Clinical Complications

In some instances, the initial presentation is catastrophic. In other cases, especially with delays in diagnosis, patients may have a course complicated by rebleeding (4%), hydrocephalus, seizures, or vasospasm.[2,3] Rebleeding is associated with a 70% mortality rate and is the most concerning immediate complication.[3]

Management

Patients with SAH require close neurologic observation in an intensive care setting, including blood pressure control and pain management, while awaiting the definitive aneurysm repair.[3] In addition, patients should receive seizure prophylaxis and calcium channel blockers for vasospasm.[3]

REFERENCES

1. Edlow JA. Diagnosis of subarachnoid hemorrhage in the emergency department. *Emerg Med Clin North Am* 2003;21:73–87.
2. Edlow JA, Caplan LR. Avoiding pitfalls in the diagnosis of subarachnoid hemorrhage. *N Engl J Med* 2000;342:29–36.
3. Fahy BG, Sivaraman V. Current concepts in neurocritical care. *Anesthesiol Clin North Am* 2002;20:441–462.

Cerebellar Hemorrhage

Cherie Mininger

Clinical Presentation

Patients with cerebellar hemorrhage (CBH) present with nonspecific complaints of headache, vomiting, and neck stiffness.[1-3] Initial findings may include nonspecific findings of altered consciousness and elevated blood pressure.[1] Findings specific to CBH include ataxia, nystagmus, and dysmetria.[1,3]

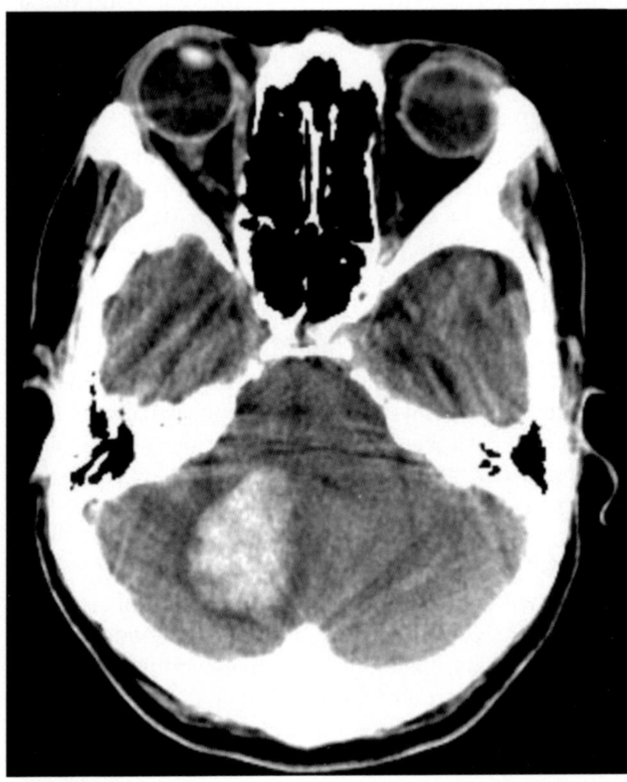

FIGURE 3–3 Computed tomogram showing large cerebellar hemorrhage. (Courtesy of Mark Silverberg, MD.)

Diagnosis

Diagnosis is made by computed tomography (CT). If there is concern for CBH, the CT scan must include thin cuts through the posterior fossa, so that small cerebellar hemorrhages are not missed.[2]

Pathophysiology

CBH is caused by bleeding from the cerebellar arteries.[3] Bleeding expands secondary to continued bleeding of the vessel and disruption of surrounding vessels. Secondary neuronal injury occurs as a result of edema and neuronal damage in the surrounding parenchyma.[3]

Clinical Complications

Complications associated with CBH include neurologic deterioration, cardiovascular instability, rebleeding, and increased intracranial pressure (ICP).[2,3] Overall, patients with CBH have a high mortality rate.[1-3]

Management

Patients with CBH require aggressive airway management, because most have a depressed mental status.[3] Urgent neurosurgical consultation should be obtained, because these patients may be candidates for emergency surgical decompression.[1-3] Intensive care unit (ICU) admission is warranted for management of the airway, blood pressure, and ICP, as well as seizure prevention.[1]

REFERENCES

1. Panagos PD, Jauch EC, Broderick JP. Intracerebral hemorrhage. *Emerg Med Clin North Am* 2002;20:631–655.
2. Gebel JM, Broderick JP. Intracerebral hemorrhage. *Neurol Clin* 2000;18:419–438.
3. Qureshi AI, Tuhrim S, Broderick JP, Batjer HH, Hondo H, Hanley DF. Spontaneous intracerebral hemorrhage. *N Engl J Med* 2001;344:1450–1460.

Cerebrovascular Accident

Rachel Haroz

Clinical Presentation

Patients experiencing a cerebrovascular accident (CVA) may present with abrupt onset of a variety of neurologic problems, including vision loss, headache, and change in mental status. Patients may also develop respiratory compromise and hemodynamic instability. Transient ischemic attacks (TIAs) are focal neurologic deficits that resolve within 24 hours. There are about 750,000 new CVAs annually in the United States, with more than 150,000 fatalities, making CVA the third leading cause of death and the leading cause of disability.[1] Risk factors include hypertension, heart disease, diabetes, high cholesterol, male gender, age older than 55 years, family history, smoking, and pregnancy. African-American race is also a risk factor.[1,2]

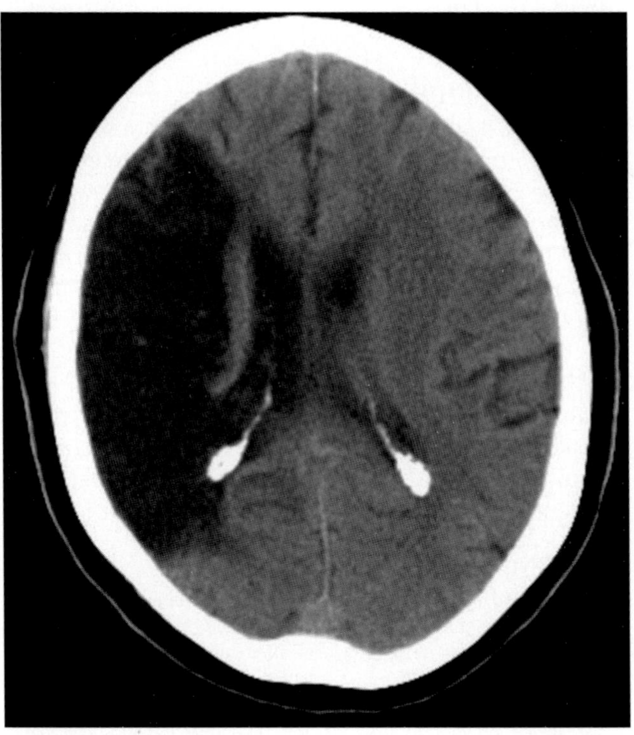

FIGURE 3–4 Computed tomogram showing large cerebral infarct. (Courtesy of Mark Silverberg, MD.)

Pathophysiology

A CVA occurs when cerebral blood flow is acutely disrupted to a focal area, leading to decreased supply of oxygen and glucose. The underlying cause may be ischemic (85%), caused by a thrombotic or embolic occlusion, or hemorrhagic (15%), creating a cascade of events that leads to decreased energy production, acidosis, and, ultimately, cell death.[2]

Diagnosis

The diagnosis is made based on examination and history. Electrocardiography (ECG) and echocardiography are helpful to rule out atrial fibrillation, thrombus, and myocardial infarction. A computed tomography (CT) or magnetic resonance imaging (MRI) scan of the head should be performed. The differential diagnosis includes seizures, brain tumors, migraines, hypoglycemia, and hypertensive encephalopathy.[1]

Clinical Complications

Potential complications include seizures, sepsis, pneumonia, deep vein thrombosis, respiratory depression, pulmonary embolus, decubitus ulcers, and urinary tract infections.[1]

Management

The cause of the CVA (hemorrhagic or ischemic) determines the treatment. Patients with significant symptoms and ischemic strokes, less than 3 hours of symptoms, and no contraindications may be candidates for thrombolytic therapy. Other treatments include heparin, aspirin, and IIB/IIIA inhibitors. Hemorrhagic strokes should be treated supportively, and consultation with a neurosurgery service should be obtained.[1,2]

REFERENCES

1. Brott T, Bogousslavsky J. Treatment of acute ischemic stroke. *N Engl J Med* 2000;343:710–722.
2. Lewandowski C, Barsan W. Treatment of acute ischemic stroke. *Ann Emerg Med* 2001;37:202–216.

Lacunar Cerebral Vascular Accident

Erica McKernan

Clinical Presentation

Lacunar cerebral vascular accidents (CVAs) (infarcts) are small (less than 15 mm in diameter), deep infarcts that result from occlusion of a penetrating artery. These subcortical infarcts are located primarily in the basal ganglia, thalamus, internal capsule, corona radiata, and brainstem.[1-3]

If a lacunar infarct is symptomatic, the patient will present complaining of a motor and/or sensory deficit. Five well-described clinical lacunar syndromes are associated with lacunar infarcts: pure motor hemiparesis, sensorimotor stroke, pure sensory stroke, dysarthria or clumsy hand syndrome, and ataxic hemiparesis. Involvement of the face, arm, and leg are characteristic of the pure motor hemiparesis, sensorimotor stroke, and pure sensory stroke syndromes.[1-3]

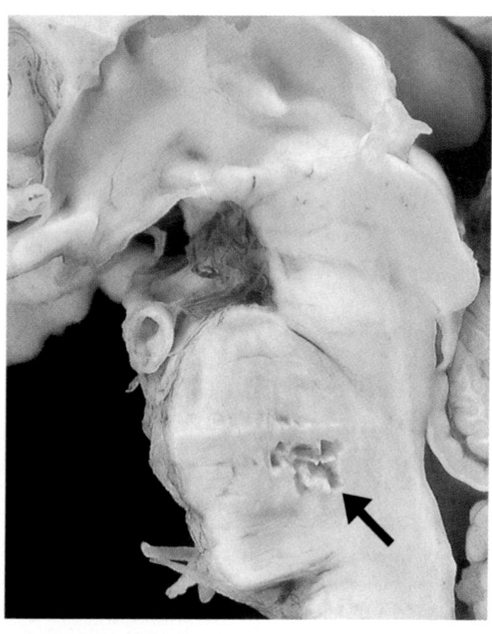

FIGURE 3–5 A median section through the pons, revealing a cluster of multiple lacunar infarcts caused by hypertension. (From Hurst, with permission.)

Pathophysiology

Lacunar infarcts account for about 25% of strokes. These infarcts are small, deep, intraparenchymal infarcts that result from occlusion of penetrating arteries. Occlusion of the vessel may be caused by intracranial atherosclerosis or lipohyalinosis secondary to chronic hypertension. Lacunar infarcts are typically located in the basal ganglia and thalamus. Risk factors include age, gender, hypertension, diabetes mellitus, smoking, previous TIA, and possibly ischemic heart disease.[2]

Diagnosis

Most lacunar infarcts are clinically silent. In patients with neurologic deficits, neuroimaging can aid in the diagnosis of lacunar stroke. Because these infarcts are small, they usually are not seen on computed tomography (CT). Magnetic resonance imaging (MRI) is the study of choice.

Clinical Complications

The risk of death immediately after stroke onset is low, and the rate of recovery is usually rapid. Lacunar strokes have the best short- and long-term prognoses, with 30-day mortality rate of 2%, and the lowest risk for early recurrence of stroke. Late recurrence of stroke is about 14% at 3 years.[3] Patients have an increased risk of developing cognitive decline and dementia.[2]

Management

Airway, breathing, and circulation must be ensured and assessment of neurologic function completed. Neurology consultation should occur immediately for further management.[1]

REFERENCES

1. Thurman RJ, Jauch EC. Acute ischemic stroke: emergent evaluation and management. *Emerg Med Clin North Am* 2002;20:609–630.
2. Norrving B. Long-term prognosis after lacunar infarction. *Lancet Neurol* 2003;2:238–245.
3. Sacco RL, Wolf PA, Gorelick PB. Risk factors and their management for stroke prevention: outlook for 1999 and beyond. *Neurology* 1999;53[7 Suppl 4]:S15–S24.

Cavernous Sinus Thrombosis

Lekha Shah

Clinical Presentation

Patients with cavernous sinus thrombosis (CST) may appear quite ill with abrupt onset of fever, headache, nuchal rigidity, nausea, vomiting, and eye pain.[1,2] Testing of the cranial nerves may reveal unilateral or bilateral palsies of nerves III, IV, and VI, as well as sensory deficits in the ophthalmic branch of the trigeminal nerve. Eye findings may include orbital edema and tenderness, retinal hemorrhages, papilledema, proptosis, and dilated or sluggish pupils.[1,2] Visual deficits may progress to blindness.[1,2]

Pathophysiology

CST is usually caused by a blood-borne infection extending from the face, ear, nasal cavity, or paranasal sinuses.[3] Seeding often occurs via the superior and inferior ophthalmic veins, which drain the middle portion of the face.[1,2] The end result is thrombosis and inflammation of structures within or surrounding the cavernous sinus: the internal carotid artery, cranial nerves III and IV, and the V1 and V2 branches of the trigeminal nerve.[1,2] *Staphylococcus aureus* is the most commonly isolated organism, followed by *Streptococcus* species.[1,2]

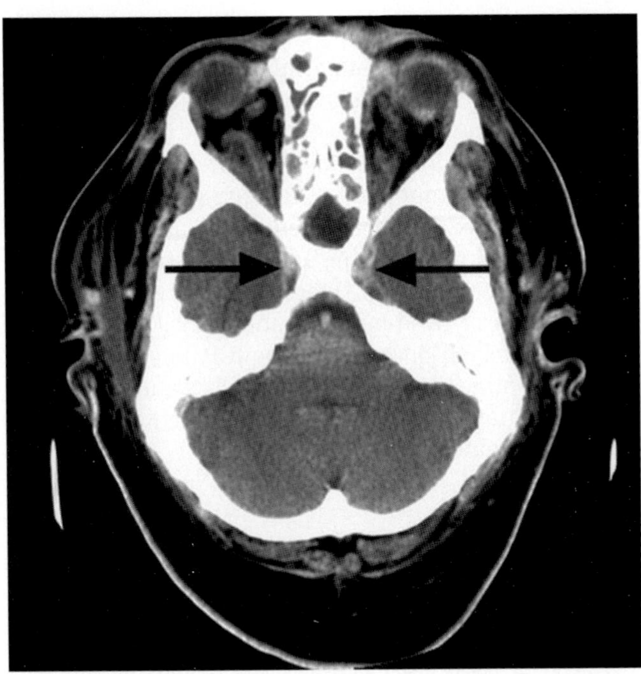

FIGURE 3–6 Computed tomogram of the head with contrast, showing cavernous sinus thrombosis *(arrows)*. (From Cannon, et al., 2004, with permission.)

Diagnosis

CST should be considered in patients with proptosis, ptosis, chemosis, and unilateral or bilateral palsies of cranial nerves III, IV, and VI.[3] Magnetic resonance imaging (MRI) is the most sensitive imaging modality for diagnosis of CST.[1] Computed tomography (CT) may aid in identifying CST.[1,2]

Clinical Complications

If CST is left untreated, the mortality rate approaches 100%.[3] Even with appropriate management, mortality ranges from 20% to 30%.[3] Nonfatal complications include permanent ophthalmoplegia, blindness, hemiparesis, and pituitary insufficiency.[1]

Management

Treatment includes broad-spectrum antibiotics with coverage for *S. aureus*, gram-negative organisms, and anaerobes.[2] Emergency surgical drainage at the primary site of infection may be required. Steroid therapy and anticoagulation with heparin are suggested but remain controversial.[1]

REFERENCES

1. Volturo GA, Repeta RJ Jr. Non-lower extremity deep vein thrombosis. *Emerg Med Clin North Am* 2001;19:877–893.
2. Goldberg AN, Oroszlan G, Anderson TD. Complications of frontal sinusitis and their management. *Otolaryngol Clin North Am* 2001;34:211–225.
3. Ebrigth JR, Pace MT, Niazi AF. Septic thrombosis of the cavernous sinuses. *Arch Intern Med* 2001;161:2671–2676.

Acute Subdural Hematoma

Treve Henwood and John Queen

Clinical Presentation

Acute subdural hematoma (ASDH) occurs in approximately 30% of severe head injuries and results in altered consciousness in almost all cases. Headache, vomiting, or lethargy (97% to 99%); hemiparesis (34% to 47%); and papillary irregularity ipsilateral to hematoma (47% to 53%) may also occur. Patients may have a lucid interval before neurologic symptoms appear (30%).[1]

Pathophysiology

Bleeding results from tearing of bridging veins between the cerebral cortex and the draining venous sinus, resulting in increased intracranial pressure, narrowing of ventricles due to clot volume, and edema secondary to brain injury.[2]

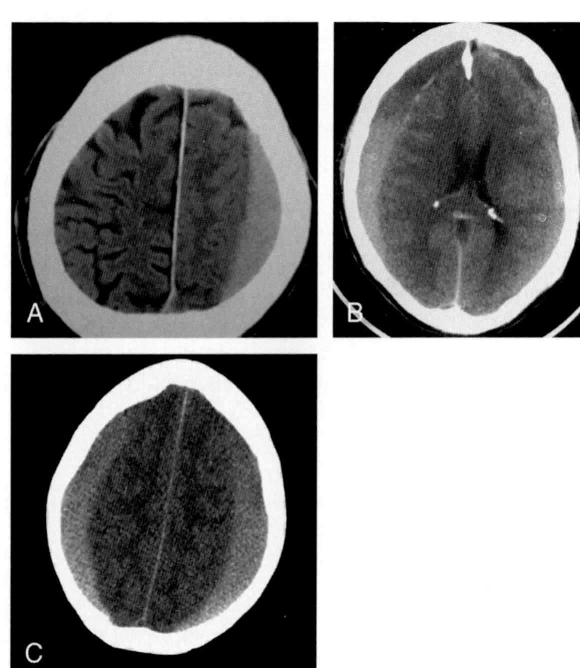

FIGURE 3–7 **A:** Acute subdural hematoma. **B:** Old chronic subdural hematoma with a new bleed that appears as white layering out at the bottom. **C:** Bilateral chronic subdural hematomas. (**A** and **B,** courtesy of Mark Silverberg, MD; **C,** courtesy of Robert Hendrickson, MD.)

Diagnosis

The history focuses on the mechanism of injury (direct versus acceleration/deceleration) and the neurologic states before and after injury. Radiographic findings from noncontrast head computed tomography (CT) include a crescent-shaped, high-density blood collection between the brain and dura. Loss of sulci and narrowing of the ventricles may be seen, and a midline shift occurs secondary to large clot volume.[2,3]

Clinical Complications

Secondary brain injury occurs after the initial trauma as a result of damage to neurons and is the leading cause of morbidity and mortality. Elevated ICP, brain edema, recurrent bleeding, and seizures are potential complications; they affect 33% of patients treated in the emergency department (ED).[3]

Management

Minimizing secondary brain injury and obtaining early neurosurgical intervention (within 4 hours) optimize outcomes. Early intervention in patients with a Glasgow Coma Scale (GCS) score lower than 8 should include rapid-sequence intubation. Short-term hyperventilation is recommended only for patients who are rapidly deteriorating. The target mean arterial pressure should be greater than 90 mm Hg. Hypertonic saline in the initial resuscitation of head-injured patients has shown some short-term benefit in lowering the ICP, but it is not currently recommended for all patients.[2–4] Patients who are triaged or transferred early to trauma centers have the best overall outcomes.[2–4]

REFERENCES

1. Klun B, Fettich M. Factors influencing the outcome in acute subdural haematoma: a review of 330 cases. *Acta Neurochir (Wien)* 1984;71:171–178.
2. Marik PE, Varon J, Trask T. Management of head trauma. *Chest* 2002;122:699–711.
3. Zink BJ. Traumatic brain injury outcome: concepts for emergency care. *Ann Emerg Med* 2001;37:318–332.
4. Servadei F. Prognostic factors in severely head injured adult patients with acute subdural haematomas. *Acta Neurochir (Wien)* 1997;139:279–285.

Epidural Hematoma

Cherie Mininger

Clinical Presentation

Patients with epidural hematoma (EH) experience a brief loss of consciousness after head trauma, followed by a lucid interval and subsequent neurologic deterioration.[1,2]

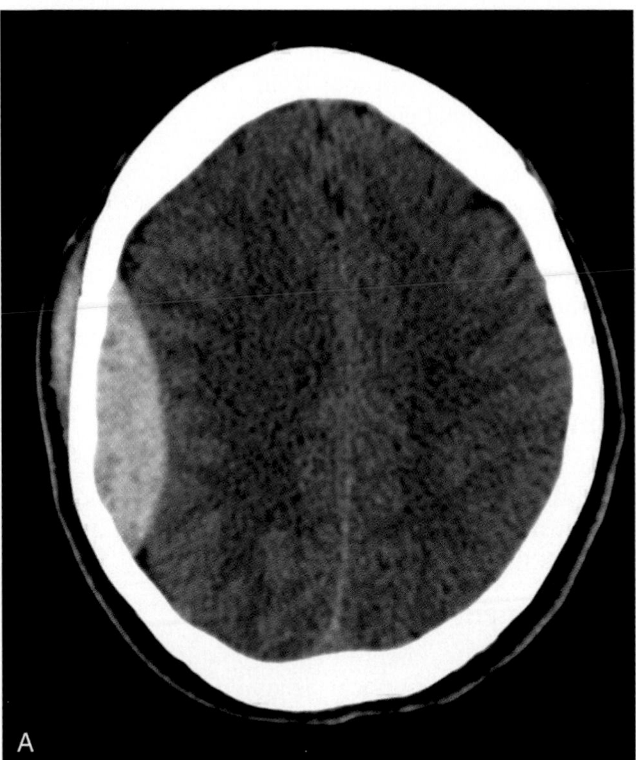

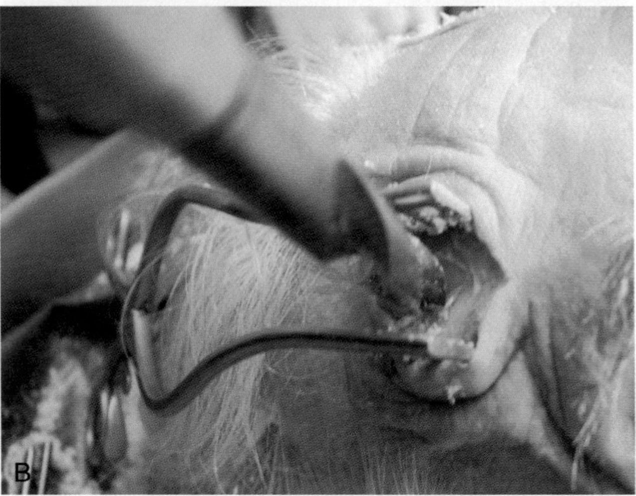

FIGURE 3–8 **A:** Epidural hematoma. (Courtesy of Robert Hendrickson, MD.) **B:** Emergency bur holes in epidural hematoma. (Courtesy of Ralph Weiche, MD.)

Diagnosis

The diagnosis is made radiographically; computed tomography (CT) shows a lenticular lesion, often in the temporal or temporoparietal region.[1]

Pathophysiology

EH is not common; it occurs in fewer than 1% of all head trauma cases.[1] The injury is caused by laceration of the middle meningeal artery, middle meningeal vein, or dural sinus,[2] with or without associated skull fracture. Bleeding from an EH can cause compression, shift, and increased intracranial pressure (ICP).[2]

Clinical Complications

Complications may be primary or secondary. Primary complications, resulting from direct mechanical injury, cause axonal injury manifested by an initial loss of consciousness or depressed mental status.[1,2] Secondary complications, resulting from the expanding hematoma, cause neurologic deterioration.[2]

Management

Patients with EH require emergency neurosurgical evaluation and evacuation of the hematoma. The priority in managing the head-injured patient focuses on limiting secondary complications. Airway, breathing, circulation, and cervical spine stabilization must be addressed immediately. Any patient with a Glasgow Coma Scale (GCS) score of 8 or less, and any patient who is unable to protect his or her airway, should be intubated early, with the use of rapid-sequence techniques to limit fluctuations in ICP.[2]

REFERENCES

1. Marik PE, Varon J, Trask T. Management of head trauma. *Chest* 2002;122:699–711.
2. Gedeit R. Head injury. *Pediatr Rev* 2001;22:118–124.

Spinal Epidural Hematomas

Matthew Warner

Clinical Presentation

Patients with a spinal epidural hematoma (SEH) present with the acute onset of local pain at the site of the hematoma. Neurologic symptoms are dependent on the location of the expanding mass.[1] Progression from radicular paresthesia to paraplegia or quadraplegia, loss of sensory function, and death can occur.[2]

Pathophysiology

SEH is a rare condition, with only 260 reported cases.[3] SEH may be secondary to trauma or an underlying medical condition (hypertension, coagulation disorders, anticoagulation medications, vascular malformations, collagen vascular disease), or it may be spontaneous, without any underlying cause. In all cases, bleeding originates from the venous plexus of the epidural space. Bleeding may also arise from hemorrhage of the epidural arteries. Bleeding from arteries is more likely to produce cord compression. Most SEHs are in the posterolateral position, the location of the epidural arteries. Traumatic SEHs are most often in the cervical region, whereas spontaneous SEHs are mostly in the lumbar region or distal to the spinal cord.[1,2]

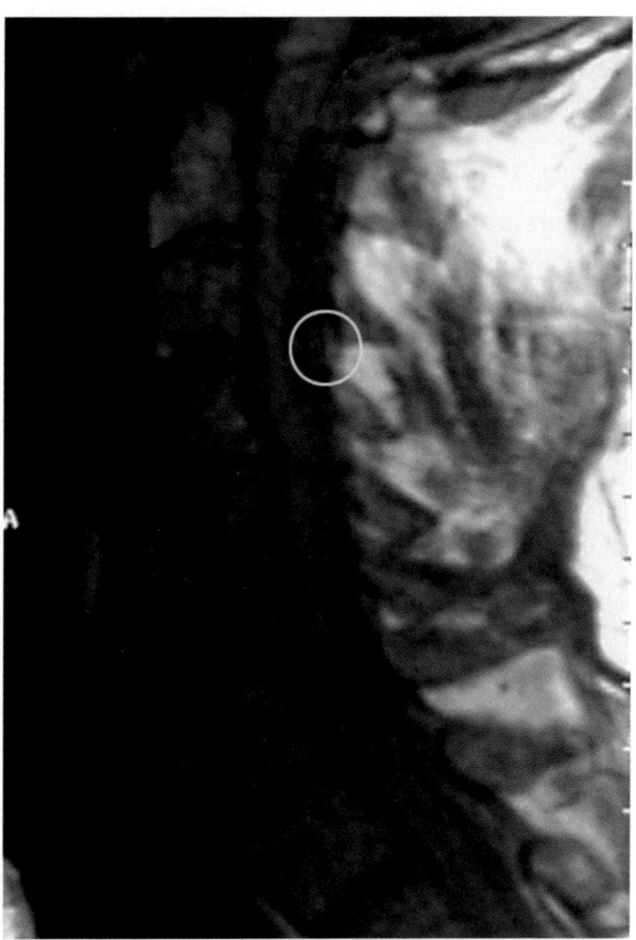

FIGURE 3–9 The hematoma has been outlined by the radiologist. (Courtesy of Todd McGrath, MD.)

Diagnosis

Magnetic resonance imaging (MRI) appears to be superior to computed tomography (CT) in the diagnosis of SEH, because MRI more clearly displays the hematoma and the extent of spread.[2,3] The differential diagnosis includes spinal abscess, tumor, ischemia, transverse myelitis, and acute vertebral disk disease.[2]

Clinical Complications

Delay in diagnosis and treatment can result in devastating and permanent neurologic dysfunction. Cervical SEH can cause respiratory failure and death within hours after onset.[1–3]

Management

The definitive treatment of spinal epidural hematoma is laminectomy with surgical decompression.[2] Permanent impairment depends on the time interval between onset of symptoms and surgery; only patients who undergo decompression within 12 hours after onset are expected to show significant improvement in neurologic function. However, there are case reports of patients with SEH managed medically. These patients all had minor neurologic deficits that were nonprogressive.[3]

REFERENCES

1. Marinella MA, Barsan WG. Spontaneously resolving cervical epidural hematoma presenting with hemiparesis. *Ann Emerg Med* 1996;27:514–517.
2. Alexiadou-Rudolf C, Ernestus RI, Nanassis K, Lanfermann H, Klug N. Acute nontraumatic spinal epidural hematomas: an important differential in spinal emergencies. *Spine* 1998;23:1810–1813.
3. Lefranc F, David P, Brotchi J, De Witte O. Traumatic epidural hematoma of the cervical spine: magnetic resonance imaging diagnosis and spontaneous resolution. Case report. *Neurosurgery* 1999;44:408–410.

Decorticate and Decerebrate Posturing

Arthur Chang

Clinical Presentation

In decorticate posturing, patients display rigidity, with the arms flexed at the elbow and held inward and close to the body; the wrists and fingers are clenched and held tightly toward the chest; the legs and feet are usually extended. In decerebrate posturing, patients are rigid, with extension and internal rotation of the arms and legs, and plantar flexion of the feet. These signs can be intermittent, can be unilateral or bilateral, or can involve the upper extremities only. They may be seen in patients with severe traumatic vascular injury to the central nervous system (CNS) and in patients with hypoglycemia, cerebral edema, or diffuse axonal injury.[1,2]

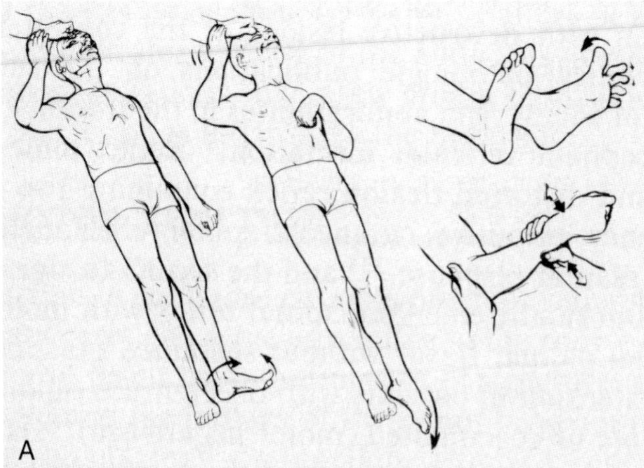

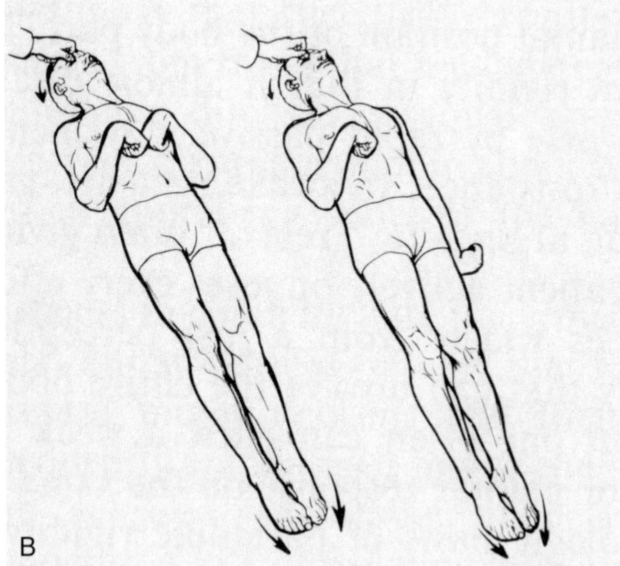

FIGURE 3–10 Decorticate posturing **(A)** is characterized by slow flexion of the arms, wrists, and fingers with adduction in the upper extremities and extension, internal rotation, and plantar flexion of the lower extremities. Decerebrate posturing **(B)** is characterized by clenched teeth; stiffly extended, adducted, hyperpronated arms; and stiffly extended legs with plantar flexion. (From Plum and Posner, with permission.)

Pathophysiology

Decorticate and decerebrate posturing result from damage to the structures that control motor tone associated with the corticospinal tract. In decorticate posturing, the lesion is rostral to the midbrain (i.e., cortex); in decerebrate posturing, the damage is at the level of the midbrain or caudal diencephalons.[1] A progression from a decorticate state to a decerebrate state is associated with progressive destruction or compression of brain structures.[1,2]

Diagnosis

Emergency noncontrast computed tomography (CT) of the head should be done after initial stabilization of the patient. Magnetic resonance imaging (MRI) may better delineate cerebral edema or tumor progression, but it should be reserved until the patient is stable.[1,2]

Clinical Complications

Patients exhibiting posturing are usually comatose and frequently have a poor prognosis. They are at risk for respiratory failure, cardiac arrhythmias, and cardiovascular collapse.[1,2]

Management

Definitive treatment depends on the underlying cause. Prompt on-site consultation by a neurosurgeon should be arranged. Hyperventilation, manitol, nimodipine, or decadron may be indicated to decrease the intracranial pressure.[2]

REFERENCES

1. Saposnik G, Caplan LR. Convulsive-like movements in brainstem stroke. *Arch Neurol* 2001;58:654–657.
2. Ayling J. Managing head injuries. *Emerg Med Serv* 2002;31:42.

Glasgow Coma Scale

John R. Queen and Treve Henwood

In 1974, physicians from the Glasgow University Department of Neurological Sciences published their scale for evaluating altered consciousness in *Lancet*.[1] Because of its simplicity and interrater reliability, the Glasgow Coma Scale (GCS) has become widely used.[2,3]

Diagnosis

The GCS has three components: eye opening, verbal response, and motor response. For each component, the patient is rated for the best response. Eye opening is scored from 1 to 4. The patient receives 4 points for spontaneous eye opening, 3 for opening to verbal commands, 2 for opening to painful stimuli, or 1 for no eye opening. The verbal response is scored from 1 to 5. The patient receives 5 points for oriented conversation, 4 points for disoriented conversation, 3 points for nonsensical words, 2 points for unintelligible sounds, or 1 point for no vocalizations. The motor response is scored from 1 to 6. Patients receive 6 points for following motor commands, 5 points for localizing pain, 4 points for withdrawal with pain, 3 points for flexion with pain, 2 points for extension with pain, or 1 point for no motor response to pain.[1,2] Note that examination of the pupil is not included in the evaluation, because it is not a reliable measure of the level of consciousness.[2]

The lower the GCS score, the more profound the deficit and the higher the mortality rate. The GCS score has been shown to be consistent across different regions and with different mechanisms and treatments. Also, it can reliably be performed in the field before transport to the hospital. The GCS score can be valuable to the emergency physician treating a patient who has been intubated. In recent years, it has become an essential part of the Revised Trauma Score.[2]

Difficulty arises in assessing a patient who has been intubated, sedated, or paralyzed before measurement of the GCS score. The GCS does not assess focal or lateralizing signs. The field GCS score does not predict outcomes as well as the score obtained in the hospital.[2]

REFERENCES

1. Teasdale G, Jennett B. Assessment of coma and impaired consciousness: a practical scale. *Lancet* 1974;2:81–84.
2. Senkowski CK, McKenney MG. Trauma scoring systems: a review. *J Am Coll Surg* 1999;189:491–503.
3. The Brain Trauma Foundation, The Joint Section on Neurotrauma and Critical Care. The Glasgow Coma Scale score. *J Neurotrauma* 2000;17:563–571.

TABLE 3–11 Glasgow Coma Scale

Parameter	Response	Score
Eyes open	Spontaneously	4
	To verbal command	3
	To pain	2
	No eye opening	1
Best motor response to verbal command	Obeys	6
Best motor response to painful stimulus	Localizes pain	5
	Flexion (withdrawal)	4
	Flexion—abnormal (decorticate rigidity)	3
	Extension (decerebrate rigidity)	2
	No response	1
Best verbal response	Oriented and converses	5
	Disoriented and converses	4
	Inappropriate words	3
	Incomprehensible sounds	2
	No response	1
Total		3–15

Cerebral Ventricular Shunt Failure

John R. Queen and Treve Henwood

Clinical Presentation

Cerebral ventricular shunt malfunctions may result in nausea, vomiting, headache, neck pain, lethargy, irritability, diplopia, and increased clumsiness.

Pathophysiology

Undiagnosed shunt malfunction is associated with an increased mortality rate.[1] Malfunction of a shunt can be caused by undershunting, most often due to obstruction, or by overshunting.[1,2] Obstruction most commonly occurs within the ventricular catheter as a result of brain debris, fragments of choroid plexus, or fibrin.[2] Overshunting can cause orthostatic hypotension, slit ventricles, loculated ventricles, subdural cerebrospinal fluid (CSF) collections, or craniosynostosis.[2]

Diagnosis

Findings may include seizure, papilledema, a bulging or sunken fontanelle, ataxia, bradycardia, abdominal pain, sixth nerve palsy, and optic atrophy.[1] A "shunt series" of radiographs includes plain films of the skull, neck, chest, and abdomen and may help to identify disconnections or fractures in the system, fluid collections, and migrated hardware. Tapping of the shunt may be done to aid in assessing shunt pressures and flow dynamics and to obtain CSF for cell count, culture, Gram staining, and chemistry studies. This should be done only by an experienced neurosurgeon.[1]

Clinical Complications

Tapping a shunt and dropping the CSF pressure too quickly can precipitate headache, mental status changes, nausea, vomiting, or intraventricular or subdural bleeding. Whenever a shunt is accessed, there is the risk of bleeding at the puncture site, introduction of infection, damage to the valve, or a CSF leak.[1] High rates of shunt failure have led to modifications to the original designs. However, these changes have resulted in a number of uncommon complications, including cor pulmonale, shunt nephritis, bowel erosion and perforation, and tonsilar herniation.[3]

Management

Surgical repair of disconnected or fractured hardware may be required. Adjustment of shunt settings is best done by a neurosurgeon.

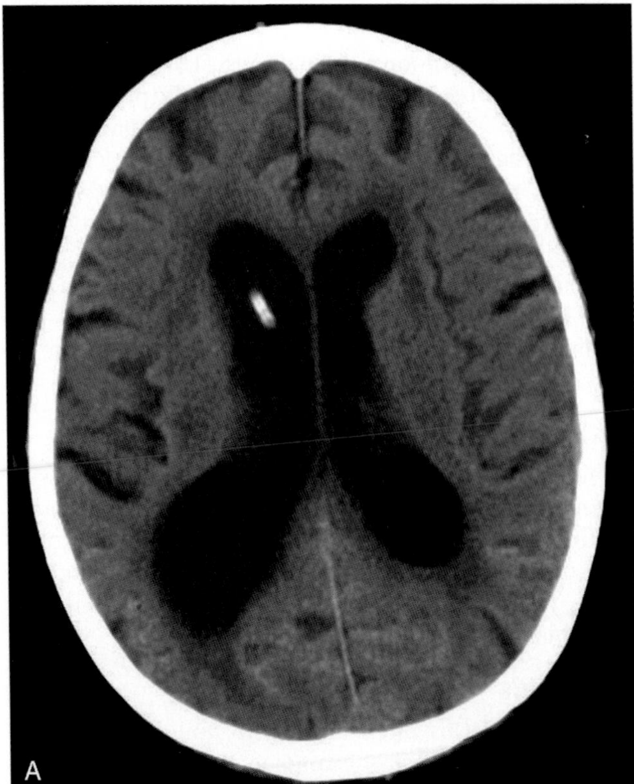

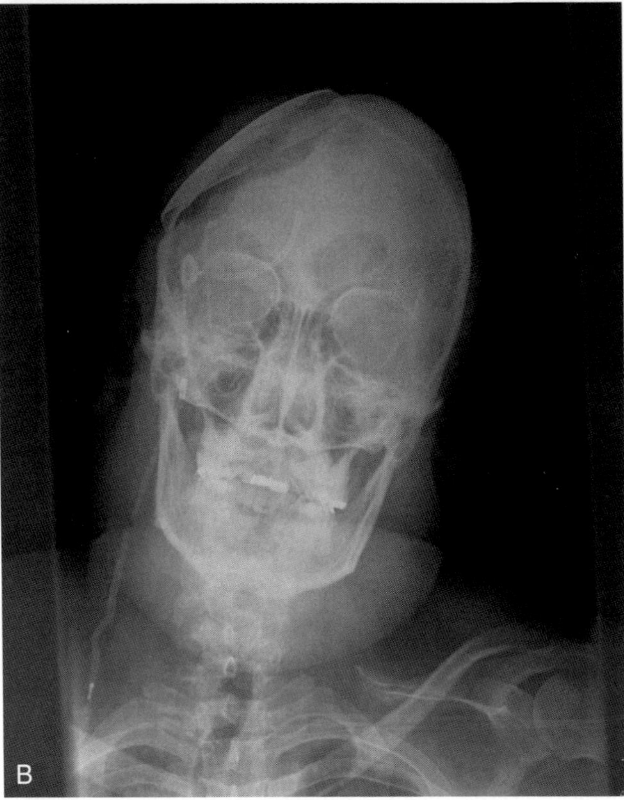

FIGURE 3–12 **A:** Hydrocephalus due to blocked shunt. (Courtesy of Mark Silverberg, MD.) **B:** Disruption of shunt due to skull fracture. (Courtesy Alfredo Sabbaj, MD.)

REFERENCES

1. Naradzay JF, Browne BJ, Rolnick MA, Doherty RJ. Cerebral ventricular shunts. *J Emerg Med* 1999;17:311–322.
2. Kang JK, Lee IW. Long-term follow-up of shunting therapy. *Childs Nerv Syst* 1999;15:711–717.
3. Drake JM, Kestle JR, Tuli S. CSF shunts 50 years on: past, present and future. *Childs Nerv Syst* 2000;16:800–804.

3–13

Seizures

Rachel Haroz

Clinical Presentation

Seizures are common presentations (1% of emergency department visits). They have a bimodal peak in incidence, during childhood/adolescence and again after 60 years of age. Seizures can be generalized or partial. Generalized seizures involve both cerebral hemispheres and may be convulsive (tonic-clonic seizures) or petit mal (absence seizures). Partial seizures can be simple or complex and may progress to a generalized seizure. Seizures lasting longer than 30 minutes and seizures that recur without reversion to baseline mental status are referred to as status epilepticus.[1]

Pathophysiology

Seizures result from sudden, abnormal and excessive discharges of neuronal electrical activity that may propagate through neuronal processes. Secondary seizures may occur as a result of toxins, infections, stroke, hypoxia, head trauma, intracranial hemorrhage, metabolic abnormalities, withdrawal, or eclampsia.[1]

Diagnosis

Seizure activity is often diagnosed clinically based on the history and physical examination. For patients with known seizure disorder who have a typical breakthrough seizure, an anticonvulsant concentration and observation may be all that is necessary. A new-onset seizure requires further workup, which may include a metabolic panel, complete blood count (CBC), blood urea nitrogen (BUN) concentration, creatinine concentration, pregnancy test, drug screen, urinalysis, head computed tomography (CT) scan, and possibly cerebrospinal fluid (CSF) analysis. An electroencephalogram (EEG) and MRI may also be performed.[1]

Clinical Complications

Seizures can cause trauma (including fractures, dislocations, and head injuries), rhabdomyolysis, apnea, hypoxia, hypotension, metabolic acidosis, and neuronal damage.[1]

Management

Oxygen should be administered, a cardiac monitor employed, reliable intravenous access gained, and a glucose determination performed. Initial pharmacologic therapy should consist of parenteral benzodiazepines. Patients with continued seizure activity should have their airway controlled and should be treated with phenytoin/fosphenytoin, followed by barbiturates or propofol.[1]

REFERENCES

1. Bradford JC, Kyriakedes CG. Evaluation of the patient with seizures: an evidence based approach. *Emerg Med Clin North Am* 1999; 17:203–220.

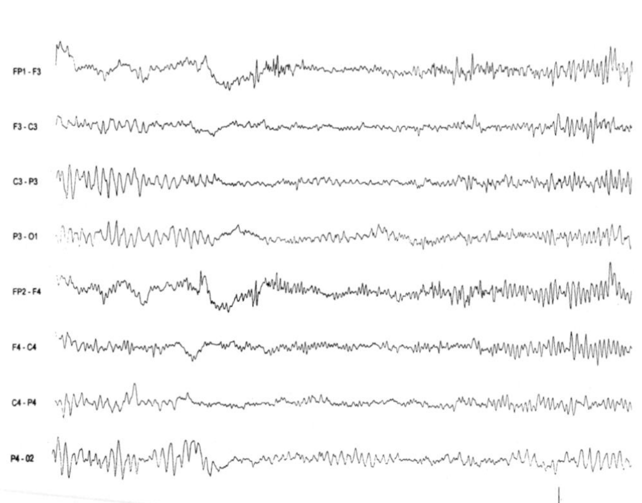

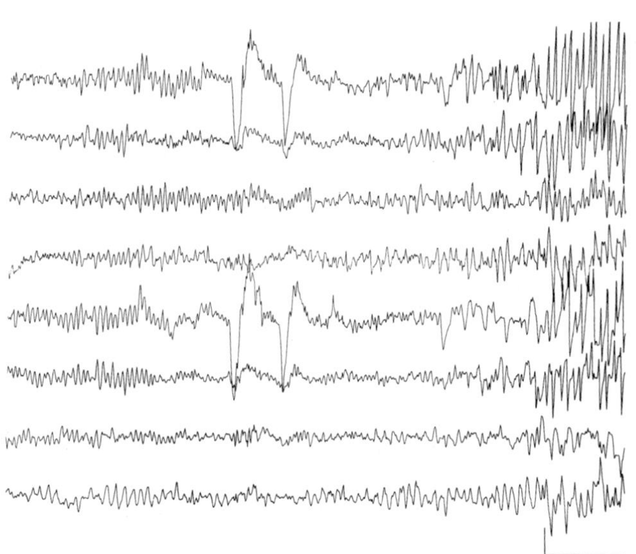

FIGURE 3–13 Electroencephalogram showing generalized tonic-clonic seizure. (From Blume, with permission.)

Brain Abscess

Lekha Shah

Clinical Presentation

There are three "classic" stages of the clinical presentation of brain abscess: (1) transient malaise, fever, and hemispheric or global headache; (2) a latent asymptomatic phase; (3) a terminal phase with focal deficits, herniation, and coma.[1] Valsalva and postural changes should aggravate the headache by raising intracranial pressure (ICP). In variance to the "classic" theory, patients are frequently afebrile. Vomiting is often present, and seizures occur in 25% to 50% of patients.[1] Papilledema may also be present. Most patients become symptomatic within 1 week after abscess formation.[1]

Pathophysiology

Brain abscesses form in areas of preexisting brain injury or necrosis from hypoxia, trauma, or ischemia. A localized area of cerebritis undergoes liquefaction necrosis in its center and becomes surrounded by a collagenous capsule of fibroblasts. Edema and reactive gliosis encircle the inflamed area. Abscesses may result from contiguous spread from chronic sinusitis, mastoiditis, otitis media, or dental infections. Hematogenous spread may result in multiple abscesses in ischemic watershed areas. Trauma and operative procedures may directly inoculate brain tissue. Disruption of local brain parenchyma and mass effect are responsible for symptoms and complications.

Diagnosis

Precontrast head computed tomography (CT), the diagnostic modality of choice, may demonstrate an evolution of brain abscess from early cerebritis to late cerebritis and capsule formation. Contrast administration highlights characteristic ring-enhancing lesions by emphasizing the surrounding edema. Lumbar puncture is contraindicated in the presence of midline shift or a space-occupying lesion in the posterior fossa because of the potential for herniation.[2]

Clinical Complications

Abscess rupture transforms localized infection into meningitis or ventriculitis. Elevated ICP may cause uncal herniation and subsequently death. Seizures occur in 40% to 50% of patients, even after treatment.[1]

Management

Treatment includes aspiration of pus, antimicrobial therapy, and decreasing mass effect.[1] Abscess drainage may be done under CT guidance. Excision is reserved for gas-containing abscesses and some fungal abscesses.[1] Antimicrobial therapy is guided by the suspected primary source of infection and, later, by culture and sensitivity results. Steroids may transiently decrease ICP to prevent impending herniation, but they may also impair capsule formation.[1] Seizures should be controlled with anticonvulsants as needed.

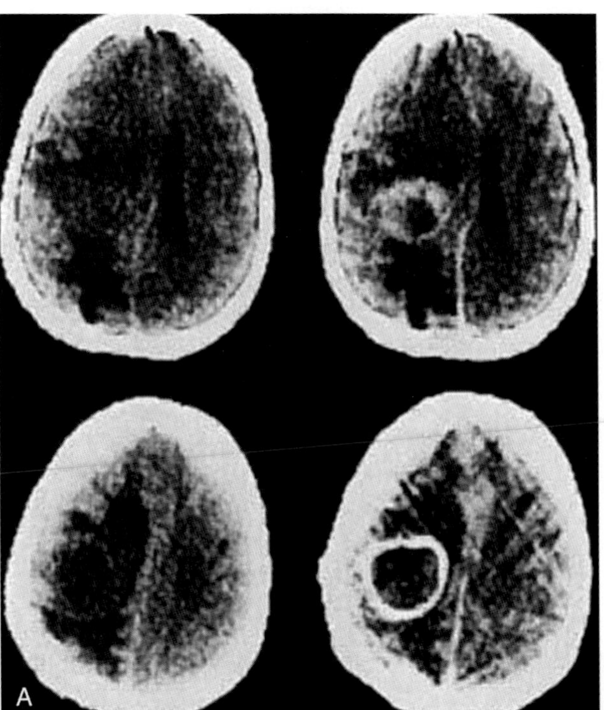

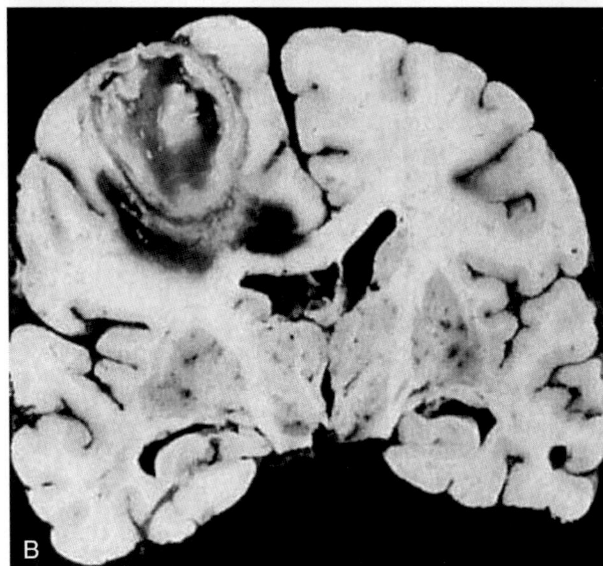

FIGURE 3–14 A: Unenhanced *(left)* and enhanced *(right)* computed tomographic scans from the same patient, with lesion in the cerebritis stage *(above)* and early capsule stage *(below)*. (From Britt RH, Enzmann DR. Clinical stages of human brain abscesses on serial CT scans after contrast infusion: computerized tomographic, neuropathological, and clinical correlations. *J Neurosurg* 1983;59:972, with permission.) **B:** Gross specimen showing a large brain abscess. (From Griggs and Joynt, with permission.)

REFERENCES

1. Cochrane DD. Consultation with the specialist: brain abscess. *Pediatr Rev* 1999;20:209–215.
2. Zunt JR. Central nervous system infection during immunosuppression. *Neurol Clin* 2002;20:1–22.

Spinal Epidural Abscess

Laura Spivak

Clinical Presentation

Patients with spinal epidural abscess usually present with fever, malaise, back pain, and, at times, focal neurologic dysfunction.[1,2] Neurologic deficits in order of disease progression include radiculopathy, paresis, bladder and bowel dysfunction, and paralysis.[1,2] Cervical spinal cord involvement leads to respiratory dysfunction.[2] Sepsis, with or without change in mental status, heralds late progression of the disease.[1]

Pathophysiology

Staphylococcus aureus is the most common infecting agent. However, streptococci and aerobic gram-negative bacilli are also seen.[1,2] Patients with human immunodeficiency virus (HIV) infection are at risk for abscess caused by *Mycobacterium tuberculosis*.[2] Actinomycosis is seen in patients with poor dentition and in those who have undergone dental procedures.[1] Risk factors for epidural abscess include immunodeficieny states (e.g., acquired immunodeficiency syndrome [AIDS]), diabetes mellitus, alcoholism, chronic renal failure, intravenous drug abuse, malignancy, and spinal trauma or surgery.[1] Most posterior abscesses originate from distant infectious foci, whereas anterior epidural abscesses are associated with osteomyelitis or discitis, or with direct spread of retropharyngeal or retroperitoneal infection.[1,2] Blunt trauma is believed to be a predisposing factor in abscess formation, because of the resultant devitalized tissue and formation of vertebral hematomas, which provide a nutrient medium for bacteria.[1,2] Neurologic sequelae are postulated to arise from a combination of mechanical compression of the spinal cord and nerve roots and cord ischemia.[1]

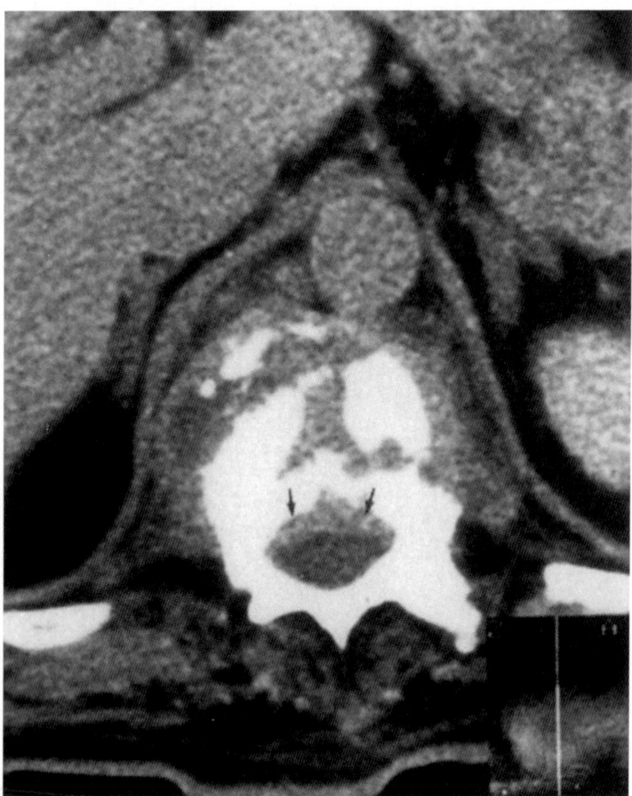

FIGURE 3–15 Computed tomographic scan demonstrating osseous destruction and epidural abscess. (From Scheld et al., with permission.)

Diagnosis

Gadolinium-enhanced magnetic resonance imaging (MRI) is the confirmatory diagnostic study of choice, because it can differentiate between an epidural abscess and other compressive lesions. With the advent of MRI as a diagnostic modality, lumbar puncture is no longer indicated.[1]

Clinical Complications

Complications include irreversible neurologic damage, respiratory failure, sepsis, and death.[1,2]

Management

Blood cultures should be drawn, and empiric antibiotic therapy with coverage against all suspected organisms should be initiated immediately in the emergency department.[1,2] Vancomycin or nafcillin provides adequate antistaphylococcal coverage.[2] A second agent with coverage against aerobic gram-negative bacilli, including *Pseudomonas aeruginosa*, is recommended.[2] Emergency, on-site neurosurgical consultation should be obtained for possible laminectomy with decompression and drainage of the abscess.[1] Serial MRI studies and neurologic evaluations are used to monitor disease progress in the medically treated patient.[1,2] Neurologic deterioration or increase in abscess size warrants immediate surgical intervention.[1,2]

REFERENCES

1. Chao D, Nanda A. Spinal epidural abscess: a diagnostic challenge. *Am Fam Physician* 2002;65:1341–1346.
2. Tunkel AR, Pradhan SK. Central nervous system infections in injection drug users. *Infect Dis Clin North Am* 2002;16:589–605.

Meningioma

Lekha Shah

Clinical Presentation

Meningiomas may be discovered in asymptomatic patients undergoing neuroimaging for unrelated reasons. Seizures are the most common presenting complaint among symptomatic patients. Tumor location determines the specific constellation of presenting symptoms and neurologic signs. Because these tumors develop slowly, they may grow for long periods and may erode through the skull, manifesting with external skin changes.[1]

Pathophysiology

Meningiomas are slow-growing tumors that arise from the arachnoid villi of the leptomeninges. They are usually benign and cause symptoms because of their space-occupying properties; however, local disruption of brain architecture in some cases gives rise to neurologic deficits. Low-dose ionizing radiation has been found to be a risk factor for meningioma development.[1]

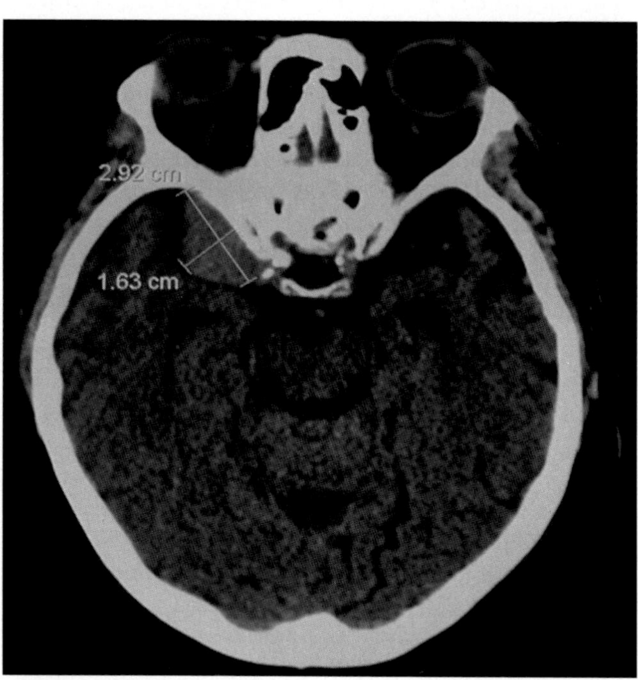

FIGURE 3–16 Computed tomogram showing meningioma. (Courtesy of Robert Hendrickson, MD.)

Diagnosis

Although contrast computed tomography (CT) delineates these tumors well, magnetic resonance imaging (MRI) with gadolinium is the diagnostic imaging modality of choice. Lesions appear as smooth, homogenously enhancing masses. Plain skull radiographs may have some utility in patients who cannot tolerate lying in the CT or MRI machine. They may show bone erosion, hyperostosis, or calcification from local tumor invasion.[1] On angiography, the rich meningeal blood supply gives the tumors a characteristic delayed vascular blush.

Clinical Complications

After resection, the rate of tumor recurrence approaches 30% at 5 years. Lesions of the medial sphenoid wing may extend into the cavernous sinus, causing thrombosis.[1] Patients may also be prone to deep vein thrombosis due to an associated hypercoagulable state. Treatment modalities such as radiotherapy can damage adjacent brain tissue.[1]

Management

In elderly and asymptomatic patients, meningiomas may be monitored with serial neuroimaging. Complete resection, if feasible, can be curative in symptomatic patients, and radiosurgery with the gamma knife is currently under investigation.[1] Stereotactic radiation may decrease recurrence rates postoperatively. Hormone manipulations with tamoxifen, mifepristone, and β-interferon are currently under investigation. Anticonvulsants are appropriate in patients who are experiencing seizures. Chemotherapy has not been found to be useful thus far.[1]

REFERENCES

1. Chozick BS, Reinert SE, Greenblatt SH. Incidence of seizures after surgery for supratentorial meningiomas: a modern analysis. *J Neurosurg* 1996;84:382–386.

3-17

Glioblastoma Multiforme

Lekha Shah

Clinical Presentation

Patients with glioblastoma multiforme (GBM) may present with headache, nausea, and vomiting caused by increased intracranial pressure (ICP). Seizures are present in 27% of patients. Focal and generalized symptoms ultimately culminate in obtundation, progressive coma, and death, often over a period of weeks to months.

Pathophysiology

GBM begins as a diffuse tumor rather than a discrete mass.[1] One third of tumors arise *de novo* in association with epidermal growth factor receptor (EGFR) amplifications. Another third are termed secondary glioblastomas because of their origin in lower-grade astrocytomas with a *TP53* mutation. These tumors display a pattern of rapid growth and invasion. In addition to the usual predilection of astrocytomas for white matter, GBM may be found in perineuronal and submeningeal spaces. A clinical picture resembling meningitis results from carcinomatous spread into the cerebrospinal fluid.

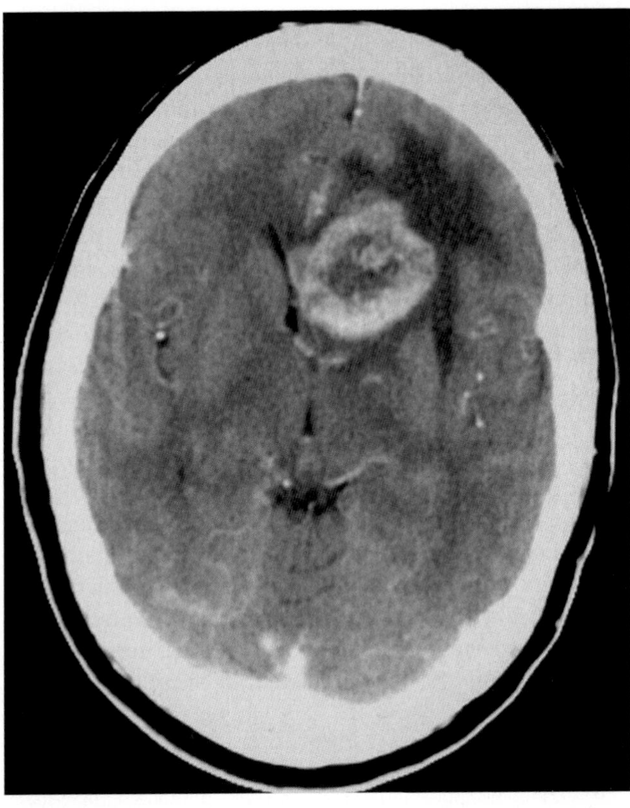

FIGURE 3–17 Computed tomogram showing glioblastoma multiforme. (Courtesy of Mark Silverberg, MD.)

Clinical Complications

GBM eventually causes obtundation, coma, and death from rising ICP. This final common pathway terminates in transtentorial, uncal, tonsillar, or cingulate herniation. Hemorrhage into the tumor may manifest as a severe headache and can precipitate herniation. Several case reports have described GBM metastatic to lung, lymph nodes, pleura, and liver.[1] GBM that is genetically distinct from the primary tumor may also recur in the contralateral hemisphere.[1]

Diagnosis

For conclusive diagnosis, brain biopsy establishes the diagnosis in a live patient. The electroencephalogram (EEG) shows nonspecific slowing in the area of the lesion. Lumbar puncture, usually contraindicated because of herniation, may reveal carcinomatous meningitis.[1]

Management

Corticosteroids, intravenous mannitol, and intubation with hyperventilation decrease ICP in the setting of impending herniation. Surgical resection remains controversial, with contradictory findings regarding survival benefit. The current standard of care holds that partial or whole resection allows for greater sensitivity to chemotherapy and radiotherapy. Chemotherapy (including nitrosoureas and procarbazine) is of limited therapeutic value.[1]

REFERENCES

1. Subramanian A, Harris A, Piggott K, Shieff C, Bradford R. Metastases to and from the central nervous system: the "relatively protected site." *Lancet Oncol* 2002;3:498–507.

Brain Metastases

Lekha Shah

Clinical Presentation

Brain metastases commonly arise from neoplasms of the lung, breast, and colorectum and from melanomas.[1] The clinical presentation depends on the anatomic location of the metastasis. Headache is the most common presenting symptom, although the "classic" morning headache secondary to increased intracranial pressure (ICP) was found in only 17% of patients.[1] Hemorrhage into the metastasis is likely to precipitate severe headache, coma, or focal neurologic deficits. Papilledema has been noted in approximately 25% of patients.[1] Other symptoms include cognitive dysfunction, weakness, ataxia, seizure, visual changes, nausea, vomiting, syncope, and sensory changes.[1,2]

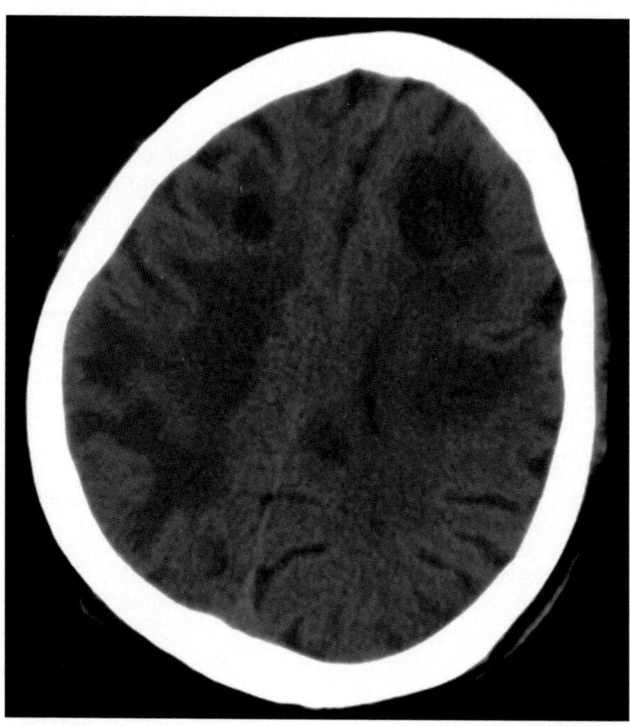

FIGURE 3–18 Computed tomogram showing multiple metastatic lesions. (Courtesy of Mark Silverberg, MD.)

Pathophysiology

Specific tumors tend to spread to specific areas of the brain. Colorectal and genitourinary cancers have a predisposition for the posterior fossa, whereas hematologic malignancies have a propensity to seed the leptomeninges.[1]

Diagnosis

The imaging modality of choice is the contrast-enhanced magnetic resonance angiogram (MRA), although computed tomography (CT) with and without contrast usually delineates most lesions, except for small masses in the posterior fossa.[1] Lumbar puncture is often contraindicated because of the risk of transtentorial herniation, but it may assist in the diagnosis of leptomeningeal seeding.[1]

Clinical Complications

The most feared complication is herniation and death. Less severe complications include focal neurologic deficits and seizures. Recurrence of metastases after chemotherapeutic or surgical therapy is common.[1,2]

Management

Temporizing measures include corticosteroids to relieve vasogenic edema, use of osmotic diuretics, hyperventilation, elevation of the head of the bed, and ventricular drains to decrease ICP in cases of impending herniation. Definitive treatment includes whole brain radiotherapy, stereotactic radiosurgery, and surgical resection, often in combination.[1] Chemotherapy has a limited and unproven role as a treatment modality.[2] Asymptomatic and treated patients should be monitored with serial magnetic resonance imaging (MRI) or CT imaging.

REFERENCES

1. Lassman AB, DeAngelis LM. Brain metastases. *Neurol Clin* 2003;21:1–23.
2. Arnold SM, Patchell RA. Diagnosis and management of brain metastases. *Hematol Oncol Clin North Am* 2001;15:1085–1107.

Pseudotumor Cerebri

Lekha Shah

Clinical Presentation

Pseudotumor cerebri (PC; idiopathic benign intracranial hypertension) is caused by increased intracranial pressure (ICP) without a space-occupying lesion or obstruction of cerebrospinal fluid (CSF) flow.[1]

The prototypical patient is an obese woman of childbearing age with a headache, nausea, vomiting, visual disturbances, pulsatile tinnitus, or vertigo.[1] Bilateral papilledema with loss of venous pulsations is a hallmark finding.

Pathophysiology

The cause of increased ICP in PC is not well understood but may involve a combination of increased CSF production and decreased CSF reabsorption.[1] Right-sided heart failure or pulmonary disease with carbon dioxide retention may contribute to increased intracranial vascular diameter, and thus the amount of vascular space occupied, leading to further elevation of the ICP.[2] PC may be associated with medications such as sulfonamides and conditions such as hypervitaminosis A and glucocorticoid withdrawal.[2] The common absence of hydrocephalus on computed tomography (CT) implies that PC is unrelated to communicating hydrocephalus.

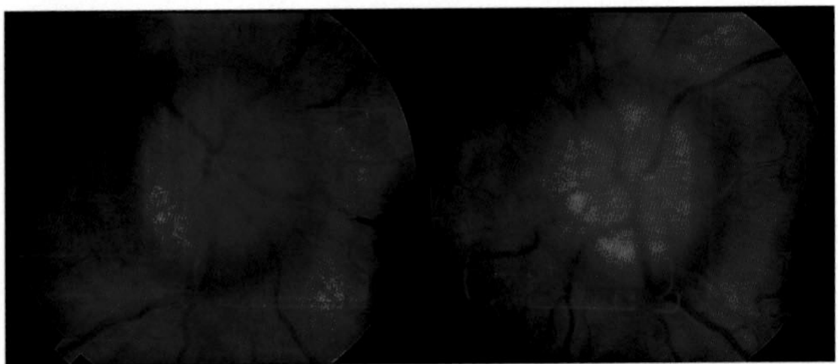

FIGURE 3–19 Papilledema in a 24-year-old, obese woman with severe headaches and obscuration of vision. (From Tasman and Jaeger, with permission.)

Diagnosis

Diagnostic criteria for PC require that the patient be alert and devoid of focal neurologic deficits.[1] In addition, a head CT or magnetic resonance imaging (MRI) study must be negative for intracranial masses or signs of obstructing hydrocephalus, the opening pressure on lumbar puncture should be greater than 250 mm of water, and the CSF should have a normal or low protein concentration, a normal glucose level, and a normal cell count.[2] Venous sinus thrombosis should be ruled out if suspected. Visual field testing may reveal blind spots followed by loss of peripheral vision.

Clinical Complications

Loss of vision is reported in a small percentage of patients.[1] Other complications include transient visual distortion as well as nausea and vomiting.

Management

Frequent lumbar punctures may relieve ICP, decreasing both the symptoms and the risk of visual complications.[2] Carbonic anhydrase inhibitors, loop diuretics, and steroids may help decrease production of CSF.[1]

REFERENCES

1. Friedman DI. Papilledema and pseudotumor cerebri. *Ophthalmol Clin North Am* 2001;14:129–147.
2. Friedman DI, Jacobson DM. Diagnostic criteria for idiopathic intracranial hypertension. *Neurology* 2002;59:1492–1495.

Horner's Syndrome

Cherie Mininger

Clinical Presentation

Horner's syndrome (HS; ipsilateral oculosympathetic paresis[1]) is a constellation of physical findings caused by disruption of the sympathetic pathway along its course from the hypothalamus to the eye.[2]

The triad of HS is ptosis, miosis, and facial anhidrosis. In some patients, the ptosis is only very subtle.[2] Because upper-lid ptosis can be overcome by muscles not innervated by the oculosympathetic system, lower-lid ptosis may be a more reliable finding.[2] Anhidrosis is an inconsistent finding that may be difficult to discern.[2] The most reliable clinical finding is anisocoria.[2]

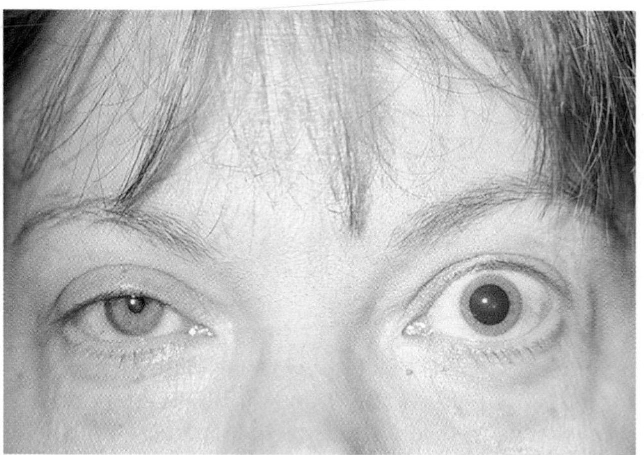

FIGURE 3–20 The right pupil does not dilate with 1% hydroxyamphetamine (Paradrine), indicating a third-order Horner's syndrome. (From Tasman and Jaeger, with permission.)

Pathophysiology

HS may be caused by a disruption of the sympathetic innervation anywhere along the pathway. Typically, lesions of the central neuron result from strokes, lesions of the preganglionic neuron from tumors, and lesions of the postganglionic neuron from vascular abnormalities.[2]

Diagnosis

The gold standard for diagnosis of HS is made by placing 10% cocaine drops in both eyes; the Horner's pupil becomes less dilated.[1,2]

Clinical Complications

Complications related to HS depend on the underlying cause. Possible causes include tumors (Pancoast), cerebral infarctions (ischemic or hemorrhagic), trauma, carotid dissection, vascular abnormalities, and idiopathic causes.[2]

Management

Further testing with hydroxyamphetamine 1% can help localize the defect.[2] Evaluation of the cause of HS requires chest radiography (if an apical abnormality is suspected) and computed tomography (CT) or magnetic resonance imaging (MRI) of the head and neck to identify lesions along the sympathetic pathway. Patients should be admitted for a full evaluation of the underlying cause.

REFERENCES

1. Leira EC, Bendixen BH, Kardon RH, Adams HP Jr. Brief, transient Horner's syndrome can be the hallmark of a carotid artery dissection. *Neurology* 1998;50:289–290.
2. Kawasaki A, Kardon RH. Disorders of the pupil. *Ophthalmol Clin North Am* 2001;14:149–168.

Migraines/Cluster Headaches

Laura Spivak

Clinical Presentation

Migraines are episodic headaches associated with nausea, photophobia, phonophobia, and aura.[1] Cluster headaches are episodic, unilateral headaches with ipsilateral cranial autonomic features.[2]

Migraineurs complain of unilateral, throbbing pain that is worsened by movement and is associated with nausea, vomiting, photophobia, or phonophobia. Cognitive function may be impaired.[1] Patients with cluster headache describe the rapid onset of a periorbital, boring pain, sometimes likened to "a hot poker in the eye." Associated findings include miosis, ptosis, conjunctival injection, lacrimation, rhinorrhea, and nasal congestion. Lying still may exacerbate the pain.[2]

Pathophysiology

Migraine pain may arise from activation of the trigeminal nerve.[1] Presumed migraine triggers include estrogen, certain food ingredients, and sleep disorders.[1] Auras, reported in 20% of migraines, arise from the cerebral cortex and include visual and other focal neurologic symptoms.[1] Bipolar disorder, anxiety, and depression are often linked with migraine.[1] Cluster headaches are believed to originate from the hypothalamus.[3] They occur most commonly in the third decade, with a male predominance of 2.1:1.[2] There may be a genetic predisposition.[2] Cluster headaches tend to recur for weeks to months at a time and then remit for months to years.[2]

TABLE 3–21 Common Prevocational Triggers for Migraine

Triggers for migraine	
Hormonal triggers	Menstruation, ovulation, oral contraceptive, hormonal replacement
Dietary triggers	Alcohol, nitrite-laden meat, monosodium glutamate, aspartame, chocolate, aged cheese, missing a meal
Psychologic triggers	Stress, period after stress (weekend or vacation), anxiety, worry, depression
Physical/environmental triggers	Glare, flashing lights, visual stimulation, fluorescent lighting, odors, weather changes, high altitude
Sleep-related triggers	Lack of sleep, excessive sleep
Miscellaneous triggers	Head trauma, physical exertion, fatigue
Drugs	Nitroglycerine, histamine, reserpine, hydralazine, ranitidine, estrogen

From Evans, with permission.

Diagnosis

Clinical presentation is the cornerstone of diagnosis in patients with migraine or cluster headaches. Magnetic resonance imaging (MRI) findings are usually normal in patients with cluster headaches.[3]

Clinical Complications

Migraine headaches cause disruptions in educational, occupational, and familial and social activities.[1] Patients with cluster headaches may have a persistent partial Horner's syndrome.[2] Attacks are so severe that some patients attempt suicide.[2]

Management

Triptans, dihydroergotamine, and ergotamine are 5-hydroxytryptamine receptor agonists used for migraine treatment.[1] Acute cluster headaches are treated with oxygen, sumatriptan, and dihydroergotamine.[2] Prophylactic medications include verapamil, sodium valproate, lithium, methysergide, and ergotamine.[2]

REFERENCES

1. Mathew NT. Pathophysiology, epidemiology, and impact of migraine. *Clin Cornerstone* 2001;4:1–17.
2. Newman LC, Goadsby P, Lipton RB. Cluster and related headaches. *Med Clin North Am* 2001;85:997–1016.
3. Silberstein SD, Niknam R, Rozen TD, Young WB. Brief communications: cluster headache with aura. *Neurology* 2000;54:219–221.

Multiple Sclerosis

Rachel Haroz

Clinical Presentation

Patients with multiple sclerosis (MS) report a relatively abrupt onset of symptoms that persist for several weeks and then slowly resolve. The symptoms are variable and involve various areas of the central nervous system (CNS). Ocular symptoms, including diplopia (internuclear ophthalmoplegia), unilateral optic neuritis, and unilateral vision loss, are the presenting feature in 30% of patients. Other symptoms include ataxia, vertigo, paresthesias, dysarthria, paralysis, incontinence, and Lhermitte's sign, which is characterized by sensations of electric shock in the limbs and trunk (e.g., with neck flexion).[1] Fatigue may worsen as the day progresses, and symptoms are exacerbated by increases in body temperature (Uhthoff's symptom).[1] On examination, increased tone, clonus, hyperreflexia, and decreased pain and temperature sensation may be observed, as well as a pale disc on funduscopic examination.[1]

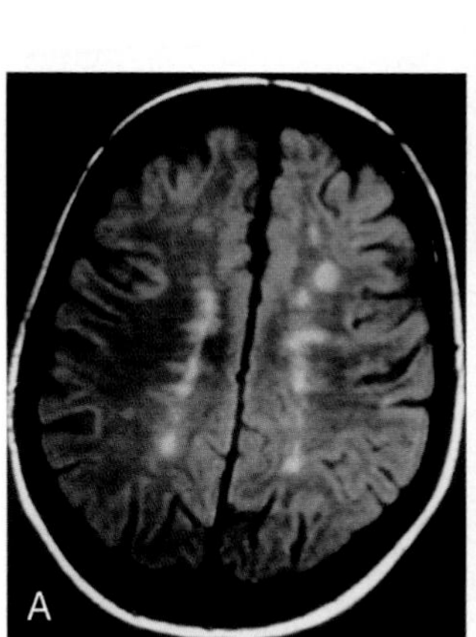

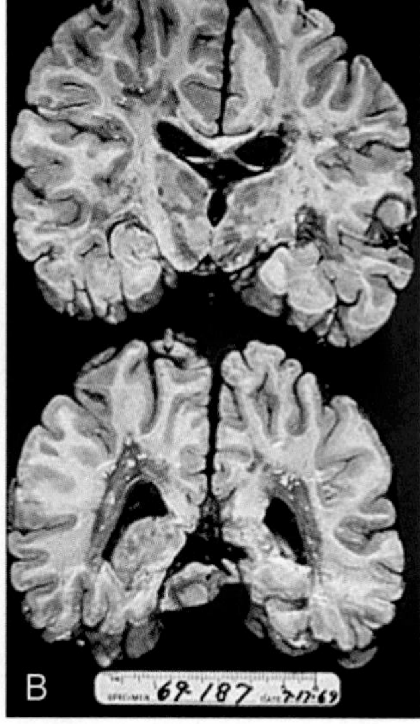

FIGURE 3–22 **A:** Axial fluid attenuated inversion recovery (FLAIR) and T2-weighted magnetic resonance image shows multiple foci of increased signal in the periventricular deep white matter perpendicular to the subependymal, compatible with Dawson's fingers and consistent with the diagnosis of demyelinating disease (multiple sclerosis). (Courtesy of José Biller, MD.) **B:** Gross postmortem specimen confirming diagnosis of multiple sclerosis via new (pink) and old (grey) lesions. (From Griggs and Joynt, with permission.)

Pathophysiology

The exact cause of MS is unknown, but demyelination may occur in the brainstem, spinal cord white matter, optic nerves, periventricular white matter, and cerebellum. Typically, there is loss of the myelin, with relative preservation of the axon and scar formation leading to decreased conduction. This disorder is believed to be immune mediated and has a genetic susceptibility.[1]

Diagnosis

The diagnosis is primarily clinical. The disease may either be relapsing-remitting (80%) or primary progressive (20%). The former commonly manifests in the third decade of life and has a female-to-male predominance of 2:1. Patients typically have at least two episodes lasting days to weeks at least 2 months apart, with symptoms affecting different regions of the CNS. Magnetic resonance imaging (MRI) may show scattered white matter lesions of the brain and spinal cord. The cerebrospinal fluid often shows increased levels of protein and gamma globulin. The differential diagnosis includes Lyme disease, HIV, neurosyphilis, systemic lupus erythematosus (SLE), and sarcoidosis.[1]

Clinical Complications

Patients may experience recurrent infections or exacerbating symptoms or both. Progressive neurologic dysfunction may lead to respiratory compromise requiring aggressive respiratory support. Patients may also experience depression with suicidal ideation, dementia, chronic pain, speech and swallowing disorders, and gait dysfunction.[1]

Management

High-dose corticosteroids are used to treat relapses. Other immunosuppressive therapies such as interferon-β-1, are currently being used to prevent relapses.[1]

REFERENCES

1. Noseworthy JH, Lucchinetti C, Rodriquez M, Weinshenker BG. Medical progress: multiple sclerosis. *N Engl J Med* 2000;343: 938–952.

Myasthenia Gravis

Rachel Haroz

Clinical Presentation

Patients with myasthenia gravis (MG) present with muscle weakness and fatigability that worsen with use and improve with rest. Muscle weakness may be generalized (85%) or localized, and it is not accompanied by sensory, cerebellar, or reflex function deficits. The most common symptoms are ptosis, blurred vision, and diplopia. Fifteen percent of patients have symptoms limited to the ocular muscles. Facial and bulbar muscles are often affected, resulting in dysarthria, dysphagia, and a characteristic flattened smile and nasal speech. Neck extensors and diaphragm weakness may occur. Limb muscles are affected, usually in a proximal and often asymmetric manner.[1,2]

Pathophysiology

MG is caused by circulating antibodies that destroy postsynaptic acetylcholine receptors (AchR). This results in fewer active binding sites and, consequently, decreased muscle contraction. Seventy-five percent of patients have thymic abnormalities; of these, 15% have thymomas and 85% have thymic hyperplasia. MG is often associated with other autoimmune diseases such as systemic lupus erythematosus (SLE) and hyperthyroidism.[1,3] MG affects men and women similarly; however, peak onset occurs during the second to third decades for women and the seventh to eighth decades for men.[1] Passive transfer of maternal antibodies to neonates can occur and results in transient symptoms.[1]

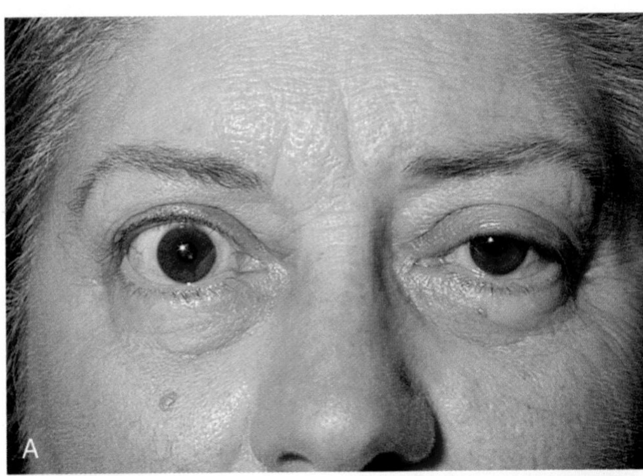

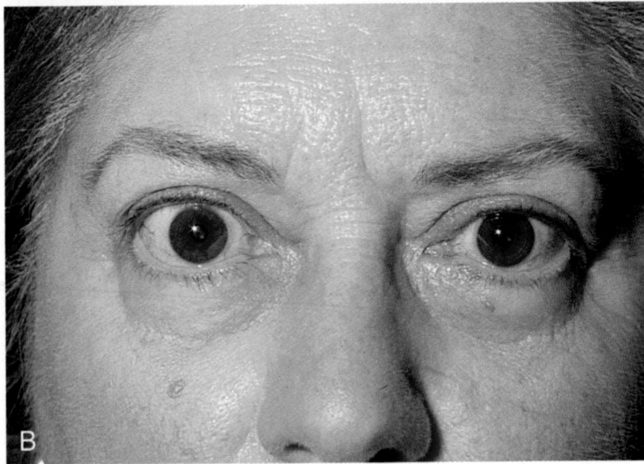

FIGURE 3–23 **A:** Myasthenia gravis can cause ptosis, as seen here. **B:** Ptosis is resolved by treatment with intravenous edrophonium chloride (Tensilon). (From Tasman and Jaeger, with permission.)

Diagnosis

The diagnosis of MG is established by physical examination, edrophonium (Tensilon) test, repetitive nerve stimulation, serum testing for AchR antibodies, and electromyographic testing. The physical examination reveals progressive weakness with repetitive movements. Tensilon is an acetylcholinesterase inhibitor that improves muscle strength transiently but dramatically. The antibody assay is very specific, but only 85% of patients have antibodies. The differential diagnosis includes drug-induced disorders, botulism, Eaton-Lambert syndrome, and amyotrophic lateral sclerosis (ALS).[2]

Clinical Complications

The primary complication of MG is respiratory failure. This results from either a myasthenic crisis, caused by a functional deficiency of acetylcholine, or a cholinergic crisis, caused by overtreatment with acetylcholinesterase inhibitors. Either crisis results in muscle weakness and may affect respiratory function.[1,2]

Management

The mainstay of treatment is pyridostigmine bromide and neostigmine bromide (anticholinesterase drugs). Patients with severe symptoms may require high-dose steroids, plasmapheresis, and intravenous immunoglobulin treatment. Other therapies include azathioprine, methotrexate, cyclophosphamide, mycophenolate mofetil, and cyclosporine A. Thymectomy has been shown to improve the clinical course and increase the remission rate.[2]

REFERENCES

1. Drachman DB. Myasthenia gravis. *N Engl J Med* 1994;330:1797–1810.
2. Palace J, Vincent A, Beeson D. Myasthenia gravis: diagnostic and management dilemmas. *Curr Opin Neurol* 2001;14:583–589.

Cranial Third Nerve Neuropathy (Oculomotor)

Treve Henwood and John R. Queen

Clinical Presentation

Patients with third cranial nerve neuropathy complain of diplopia and unilateral, supraorbital, or retrobulbar pain. Hypertension and diabetic complications account for 58% of third cranial nerve mononeuropathies. Migraines have been a noted cause of isolated oculomotor neuropathy in younger patients. Other causes include trauma, migraine, intracranial aneurysm and intracranial hemorrhage (ICH), vertebrobasilar ischemia, and tumor. Individual case reports of myasthenia gravis (MG) and multiple sclerosis (MS) have been noted.[1–3]

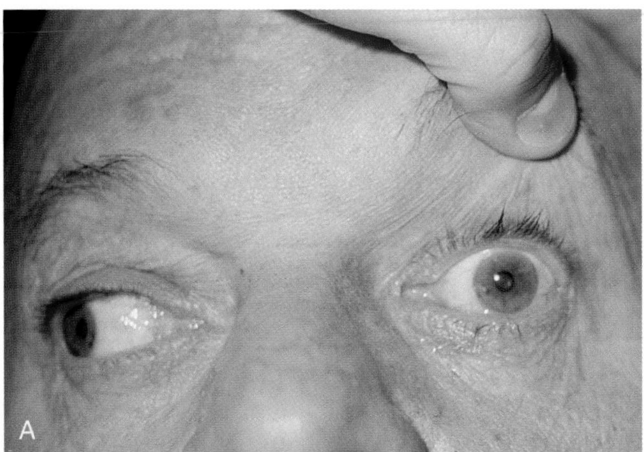

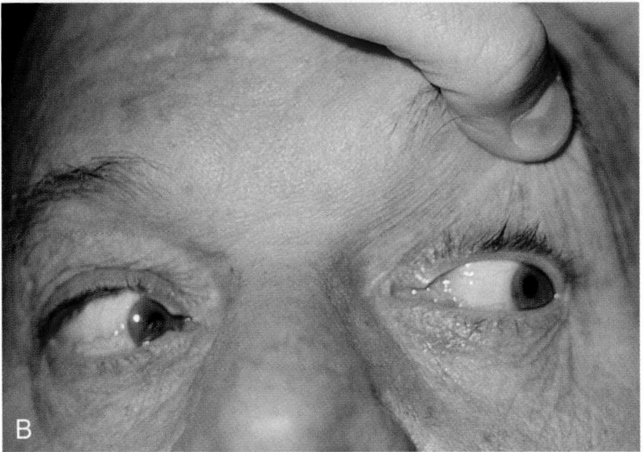

FIGURE 3–24 **A:** Palsy of cranial nerve III with relative pupil sparing. The patient is unable to adduct the eye. **B:** Third nerve palsy with relative pupil sparing. Abduction remains normal. (From Tasman and Jaeger, with permission.)

Pathophysiology

Diabetic mononeuropathy is thought to result from ischemia of the cranial nerve with preservation of circumferentially located parasympathetic fibers, which explains pupillary sparing.[1]

Diagnosis

Isolated cranial nerve neuropathy is a diagnosis of exclusion. A complete history and physical examination, with emphasis on neurologic and ophthalmologic function, and cranial nerve imaging with magnetic resonance imaging (MRI) are recommended. Other testing modalities to consider include a complete blood count (CBC) and lumbar puncture for infection, blood glucose for diabetes, erythrocyte sedimentation rate (ESR) or C-reactive protein determination for autoimmune diseases, and a Tensilon test for MG. Examination findings include external strabismus, with inability to move the eye superiorly and medially, and complete ptosis. Pupillary dilation may or may not be present, because the light reflex is most often spared.[1–3]

Clinical Complications

Other underlying causes of oculomotor neuropathy, such as sacular aneurysms and brainstem lesions, must be addressed and treated as indicated. For patients with oculomotor neuropathy caused by diabetes or hypertension, resolution of symptoms usually occurs within 2 weeks to 3 months. However, symptoms may last as long as 1 year.[1–3]

Management

Eye patching of the affected eye for diplopia, administration of analgesics, and antiplatelet therapy may be helpful in neuropathy of ischemic origin.[1–3]

REFERENCES

1. Brown MJ, Asbury AK. Diabetic neuropathy. *Ann Neurol* 1984; 15:2–12.
2. Wortham E, Blumenthal H. Diplopia: a review of 48 cases of isolated ocular cranial neuropathy. *J Okla State Med Assoc* 1985; 78:99–103.
3. Lance JW, Zagami AS. Ophthalmoplegic migraine: a recurrent demyelinating neuropathy? *Cephalalgia* 2001;21:84–89.

Cranial Fourth Nerve Neuropathy (Trochlear)

Treve Henwood and John R. Queen

Clinical Presentation

Isolated fourth cranial nerve neuropathy is rare, and the most common cause is trauma. Other causes can be categorized by age. Older patients may be affected by diabetes, hypertension, herpes zoster, myasthenia gravis (MG), or multiple sclerosis (MS), with diabetes being the most common cause in this group.[1–3]

Patients are unable to look medially and down; the eye is passively directed down and outward. Patients often complain of diplopia and present with the head tilted away from the affected eye to maintain binocular vision.[1–3]

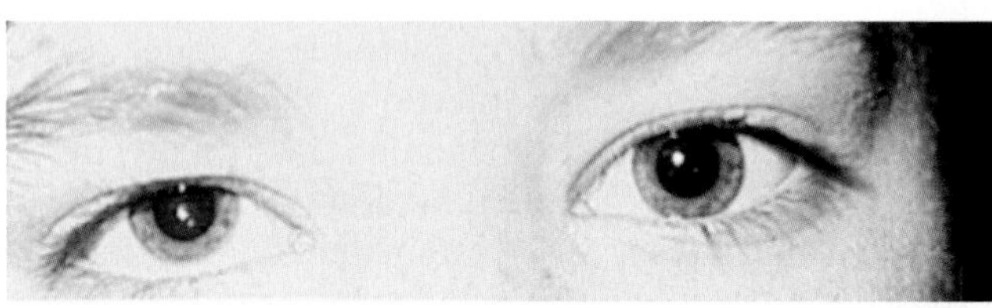

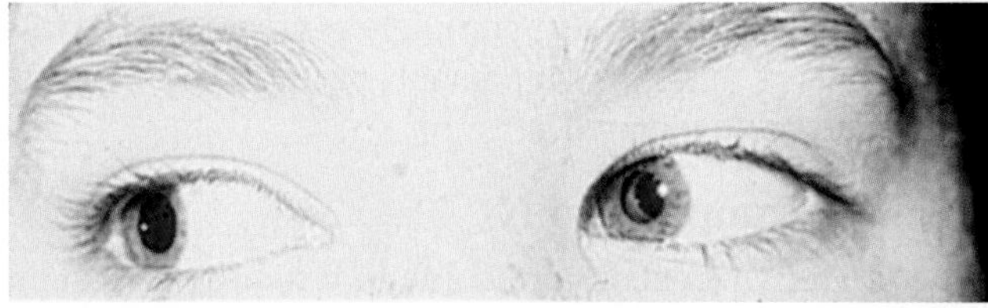

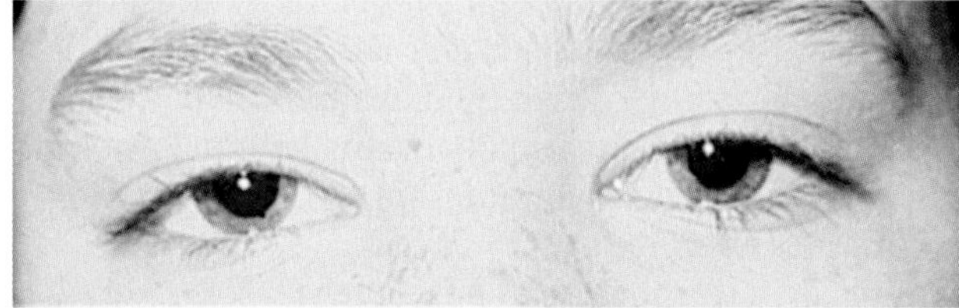

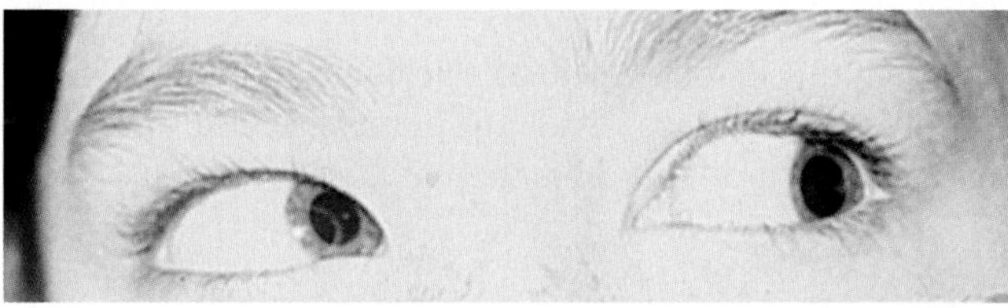

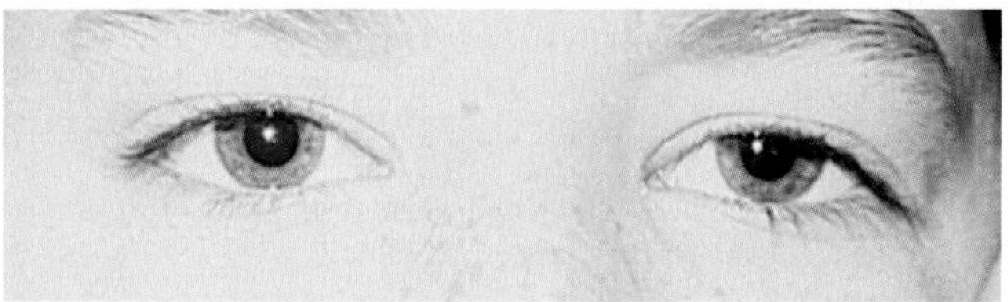

FIGURE 3–25 Right cranial nerve IV palsy. On right head tilt *(top),* the right eye elevates and the sclera below the inferior limbus is visible. On left head tilt *(bottom),* the patient is orthotopic. (From Tasman and Jaeger, with permission.)

Pathophysiology

The trochlear nerve innervates the superior oblique muscle. Diabetic mononeuropathy is thought to be a result of centrofascicular ischemia of the cranial nerve. Neuropathies can also be caused by inflammation of local orbital muscle and nerve.[1]

Diagnosis

Isolated cranial nerve neuropathy is a diagnosis of exclusion. A complete history and physical examination, with emphasis on neurologic and ophthalmologic function, and cranial nerve imaging with magnetic resonance imaging (MRI) are recommended. Other testing modalities to consider include a complete blood count (CBC), lumbar puncture for infection, blood glucose for diabetes, erythrocyte sedimentation rate (ESR) or C-reactive protein determination for autoimmune diseases, and a Tensilon test for MG.[1–3]

Clinical Complications

Other underlying causes of trochlear neuropathy, such as sacular aneurysms and brainstem lesions, must be addressed and treated as indicated. For patients with trochlear neuropathy caused by diabetes or hypertension, resolution of symptoms usually occurs within 2 weeks to 3 months. However, symptoms may last as long as 1 year. If symptoms do not improve within 3 to 6 months, another cause should be investigated.[1–3]

Management

Eye patching of the affected eye for diplopia, administration of analgesics, and antiplatelet therapy may be indicated for neuropathy of ischemic origin.[1–3]

REFERENCES

1. Brown MJ, Asbury AK. Diabetic neuropathy. *Ann Neurol* 1984;15:2–12.
2. Grimson BS, Glaser JS. Isolated trochlear nerve palsies in herpes zoster ophthalmicus. *Arch Ophthalmol* 1978;96:1233–1235.
3. Wortham E, Blumenthal H. Diplopia: a review of 48 cases of isolated ocular cranial neuropathy. *J Okla State Med Assoc* 1985; 78:99–103.

Cranial Sixth Nerve Neuropathy (Abducens)

Matthew Warner

Clinical Presentation

The sixth cranial nerve innervates the extraocular lateral rectus muscle, which provides lateral movement to the eye. Abducens neuropathy prevents lateral gaze on the affected side.[1]

Patients may present with double vision or with esotropia secondary to unopposed action of the medial rectus.[1,2] Concurrent involvement of other cranial nerves, especially nerves V and VII, is possible. Bilateral abducens nerve palsy is rare (less than 10% of cases).[1] Additional symptoms are present depending on the underlying cause (e.g., headache and nuchal rigidity with meningitis).[1,2]

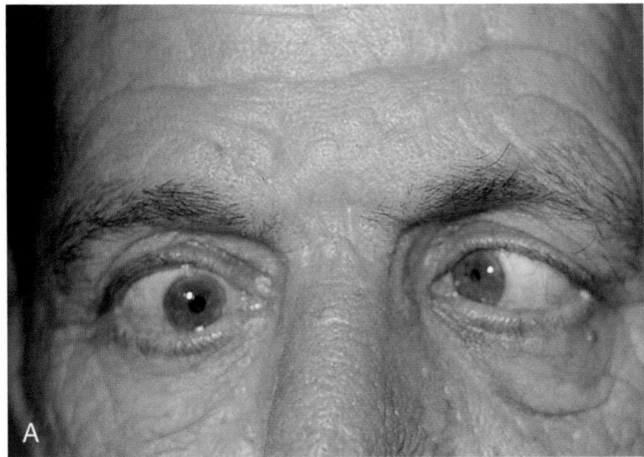

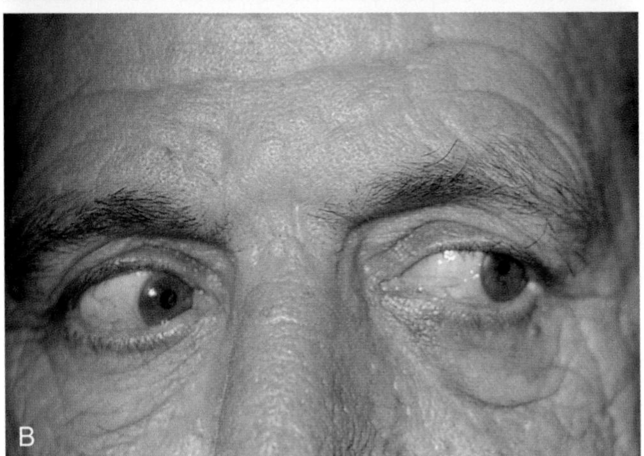

FIGURE 3–26 **A:** Right cranial nerve VI palsy. Right gaze reveals complete abduction deficit. **B:** Right cranial nerve VI palsy. The patient was orthotopic on left gaze. (From Tasman and Jaeger, with permission.)

Pathophysiology

The original location of injury can be the nerve nucleus, the intracranial or extracranial course, the neuromuscular junction, or the latereral rectus muscle.[2] The long intracranial course of the abducens nerve makes it particularly vulnerable to insult.[1] Any process that increases intracranial pressure (ICP) may produce neuropathy. Abducens palsy may be associated with vascular events, trauma, tumor, ischemia, meningitis, botulism, Lyme disease, myasthenia gravis (MG), multiple sclerosis (MS), pseudotumor cerebri (PC), demyelinating disorders, Wernecke's encephalopathy, or abuse of methylenedioxymethamphetamine (MDMA).[1]

Diagnosis

It is necessary to determine whether the diplopia is monocular or binocular.[2] A neurologic examination should be performed to localize the affected area. Computed tomography (CT) may help to determine the location of an intracranial source.

Clinical Complications

Abducens palsy may persist after the source has been removed. Traumatic abducens palsy demonstrated a recovery rate of only 73%.[1]

Management

The management of acute abducens palsy is conservative.[3] Eye patches may limit diplopia, and frequent follow-up visits with an ophthalmologist are required to assess resolution.[1] If there is no resolution of symptoms within 4 to 6 months, administration of botulinum toxin to the medial rectus muscle of the affected eye may restore binocular vision and improve esotropia.[3]

REFERENCES

1. Caldicott DG, Wurm A, Edwards NA. The eyes have it: an uncommon but useful sign after serious craniocervical trauma. *J Trauma* 2002;53:1001–1005.
2. Feuer H, Jogoda A. Myasthenia gravis presenting as unilateral abducens nerve palsy. *Am J Emerg Med* 2001;19:410–412.
3. Achesan JF, Bentley CR, Shallo-Hoffmann J, Gresty MA. Dissociated effects of botulinum toxin chemodenervation on ocular deviation and saccade dynamics in chronic lateral rectus palsy. *Br J Ophthalmol* 1998;82:67–71.

3-27

Bell's Palsy

Matthew Warner

Clinical Presentation

Patients with Bell's palsy present with a nonprogressive facial hemiparalysis. Sixty percent of patients have had a preceding viral illness.[1] Other symptoms may include ipsilateral ear pain; ear, tongue, and facial numbness; and taste disturbances.[1-3]

Pathophysiology

The cause of Bell's palsy is unknown, although there may be an association with viral infection, especially herpes simplex virus (HSV).[1-3] It is theorized that palsy may occur secondary to reactivation of HSV in the geniculate ganglion and subsequent migration to the facial nerve.[2]

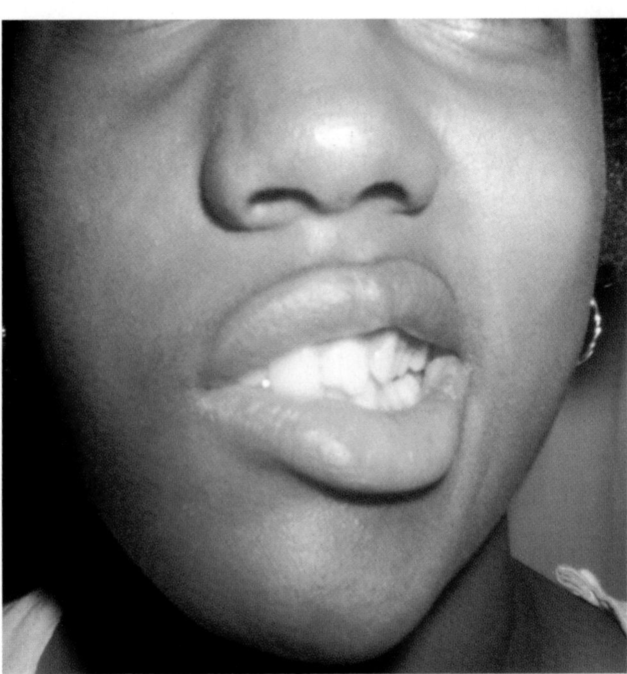

FIGURE 3–27 Paralysis of peripheral cranial nerve VII (Bell's palsy). (Courtesy of David K. Wagner, MD.)

Diagnosis

The diagnosis, based on history and physical examination, is one of exclusion. The differential diagnosis includes stroke, tumor, otitis media, trauma, Guillain-Barré syndrome, HIV infection, Lyme disease, and Ramsay Hunt syndrome.[2] Laboratory and imaging studies are not helpful in making this diagnosis. It is still recommended that patients with Bell's palsy be referred to a neurologist or otolaryngologist.[1]

Clinical Complications

Most patients recover completely. However, up to 30% are left with partial palsy, involuntary movements, and persistent lacrimation.[2,3] Recurrence is seen in 12% of patients, with 36% experiencing paralysis on the same side.[2]

Management

There is no prevention or cure for Bell's palsy.[2] Combined prednisone and acyclovir, especially in adults, has been recommended.[1,3] To reduce the chance of corneal abrasion, patients should use eye lubrication and an eye patch.

REFERENCES

1. Benecke JE Jr. Facial paralysis. *Otolaryngol Clin North Am* 2002;35:357–365.
2. Shannon S, Meadow S, Horowitz SH. Are drug therapies effective in treating Bell's palsy? *J Fam Pract* 2003;52:156,159.
3. Schirm J, Mulkens PS. Bell's palsy and herpes simplex virus. *APMIS* 1997;105:815–823.

Central Cord Syndrome

Arthur Chang

Clinical Presentation

Central Cord Syndrome (CCS) usually occurs after a cervical spine injury and is characterized by bilaterally symmetric motor paresis, with upper extremities affected more severely than lower extremities, and distal more than proximal muscle groups. Sensation is usually intact proximal to the spinal cord lesion, and variably impaired distal to the lesion. Bladder and rectal function may be affected.[1,2]

Pathophysiology

CCS occurs after injury to the central gray matter and inner section of the corticospinal and spinothalamic tracts of the cervical spinal cord. It usually results from cervical hyperextension, wherein the spinal cord is "pinched" by an intrusion of the ligamentum flavum. Patients with preexisting cervical canal narrowing are at a greater risk for development of CCS.[1]

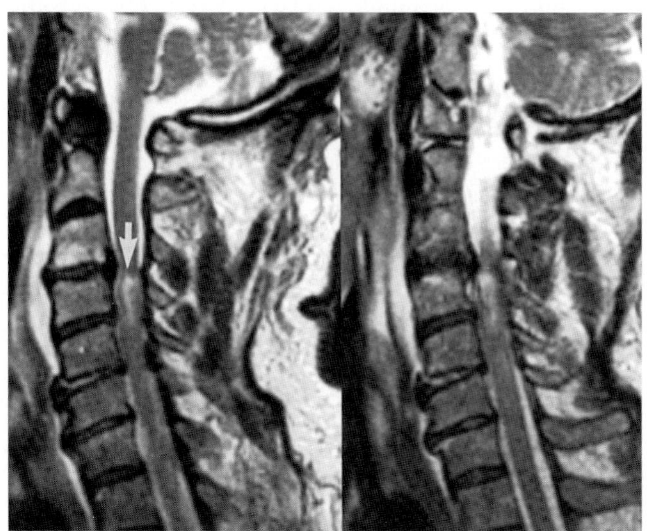

FIGURE 3–28 Sagittal T2-weighted magnetic resonance image shows high-intensity signal of edema in the central portion of the cervical cord, posterior to C4. (From Harris and Harris, with permission.)

Diagnosis

Diagnosis is clinical. Lateral radiographic films and unenhanced computed tomography (CT) of the cervical spine may show vertebral fractures at the level of the spinal cord lesion. Magnetic resonance imaging (MRI) is the study of choice to image the cervical spinal cord.[1,2]

Clinical Complications

Prognosis is favorable for patients younger than 50 years of age; 80% to 90% of these patients regain ambulatory status and bladder control. Patients older than 50 years of age have a worse prognosis.[1] The most frequent sequela is neurogenic bladder dysfunction.[2]

Management

Cervical spine immobilization is the first and most important aspect of management in the emergency department for patients with cervical spine injury. After resuscitation, patients should be given intravenous methylprednisolone.[1,2] Maximal benefit has been shown in patients who received methylprednisolone within the first 8 hours after injury. Surgical stabilization may be required for patients with an unstable cervical spine. Consultation with a neurosurgeon should be arranged promptly.

REFERENCES

1. Newey ML, Sen PK, Fraser RD. The long-term outcome after central cord syndrome: a study of the natural history. *J Bone Joint Surg Br* 2000;82:851–855.
2. Smith CP, Kraus SR, Nickell KG, Boone TB. Video urodynamic findings in men with the central cord syndrome. *J Urol* 2000; 164:2014–2017.

Anterior Cord Syndrome

Arthur Chang

Clinical Presentation

Anterior cord syndrome (ACS) involves a partial lesion of the spinal cord and is characterized by loss of motor function, decreased fine touch, and decreased pain and temperature sensation, with preservation of sensory vibration, proprioception and crude touch below the level of the injury.[1,2]

Pathophysiology

ACS results from an injury to the anterior portion of the spinal cord. Traumatic causes of ACS include hyperflexion injuries that result in a burst fracture, with protrusion of the anterior bony fragment into the spinal canal. Nontraumatic causes include acute disk herniation and spinal cord infarction from diminished vascular supply via the anterior spinal artery.[1] The descending pathways in that area (e.g., corticospinal tract) carry impulses from the cortex for motor control. Some ascending pathways are also affected, including the spinothalamic tract, which carries fine touch, pain, and temperature information to the brain. Posterior structures remain unaffected in ACS, and therefore vibratory, proprioceptive, and crude touch sensation are preserved.[1,2]

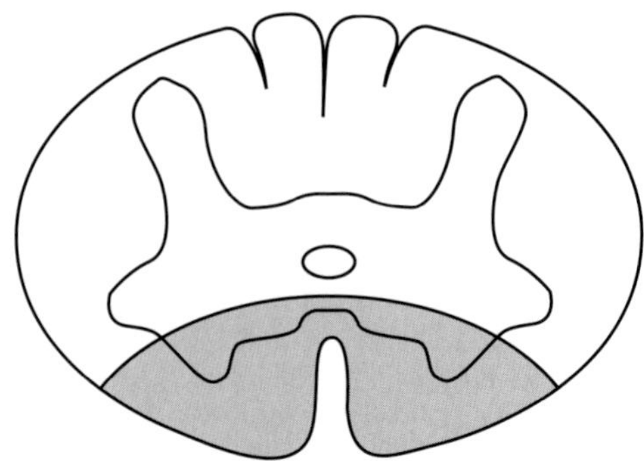

FIGURE 3–29 Zone of injury for anterior cord syndrome. (From Bucholz, with permission.)

Diagnosis

The diagnosis is made by clinical examination. Lateral cervical/thoracic spinal radiographic films and unenhanced computed tomography (CT) scans may show vertebral fractures at the level of the spinal cord lesion. Magnetic resonance imaging (MRI) of the spine is the study of choice to image both osseous structures and the spinal cord itself.[2]

Clinical Complications

Prognosis is variable, but up to 50% of patients with acute spinal cord injury sustain complete paralysis below the level of the lesion. If the lesion occurs in the lower cervical or upper thoracic spine, neurogenic shock, including bradycardia and hypotension, may result from the interruption of the sympathetic chain ganglia. Volume resuscitation and vasopressor support using phenylephrine may be indicated.[1]

Management

Cervical spine immobilization is the first and most important aspect of management in the emergency department. After initial resuscitation (including intubation if respiratory muscles are paralyzed), an intravenous methylprednisolone protocol for acute spinal injury should be started. Maximal benefit has been shown in patients who received methylprednisolone within the first 8 hours after injury. Emergency surgical intervention may be required for some patients, so on-site consultation with a neurosurgeon is required.

REFERENCES

1. King BS, Gupta R, Narayan RK. The early assessment and intensive care unit management of patients with severe traumatic brain and spinal cord injuries. *Surg Clin North Am* 2000;80:855–870.
2. Takhtani D, Melhem ER. MR imaging in cervical spine trauma. *Clin Sports Med* 2002;21:49–75.

Brown-Séquard Syndrome

Arthur Chang

Clinical Presentation

Brown-Séquard syndrome (BSS; spinal cord hemisection) produces characteristic neurologic deficits, including ipsilateral motor weakness and loss of sensory proprioception and vibration, as well as contralateral loss of fine touch, pain, and temperature sensation distal to the affected spinal cord level.[1,2]

Pathophysiology

BSS is the result of an injury to a lateral transverse half of the spinal cord. Involvement of the corticospinal tract results in spastic hemiparesis. Ipsilateral dorsal columns are also affected, producing loss of proprioception and vibratory sensation. Because the spinothalamic tract crosses within the spinal cord, this results in *contralateral* loss of fine touch, pain, and temperature sensation one or two levels below the lesion. Traumatic causes of BSS include penetrating trauma to the spine by a gunshot or stab wound. Other causes include spinal epidural hematoma, epidural abscess, extramedullary tumor causing spinal cord compression, and spinal herniation.[1,2]

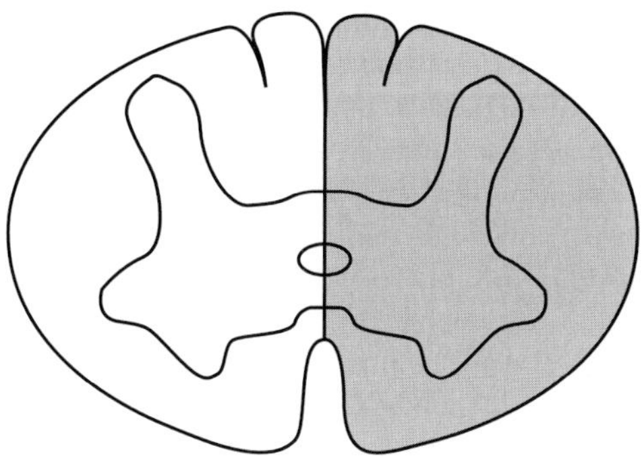

FIGURE 3–30 Potential zone of injury in Brown-Séquard syndrome. (From Bucholz, with permission.)

Diagnosis

Diagnosis is clinical. Unenhanced computed tomography (CT) of the spine may show foreign bodies (e.g., bullets, knife) or bony tumor involvement. MRI of the spine is the study of choice for evaluating the spinal cord itself, as well as surrounding bony and soft tissue.[1,2]

Clinical Complications

Patients with incomplete spinal cord lesions, specifically BSS, have a favorable prognosis for recovery.[1] As with any injury to the spinal cord, these patients may develop transverse myelopathy or spinal shock, which usually resolves in 1 to 2 days. Extreme fluctuations in heart rate, blood pressure, and temperature may occur because of autonomic dysfunction.[1,2]

Management

After initial resuscitation and stabilization, patients may benefit from intravenous methylprednisolone. Immediate on-site neurosurgical consultation should be sought for evaluation of surgically reversible causes of BSS, including spinal epidural abscess, hematoma, and herniation.[2]

REFERENCES

1. Pollard ME, Apple DF. Factors associated with improved neurologic outcomes in patients with incomplete tetraplegia. *Spine* 2003; 28:33–39.
2. Iyer RV, Countinho C, Lye RH. Spontaneous spinal cord herniation. *Br J Neurosurg* 2002;16:507–510.

4

Ophthalmologic

Corneal Abrasion

Anthony S. Mazzeo

Clinical Presentation

Patients with corneal abrasion (CA) present with eye pain, tearing, foreign body sensation, photophobia, blurry vision, and, occasionally, headache.

Pathophysiology

Any mechanism that disrupts the corneal epithelium may leave a residual defect. Common mechanisms include scratches from fingernails, sports-related eye trauma, dust or debris from a blast, and other accidental instillations of foreign bodies. Contact lens wearers are at risk because of the frequency of ocular instrumentation.

Diagnosis

A complete eye examination with adequate ocular anesthesia is imperative to confirm the diagnosis and evaluate for more serious injury. Visual acuity should be tested and documented. The globe should be inspected with eyelid eversion to evaluate for an existing foreign body. Fluorescein staining of the eye and subsequent cobalt-blue light and slit-lamp inspection will reveal the CA. The dimensions and location of the abrasion should be documented so that follow-up examinations can accurately monitor healing.

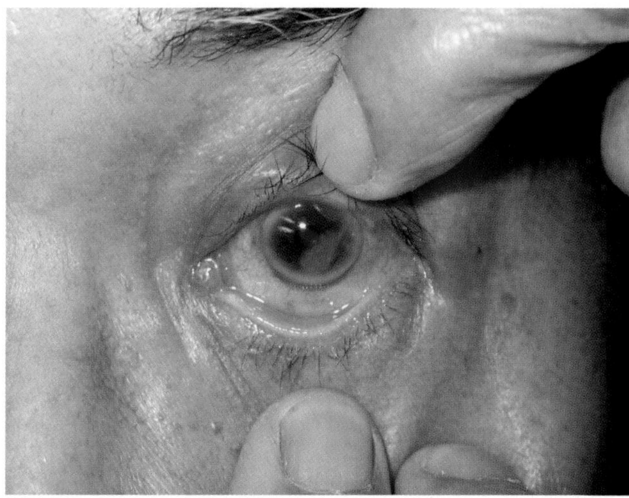

FIGURE 4–1 Fluorescein-stained large central corneal abrasion. (Courtesy of Anthony Morocco, MD.)

Clinical Complications

Complications include superinfection, corneal ulcer (CU) formation, scarring, and recurrence.

Management

Prophylactic topical antibiotics are usually prescribed, with expected healing in 1 to 3 days. Patients at risk for *Pseudomonas* infection (contact lens wearers) should be given aminoglycoside or quinolone drops and told not to use a contact lens in the affected eye until seen by an ophthalmologist. Oral narcotic analgesia may be necessary. Of note, topical ophthalmic nonsteroidal antiinflammatory drugs (NSAIDs) such as ketorolac 0.5%, diclofenac 0.1%, or indomethacin 0.1% can be used as an alternative or in conjunction with oral medication.[1] Patching of the affected eye was done in the past, but the medical literature has documented no clear benefit to patching.[2] Similarly, although instillation of cycloplegic/mydriatic agents is routinely practiced for pain relief (especially for larger abrasions), there is no convincing evidence to support the use of this therapy.[3] CAs can predispose to tetanus, so a tetanus booster should be considered. All patients with CA should be seen for follow-up within 24 hours to evaluate proper healing and for early detection of complications.

REFERENCES

1. Weaver CS, Terrell KM. Evidence based emergency medicine. Update: do ophthalmic NSAIDs reduce the pain associated with simple corneal abrasion without delaying healing? *Ann Emerg Med* 2003;41:134–140.
2. Le Sage N, Verreault R, Rochette L. Efficacy of eye patching for traumatic corneal abrasions: a controlled clinical trial. *Ann Emerg Med* 2001;38:129–134.
3. Carley F, Carley S. Towards evidence based emergency medicine: best BETs from the Manchester Royal Infirmary. Mydriatics in Corneal Abrasion. *Emerg Med J* 2001;18273.

Corneal Laceration

Rachel Haroz

Clinical Presentation

Patients with corneal laceration present with pain, decreased vision, and often other injuries due to the trauma event that caused the corneal injury. The presentation varies based on the severity of the laceration.

Pathophysiology

Corneal lacerations occur more commonly in men younger than 40 years of age. Blunt trauma accounts for about one third of these injuries; in younger patients, 12% are caused by motor vehicle accidents.[1] Superficial corneal lacerations include partial-thickness injuries and full-thickness lacerations that are self-healing. Severe lacerations are those with scleral involvement, posterior scleral rupture, intraocular foreign body, or intraocular damage and those lacerations that are extensive or large.[2]

Diagnosis

Superficial lacerations can have minimal to no symptoms and no obvious abnormalities on examination. In severe lacerations, blood in the anterior chamber and decreased anterior chamber depth may be observed. A teardrop-shaped pupil may be present secondary to prolapse of the iris. An abnormally shaped pupil and anterior chamber abnormalities should alert the examiner to a possible corneal laceration or globe rupture. To determine the presence of a laceration, the placement of a fluorescein strip in the corneal region (Seidel test) may be helpful. Aqueous humor leakage turns fluorescent green-blue and can easily be visualized. Other ophthalmologic testing modalities include retroillumination, sclerotic scatter, and indirect illumination. Ocular tonometry is contraindicated in the emergency department for cases of suspected corneal laceration, because of the possible presence of an occult globe rupture.[1]

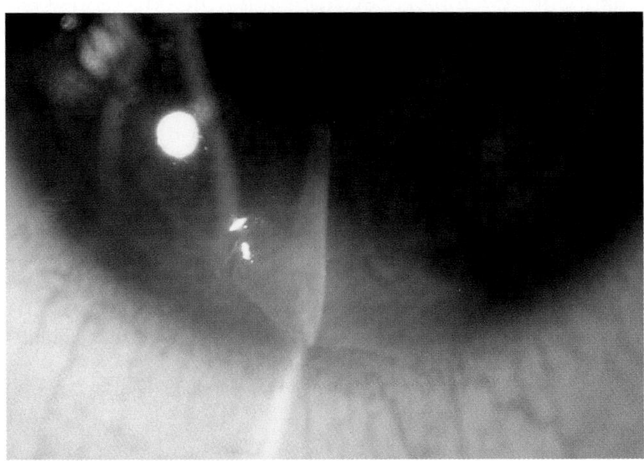

FIGURE 4–2 A corneal laceration with a formed anterior chamber. (From Tasman and Jaeger, with permission.)

Clinical Complications

Complications include visual disability due to astigmatism, infection, and retained foreign bodies.

Management

An ophthalmologist should be consulted for all cases of corneal laceration. Nonsevere (small or partial-thickness) lacerations may be managed with the use of cyanoacrylate tissue adhesive and bandage soft contact lenses.[1] Pressure patching may be used. Severe lacerations require surgical intervention. In such cases, a protective rigid eye cover should be secured in place until the surgery is performed. Tetanus immunization should be updated in all cases, and intravenous antibiotics may be necessary for severe lacerations.[2] Topical antibiotics and cycloplegics may be sufficient for nonsevere lacerations.[2]

REFERENCES

1. Hamill MB. Corneal and scleral trauma. *Ophthalmol Clin North Am* 2002;15:185–194.
2. Hamill MB, Thompson WS. The evaluation and management of corneal lacerations. *Retina* 1990;10[Suppl 1]:S1–S7.

4-3

Traumatic Iritis

Roger D. Tillotson

Clinical Presentation

Patients with traumatic iritis present after facial or ocular trauma with complaints of eye pain, redness, photophobia, blurred vision, and tearing.[1,2] These symptoms usually begin hours to days after the injury.[2]

Pathophysiology

Blunt trauma to the eye may give rise to structural damage to the iris secondary to a sudden and transient elevation in anterior chamber pressure, which incites a localized inflammatory response.[2] This injury may also tear the iris and cause local vascular damage, further increasing inflammation. The iris sphincter constricts in response to the presence of prostaglandins, leading to a miotic pupil.[2]

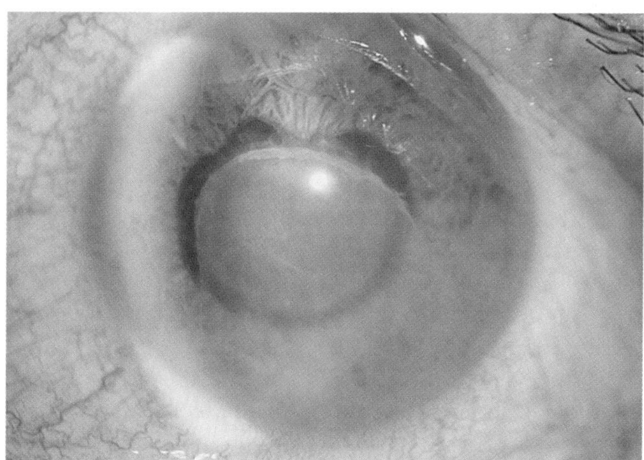

FIGURE 4–3 Rapid onset of pain, photophobia, redness, tearing, and diminished vision are classic features of acute traumatic iritis. A fibrin membrane generated by transudation from acutely inflamed tissues and synechiae involving most of the lens are seen. (From Tasman and Jaeger, with permission.)

Diagnosis

History of trauma to the eye, accompanied by classic clinical findings, implies the diagnosis of traumatic iritis. Fluorescein staining should be used to assess concomitant corneal injury.[3] Measurement of intraocular pressure (IOP) enables the physician to exclude the presence of glaucoma and should be performed in all patients with ocular trauma.[3] Physical findings may include decreased visual acuity, circumcorneal injection (ciliary flush), and a miotic, sluggish pupil.[1–3] Slit-lamp examination usually reveals "cells and flare" in the anterior chamber, which may settle into a hypopyon.[2]

Clinical Complications

Complications include posttraumatic glaucoma and posterior synechiae (fibrous adhesions of the iris to the lens). Severe cases may, on occasion, progress to involve the posterior uvea and retina, with the potential for permanent visual impairment.[2]

Management

Mild cases may resolve within 1 to 2 weeks with no treatment.[2] Cycloplegic eye drops may help to reduce ciliary muscle spasm, reduce synechiae formation, and improve patient comfort. In cases with moderate to severe inflammation, a short course of topical corticosteroids may be considered after consultation with an ophthalmologist.[1] In all cases, follow-up with an ophthalmologist should be provided within 24 hours.

REFERENCES

1. Patel H, Goldstein D. Pediatric uveitis. *Pediatr Clin North Am* 2003;50:125–136.
2. Dalma-Weiszhausz J, Dalma A. The uvea in ocular trauma. *Ophthalmol Clin North Am* 2002;15:205–213.
3. Liebowitz HM. The red eye. *N Engl J Med* 2000;343:345–351.

Ruptured Globe

Michael Horowitz

Clinical Presentation

Ruptured globe describes any eye in which the full thickness of either the sclera or the cornea has been disrupted.

Patients present with complaints of eye pain and decreased vision. The rupture is typically secondary to a blunt trauma or a penetrating injury. The affected eye may show chemosis, subconjunctival hemorrhage (SH), visible intraocular contents, decreased anterior chamber depth, decreased intraocular pressure (IOP), and hyphema.

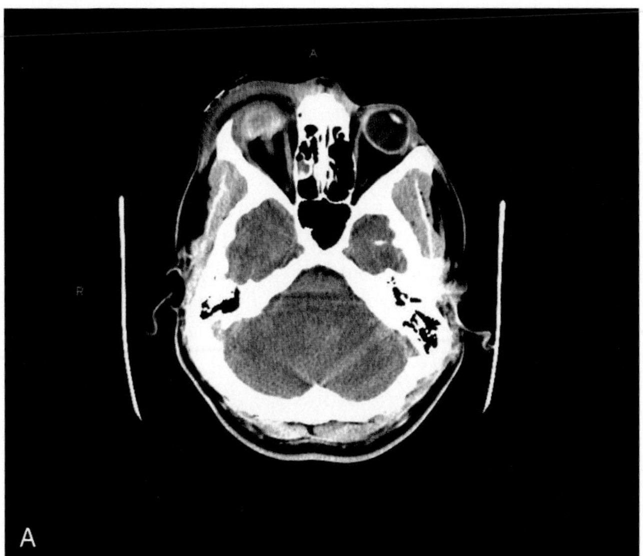

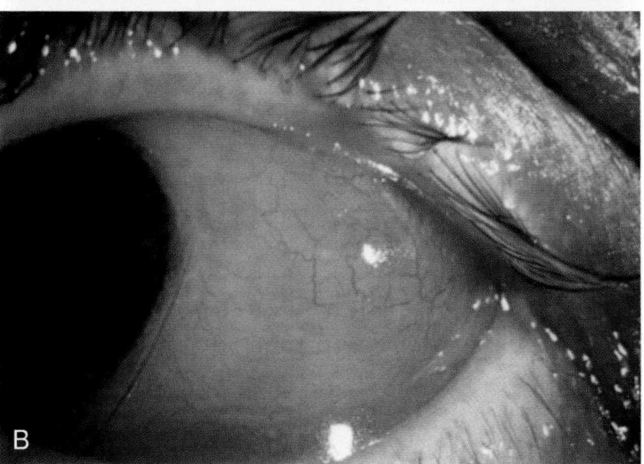

FIGURE 4–4 **A:** Computed tomogram of right globe rupture. (Courtesy of Sarah Paris, MD.) **B:** Subconjunctival edema signals a ruptured globe. (From Duane's, with permission.)

Pathophysiology

In blunt trauma, the scleral rupture is secondary to a sudden increase in IOP; this usually causes rupture in the thinnest portions of the sclera, where the intraocular muscles attach or at the limbus. In patients with prior surgery, the rupture usually occurs at an old surgical site. The full thickness of the cornea or sclera can also be penetrated by a foreign object.[1,2]

Diagnosis

Ruptured globe should be suspected in any patient with a lid or orbit injury. There may be obvious signs of rupture, such as extrusion of intraocular contents, or the signs may be very subtle, such as a decreased anterior chamber depth or a tented pupil. A modified Seidel test (instillation of fluorescein and observation for streaming) can be used to look for fluid leaks. Decreased IOP is a good indication of ruptured globe, but measurement of IOP should be avoided, because it can worsen the condition. Imaging studies such as computed tomography (CT) for metal objects, magnetic resonance imaging (MRI) for wood or glass, and ultrasonography can be very useful in making the diagnosis.[1,2]

Clinical Complications

The risk of infectious endophthalmitis is increased if a foreign body is present. Other complications include permanent changes in vision, traumatic cataracts, and various other conditions associated with severe trauma to the eye.

Management

A rigid shield should be kept over the eye at all times. Activities that can increase the IOP (e.g., control emesis, coughing) must be avoided. If the patient needs to be intubated, a nondepolarizing agent should be used first, to avoid the increase in IOP seen with succinylcholine. Systemic antibiotics should be used as prophylaxis for infectious endophthalmitis. Tetanus prophylaxis should be brought up to date, and topical medications should be avoided. The emergency physician should not remove any foreign bodies but should seek early consultation with an ophthalmologist.[1,2]

REFERENCES

1. Navon SE. Management of the ruptured globe. *Int Ophthalmol Clin* 1995;35:71–91.
2. Harlan JB Jr, Pieramici DJ. Evaluation of patients with ocular trauma. *Ophthalmol Clin North Am* 2002;15:153–161.

Penetrating Foreign Body of the Globe

Michael Greenberg

Clinical Presentation

Patients present after injuries involving particles of metal or other materials projected against unprotected ocular surfaces at high speeds. Although most patients with penetrating foreign body of the globe (PFBG) present with eye pain, 20% have no pain.[1-3]

Pathophysiology

PFBG is involved in up to 40% of open globe injuries, with 90% to 100% of cases occurring in men. Most cases of PFBG result from work-related injury; hammering (usually metal on metal) is the source for up to 80% of all cases. Multiple foreign bodies are always a possibility and should be assumed in cases of explosion, ballistic injury, or motor vehicle accident. Most penetrating foreign bodies come to rest in the posterior segment, and more than half lodge in the retina and choroid.[3] Injuries involving early signs of endophthalmitis; penetration by objects made of vegetable matter or with copper content; and penetration with possible soil contamination are associated with extraordinarily high risks of permanent visual loss and loss of the globe.[3]

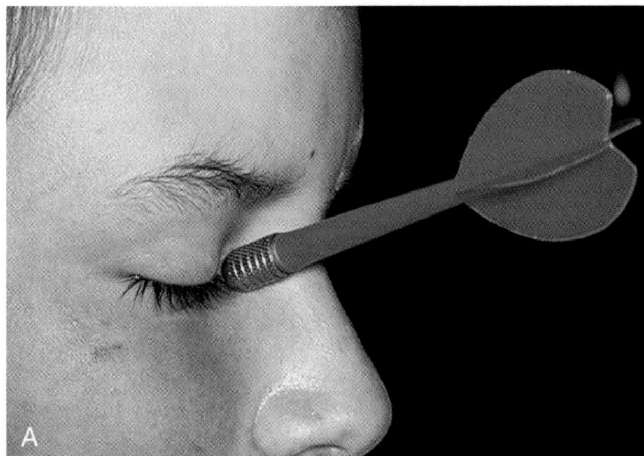

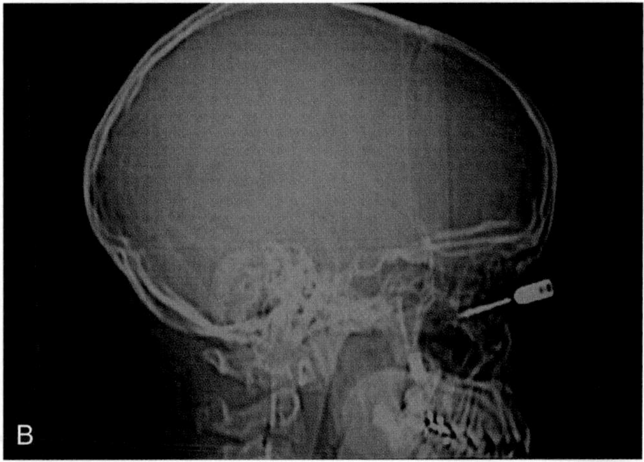

FIGURE 4–5 Penetrating foreign body of the globe seen clinically **(A)** and on computed tomogram **(B).** The entry site of the dart was inferior to the canaliculus, and the eye examination was normal. (From Tasman and Jaeger, with permission.)

Diagnosis

PFBG should be assumed in all cases of laceration of the globe. Diagnostic clues include scleral hemorrhage, localized corneal edema, and an obvious rent in the iris. Ultrasonography may be a useful diagnostic adjunct but can give falsely negative results. Plain radiographs are not reliable for the detection of small or nonmetallic foreign bodies. Computed tomography (CT) has a sensitivity of approximately 65%, but many plastic and other foreign bodies may be missed. Magnetic resonance imaging (MRI) is extremely sensitive, but the associated magnetic fields can cause movement of metallic foreign bodies, resulting in secondary damage. Metal detector devices are of virtually no use in diagnosis of PFBG.

Clinical Complications

Complications include missed diagnosis, siderosis (caused by iron-containing foreign bodies), chalcosis (related to copper-containing foreign bodies), retinal damage, hyphema, infection (endophthalmitis), and partial or complete visual loss.[1-3]

Management

Emergency on-site ophthalmology consultation is mandatory, because a rapid decision regarding surgical intervention is necessary. It is appropriate to transfer stable patients in order to obtain such consultation in a timely fashion. The benefit of intravenous antibiotics remains unproven, but they should be considered in the discussion with the consulting ophthalmologist. Care must be taken to protect the injured globe from further damage; the use of protective eye shields that do not put pressure on the globe is appropriate.

REFERENCES

1. Harlan JB Jr, Pieramici DJ. Evaluation of patients with ocular trauma. *Ophthalmol Clin North Am* 2002;15:153–161.
2. Hamill MB. Corneal and scleral trauma. *Ophthalmol Clin North Am* 2002;15:185–194.
3. Mester V, Kuhn F. Intraocular foreign bodies. *Ophthalmol Clin North Am* 2002;15:235–242.

Hordeolum

Michael Greenberg

Clinical Presentation

Hordeola, sometimes called "styes," manifest as acute and focal eyelid abscesses.

Pathophysiology

So-called internal hordeola form by infection of a meibomian gland in the eyelid. External hordeola form by infection of a Zeis gland (hair follicle) in the lid. Most cases are caused by infection with *Staphylococcus aureus.*[1]

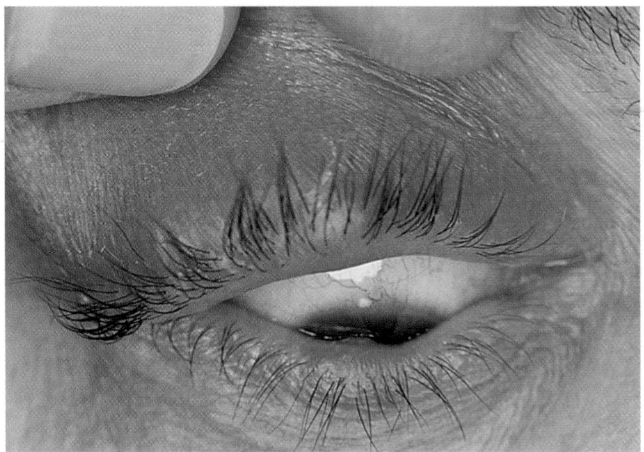

FIGURE 4–6 Hordeolum evidenced by a tender mass of the upper lid with surrounding cellulitis. A chalazion of the central lower lid is also present. (From Tasman and Jaeger, with permission.)

Diagnosis

The diagnosis is based on clinical recognition.

Clinical Complications

Complications are rare but may include infectious spread to contiguous tissue with the establishment of cellulitis. It is possible for systemic bacteremia to begin from a hordeolum.

Management

Warm, wet compresses applied to the area every 2 to 3 hours help the infection localize.[1] Topical antibiotics (e.g., erythromycin) may be added if there is coexistent blepharitis. Systemic antibiotics are rarely needed. Plucking of the eyelashes at the site of a pointing abscess facilitates drainage. Patients should be cautioned against squeezing or puncturing hordeola, because doing so may facilitate the spread of infection. Persistent cases may require incision and drainage.[1]

REFERENCES

1. Lederman C, Miller M. Hordeola and chalazia. *Pediatr Rev* 1999;20:283–284.

Optic Nerve Avulsion

Michael Greenberg

Clinical Presentation

Patients with optic nerve avulsion (ONA) present with acute and complete visual loss coincident with trauma to the orbit.

Pathophysiology

ONA usually occurs after major trauma to the orbit but result from seemingly minor injuries to the globe. Common events associated with ONA include high-speed facial trauma, martial arts injuries, and autoenucleations in psychiatric patients.[1] ONA may result from shearing forces that develop when forces applied to the globe cause its rotation; these rotational forces can cause a tearing of the nerve and partial or complete avulsion. In other cases, the globe is forced posteriorly, with a sudden rebound to the anterior position, which can tear the nerve. In most cases, some combination of rotational and retropulsive forces is the most likely mechanism for ONA. In addition, sudden extreme increases in intraocular pressure (IOP) may play a role. ONAs typically occur at one of three anatomic locations: the optic disc, the orbital apex, and the optic chiasm.[1] Most ONAs occur at the orbital apex.[1]

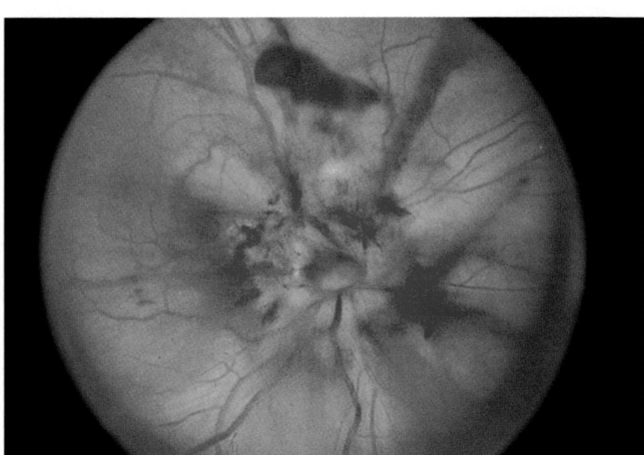

FIGURE 4–7 Avulsion of the optic nerve head, showing a pit at the site of the papilla, surrounded by a ring of hemorrhage. (From Tasman and Jaeger, with permission.)

Diagnosis

The clinical ocular examination is often diagnostic for ONA. Indirect ophthalmoscopy may reveal absence of the optic disc. In addition, retinal bleeding is often evident. The diagnosis can be confirmed with advanced imaging studies such as computed tomography (CT) or magnetic resonance imaging (MRI), which typically demonstrate avulsion of the nerve. In these cases, the optic nerve sheath usually remains intact. Ocular ultrasonography may be helpful in determining the diagnosis of ONA.

Clinical Complications

Complications include permanent blindness, endocrine abnormalities due to pituitary injury, leaks of cerebrospinal fluid (CSF), meningitis, subarachnoid bleeding, and development of carotid-cavernous fistulae.[1]

Management

In cases involving the sudden and severe accumulation of orbital blood, emergency decompression by lateral canthotomy may be necessary. Surgical decompression may be helpful in some cases in which optic nerve sheath hematoma is a problem. High-dose corticosteroids may be helpful. There is no effective treatment for ONA at the chiasm, and, in fact, most treatments have not met with good results for ONA at any anatomic location.[1,2]

REFERENCES

1. Arkin MS, Rubin PA, Bilyk JR, Buchbinder B. Anterior chiasmal optic nerve avulsion. *AJNR Am J Neuroradiol* 1996;17:1777–1781.
2. Thakar A, Mahapatra AK, Tandon DA. Delayed optic nerve decompression for indirect optic nerve injury. *Laryngoscope* 2003;113:112–119.

Corneal/Conjunctival Foreign Body

Michael Greenberg

Clinical Presentation

Patients with corneal/conjunctival foreign body (CCFB) present with eye discomfort and a sensation of foreign material in the eye, excessive tearing, sensitivity to light, and redness. Some patients are able to indicate what the specific foreign material might be.[1]

Pathophysiology

CCFBs can result from minor or serious trauma. In most cases, foreign material is inadvertently introduced into the eye by rubbing with unclean hands. Some CCFBs are introduced as a result of movement of foreign particles by high-speed equipment. Other CCFBs are simply suspended in the air as particulates and come into contact with the eye randomly.[1]

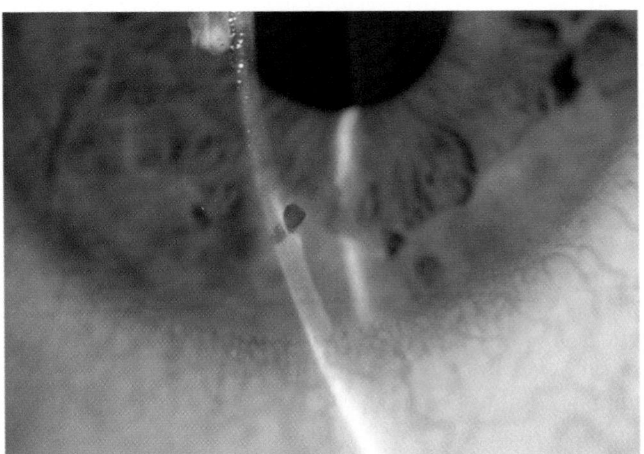

FIGURE 4–8 The end of a thorn is apparent deep in the corneal stroma. Because it did not perforate Descemet's membrane, the eye was not Seidel positive. (From Tasman and Jaeger, with permission.)

Diagnosis

Although the diagnosis is suspected based on the history, confirmation requires a careful physical examination, including triple eversion of the upper lid and eversion of the lower lid. In addition, all patients with suspected CCFBs must be examined with the use of a slit-lamp microscope to identify, locate, and remove the CCFBs.[1]

Clinical Complications

Complications include corneal abrasions, conjunctivitis, deep ocular infection, retained intraocular foreign body, and permanent corneal damage.

Management

All CCFBs must be removed. Removal technique depends on the location of the CCFB. The slit-lamp microscope vastly facilitates removal by providing adequate magnification and visualization. If the emergency physician is unable to perform this procedure, an ophthalmologist should be consulted for timely CCFB removal. After removal, underlying corneal or conjunctival damage or injury should be evaluated. Cycloplegia and the instillation of topical ophthalmic antibiotics is reasonable in most cases. Patching usually is not needed. All patients should be reevaluated 24 hours after CCFB removal.[1]

REFERENCES

1. Leibowitz HM. The red eye. *N Engl J Med* 2000;343:345–351.

4–9

Tarsal Plate Foreign Body

Michael Greenberg

Clinical Presentation

Patients with tarsal plate foreign body (TPFB) invariably present complaining of the sensation of a foreign body in the eye, or of a painful eye with tearing and photophobia, or both. Some complain of a scratching sensation or a feeling that the eye is being abraded every time the upper lid closes over the eye.

Pathophysiology

TPFBs are foreign bodies that have not penetrated the globe and have come to rest beneath the upper eyelid. They may be small particles from virtually any source of airborne particulates or materials inadvertently instilled into the eyes by unclean hands, clothing, or the work or recreational environment. They may be made of metal, wood, glass, plant materials, plastic, or other materials.

Diagnosis

As a result of pain and tearing, patients may be unable to cooperate for an adequate physical examination. On fluorescein staining, multiple superficial vertical corneal abrasions (CAs)provide a clue that a TPFB may be present, and a lid eversion examination should be carried out.

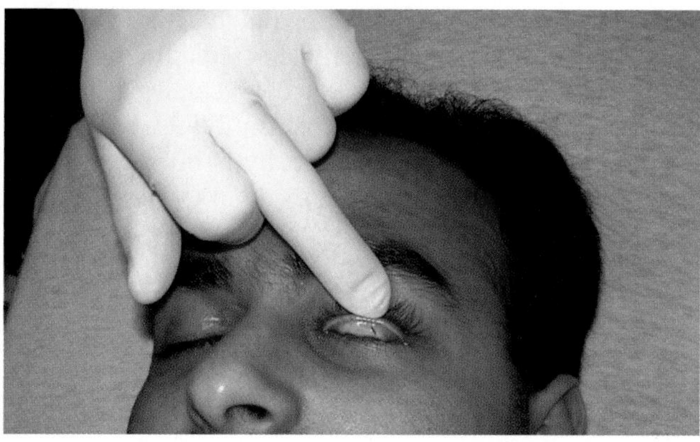

FIGURE 4–9 Tarsal plate foreign body. (Courtesy of Mridul Kumar, MD.)

Clinical Complications

Complications include CAs, infection, and foreign body penetration into the cornea, as well as the potential for missed associated ocular injuries (e.g., penetrating foreign bodies). The failure to diagnose an ocular penetrating foreign body has the potential to result in devastating intraocular infection.[1]

Management

All patients should be treated with a short-acting topical ocular anesthetic to facilitate the examination. Anesthesia is appreciated by the patient and allows the examiner to perform double lid eversion, typically by gently pulling the upper lid out and over a sterile wooden applicator stick, to reveal its underside. Although most TPFBs are visible to the naked eye, it is advisable to perform this examination under slit-lamp microscopy. The TPFB is then easily visualized in almost 100% of cases and can be removed with the moistened cotton tip of another applicator stick. After TPFB removal, fluorescein staining should be performed to check for CAs induced by the TPFB. Superficial CAs may be allowed to heal without treatment, whereas deeper abrasions may benefit from cycloplegia and topical antibiotic drops. Abrasions should be reevaluated in 24 hours to check for adequate healing. At no time should patients be given topical analgesics to go home with, because they may mask the development of serious corneal disease, including destructive infection.

REFERENCES

1. Mester V, Kuhn F. Intraocular foreign bodies. *Ophthalmol Clin North Am* 2002;15:235–242.

Subconjunctival Hemorrhage

Michael Greenberg

Clinical Presentation

Patients with subconjunctival hemorrhage (SH) present with painless hemorrhagic areas of varying size in the conjunctiva. Some patients present after ocular trauma and may have pain related to their injury or to other ocular or facial injuries. Often, patients are unaware of the conjunctival bleeding and are alerted to its existence by family members or coworkers.

Pathophysiology

SH is usually spontaneous and in most cases unilateral. SH results when the small vessels bridging the potential space between the conjunctival tissues and episcleral blood vessels tear, as a result of either direct forces applied to the globe or intermittent increased intrathoracic pressure. Other causes include forceful and frequent vomiting (as in bulimia), prolonged extremes of patient positioning (head in dependent position), blunt ocular trauma, forceful and frequent coughing (as may occur in pertussis, influenza, or viral upper respiratory tract infections), heavy exercise, straining at stool, forceful sneezing, Valsalva maneuver, systemic hypertension, ocular amyloidosis, salicylate overuse, idiopathic thrombocytopenic purpura, acute conjunctivitis, and as a complication of gastrointestinal endoscopy.[1]

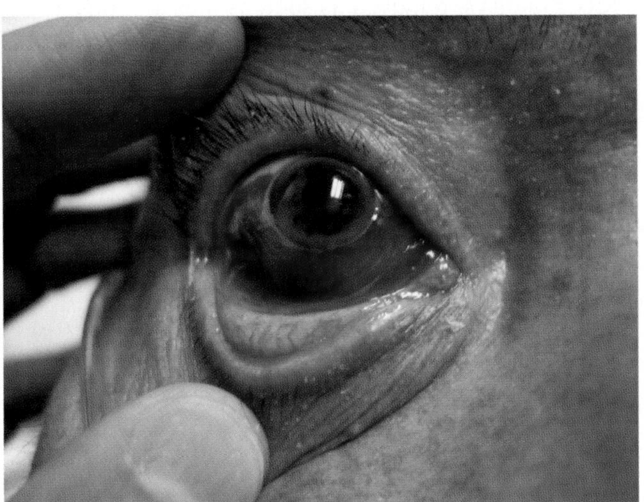

FIGURE 4–10 Subconjunctival hemorrhage. (Courtesy of Anthony Morocco, MD.)

Diagnosis

The diagnosis is based on the clinical examination. A complete examination, including a slit-lamp evaluation, should be performed in cases of trauma to the globe, or if penetration of the globe is a possibility.

Clinical Complications

Most SHs resolve spontaneously with no special complications.

Management

Most SHs resolve over a period of 3 to 4 weeks and require no treatment other than reassurance to the patient. However, because SH may represent a manifestation of disease, a complete history and physical examination should be provided, both at the initial presentation and at follow-up. Bilateral involvement should prompt a search for a systemic cause.[1]

REFERENCES

1. Fukuyama J, Hayasaka S, Yamada K, Setogawa T. Causes of subconjunctival hemorrhage. *Ophthalmologica* 1990;200:63–67.

Corneal Rust Ring

Michael Greenberg

Clinical Presentation

Patients with corneal rust ring (CRR) present with the presence of a metallic foreign body on the surface of the cornea.

Pathophysiology

Iron-containing foreign bodies may oxidize if they remain in contact with the moist microenvironment of the cornea. The portion of the foreign body that is in contact with the cornea rusts and leaves a circular ring of rust embedded in the corneal tissue. The longer the object has been in contact with the cornea, the larger and deeper the rust ring.[1]

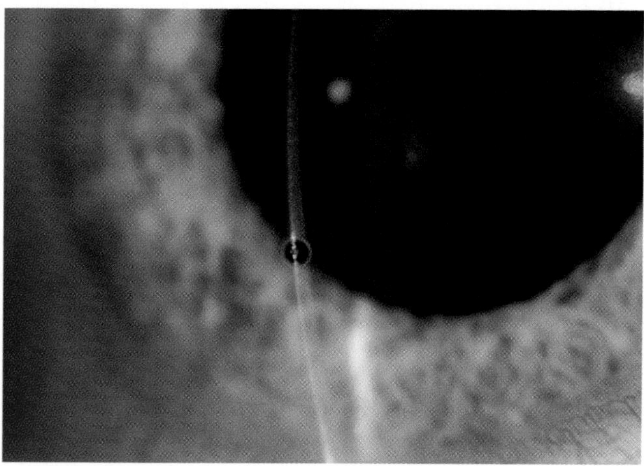

FIGURE 4–11 Corneal rust ring. (From Tasman and Jaeger, with permission.)

Diagnosis

CRRs are diagnosed by physical examination, usually immediately after the removal of a corneal/conjunctival foreign body (CCFB). At times, a CRR is easily visible to the naked eye. However, a slit-lamp examination is in order for patients who may have residual CRRs after foreign body removal.

Clinical Complications

Untreated CRR may predispose to deep ocular infection, as well as conjunctivitis and ocular irritation. CRRs that remain in the cornea may retard healing of the corneal defect left by the removal of the associated foreign body.[1]

Management

CRRs should be removed as soon as they are diagnosed. Frequently, they can be removed by the emergency physician with the use of a slit-lamp microscope and a bur or small-gauge needle with appropriate topical anesthesia. It is essential to remove the majority of the rust ring, but it is not necessary to remove 100% of it. Difficult cases and those in which the majority of the CRR cannot easily be removed should be referred to an ophthalmologist as soon as possible. After removal of the CRR, some authorities recommend application of topical antibiotics and daily reevaluation until the corneal defect has healed.[1]

REFERENCES

1. Newell SW. Management of corneal foreign bodies. *Am Fam Physician* 1985;31:149–156.

Chalazion

Michael Greenberg

Clinical Presentation

Chalazia present as a swollen, minimally tender mass at the eyelid margin or within the body of the lid itself.[1]

Pathophysiology

Chalazia are lipid-containing granulomatous masses that represent foreign body reactions surrounding a meibomian gland. These are essentially reactions to lipid produced by the gland. The inflammatory exudates contain histiocytes, multinucleated giant cells, plasma cells, eosinophils, lymphocytes, and polymorphonuclear leukocytes.[1]

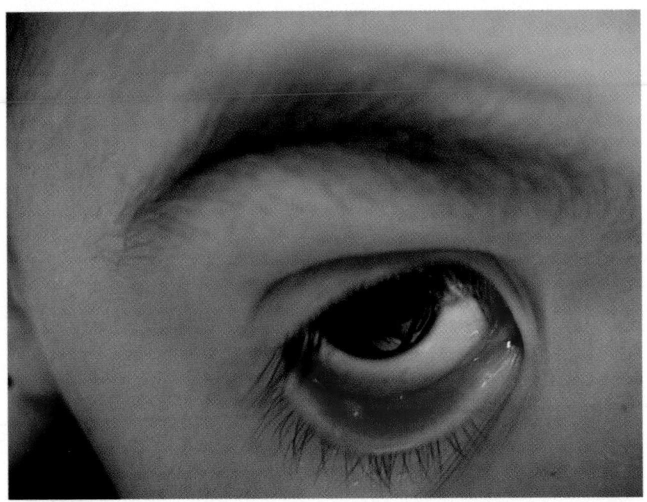

FIGURE 4–12 Lower lid chalazion. (Courtesy of Christy Salvaggio, MD.)

Diagnosis

Chalazia are diagnosed based on clinical recognition.

Clinical Complications

Complications include the potential for superinfection if the chalazion is manipulated by the patient or other nonmedical personnel. The most common complication of chalazia is recurrence.

Management

Some chalazia resolve without treatment. Most authors recommend frequent application of warm, moist compresses, which serve to facilitate drainage of the chalazion.[1] If blepharitis coexists, topical antibiotics may be helpful. If the problem does not resolve after 1 month of conservative therapy, the patient should be referred to an ophthalmologist for incision and curettage. Some ophthalmologists advocate the administration of intralesional steroids by injection. Recurrent chalazia may require the use of oral antibiotics.[1]

REFERENCES

1. Lederman C, Miller M. Hordeola and chalazia. *Pediatr Rev* 1999;20:283–284.

Dacryoadenitis/Dacryocystitis

Michael Greenberg

Clinical Presentation

Patients with dacryoadenitis/dacryocystitis present with pain, periorbital swelling, and redness in and near the medial canthus. In addition, some patients complain of excessive tearing, diminished vision, and lid swelling. Low-grade to high fever may be present.[1,2]

Pathophysiology

Dacryocystitis can be acute or chronic. In cases of acute dacryocystitis, there is acute blockage of the nasolacrimal duct as a result of inflammation, swelling, and debris accumulation in that duct.[1,2] Secondary infection results in acute dacryocystitis as a preseptal infection that may be of viral, bacterial, or fungal origin. Most cases of bacterial origin involve staphylococcal organisms.[1,2] Prior dacryocystitis is a substantial risk factor for the development of orbital extension.[2]

Diagnosis

The diagnosis is based on clinical examination and history. Orbital computed tomography (CT) may confirm the diagnosis and rule in or out various clinical complications, including abscess formation and malignancy.

Clinical Complications

Complications include reoccurrence, orbital cellulitis, orbital abscess formation, necrotizing fasciitis, central nervous system extension, and death.[1,2]

Management

Patients who appear to be systemically ill or are febrile, diabetic, immunocompromised, suffering a reoccurrence of dacryocystitis, homeless, or noncompliant should be admitted to the hospital for local care and administration of intravenous antibiotics.[1,2] Other patients may be treated as outpatients with hourly warm compresses, oral antibiotics, and follow-up with an ophthalmologist within 24 hours. Despite therapy, most patients require surgical intervention for drainage procedures.

REFERENCES

1. Ataullah S, Sloan B. Acute dacryocystitis presenting as an orbital abscess. *Clin Exp Ophthalmol* 2002;30:44–46.
2. Kikkawa DO, Heinz GW, Martin RT, Nunery WN, Eiseman AS. Orbital cellulitis and abscess secondary to dacryocystitis. *Arch Ophthalmol* 2002;120:1096–1099.

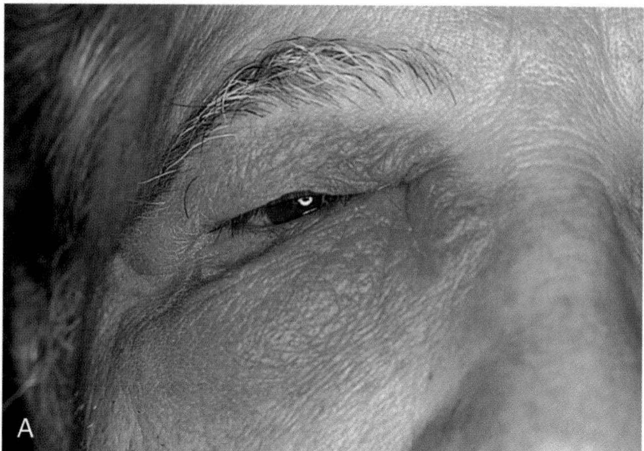

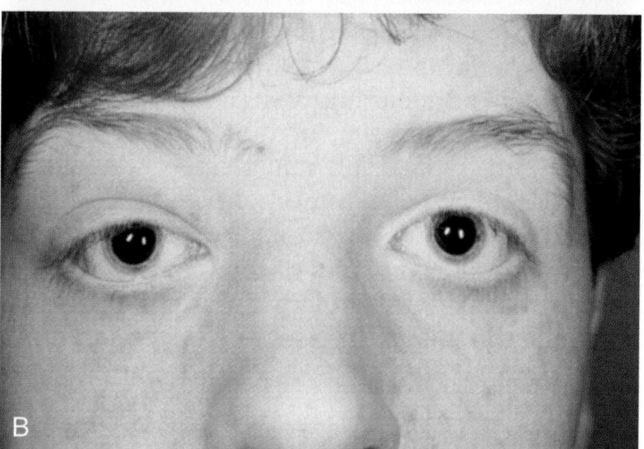

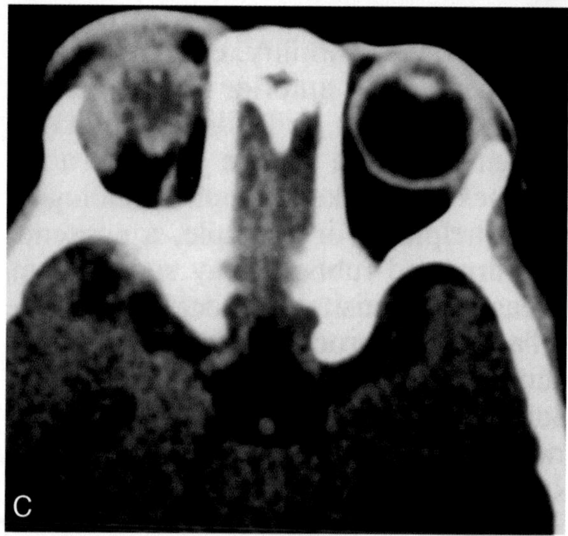

FIGURE 4–13 **A:** Inflammation of right lacrimal gland with minimal redness and swelling. (From Tasman and Jaeger, with permission.) **B:** Acute dacryocystitis evidenced by a large, tender, swollen, fluctuant erythematous mass in the medial canthal area. (From Duane, with permission.) **C:** Axial computed tomogram demonstrating the poorly demarcated, oblong lesion associated with lacrimal gland inflammation. (From Duane, with permission.)

Blepharitis

Michael Greenberg

Clinical Presentation

Patients with blepharitis present with acute or chronic inflammatory changes of the eyelids, often accompanied by ocular foreign body sensation, light sensitivity, redness and swelling of the eyelids, loss of eyelashes, and conjunctival redness.[1]

Pathophysiology

Blepharitis usually arises from local staphylococcal infection; however, seborrhea, acne rosacea, and *Demodex folliculorum* infection may also be causative. Seborrheic blepharitis is similar but less severe than staphylococcal blepharitis. Seborrheic blepharitis involves dysfunction of the glands of Zeis; it occurs in patients who already have seborrheic dermatitis. Dysfunction of the meibomian glands is characterized by excess lipid secretion. Staphylococcal infection occurs at the base of the lashes and results in chronic irritation, itching, soreness, photophobia, and tearing. Dry, scaly concretions called collarettes build up at the base of the lashes. Hypersensitivity to staphylococcal exotoxins may cause inflammation of the conjunctiva. Seborrhea can be oily or dry, and it is thought that the excessive amounts of neutral lipids produced in this condition are broken down into irritating fatty acids by *Corynebacterium acnes*. In some cases, it is possible to see globules of oil on the posterior lid margin.

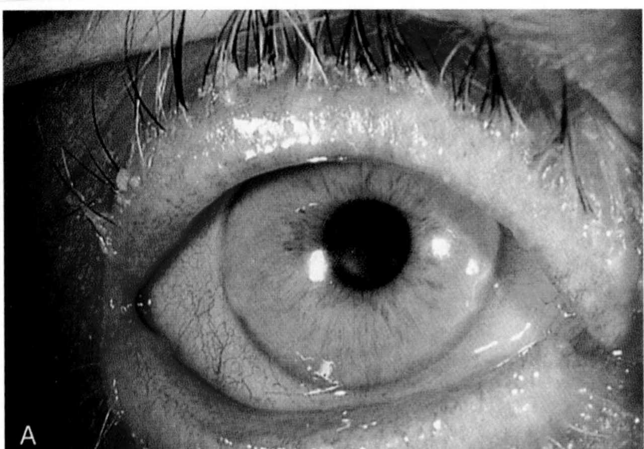

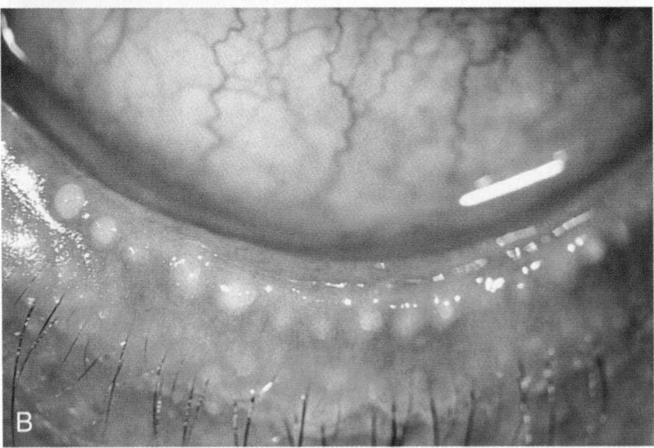

FIGURE 4–14 **A:** Blepharitis is associated with eyelash crusting, thickened eyelids, and telangiectatic vessels along lid margins. **B:** The meibomian glands become plugged in chronic blepharitis. (From Tasman and Jaeger, with permission.)

Diagnosis

The diagnosis is based on physical examination. Slit-lamp examination is essential to identify inverted lashes, corneal inflammation, and associated foreign material. Blepharitis symptoms tend to be worse in the morning.

Clinical Complications

Complications include hordeola, meibomian cysts, and keratitis.[1]

Management

Frequent lid cleansing is essential and is directed at removal of debris and secretions from the lid margins. This can be accomplished with the use of a clean cloth and a dilute solution of baby shampoo. Lid cleansing should be done twice daily until the symptoms are under control, and the patient should be cautioned that this may take months. If staphylococcal infection is suspected, topical antibiotic ointment should be applied to the eyelids and lid margins. In severe cases, topical steroids may be helpful, but they should be used in consultation with an ophthalmologist, because prolonged ocular exposure to steroids increases the risk of iatrogenic glaucoma and cataract induction. Artificial tears may be helpful in alleviating ocular irritation from inflamed lid margins. All cases not responding to basic therapy should be referred to the care of an ophthalmologist.[1,2]

REFERENCES

1. Leibowitz HM. The red eye. *N Engl J Med* 2000;343:345–351.
2. McCulley JP, Shine WE. Changing concepts in the diagnosis and management of blepharitis. *Cornea* 2000;19:650–658.

4-15

Gonococcal Conjunctivitis

Benjamin Roemer

Clinical Presentation

Patients with this hyperacute conjunctivitis present with purulent discharge, erythema, and irritation of the eye. Additional complaints may include foreign body sensation, eyelids "stuck together," and genital symptoms.[1]

Pathophysiology

Gonococcal conjunctivitis is caused by *Neisseria gonorrhoeae* via direct inoculation of the organism into the eye. This conjunctivitis is seen in two patient populations: sexually active adults and neonates. Hand-eye inoculation occurs most commonly in the adult. Neonatal inoculation occurs via direct contact during passage through an infected birth canal. Neonatal infection usually manifests within the first 48 hours of life.

The conjunctiva is a thin, translucent layer composed of nonkeratinizing squamous epithelium and the substantia propria. Much of the inflammatory reaction to gonococcus occurs due to the activity of lymphocytes, plasma cells, macrophages, and mast cells in the substantia propria. The incidence of gonococcal ophthalmia neonatorum is 3 per 1,000 live births in the United States, and it is higher in countries without routine silver nitrate prophylaxis.[2] The exact incidence in adults is not known. Gonococcal conjunctivitis appears to be more prevalent among the urban poor.

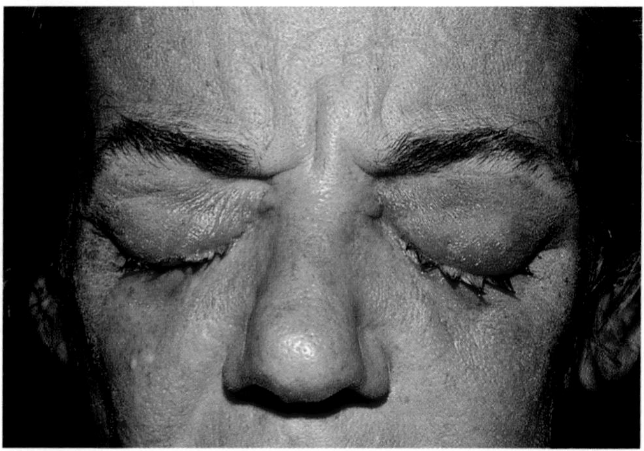

FIGURE 4–15 Hyperacute gonococcal conjunctivitis, with copious mucopurulent discharge and lid swelling. (From Tasman and Jaeger, with permission.)

Diagnosis

Diagnosis is made by clinical examination, Gram staining for intracellular gram-negative diplococci, and culture of conjunctival discharge.[2] The clinical presentation includes severe purulent discharge, punctate keratitis, chemosis, and conjunctival papillae. Membrane formation, subconjunctival hemorrhage (SH), and preauricular lymph nodes usually are present. Corneal infiltrates and ulceration occur in severe cases.[3]

Clinical Complications

Complications include permanent partial or total blindness and disseminated disease.

Management

Treatment consists of administration of topical chloramphenicol eye drops and intramuscular benzylpenicillin or a cephalosporin. Prophylactic treatment is required for neonates born to mothers with known gonorrhea within the first hour of life.

REFERENCES

1. Greenberg MF, Pollard ZF. The red eye in childhood. *Pediatr Clin North Am* 2003;50:105–124.
2. Rapoza PA, Quinn TC, Kiessling LA, Taylor HR. Epidemiology of neonatal conjunctivitis. *Ophthalmology* 1986;93:456–461.
3. Wan WL, Farkas GC, May WN, Robin JB. The clinical characteristics and course of adult gonococcal conjunctivitis. *Am j Ophthalmol* 1986;102:575–583.

Bacterial Conjunctivitis

Nick Gorton

Clinical Presentation

Patients with bacterial conjunctivitis (BC) present with a painful, red eye and mucopurulent discharge. Severe discharge and a hyperacute presentation suggest neisserial disease. A subacute presentation with concomitant genital symptoms suggests chlamydial disease. Infections are unilateral initially but spreads to the contralateral eye in up to 80% of cases. Patients may complain of a foreign body sensation. Mild pruritus may be present, but if it is a prominent symptom, allergic conjunctivitis should be suspected.[1–3]

Pathophysiology

Pathogenic bacteria overwhelm conjunctival defenses, resulting in inflammation followed by purulent infection. Hyperacute and hyperpurulent disease is generally *N. gonorrhoeae* or *Neisseria meningitidis,* although staphylococcal and streptococcal species may also be present. Chronic infections are frequently secondary to repeated bacterial contamination of the conjunctiva from blepharitis or dacryocystitis. Three fourths of acute childhood conjunctival infections are bacterial, with *Haemophilus influenzae* comprising the majority. *Streptococcus pneumoniae, S. aureus,* and *Moraxella catarrhalis* are also common. Only half of acute adult conjunctival infections are bacterial in nature, with *S. aureus* being the most common cause, followed by pneumococcus, *H. influenzae,* and *Moraxella* species.[1]

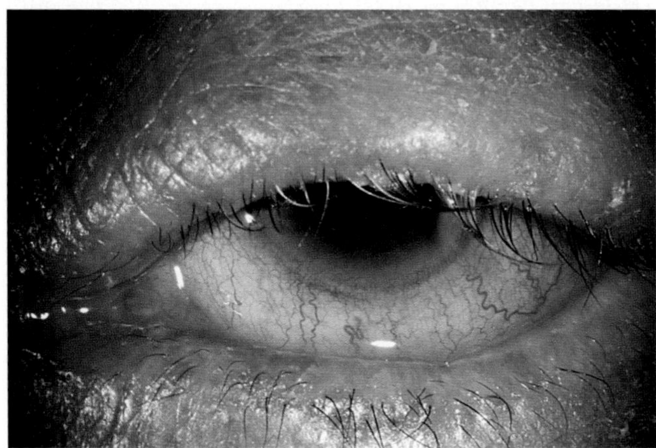

FIGURE 4–16 Acute bacterial conjunctivitis, with mild lid swelling, conjunctival injection, and discharge along the lid margin. (From Tasman and Jaeger, with permission.)

Diagnosis

It is impossible to clinically differentiate between bacterial and viral conjunctivitis. In patients who are debilitated, if severe discharge is present, or if clinical suspicion exists for sexually transmitted diseases, samples should be collected for culture. Physical examination with and without fluorescein staining is recommended. In simple conjunctivitis, the corneal epithelium is intact and no corneal ulcers are revealed with fluorescein stain. Cell and flare in the anterior chamber suggests uveitis.[1–3]

Clinical Complications

Most BC is self-limited even without treatment, and ocular complications are rare. However, complications of concomitant systemic infections can be significant. In addition to the sequelae of untreated genital infections, *N. meningitidis* conjunctivitis is accompanied by meningitis in 18% of cases, and *H. influenzae* conjunctivitis is complicated by otitis media in 25% of children.[3]

Management

Uncomplicated cases are self-limited, but topical antibiotics shorten the average duration of clinical disease.[3] Prompt referral to an ophthalmologist is advisable. Adults with suspected gonococcal disease should have a follow-up visit with an ophthalmologist within 24 hours. Children with suspected gonococcal disease must be admitted for intravenous antibiotic therapy. Other patients should be rechecked within 2 days.[1]

REFERENCES

1. Diamant JI, Hwang DG. Therapy for bacterial conjunctivitis. *Ophthalmol Clin North Am* 1999;12:15–20.
2. Chung C, Cohen E, Smith J. Bacterial conjunctivitis. *Clin Evid* 2002;(7):574–579.
3. Sheikh A, Hurwitz B, Cave J. Antibiotics for acute bacterial conjunctivitis. *Cochrane Database Syst Rev* 2000;(2):CD001211.

Viral Conjunctivitis

Roger D. Tillotson

Clinical Presentation

Patients with viral conjunctivitis (VC) may present with only ocular symptoms or with a concomitant upper respiratory tract infection.[1,2] VC usually begins unilaterally, but contralateral involvement often develops after the patient touches the disease-free eye without washing.[1,2] These patients classically complain of conjunctival injection, discharge, and pruritus. Transient blurry vision may occur because of the ocular discharge, but persistent blurry vision should prompt consideration of an alternative diagnosis.[2] On physical examination, scleral injection, epiphora, chemosis, subconjunctival hemorrhage (SH), and eyelid erythema and edema may all be present. Preauricular adenopathy is also common, but it is a nonspecific finding.[2]

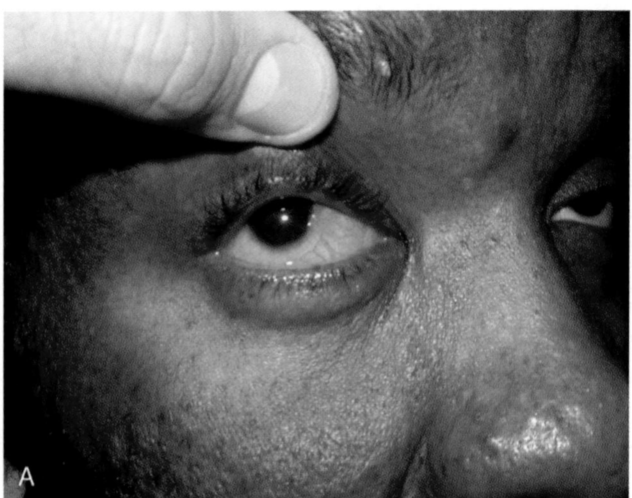

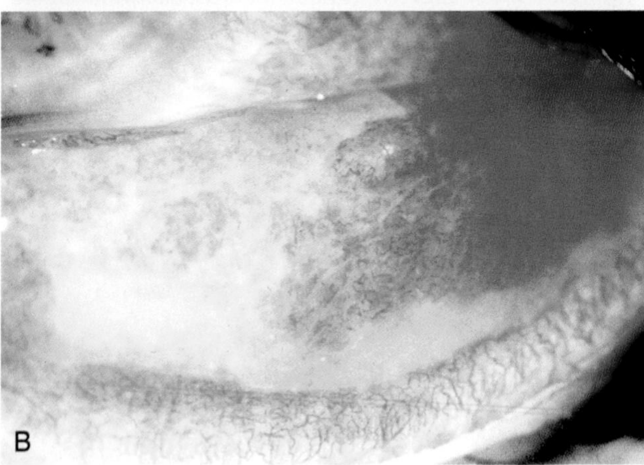

FIGURE 4–17 **A:** Viral conjunctivitis. (Courtesy of Mark Silverberg, MD.) **B:** Note subconjunctival hemorrhage and pseudomembrane formation. (From Tasman and Jaeger, with permission.)

Pathophysiology

All age groups are susceptible to viral conjunctivitis.[1] Because of the highly contagious nature of this disease, the patient may report recent exposure to another individual with similar symptoms. Adenovirus is the most common cause, but a variety of other viruses, such as herpes simplex virus (HSV), enterovirus, coxsackievirus, poxvirus, and human immunodeficiency virus (HIV) can all cause viral conjunctivitis.[1] Viral transmission is through direct contact or via fomites.

Diagnosis

The diagnosis usually is based on clinical findings. There is little or no role for sending swabs for culture and smear in uncomplicated cases of viral conjunctivitis. Fluorescein staining should be performed if corneal abrasion (CA) or herpetic keratitis is suspected.[1,2]

Clinical Complications

Complications include superinfection with bacteria, ulcer formation, and other consequences of bacterial conjunctivitis (BC).

Management

VC is self-limited in most cases.[1] Cold compresses and eye lubricants may provide symptomatic relief. Broad-spectrum antibiotic eye drops should be prescribed if bacterial superinfection is suspected. Referral to an ophthalmologist should be considered for severe cases or if symptoms persist.[2]

REFERENCES

1. Greenberg MF, Pollard ZF. The red eye in childhood. *Pediatr Clin North Am* 2003;50:105–124.
2. Liebowitz HM. The red eye. *N Engl J Med* 2000;343:345–351.

Herpes Simplex Keratitis

Roger D. Tillotson

Clinical Presentation

Herpes simplex keratitis (HSK) can occur in the context of primary infection by herpes simplex virus (HSV); however, it is observed more frequently in secondary or recurrent disease.[1] Patients present with a painful, red eye accompanied by tearing, blurred vision, and photophobia. The patient may reveal a history of prior episodes of HSK, because approximately 25% of patients with prior episodes of HSK experience a recurrence within 1 to 2 years.[1]

Pathophysiology

HSV is a DNA virus with worldwide distribution.[2] HSK is among a spectrum of eye diseases caused by HSV; blepharitis, conjunctivitis, and retinitis are also well documented.[1,2] HSK may be classified into four main forms: infectious epithelial keratitis, neurotrophic keratopathy, stromal keratitis, and endotheliitis.[3] Infectious epithelial keratitis is the most common form; it results from viral replication in the corneal epithelium with subsequent cell lysis. Stromal keratitis and endotheliitis result from a combination of infectious and immune-mediated effects.[3]

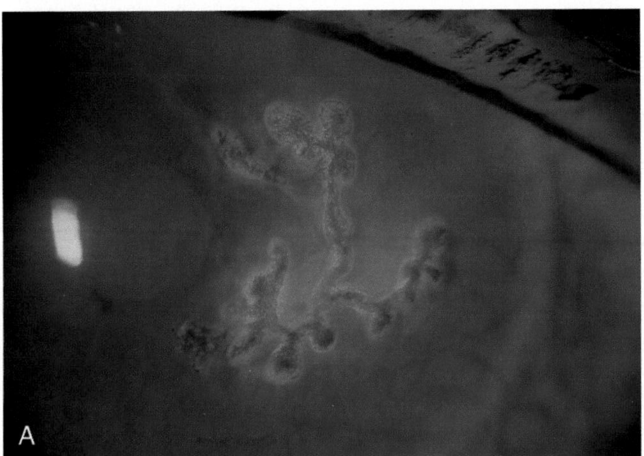

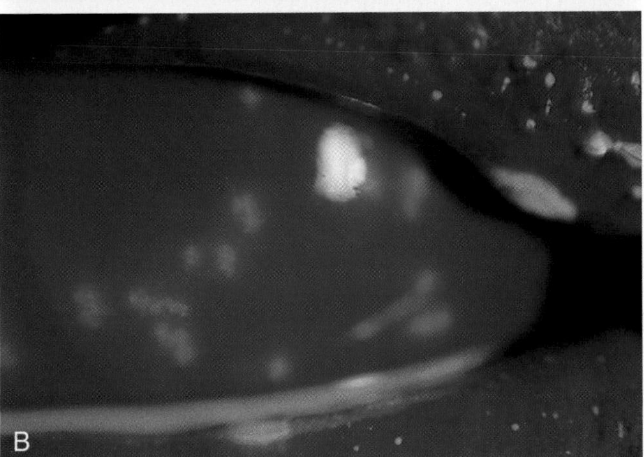

FIGURE 4-18 **A:** The hallmark of herpes simplex keratitis is the dendrite—a branching, epithelial ulceration with swollen, raised edges and terminal bulbs. **B:** Multiple small dendrites may develop. (From Tasman and Jaeger, with permission.)

Diagnosis

Fluorescein staining reveals the characteristic dendritic pattern of ulcers, which represent areas of denuded corneal epithelium.[1] Geographic ulcers occur as the dendrites enlarge and lose their linear, tree-like morphology.[1] The cornea and anterior chamber should be inspected by slit-lamp microscopy, carefully searching for signs of inflammation, which may indicate the presence of stromal keratitis or endotheliitis.[3] Viral cultures may be sent to confirm clinical suspicion.

Clinical Complications

Ocular HSV infection is one of the most common causes of corneal blindness in developed countries.[1,2] Untreated or frequent recurrences of HSK result in corneal scarring and subsequent decline in visual acuity.[1]

Management

Both oral and topical antiviral therapy are options. Use of topical therapy is effective; however, corneal toxicity is a common side effect.[1] Oral acyclovir is known to be equivalent to topical treatment in efficacy.[1] The modality of medication delivery should be determined in consultation with an ophthalmologist, because the patient will need close follow-up.

REFERENCES

1. Kaufman HE. Treatment of viral diseases of the cornea and external eye. *Prog Retin Eye Res* 2000;19:69–85.
2. Liesegang TJ. Herpes simplex virus epidemiology and ocular importance. *Cornea* 2001;20:1–13.
3. Hollander EJ, Schwartz GS. Classification of herpes simplex virus keratitis. *Cornea* 1999;18:144–154.

Herpes Zoster Ophthalmicus

Wendymarie Gejer

Clinical Presentation

Patients with herpes zoster ophthalmicus (HZO) present with an erythematous, macular rash around the eye of the affected dermatome, and this rash does not cross the midline. The rash progresses through varying stages including vesicles, papules, pustules, and, finally, crusting lesions. The rash can be very painful, is usually preceded by a week of flu-like symptoms, and can last for several weeks.[1]

Pathophysiology

HZO is caused by the reactivation of latent human herpesvirus 3 in the ganglia of the ophthalmic division of the trigeminal nerve. The reactivation can be caused by emotional or physical stress, an immunocompromised state, aging, or malnutrition.[1]

Diagnosis

The diagnosis is made clinically, based on the presence of the characteristic erythematous rash with vesicles affecting only the dermatome associated with the ophthalmic division of cranial nerve V. If the cornea is affected, a slit-lamp examination must be performed to look for the presence of dendrites. Some patients have Hutchinson's sign, which is a rash or blistering of the tip of the nose caused by involvement of the external nasal nerve, a smaller branch of the ophthalmic division of the trigeminal nerve.[1]

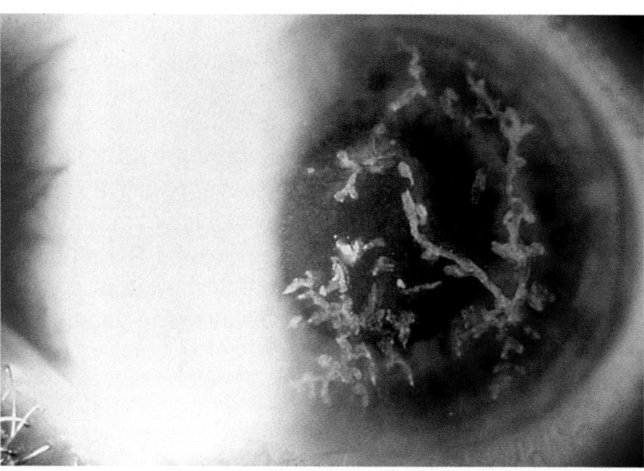

FIGURE 4–19 Classic zoster pseudodendrites are elevated mucous plaques with tapered ends. (From Tasman and Jaeger, with permission.)

Clinical Complications

Complications include conjunctivitis (most common), vision loss (if the cornea is involved), epithelial keratitis, uveitis, episcleritis, scleritis, postherpetic neuralgia, and glaucoma. Less common complications include extraocular muscle palsies and retinal necrosis.[2]

Management

Immunocompetent patients should receive oral acyclovir, valacyclovir, or famciclovir as well as oral analgesia for discomfort. Topical anesthetics should not be given to the patient to take home, because important symptoms may be masked.[1] Immunocompromised patients should be admitted to the hospital and treated with intravenous acyclovir. In some cases, topical steroids, oral steroids, or topical antibiotics are indicated, but they should be initiated only in conjunction with on-site ophthalmologic consultation.[1] Optimally, antiviral medication should be initiated within 72 hours after onset of the rash. Early intervention results in more rapid healing and may lead to a decrease in the frequency and severity of complications.[2] All patients presenting with HZO should be seen by an on-site ophthalmologist on an emergency basis.[3]

REFERENCES

1. Shaikh S, Ta CN. Evaluation and management of herpes zoster ophthalmicus. *Am Fam Physician* 2002;66:1723–1730.
2. Severson EA, Baratz KH, Hodge DO, Burke JP. Herpes zoster ophthalmicus in Olmsted County, Minnesota: have systemic antivirals made a difference? *Arch Ophthalmol* 2003;121:386–390.
3. Gnann JW Jr, Whitley RJ. Clinical practice. Herpes zoster. *N Engl J Med* 2002;347:340–345.

Corneal Ulcer

Anthony S. Mazzeo

Clinical Presentation

Patients with corneal ulcer (CU) present with eye pain, tearing, foreign body sensation, and photophobia.

Pathophysiology

CUs develop from a defect in the corneal epithelium that develops into an ulceration, usually as a result of infection.[1] Ulcers are often seen in patients who use soft contact lenses, in whom *Pseudomonas* may cause aggressive superinfection. Staphylococci and streptococci are also common pathogens, especially in patients who do not use contact lenses. Fungal ulcers may develop in individuals with vegetable or agricultural traumatic inoculation.[2] The primary infection may seed deeper than the corneal epithelium to involve multiple layers.

Diagnosis

A complete eye examination must be performed, as in the workup for corneal abrasion (CA). The initial examination reveals hyperemic conjunctiva and a whitish, hazy area at the site of the ulcer. When fluorescein is applied, an irregular, nonlinear area of uptake is seen. On slit-lamp examination, there may also be signs of iritis, such as miosis, cells and flare, or an associated hypopyon if an infected CU is present.

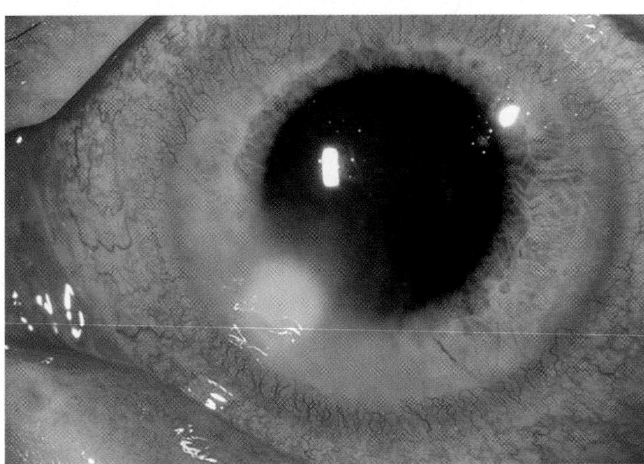

FIGURE 4–20 Infected corneal ulcers are characterized by corneal infiltrates associated with overlying epithelial defects and an anterior chamber reaction. (From Tasman and Jaeger, with permission.)

Clinical Complications

Decreased corneal sensation from denervation can lead to corneal melting or perforation.[1] Pseudomonal infection can destroy the cornea in 12 to 24 hours. Without appropriate treatment, CU can lead to blindness.[2]

Management

CU is a true ocular emergency, requiring immediate onsite ophthalmologic consultation. In conjunction with an ophthalmologist, the ulcer can be cultured and broad-spectrum antibiotics initiated. Current literature recommends topical antimicrobial therapy, either dual therapy with cefazolin and an aminoglycoside or monotherapy with a quinolone.[3] Initially, the dosing regimen is as frequent as every 15 to 30 minutes. In severe cases, hospital admission with intravenous as well as topical antibiotics may be required. Oral narcotics are often necessary for pain control. Unlike simple CAs, topical anesthetics and nonsteroidal antiinflammatory drugs (NSAIDs) should be avoided unless prescribed by the ophthalmologist. Eye patching is contraindicated and may worsen the condition. Patients should not wear contact lenses until determined by an ophthalmologist. Because of the potential for serious complications, it is imperative that the patient be seen in follow-up by an ophthalmologist as soon as possible, but not longer than 12 to 24 hours. Tetanus prophylaxis should be considered.

REFERENCES

1. Ma JJ, Dohlman CH. Mechanisms of corneal ulceration. *Ophthalmol Clin North Am* 2002;15:27–33.
2. Whitcher JP, Srinivasan M, Upadhyay MP. Prevention of corneal ulceration in the developing world. *Int Ophthalmol Clin* 2002;42: 71–77.
3. Benson WH, Lanier JD. Current diagnosis and treatment of corneal ulcers. *Curr Opin Ophthalmol* 1998;9:45–49.

Hyphema

Michael Greenberg

Clinical Presentation

Patients with hyphema present with diminished vision and ocular pain after blunt force or penetrating trauma to the globe. However, hyphemas may also develop atraumatically, in conjunction with anticoagulant use, bleeding disorders, melanoma, or leukemia.[1,2]

Pathophysiology

More than 50% of hyphemas are sports related; lack of protective eyewear is a predisposing factor. Other causes include fists, airbags, snowballs, explosions, lawnmower injuries, firecrackers, sticks, and wood chips.[1,2] Blunt force to the eye deforms the globe, increasing intraocular pressure (IOP) and displacing the lens-iris diaphragm posteriorly. This causes bleeding by tearing and disruption of these vascular structures. As IOP increases, the bleeding tends to cease and a clot forms, which may project from the anterior into the posterior chamber. This clot becomes maximally stable after 3 to 7 days. Hyphemas tend to break down within the anterior chamber by fibrinolysis and are dissipated through the trabecular meshwork.

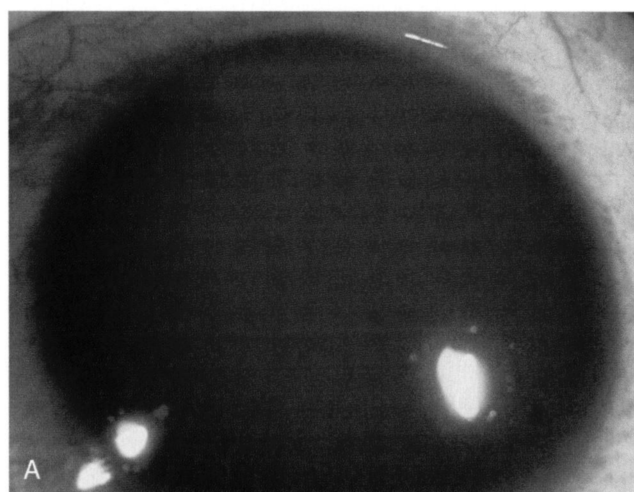

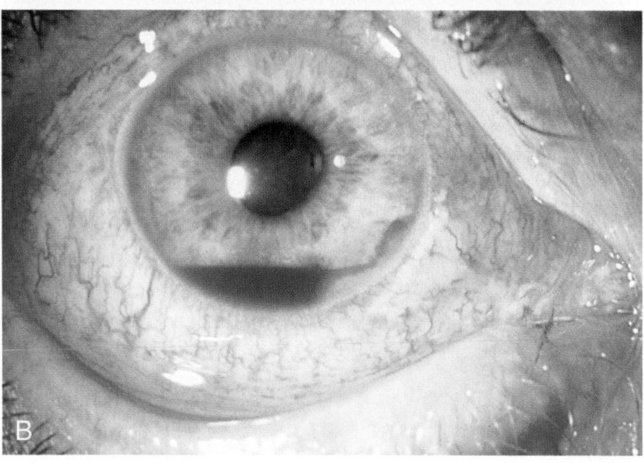

FIGURE 4–21 **A:** Total hyphema. **B:** Spontaneous hyphema due to iris metastasis from lung cancer. (From Tasman and Jaeger, with permission.)

Diagnosis

Hyphemas are clinically graded based on the amount of anterior chamber filling: grade I (less than one-third filling), grade II (one-third to one-half filling), grade III (one-half to near-total filling), and grade IV, known as "eight-ball hyphema" (total anterior chamber filling).[1,2] It is important to assess bleeding parameters and liver function in patients with hyphema. Visual acuity and IOP should be assessed as well.[1,2]

Clinical Complications

Recurrence of bleeding is the most common complication (up to 38% of cases).[1,2] The most common time for rebleeding is 2 to 5 days after the initial injury. Rebleeding is more common in larger hyphemas, in African-Americans (related to sickle cell disease or trait), and in patients with initially elevated IOP.[1,2] Other complications include corneal blood staining, glaucoma, cataract formation, synechiae, optic atrophy, and permanent visual loss.[1,2]

Management

Patients who are at risk for rebleeding and those who are unable to comply with instructions must be hospitalized. Most authorities recommend bed rest with the head of the bed elevated.[1,2] The eye should be shielded. Anticoagulant medications (aspirin, Coumadin, and nonsteroidal antiinflammatory drugs [NSAIDs]) should be discontinued. Ophthalmology consultation should be obtained in all cases, and steroids (topical, systemic, or both) should be used based on the consultant's recommendations. Some recommend the use of antifibrinolytics such as aminocaproic acid or tranexamic acid.[1,2]

REFERENCES

1. Walton W, Von Hagen S, Grigorian R, Zarbin M. Management of traumatic hyphema. *Surv Ophthalmol* 2002;47:297–334.
2. Brandt MT, Haug RH. Traumatic hyphema: a comprehensive review. *J Oral Maxillofac Surg* 2001;59:1462–1470.

Chemosis

Michael Greenberg

Clinical Presentation

Chemosis is a nonspecific term denoting the presence of conjunctival edema.[1,2]

Patients present with localized or generalized conjunctival edema.

Pathophysiology

Chemosis is an irritative and inflammatory phenomenon associated with a variety of conjunctival and ocular insults. The introduction of foreign matter, chemicals, mechanical irritation, virus or bacterial infection, or allergens may induce conjunctival edema. Immunoglobulin E–mediated hypersensitivity may be involved in the production of chemosis in some cases.[1,2]

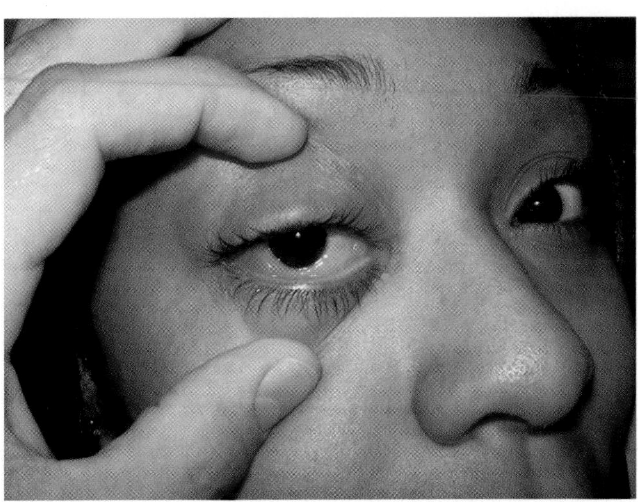

FIGURE 4–22 Chemosis. Note scleral swelling and injection. (Courtesy of Mark Silverberg, MD.)

Diagnosis

Chemosis is diagnosed by clinical observation of conjunctival swelling, which may be bilateral or unilateral. Chemosis can manifest with what appear to be multiple tiny bubbles in and around the conjunctiva.

Clinical Complications

Chemosis tends to be self-limited with no substantial complications.

Management

Chemosis usually resolves after the underlying cause is alleviated. Therefore, treatment for bacterial or viral causes is essential. Other helpful modalities include cool compresses applied frequently. The avoidance of allergens is essential in allergen-induced chemosis. Vasoconstrictors, antihistamines, H_1 receptor antagonists, topical nonsteroidal antiinflammatory drugs (NSAIDs), and mast cell stabilizers such as iodoxamide, nedocromil, or pemirolast have proved helpful in some cases.[2]

REFERENCES

1. Kalin NS, Orlin SE, Wulc AE, et al. Chronic localized conjunctival chemosis. *Cornea* 1996;15:295–300.
2. Teoh DL, Reynolds S. Diagnosis and management of pediatric conjunctivitis. *Pediatr Emerg Care* 2003;19:48–55.

Episcleritis and Scleritis

Michael Greenberg

Clinical Presentation

Patients with scleral inflammatory disease present with the acute onset of red eye associated with dull, achy, ocular pain and tenderness.[1–3] In addition, a watery, nonpurulent discharge may be present. Scleritis is associated with decreased visual acuity in up to 16% of patients, whereas visual acuity is normal in episcleritis.[2]

Pathophysiology

Episcleritis is a self-limited disorder, usually of young adults, that is probably autoimmune in origin. Scleritis may be associated with severe (even life-threatening) vascular or connective tissue disease, such as rheumatoid arthritis. Both disorders are more common in women.[2]

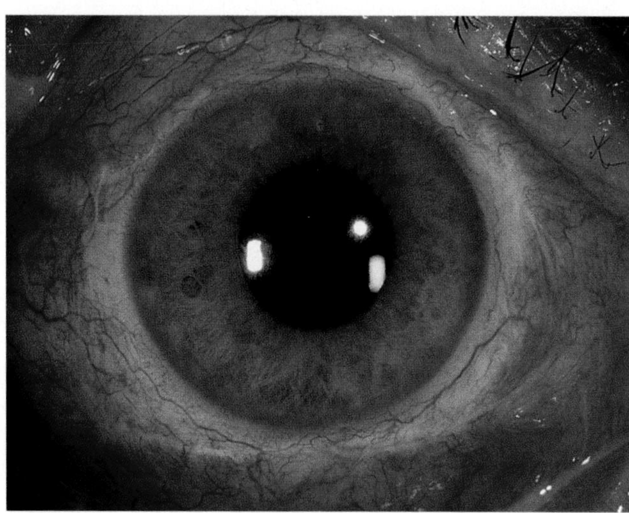

FIGURE 4–23 Anterior scleritis. The sectorial, diffuse area of scleral inflammation was moderately painful and did not blanch in response to instillation of a 2.5% phenylepinephrine solution. (From Tasman and Jaeger, with permission.)

Diagnosis

The diagnosis for both entities depends on a careful history and thorough physical examination, including slit-lamp microscopy.

Clinical Complications

Complications of scleritis include glaucoma, uveitis, keratitis, and retinal detachment (RD). Both scleritis and episcleritis may be complicated by recurrence.

Management

The differentiation of episcleritis from scleritis is critical, because episcleritis usually resolves without treatment or responds to topical antiinflammatory drugs, whereas scleritis typically requires systemic therapy, and most patients require oral corticosteroids or immunosuppressive drugs. Emergency on-site ophthalmology consultation is required if there is a question of differentiating episcleritis from scleritis or if the diagnosis of scleritis is clear.[1,2]

REFERENCES

1. Leibowitz HM. The red eye. *N Engl J Med* 2000;343:345–351.
2. Jabs DA, Mudun A, Dunn JP, Marsh MJ. Episcleritis and scleritis: clinical features and treatment results. *Am J Ophthalmol* 2000;130:469–476.
3. Pavesio CE, Meier FM. Systemic disorders associated with episcleritis and scleritis. *Curr Opin Ophthalmol* 2001;12:471–478.

Periorbital Cellulitis

Gregory P. Conners

Clinical Presentation

Periorbital cellulitis, also known as preseptal cellulitis, is an infection of the eyelids and adjacent tissues anterior to the orbital septum.[1]

Patients present with redness, pain, and swelling of the eyelid. Fever and conjunctival injection are common, often with an associated discharge. The degree of severity varies, from mild erythema of one lid to beefy erythema in both lids of both eyes that cannot be opened. Visual acuity and extraocular movements should not be affected. Bilateral disease is possible but uncommon.[1,2]

Pathophysiology

Infection of the preseptal tissues may be attributable to direct extension of an upper respiratory tract or sinus infection, superinfection of a periorbital cutaneous injury, or an insect bite. Pathogens include *S. aureus, S. pneumoniae* and other *Streptococcus* species; *M. catarrhalis* and nontypeable *H. influenzae* are occasionally cultured.[2]

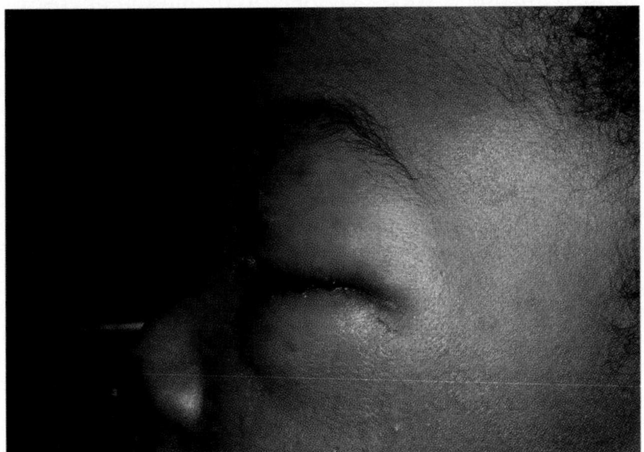

FIGURE 4–24 Left periorbital cellulitis. (Courtesy of Madelyn Garcia, MD.)

Diagnosis

The diagnosis is made clinically, with the key factor being the differentiation of periorbital cellulitis from the more severe orbital cellulitis. In periorbital cellulitis, the globe itself exhibits normal function and appearance, although conjunctivitis may be present. The two entities can be difficult to distinguish, and computed tomography (CT) scanning of the orbit and sinuses may be necessary.[1,2] Periorbital cellulitis is primarily seen in children younger than 5 years of age.[1,2]

Clinical Complications

Complications include orbital cellulitis, orbital abscess, cavernous sinus thrombosis, meningitis, permanent eye injury, visual deficits, sepsis, and bacteremia.[1]

Management

Broad-spectrum antibiotics are integral to treatment. Patients who are very young, ill-appearing, severely infected, or immunosuppressed or have other complicating factors should be admitted for intravenous antibiotic therapy. Ophthalmology and ear, nose, and throat (ENT) consultations are helpful for patients with concurrent sinusitis.[1] Once orbital cellulitis has been ruled out, more mildly affected children may be treated as outpatients with either oral or serial parenteral antibiotics, but early follow-up must be assured.[1]

REFERENCES

1. Givner LB. Periorbital versus orbital cellulitis. *Pediatr Infect Dis J* 2002;21:1157–1158.
2. Ambati BK, Ambati J, Azar N, Stratton L, Schmidt EV. Periorbital and orbital cellulitis before and after the advent of *Haemophilus influenzae* type B vaccination. *Ophthalmology* 2000;107:1450–1453.

Orbital Cellulitis

Gregory P. Conners

Clinical Presentation

Orbital cellulitis is predominantly, but not exclusively, a disease of childhood. Patients typically present with fever and an erythematous, swollen, tender eyelid.[1,2] The patient may be unable to voluntarily open the eye, which may be proptotic or bulging outward.[2] Patients with orbital, but not periorbital, cellulitis may complain of pain with extraocular muscle motion in addition to visual changes. Bilateral disease is uncommon.

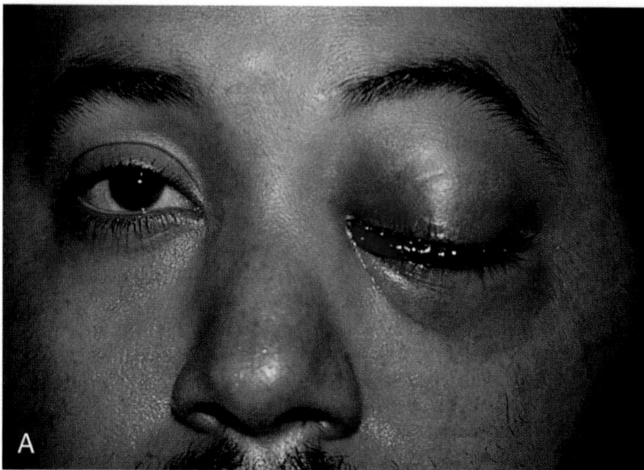

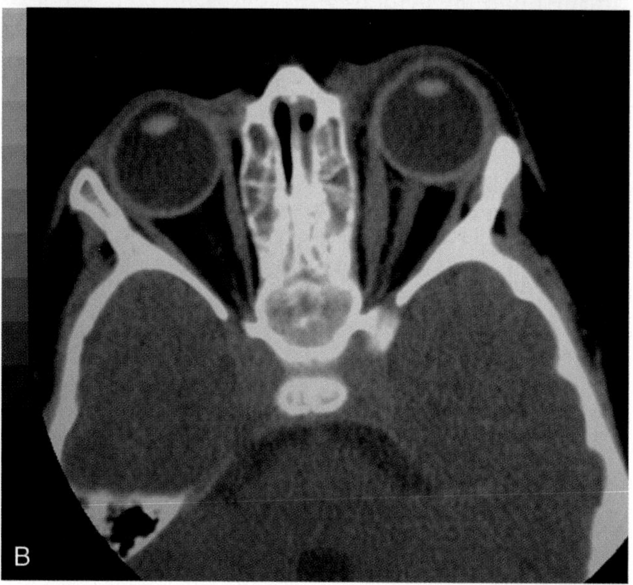

FIGURE 4–25 **A:** Orbital cellulitis manifesting with massive swelling, chemosis, erythema, and poor ocular motility. (From Tasman and Jaeger, with permission.) **B:** Computed tomogram showing left-sided orbital cellulitis. (Courtesy of Mark Silverberg, MD.)

Pathophysiology

Orbital cellulitis is typically caused by direct extension of an adjacent infection, often ethmoid sinusitis, periorbital cellulitis, or other orofacial infections.[1,2] Common bacterial causes include *S. aureus, S. pneumoniae, M. catarrhalis,* and nontypeable *H. influenzae.*[1,2]

Diagnosis

Differentiation between orbital and periorbital cellulitis is crucial. Proptosis, tenderness, resistance to the examiner's pressure on the eye, limitation of extraocular movements, and visual changes such as double vision or decreased acuity each suggest orbital cellulitis. Because of the frequent association of orbital cellulitis with sinusitis, nasal discharge is common. Computed tomography (CT) is mandatory in patients with suspected orbital cellulitis.[2] Patients who have normal CT findings but signs and symptoms suggesting orbital cellulitis should still be considered to have orbital cellulitis. Magnetic resonance imaging (MRI) may help to define the degree of involvement.

Clinical Complications

If left untreated, orbital cellulitis carries a substantial risk of death or blindness. Sepsis, orbital or subperiosteal abscess, meningitis, cavernous sinus thrombosis, and intracranial abscess are possible complications.[2]

Management

Parenteral, broad-spectrum antibiotics should be initiated immediately. Patients require hospitalization and emergency ophthalmologic and/or ear, nose, and throat consultation, because surgical drainage may be necessary.[2]

REFERENCES

1. Ambati BK, Ambati J, Azar N, Stratton L, Schmidt EV. Periorbital and orbital cellulitis before and after the advent of *Haemophilus influenzae* type B vaccination. *Ophthalmology* 2000;107:1450–1453.
2. Givner LB. Periorbital versus orbital cellulitis. *Pediatr Infect Dis J* 2002;21:1157–1158.

Ocular Alkali Injury

Judith Eisenberg

Clinical Presentation

Patients with ocular alkali injury (OAI) present after accidental or intentional splash (or more extensive) exposure of the eyes to a substance with a pH in the alkaline range. OAI is usually immediately painful, with concurrent blepharospasm, tearing, and visual impairment.[1–3]

Pathophysiology

Alkali ocular exposures result in a broad spectrum of injuries, ranging from superficial damage to destruction of the deep intraocular structures. Common alkaline substances involved in ocular exposures include aluminum hydroxide, sodium hydroxide, and calcium hydroxide. On exposure to water, these substances release hydroxyl ions, which are responsible for cell membrane disruption and cell death. In addition, cations are produced, and they are the determining factor for the degree of stromal penetration of the alkali.[1] The burned tissue releases collagenases and proteases, which cause further corneal injury with a risk of corneal perforation.[2] The stronger the alkali (i.e., the higher the pH), the deeper the penetration, with an increased potential risk of damage to deep intraocular structures.[1]

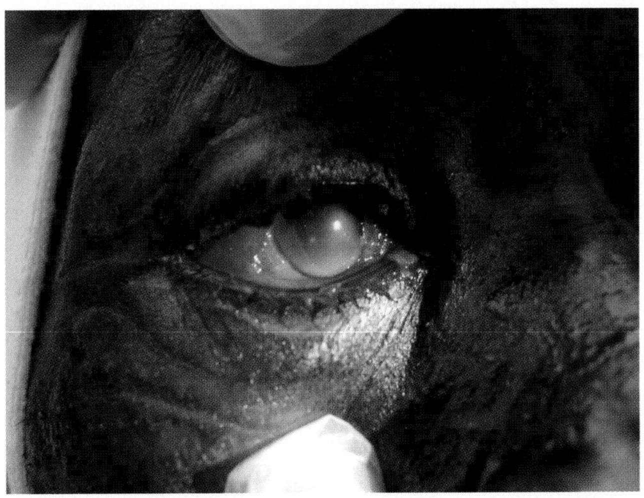

FIGURE 4–26 Severe corneal alkali injury. Note corneal opacification. (Courtesy of John Fojtik, MD.)

Diagnosis

The diagnosis is based on a history of exposure to an alkali substance. The degree of injury is defined by the results of visual acuity testing, pH testing, fluorescein staining, and slit-lamp examination.

Clinical Complications

Complications include permanent partial or total loss of vision.

Management

Immediate and aggressive irrigation of the eye must be performed, with an aim to return the ocular tissue to a neutral pH. Topical anesthetics such as tetracaine may be needed to overcome pain and blepharospasm and to allow for irrigation and proper examination of the eye. The patient should be instructed to look in all directions during irrigation, to ensure that all portions of the ocular surface are flushed. The corneal stroma has an osmolarity of 420 mOsm/L. Therefore, irrigation solutions with higher osmolarities, such as lactated Ringer's solution, are preferred over water or saline.[1] Prompt ophthalmologic evaluation is needed for a more complete initial assessment of the degree of injury and for treatment with topical steroids.[2] These patients require close ophthalmologic follow-up for prolonged periods.

REFERENCES

1. Kuckelkorn R, Schrage N, Keller G, Redbrake C. Emergency treatment of chemical and thermal eye burns. *Acta Ophthalmol Scand* 2002;80:4–10.
2. Davis AR, Ali QK, Aclimandos WA, Hunter PA, Ali QH. Topical steroid use in the treatment of ocular alkali burns. *Br J Ophthalmol* 1997;81:732–734.
3. Brodovsky SC, McCarty CA, Snibson G, et al. Management of alkali burns: an 11-year retrospective review. *Ophthalmology* 2000;107: 1829–1835.

Hypopyon

Colleen Campbell

Clinical Presentation

A hypopyon is a purulent collection of fluid located within the anterior chamber of the eye.

Most patients present with pain, irritation, or itching in the affected eye. Some have decreased visual acuity or visual field deficits, depending on the severity of the infection. Some patients have photophobia as well. Lid edema and chemosis may be present in severe infections.

Pathophysiology

Hypopyon may develop after surgery or trauma or as a result of spread from other infections (e.g., keratitis). Bacteria, fungi, amoebae, syphilis, brucellosis, and herpes simplex virus (HSV) may be responsible for hypopyon formation. Common bacterial pathogens include staphylococci and streptococci. Less common causes include fungal infections. Noninfectious uveitis may be associated with "pseudohypopyon," which can be caused by Behçet's syndrome, Reiter's syndrome, other disorders associated with the human leukocyte antigen (HLA) B27 allele, rifabutin, or malignancy. Pseudohypopyon appears identical to hypopyon on examination, but by the strictest definition it represents a distinct entity.[1] Microscopically, hypopyon consists of leukocyte collections, fibrin, and debris.

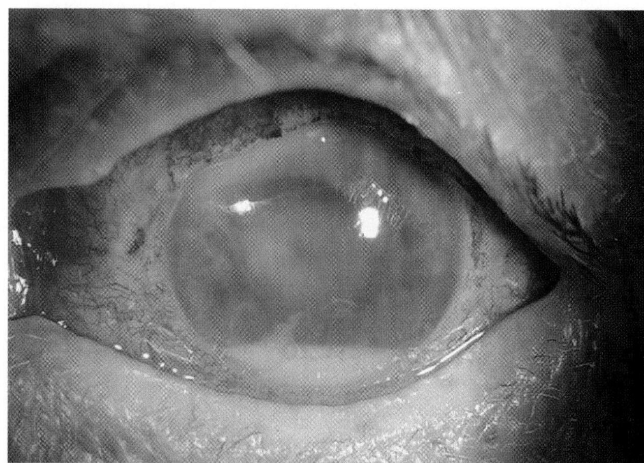

FIGURE 4–27 Hypopyon in acute endophthalmitis. Note hazy cornea and fluid level of pus. (From Tasman and Jaeger, with permission.)

Diagnosis

The diagnosis of hypopyon is made on the basis of history and slit-lamp examination. Needle aspiration of the anterior chamber by an ophthalmologist may be necessary to identify the causative organism in resistant infections.[2] On slit-lamp examination, there usually is a visible layering of white or opaque material at the inferior aspect of the anterior chamber. Rarely, the collection is in another region of the anterior chamber.[1]

Clinical Complications

Complications include chronic endophthalmitis and permanent loss of vision.

Management

Treatment of hypopyon requires immediate on-site ophthalmologic consultation. Treatment options include drainage and topical antibiotics, parenteral antibiotics, and intravitreal antibiotic injections.

REFERENCES

1. Ramsay A, Lightman S. Hypopyon uveitis. *Surv Ophthalmol* 2001; 46:1–18.
2. Sridhar MS, Sharma S, Savitri G, Gopinathan U, Rao GN. Anterior chamber tap: diagnostic and therapeutic indications in the management of ocular infections. *Cornea* 2002;21:718–722.

Macular Degeneration

Nick Gorton

Macular degeneration (MD) is an age-related, gradual degeneration of the macular area of the retina; it occurs in "wet" and "dry" forms.[1,2] If choroidal neovascularization (CNV) is present, the MD is considered to be exudative or "wet." If CNV is not present, it is defined as nonexudative or "dry" MD.[1]

Clinical Presentation

Patients usually are older than 50 years of age, and the incidence of MD increases with advancing age.[1,2] Individuals with dry MD complain of a gradual decrease in vision, whereas patients with wet MD may experience more acute vision losses. MD can manifest clinically in one or both eyes, but if it is present in a symptomatic eye, it almost always exists subclinically in the contralateral eye. The patient may report that straight lines or edges appear "bent" or "wavy." Central vision usually is affected more profoundly than peripheral vision.[1]

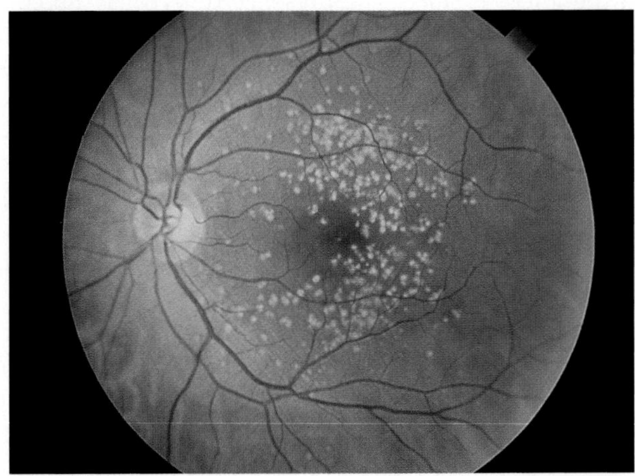

FIGURE 4–28 Multiple, hard drusen in early-stage, age-related macular degeneration. (From Tasman and Jaeger, with permission.)

Pathophysiology

The precise pathophysiology of MD remains unknown. There appears to be both a genetic predisposition and some role for the negative effect of photo-oxidative stress (e.g., tobacco use, macular sunlight exposure, Western diet).[1]

Diagnosis

The diagnosis should be suspected in any patient older than 50 years of age who complains of gradual vision loss. Every patient with a visual deficit should receive a complete ocular examination, including intraocular pressure (IOP) determination. In dry MD, funduscopy reveals drusen (light-colored patches on the retina, found most frequently near the macula), as well as atrophy and mottling of the retinal-pigmented epithelium. Whereas the CNV of wet MD usually is seen only with fluorescein angiography, the secondary manifestations of wet MD may be visualized on funduscopy. These manifestations include retinal detachment or retinal edema, subretinal hemorrhages, and hard exudates.[2]

Clinical Complications

The primary complication of MD is irreversible blindness, either partial or complete.[1,2]

Management

The most important role for the emergency physician in caring for patients with MD is prompt referral to an ophthalmologist for evaluation of vision loss. Currently, there are no specific therapies for dry MD. Wet MD can be treated with photocoagulation or photodynamic therapy, in an attempt to preserve remaining vision.[1]

REFERENCES

1. La Cour M, Kiilgaard JF, Nissen MH. Age-related macular degeneration: epidemiology and optimal treatment. *Drugs Aging* 2002;19:101–133.
2. Mittra RA, Singerman LJ. Recent advances in the management of age-related macular degeneration. *Optom Vis Sci* 2002;79:218–224.

Vitreous Hemorrhage

Colleen Campbell and Michael Greenberg

Clinical Presentation

Patients with vitreous hemorrhage (VH) present with complaints of "hazy" vision; the perception of shadows, floaters, or lines in the visual field; photophobia; "smoke signals"; and seeing "cobwebs."[1] These complaints may be more noticeable with eye movement. In addition, patients may complain of blurry vision with diminished visual acuity that is notable on examination if hemorrhage is significant.[1,2] Symptoms may begin after head or orbital trauma, or there may be no preceding trauma in patients with retinal disease or diabetes.[1,2]

Pathophysiology

Three general pathophysiologic mechanisms have been identified: bleeding from diseased or abnormal retinal vessels, rupture of normal vessels, and extension of bleeding from other sources.[1] Occasionally, VH is related to coagulopathies or anticoagulant therapy. Spontaneous VH occurs as a common complication of proliferative diabetic retinopathy, blunt or sharp ocular trauma, retinal detachment (RD), retinal tears, retinal vein occlusion, sickle cell retinopathy, age-related macular degeneration (MD), or vitreous detachment. VH can also occur in response to inflammation, as may be present in intermediate uveitis.[1] VH occurs in premature infants as a result of retinal disease of prematurity. VH associated with subarachnoid or intracranial hemorrhage, also known as Terson's syndrome, is characterized by headache, altered mental status, and decreased visual acuity.[2] Most bilateral VH is related to proliferative diabetic retinopathy.[1] Regardless of the mechanism of hemorrhage into the vitreous, clot formation occurs rapidly and is then followed by slow clearance at the rate of approximately 1% per day.[1]

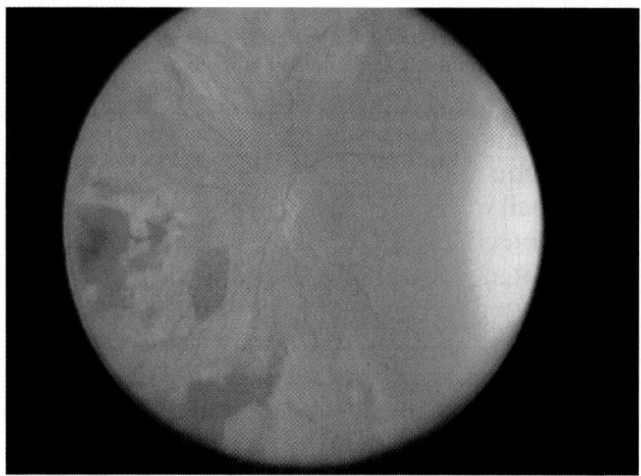

FIGURE 4–29 Vitreous hemorrhage. (From Duane's, with permission.)

Diagnosis

The diagnosis of VH is made on examination with the use of indirect funduscopy. The ocular examination is characterized by the finding of a decreased red reflex and inability to obtain a clear funduscopic examination on the affected side.[3] The presence of VH may be confirmed with the visualization of point-like and linear echoes, seen in the usually echo-free vitreous with the use of a 10-Mhz ultrasound probe.[2]

Clinical Complications

Complications include permanent partial or complete vision loss, recurrent hemorrhage, and glaucoma.

Management

Immediate on-site ophthalmologic consultation is warranted for any patient with suspected VH. Immediate treatment includes elevation of the head and avoidance of measures that increase intraocular pressure (IOP). Vitrectomy is indicated in cases involving severe hemorrhage and in those patients with substantially diminished visual acuity.[2]

REFERENCES

1. Spraul CW, Grossniklaus HE. Vitreous hemorrhage. *Surv Ophthalmol* 1997;42:3–39.
2. Ogawa T, Kitaoka T, Dake Y, Amemiya T. Terson syndrome: a case report suggesting the mechanism of vitreous hemorrhage. *Ophthalmology* 2001;108:1654–1656.

Central Retinal Artery Occlusion

Nick Gorton

Clinical Presentation

Patients with central retinal artery occlusion (CRAO) complain of sudden, painless visual loss, sometimes preceded by temporary visual loss that resolves spontaneously. Most patients present in their early sixties, although the disease does occur in young adults and children.[1]

Pathophysiology

Most cases are caused by emboli, atherosclerosis, vasculitis, vascular spasm, dissecting aneurysm, systemic hypoperfusion, hypertensive arterial necrosis, or coagulopathy.[1]

Diagnosis

Early on, the fundus may appear normal. If the obstruction is at the level of the central retinal artery rather than a branch of the retinal artery, an afferent pupillary defect is almost universally present within seconds after the occlusion. If the initial obstruction is not relieved, the retina develops cloudy swelling followed by whitening of the retina. This can be seen as early as 15 minutes after the obstruction occurs, and it corresponds to ischemic necrosis of the retina. When this whitening occurs, a "cherry-red spot" can be found at the fovea. Emboli can be visualized in up to 40% of cases.[1]

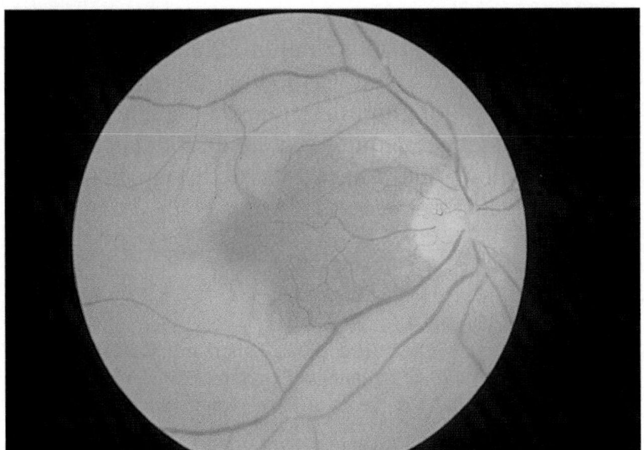

FIGURE 4–30 Acute central retinal artery obstruction with cilioretinal sparing and retained retinal perfusion of the foveola. (From Tasman and Jaeger, with permission.)

Clinical Complications

If left untreated, CRAO usually leads to permanent visual loss. Although they are not a direct complication of ocular pathology, patients with CRAO or branch retinal artery occlusion (BRAO) are at much greater risk for further thromboembolic diseases, such as cerebrovascular accident and acute myocardial infarction. For this reason, they have a significantly higher mortality rate than aged-matched controls.[1]

Management

Patients require a thorough evaluation, because 90% have evidence of systemic disease. Echocardiography reveals structural pathology in up to 50% of patients. Adult patients require carotid ultrasonography and a determination of the erythrocyte sedimentation rate (ESR) to rule out giant cell arteritis. Coagulation studies, including protein C, protein S, and antithrombin III assays, should be considered.[1]

Acute interventions include dilation of the central retinal artery by rebreathing of expired carbon dioxide, breathing of carbogen (5% CO_2 with 95% O_2,), or sublingual isosorbide dinitrate. These interventions should be attempted with caution, because systemic vasodilation occurs with all three. Gentle massage through a closed lid (steady pressure for 10 to 15 seconds, followed by sudden release) may move the embolus distally into the smaller-caliber vasculature. Other treatments include intravenous acetazolamide or mannitol, anterior chamber paracentesis, and trabeculectomy. Antiplatelet therapy with aspirin is reasonable in patients without contraindications.[2]

REFERENCES

1. Sharma S, Brown M, Brown GC. Retinal artery occlusions. *Ophthalmol Clin North Am* 1998;11:591–600.
2. Fraser S, Siriwardena D. Interventions for acute non-arteritic central retinal artery occlusion. *Cochrane Database Syst Rev* 2002;(1):CD001989.
3. Beatty S, Au Eong KG. Local intra-arterial fibrinolysis for acute occlusion of the central retinal artery: a meta-analysis of the published data. *Br J Ophthalmol* 2000;84:914–916.

Central Retinal Vein Occlusion

Nick Gorton

Clinical Presentation

Central retinal vein occlusion (CRVO) involves the formation of an *in situ* thrombus in the venous drainage system of the retina. CRVO can be divided into two major subtypes: nonischemic (NICRVO) and ischemic (ICRVO).[1]

Patients with NICRVO may be asymptomatic, with the occlusion discovered only on routine funduscopic examination. Symptoms may develop if the foveal region becomes involved through the development of macular edema or hemorrhage. Visual symptoms of NICRVO range from none to visual blurring that is usually central and may be more pronounced in the morning, just after awakening. Patients may also complain of prior episodic blurring (amaurosis fugax) before the constant visual changes occurred. However, ICRVO always involves a marked decrease in vision, which most often is first discovered on wakening in the morning. Neither ICRVO nor NICRVO should be painful.[1]

Pathophysiology

Hypercoagulability and endothelial damage predispose to thrombus formation. Patients with glaucoma have a greater risk owing to sluggish venous outflow caused by increased intraocular pressure (IOP). Patients with arterial hypertension, diabetes, coronary artery disease, hyperlipidemia, or a higher blood viscosity are all at increased risk. Eighty percent of CRVO cases are nonischemic.[1]

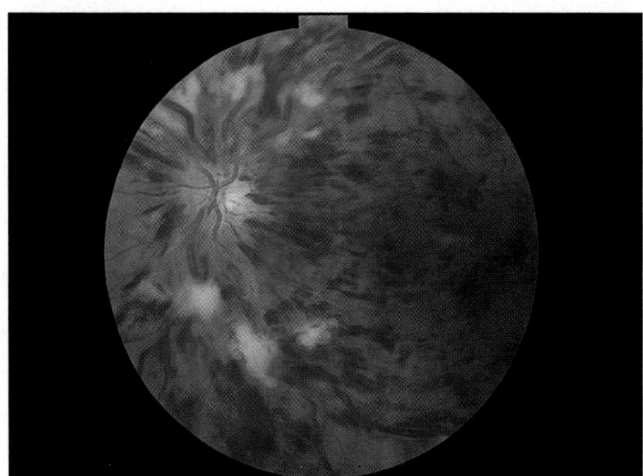

FIGURE 4–31 Central retinal vein obstruction. (From Tasman and Jaeger, with permission.)

Diagnosis

Diagnosis is based on the characteristic retinal findings. On funduscopy, retinal hemorrhages extending outward from the optic disk are a common finding. With branch retinal vein occlusion (BRVO), the entire retina is not involved; only the portion of the retina drained by the branch vein reveal the characteristic hemorrhages.[1,2]

Clinical Complications

The main complications of CRVO are visual impairment from macular edema and resultant macular degeneration (MD), ocular neovascularization, and vitreous hemorrhage (VH). Although macular edema and VH occur with both types of CRVO, neovascularization is seen only with ICRVO.[1]

Management

Some patients can be safely discharged to follow-up with an ophthalmologist. Those with new bilateral blindness, patients who live alone, and elderly patients are all at increased risk due to visual loss, and admission should be considered. Acute treatment may include surgical decompression, fibrinolytic or thrombolytic agents, systemic corticosteroids, hemodilution, Diamox, and watchful waiting.[1] The decision to institute therapy should be left to the consulting ophthalmologist. Patients younger than 55 years of age require evaluation for genetic or acquired thrombophilias; up to 25% of these patients have a hypercoagulable state.[2]

REFERENCES

1. Hayreh SS. Central retinal vein occlusion. *Ophthalmol Clin North Am* 1998;11:559–590.
2. Lahey JM, Tunc M, Kearney J, et al. Laboratory evaluation of hypercoagulable states in patients with central retinal vein occlusion who are less than 56 years of age. *Ophthalmology* 2002;109: 126–131.

Hypertensive Retinopathy

Nick Gorton

Clinical Presentation

The retinal vascular changes associated with chronic hypertension are usually asymptomatic. Occasionally, patients with malignant hypertension present with acute visual disturbances, but these are probably related to optic disk edema.[1]

Pathophysiology

Both chronic, poorly controlled hypertension and acute malignant hypertension can produce changes within the retina.[1,2] These lesions develop when the mean arterial pressure exceeds a critical range, resulting in failure of the blood-retinal barrier. This leads to increased vascular permeability, edema, and exudative changes.[1]

Diagnosis

Although systemic hypertension is often revealed at triage, a funduscopic examination is necessary to diagnose hypertensive retinopathy (HR). In chronic disease, arteriolosclerosis is evidenced by arteriolar narrowing, described as having a "copper wire" appearance. Chronic hypertensive venous changes may be seen, such as dilation and tortuosity of retinal veins proximal to arteriovenous (AV) crossings and narrowing of the veins at the crossings themselves (AV nicking).[1] Cotton-wool spots and hard exudates are also typical retinal findings in hypertensive patients. Flame-shaped hemorrhages are sometimes noted and are the result of capillary or venous bleeding.[1] Disk edema is sometimes seen and is usually the result of acute disease caused by malignant hypertension.[2]

Clinical Complications

Complications of long-standing HR include central or branch retinal artery or vein occlusions, macular edema, and proliferative vitreoretinopathy.[2] All of these changes eventually lead to decreased visual acuity and blindness.

Management

The main issue in the management of HR is chronic control of blood pressure in an outpatient setting. Initial therapy for patients with more severe essential hypertension may be started in the emergency department but is best coordinated with the patient's primary care physician. Patients with severely elevated blood pressure who manifest funduscopic changes consistent with malignant hypertension have, by definition, a hypertensive emergency, because these ocular findings represent acute end-organ damage. These patients merit emergency lowering and tight control of their blood pressure, as well as complete evaluation for other end-organ damage in an inpatient setting.

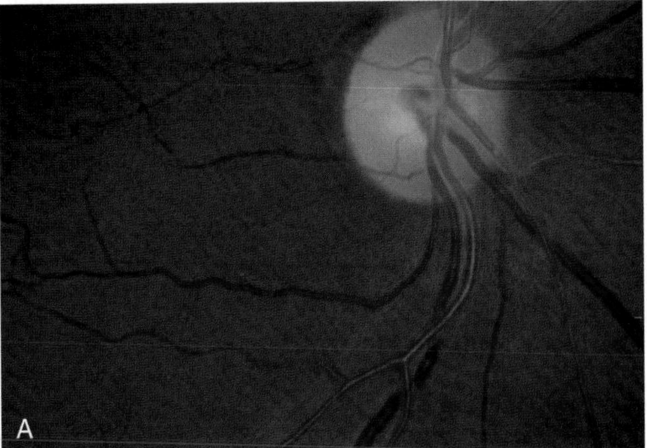

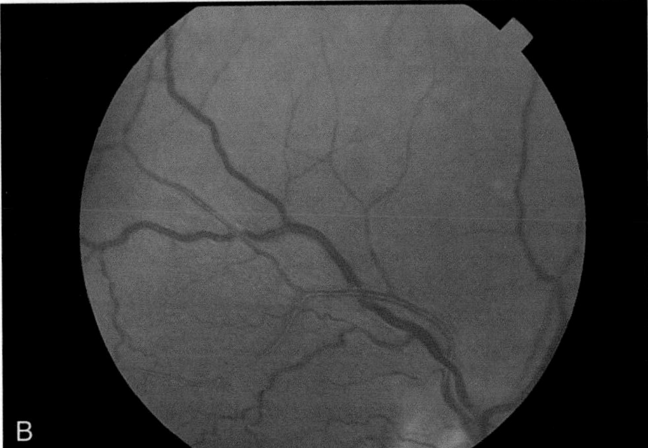

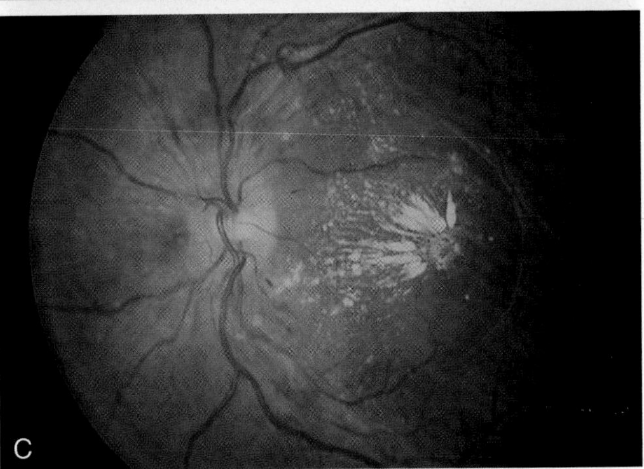

FIGURE 4–32 **A:** In grade I hypertensive retinopathy, the retinal arteries and arterioles have become narrowed. **B:** In grade II hypertensive retinopathy, the retinal arteries are narrowed, and arteriovenous nicking is evident. **C:** Grade III hypertensive retinopathy. The eye has retinal hemorrhages and hard exudates in the form of a hemimacular star. (From Tasman and Jaeger, with permission.)

REFERENCES

1. Hayreh SS. Hypertensive retinopathy. *Ophthalmol Clin North Am* 1998;11:535–558.
2. Wong TY, Klein R, Klein BE, Tielsch JM, Hubbard L, Nieto FJ. Retinal microvascular abnormalities and their relationship with hypertension, cardiovascular disease, and mortality. *Surv Ophthalmol* 2001;46:59–80.

Diabetic Retinopathy

Nick Gorton

Clinical Presentation

Patients with established diabetic retinopathy (DR) are often asymptomatic or have chronic progressive visual changes. Retinopathy is almost universal in persons who have had diabetes mellitus for longer than 2 decades.[1] Patients may present with abrupt changes in vision due to the complications of proliferative diabetic retinopathy (PDR) or advanced diabetic eye disease (e.g., vitreous hemorrhage [VH], retinal detachment [RD]).[2]

Pathophysiology

Prolonged elevation in serum glucose, coupled with systemic hypertension, renal disease, or elevated serum lipid concentrations, damages the ocular microvascular circulation, resulting in hemorrhages, edema, neovascularization, microaneurysms, and retinal ischemia.[2,3]

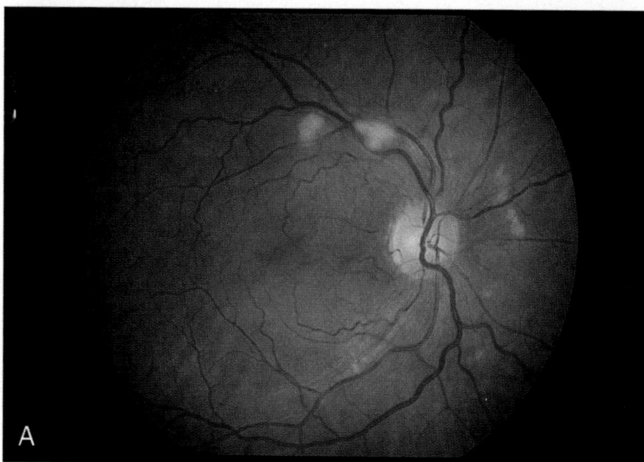

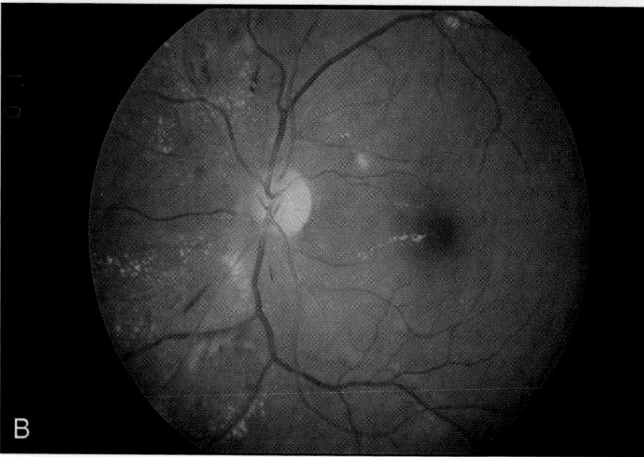

FIGURE 4–33 **A:** Cotton-wool spots located supertemporal to the optic nerve head. **B:** Multiple, discrete, yellow, hard exudates in the posterior pole of an eye with background diabetic retinopathy. (From Tasman and Jaeger, with permission.)

Diagnosis

The most sensitive way to diagnose DR is by skilled fundus photography through a dilated pupil, interpreted by a qualified ophthalmologist. Alternatively, dilated funduscopy is often performed. However, if retinal pathology suggestive of DR is detected on *any* examination in a diabetic patient, the diagnosis is likely, and the appropriate referral should be made.

Clinical Complications

If left untreated, DR causes progressive bilateral visual loss that often results in blindness. Legal blindness is estimated to be 25 times more prevalent among diabetics compared with nondiabetics.[1] However, 90% of such blindness is preventable with appropriate treatment.[2]

Management

Diabetic patients presenting with acute visual changes should be fully evaluated for complications of DR, as well as other causes of acute visual changes. They should also be evaluated by an ophthalmologist on an urgent basis. Patients with suspected macular edema or proliferative retinopathy may be evaluated by an ophthalmologist at an urgent outpatient follow-up visit. Those patients with advanced disease who have suspected RD should be seen on the same day, because retinal reattachment with some visual recovery is possible with prompt treatment.[2] In addition to intensive blood glucose and blood pressure control, which slows the progression of DR, laser photocoagulation is the mainstay of care for patients with more severe disease.[1] Vitrectomy may preserve some vision in patients with VH or severe PDR.[2]

REFERENCES

1. Aiello LP, Cahill MT, Wong JS. Systemic considerations in the management of diabetic retinopathy. *Am J Ophthalmol* 2001;132: 760–776.
2. Skyler JS. Microvascular complications: retinopathy and nephropathy. *Endocrinol Metabol Clin North Am* 2001;30:833–856.
3. Pelzek C, Lim JI. Diabetic macular edema: review and update. *Ophthalmol Clin North Am* 2002;15:555–563.

Cytomegalovirus Retinitis

Nick Gorton

Clinical Presentation

Patients with cytomegalovirus retinitis (CMVR) are uniformly immunocompromised and present with complaints of blurred vision, floaters, or flashes of light.[1] Redness and pain usually are not present.[2]

Pathophysiology

CMVR is caused by cytomegalovirus (CMV), a herpesvirus that is spread by sexual activity or other intimate contact, as well as through vertical transmission.[1,2] After primary infection, the virus becomes dormant in the secretory glands and lymphoreticular cells until the T-cell–mediated immune response is damaged (e.g., by HIV infection). Seroprevalence in adults is approximately 50%, and it approaches 100% in homosexual men.[1,2]

Diagnosis

CMVR should be suspected in any immunosuppressed patient with visual complaints. The retinitis begins as small, white, perivascular infiltrates known as "dot" or "blot" hemorrhages. CMVR causes a hemorrhagic necrotizing retinitis along the course of retinal vessels. If left untreated, the lesion spreads slowly, with large areas of retinal necrosis leading to retinal tears and detachments. CMVR may also manifest in the "brushfire" pattern, with an enlarging white geographic lesion and central clearing.[1]

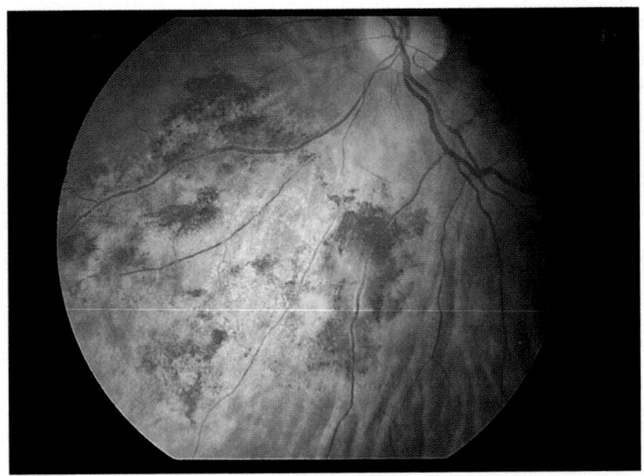

FIGURE 4–34 The characteristic findings of cytomegalovirus retinopathy include yellowish retinitis with secondary hemorrhage along the edge, seen off the inferior nasal areas in this example. (From Tasman and Jaeger, with permission.)

Clinical Complications

Complications include progressive and irreversible visual loss.[1,2]

Management

Treatment of CMVR involves specific anti-CMV therapy as well as treatment to bolster the immune response. In patients not receiving highly active antiretroviral therapy (HAART), institution of HAART may sufficiently reconstitute the T-cell response to effectively suppress viral reactivation. However, HAART is best instituted by the patient's primary care provider or infectious disease specialist. In both HAART-naive patients and those already receiving this therapy, CMVR should be treated with CMV-specific therapy. Until recently, this involved prolonged intravenous induction with ganciclovir, cidofovir, or foscarnet, followed by oral or intravitreal therapy. The recent development of valganciclovir, a prodrug of ganciclovir, allows for oral induction therapy. Patients with CMVR should be admitted to the hospital and should have an ophthalmologic evaluation on an urgent basis.[1]

REFERENCES

1. See RF, Rao NA. Cytomegalovirus retinitis in the era of combined highly active antiretroviral therapy. *Ophthalmol Clin North Am* 2002;15:529–536.
2. Dunn JP. Viral retinitis. *Ophthalmol Clin North Am* 1999;12: 109–121.

Optic Neuritis

Nick Gorton

Clinical Presentation

Optic neuritis (ON) is an inflammatory process that involves the optic nerve.[1,2] It may occur as an isolated event or as a part of an established diagnosis of multiple sclerosis (MS).

Patients may present with unilateral and subacute vision loss. Eye pain is present in 90% to 95% of cases and is aggravated by ocular movement.[1,2] Often, an afferent pupillary defect can be elicited. On funduscopic examination, the optic disk may appear normal or may evidence edema. A thorough history may reveal a prior diagnosis of MS or previous neurologic events that are suggestive of MS.[1]

Pathophysiology

The precise pathogenesis of ON (and MS) remains controversial. However, the disease is thought to be immune mediated, with exaggerated B- and T-cell responses within the central nervous system.[1,2] An association with certain human leukocyte antigen (HLA) genotypes has also been identified.[1] The disease process itself is an acute neuropathy caused by focal inflammation and demyelination of the optic nerve.[1,2] Patients with isolated ON have a substantially greater risk of developing MS (50% of cases).[1]

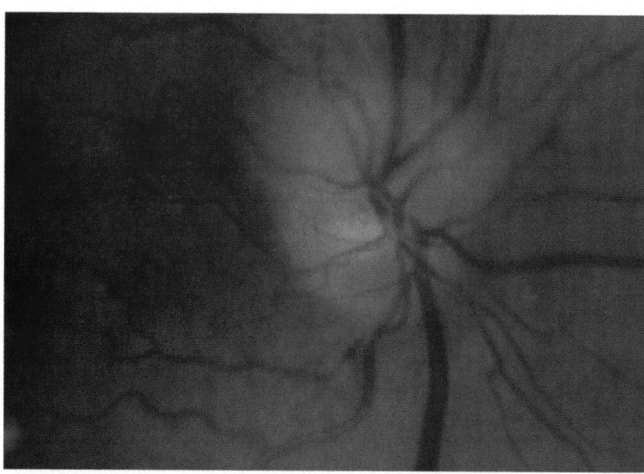

FIGURE 4–35 Nonarteritic anterior ischemic optic neuropathy showing swelling of the right optic disk with acute superior segmental swelling. (From Tasman and Jaeger, with permission.)

Diagnosis

The diagnosis of ON is suggested in a young to middle-aged person (often female) with the above-mentioned signs and symptoms. No specific test exists for either ON or MS, so the diagnosis remains a clinical one. However, a myriad of other causes, including infectious, inherited, malignant, ischemic, and autoimmune disorders, must be ruled out.[2] The definitive diagnosis should be made in conjunction with neurology or ophthalmology consultantation.[2]

Clinical Complications

The only significant complication of ON is persistent visual disturbances, with blindness being a rare possibility.

Management

Even if untreated, ON usually resolves within 6 weeks, although some residual visual deficits may persist.[2] Steroid or interferon-β therapy may hasten visual recovery and reduce the risk or delay the onset of MS, but this is controversial. Oral analgesics are beneficial in decreasing eye pain. Neurology or ophthalmology consultation should be obtained to help deliver acute and follow-up care.[2]

REFERENCES

1. Soderstrom M. Optic neuritis and multiple sclerosis. *Acta Ophthalmol Scand* 2001;79:223–227.
2. Hickman SJ, Dalton CM, Miller DH, Plant GT. Management of acute optic neuritis. *Lancet* 2002;360:1953–1962.

Papilledema

Jennifer Wiler

Clinical Presentation

Papilledema ("choked disk") is optic disk swelling secondary to increased intracranial pressure (ICP) and subsequent optic nerve compression.[1-3]

Early on, the patient may present with an enlarged blind spot or a subtle change in vision. As the condition persists, intermittent, temporary loss of vision may occur in one or both eyes (known as amaurosis fugax). Patients may also complain of headache, nausea, and vomiting.

Pathophysiology

Papilledema may be associated with intracranial infections, intracranial tumors, hydrocephalus, pseudotumor cerebri (idiopathic intracranial hypertension), cerebral trauma, meningitis, encephalitis, space-occupying lesions, venous sinus obstruction, malignant hypertension, arteriovenous (AV) shunts, atherosclerosis, subarachnoid hemorrhage, salicylate poisoning, or polycythemia.[1-3]

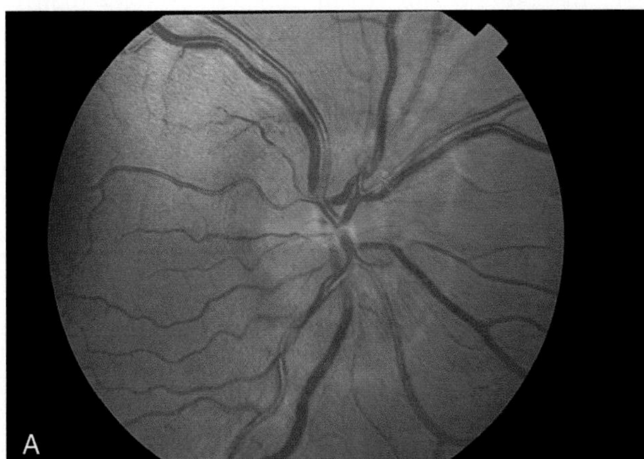

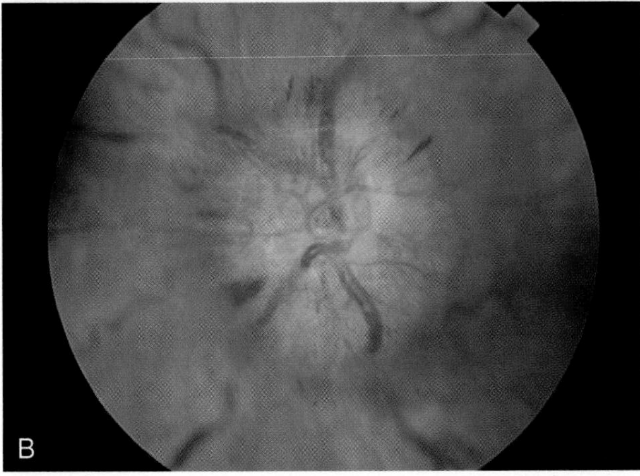

FIGURE 4–36 **A:** Early papilledema, with disk elevation, blurring of the margins, hyperemia, and venous engorgement in the right eye. **B:** Chronic papilledema, showing elevation and residual hemorrhages. (From Tasman and Jaeger, with permission.)

Diagnosis

Papilledema causes bilateral and symmetric loss of optic disk cupping and blurring of the previously sharp disk margins, with marked disk elevation visible on funduscopic examination. Disks may appear hyperemic with tortuous retinal vessels, absent venous pulsations, and increased vessel diameter. Surrounding flame hemorrhages and exudates may also be appreciated. Papilledema has numerous causes; the clinical picture will direct the clinician to identify the likely cause.[1-3]

Clinical Complications

If the ICP is not reduced, vision may be permanently impaired secondary to optic nerve atrophy.

Management

Because papilledema is associated with increased ICP, an immediate workup is warranted. Definitive treatment is focused on alleviating the underlying cause of the increased ICP. Computed tomography (CT) or magnetic resonance imaging (MRI) can be helpful in identifying the underlying cause. If neuroradiologic studies show no midline shift or obvious space-occupying lesion, a lumbar puncture should be performed to measure the subarachnoid opening pressure. Treatment modalities include serial lumbar punctures to temporize the evolution of optic disk compression. Occasionally, emergency surgical intervention is required to preserve the patient's vision. This includes optic nerve sheath fenestration and lumboperitoneal shunting. Disposition depends on the underlying cause.[1-3]

REFERENCES

1. McCulley TJ, Lam BL, Bose S, Feuer WJ. The effect of optic disk edema on spontaneous venous pulsations. *Am J Ophthalmol* 2003;135:706–708.
2. Almog Y, Goldstein M. Visual outcome in eyes with asymptomatic optic disc edema. *J Neuroophthalmol* 2003;23:204–207.
3. Biousse V, Rucker JC, Vignal C, Crassard I, Katz BJ, Newman NJ. Anemia and papilledema. *Am J Ophthalmol* 2003;135:437–446.

Arcus Senilis

Michael Greenberg

Clinical Presentation

Arcus senilis (AS) is a benign, white-grey discoloration of the cornea.[1,2]

AS is usually an incidental finding on physical examination. It is unlikely to be the primary presenting complaint for emergency department patients.

Pathophysiology

AS represents a deposition of cholesterol, triglycerides, phospholipids, and apolipoprotein B at and around the margins of the cornea.[1,2] It has been suggested that AS may be an indicator of arthrosclerosis and therefore may be of some prognostic value regarding premature coronary disease. However, recent work has dispelled this theory and verified that AS provides no more information about mortality risk than does the chronologic age. AS in patients younger than 60 years of age has been associated with enhanced thickness of the intima media in the carotid arteries of men with hypercholesterolemia. AS is more prevalent in men and is not related to diabetes, hypertension, obesity, hypertriglyceridemia, or family history of coronary artery disease.[1,2]

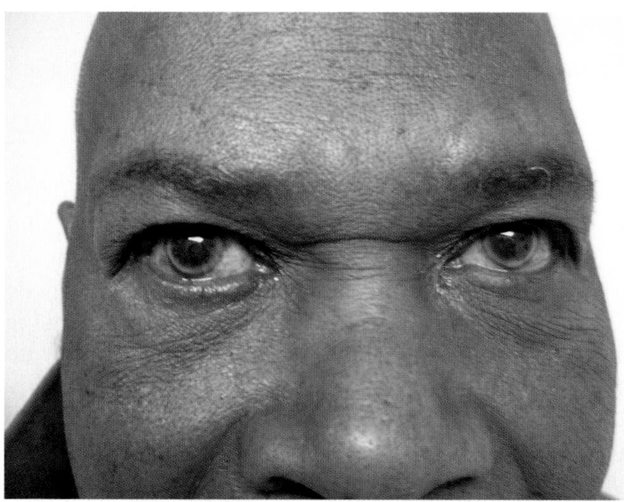

FIGURE 4–37 Bilateral arcus senilis. (Courtesy of Mark Silverberg, MD.)

Diagnosis

The diagnosis is usually obvious on gross examination of the cornea without magnification.

Clinical Complications

There are no specific complications related directly to AS. In white Americans with symptoms of coronary disease, the presence of AS in patients younger than 60 years of age indicates a high risk for multivessel coronary atherosclerosis.[1]

Management

Specific therapy for AS is not indicated. However, the finding of premature or heavy AS should prompt the emergency physician to obtain a lipid profile or to refer the patient to a primary care provider for lipid evaluation.

REFERENCES

1. Hoogerbrugge N, Happee C, van Domburg R, Poldermans D, van den Brand MJ. Corneal arcus: indicator for severity of coronary atherosclerosis? *Neth J Med* 1999;55:184–187.
2. Moss SE, Klein R, Klein BE. Arcus senilis and mortality in a population with diabetes. *Am J Ophthalmol* 2000;129:676–678.

Retinal Detachment

David Fintak

Clinical Presentation

Patients with retinal detachment (RD) may present complaining of flashes of light, floaters in the form of "flying insects" or "spider webs," a curtain or shadow moving over the field of vision, and peripheral or central visual loss (or both).[1,2] Pain is typically absent.

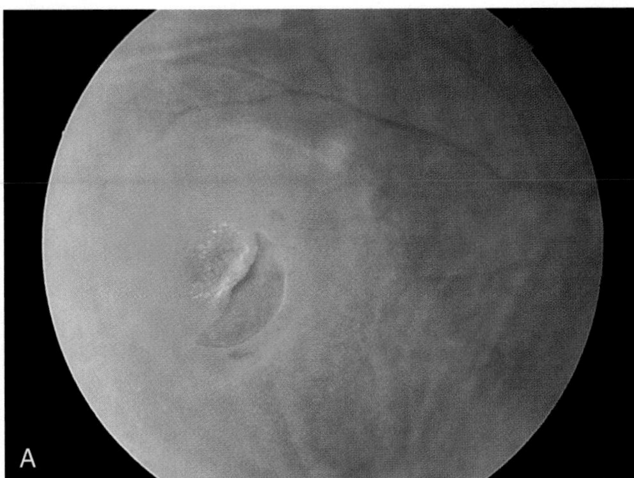

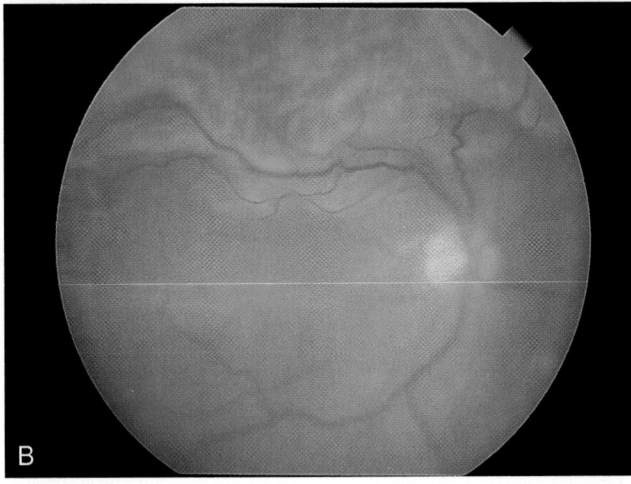

FIGURE 4–38 **A:** Flap ("horseshoe") retinal tear surrounded by subretinal fluid. **B:** Corrugated, opaque appearance of the detached retina in a patient with rhegmatogenous retinal detachment. (From Tasman and Jaeger, with permission.)

Pathophysiology

Rhegmatogenous RD occurs as a result of a tear or hole in the neuronal layer. This typically occurs in patients older than 45 years of age and is more common in men than in women. It is associated with degenerative myopia, lattice degeneration, previous cataract surgery, and trauma.[3] Exudative RDs are produced by retinal and choroidal conditions that damage the blood-retina barrier. Conditions leading to this type of RD include central retinal vein occlusion (CRVO), papilledema, hypertension, toxemia of pregnancy, glomerulonephritis, vasculitis, and choroidal tumor. Traction RD is a consequence of fibrous band formation in the vitreous; contraction of the bands pulls the retina away from the pigmented retinal epithelium. Conditions leading to this type of RD include proliferative diabetic retinopathy, retinopathy of prematurity, toxocariasis, sickle cell retinopathy, trauma, and previous giant retinal tear.[2]

Diagnosis

RDs are suspected based on the history and are diagnosed clinically by means of direct and indirect ophthalmoscopy. Pigmented cells in the anterior vitreous, vitreous hemorrhage (VH), posterior vitreous detachment, and elevation of the retina with or without an accompanying retinal break are observed. An afferent pupillary defect may be present.[2] Any patient with suspected RD requires emergency ophthalmologic evaluation.

Clinical Complications

Depending on the type of RD, progressive visual field and visual acuity loss may occur if treatment is not received in a timely fashion.

Management

Emergency ophthalmology consultation is essential if the diagnosis of RD is suspected.

REFERENCES

1. Banker AS, Freeman WR. Retinal detachment. *Ophthalmol Clin North Am* 2001;14:695–704.

Kayser-Fleischer Rings

Michael Greenberg

Clinical Presentation

Kayser-Fleischer rings (KFRs) may be present in patients with Wilson's disease (WD), cholestatic liver disease, primary biliary cirrhosis, or autoimmune hepatitis.

Pathophysiology

KFRs are brown-yellow discolorations found in Descemet's membrane that result from deposition of copper in the limbic zone of the cornea.[1,2]

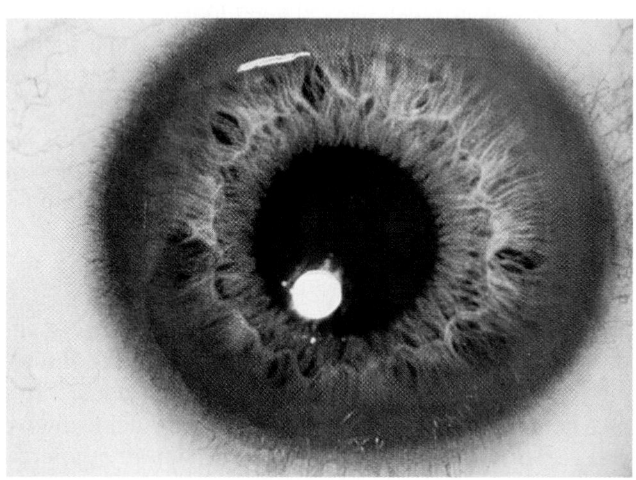

FIGURE 4–39 Kayser-Fleischer rings: copper deposits in the periphery of Descemet's membrane. (From Tasman and Jaeger, with permission.)

Diagnosis

KFRs are best visualized with the use of the slit-lamp microscope. However, in many cases, they may be seen with the naked eye without magnification. Although they are frequently associated with WD, KFRs are not pathognomonic for WD. It is thought that KFRs are present in almost 100% of WD patients with neuropsychiatric signs.[1,2]

Clinical Complications

No specific ocular complications are associated with KFRs.

Management

Specific treatment is not indicated for KFRs. However, the finding of KFR should prompt a diagnostic search for liver disease or WD, or both.[1,2]

REFERENCES

1. Pfeil SA, Lynn DJ. Wilson's disease: copper unfettered. *J Clin Gastroenterol* 1999;29:22–31.
2. El-Youssef M. Wilson disease. *Mayo Clin Proc* 2003;78:1126–1136.

Anisocoria

Michael Greenberg

Clinical Presentation

Some patients present with the knowledge that they have benign physiologic anisocoria. Others present for a variety of unrelated reasons, and previously unrecognized anisocoria is uncovered in the course of the physical examination.[1]

Pathophysiology

Anisocoria is defined as unequal-sized pupils from any cause. As much as 25% of the population has physiologic anisocoria manifested by a difference in pupillary size of as much as 2 mm.[1] Other causes of anisocoria may involve serious underlying ocular or intracranial pathology or unilateral ocular exposure to specific chemicals or drugs that affect pupillary size.[1,2]

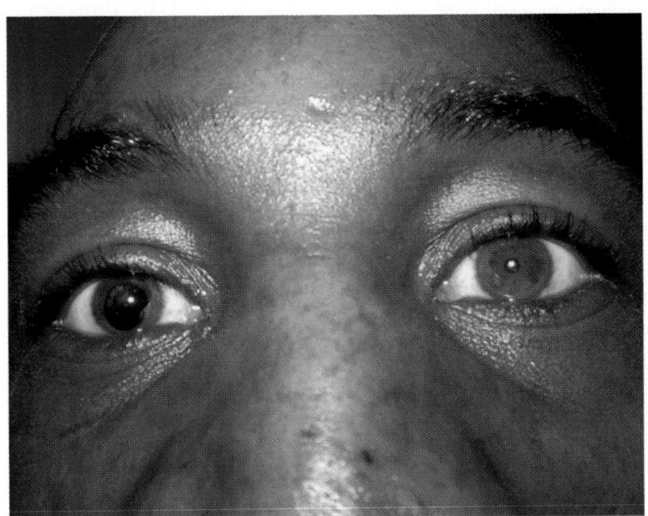

FIGURE 4–40 Anisocoria related to right-sided ocular trauma. (Courtesy of Michael Lucchesi, MD.)

Diagnosis

If the anisocoria is physiologic, the relative difference in pupillary size remains constant in both reduced light and bright light.[1] For example, if one pupil is measured at 4 mm and the other at 5 mm, the pupil sizes would be expected to retain the same respective percentage difference in both dim and bright light. Individuals with anisocoria demonstrate round, normal-appearing, and appropriately reactive pupils. Most cases of benign anisocoria involve pupillary differences of only about 1 mm and may be more apparent in reduced light than in normal room light.[1]

Clinical Complications

Complications involve misdiagnosis of intracranial or ocular disease.

Management

Specific treatment is unnecessary for physiologic anisocoria beyond confirming its physiologic nature (i.e., ruling out possible underlying pathology). Newly diagnosed anisocoria may indicate a serious ocular or intracranial disorder, and prompt ophthalmologic consultation is recommended.

REFERENCES

1. Kawasaki A, Kardon RH. Disorders of the pupil. *Ophthalmol Clin North Am* 2001;14:149–168.
2. Lin YC. Anisocoria from transdermal scopolamine. *Pediatr Anaesth* 2001;11:626–627.

Sympathetic Ophthalmia

David Fintak

Clinical Presentation

Patients with sympathetic ophthalmia (SO) present with bilateral eye pain, photophobia, decreased visual acuity, and red eyes.

Pathophysiology

SO is a rare, bilateral inflammatory reaction that develops weeks to months after penetrating injury to one eye. The incidence of SO is less than 1% in penetrating wounds and less than 1 in 10,000 surgically related penetrating wounds.[1] SO may be an autoimmune response to the normally sequestered uveal tissues that become exposed with eye injury. Although the specific antigens involved in SO have not been identified, cell-mediated immune responses have been implicated in some studies.[2] A penetrating wound, causing uveal prolapse, appears to be essential for SO development. This prolapse permits tolerated ocular antigens to reach dendritic antigen-presenting cells outside the eye, producing an immunogenic stimulus.[1]

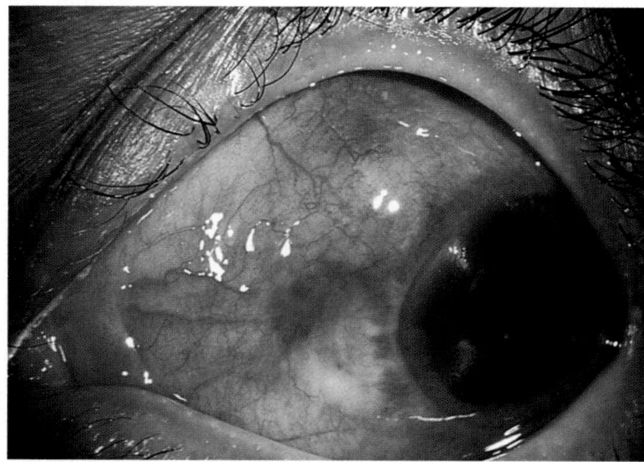

FIGURE 4–41 Sympathetic ophthalmia with scleral rupture, low-grade inflammation, and irregular healing. (From Tasman and Jaeger, with permission.)

Diagnosis

Most cases are clinically evident within 3 months, with the earliest reported cases occurring 9 days after injury.[1] Possible studies include a complete ophthalmic examination with a dilated retinal examination, complete blood count (CBC), rapid plasma reagin test (RPR), and angiotensin-converting enzyme concentration (if sarcoidosis is a consideration). A chest radiograph may also be considered to evaluate for tuberculosis or sarcoidosis. Fluorescein angiography or ultrasonography (or both) helps to confirm the diagnosis.[1,2] Any inflammation in the uninvolved eye should raise clinical suspicion of the diagnosis.

Clinical Complications

Poor visual acuity is associated with delayed or suboptimal treatment modalities. These patients require lifelong periodic checkups because of the possibility of recurrence.

Management

The risk of SO may be significantly reduced with enucleation of the injured eye before a sympathetic reaction can develop (usually within 7 to 14 days).

The objective of antiinflammatory treatment is to suppress the inflammatory response completely and as soon as possible. This may be accomplished with the use of topical, periocular, and systemic steroids. Steroids or immunosuppressive therapy should be maintained for 3 to 6 months after all signs of inflammation have resolved.

REFERENCES

1. Chan CC, Benezra D, Rodrigues MM, et al. Immunochemistry and electron microscopy of choroidal infiltrates and Dalen-Fuchs nodules in sympathetic ophthalmia. *Ophthalmology* 1985;92:580–590.
2. Gurdal C, Erdener U, Irkec M, Orhan M. Incidence of sympathetic ophthalmia after penetrating eye injury and choice of treatment. *Ocul Immunol Inflamm* 2002;10:223–227.

Pterygium

Colleen Campbell

Clinical Presentation

Pterygium is an overgrowth of vascularized conjunctiva or stroma on the sclera that extends over the cornea.

Patients may present with dry eyes or complaints regarding either the existence or the cosmetic appearance of a pterygium. An early pterygium may manifest as a localized chronic conjunctivitis.

Pathophysiology

Because pterygia occur most commonly in tropical climates, they are thought to be a response to excessive ultraviolet sunlight, although their appearance is often delayed by many years after the peak period of sun exposure. The risk of pterygium increases with increased age and outdoor occupations.[1,2] The more extensive the lesion, the more obvious the episcleral vascularity. The nasal aspect of the eye is most commonly affected. Pterygia may extend to the limbus, causing dry eyes as well. It is unclear whether a pterygium is simply an extension of a pinguecula or if it is a distinct entity.

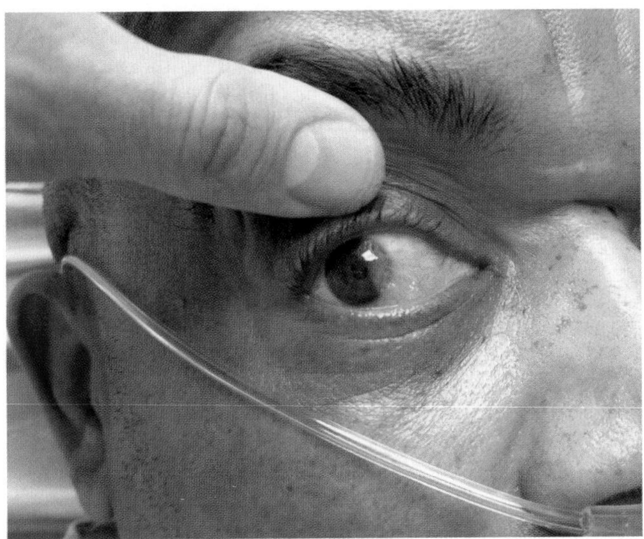

FIGURE 4–42 Right-sided pterygium. (Courtesy of Mark Silverberg, MD.)

Diagnosis

The diagnosis is made on the basis of physical examination. The pterygium appears as a wedge-shaped, fibrous growth on the cornea that is best seen on slit-lamp examination of the eye. Pterygia are graded according to the extent of episcleral vascularization.[2] The growth appears as connective tissue that grows over the margin of the iris. The overgrowth may appear opaque, fibrous, or yellowish on slit-lamp examination.[3]

Clinical Complications

Complications include postsurgical reoccurrence, astigmatisms, cosmetic deformities of the globe, diminution or loss of vision, dry eyes, and secondary infection or inflammation.[1,2]

Management

Pterygium does not require emergency treatment. Emergency department patients can be given a referral for outpatient ophthalmology follow-up. For patients with persistent irritation from a pterygium and those with invasion of the visual axis, surgery may be required. Incision with conjunctival autografting or combined with mitomycin C application has yielded good results, with recurrence rates of only about 10%.[2] Perioperative radiation or strontium has also been employed to reduce recurrences.[3]

REFERENCES

1. Gazzard G, Saw SM, Farook M, et al. Pterygium in Indonesia: prevalence, severity and risk factors. *Br J Ophthalmol* 2002;86:1341–1346.
2. Kammoun B, Kharrat W, Zouari K. Pterygium: surgical treatment. *J Fr Ophtalmol* 2001;24:823–828.
3. Scheiderman H. What is your diagnosis?: sharpen your diagnostic skills. *Consultant* 2002;42:210–212.

Entropion

Michael Greenberg

Clinical Presentation

Patients with entropion may present with the sensation of an ocular foreign body, eye pain, or irritation. The pain may be relieved by manually pulling the lid away from the eye.[1]

Pathophysiology

Five categories of entropion have been identified: congenital, acute spastic, involutional, mechanical, and cicatricial.[1] Involutional entropion is the most common form; it is caused primarily by age-related changes and increased laxity in the tissues surrounding the eye. Congenital entropion is the rarest form and may be caused by "disinsertion of the eyelid retractors."[1] Acute spastic entropion is a transient condition caused by blepharospasm, usually after ocular surgery. Mechanical entropion is often caused by morbid obesity and is a common form of entropion found in the Asian population. Cicatricial entropion is associated with a variety of diseases, including trachoma, Stevens-Johnson syndrome, ocular cicatricial pemphigoid, and chemical injuries, as well as the prolonged use of certain topical ocular medications.[1]

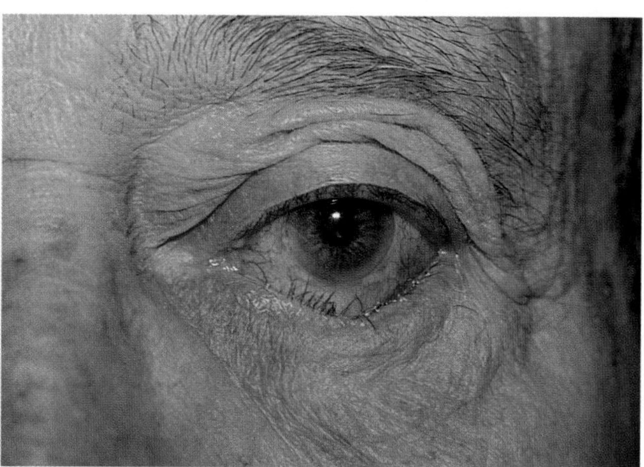

FIGURE 4–43 Involutional entropion. (From Tasman and Jaeger, with permission.)

Diagnosis

The diagnosis is based on visual identification of the entropion.

Clinical Complications

Complications include epithelial breakdown of the cornea, corneal ulcers (CUs), corneal scar formation, and decreased visual acuity.[1]

Management

Definitive treatment for entropion depends on the specific cause. In most cases, no special treatment in the emergency department (ED) is necessary except arranging ophthalmology follow-up. The provision of artificial tears for ocular lubrication and the removal of eyelashes that are irritating the ocular surface may be necessary in the ED.

REFERENCES

1. Choo PH. Distichiasis, trichiasis and entropion: advances in management. *Int Ophthalmol Clin* 2002;42:75–87.

Closed-Angle Glaucoma

Nick Gorton

Clinical Presentation

Patients with closed-angle glaucoma (CAG) may present with acute onset of monocular pain, red eye, mid-dilated pupil, photophobia, nausea, vomiting, and visual changes such as blurred vision or seeing halos or starbursts around lights. CAG may occur in patients with few or only one of these symptoms. A nonspecific headache may be the only presenting symptom.[1–3]

Pathophysiology

Numerous anatomic and physiologic variants predispose to the final common pathway, which is disruption of aqueous humor outflow through the canal of Schlemm. The majority of cases are caused by pupillary block.[2] Angle closure is more commonly seen in patients 55 years of age or older and may indicate an age-related decline in the depth of the anterior chamber. Patients of Asian descent, women with hyperopia, and patients with a positive family history are at greater risk for development of CAG.[1,3]

Diagnosis

Intraocular pressure (IOP) should be measured in both eyes by applanation tonometry, a Shiotz tonometer, or a TonoPen. Normal IOP is between 10 and 22 mm Hg. Typically, IOP rises to 40 mm Hg or more with acute attacks of CAG.[2]

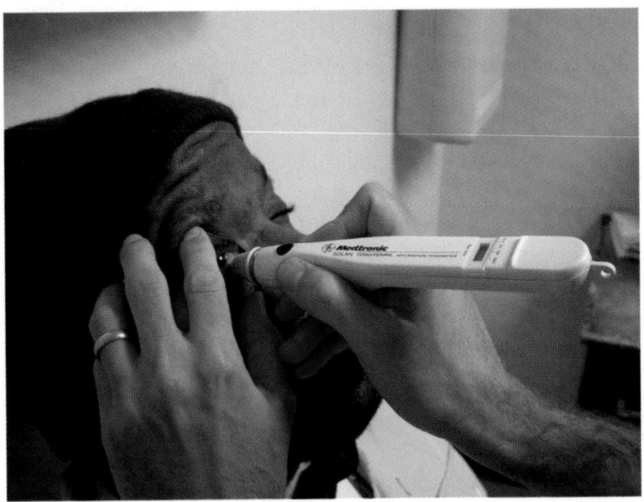

FIGURE 4–44 Glaucoma can be diagnosed with the use of various devices, including the TonoPen seen here. (Courtesy of Mark Silverberg, MD.)

Clinical Complications

Irreversible blindness may result in severe or untreated cases.

Management

Strategies to acutely decrease IOP use three mechanisms: decreasing the production of aqueous humor, reestablishing the outflow of aqueous humor through the canal of Schlemm, and decreasing the volume of the existing aqueous humor through osmotic shifts. Decreasing the production of aqueous humor is accomplished through the use of topical β-adrenergic blockers (e.g., timolol 0.5%), topical α-adrenergic agonists (e.g., apraclonidine 1%, brimonidine 0.2%), and oral carbonic anhydrase inhibitors (acetazolamide 500 mg initially). Reestablishing the outflow through the canal of Schlemm is accomplished through the use of a topical mydriatic. Generating osmotic shifts to decrease the volume of existing aqueous humor may be accomplished with oral glycerol or isosorbide or with intravenous mannitol. A reasonable initial approach after calling an ophthalmologist is to instill 1 drop each of 0.5% timolol, 1% apraclonidine, and 2% pilocarpine into the affected eye, waiting 1 minute between drops. Patients should receive acetazolamide by mouth. IOP should be reassessed every 15 to 30 minutes. If the IOP has not fallen to less than 35 mm Hg after 30 minutes, timolol, apraclonidine, and pilocarpine drops should be repeated and an osmotic agent should be started.[2]

REFERENCES

1. Tello C, Rothman R, Ishikawa H, Ritch R. Differential diagnosis of the angle-closure glaucomas. *Ophthalmol Clin North Am* 2000;13:443–453.
2. Ritch R. Directed therapy for specific glaucomas. *Ophthalmol Clin North Am* 2000;13:429–441.
3. Coleman AL. Glaucoma. *Lancet* 1999;354:1803–1810.

Marcus Gunn Pupil

Rachel Haroz

Clinical Presentation

Patients with Marcus Gunn pupil (MGP) may present with a wide variety of ocular symptoms, including loss of vision, decreased vision, visual field defects, dimming, loss of color vision, and diplopia.[1] A light stimulus, rather than causing both pupils to constrict, elicits bilateral pupil constriction if shone into the unaffected eye and no constriction bilaterally if shone into the affected eye. Depending on the extent of the defect, the constriction may be partial or absent.

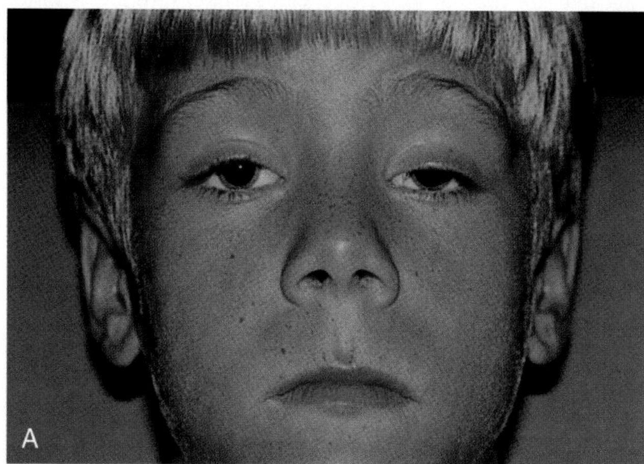

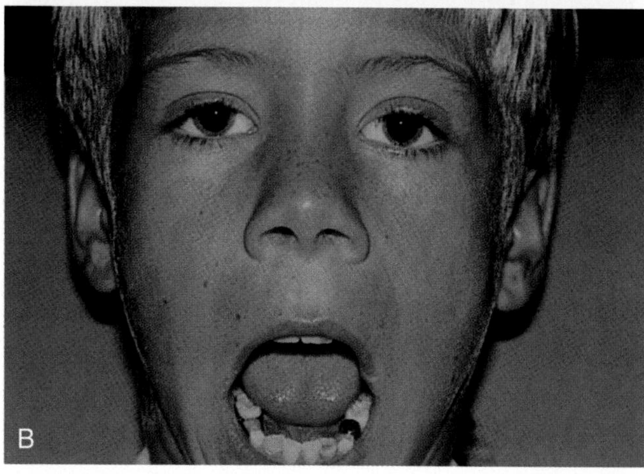

FIGURE 4-45 **A:** Marcus Gunn jaw winking, showing ptosis of the left eye at rest. **B:** Marcus Gunn jaw winking; lid elevates with jaw movement, reflecting synkinesis between pterygoid and levator muscles. (From Tasman and Jaeger, with permission.)

Pathophysiology

MGP involves a relative afferent pupillary defect caused by interference with light transmission into the pupillomotor system. The defect indicates injury in the afferent limb of the pupillary reflex, between the pretectal nucleus and the retina. The defect may be located in the retina, optic nerve, chiasm, optic tract, or midbrain.[2]

Diagnosis

Diagnosis of MGP requires performing an alternating light test (a so-called "swinging flashlight" test). This test involves directing a bright light source into one pupil for 3 seconds and then rapidly swinging it to the other pupil for 2 to 4 seconds. This should be repeated several times without variation of distance, time, or speed. The final diameter and speed of constriction should be measured. In a positive test, the unaffected pupil appears to dilate when the light is shone into the affected eye, due to a relative decrease in light intensity.[3]

Clinical Complications

Differential causes for MGP include retinal vein occlusion, retinal artery occlusion, optic tract lesion, intraocular hemorrhage, optic neuropathy, central serous retinopathy, chiasmal compression, optic neuritis, midbrain lesion, postgeniculate damage, and retinal detachment (RD).[2]

Management

MGP may indicate concerning underlying pathology. This should be further investigated with radiologic modalities such as computed tomography (CT) and magnetic resonance imaging (MRI). Ophthalmology and neurology consultations may be indicated. Treatment depends on the specific underlying clinical problem.

REFERENCES

1. Murtha T, Stasheff SF. Visual dysfunction in retinal and optic nerve disease. *Neurol Clin* 2003;21:445–481.
2. Kawasaki A, Kardon RH. Disorders of the pupil. *Ophthalmol Clin North Am* 2001;14:149–168.
3. Girkin CA. Evaluation of the pupillary light response as an objective measure of visual function. *Ophthalmol Clin North Am* 2003;16:143–153.

Retinoblastoma

Gregory P. Conners

Clinical Presentation

Retinoblastoma is usually seen in children younger than 5 years of age (average age at diagnosis, 18 months) and typically manifests with strabismus or decreased visual acuity.[1-3]

Pathophysiology

Two forms of retinoblastoma have been identified; both are caused by the loss of function of both alleles of the cancer-preventing *Rb* gene.[2] The nonfamilial (noninheritable) form is caused by a somatic mutation in one cell, which then proliferates. This is typically a single, unilateral tumor. The familial (inheritable) form is caused by an inborn inactivation of one of the alleles, leading to a propensity to develop retinoblastoma and other tumors. These tumors are often bilateral (85%) and multifocal.[2]

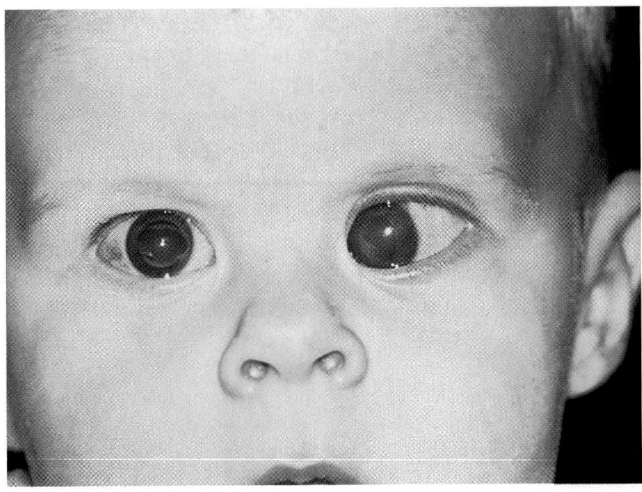

FIGURE 4–46 External photograph showing glaucoma caused by retinoblastoma. (From Tasman and Jaeger, with permission.)

Diagnosis

A white papillary reflex (leukocoria), also called a "cat's eyes" reflex, is a common finding. Diagnosis is based on the physical examination and confirmed with computed tomography (CT), ultrasonography, or magnetic resonance imaging (MRI). Genetic blood testing exists but is currently unreliable.[2] Such tumors occasionally simulate an inflammatory condition such as orbital cellulitis, but these unusual presentations are more common in older children.[1]

Clinical Complications

Retinoblastoma was at one time uniformly fatal, but survival rates in the United States currently exceed 90%.[1,2] Blindness may occur due to enucleation or the effects of the tumor or its treatment. Second tumors are often found in patients with familial retinoblastoma. Because the familial form has an autosomal dominant inheritance pattern, family members should be counseled.[2]

Management

Combinations of chemotherapy, cryotherapy, thermotherapy, laser photocoagulation, and radiotherapy are used to avoid enucleation surgery if possible.[2,3] Enucleation remains a mainstay treatment for severe forms of retinoblastoma.[3] If the disease is metastatic, autologous bone marrow transplantation may be required after chemotherapy.[3]

REFERENCES

1. Tsai T, O'Brien JM. Masquerade syndromes: malignancies mimicking inflammation in the eye. *Int Ophthalmol Clin* 2002;42:115–131.
2. Castillo BV Jr, Kaufman L. Pediatric tumors of the eye and orbit. *Pediatr Clin North Am* 2003;50:149–172.
3. DePotter P. Current treatment of retinoblastoma. *Curr Opin Ophthalmol* 2002;13:331–336.

Xanthelasma Palpebrarum

Michael Greenberg

Clinical Presentation

Xanthelasma palpebrarum (XP) is seen in middle-aged and older individuals who are concerned about yellowish, plaque-like lesions on the upper eyelids.

Pathophysiology

XP may be a marker for hyperlipidemia, because at least 50% of patients with XP are expected to have elevated blood lipids.[1] XP lesions consist of xanthoma cells that are actually lipid-containing histiocytes.[1] These cells may accumulate in the superficial layers of the dermis in "perivascular and periadnexal locations" and are associated with inflammation and fibrosis.[1] XP lesions are most frequently associated with familial dysproteinemia type IIa.[1] Xanthomas involving extensor tendons and AS may also be associated with XP lesions.[1] XP lesions in persons younger than 40 years of age carry an increased probability of associated familial hypercholesterolemia.[1]

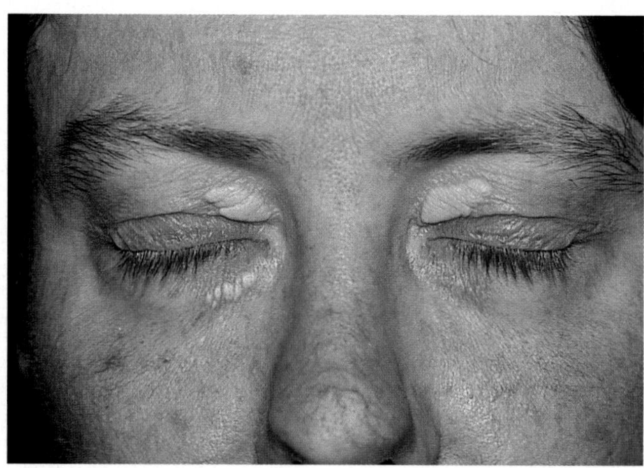

FIGURE 4–47 Creamy yellow plaques in the dermis of all four lids, typical of xanthelasma. (From Tasman and Jaeger, with permission.)

Diagnosis

The diagnosis is based on the physical examination and identification of the typical lesions.

Clinical Complications

If XP lesions enlarge substantially, they can cause mechanical interference with normal vision. However, short of this eventuality, there are no complications related to XP lesions *per se* beyond issues of cosmesis. XP lesions may reoccur (40% to 60% of cases) despite the modality chosen for cosmetic removal.

Management

No specific therapy is indicated in the emergency department. Patients should be referred to their primary care provider for assessment of their lipid profile. Patients who are concerned about cosmesis may be referred to a facial plastic surgeon or dermatologist, who may excise the lesions or perform laser ablation.[1] In the past, some surgeons applied dichloroacetic or trichloroacetic acid to dissolve the lesions; however, this is mentioned simply to discourage emergency physicians from providing any such primary cosmetic therapy.[1]

REFERENCES

1. Rohrich RJ, Janis JE, Pownell PH. Xanthelasma palpebrarum: a review and current management principles. *Plast Reconstr Surg* 2002;110:1310–1314.

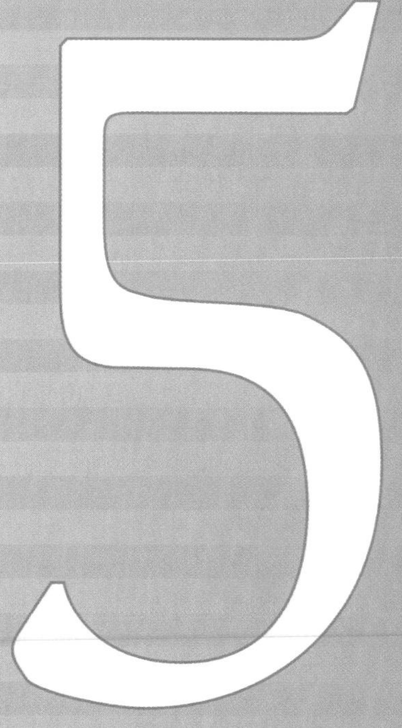

Ear, Nose, and Throat

Sinusitis

Matthew Spencer

Clinical Presentation

Acute sinusitis consists of persistent purulent nasal discharge, cough, unilateral facial pain and fullness, fever, nasal congestion, maxillary or periorbital swelling, and headache.[1] Patients who are ill-appearing, with a fever of at least 39°C and purulent nasal discharge for 3 to 4 days, are considered to be more severely affected.[1] On physical examination, there is often sinus tenderness and opacification of the affected sinus with transillumination, but these findings are considered unreliable.[2]

Pathophysiology

Sinusitis is a bacterial infection of the paranasal sinuses. Sinusitis is classified as acute, subacute, or chronic, based on the duration of symptoms. Sinusitis is acute if the infection has been present for less than 4 weeks.[1,3] In subacute sinusitis, symptoms have been present for 1 to 3 months. Sinusitis is considered to be chronic if symptoms have been present for longer than 3 months.[1] Sinusitis develops when there is inflammation of the paranasal sinus mucosa, usually secondary to allergies or viral infection. Inflammation leads to mucosal edema, excessive mucus production, decreased fluid clearance, and then bacterial overgrowth.[1,2,4] Bacterial overgrowth usually consists of the normal respiratory flora, with *Streptococcus pneumoniae* present in 30% to 66% of cases, *Haemophilus influenzae* in 20% to 30%, *Moraxella catarrhalis* in 12% to 30%, and *Streptococcus pyogenes* in 3% to 7%.[1,2,4] Fungal organisms occasionally are the etiologic cause of acute sinusitis in diabetics and patients with other types of immunocompromise.[2,4]

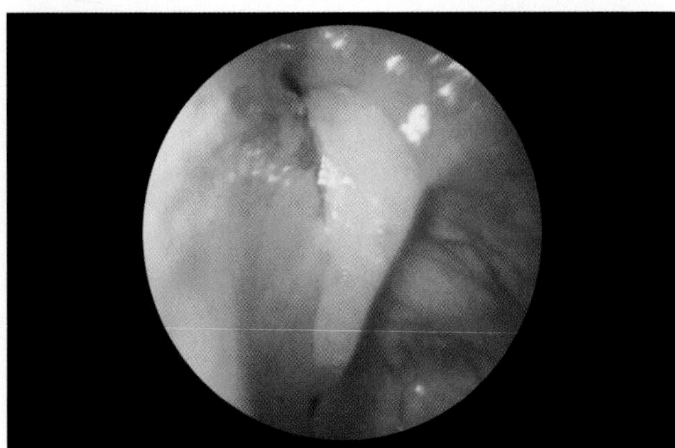

FIGURE 5–1 Accessory maxillary sinus ostium with purulent drainage. (From Benjamin, with permission.)

Diagnosis

Acute sinusitis usually is a clinical diagnosis. However, the gold standard requires needle aspiration of the maxillary sinus, although this procedure is not usually performed in the emergency department.[1]

Various clinical criteria may differentiate bacterial from viral sinusitis. Some consider purulent nasal discharge and cough that persists for 10 to 14 days, with a history of preceding upper respiratory tract infection, to be diagnostic.[1] Others use a combination of major and minor clinical criteria. Major criteria are facial pain or pressure, facial fullness, nasal obstruction, purulent nasal discharge, decreased sense of smell, and fever.[2] Minor criteria are headache, halitosis, fatigue, dental pain, cough, ear pain, ear pressure, and ear fullness.[2] The presence of any two major criteria or one major plus two minor criteria is considered diagnostic.[2] Another group found four clinical criteria that correlated significantly with computed tomography (CT)-confirmed sinusitis: acute worsening of symptoms after some improvement, a history of purulent nasal secretions, purulent nasal secretions present on examination, and an elevated erythrocyte sedimentation rate (ESR).[2-4] None of these methods is perfect, but the diagnosis is highly likely if symptoms have persisted for longer than 10 days with an acute worsening at some time during this period, if purulent nasal secretions are present, if there has been no response to decongestants, or if fever or other severe symptoms are present.[4]

Plain radiographs are not considered to be of value in most patients with possible sinusitis, and CT has been shown to overdiagnose the disease.[4] However, despite the risk of overdiagnosis, CT is the radiographic modality of choice; it should be used primarily for patients in whom the diagnosis is uncertain, for those with suspected orbital or intracranial complications, for those with no response to adequate therapy, and to define anatomy in preparation for surgery.[1,2,4]

Clinical Complications

The complications of acute sinusitis are brain abscess, orbital or periorbital cellulitis, orbital abscess, subperiosteal abscess, osteomyelitis, and meningitis.[2,4]

Sinusitis

Matthew Spencer

Management

Treatment consists of antibiotics, decongestants, and symptomatic therapies. First-line antibiotics should be inexpensive, with high-dose amoxicillin the drug of choice and trimethoprim-sulfamethoxazole, azithromycin, and clarithromycin possible agents for penicillin-allergic patients.[1,2,4] Common second-line agents are amoxicillin/clavulanate, cefpodoxime, cefuroxime, cefdinir, cefprozil, and the fluoroquinolones.[1,2,4] All antibiotics should be continued for 10 to 14 days.[1] Patients with complications, frequent recurrences, or treatment failures should be referred to an ear, nose, and throat (ENT) specialist.[2,4]

REFERENCES

1. Conrad DA, Jenson HB. Management of acute bacterial rhinosinusitis. *Curr Opin Pediatr* 2002;14:86–90.
2. Brook I, Gooch WM 3rd, Jenkins SG, et al. Medical management of acute bacterial sinusitis: recommendations of a clinical advisory committee on pediatric and adult sinusitis. *Ann Otol Rhinol Laryngol Suppl* 2000;182:2–20.
3. Lindbaek M, Hjortdahl P. The clinical diagnosis of acute purulent sinusitis in general practice: a review. *Br J Gen Pract* 2002;52:491–495.
4. Poole MD. A focus on acute sinusitis in adults: changes in disease management. *Am J Med* 1999;106:38S–47S.

Allergic Rhinitis

Andrew Gorlin

Clinical Presentation

In the acute phase (within 5 minutes after exposure to the allergen), allergic rhinitis manifests as sneezing, nasal itching, and watery rhinorrhea. During the late phase (4 to 8 hours after exposure), the main symptom of allergic rhinitis is nasal congestion.[1,2] Chronic allergic rhinitis results in postnasal drip with chronic cough, headache, nasal voice, and systemic symptoms such as malaise, irritability, and decreased appetite.[2] On physical examination, a boggy, pale-blue nasal mucosa, clear secretions, and swollen turbinates are found. More subtle symptoms include the "allergic salute," in which the patient repetitively rubs his nose upward with his palm, and the resultant "allergic crease," a transverse skin line below the bridge of the nose.[1]

Pathophysiology

Seasonal allergic rhinitis is caused by airborne allergens released by seasonal vegetation such as ragweed, grass, and tree pollen. Perennial allergic rhinitis results from exposure to allergens such as animal dander, molds, and dust. Regardless of the type of allergen, the precipitating event is immunoglobulin E binding of the allergen, with subsequent mast cell and basophil activation. Activated mast cells and basophils in the nasal mucosa release histamine, leukotrienes, prostaglandins, and other inflammatory mediators that cause local edema, increased mucus secretion, and cellular infiltration.[2]

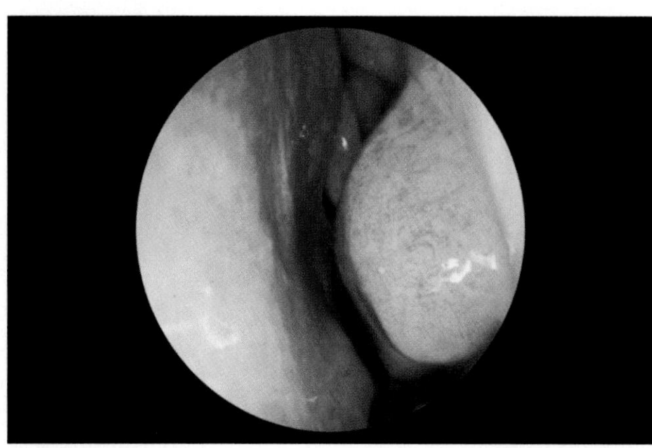

FIGURE 5–2 This swollen, bluish, left inferior turbinate is pathognomonic for allergic rhinitis. (From Benjamin, with permission.)

Diagnosis

The history and physical examination are key to the diagnosis of allergic rhinitis. Eosinophilia identified on a nasal smear can aid diagnosis; a positive smear is defined as greater than 10% eosinophils (normal, 2% to 3%). Definitive diagnosis requires skin testing.[1]

Clinical Complications

Common sequelae include otitis media (OM) and sinusitis secondary to obstruction of the eustachian tube and sinus ostia, respectively. Other sequelae include decreased olfaction and taste, snoring, sleep apnea, and, in developing children, facial abnormalities such as high-arched palate and dental malocclusion due to chronic mouth breathing.

Management

Allergic rhinitis is managed in the outpatient setting. Removal of the inciting allergen and use of allergen-proof products in the home is an important first step in treatment. Oral antihistamines, topical corticosteroids, and oral and topical α-adrenergic agents are the mainstays of pharmacologic therapy. Severe refractory cases may be treated with immunotherapy.[1,2]

REFERENCES

1. McNamara RM. Approach to rhinitis. *Emerg Med Clin North Am* 1987;5:279–292.
2. Berger WE. Overview of allergic rhinitis. *Ann Allergy Asthma Immunol* 2003;90[6 Suppl 3]:7–12.

Viral Rhinitis

Andrew Gorlin

Clinical Presentation

Patients with viral rhinitis, also known as the "common cold," present with rhinorrhea, sneezing, nasal congestion, sore throat, and low-grade fever.

Pathophysiology

Human rhinovirus causes more than 50% of cases of viral rhinitis, followed by coronavirus (20%), influenza, adenovirus, and respiratory syncytial virus.[1–3] Infection starts with local invasion of the epithelial surface of the nasal mucosa. Viral replication ensues, with cell death and subsequent viral spread. Infection triggers the cellular release of cytokines and chemotactic factors, resulting in local edema, mucus secretion, and influx of neutrophils and lymphocytes.[2,3]

Diagnosis

The history and physical examination usually are sufficient to diagnose viral rhinitis. Diagnostic testing is rarely indicated. A nasal smear may distinguish viral rhinitis from allergic rhinitis by the lack of eosinophilia. Viral culture can provide a definitive diagnosis.[1] Physical examination findings include a red, edematous nasal mucosa, with nasal secretions varying from watery and clear to thick and mucoid. Patients also may have injected conjunctivae and oropharynx, as well as sinus tenderness. The condition is self-limited, with symptoms usually peaking 2 to 4 days after viral inoculation.[1]

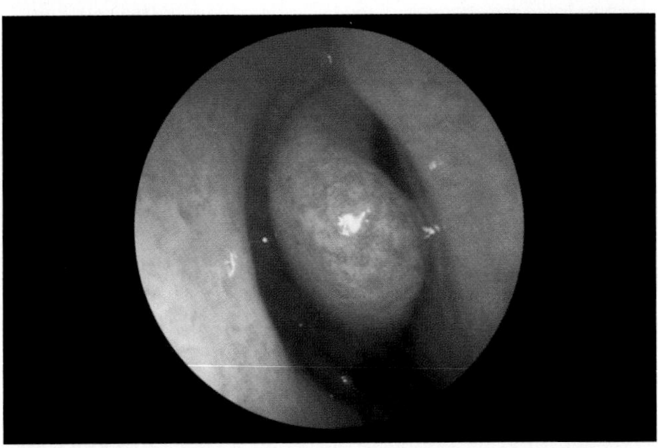

FIGURE 5–3 During the prodromal phase of acute viral rhinitis, the mucous membranes lining the nasal cavity are reddened, the nose is often abnormally patent, and the patient usually complains of an itching or burning inside the nose. (From Benjamin, with permission.)

Clinical Complications

The most frequent complication of viral rhinitis is bacterial sinusitis, which occurs secondary to inflammatory obstruction of the sinus ostia. Bacterial superinfection of the nasal mucosa may also occur. Streptococcal species are noted to be the predominate bacteria in these conditions.[1]

Management

Most cases of viral rhinitis are mild and self-limited and can be managed in the outpatient setting. Hand washing and basic hygiene are sensible preventative measures. Oral and topical α-adrenergic agents are the most commonly used agents for symptomatic relief. Topical steroids are also effective, but they are not universally recommended because of potential immunosuppression. There is no role for antihistamines in viral rhinitis. Antibiotics are indicated only for secondary bacterial infections.[1,2]

REFERENCES

1. McNamara RM. Approach to rhinitis. *Emerg Med Clin North Am* 1987;5:279–292.
2. Winther B, Gwaltney JM Jr, Mygind N, Hendley JO. Viral-induced rhinitis. *Am J Rhinol* 1998;12:17–20.
3. van Cauwenberge P, Ingels K. Effects of viral and bacterial infection on nasal and sinus mucosa. *Acta Otolaryngol* 1996;116:316–321.

Anterior Epistaxis

Matthew Spencer

Clinical Presentation

Patients with anterior epistaxis (AE) present with bleeding from one or both nostrils. AE is more common in younger patients but can be seen in all age groups. The bleeding is usually less profuse than in posterior epistaxis, and a source is often visible on the nasal septum.

Pathophysiology

AE originates from Kiesselbach's plexus, an area of convergence of multiple blood vessels located on the anterior of the nasal septum.[1,2] Bleeding has been associated with various causes, including low humidity, trauma, inflammation, allergies, hypertension, coagulation abnormalities, and anticoagulant or antiplatelet medications.[2] Most adult cases are idiopathic, whereas those in children usually are caused by digital trauma.[2,3]

Diagnosis

The diagnosis of AE is clinical. However, it is difficult to distinguish posterior epistaxis from AE; severity of bleeding, lack of response to initial treatment modalities, and quantity of blood in the oropharynx should be considered.[3]

Clinical Complications

Complications include persistent bleeding, hypotension, septal perforation, sinusitis, otitis media (OM), staphylococcal toxic shock syndrome, dislodgement of the packing material, aspiration of secretions, and hypoxia.[1,2]

Management

Initial treatment includes digital pressure to the nose.[2,3] If direct pressure succeeds but a point source is not identified, the patient is observed for 60 minutes for rebleeding and discharged with instructions to use saline nasal spray three times per day and to apply a petroleum-based antibiotic ointment daily. A point source of bleeding should be identified for cautery, if possible.[1]

If bleeding persists, the nose should be packed. Use of packing soaked with agents such as oxymetazoline 0.5%, phenylephrine HCl 1%, pseudoephedrine, or epinephrine (1:10,000), plus either lidocaine 2% to 4% or Pontocaine (tetracaine), is approriate.[1,2] Cocaine 4% may be used, because it is both an anesthetic and a vasoconstrictor.[1-3] If an anterior source is identified after the nasal mucosa is anesthetized, it should be cauterized with silver nitrate.[1-3] One should never cauterize both sides of the nasal septum, because this may lead to a perforation.

If anterior nasal packing successfully stops the bleeding, it should be left in place for 2 to 3 days, the patient should be prescribed oral antibiotics to cover staphylococcal and streptococcal species, and follow-up should be arranged within 1 to 3 days.[1,2] If anterior nasal packing is unsuccessful, then a posterior source should be suspected.

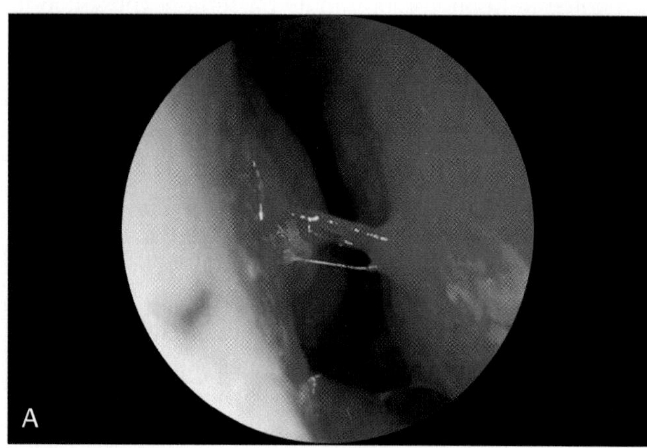

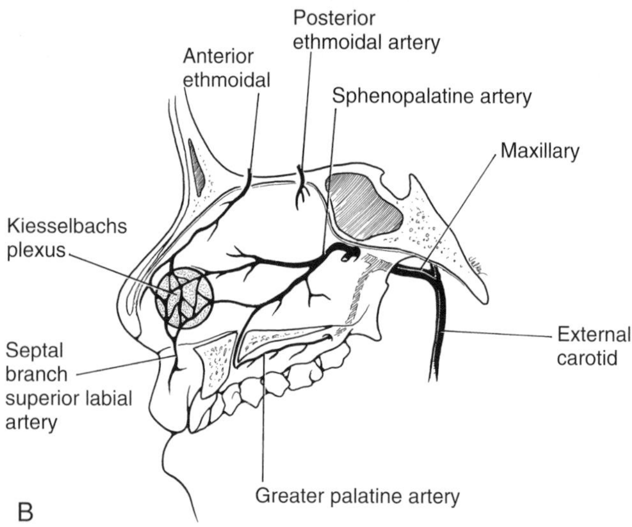

FIGURE 5–4 **A:** Anterior-nasal-septum with active bleeding. (From Benjamin, with permission.) **B:** Note location of Kiesselbach's plexus, the most common site of anterior bleeding. (From Cotton, with permission.)

REFERENCES

1. Tan LK, Calhoun KH. Epistaxis. *Med Clin North Am* 1999;83:43–56.
2. Pashen D, Stevens M. Management of epistaxis in general practice. *Aust Fam Physician* 2002;31:717–721.
3. Chopra R. Epistaxis: a review. *J R Soc Health* 2000;120:31–33.

Posterior Epistaxis

Matthew Spencer

Clinical Presentation

Patients with posterior epistaxis present with profuse bleeding from one or both nostrils, with the large amount of swallowed blood and blood visible in oropharynx.[1-3] In one study, 88% of clinicians reported the bleeding as moderate or severe.[3] Occasionally, brisk anterior nosebleeds produce similar findings.

Pathophysiology

Posterior epistaxis is bleeding that originates from the posterior nasopharynx, usually the sphenopalatine artery or Woodruff's plexus. Epistaxis may result from damage to the nasal epithelium caused by a variety of factors, including low humidity, trauma, inflammation, allergies, hypertension, bleeding abnormalities, and anticoagulant or antiplatelet medications.[2-4]

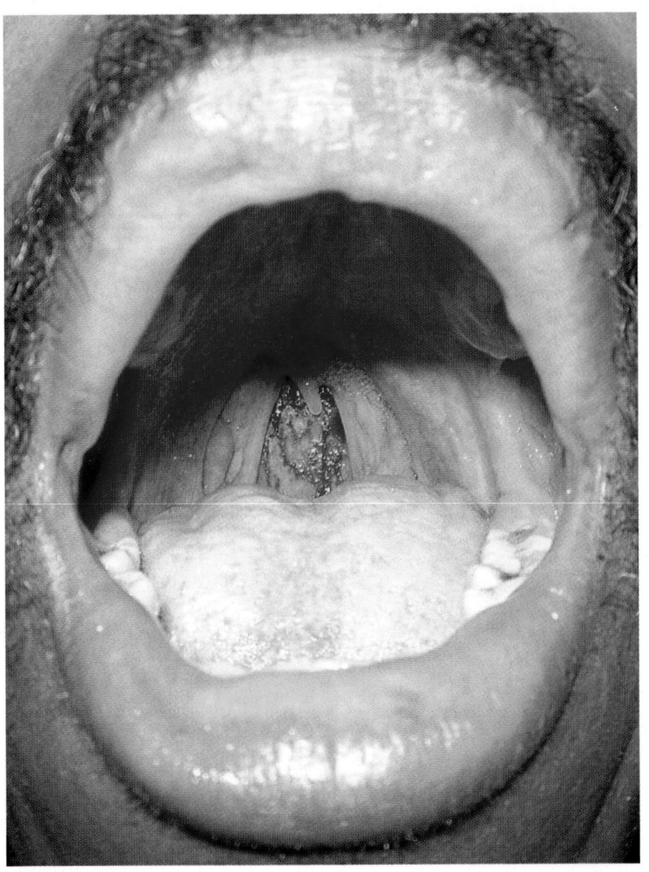

FIGURE 5–5 Active bleeding from the posterior septum is visible in the posterior pharynx. (Courtesy of Mark Silverberg, MD.)

Diagnosis

The diagnosis is clinical. However, it is difficult to distinguish posterior epistaxis from AE; the severity of bleeding, lack of response to initial treatment modalities, and quantity of blood in the oropharynx must all be taken into consideration.[3]

Clinical Complications

Common complications include persistent bleeding, hypotension, and aspiration of blood.[2] Cauterization can cause pain or septal perforation. Complications from posterior nasal packing include sinusitis, otitis media (OM), nasal trauma, bradycardia, hypotension, hypoxia, apnea, and aspiration.[1-3]

Management

Initial treatment includes digital pressure, cotton or tissue packing, having the patient lean forward so that the blood runs out of the mouth instead of down the throat, and cold compresses to the bridge of the nose.[2,5] If a posterior source is suspected, posterior nasal packing must be performed as quickly as possible. One method is to insert a Foley catheter through the nostril into the oropharynx, inflate the balloon, and then withdraw the catheter to exert pressure from the balloon against the choana.[1] Other catheters are available for this purpose, such as balloon catheters made by Brighton and Simpson (West Sussex, U.K.) that are specifically designed for posterior nasal packing.[2,4] These patients should all be admitted to the intensive care unit (ICU) for sedation, intravenous fluid therapy, and oxygen administration, because the complications from posterior nasal packing are severe. The packing material must be left in place for 48 to 72 hours.[3] Emergency, on-site consultation with an otolaryngologist must be obtained in all cases of posterior bleeding.[1,2,4]

REFERENCES

1. Sparacino LL. Epistaxis management: what's new and what's noteworthy. *Lippincott's Prim Care Pract* 2000;4:498–507.
2. Tan LK, Calhoun KH. Epistaxis. *Med Clin North Am* 1999;83:43–56.
3. Viducich RA, Blanda MP, Gerson LW. Posterior epistaxis: clinical features and acute complications. *Ann Emerg Med* 1995;25:592–596.
4. Chopra R. Epistaxis: a review. *J R Soc Health* 2000;120:31–33.

Zygomatic Arch Fracture

Matthew Spencer

Clinical Presentation

Patients with zygomatic arch fracture present with a history of facial trauma, trismus, facial ecchymosis, and edema. In many cases, facial asymmetry due to flattening of the malar eminence and tenderness over the zygoma are clearly present.[1,2] Isolated arch fractures often produce only severe swelling and pain; without radiographic studies, the condition may not be apparent for up to 1 week, after local swelling has diminished.[1] If there is associated diplopia, enophthalmos, ptosis, or infraorbital nerve hypoesthesia or anesthesia, a zygomaticomaxillary (ZMC) fracture should be suspected.[1,3]

Pathophysiology

Zygomatic arch fractures result from trauma, most commonly secondary to motor vehicle collisions, assaults, or athletics.[2] Zygomatic fractures are the third most common facial fractures.[2] ZMC fractures, which are more common than isolated arch fractures, involve the body of the zygoma, orbital floor, and maxillary sinus wall.[1,2]

Diagnosis

The diagnosis should be suspected if a patient presents with a history of facial trauma and a characteristic clinical examination. However, the diagnosis must be confirmed radiographically. A Waters view and a submentovertex (SMV) view usually are adequate to diagnose an isolated zygomatic arch fracture, but if more extensive fractures are suspected, axial and coronal computed tomography (CT) with 2- to 3-mm cuts is necessary.[1,2]

Clinical Complications

Complications resulting from isolated zygomatic arch fractures are usually cosmetic; the more complicated ZMC fractures commonly result in ocular injury, infraorbital nerve dysfunction, sinusitis, malar asymmetry, and persistent enophthalmos and diplopia.[2,4]

Management

The treatment in the emergency department consists of analgesics, ice packs to reduce swelling, and prompt consultation with an otolaryngologist or plastic or oral surgeon, because these fractures usually are repaired by open reduction and internal fixation.[2,3] Fracture reduction does not have to be immediate; it may be delayed 4 to 7 days to allow the edema to subside.[2]

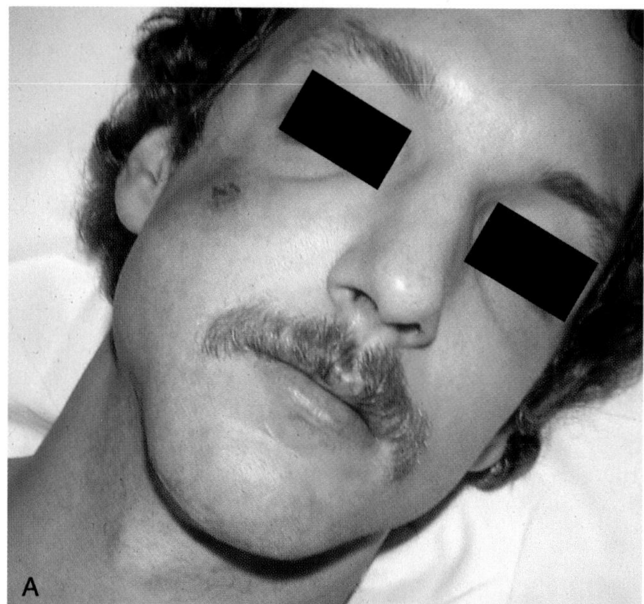

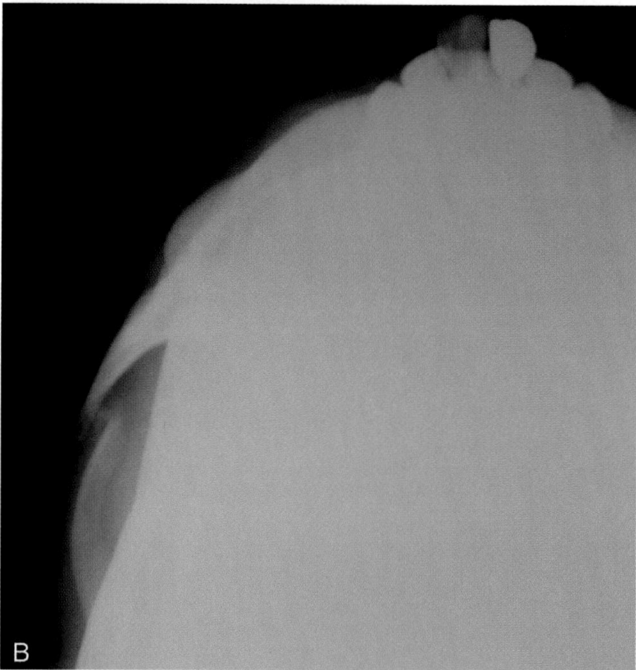

FIGURE 5-6 **A:** Facial depression indicative of zygomatic arch fracture. (Courtesy of Michael Greenberg, MD.) **B:** X-ray film showing "jug-handle" view of zygomatic arch. (Courtesy of Mark Silverberg, MD.)

REFERENCES

1. Ellis E III, Scott K. Assessment of patients with facial fractures. *Emerg Med Clin North Am* 2000;18:411–448.
2. Carithers JS, Koch BB. Evaluation and management of facial fractures. *Am Fam Physician* 1997;55:2675–2682.
3. Greenberg AM. Management of facial fractures. *N Y State Dent J* 1998;64:42–47.
4. Zingg M, Laedrach K, Chen J, et al. Classification and treatment of zygomatic fractures: a review of 1,025 cases. *J Oral Maxillofac Surg* 1992;50:778–790.

Orbital Floor Fracture

Matthew Spencer

Clinical Presentation

Patients with orbital floor fracture present after facial trauma with periorbital edema and ecchymosis associated with tenderness to palpation along the inferior orbital rim.[2–4] Subconjunctival hemorrhage, enophthalmos, or a palpable step-off of the orbital rim may also be present.[1–4] Diplopia may be present, or the patient may experience limited globe mobility if entrapment of one or more of the extraocular muscles also exists.[3]

Pathophysiology

Orbital floor fractures are more common in adults and are seen in 10% of head injuries.[1–3] The classic "blowout fracture" is hypothesized to result from a hard object striking the orbit anteriorly and pushing its contents backward, leading to increased intraorbital pressure and a break in the weakest portion of the bony orbit, the medial floor.[3,4]

Diagnosis

The diagnosis should be suspected in the setting of trauma with periorbital edema and tenderness, and it is more likely if entrapment is clinically evident. The Waters view of facial plain films often reveals such a fracture or shows a "teardrop sign." The diagnostic modality of choice is the orbital computed tomography (CT).[1–4]

Clinical Complications

Complications include infraorbital anesthesia, ptosis or pseudoptosis, diplopia, lacrimal duct injury, medial and lateral canthus injuries, and corneal abrasions or lacerations. More severe injuries associated with orbital floor fractures are hyphema, retinal hemorrhages, retrobulbar and vitreous hemorrhages, globe displacement or injury, glaucoma, and blindness.[1,3]

Management

The mainstay of therapy in the emergency department is analgesics, ice to reduce swelling, and consultation with an ophthalmologist; ear, nose, and throat (ENT); or plastic surgery specialist. Treatment in both adults and children is controversial and varies depending on the consultant. Antibiotic therapy is controversial with these injuries and should be considered in the consultations.[4]

REFERENCES

1. McDonald WS, Thaller SR. Priorities in the treatment of facial fractures for the millennium. *J Craniofac Surg* 2000;11:97–105.
2. Koltai PJ, Rabkin D. Management of facial trauma in children. *Pediatr Clin North Am* 1996;43:1253–1275.
3. Roncevic R, Roncevic D. Extensive, traumatic fractures of the orbit in war and peace time. *J Craniofac Surg* 1999;10:284–300.
4. Carithers JS, Koch BB. Evaluation and management of facial fractures. *Am Fam Physician* 1997;55:2675–2682.

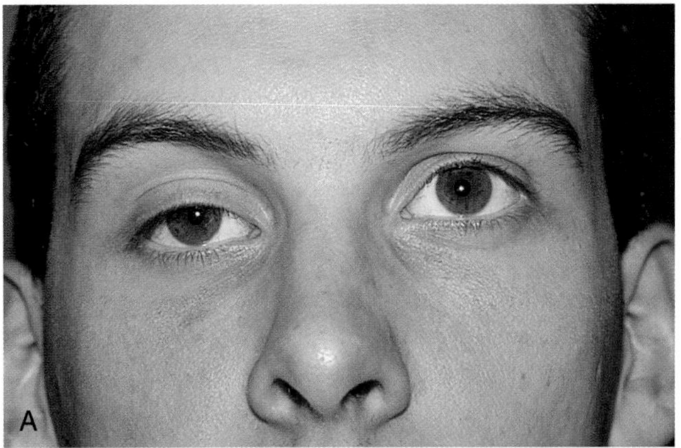

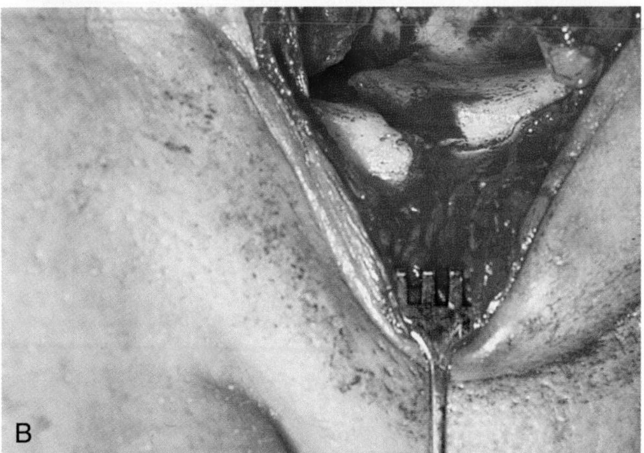

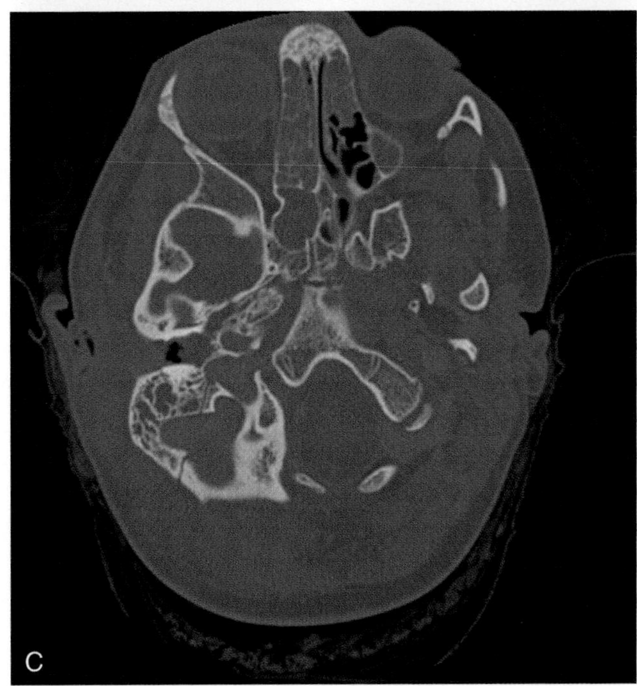

FIGURE 5–7 **A:** Pseudoptosis: enophthalmos secondary to an orbital blowout fracture. (From Tasman, with permission.) **B:** A direct fracture of the orbital floor extends from the infraorbital rim. (From Tasman, with permission.) **C:** Computed tomogram showing right orbital fracture. (Courtesy of Robert Hendrickson, MD.)

5-8

Nasal Septal Hematoma

Matthew Spencer

Clinical Presentation

Patients with nasal septal hematoma typically present to the emergency department complaining of nasal pain after facial trauma. They may occasionally report unilateral nasal obstruction.[1] On physical examination, the hematoma appears as a purple swelling of the nasal mucosa that arises from the septum, bulges into the nostril, and may cause either partial or complete obstruction.[1,2] The hematoma usually feels soft when palpated with a cotton swab or finger and should not change size with topical vasoconstrictors.[1,2]

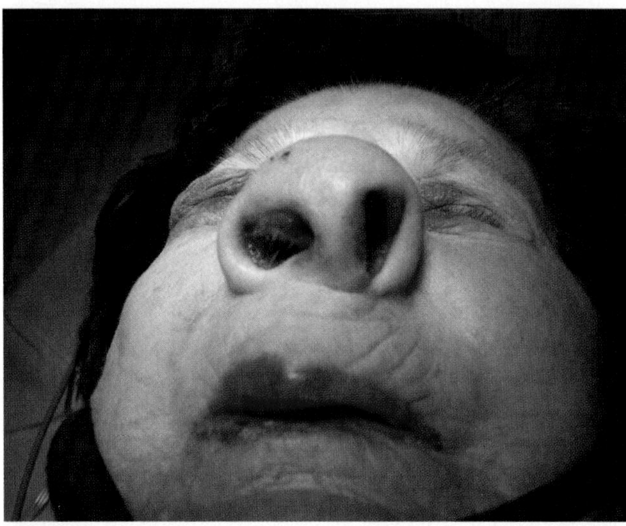

FIGURE 5–8 Large right-sided septal hematoma causing septal deviation to the left. (© Philip Mead, MD. Used with permission.)

Pathophysiology

A nasal septal hematoma results from accumulation of blood between the perichondrium and the cartilage of the nasal septum after nasal trauma.[2] Nasal septal hematomas accumulate after injury to the internal lining of the septal perichondrium, resulting in blood accumulation between the perichondrium and the cartilage.[1,2]

Diagnosis

The diagnosis usually is made based on clinical findings in the setting of trauma. A nasal speculum may be necessary to properly visualize the nasal septum.[1]

Clinical Complications

Complications of a septal hematoma are often severe and include abscess formation (most common), aseptic septal necrosis, intracranial infection, and septum perforation with saddle deformity.[1]

Management

Treatment consists of incision and drainage of the hematoma, followed by nasal packing to prevent reaccumulation.[1,2] Children may require sedation or general anesthesia for this procedure.[1]

REFERENCES

1. Koltai PJ, Rabkin D. Management of facial trauma in children. *Pediatr Clin North Am* 1996;43:1253–1275.
2. Ginsburg CM. Nasal septal hematoma. *Pediatr Rev* 1998;19:142–143.

Parotitis

Matthew Spencer

Clinical Presentation

Patients with parotitis present with fever and unilateral erythema, swelling, and warmth lateral to the angle of the mandible.[1]

Pathophysiology

Acute suppurative parotitis results from bacterial infection of the parotid gland.[1] Risk factors for infection include dehydration, recent surgery or anesthesia, advanced age, prematurity, radiation therapy, immune compromise, sialolithiasis, and oral neoplasm.[1] The most common bacterial cause is *Staphylococcus aureus,* but *S. pyogenes* and α-hemolytic *Streptococcus* species are also encountered.[1] The most common viral causes are mumps and paramyxovirus, but other species have been implicated.[1]

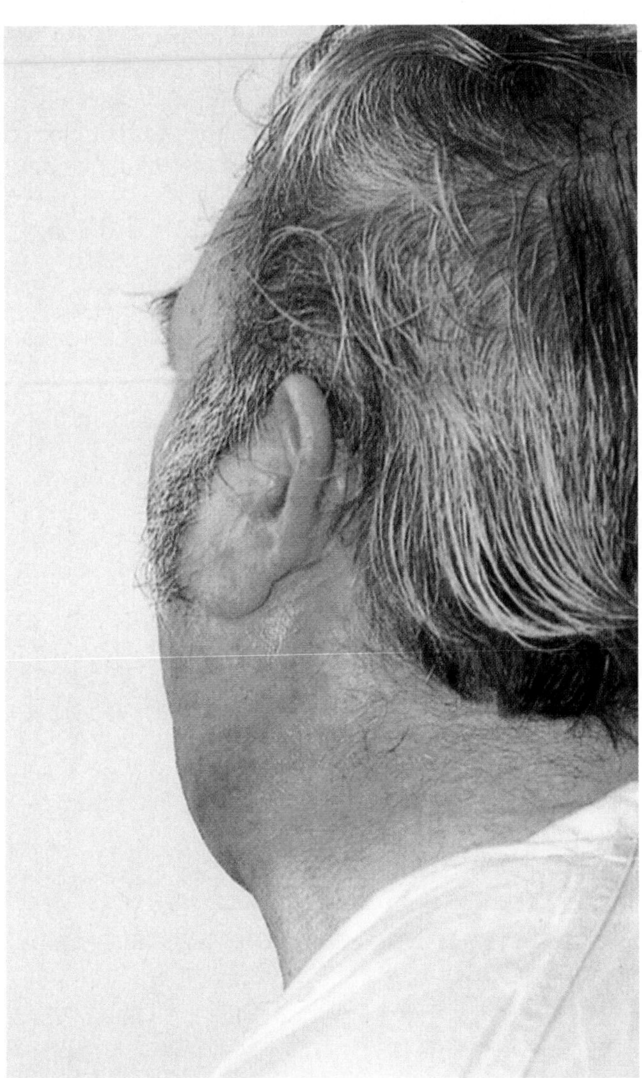

FIGURE 5–9 Left-sided parotid abscess with swelling and redness. (From Benjamin, with permission.)

Diagnosis

The diagnosis of suppurative parotitis can be made clinically with the expression of pus from Stensen's duct or by needle aspiration.[1] The diagnosis of viral parotitis may be assumed if the patient exhibits the classic prodromal history in conjunction with localized parotid inflammation. Viral parotitis usually manifests after a 1- to 5-day prodrome of low-grade fever, headache, myalgias, and malaise.[1] The gland then becomes swollen and painful, and ear pain, trismus, and dysphagia may also develop. Pus should not be expressible from the duct (in contrast to bacterial parotitis).[1] Viral parotitis is bilateral 75% of the time.[1]

Clinical Complications

Complications include septicemia, mandibular osteomyelitis, fascial extension, airway obstruction, mediastinitis, internal jugular vein thrombosis, and facial nerve dysfunction.[1] Mumps has been reported to lead to meningoencephalitis, pancreatitis, orchitis, myocarditis, pericarditis, arthritis, and nephritis.[1]

Management

Patients with parotitis should be treated with warm compresses, sialagogues such as lemon drops, and external parotid massage.[1] Intravenous fluids may be necessary to prevent dehydration due to limited oral intake. Broad-spectrum oral antibiotics covering *Staphylococcus* and *Streptococcus* species should be initiated if bacterial infection is suspected and the patient is stable and nontoxic in appearance.[1] First-line agents include dicloxacillin and cephalexin.[1] If the response is suboptimal or the patient is ill and dehydrated, intravenous antibiotics may be more appropriate.[1] Ampicillin-sulbactam, oxacillin, methicillin, and the second-generation cephalosporins are adequate single agents.[1] Incision and drainage should be considered if an abscess is present, if there is facial nerve involvement, or if there is lateral neck extension. The treatment for viral parotitis is supportive.[1]

REFERENCES

1. McQuone SJ. Acute viral and bacterial infections of the salivary glands. *Otolaryngol Clin North Am* 1999;32:793–811.

Temporomandibular Joint Syndrome

Matthew Spencer

Clinical Presentation

Patients with temporomandibular joint (TMJ) syndrome complain of unilateral (90%), deep, dull, aching pain that may become sharp and radiate across the face or temple.[1] On physical examination, there may be trismus, TMJ "clicking," limitation of jaw movement, deviation of the jaw to the side with opening, and tenderness at the insertion of the lateral pterygoid muscle.[1,2]

Pathophysiology

TMJ syndrome is thought to be caused by spasm of the pterygoid muscles.[1] Risk factors include a history of bruxism, trauma, recent dental work, anxiety, cradling of the telephone between the jaw and shoulder, and malocclusion.[1]

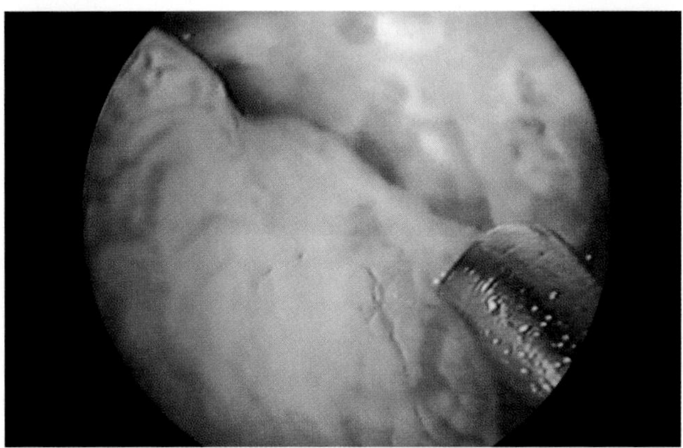

FIGURE 5–10 Synovitis of the temporomandibular joint may be treated with laser synovectomy, as shown here. (From Benjamin, with permission.)

Diagnosis

The diagnosis is made from the history and physical examination. Radiographs are rarely helpful except in cases of suspected arthropathy.[1]

Clinical Complications

Complications include chronic pain and difficulty eating.[1,2]

Management

Treatment is multifactorial and includes stress reduction, decrease in intake of caffeine and nicotine, muscle massage, jaw muscle exercises, and regular aerobic exercise.[2] In the emergency department, patients should be treated with analgesics and muscle relaxants, with recommendations for several days of soft diet, heat to the affected areas, and referral to an oral surgeon or otolaryngologist within 1 to 2 weeks.[2]

REFERENCES

1. Jones NS. Classification and diagnosis of facial pain. *Hosp Med* 2001;62:598–606.
2. Blank LW. Clinical guidelines for managing mandibular dysfunction. *Gen Dent* 1998;46:592–597.

Acute Mastoiditis

Matthew Spencer

Clinical Presentation

Before antibiotic therapy for acute otitis media (OM) became widely available, mastoiditis was the most common complication of OM (up to 20% of patients).[1–3] In the postantibiotic era, mastoiditis has become uncommon, with an incidence of only 0.2% to 2%.[2] It primarily affects young children, with the peak age at onset being 6 to 36 months. Patients usually present with pain and tenderness of the postauricular area, followed by swelling and erythema. The pinna of the ear is often displaced forward, and the tympanic membrane (TM) is usually thickened, inflamed, dull, and immobile.[1–3]

Pathophysiology

Mastoiditis results from a middle ear infection that causes mucosal swelling and blockage of the passage between the middle ear and the mastoid air cells (the aditus ad antrum).[1,2] This inflammation leads to impaired mastoid drainage, fluid accumulation in the air cells that provides a hospitable environment for bacterial growth, and eventually infection.[1,2] There appears to be a spectrum of disease. In the first stage, known as acute mastoiditis with periostitis, the infection is confined to the periosteum and mucosa of the mastoid air cells. The second stage, acute coalescent mastoiditis, occurs when the infection extends beyond the periosteum and bony destruction of the air cells develops.[1] The most common cause is *S. pneumoniae,* followed by *H. influenzae* and *S. pyogenes.*[1,2] Other, less commonly implicated organisms include *Proteus mirabilis, Streptococcus hominis, M. catarrhalis,* and *S. aureus.*[2,3]

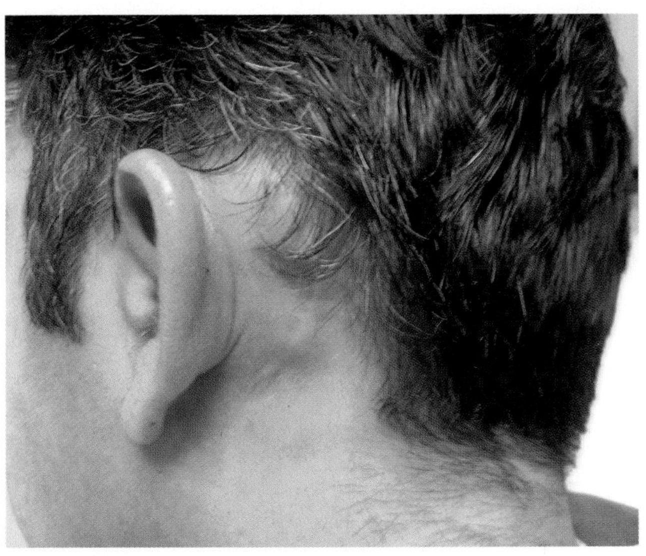

FIGURE 5–11 Swelling, redness, and adenopathy in the area of the left mastoid. (Courtesy of Mark Silverberg, MD.)

Diagnosis

The diagnosis is a clinical one, with confirmation by radiographic imaging studies. Plain radiographs of the mastoid region generally are not useful.[2] Computed tomography (CT) is the preferred means for determining the presence or absence of fluid or pus collections in the mastoid cells.

Clinical Complications

Complications include facial paralysis, meningitis, lateral sinus thrombosis, sepsis, hearing loss, bony erosion, osteomyelitis, and brain abscess.[2,3]

Management

Mastoiditis requires prompt ear, nose, and throat (ENT) consultation and hospitalization for intravenous antibiotic therapy. Surgical drainage procedures may be necessary.[1–3] The antibiotics of choice for mastoiditis are the third-generation cephalosporins.[1–3]

REFERENCES

1. Fliss DM, Leiberman A, Dagan R. Acute and chronic mastoiditis in children. *Adv Pediatr Infect Dis* 1997;13:165–185.
2. Spratley J, Silveira H, Alvarez I, Pais-Clemente M. Acute mastoiditis in children: review of current status. *Int J Pediatr Otorhinolaryngol* 2000;56:33–40.
3. Wang NE, Burg JM. Mastoiditis: a case-based review. *Pediatr Emerg Care* 1998;14:290–292.

Perichondritis

Matthew Spencer

Clinical Presentation

Patients with perichondritis present with pain, redness, swelling, warmth, and tenderness of the involved ear.[1,2] Often the ear lobe, which does not contain cartilage, is not involved; this finding can be helpful in distinguishing perichondritis from cellulitis.[2]

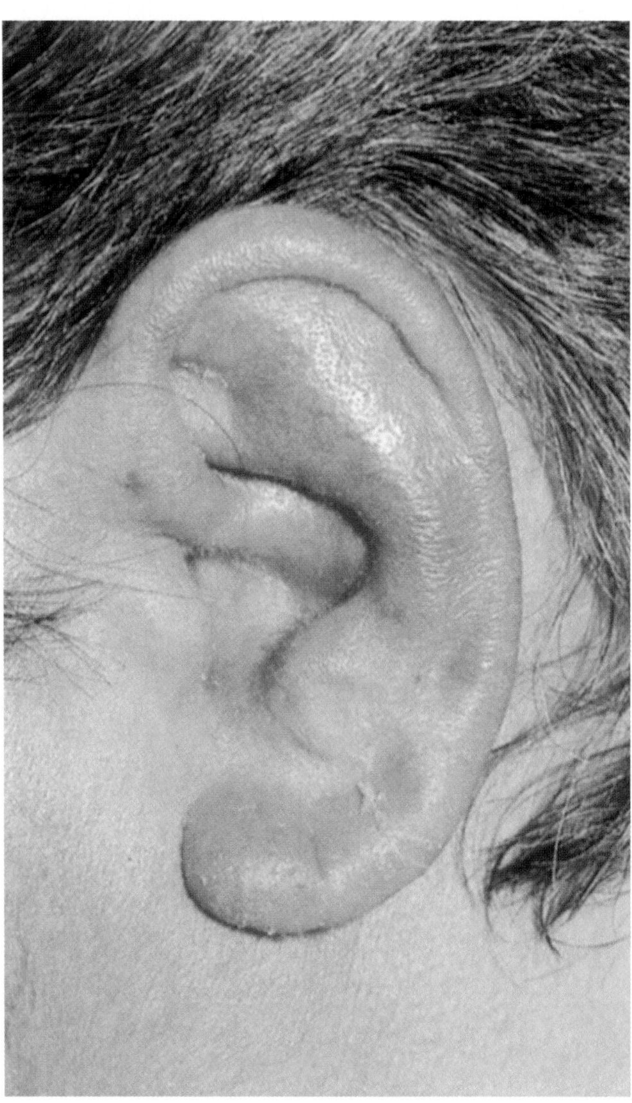

FIGURE 5–12 Acute perichondritis secondary to pinna trauma. (From Benjamin, with permission.)

Pathophysiology

Perichondritis is often seen as a complication of ear piercing or surgical ear repair after trauma.[1,2] The most common etiologic organisms are *S. aureus* and *Pseudomonas aeruginosa.*[1,2]

Diagnosis

The diagnosis is made by history and physical examination; no radiographic studies are necessary.

Clinical Complications

Complications of perichondritis include abscess formation, cartilage loss, and ear deformity.[1,2]

Management

All patients require antibiotic therapy to cover *S. aureus* and *P. aeruginosa.* Fluoroquinolone antibiotics are appropriate. Prompt consultation with an otolaryngologist is recommended.[1,2] If the infection progresses, surgical intervention may be necessary.[2,3]

REFERENCES

1. Templer J, Renner GJ. Injuries of the external ear. *Otolaryngol Clin North Am* 1990;23:1003–1018.
2. Yahalom S, Eliashar R. Perichondritis: a complication of piercing auricular cartilage. *Postgrad Med J* 2003;79:29.
3. Bassiouny A. Perichondritis of the auricle. *Laryngoscope* 1981;91: 422–431.

Cauliflower Ear

Matthew Spencer

Clinical Presentation

Patients with cauliflower ear (CE) present with painful swelling of the anterior or lateral contour of the ear, which develops within minutes to hours after direct trauma.[1,3]

Pathophysiology

The term *cauliflower ear* is used to describe a deformity of the external ear that results from an improperly or incompletely treated perichondral hematoma.[1-3] This injury is commonly seen in wrestlers and boxers at the high school and college level, who may sustain repeated trauma to the ear.[3] CE develops secondary to hematoma formation between the perichondrium and the underlying cartilage. As the locally accumulated blood clot resolves, the perichondrium is stimulated to produce new cartilage in an irregular pattern as it heals.[1,2] These deformities are more commonly associated with blunt and tractional trauma, but they can develop after penetrating injuries (as a result of persistent subcutaneous bleeding after laceration repair).[2]

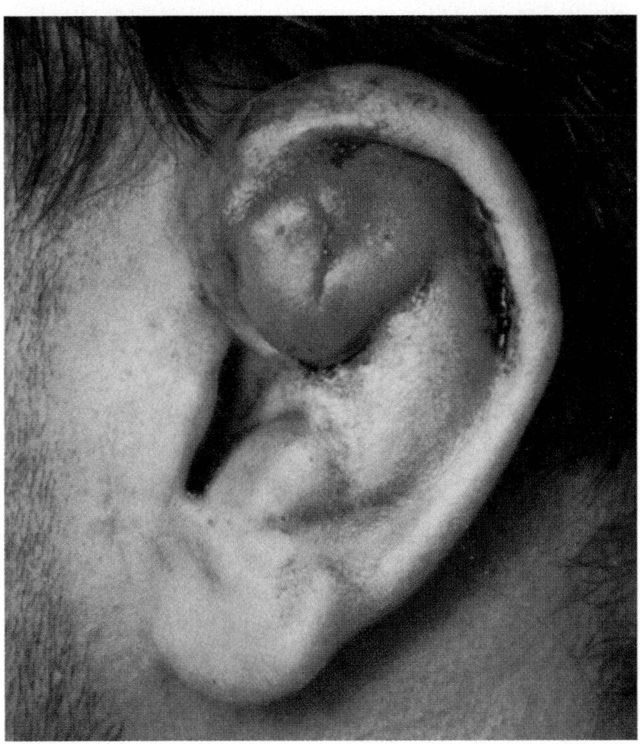

FIGURE 5–13 Cauliflower ear. (From Khalak R. Images in clinical medicine: cauliflower ear. *N Engl J Med* 1996;335:399.)

Diagnosis

The diagnosis of CE is made clinically. The ear is usually tender to palpation and may be ecchymotic. If the ear injury is old, CE may be an incidental finding on physical examination. The diagnosis of CE is based on a history of ear trauma in conjunction with the development of a characteristic deformity, ranging from a mild cartilaginous thickening to severe irregular deformity of the pinna. This may eventually result in the development of a fleshy growth of the ear that resembles a piece of cauliflower.

Clinical Complications

There are no specific complications associated with CE except for a generally poor cosmetic appearance. However, the initial perichondral hematoma may also lead to cartilage necrosis and perichondritis.[1-3]

Management

To prevent the development of a CE, the initial perichondral hematoma must be drained and a pressure dressing applied to prevent its reaccumulation.[1] Drainage of the hematoma may be performed by either incision and drainage or needle aspiration performed under local anesthesia.[1-3] If the hematoma needs to be aspirated on more than one occasion, it should be incised and drained.[2] Oral antibiotics are not routinely necessary. However, antibiotic coverage is clearly indicated in the immunocompromised patient.[1]

REFERENCES

1. Lee D, Sperling N. Initial management of auricular trauma. *Am Fam Physician* 1996;53:2339–2344.
2. Chudnofsky CR, Sebastian S. Special wounds: nail bed, planter puncture, and cartilage. *Emerg Med Clin North Am* 1992;10: 801–822.
3. Templer J, Renner GJ. Injuries of the external ear. *Otolaryngol Clin North Am* 1990;23:1003–1018.

Otitis Externa

Matthew Spencer

Clinical Presentation

Patients with otitis externa (OE) present with otalgia, otorrhea, pruritus, redness, and swelling of the auditory canal.

Pathophysiology

OE consists of three clinical stages.[1] The preinflammatory stage develops when the lipid layer of the external auditory canal is removed by moisture or trauma, leading to swelling that causes obstruction, ear fullness, and pruritus.[1] The inflammatory stage ranges from mild to severe and progresses from only slight edema, erythema, and clear discharge to total canal obstruction with large amounts of purulent discharge and debris.[1] The chronic stage consists of low-grade inflammation and infection that persists despite therapy.[1] Causes for OE range from bacterial and fungal infection to eczema. The most common causative bacteria are *S. aureus, P. aeruginosa, Proteus vulgaris,* and streptococci. Fungal infections are common in diabetics, and *Aspergillus* and *Candida* are the common causative strains.[1–4] Risk factors for OE include persistent moisture, local irritants, systemic diseases, and local trauma.[1,4]

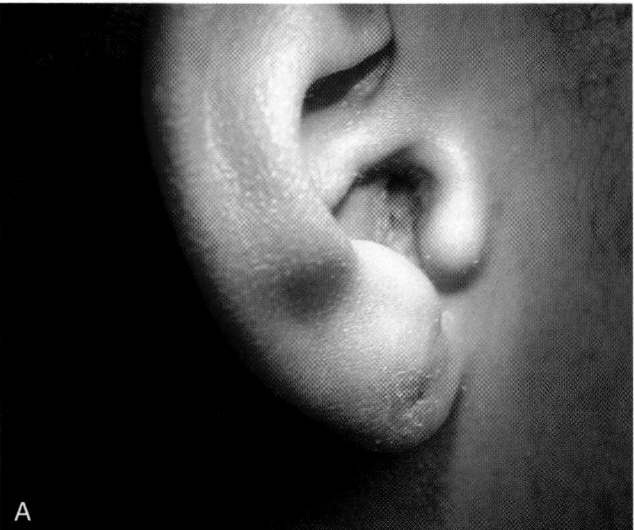

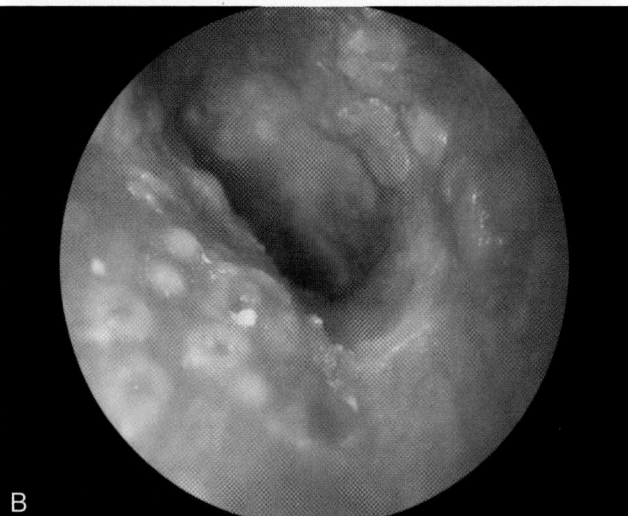

FIGURE 5–14 Otitis externa. **A:** View of infected ear. (Courtesy of Christy Salvaggio, MD.) **B:** View of macerated external canal. (From Benjamin, with permission.)

Diagnosis

OE is a clinical diagnosis. Swab cultures may provide diagnostic confirmation but are not useful in acute treatment.

Clinical Complications

Complications include chondritis, parotitis, ear canal stenosis, chronic otitis, hearing deficits, and malignant OE.

Management

Treatment consists of local cleaning and debris removal, topical medication, oral analgesics, and education on methods of prevention. Various ear drops are available, including 2% acetic acid preparations, polymyxin B/neomycin/hydrocortisone, ciprofloxacin/hydrocortisone, and ofloxicin.[1–4] Quinolone or aminoglycoside ophthalmic solutions should be used if other otic preparations are not tolerated, because they are less acidic and less irritating. Ear drops should be administered as 3 to 4 drops four times per day for 3 days beyond the resolution of symptoms, or for a total of 7 to 10 days, whichever is longer. More severe infections may require 10 to 14 days of therapy.[1] Ear drops should be placed directly into the ear canal, or on a cotton wick inserted into the canal if there is severe swelling of the canal. Fungal OE requires treatment with clotrimazole, tolnaftate, or natamycin.[1–3] Oral analgesics such as acetaminophen, ibuprofen, or acetaminophen/narcotic combinations are commonly required. Referral to an otolaryngologist should be considered for recurrent or resistant cases.[4]

REFERENCES

1. Hughes E, Lee JH. Otitis externa. *Pediatr Rev* 2001;22:191–197.
2. Biedlingmaier JF. Two ear problems you may not need to refer: otitis externa and bullous myringitis. *Postgrad Med* 1994;96:141–145,148.
3. Schapowal A. Otitis externa: a clinical overview. *Ear Nose Throat J* 2002;81[8 Suppl 1]:21–22.
4. Sander R. Otitis externa: a practical guide to treatment and prevention. *Am Fam Physician* 2001;63:927–936,941–942.

Malignant Otitis Externa

Matthew Spencer

Clinical Presentation

Most patients with malignant otitis externa (MOE) present with acute onset of severe otalgia (often worse at night), otorrhea, a feeling of ear fullness, and loss of hearing.[1]

Pathophysiology

MOE, also called necrotizing otitis externa (OE), is a severe infection of the external auditory canal that usually is caused by infection with *P. aeruginosa.*[1,2] It is often a disease of elderly diabetic patients, with an average age of 65 years. However, it has also been described in middle-aged and pediatric patients with immune system compromise.[1-3] Bacterial invasion occurs through clefts in the cartilage of the external auditory canal, leading to infection of the soft tissues at the base of the skull.[3]

Diagnosis

The diagnosis usually is clinical and should be suspected if there is no improvement or a worsening of symptoms in a patient with adequately treated OE, or if the pain is out of proportion to the findings on clinical examination. The external auditory canal usually is swollen and erythematous, with a purulent discharge, and the pinna of the ear often is inflamed and tender.[3] Granulation tissue may be present at the bony cartilaginous junction of the ear. Fever and lymphadenopathy are not common, and the white blood cell count usually is normal. computed tomography (CT), magnetic resonance imaging (MRI), and radionuclide imaging are useful in confirming the diagnosis and delineating the extent of infection.[1,3] Radionuclide imaging and the erythrocyte sedimentation rate (ESR) are also frequently used to monitor the response to therapy.

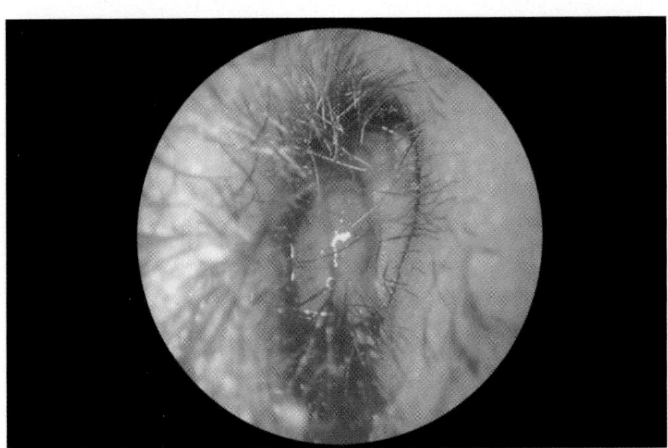

FIGURE 5–15 In malignant otitis externa, exuberant granulation tissue may arise from the floor of the external auditory canal at the junction of the bony and cartilaginous portions. (From Benjamin, with permission.)

Clinical Complications

Facial nerve palsies have been described secondary to MOE.[1,3] Other complications include temporal bone osteomyelitis, mastoiditis, sinus thrombosis, and septicemia.[1] There is an overall mortality rate of 20% to 53% in adults, with neurologic symptoms predictive of a poor prognosis.[1,3]

Management

Treatment includes 2 to 4 weeks of intravenous antibiotics, good control of diabetes, analgesics, and, occasionally, surgical débridement of granulation tissue.[1-3] Antibiotics should cover *P. aeruginosa,* with the fluoroquinolones as first-line agents and an antipseudomonal penicillin plus an aminoglycoside as the second-line choice.[3] An ear, nose, and throat (ENT) consultation should be obtained as soon as the diagnosis is suspected.

REFERENCES

1. Hughes E, Lee JH. Otitis externa. *Pediatr Rev* 2001;22:191–197.
2. Schapowal A. Otitis externa: a clinical overview. *Ear Nose Throat J* 2002;81[8 Suppl 1]:21–22.
3. Ramsey PG, Weymuller EA. Complications of bacterial infection of the ears, paranasal sinuses, and oropharynx in adults. *Emerg Med Clin North Am* 1985;3:143–160.

Otitis Media

Matthew Spencer

Clinical Presentation

Patients with otitis media (OM) present with ear pain, fever, and flu-like symptoms.[1] Additional complaints may include vertigo, nausea, vomiting, and hearing loss.[1]

Pathophysiology

OM often occurs after a viral upper respiratory tract infection that causes mucosal inflammation, impairing middle ear drainage and leading to the accumulation of sterile fluid.[1] Bacteria or viruses then enter the middle ear via reflux through the eustachian tube, resulting in a middle ear infection.[1] The most common bacteria involved in OM are *S. pneumoniae, H. influenzae,* and *M. catarrhalis.*[1,2] Less common bacterial pathogens include group A *Streptococcus* spp., *S. aureus,* and gram-negative species.[2] No bacterial pathogens are isolated in up to 30% of cases, and viruses are the only organisms found in as many as 44% of cases.[1,2] The peak incidence of OM occurs at 6 to 12 months of age, with a seasonal variation demonstrating the highest incidence during the winter months.[2]

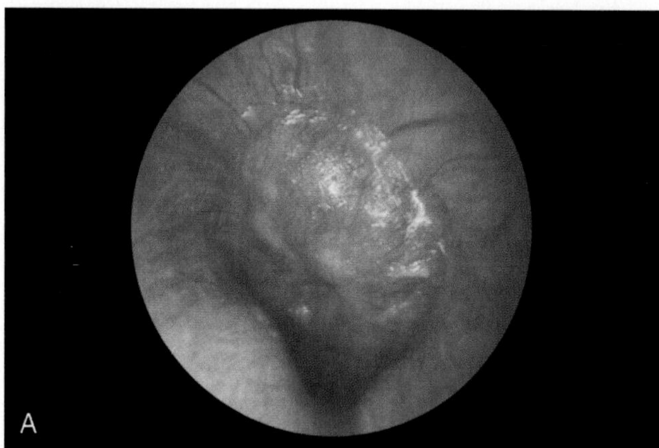

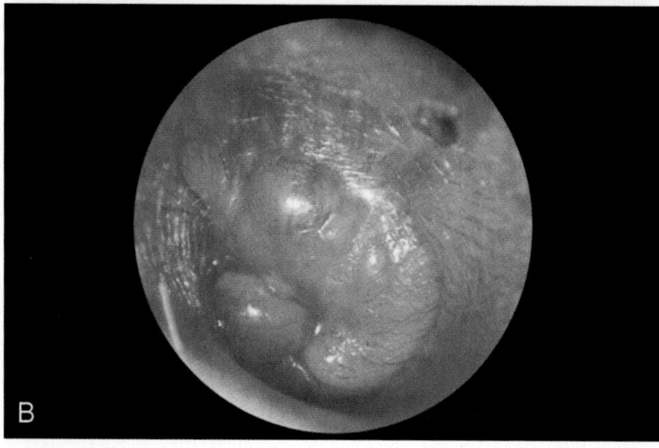

FIGURE 5–16 Otitis media. **A:** Early infection showing redness, edema, and marked outward bulging. **B:** Late infection showing bulging membrane and purulent debris. (From Benjamin, with permission.)

Diagnosis

The diagnosis usually is made clinically. On physical examination, the tympanic membrane (TM) on the affected side is often bulging and abnormal in color, and the malleus may be obscured.[2] On pneumatic otoscopic examination, decreased mobility of the TM may indicate the presence a middle ear effusion.[2] Decreased TM mobility is the best method for determining the presence of middle ear fluid. Other techniques for diagnosing OM include tympanometry, spectral gradient acoustic reflectometry, and diagnostic tympanocentesis and myringotomy, but these modalities are not routinely applied in the emergency department.[2]

Clinical Complications

The complications of OM include perforation of the TM, mastoiditis, chronic hearing loss, labyrinthitis, petrositis, cholesteatoma, cranial nerve palsies, cranial osteomyelitis, lateral sinus thrombosis, brain abscess, and meningitis.[1]

Management

Treatment includes antibiotics, antihistamines, antipyretics, and analgesics. In suspected bacterial OM, the first-line antibiotic of choice remains oral amoxicillin.[1] For penicillin-allergic patients, azithromycin or intramuscular ceftriaxone as a single dose can be substituted.[1,2] Resistant OM should be treated with amoxicillin/clavulanate, cefuroxime, axetil, or a macrolide in a penicillin-allergic patient.[1,2]

REFERENCES

1. Hendley JO. Clinical practice: otitis media. *N Engl J Med* 2002;347: 1169–1174.
2. Hoberman A, Paradise JL. Acute otitis media: diagnosis and management in the year 2000. *Pediatr Ann* 2000;29:609–620.

Serous Otitis Media

Matthew Spencer

Clinical Presentation

The most common symptom of serous otitis media (OM) is hearing loss, although this often is not recognized in young children.[2] On otoscopic examination, the tympanic membrane (TM) often is abnormal in color and has decreased mobility, with bubbles or an air–fluid level behind it.[2]

Pathophysiology

Serous OM, or otitis media with effusion (OME), results when there is nonpurulent fluid accumulation behind the TM without any local or systemic symptoms.[1,2] Serous OM often occurs after a viral nasopharyngeal infection that causes mucosal inflammation, which impairs middle ear drainage through the eustachian tubes.[1,3] Impaired drainage leads to sterile fluid accumulation and increased middle ear pressures.

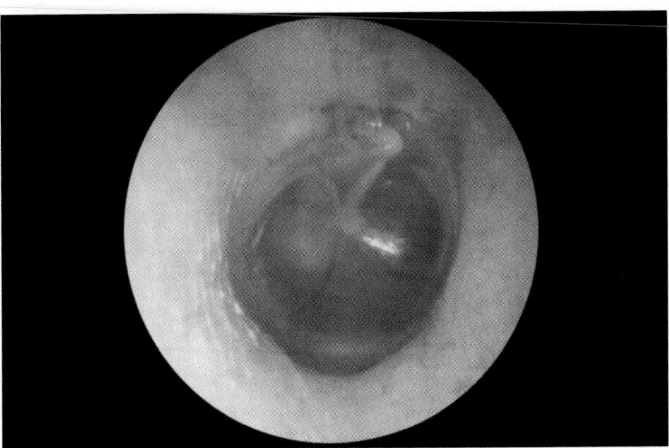

FIGURE 5–17 Serous otitis media: a well-defined air–fluid level is present. (From Benjamin, with permission.)

Diagnosis

The diagnosis is made clinically on otoscopic examination, usually during a routine physical examination. Two of the following three TM abnormalities are required for the diagnosis: color, opacification, or decreased motility. The diagnosis also may be made based on visual observation of bubbles or an air–fluid level behind the TM.[2]

Clinical Complications

Serous OM may progress to acute purulent OM through secondary bacterial infection of the middle ear effusion.[1]

Management

Specific therapy usually is not indicated for uncomplicated serous OM, because most patients are asymptomatic.[1] If hearing impairment is present, the patient should be referred to an otolaryngologist for formal auditory testing and possible tympanocentesis or myringotomy tube placement.[1]

REFERENCES

1. Hendley JO. Clinical Practice. Otitis media. *N Engl J Med* 2002;347: 1169–1174.
2. Hoberman A, Paradise JL. Acute otitis media: diagnosis and management in the year 2000. *Pediatr Ann* 2000;29:609–620.
3. Ramsey PG, Weymuller EA. Complications of bacterial infection of the ears, paranasal sinuses, and oropharynx in adults. *Emerg Med Clin North Am* 1985;3:143–160.

Bullous Myringitis

Matthew Spencer

Clinical Presentation

Patients with bullous myringitis present after the sudden onset of ear pain with a serosanguineous discharge.[1,2] Many patients report symptoms of an upper respiratory tract infection in the preceding week.[2]

Pathophysiology

Bullous myringitis may involve infection with *Mycoplasma pneumoniae.* However, the majority of organisms isolated appear to be those most commonly associated with otitis media (OM): *S. pneumoniae, H. influenzae,* or β-hemolytic *Streptococcus* spp.[1,2]

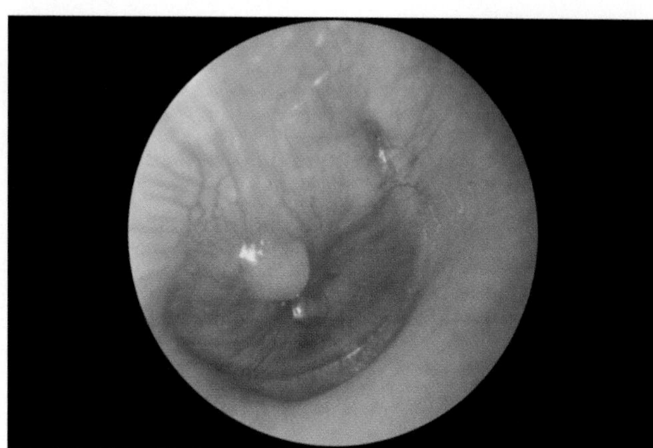

FIGURE 5–18 Myringitis bullosa. Blebs can be seen on the tympanic membrane. (From Benjamin, with permission.)

Diagnosis

The diagnosis is made by otoscopic examination.[1] Multiple small, vesicular lesions are present on the tympanic membrane (TM).[1–3] Occasionally, the TM is inflamed and harbors a middle ear effusion. Posterior cervical lymphadenopathy is also common.[1–3]

Clinical Complications

The most common reported complication is sensorineural hearing loss, which usually resolves over several weeks. Perforation of the TM may occur.[2]

Management

Treatment depends on the condition of the TM. If the nonblistered portion of the TM appears normal, symptomatic care is all that is necessary.[1] However, if the TM is inflamed, the patient should be treated with oral antibiotics, as for OM.[1,2]

REFERENCES

1. Roberts DB. The etiology of bullous myringitis and the role of mycoplasmas in ear disease: a review. *Pediatrics* 1980;65:761–766.
2. Biedlingmaier JF. Two ear problems you may not need to refer: otitis externa and bullous myringitis. *Postgrad Med* 1994;96:141–145,148.
3. Merifield DO, Miller GS. The etiology and clinical course of bullous myringitis. *Arch Otolaryngol* 1966;84:487–489.

Ramsay Hunt Syndrome

Matthew Spencer

Clinical Presentation

Patients with Ramsay Hunt syndrome (RHS) develop ear or facial pain, sometimes associated with a prodrome of vomiting, diarrhea, and fever.[1] Within 1 week, facial palsy in a lower motor neuron distribution develops.[1] Patients may also complain of abnormal taste, dry eye, hearing loss, tinnitus, vertigo, sensitivity to sound, or cranial nerve V, VIII, IX, or X symptoms.[1,2] A vesicular rash over the ear, mastoid process, face, neck, shoulder, tongue, buccal mucosa, palate, uvula, or larynx is usually present at the same time as the facial palsy but may be delayed up to 10 days.[1,2]

Pathophysiology

RHS is the second most common cause of facial palsy, accounting for 3% to 12% of all cases.[1,2] It results from reactivation of varicella-zoster virus in the geniculate ganglion, leading to inflammation of the seventh and eighth cranial nerves.[1] Adults are affected more often than children, and women more often than men, with the highest incidence in the fifth decade of life.[1,2] Facial weakness progresses to maximum intensity at 11 to 21 days, and most patients show some amount of recovery by 6 to 12 months; the rash resolves quickly over 10 to 14 days.[1]

Diagnosis

The diagnosis is a clinical one, based on history and physical examination. Some propose the use of gadolinium-enhanced magnetic resonance imaging (MRI) to detect inflammation of the facial and vestibulocochlear nerves in patients without a characteristic rash.[3]

Clinical Complications

Complications include hearing loss, persistent facial palsy, tearing, facial spasm, ptosis, dry eye, and postherpetic neuralgia.[1,2] Facial palsy from RHS has a worse outcome than all other types of Bell's palsy. Complete neurologic recovery occurs in 10% of patients exhibiting complete facial palsy, and 66% of those exhibiting a partial facial palsy.[1,3]

Management

Treatment consists of analgesics, acyclovir, prednisone, and appropriate eye care.[1,2] Patients who are unable to close the affected eye completely should be provided with saline eye drops, ointments, or instructions on taping the eye closed at night to prevent drying.[1] Patients may be discharged from the emergency department to follow-up with an otolaryngologist in 1 to 2 weeks.[1]

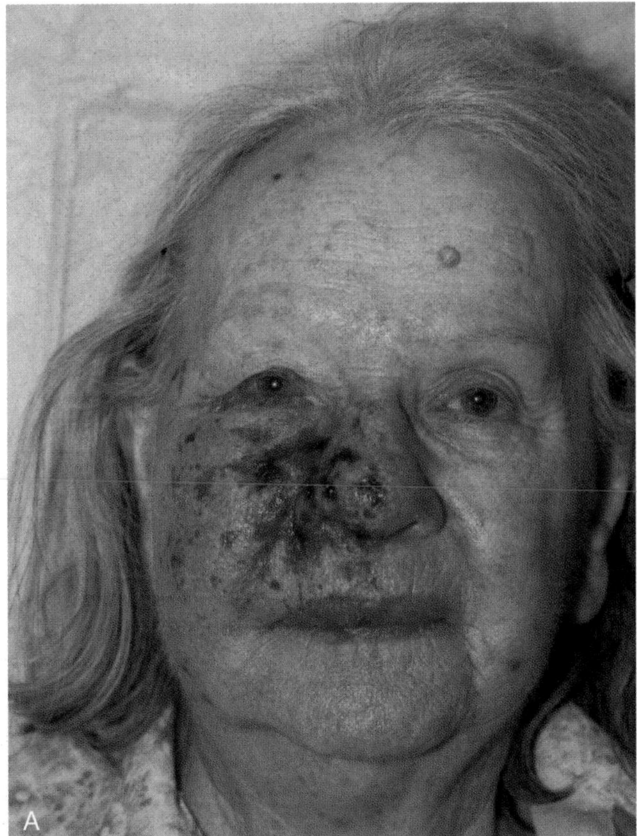

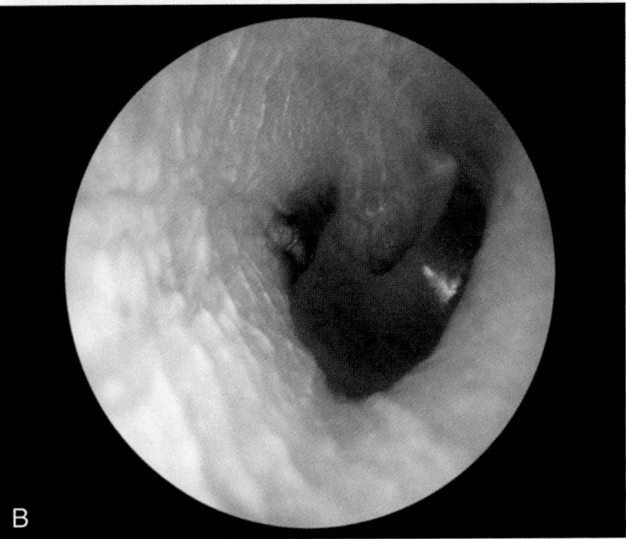

FIGURE 5–19 Ramsey Hunt syndrome **A:** Facial paralysis due to herpes zoster. (© David Effron, MD. Used with permission.) **B:** Herpes zoster of the tympanic membrane. (From Benjamin, with permission.)

REFERENCES

1. Birinyi F. Facial weakness and rash: Ramsay Hunt syndrome (herpes zoster cephalicus, herpes zoster oticus, herpes zoster auricularis). *Acad Emerg Med* 1996;3:1144–1145,1153–1155.
2. Hato N, Kisaki H, Honda N, Gyo K, Murakami S, Yanagihara N. Ramsay Hunt syndrome in children. *Ann Neurol* 2000;48:254–256.
3. Kuo MJ, Drago PC, Proops DW, Chavda SV. Early diagnosis and treatment of Ramsay Hunt syndrome: the role of magnetic resonance imaging. *J Laryngol Otol* 1995;109:777–780.

Cholesteatoma

Matthew Spencer

Clinical Presentation

Cholesteatoma includes two subtypes, congenital and acquired. Patients with congenital cholesteatoma are usually asymptomatic, except for a conductive hearing deficit and a white mass located behind the tympanic membrane (TM).[1,2] Acquired cholesteatoma manifests with persistent otorrhea and hearing loss and a TM defect marked by collections of fluid and debris.[1]

Pathophysiology

Cholesteatoma is an abnormal collection of keratin-producing epithelium in the middle ear, mastoid, or petrous apex.[1,2] Congenital cholesteatoma is thought to result from persistence of an epithelial rest within the inner ear during development.[1,2] Acquired cholesteatoma is thought to develop by several possible mechanisms, such as immigration, implantation, retraction, or metaplasia.[1,2] The incidence of cholesteatoma is 1 to 6 cases per 100,000 people, with higher rates seen in Native Americans and in patients with chronic ear infections, cleft lip and palate, or other craniofacial syndromes.[1,2]

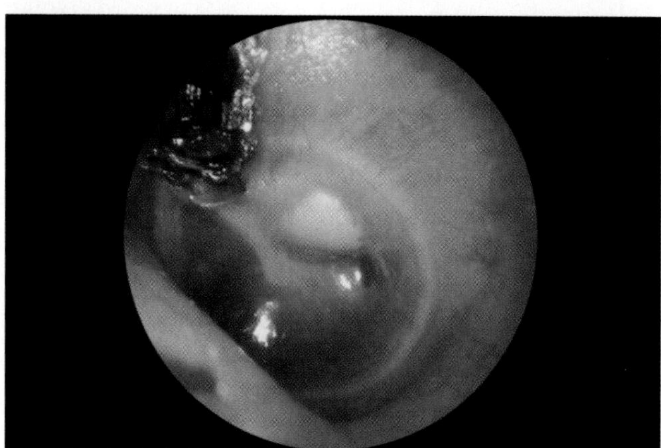

FIGURE 5–20 Attic crust and white mass of cholesteatoma behind the posterior quadrant of the tympanic membrane. (From Benjamin, with permission.)

Diagnosis

The diagnosis is based on history and physical examination, with radiographic testing such as computed tomography (CT) and magnetic resonance imaging (MRI) helpful for operative planning.[2]

Clinical Complications

Complications occur in 5% of children and 13% of adults; recurrent disease is more common in children.[1] Complications include sensorineural hearing loss, labyrinthine fistula, facial nerve paralysis, ossicular fallopian canal, and scutal or tegmental erosions.[1,2]

Management

Emergency department treatment consists of antibiotic therapy to cover *Pseudomonas* and prompt referral to an otolaryngologist.[1,2] Definitive therapy involves surgical resection of the cholesteatoma.[1]

REFERENCES

1. De la Cruz A, Fayad JN. Detection and management of childhood cholesteatoma. *Pediatr Ann* 1999;28:370–373.
2. Shohet JA, de Jong AL. The management of pediatric cholesteatoma. *Otolaryngol Clin North Am* 2002;35:841–851.

Tympanosclerosis

Matthew Spencer

Clinical Presentation

The two types of tympanosclerosis, myringosclerosis and intratympanic tympanosclerosis, manifest in different ways.[1] In myringosclerosis, the tympanic membrane (TM) is the only structure involved.[1] Patients usually are asymptomatic unless large areas of the TM are calcified or the plaques are adherent to the ossicles, which results in a conductive hearing deficit.[1] The chalky white plaques are easily visualized on otoscopic examination.[1,2] The intratympanic type of tympanosclerosis usually causes marked conductive hearing loss, but plaques are not visualized externally.[1]

Pathophysiology

Tympanosclerosis is a condition in which there are calcified deposits within the TM, ossicular chain, tympanic cavity, and mastoid.[1,2] Tympanosclerosis is thought to result from persistent inflammation and is usually associated with chronic middle ear infections. It is believed that fibroblast proliferation leads to the deposition of excessive amounts of collagen fibers, which causes hyaline mass formation and subsequent calcium deposition.[1] The incidence of this disease has been reported to range from 7% to 33% among patients with chronic middle ear infections.[1]

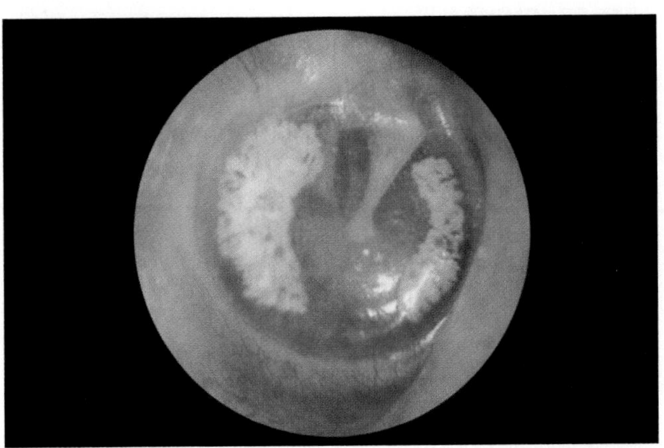

FIGURE 5–21 Crescent-shaped plaque of tympanosclerosis. (From Benjamin, with permission.)

Diagnosis

The diagnosis is made easily on otoscopic examination in those with myringosclerosis, but a computed tomography (CT) scan of the middle ear is often necessary for those with the intratympanic type.[1]

Clinical Complications

The most common complication is conductive hearing loss.[1]

Management

Patients should be referred to an otolaryngologist. Ongoing treatment is focused on augmenting hearing, either with surgery (which is controversial) or through the use of a hearing aid.[1]

REFERENCES

1. Asiri S, Hasham A, al Anazy F, Zakzouk S, Banjar A. Tympanosclerosis: review of literature and incidence among patients with middle-ear infection. *J Laryngol Otol* 1999;113:1076–1080.
2. Fitzgerald DC. The aging ear. *Am Fam Physician* 1985;31:225–232.

Tympanic Membrane Rupture

Matthew Spencer

Clinical Presentation

Patients with tympanic membrane (TM) rupture present with ear pain, with or without blood from the affected ear, often associated with tinnitus and a conductive hearing loss.[2,3] Most patients with an infectious cause have a history of otitis media (OM) that is often followed by a rush of pus and blood from the ear and immediate relief of pain.[1]

Traumatic TM rupture may occur in a dry or wet environment.[1] Dry TM rupture results in ear pain secondary to trauma from any dry source. It is classically a result of a blow to the side of the head with the flat of the hand, which is often associated with bloody discharge from the affected ear.[1] Wet TM rupture results in ear pain usually after a fall during water-skiing, surfing, or other water sports.[1]

Pathophysiology

TM rupture is a defect of the TM from any cause, usually infection or trauma.[1,2] Approximately 1% to 3% of the U.S. population develop ruptured TMs from infection, whereas 0.14% to 0.86% develop them from trauma.[2,3] An infectious cause is more common in developing countries and in lower socioeconomic populations of developed countries.[2]

Traumatic TM rupture occurs as a result of blunt or penetrating trauma or rapid changes in barometric pressure.[2] The most common cause of penetrating rupture is self-inflicted injury secondary to overly aggressive ear cleaning.[2] Infectious TM rupture develops after a middle ear infection leads to pus accumulation in the middle ear, which exerts pressure on the TM, forcing it outward. The middle of the TM becomes ischemic, then necrotic, and eventually ruptures.[2] Traumatic TM rupture develops after 0.5 to 2 atmospheres of pressure is exerted against the TM. If it occurs in a wet environment, there is a risk of secondary infection with *Pseudomonas.*[1,2]

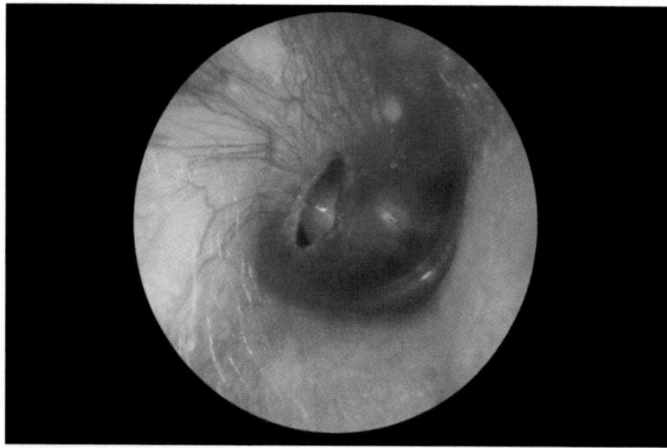

FIGURE 5–22 Traumatic perforation of the tympanic membrane. (From Benjamin, with permission.)

Diagnosis

The diagnosis of ruptured TM is made by finding a defect in the TM on otoscopic examination of a patient with a characteristic history.[1]

Clinical Complications

Complications from ruptured TM include OM, cholesteatoma, conductive hearing loss, and perilymphatic fistulas.[3]

Management

The treatment for a ruptured TM depends on its cause. If there is an infectious etiology, then the underlying infection must be treated and the defect should heal spontaneously.[1] Recommendations include topical agents such as ciprofloxacin or chloramphenicol, which are not considered ototoxic in the setting of perforation with discharge, as well as oral antibiotics.[1] Topical antibiotics are not necessary unless the rupture is secondary to an infectious process. Corticosteroids should be avoided under all circumstances, because they may impede healing.[1-3] Traumatic TM rupture in a dry environment requires no therapy, whereas ruptures that occur in a wet environment should be treated with ear drops that cover *Pseudomonas.* The patient should be instructed to keep the ear dry.[1] All patients should be referred to an otolaryngologist within 2 to 3 days for follow-up, because some TM ruptures take up to 9 months to heal, although most heal spontaneously in a short time.[1]

REFERENCES

1. Fagan P, Patel N. A hole in the drum: an overview of tympanic membrane perforations. *Aust Fam Physician* 2002;31:707–710.
2. Gladstone HB, Jackler RK, Varav K. Tympanic membrane wound healing: an overview. *Otolaryngol Clin North Am* 1995;28:913–932.
3. Kristensen S, Juul A, Gammelgaard NP, Rasmussen OR. Traumatic tympanic membrane perforations: complications and management. *Ear, Nose, Throat J* 1989;68:503–516.

Mandibular Dislocation

Matthew Spencer

Clinical Presentation

Each type of mandibular dislocation has a slightly different presentation. However, most signs and symptoms are shared, making it difficult to differentiate the dislocation direction on physical examination alone. An inability to close the mouth, limited range of motion of the mandible, difficulty speaking, and temporomandibular joint (TMJ) pain are common manifestations of all mandible dislocations.[1,2]

Pathophysiology

Dislocation of the jaw involves displacement of the mandibular condyle completely out of the maxillary glenoid fossa.[1] Four different types of mandibular dislocation exist—anterior, posterior, lateral, and superior—with anterior dislocations being the most common variety.[1] Superior dislocations result in the condyle's being forced into the middle cranial fossa through the glenoid fossa.[1] Posterior dislocations are associated with the application of very strong forces and are usually seen in victims of high-speed accidents.[2] Posterior dislocations are more common in children and young adults and are usually the result of the mouth being open at the time of impact.[1,2]

There are three general risk factors for mandibular dislocations. The first is reduced capsular integrity secondary to seizures, intubations, prolonged operative procedures, or chronic mild hyperextension.[1] The second risk factor is the presence of an anatomically shallow articular eminence. The third risk factor is hypertonic masticator muscles, often seen in patients with chronic bruxism.[1] Acute dislocations are usually bilateral and have been reported after coughing, oral sex, taking a large bite of food, trauma, tooth extraction, tonsillectomy, seizures, yawning, or vomiting.[1]

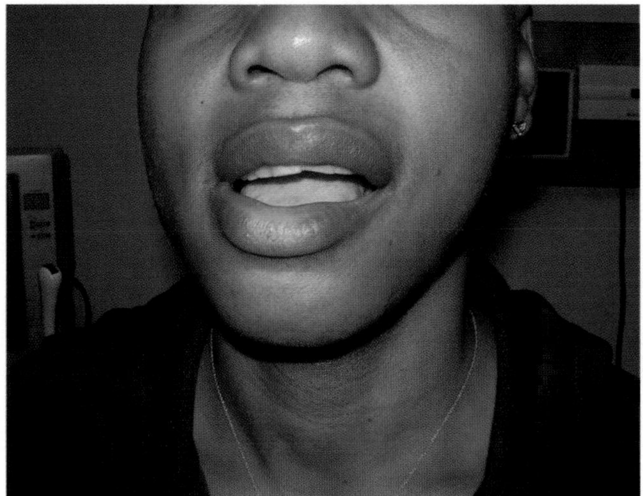

FIGURE 5–23 Mandibular dislocation. Note inability to close mouth. (Courtesy of Mark Silverberg, MD.)

Diagnosis

The diagnosis must be suspected in any patient with jaw pain and reduced jaw mobility. It may be confirmed radiographically with temporomandibular joint (TMJ) views, a Panorex, or computed tomography (CT).[1] If a superior dislocation is suspected, CT is essential to both confirm the diagnosis and check for an associated intracranial injury.[2]

Clinical Complications

Most dislocations are easily reduced without complications. However, cerebral contusion, facial nerve paralysis, deafness, external auditory canal laceration, crossbite, recurrent dislocation, chronic TMJ pain, growth disturbance, and cerebrospinal fluid otorrhea have all been described. Most of these complications are more common with superior dislocations.[1,2]

Management

The mainstay of treatment is analgesics and dislocation reduction.[1] There are two generally accepted reduction techniques, one with the patient seated and the other with the patient supine.[1] In the seated method, the patient should be positioned with the head braced against a wall or a firm chair headrest, with the mandible at or below the level of the physician's forearm when the elbow is flexed to 90 degrees. The physician should wrap his or her thumbs in gauze (to prevent being bitten at the time of relocation), and place them intraorally over the molars. The other fingers should then grasp the angle of the mandible and apply gentle pressure downward and backward until the jaw is reduced.[1] The supine method is performed by applying pressure in a similar manner, except the patient is lying on a stretcher with the physician standing at the head of the bed.[1] Conscious sedation or local anesthesia may be needed to facilitate reduction. Most dislocations can be reduced in the emergency department, and patients are discharged with instructions to support the chin with the hand while yawning, avoid wide opening of the mouth for 3 weeks, consume a soft diet for 2 to 3 days, use nonsteroidal antiinflammatory pain medications, and follow-up with the primary care physician or dentist in 2 to 3 days.[1] Mandible fracture/dislocations and superior dislocations require an immediate oral surgery consultation.[1,2]

REFERENCES

1. Luyk NH, Larsen PE. The diagnosis and treatment of the dislocated mandible. *Am J Emerg Med* 1989;7:329–335.
2. Koretsch LJ, Brook AL, Kader A, Eisig SB. Traumatic dislocation of the mandibular condyle into the middle cranial fossa: report of a case, review of the literature, and a proposal management protocol. *J Oral Maxillofac Surg* 2001;59:88–94.

Mandible Fracture

Matthew Spencer

Clinical Presentation

Patients with mandible fracture present after direct trauma with jaw pain and tenderness associated with extraoral or intraoral swelling and ecchymoses. Often the patient expresses the sensation of an uneven bite, trismus, or the inability to open or close the mouth. Some patients have an obvious jaw deformity, with widely separated teeth, a palpable fracture line, or crepitus.[1–3] Other symptoms that may be present are anesthesia in the inferior alveolar or mental nerve distribution and preauricular or anterior external auditory canal tenderness.[2]

Pathophysiology

Mandible fractures are extremely common, accounting for 48% to 78% of all facial fractures.[1] They are seen three to five times more often in men than in women, with the highest incidence occurring between 20 and 40 years of age.[1] The most frequently broken portion of the mandible is the condyle, followed by the angle, and then the body.[1] Mandible fractures are usually a result of direct trauma, with assault and motor vehicle collisions being the most commonly reported mechanisms.[1,2] Because of its somewhat "crescent" shape, the mandible is fractured in two places in more than 50% of the cases.[2]

Diagnosis

The diagnosis is either clinically obvious or suspected based on history and physical examination; it should be confirmed by radiographic examination.[1,3] Panorex is the first choice, followed by computed tomography (CT), and then a plain mandible series consisting of right and left lateral obliques, a posteroanterior view, and a Towne view.[1–3]

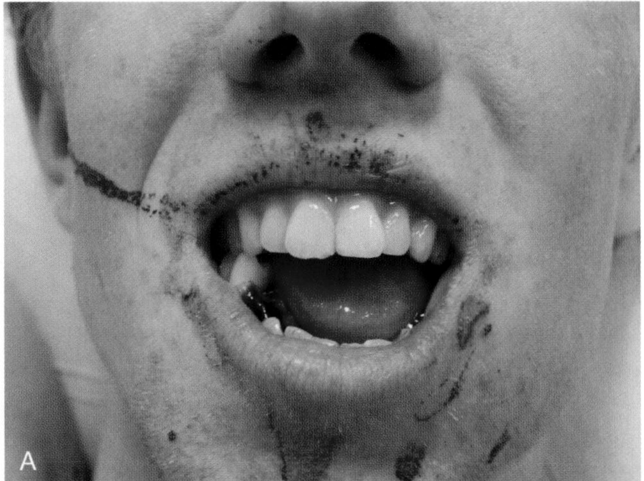

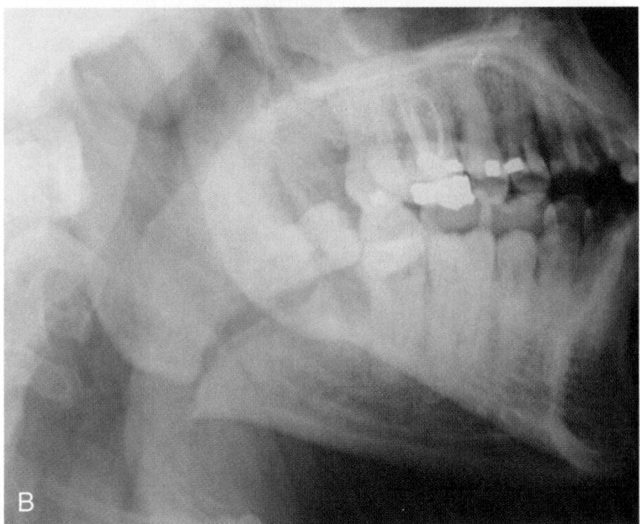

FIGURE 5–24 Open mandibular fracture as seen clinically **(A)** and radiographically **(B)**. (**A,** Courtesy of Madelyn Garcia, MD; **B,** Courtesy of Robert Hendrickson, MD.)

Clinical Complications

Possible complications include persistent malocclusion, temporomandibular joint (TMJ) disease, periodontal problems, cosmetic deformity, nonunion, permanent facial numbness, and growth disturbances.[1,3]

Management

The standard ABCs (airway, breathing, and circulation) should always be addressed initially in any trauma case. The examining physician should be particularly aware that a bilateral mandible fracture can allow the tongue to fall into the back of the throat and compromise the airway when the patient is in a supine position.[1,2] Pain control can be attended to once all life- and limb-threatening issues have been evaluated. The majority of mandible fractures require surgical repair, so consultants such as otolaryngology, oral surgery, or plastic surgery specialists should be called as soon as the diagnosis is apparent.[1,3] If there is an intraoral laceration at the fracture site, it should be considered an open fracture, and antibiotics covering the oral flora should be administered. Intravenous penicillin is the drug of choice, but clindamycin should be considered in penicillin-allergic patients.[2]

REFERENCES

1. Oikarinen KS. Clinical management of injuries to the maxilla, mandible, and alveolus. *Dent Clin North Am* 1995;39:113–131.
2. Ellis E III, Scott K. Assessment of patients with facial fractures. *Emerg Med Clin North Am* 2000;18:411–448.
3. McDonald WS, Thaller SR. Priorities in the treatment of facial fractures for the millennium. *J Craniofac Surg* 2000;11:97–105.

Sialolithiasis (Parotid Duct Stone)

Matthew Spencer

Clinical Presentation

The most common symptoms of sialolithiasis are recurrent pain and spasm while eating.[1,2] Frequently, the gland becomes tense, painful, and tender after meals and the swelling slowly decreases after finishing.[3] Most patients (59%) present with both salivary gland pain and swelling; 29% present with swelling alone, and 12% present with pain alone.[1] Often the stone is palpable in the submandibular gland or its duct on bimanual examination of the gland.[1,3]

Pathophysiology

Sialolithiasis involves the development of salivary gland calculi.[1,3] Approximately 1% of the population develop these stones, usually in the third through sixth decades of life.[1] There is a male predominance, and the condition is very rare in children.[1] The submandibular gland is the most common site, accounting for 80% to 92% of all cases, whereas the parotid is involved in 6% to 20% of cases.[1–3] Single stones are found 70% to 80% of the time; fewer than 5% of patients have three or more stones at once. The largest documented stone was 55 mm in diameter.[1]

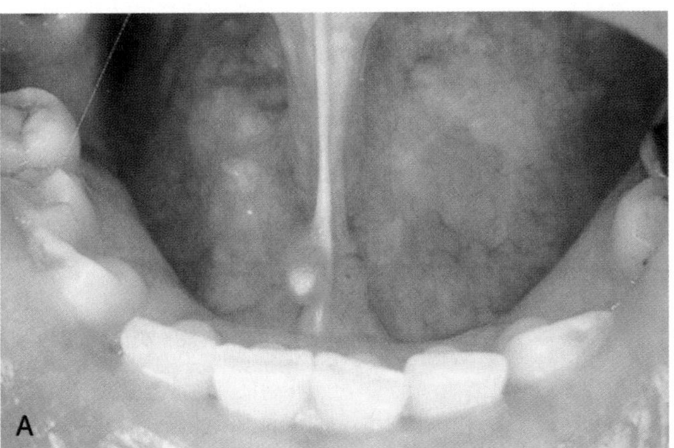

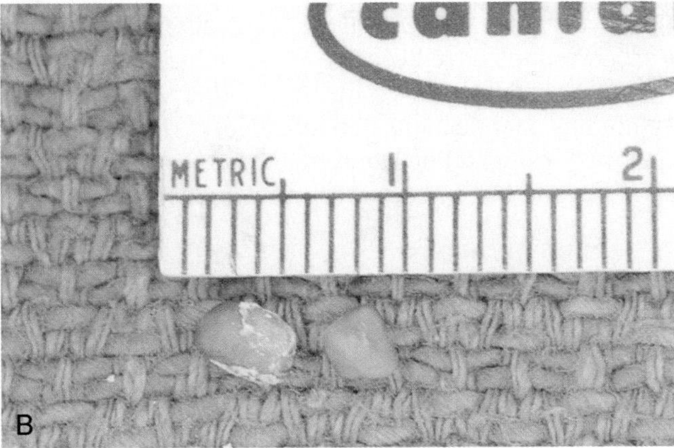

FIGURE 5-25 **A:** Impacted submandibular duct calculus. **B:** Characteristic yellow submandibular duct stones. (From Benjamin, with permission.)

Diagnosis

The diagnosis is primarily clinical, but radiography and fine-needle aspiration may be useful.[1] Because 80% to 95% of stones are radiopaque, intraoral and occlusal radiographs of the salivary glands and mouth floor can be diagnostic, and an anteroposterior view with the mouth open is preferred before sialography.[1–3] Sialography is considered to be 100% diagnostic for intraductal or glandular stones, and it is the gold standard for diagnosis. Contraindications include dye allergy and sialoadenitis.[1,2]

Clinical Complications

Complications include acute and chronic sialadenitis, salivary gland fibrosis, salivary duct stricture, salivary duct stenosis, and abscess formation.[1,2] Complications after therapy include xerostomia, stone recurrence, facial nerve injury, and marginal mandibular nerve injury.[1,3] Approximately 18% recur after simple removal.[1,2]

Management

Emergency department therapy includes recommendations for local heat, gland massage, sialagogues such as lemon drops or orange juice, and analgesics.[1] If the gland is swollen and inflamed, it is assumed to be infected and is treated with antibiotics to cover *S. aureus.*[1] All patients should be referred to an otolaryngologist within 2 to 3 days, because stones that do not pass on their own must be removed surgically via transoral ductoplasty or gland excision, depending on their location.[1–3]

REFERENCES

1. Williams MF. Sialolithiasis. *Otolaryngol Clin North Am* 1999;32:819–834.
2. Bradley PJ. Benign salivary gland disease. *Hosp Med* 2001;62:392–395.
3. Bull PD. Salivary gland stones: diagnosis and treatment. *Hosp Med* 2001;62:396–399.

Exudative Pharyngitis

Matthew Spencer

Clinical Presentation

Patients with exudative pharyngitis (EP) present with sore throat, fever, and malaise.

Pathophysiology

Viruses are the most common causative agents for EP, with adenovirus species being most common, followed by rhinoviruses and coronaviruses.[1] Streptococcal pharyngitis is the most common bacterial EP; it is caused by group A, β-hemolytic *Streptococcus* species.[1] The cause of infectious mononucleosis is the Epstein-Barr virus, a large DNA-containing virus of the Herpesviridae family.[2]

Diagnosis

The diagnosis is clinical, and all patients should undergo a workup for streptococcal infection and infectious mononucleosis. Only after these diagnoses are excluded can a viral cause be presumed. Rapid antigen detection tests (RADT) are useful for identifying streptococcal pharyngitis. A positive RADT is as reliable as a positive culture; however, a negative test should be followed by throat culture, which is still considered the gold standard.[1] The diagnosis of infectious mononucleosis can be confirmed with the Monospot test. Examination reveals tonsillopharyngeal erythema and swelling with white or grey exudates. Patients with "strep" infections usually have enlarged, tender anterior cervical lymph nodes, whereas viral pathogens are usually associated with cough and rhinorrhea.[1] Infectious mononucleosis has a brief prodrome of malaise, anorexia, and chills, followed by fever that lasts up to 2 weeks and lymphadenopathy involving both anterior and posterior cervical lymph nodes.[2]

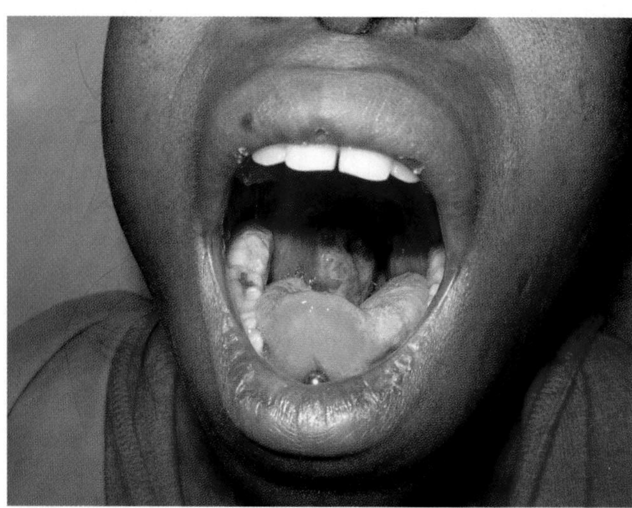

FIGURE 5-26 Streptococcal pharyngitis with extensive swelling and grey/white exudate. (Courtesy of Mark Silverberg, MD.)

Clinical Complications

Most cases of viral pharyngitis resolve without complication. There are both suppurative (otitis media, sinusitis) and nonsuppurative (acute rheumatic fever, post-streptococcal glomerulonephritis) complications of "strep throat."[1] The most common complications of infectious mononucleosis are upper airway obstruction, thrombocytopenia, and splenic rupture.[2]

Management

The treatment for EP is supportive, consisting of rest, fluids, analgesics, and antipyretics. Antibiotic therapy is indicated for cases of streptococcal pharyngitis, because it reduces the duration of symptoms and the length of contagiousness while preventing the development of acute rheumatic fever.[1,2] Antibiotics do not, however, prevent poststreptococcal glomerulonephritis.[1] The antibiotic of choice is penicillin for 10 days, or erythromycin may be substituted in allergic patients.[1] Corticosteroids have been proven to reduce the duration of fever, lymphadenopathy, and other constitutional symptoms in infectious mononucleosis, but otherwise they are recommended only if there is severe tonsillar swelling and impending upper airway obstruction.[2]

REFERENCES

1. Stephenson KN. Acute and chronic pharyngitis across the lifespan. *Lippincott's Prim Care Pract* 2000;4:471–489.
2. Hickey SM, Strasburger VC. What every pediatrician should know about infectious mononucleosis in adolescents. *Pediatr Clin North Am* 1997;44:1541–1556.

Viral Pharyngitis

Matthew Spencer

Clinical Presentation

The clinical manifestation of viral pharyngitis is most often a sore throat, usually associated with fever, cough, coryza, conjunctivitis, malaise, myalgias, and arthralgias, which may be accompanied by vomiting and diarrhea.[1,2] Symptoms usually begin gradually and last an average of 7 days.[1] Rhinorrhea and nasal congestion are common findings in viral infections of the pharynx. The tonsils usually are enlarged and erythematous and occasionally demonstrate exudates. Other findings on examination are petechiae on the soft palate and aphthous ulcers on the lips, gingiva, soft palate, mucosa, and tonsils.

Pathophysiology

Viruses account for 90% of cases of tonsillopharyngitis in adults and up to 60% to 75% of cases in children.[1] Various species propagate pharyngitis year round. Person-to-person spread is by respiratory droplet inhalation and hand-to-hand transmission.[1] There are many viral etiologies, but the most common involve adenovirus species, followed closely by rhinoviruses and coronaviruses.[1,2]

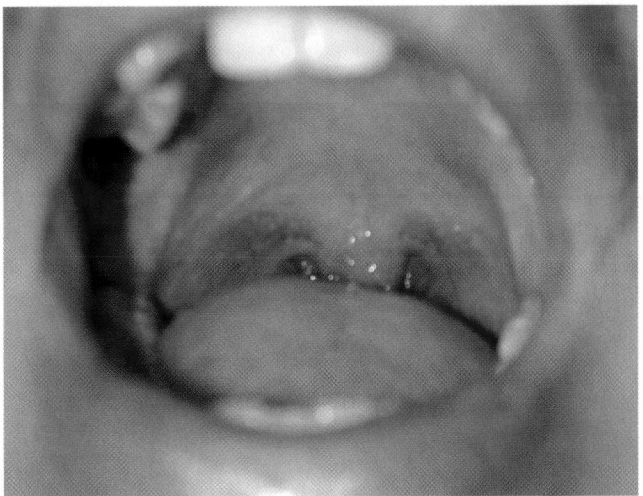

FIGURE 5–27 Viral pharyngitis. Note mild redness and minimal soft tissue swelling. (Courtesy of Robert Hendrickson, MD.)

Diagnosis

The diagnosis of viral tonsillopharyngitis is made clinically by the exclusion of streptococcal infection and infectious mononucleosis. Viral cultures are available, but they are not useful in the emergency department setting.

Clinical Complications

Complications include bacterial superinfection of the pharynx, lymphoid tissues, conjunctivae, or sinuses.

Management

Treatment is supportive and includes the use of analgesics, antipyretics, antihistamines, anesthetic throat sprays, gargling, cough suppressants, and decongestants.[1] Decongestants should be used cautiously in patients with hypertension. Decongestant nasal sprays are preferable to oral medications, but their use should be limited to 3 or 4 days to prevent systemic toxicity and tachyphylaxis. Patients should be encouraged to drink copious amounts of fluids to prevent dehydration. Use of a room humidifier may be helpful.

REFERENCES

1. Stephenson KN. Acute and chronic pharyngitis across the lifespan. *Lippincott's Prim Care Pract* 2000;4:471–489.
2. White CB, Foshee WS. Upper respiratory tract infections in adolescents. *Adolesc Med* 2000;11:225–249.

Peritonsillar Abscess

Matthew Spencer

Clinical Presentation

Patients with peritonsillar abscess present with severe tonsillopharyngitis, fever, sore throat, dysphagia, muffled or "hot potato" voice, trismus, and often drooling, usually after the symptoms have persisted 2 to 4 days.[1-3] On examination, there is a unilaterally swollen, fluctuant tonsil displacing the uvula to the opposite side.[1-3]

Pathophysiology

Peritonsillar abscess is an infection usually preceded by severe tonsillopharyngitis.[1] This infection occurs primarily in adolescents and young adults.[1,2] Peritonsillar cellulitis is infection and inflammation of the peritonsillar region without an abscess and may precede abscess formation.[1] Peritonsillar abscess formation usually results from progression of an acute pharyngitis to pharyngeal cellulitis and then to abscess.[2,3] The most commonly isolated organism is group A *Streptococcus,* but most infections are polymicrobial, involving both anaerobic and aerobic organisms of the upper respiratory tract.[1-3]

Diagnosis

The diagnosis is clinical and may be confirmed by needle aspiration, which differentiates peritonsillar abscess from cellulitis.[1,3]

Clinical Complications

Complications include spontaneous abscess rupture with aspiration of pus, retropharyngeal abscess, airway obstruction, thrombophlebitis, chronic peritonsillitis, epiglottitis, septicemia, endocarditis, myocarditis, rheumatic fever, and poststreptococcal glomerulonephritis.[1,2] Carotid artery puncture during needle aspiration or incision has been reported.[1-3]

Management

The treatment for peritonsillar abscess consists of drainage, analgesics, hydration, and antibiotics.[1-3] There are three generally accepted methods of drainage: needle aspiration, intraoral incision and drainage, and abscess tonsillectomy.[3] Needle aspiration is the most common method performed in the emergency department. A 10% to 15% failure rate with needle aspiration was documented in one study.[2] Antibiotics should cover both anaerobic and aerobic organisms infecting the upper respiratory tract. Clindamycin, penicillin, and penicillin plus a β-lactamase inhibitor are acceptable agents, but penicillin is recommended as first-line therapy in children.[1,3] Mildly symptomatic patients may be treated on an outpatient basis, and severely ill patients should be admitted.

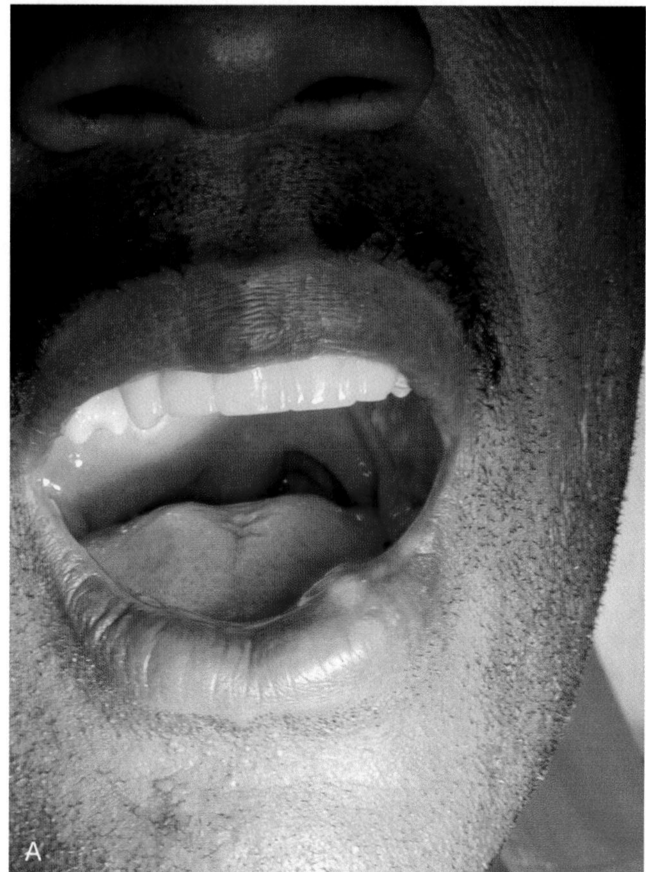

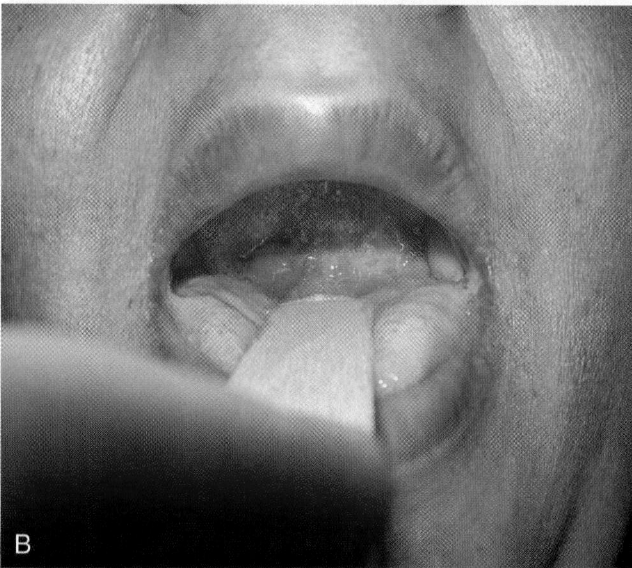

FIGURE 5–28 **A:** Right-sided peritonsillar abscess. (Courtesy of Robert Hendrickson, MD.) **B:** Left-sided peritonsillar abscess crossing the midline, with early partial upper airway obstruction. (Courtesy of Anthony Forestine, MD.)

REFERENCES

1. White CB, Foshee WS. Upper respiratory tract infections in adolescents. *Adolesc Med* 2000;11:225–249.
2. Epperly TD, Wood TC. New trends in the management of peritonsillar abscess. *Am Fam Physician* 1990;42:102–112.
3. Herzon FS, Nicklaus P. Pediatric peritonsillar abscess: management guidelines. *Curr Probl Pediatr* 1996;26:270–278.

Uvulitis

Matthew Spencer

Clinical Presentation

Patients with uvulitis may complain of a sore throat, difficulty swallowing, or the sensation of a foreign body in the throat.[1-3] A fever may or may not be present, and patients are often gagging, spitting, or choking because of discomfort when they swallow saliva.[1-3] On examination, the uvula is usually noted to be swollen and erythematous, but in some cases it actually appears to be pale.[1-3]

Pathophysiology

Uvulitis is a relatively uncommon disorder of both children and adults that develops from a variety of different causes. Inflammation of the uvula may develop as a result of infection, overuse of the voice, allergy, hereditary angioneurotic edema, angiotensin-converting enzyme inhibitor–related angioedema, local trauma, or inhalant use or abuse.[1-3] In children, uvulitis has been associated with *H. influenzae* type b bacteremia.[2]

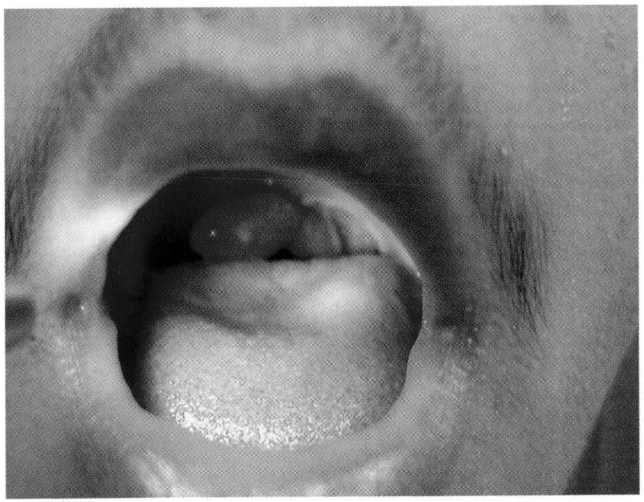

FIGURE 5–29 Edematous, erythematous, elongated uvula. (Courtesy of Christy Salvaggio, MD.)

Diagnosis

The diagnosis is made by history and physical examination. Patients with uvulitis who have fever, difficulty swallowing, or difficulty breathing should be evaluated for concomitant epiglottitis by soft tissue neck radiography, indirect or direct laryngoscopy, or fiberoptic nasolaryngoscopy.[1,2]

Clinical Complications

Local extension to involve the epiglottis and airway obstruction may complicate this problem in the most severe cases.[1-3]

Management

Patients with uvulitis secondary to allergy or angioedema should be treated with β-adrenergic agonists, antihistamines, and steroids. All pediatric patients, as well as adults with associated fever, should receive a workup for epiglottitis and should receive antibiotics that cover group A β-hemolytic *Streptococcus* and *H. influenzae* type b.[1,2] For patients without fever or other signs of airway compromise, the evidence for specific therapy is sparse and most patients improve with symptomatic care alone.[3] Emergency uvulectomy may be appropriate in some cases but should not be routinely performed. In the past, some physicians painted the swollen uvula with epinephrine solutions; however, this practice has never been validated as clinically efficacious.

REFERENCES

1. Kotloff KL, Wald ER. Uvulitis in children. *Pediatr Infect Dis* 1983;2:392–393.
2. McNamara RM, Koobatian T. Simultaneous uvulitis and epiglottitis in adults. *Am J Emerg Med* 1997;15:161–163.
3. McNamara RM. Clinical characteristics of acute uvulitis. *Am J Emerg Med* 1994;12:51–52.

Retropharyngeal Abscess

Matthew Spencer

Clinical Presentation

Retropharyngeal abscesses usually are seen in children younger than 5 years of age, and a preceding mild upper respiratory tract infection is present in 45% of patients.[1,2] Patients usually present with fever, irritability, dysphagia, drooling, and neck pain.[2,3] Other symptoms that may be present are nuchal rigidity, hyperextension of the neck, torticollis, feeding difficulties, spitting up, and stridor.[1-3] Younger children may present with respiratory distress.[2] In adults, sore throat, odynophagia, dysphagia, and neck pain are the predominant symptoms.[3] Cervical lymphadenopathy is present in 69% of patients.[1]

Pathophysiology

Retropharyngeal abscess is a pharyngeal infection that results in pus accumulation in the retropharyngeal space. Retropharyngeal abscess develops primarily from a preceding viral upper respiratory tract infection, pharyngitis, or otitis media (OM) that leads to inflammation and subsequent suppuration and necrosis of the retropharyngeal lymph nodes.[3] There is a mixed anaerobic and aerobic flora, with group A *Streptococcus* and *S. aureus* the most common organisms. *H. influenzae, Bacteroides* species, *Peptostreptococci,* and *Fusobacterium* species are also present.[1-4]

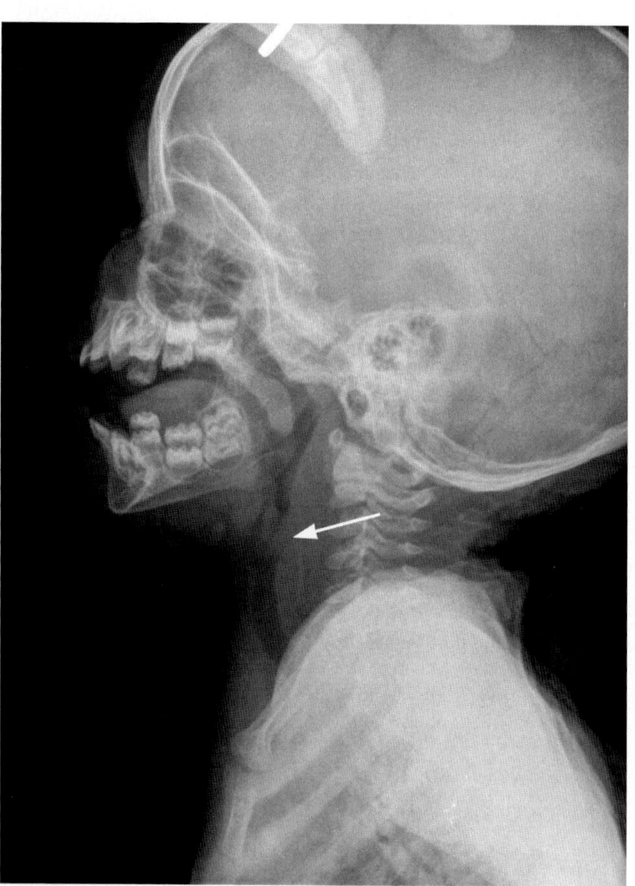

FIGURE 5-30 Radiograph showing retropharyngeal swelling due to an abscess in a child. (Courtesy of Robert Hendrickson, MD.)

Diagnosis

The diagnosis is made clinically and confirmed with lateral soft tissue neck radiographs.[1-4] Computed tomography (CT) of the neck may be useful in differentiating retropharyngeal abscess from cellulitis.[1-4]

Clinical Complications

Complications of retropharyngeal abscess include spontaneous rupture with resultant aspiration pneumonia, parapharyngeal extension, mediastinitis, airway obstruction, sepsis, empyema, psoas abscess, internal jugular thrombosis, internal carotid erosion, and atlantoaxial dislocation.[1,2] Retropharyngeal abscess carries a mortality rate of 10% and a complication rate of up to 43%.[4]

Management

Treatment for retropharyngeal abscess includes hospital admission for intravenous antibiotic therapy and immediate ear, nose, and throat (ENT) consultation for possible surgical drainage.[1,2] Antibiotics should cover both anaerobic and aerobic upper respiratory flora, and there are many suitable agents. Clindamycin, ampicillin/sulbactam, and second-generation cephalosporins are the most common single agents used.[4]

REFERENCES

1. Gaglani MJ, Edwards MS. Clinical indicators of childhood retropharyngeal abscess. *Am J Emerg Med* 1995;13:333–336.
2. White CB, Foshee WS. Upper respiratory tract infections in adolescents. *Adolesc Med* 2000;11:225–249.
3. Tannebaum RD. Adult retropharyngeal abscess: a case report and review of the literature. *J Emerg Med* 1996;14:147–158.
4. Lalakea M, Messner AH. Retropharyngeal abscess management in children: current practices. *Otolaryngol Head Neck Surg* 1999;121:398–405.

Herpes Gingivostomatitis

Matthew Spencer

Clinical Presentation

Patients present with painful, grouped vesicles on the buccal and gingival mucosa and tongue. These lesions often develop first on the gingival papillae before spreading to the rest of the oral mucosa.[1-4] Although most lesions are mucosal, up to two thirds of patients may also have extraoral lesions on their lips and face.[1] The vesicles are filled with clear or yellow fluid and have an erythematous base.[2] They rupture to form 2- to 3-mm flat ulcers and are associated with severe pain that often leads to difficulty eating and drinking, fever, malaise, and cervical lymphadenopathy.[1-5] The lesions tend to last for 1 to 3 weeks and usually heal without scarring.[1,2-5]

Pathophysiology

Herpes gingivostomatitis is a herpes simplex virus-1 (HSV-1) infection of the oral mucosa that is seen primarily in children but has also been described in adults.[1,5] It is the most common symptomatic infection of primary HSV-1 in children, with a peak incidence at 6 months to 5 years of age.[1,2,5] It is highly contagious, with an incubation period ranging from 2 to 12 days (mean, 4 days).[1,3,5] HSV-1 is transmitted by contact with open lesions or virally infected saliva.[1,2] Infection results after exposure to HSV-1 from an individual with virus-shedding lesions. The virus first infects the mucosal cells of the gingiva and anterior oropharynx, leading to symptomatic gingivostomatitis.[5]

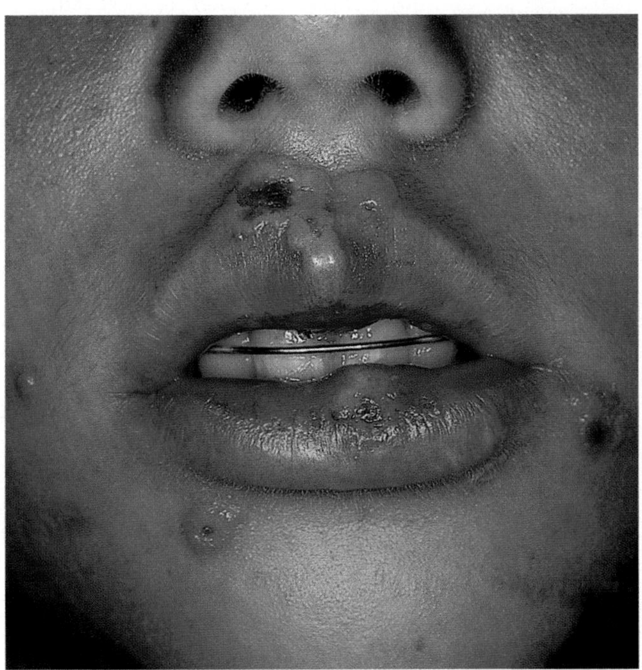

FIGURE 5–31 Primary herpes gingivostomatitis with perioral, labial, and intraoral vesiculopustular and bullous lesions. (From Ostler, with permission.)

Diagnosis

The diagnosis is made clinically by identification of the characteristic lesions and associated symptoms.[1,5] Viral culture of the active lesions is the gold standard and can be used to confirm the diagnosis, but it is not recommended for use in the emergency department.[1,4]

Clinical Complications

The most common complication of herpetic gingivostomatitis is dehydration resulting from an inability to eat or drink because of pain.[1] Other, less common complications include secondary bacterial infection from *S. pyogenes* or *Kingella kingae* and HSV encephalitis.[1,2]

Management

Emergency department treatment of herpetic gingivostomatitis is primarily supportive through the use of antipyretics, topical and systemic analgesics, warm saline mouth rinses, and intravenous fluids if the patient is dehydrated.[2,3,5] Mild cases require no additional therapy, but in severe cases, oral acyclovir should be started.[1] Acyclovir has been shown to reduce the severity and duration of disease, especially if it is started within 72 hours after symptom onset.[1,3,5] Immunocompromised patients should be admitted and treated with intravenous acyclovir until all lesions have dried and crusted.[3]

REFERENCES

1. Amir J. Clinical aspects and antiviral therapy in primary herpetic gingivostomatitis. *Paediatr Drugs* 2001;3:593–597.
2. Fenton SJ, Unkel JH. Viral infections of the oral mucosa in children: a clinical review. *Pract Periodont Aesthet Dent* 1997;9:683–692, quiz 692.
3. Rogers RS. Common lesions of the oral mucosa: a guide to diseases of the lips, cheeks, tongue, and gingivae. *Postgrad Med* 1992;91: 141–148,151–153.
4. Birek C. Herpesvirus-induced diseases: oral manifestations and current treatment options. *J Calif Dent Assoc* 2000;28:911–921.
5. Leigh IM. Management of non-genital herpes simplex virus infections in immunocompetent patients. *Am J Med* 1988;85:34–38.

Herpangina

Matthew Spencer

Clinical Presentation

Herpangina is diagnosed in children much more frequently than in adults.[1,2] There is a summer-time predominance, and most cases are mild, with the patient never seeing a physician.[1,2] If patients do seek care, they typically complain of rapid onset of sore throat, headache, fever, dysphagia, myalgias, anorexia, and, occasionally, vomiting or a stiff neck.[1,2] On examination, there are usually 2 to 10 painful, yellowish-white vesicles or ulcers located primarily on the tonsils, uvula, and soft palate, sparing the gingiva and tongue.[1,2] The vesicles are 1 to 2 mm in diameter and lie on an erythematous base. The vesicles eventually rupture to form 2- to 4-mm shallow, painful ulcers, which last 5 to 10 days. In contrast, the systemic symptoms usually last 1 or 2 days.[1]

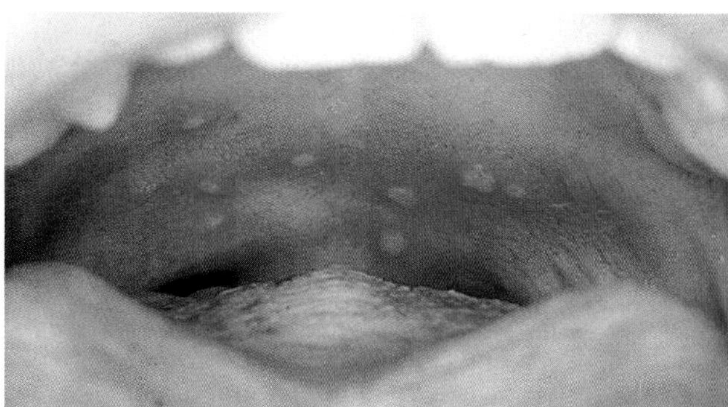

FIGURE 5-32 The classic pharyngeal lesions of herpangina. (Courtesy of Mark Silverberg, MD.)

Pathophysiology

Herpangina is an infection of the oral mucosa associated with a variety of coxsackieviruses and echoviruses.[1] It is highly contagious, with an incubation period of 4 to 6 days. Many varieties of enteroviruses can invade and infect the oral mucosa. The coxsackieviruses are the most common culprits, with coxsackievirus A being the most frequent and coxsackievirus B a close second.[1] Infection conveys immunity, but patients may become symptomatic again with infection by a different strain.[1]

Diagnosis

Diagnosis is purely clinical, based on the classic pharyngeal findings.

Clinical Complications

Dehydration may occur if the patient refuses to eat or drink due to dysphagia.

Management

Treatment for herpangina is symptomatic, with analgesics and antipyretics being most important. Often, the symptoms are so mild that no treatment is required.[1]

REFERENCES

1. Fenton SJ, Unkel JH. Viral infections of the oral mucosa in children: a clinical review. *Pract Periodont Aesthet Dent* 1997;9:683–692.
2. Rogers RS. Common lesions of the oral mucosa: a guide to diseases of the lips, cheeks, tongue, and gingivae. *Postgrad Med* 1992;91: 141–148,151–153.

Leukoplakia

Matthew Spencer

Clinical Presentation

Leukoplakia lesions consist of a single, elevated grayish/white plaque that may or may not have well-defined margins.[1] Leukoplakia may be located anywhere on the oral mucosa, but the most common locations are the buccal and alveolar mucosa and the lower lip.[1]

Pathophysiology

Leukoplakia is a precancerous lesion involving the oral mucosa. It is defined by the World Health Organization (WHO) as "a white patch or plaque that cannot be characterized clinically or pathologically as any other disease."[1,2] It is a diagnosis of exclusion that is most often seen in middle-aged and elderly men who smoke. However, women and nonsmokers with this disease have a higher rate of malignant transformation of the lesion.[1,2] Overall, leukoplakia affects approximately 1% to 5% of the U.S. population.[1] Smoking and oral tobacco use are the major risk factors for development of leukoplakia.[1,2] Although various theories exist regarding the origin of leukoplakia, they are probably caused by hyperkeratosis of the oral mucosa.[3]

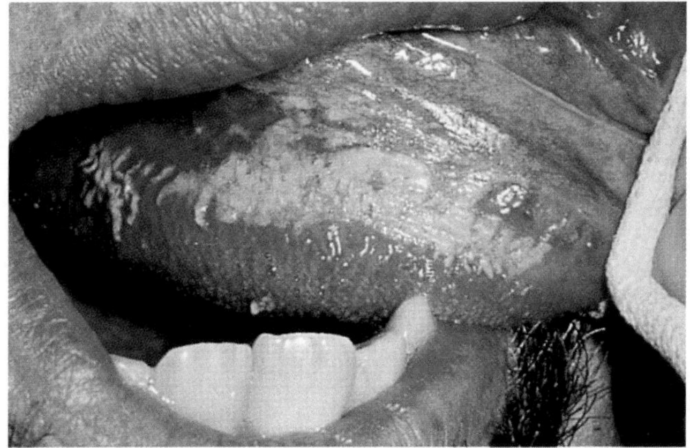

FIGURE 5–33 Painless, whitish, verrucous excrescences along the lateral aspects of the tongue are characteristic of oral hairy leukoplakia. (From Yamada, with permission.)

Diagnosis

The diagnosis is made clinically and confirmed by tissue biopsy.[1,3]

Clinical Complications

Malignant progression to squamous cell carcinoma is the most serious complication. Certain locations (floor of the mouth, tongue, and lip) have been found to have a higher risk of malignant transformation.[1] Nodular or speckled leukoplakias have the highest rate of malignant transformation.[1,3]

Management

In the early dysplastic stages, the goal is to treat the underlying cause and reduce or eliminate risk factors, including all forms of tobacco use.[1,3] Lesions of moderate to severe epithelial dysplasia must be removed surgically.[1] Dysplastic lesions are excised by laser or conventional surgery. The patient should go for follow-up every 6 months to watch for recurrence.[3] Other treatment modalities include topical bleomycin, topical or systemic 13-*cis*-retinoic acid, and systemic β-carotene and vitamin A. Leukoplakia is a chronic condition that does not require acute treatment in the emergency department. However, once it is diagnosed, patients should be referred to primary care physicians or otolaryngologists for prompt follow-up evaluation.

REFERENCES

1. Neville BW, Day TA. Oral cancer and precancerous lesions. *CA Cancer J Clin* 2002;52:195–215.
2. Lodi G, Sardella A, Bez C, Demarosi F, Carrassi A. Systematic review of randomized trials for the treatment of oral leukoplakia. *J Dent Edu* 2002;66:896–902.
3. Scully C, Porter S. ABC of oral health: swellings and red, white, and pigmented lesions. *BMJ* 2000;321:225–228.

5–34

Geographic Tongue

Matthew Spencer

Clinical Presentation

Most patients with geographic tongue are asymptomatic, but some experience mild pain, burning, a foreign body sensation, sensitivity to hot or spicy food, or pain in the ears or submandibular glands.[1] Lesions change location, size, and shape frequently but tend to remain on the dorsal and lateral surface of the tongue.[1] They may persist for days to years and usually heal on their own without scarring.[1]

Pathophysiology

Geographic tongue, or benign migratory glossitis, is a common asymptomatic inflammatory disorder of the tongue mucosa.[1,2] The prevalence of geographic tongue is approximately 1% to 2.5%, and it is seen more commonly in children.[1,2] Its cause is unknown, but it has been associated with pustular psoriasis, allergy, hormonal disturbances, juvenile diabetes, Reiter's syndrome, Down syndrome, nutritional deficiencies, psychological upsets, fissured tongue, and lichen planus.[1,2] The lesions resemble those of pustular psoriasis histologically and represent areas where the filiform papillae of the tongue have been lost.[1,2]

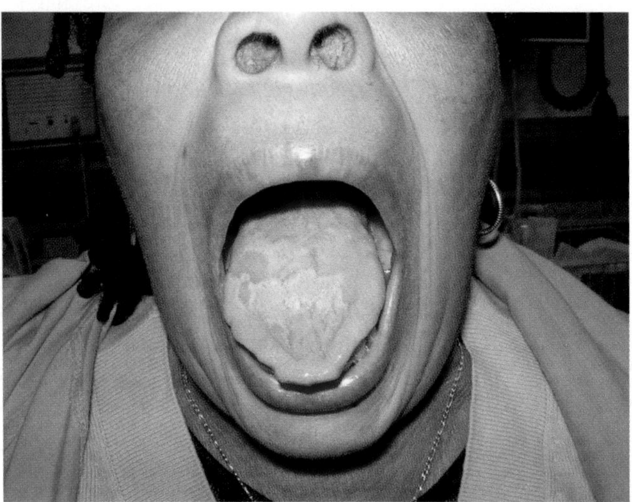

FIGURE 5–34 The classic appearance of randomly denuded patches of geographic tongue. (Courtesy of Teresa Liu, MD.)

Diagnosis

The diagnosis is made by history and physical examination and can be confirmed with tissue biopsy.[1,2]

Clinical Complications

There are no known complications of geographic tongue except the anxiety that is associated with it.[1]

Management

Various treatment regimens have been suggested, but none has proved effective.[1] Symptomatic treatment with acetaminophen, anesthetic mouth rinses, antihistamines, anxiolytics, and steroids have all been suggested, as well as topical tretinoin, systemic etretinate or acitretin, vitamin A, and cytotoxic therapy.[1] Most patients do well with reassurance and education to avoid hot, spicy, salty, or acidic foods.[1,2]

REFERENCES

1. Assimakopoulos D, Patrikakos G, Fotika C, Elisaf M. Benign migratory glossitis or geographic tongue: an enigmatic oral lesion. *Am J Med* 2002;113:751–755.
2. Brooks JK, Balciunas BA. Geographic stomatitis: review of the literature and report of five cases. *J Am Dent Assoc* 1987;115:421–424.

Aphthous Stomatitis

Matthew Spencer

Clinical Presentation

Patients with aphthous stomatitis present with painful oral ulcers that are round or oval shaped; are located on the tongue, buccal mucosa, vestibules, inner lips, or soft palate; and may be covered by a whitish-yellow, fibrinous membrane with a small ring of erythema.[1]

Pathophysiology

The cause of aphthous stomatitis is unknown, but it is thought to result from a combination of genetic predisposition, allergy, medications, hormones, stress, and immunologic factors.[1,2] Specific allergens include benzoic acid, cinnamaldehyde, nickel, mercury, fragrance mix, sorbic acid, phosphorus, and methyl methacrylate.[1] Local factors that affect the frequency of recurrence include local trauma, inadequate saliva production, tobacco use, and exposure to sodium lauryl sulfate, which is found in many oral health care products.[1] Ulcers may be classified as minor, major, or herpetiform, with minor aphthae consisting of a single shallow ulcer, less than 1 cm in diameter.[1,2] Major aphthae are generally larger, deeper, and more likely to scar. Herpetiform aphthae consist of multiple smaller lesions that usually are vesicular in character.[1,2]

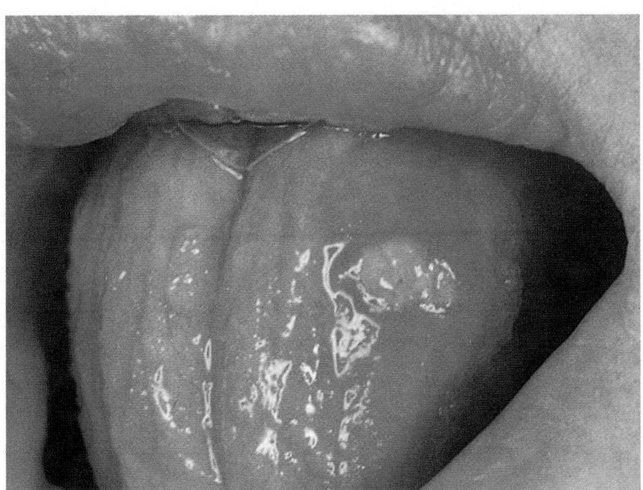

FIGURE 5-35 Aphthous ulcer on the tongue. (From Yamada, with permission.)

Diagnosis

The diagnosis is made by history and physical examination, with biopsy, culture, and cytology occasionally being useful to differentiate it from other oral lesions.[1]

Clinical Complications

The most common complication is pain, but scarring may rarely occur.[1]

Management

Treatment focuses on pain control and reduction in the rate of recurrence.[1] Over-the-counter local anesthetics, oxygenating agents, antiseptics, and chemical cautery agents may be useful, in addition to antiinflammatory medications.[1,2] Oral tetracycline rinses and pastes and magnesium hydroxide plus diphenhydramine liquid have been used with some success; severe disease may require oral prednisone therapy.[1,2] Various other therapies (zinc lozenges, vitamin C, vitamin B, and echinacea) have been reported to speed healing, but appropriate scientific confirmation is lacking.[2]

REFERENCES

1. Zunt SL. Recurrent aphthous stomatitis. *Dermatol Clin* 2003;21: 33–39.
2. McBride DR. Management of aphthous ulcers. *Am Fam Physician* 2000;62:149–154,160.

Black Hairy Tongue

Matthew Spencer

Clinical Presentation

Patients with black hairy tongue (BHT) present with brownish-black to yellowish-brown discoloration of the tongue and elongated filiform papillae that are mistaken for hair.[1,2]

Pathophysiology

BHT, also known as hyperkeratosis of the tongue, lingua villosa nigra, and melanotrichia linguae, is a benign condition of the tongue resulting from hypertrophy of the filiform papillae.[1,2] BHT has an incidence of 0.15% and is more common in the elderly and in cancer patients.[1] Filiform papillae elongation is thought to be the result of accumulated layers of keratin.[1,2] The cause is unknown but is hypothesized to be a result of reduced tongue movement and friction, leading to poor desquamation, or a tongue that is hypersensitive to irritants and then becomes discolored from pigments when eating.[1] Conditions associated with BHT include oxidizing agents, excessive tobacco use, oral or parenteral antibiotics, phenothiazines, griseofulvin, vitamin deficiency, and poor oral hygiene.[1]

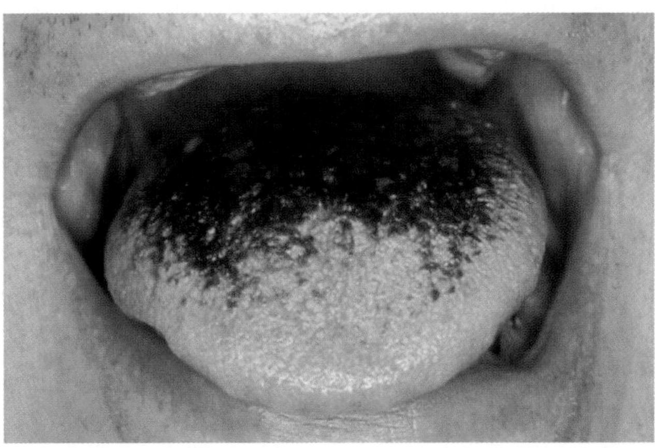

FIGURE 5–36 A velvety, hair-like thickening of the tongue; color can range from a yellowish-brown to green to jet black. (From Benjamin, with permission.)

Diagnosis

The diagnosis is made by history and physical examination.[1] Findings are restricted to the dorsum of the tongue, and patients usually have no other symptoms except an occasional metallic taste or foul odor.[1]

Clinical Complications

This condition has no known complications other than cosmetic concerns.

Management

Treatment requires elimination of predisposing factors such as tobacco, mouthwashes, or antibiotics, if possible.[1] Patients should be instructed to brush the tongue twice daily with a soft toothbrush and a 3% hydrogen peroxide solution or baking soda.[1] Oral triamcinolone applied twice daily after wiping the tongue dry has also been used successfully, as have multivitamins, B-complex vitamins, and topical antifungal agents.[1]

REFERENCES

1. Sarti GM, Haddy RI, Schaffer D, Kihm J. Black hairy tongue. *Am Fam Physician* 1990;41:1751–1755.
2. Harada Y, Gaafar H. Black hairy tongue: a scanning electron microscopic study. *J Laryngol Otol* 1977;91:91–96.

Branchial Cleft Cyst

Matthew Spencer

Clinical Presentation

Patients with branchial cleft cyst usually present with painless swelling of the neck at the anterior border of the sternocleidomastoid muscle but may also present with an abscess in the same location.[1-3]

Pathophysiology

Branchial cleft cysts are cystic congenital anomalies of the neck or face that develop from remnants of embryologic branchial clefts.[1,2] During the fourth to eighth weeks of gestation, six pairs of mesodermal arches (branchial arches) form the branchial apparatus.[2,3] These arches are separated by external folds lined by ectodermal tissue, called the branchial clefts.[2,3] Each arch develops into separate neural, muscular, and skeletal structures. All of the branchial clefts regress except part of the first cleft, which forms the external auditory canal.[2,3] Occasionally, other brachial clefts fail to resolve, resulting in cysts or fistulas. Second branchial cleft anomalies are the most common, comprising 95% of cases.[2,3] Cysts usually manifest in childhood or early adulthood, whereas sinuses, fistulas, and cartilaginous remnants manifest most often during infancy.[1-3]

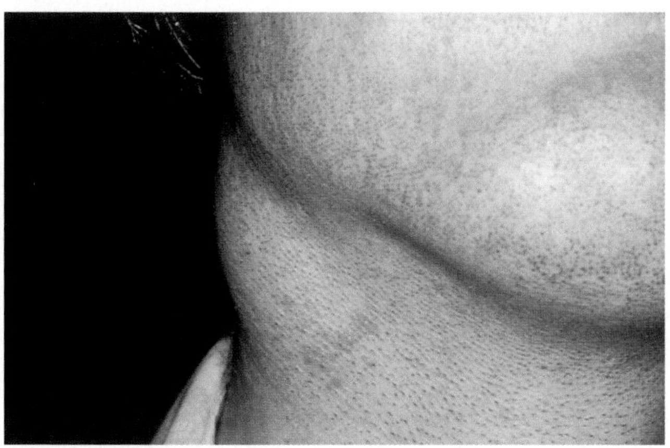

FIGURE 5–37 Branchial cyst in a typical location at the anterior border of the sternomastoid. (From Benjamin, with permission.)

Diagnosis

The diagnosis can be confirmed by fine-needle aspiration of the cystic fluid, which often has a high concentration of cholesterol crystals.[1] Ultrasonography usually identifies a deep neck cyst but may not provide enough information to diagnose the cleft from which it has originated.[2] Most practitioners recommend a barium swallow as the first radiographic study to identify the cyst's pharyngeal opening.[3] If the barium swallow is indeterminate, it should be followed by computed tomography (CT), and ultimately by direct laryngoscopy at the time of exploration.[3]

Clinical Complications

The complications of branchial cleft cysts include recurrent neck abscesses, recurrent suppurative thyroiditis, respiratory distress, and, occasionally, retropharyngeal abscess.[3]

Management

If the cyst is infected, but no abscess has formed, it should be treated with antibiotics, warm compresses, and nonemergency referral to an otolaryngologist or plastic surgeon.[2] Abscesses should be drained and packed, and the patient should be prescribed antibiotics with prompt follow-up.[2] In the absence of airway compromise, emergency consultation usually is not needed. Definitive treatment involves surgical excision of the cyst.[1-3]

REFERENCES

1. Mady SM. Managing lumps in the neck. *Practitioner* 1998;242: 472–475.
2. Brown RL, Azizkhan RG. Pediatric head and neck lesions. *Pediatr Clin North Am* 1998;45:889–905.
3. Yang C, Cohen J, Everts E, Smith J, Caro J, Andersen P. Fourth branchial arch sinus: clinical presentation, diagnostic workup, and surgical treatment. *Laryngoscope* 1999;109:442–446.

Lymphadenitis

Matthew Spencer

Clinical Presentation

The lymph nodes often involved in lymphadenitis are the submandibular nodes and the anterior and posterior cervical nodes that drain most of the face, nasopharynx, mouth, and oropharynx.[1,2] Patients are often children who present with acute onset of tender lymphadenopathy with fever, malaise, warmth, and erythema in the region.[1-3] The nodes enlarge in response to a pathogen collected from the region drained by its lymphatics. Bacterial causes of lymphadenitis are usually unilateral, and lymph nodes may range from 2 to 6 cm in diameter.[1-3] *Mycobacterium tuberculosis* cervical lymphadenitis (scrofula) manifests in older children and adolescents as a painless, nontender, slowly increasing enlargement of the anterior cervical nodes.[1,3] Nontuberculous mycobacterial lymphadenitis manifests in a similar manner but usually affects younger children.[1,2]

Pathophysiology

Lymphadenitis describes a nonspecific inflammatory enlargement of one or more lymph nodes, most commonly with a viral origin.[1,2] Bacterial lymphadenitis usually develops as secondary suppuration after an upper respiratory tract infection, and the bacteria most commonly involved are *Staphylococcus* and *Streptococcus* species.[1-3] Other, less common causes include *Bacteroides* spp., *Peptococcus* spp., *Peptostreptococcus* spp., *Propionibacterium acnes, Fusobacterium nucleatum, H. influenzae, Actinomyces israelii, Toxoplasmosa gondii, Francisella tularensis, Blastomyces dermatitidis,* and *Candida albicans.*[1,2] Mycobacterial species such as *M. tuberculosis, Mycobacterium avium-intracellulare,* and *Mycobacterium scrofulaceum* have also been found to lead to lymphadenitis, as has *Rochalimaea henselae,* which is the primary (but not sole) causative agent for cat-scratch disease.[1,2]

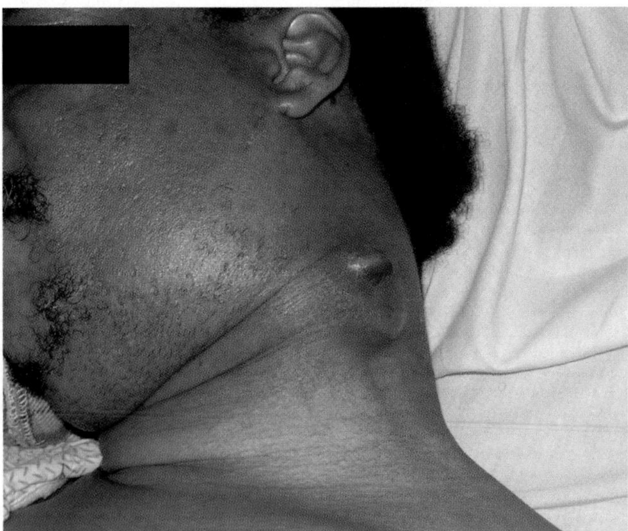

FIGURE 5–38 Pointing abscess derived from infected cervical lymph nodes. (Courtesy of Mark Silverberg, MD.)

Diagnosis

The diagnosis of lymphadenitis is made clinically and is supported by the use of biopsy, the purified protein derivative (PPD) test, and chest radiography only if the symptoms are chronic and do not respond to initial therapy.[1,2]

Clinical Complications

The potential clinical complications include local extension of infection and the development of septicemia. In the case of cat-scratch disease, osteomyelitis, encephalitis, or retinitis may occur very rarely.[1]

Management

In all cases, the treatment of lymphadenitis should include the frequent application of moist heat in the form of compresses. In addition, immobilization and elevation should be considered as treatment adjuncts. In the emergency department, it is important to consider the possibility of a bacterial origin if the lymphadenitis is of acute onset. In the case of a bacterial infection causing lymphadenitis, β-lactamase–resistant antibiotics such as dicloxacillin, cloxacillin, amoxicillin/clavulanate, and cephalexin should be considered. Macrolides and clindamycin are acceptable alternatives for penicillin-allergic patients.[1,2] If the infected lymph node is fluctuant, it should be treated similarly to any abscess, with incision and drainage, and consideration should be given to starting oral antibiotic therapy.[2]

Although the diagnosis of tuberculous lymphadenitis is unlikely to be made in the emergency department, suspected cases should be treated with rifampin and isoniazid for 12 to 18 months as one of several possible regimens.[1,2] Nontuberculous mycobacterial lymphadenitis is not responsive to pharmacologic therapy, and the involved nodes must be excised surgically.[1,2] Cat-scratch disease is self-limited and usually requires no treatment as it resolves over the following months.[1,3]

REFERENCES

1. Bodenstein L, Altman RP. Cervical lymphadenitis in infants and children. *Semin Pediatr Surg* 1994;3:134–141.
2. Brook I. The swollen neck: cervical lymphadenitis, parotiditis, thyroiditis, and infected cysts. *Infect Dis Clin North Am* 1988;2: 221–236.
3. Ortiz JA, Hudkins C, Kornblut A. Adenitis, adenopathy, and abscesses of the head and neck. *Emerg Med Clin North Am* 1987;5: 359–370.

Thyroid Mass

Matthew Spencer

Clinical Presentation

The prevalence of thyroid nodules is 0.22% to 1.5% in children and increases at a rate of 0.08% per year into the eighth decade.[1] Palpable nodules are present in 4% to 7% of all adults in the United States and are more common in women, affecting approximately 50% of middle-aged women.[1,2] Most patients present with a palpable asymptomatic thyroid mass found by themselves or their physicians.[2] If the nodule is fixed and hard with associated lymphadenopathy, recurrent laryngeal nerve palsy, obstruction, dysphagia, hoarseness, or rapid growth, then malignancy must be suspected.[1,2] However, fewer than 5% of patients with thyroid cancer have any local symptoms.[1]

Pathophysiology

Most thyroid nodules are benign thyroid adenomas. These arise from the epithelium of the thyroid follicle and contain homogeneous tissue within a fibrous capsule.[1]

Diagnosis

The diagnosis is usually clinical, in which the patient or the physician notices some degree of neck swelling or feels a small thyroid mass on examination.

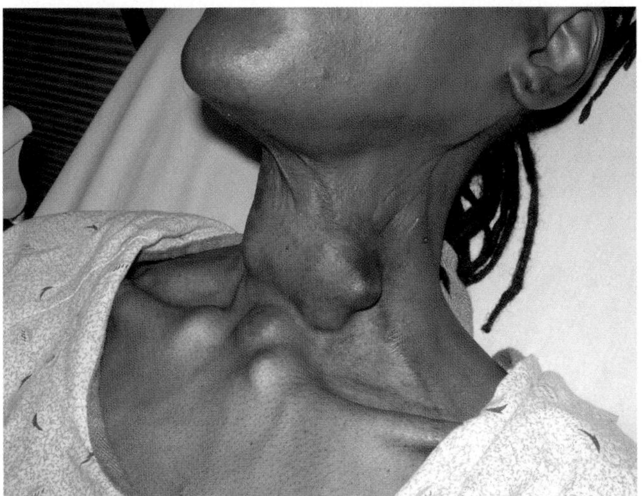

FIGURE 5–39 Multiple nodular masses of thyroid. (Courtesy of Mark Silverberg, MD.)

Clinical Complications

The most serious complication is malignancy; however, patients may also experience recurrent laryngeal nerve palsy, dysphagia, hoarseness, or upper airway obstruction due to an appropriately located mass.[1,2] Patients with a single nodule have the same risk of malignancy as those with multiple nodules.[2] Radiation exposure is a major risk factor for malignancy, with only 10% to 20% of nodules in patients without radiation exposure being malignant, as opposed to 30% to 50% of those in patients with radiation exposure.[1]

Management

In the emergency department, all acute airway issues must be addressed first. If severe airway obstruction due to a thyroid mass is present, an immediate surgical consultation should be sought while all efforts are exerted to maintain the patient's airway.[2] Patients with multinodular goiters and signs of upper airway obstruction should be admitted for treatment and further evaluation, because they will benefit from surgical resection or radioactive iodine therapy.[2] There is no need for radiographic evaluation if no signs of upper airway obstruction are present; if such signs are present and mild, plain radiographs of the thoracic inlet, computed tomography (CT), magnetic resonance imaging (MRI), or, ideally, a respiratory flow volume loop should be obtained.[2] If patients have signs of thyrotoxicosis, then it is recommended that the levels of thyroid-stimulating hormone (TSH), thyroxine (T_4), and triiodothyronine (T_3) be checked.[2] Otherwise, patients should be referred to their primary care physicians for fine-needle biopsy, which is the best initial test to differentiate benign from malignant nodules. Thyroid scintigraphy or ultrasonography may also be helpful.[1,2] Nonpalpable thyroid nodules found incidentally by MRI or CT usually do not require therapeutic intervention if they are less than 1.5 cm in size and the patient has no risk factors for thyroid malignancy.[2]

REFERENCES

1. Rojeski MT, Gharib H. Nodular thyroid disease: evaluation and management. *N Engl J Med* 1985;313:428–436.
2. Lane H, Jones MK. Management of nodular thyroid disease. *Practitioner* 2002;246:266–269.

5-40

Thyroglossal Duct Cyst

Matthew Spencer

Clinical Presentation

Patients with thyroglossal duct cyst present with a midline, nontender, palpable neck mass, which often fluctuates in size and usually moves with swallowing or movement of the tongue.[1-3] Occasionally there is associated dysphagia, midneck tenderness, or cough.[1]

Pathophysiology

A thyroglossal duct cyst is a congenital neck mass that develops as a result of the failure of a portion of the thyroglossal duct to regress normally by 8 to 10 weeks of gestation.[1,2] The thyroglossal duct is an epithelial tract that forms during the fourth through seventh weeks of gestation, as the thyroid descends to its normal anatomic position in the neck.[1] This duct normally regresses between the sixth and eighth weeks of gestation, after the thyroid has completed its descent.[1,2] A cyst forms when epithelial cells within the tract remain active, thereby preventing that portion of the tract from regressing as it should.[1]

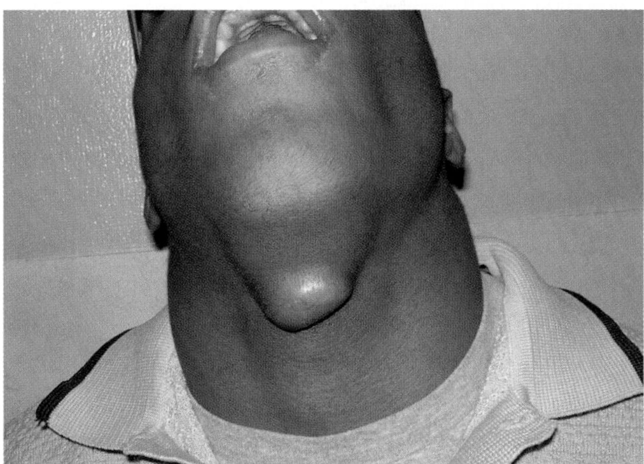

FIGURE 5–40 Infected thyroglossal duct cyst. (Courtesy of Raffi Kapitanyan, MD)

Diagnosis

Thyroglossal duct cyst should be suspected in any patient with a nontender, midline neck mass, because this is the most common presentation.[1,3] It can be confirmed radiographically with thyroid ultrasonography, computed tomography (CT), magnetic resonance imaging (MRI), or thyroid scanning, but plain radiographs are not useful.[1]

Clinical Complications

Complications from thyroglossal duct cysts are primarily infection and malignant transformation. Up to 50% of the cysts eventually become infected if they are not removed.[1,3]

Management

Elective surgical resection is the treatment of choice; however, other less common modalities have been proposed, such as ethanol-injection sclerotherapy.[1] If the patient is asymptomatic, there is no need for immediate therapy in the emergency department, and the patient should be referred to an otolaryngologist in 1 to 2 weeks. An infected cyst should be treated with warm compresses and antibiotics such as penicillin or clindamycin, to cover the normal oropharyngeal flora. The patient should be referred to an otolaryngologist within 2 to 3 days.[2]

REFERENCES

1. Josephson GD, Spencer WR, Josephson JS. Thyroglossal duct cyst: the New York Eye and Ear Infirmary experience and a literature review. *ENT J* 1998;77:642–647,651.
2. Brown RL, Azizkhan RG. Pediatric head and neck lesions. *Pediatr Clin North Am* 1998;45:889–905.
3. Ghaneim A, Atkins P. The management of thyroglossal duct cysts. *Int J Clin Pract* 1997;51:512–513.

Cleft Lip and Palate

Matthew Spencer

Clinical Presentation

Patients with cleft lip have a distinctive deformity of the lip, nose, and alveolus, which varies in severity from a simple notching of the vermilion border to complete extension through the maxillary portion of the alveolus.[1]

Pathophysiology

Cleft lip results when there is failure of the maxillary prominences to merge properly with the medial nasal prominences during the fifth week of gestation. The incidence of cleft lip with or without cleft palate varies by ethnic group, with a rate of approximately 1 per 1,000 in the white population, 2 per 1,000 in Asian populations, and 0.41 per 1,000 in African-Americans. Cleft lip with or without cleft palate is more common in males, who make up 60% to 80% of those affected.[1] Isolated bilateral cleft lips are extremely rare; in 86% of cases, there is an associated cleft palate.[1] Phenytoin use during pregnancy is the only teratogenic agent linked directly to isolated cleft lip; it results in a tenfold increase in incidence.[1]

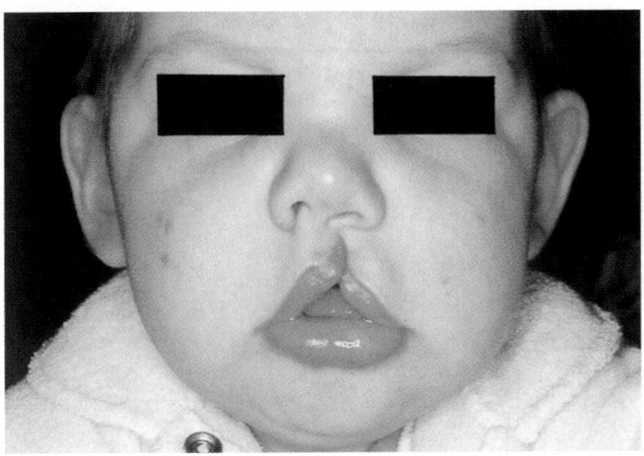

FIGURE 5–41 Cleft lip. Note the flattening of the right lower lateral cartilage and deviation of the nasal septum. (From Benjamin, with permission.)

Cleft palate occurs with failure of the lateral palatine processes to fuse properly with each other, the nasal septum, or the median palatine process between the fifth and twelfth weeks of gestation.[1] Isolated cleft palate deformities occur with an incidence of approximately 0.5 per 1,000 births, are more common in females, make up 33% of all cleft deformities, and are equally distributed across ethnic groups.[1]

Diagnosis

The diagnosis is made at birth. On physical examination, there is a wide range in severity of cleft palates, ranging from simple bifurcation of the uvula to complete extension through the hard and soft palate and the alveolar portion of the maxilla and lips bilaterally.[1]

Clinical Complications

The primary complications associated with cleft lip are cosmetic, except for feeding-related difficulties in newborns. Complications associated with cleft palate include feeding difficulties in newborns and infants, nasopharyngeal reflux, airway compromise, recurrent otitis media (OM), hearing loss, dental problems, orthodontic problems, midfacial growth impairment, and impaired speech development.[1]

Management

Definitive treatment involves surgical repair. The best results are obtained when the patient is 2 to 6 months of age. The treatment for a cleft palate deformity is surgical repair and reconstruction, usually before 12 months of age, but the optimal timing of repair is controversial.[1]

REFERENCES

1. Kirschner RE, LaRossa D. Cleft lip and palate. *Otolaryngol Clin North Am* 2000;33:1191–1215.

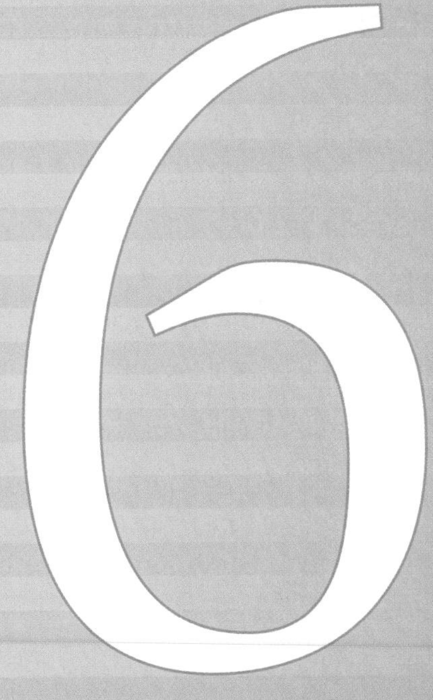

Dental

6–1

Acute Necrotizing Ulcerative Gingivitis

Matthew Spencer

Clinical Presentation

The three most common features of acute necrotizing ulcerative gingivitis (ANUG) are papillar ulcerations, gingival pain, and gingival bleeding.[1,2] It is usually of relatively acute onset, with a grayish-white exudate covering the interdental papilla and accompanying halitosis. Symptoms of severe disease include the systemic manifestations of fever and lymphadenopathy.

Pathophysiology

ANUG is an acute bacterial infection of the gingiva also known as "trench mouth," Vincent's disease, or fusospirochetal gingivitis.[1,3] ANUG is thought to be the result of gingival infection secondary to overgrowth of oral bacteria. Specifically, anaerobes of *Treponema, Selenomonas, Prevotella, Porphyromonas,* and *Fusobacterium* species have been implicated.[1,4] Predisposing risk factors include smoking, stress, poor diet, and systemic immune deficiency in the setting of chronic gingival inflammation from poor dental hygiene.[1-3]

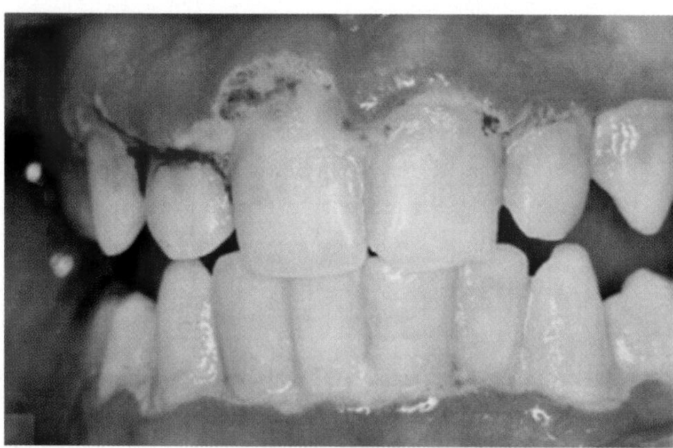

FIGURE 6–1 Generalized severe view of acute necrotizing ulcerative gingivitis (ANUG). (From Mandell, with permission.)

Clinical Complications

Acute necrotizing periodontitis, which involves the spread of infection to the periodontal ligament and surrounding alveolar bone, may complicate some cases of ANUG.

Management

First-line therapy includes instrumentation and cleaning by a dental professional, antimicrobial mouth rinses, improved personal oral hygiene, and possibly systemic oral antibiotics.[2,5] The emergency physician should prescribe penicillin, clindamycin, or metronidazole and refer the patient to a dentist within 24 to 48 hours.

REFERENCES

1. Rowland RW. Necrotizing ulcerative gingivitis. *Ann Periodontol* 1999;4:65–73.
2. Ahl DR, Hilgeman JL, Snyder JD. Periodontal emergencies. *Dent Clin North Am* 1986;30:459–472.
3. Hirsch RS, Clarke NG. Infection and periodontal diseases. *Rev Infect Dis* 1989;11:707–715.
4. Novak MJ. Necrotizing ulcerative periodontitis. *Ann Periodontol* 1999;4:74–78.
5. Pihlstrom BL, Ammons WF: Position paper: the American Academy of Periodontology. Treatment of gingivitis and periodontitis. *J Periodontol* 1997;68:1246–1253.

Dental Abscess

Matthew Spencer

Clinical Presentation

Periapical and periodontal abscesses have similar clinical presentations of local tooth pain, thermal sensitivity, and soft tissue swelling and redness.[1–4] Systemic symptoms of fever, malaise, regional lymphadenopathy, and occasionally trismus are often present as well. Periodontal abscesses generally drain through the deep gingival pocket into the oral cavity, whereas periapical abscesses form fistulas through the bone and develop many different drainage sites, depending on the abscess location and thickness of the surrounding alveolar bone.[1]

Pathophysiology

Dental abscesses are oral infections that result in localized accumulations of pus; they are classified according to the location of the infection source. An endodontic or periapical abscess develops from an infection of the root canal after pulp necrosis and expands through the apical foramen to form a pocket at the base of the tooth.[1,2] A periodontal abscess forms from an infection of the surrounding periodontal tissues: the gingiva, mucosa, periodontal ligament, or bone.[1,2] Endodontic and periodontal abscesses are commonly encountered emergency dental infections; they account for between 14% and 25% and between 7% and 14% of oral infections, respectively.[2]

Periapical abscesses are a result of severe dental caries, trauma, root fracture, or multiple dental procedures resulting in pulp necrosis and subsequent polymicrobial infection with anaerobic oral flora.[1,3] Periodontal abscesses form after debris is trapped between the gingiva and the tooth, resulting in inflammation of the periodontal tissues and secondary infection with anaerobic bacteria.[1–3]

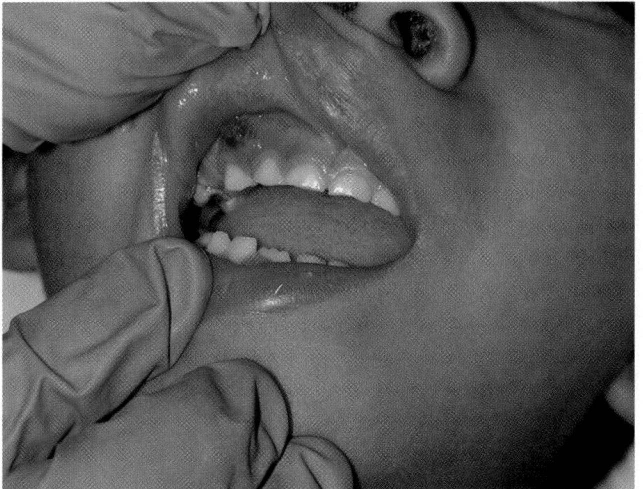

FIGURE 6–2 Dental abscess. (Courtesy of Robert Hendrickson, MD.)

Diagnosis

The diagnosis of dental abscess is primarily based on clinical examination, with confirmation of periapical abscesses by intraoral periapical or Panorex radiographs if available.

Clinical Complications

The most common complications of these infections are tooth and bone loss, osteomyelitis, and chronic pain. However, if they are left untreated, these infections can spread through the soft tissue fascial planes of the head and neck, leading to life-threatening conditions such as mediastinitis, Ludwig's angina, and cavernous sinus thrombosis.

Management

Emergency department (ED) management of these abscesses is essentially the same as for any other abscess. After incision and drainage of the purulent collection and irrigation with warm saline, packing material is placed in the wound to ensure adequate drainage.[1–3] Because of continual recontamination from oral flora, systemic antibiotics should be initiated.[1–3] The cause of these lesions is usually anaerobic oral flora of the mouth, so penicillin is the drug of choice. In case of penicillin allergy, metronidazole or clindamycin may be substituted. Patients should be treated with antibiotics for 10 to 14 days and referred to a dentist or oral surgeon within 24 hours.

REFERENCES

1. Dahlen G. Microbiology and treatment of dental abscesses and periodontal-endodontic lesions. *Periodontology 2000* 2002;28: 206–239.
2. Herrera D, Roldan S, Sanz A. The periodontal abscess: a review. *J Clin Periodontol* 2000;27:377–386.
3. Kretzschmar JL, Kretzschmar DP. Common oral conditions. *Am Fam Physician* 1996;54:225–234.
4. Flynn TR. The swollen face: severe odontogenic infections. *Emerg Med Clin North Am* 2000;18:481–519.

Dental Caries

Matthew Spencer

Clinical Presentation

The typical clinical presentation of tooth decay in the emergency department (ED) is tooth pain derived from a carious lesion or fracture of a severely decayed tooth. The classification of carious lesions is based on a scoring system from 0 to 4. Zero (0) involves a slight discoloration of the tooth's enamel, visible only after drying. One (1) is a moderate white discoloration, and 1a is a brown discoloration of the tooth; both conditions are visible only after drying of the tooth and not when the tooth is wet. Scores of 2 and 2a are, respectively, white and brown discolorations of enamel that are clearly visible on the wet tooth without drying. A score of 3 indicates localized breakdown of enamel resulting in an opaque or grayish color to the tooth. A score of 4 is an actual cavitation exposing the underlying dentin.[1] Hidden lesions are found on the occlusal tooth surface, and there may be a large lesion underneath a normal-appearing fissure.[1,2] Lesions often are missed on clinical examination. Pain indicates that there is some irritation of the pulp tissues.

Pathophysiology

Dental caries, or tooth decay, is erosion and demineralization of the enamel and other hard tissues of the teeth. According to epidemiologic data, 60% of tooth decay is found in only 20% to 25% of the population, although 70% of individuals 35 to 44 years of age have had at least one tooth extracted because of a carious lesion.[2,3] The cause of tooth decay is multifactorial.[2] The first step is the formation of dental plaque, which is a thin layer of food debris, bacteria, mucus, and dead epithelial cells that covers the tooth. Plaque forms a hospitable environment for the adherence and growth of the bacteria on the tooth surface. These oral bacteria species produce inorganic acids, leading to demineralization of the enamel and dentin. The entire process is dynamic, with the pulp constantly trying to remineralize the affected area.[1,4]

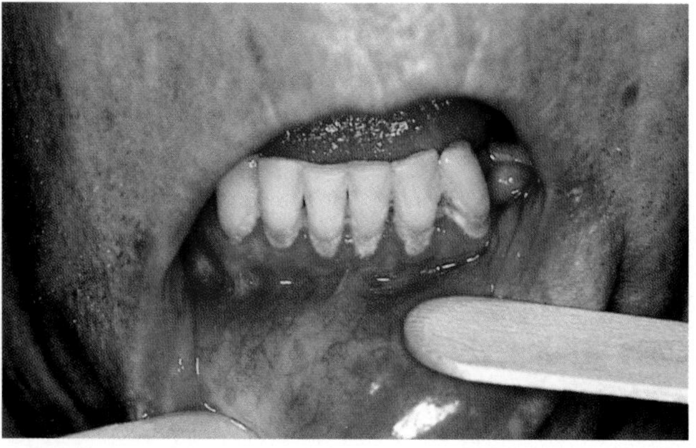

FIGURE 6–3 Dental caries is the gradual decay and disintegration of a tooth with progressive decalcification of the enamel and dentin. Moderate caries in this adult is visible around the roots of the teeth. (From Benjamin, with permission.)

Diagnosis

The diagnosis is primarily clinical, made by a thorough examination of the involved teeth. Intraoral periapical or bite-wing radiographs may be necessary to diagnose small or hidden lesions in the setting of tooth pain and a normal examination.

Clinical Complications

Complications resulting from dental caries are pain, gingivitis, dental abscess, pulpitis, pulp necrosis, dental fractures, and tooth loss.

Management

The treatment of dental caries is primarily preventive and is aimed at eradication of the plaque through good oral hygiene using a fluoride-containing toothpaste, regular professional cleaning, and a balanced diet. Lesions with a score of 0, 1, or 2 require either no therapy or plaque control alone. Lesions with a score of 3 require restoration with a sealant, whereas a score of 4 requires a temporary restoration and possible removal of all affected dentine.[1] Most patients present to the emergency department (ED) with dental pain, and analgesics are the mainstay of therapy for these individuals. Oral nonsteroidal antiinflammatory drugs (NSAIDs), narcotics, or narcotic combinations are the therapy of choice, as well as regional anesthesia with an appropriate nerve block or local alveolar infiltration. Emergency department patients who complain of dental pain usually have advanced disease with pulpal irritation causing pain and should be referred to a dentist within 24 hours. Antibiotics are not necessary unless the ED physician suspects a dental abscess or cellulitis of the surrounding gingival tissues. The antibiotic of choice for these patients is penicillin, metronidazole, or clindamycin, depending on the patient's allergy profile.

REFERENCES

1. Ekstrand KR, Ricketts DN, Kidd EA. Occlusal caries: pathology, diagnosis, and logical management. *Dent Update* 2001;28:380–387.
2. Charland R, Voyer R, Cudzinowski L, Salvail P, Abelardo L. Dental caries diagnosis and treatment. *N Y State Dent J* 2002;68:38–40.
3. Truman BI, Gooch BF, Sulemana I, Gift HC, Horowitz AM, Evans CA, et al. Reviews of evidence on interventions to prevent dental caries, oral and pharyngeal cancers, and sports related craniofacial injuries. *Am J Prev Med* 2002;23:21–54.
4. Lenander-Lumikari M, Loimaranta V. Saliva and dental caries. *Adv Dent Res* 2000;14:40–47.

Postextraction Bleeding

Matthew Spencer

Clinical Presentation

The clinical presentation involves bleeding from an extraction site that persists despite direct pressure application.[1-3]

Pathophysiology

Postextraction bleeding involves persistent bleeding after a tooth has been extracted that continues after discharge from the dental office.[1-3] Tooth extraction creates an open wound in the highly vascular gingival and alveolar bone. Persistent bleeding can be caused by salivary lysis of the blood clot, failure to obey discharge instructions, anticoagulant or antiplatelet medications, alcohol, anticancer agents, or inherited coagulation defects.[1-3]

Clinical Complications

Uncontrolled bleeding that results in anemia, requiring blood product administration or respiratory distress after aspiration of blood, may complicate postextraction bleeding.[1-3]

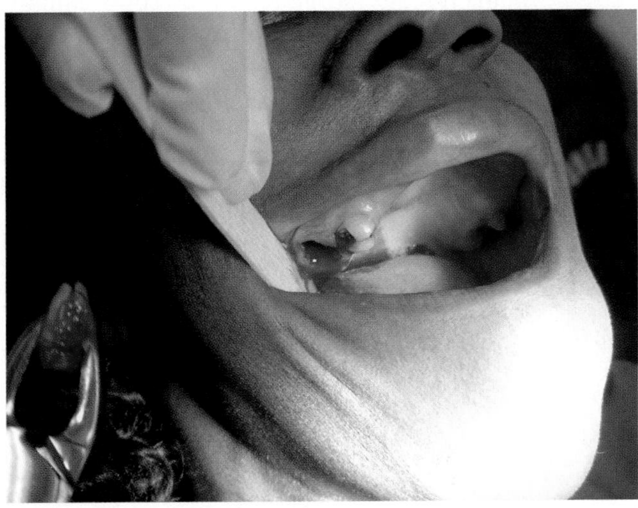

FIGURE 6–4 Bleeding from the socket of a tooth that was removed. (Courtesy of Mark Silverberg, MD.)

Management

The first step is to insert gauze into the extraction site and have the patient apply direct pressure for 15 to 30 minutes by biting down gently. If direct pressure fails to curtail the bleeding, more aggressive local therapy, consisting of absorbable suture placement and topical hemostatic agents, should be employed. Common topical hemostatic agents include Gelfoam,® Surgicel,® Oxycel,® and bovine collagen products such as Avitene,® CollaTape,® CollaCote,® and CollaPlug.® All can be applied directly to the bleeding socket, and many can be sutured in place. Both Surgicel® and Oxycel® have some bacteriocidal properties and therefore should be chosen in the setting of a concomitant infection. If bleeding still persists, the emergency physician must consider systemic causes of excessive bleeding, such as pharmacologic or inherited coagulation defects. Systemic treatment with fresh-frozen plasma or vitamin K should be used in the setting of an elevated International Normalized Ratio (INR). Factor replacement, desmopressin acetate (DDAVP), cryoprecipitate, or desmopressin should be used for the appropriate factor deficiencies.[1-3]

REFERENCES

1. Matocha DL. Postsurgical complications. *Emerg Med Clin North Am* 2000;18:549–564.
2. Leonard MS. An approach to some dilemmas and complications of office oral surgery. *Aust Dent J* 1995;40:159–163.
3. Roberts G, Scully C, Shotts R. ABC of oral health: dental emergencies. *BMJ* 2000;321:559–562.

6–5

Alveolar Osteitis

Matthew Spencer

Clinical Presentation

A dry, empty socket manifests with pain, tenderness, odor, and an unpleasant taste. Patients most commonly present 2 to 5 days after a tooth extraction. Swelling, lymphadenopathy, and bacteremia should not be associated with this syndrome.

Pathophysiology

Alveolar osteitis is a postextraction clinical syndrome that occurs in 0.5% to 5% of all tooth extractions but is seen much more frequently (9% to 30%) in mandibular third molar extractions.[1-3] There is no proven cause for alveolar osteitis, but increased fibrinolysis of the postextraction blood clot, leading to alveolar bone exposure, is the generally accepted theory.[1-3] Risk factors for the development of alveolar osteitis include traumatic extraction, oral contraceptives, smoking, older age, and preexisting local infection.[1-3]

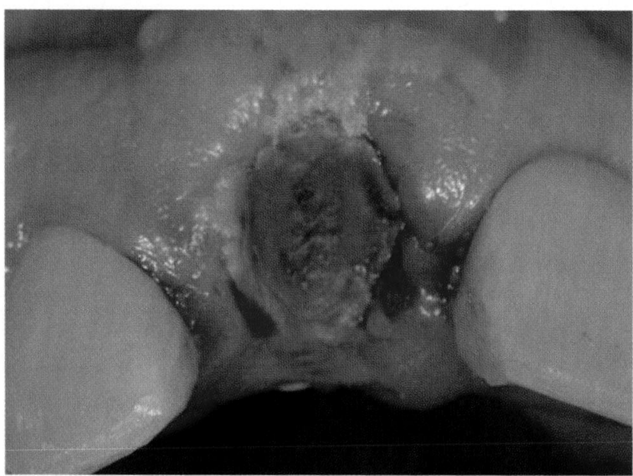

FIGURE 6–5 The classic gray-brown membrane of alveolar osteitis, or dry socket. (Courtesy of Anthony Polimeni, DDS.)

Clinical Complications

Prolonged pain and osteomyelitis are potential complications of alveolar osteitis.

Management

Dental radiographs may be taken to ensure that a root fragment or foreign body has not been retained in the empty socket. The best radiographic views to identify such retained fragments are intraoral periapical films, but they are not readily available in many emergency departments (EDs). The best extraoral film is a Panorex, if available, or a simple mandible or maxilla radiograph will suffice. The emergency physician should irrigate the socket with warm saline or chlorhexidine solution and then apply a dressing to the socket.[1,2,4] The two most commonly used dressings are iodoform gauze and Gelfoam® soaked with eugenol, but there are many other options. The patient should then receive analgesics and prompt dental follow-up. The dressing should be changed every 24 hours for the first 2 to 3 days, and then every 48 to 72 hours until granulation tissue forms in the socket.[1] Antibiotics are recommended by some authorities, but they probably should be reserved for patients who develop osteomyelitis.[1-4]

REFERENCES

1. Matocha DL. Postsurgical complications. *Emerg Med Clin North Am* 2000;18:549–564.
2. Alexander RE. Dental extraction wound management: a case against medicating postextraction sockets. *J Oral Maxillofac Surg* 2000;58:538–551.
3. Vezeau PJ. Dental extraction wound management: medicating postextraction sockets. *J Oral Maxillofac Surg* 2000;58:531–537.
4. Roberts G, Scully C, Shotts R. ABC of oral health: dental emergencies. *BMJ* 2000;321:559–562.

Dental Fracture

Matthew Spencer

Clinical Presentation

Crown fractures typically manifest as tooth pain after facial or oral trauma. A broken tooth is visualized on examination, and blood may be seen within the tooth fracture, indicating exposed pulp. Root fractures also manifest with tooth pain, but the examination reveals tooth tenderness, occasionally mobility, and gingival bleeding. The diagnosis of a root fracture can be confirmed with periapical intraoral radiographs or a Panorex view.

Pathophysiology

Any fracture of a tooth may involve either the crown or the root. Crown fractures are the most common dental injury treated in the emergency department (ED).[1] There are two classification systems for crown fractures, the more commonly used one being the Ellis classification system. An Ellis I fracture extends only through the enamel of the tooth. An Ellis II fracture involves both the enamel and the dentin. An Ellis III fracture enters the enamel, dentin, and pulp of the tooth and causes bleeding.

Dental fractures result from blunt trauma, such as a fall, motor vehicle collision, assault, or athletics, or from penetrating trauma.[2] Nutrition for the dentin of the tooth is provided by the pulp through small, communicating openings called the dentinal tubules. If these tubules are exposed to the oral cavity through trauma, they provide a route for bacteria from the oral cavity to enter the tooth pulp, increasing the risk of pulpal infection.[1,2]

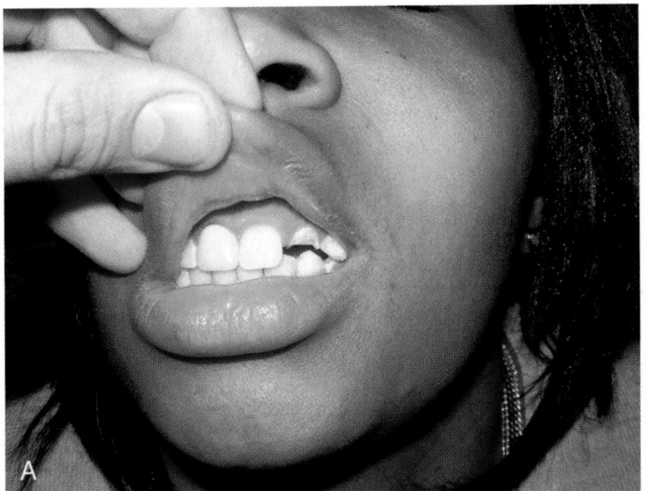

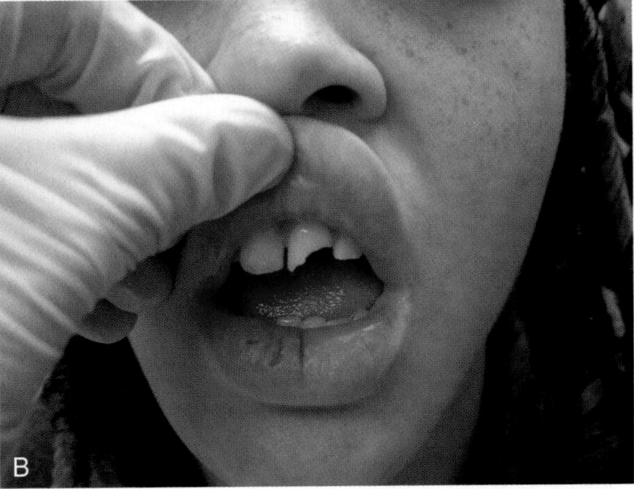

FIGURE 6–6 **A:** An Ellis class III fracture of tooth no. 10. (Courtesy of Mark Silverberg, MD.) **B:** An Ellis class II fracture of tooth no. 9. (Courtesy of Mark Silverberg, MD.)

Clinical Complications

The most common complication of dental fractures is pulp necrosis secondary to infection. It occurs in approximately 0% to 3.5% of Ellis I fractures, in 1% to 7% of Ellis II fractures, in the majority of Ellis III fractures, and in 20% of root fractures.[1,3] The risk of pulp necrosis can be minimized if the injury is addressed within 3 hours.

Management

Ellis I fractures require no specific therapy except for cosmetic concerns.[4] Ellis II and Ellis III fractures should be covered with calcium hydroxide–containing material, and the patient referred to a dentist within 24 hours.[1–5] Root fractures of the permanent teeth require manual reduction followed by rigid splinting to the adjacent teeth and prompt dental referral. Management of root fractures in primary teeth depends on the location of the fracture.[1,2–4] Apical third fractures of the primary dentition require no therapy if they are not mobile, whereas teeth with coronal third fractures or apical third fractures with mobility should be extracted, leaving the apical portion in place to resorb on its own.[1,4] Systemic antibiotics are not necessary for these fractures unless an alveolar ridge fracture also exists.

REFERENCES

1. Dale RA. Dentoalveolar trauma. *Emerg Med Clin North Am* 2000;18:521–538.
2. Rauschenberger CR, Hovland EJ. Clinical management of crown fractures. *Dent Clin North Am* 1995;39:25–51.
3. Antrim DD, Bakland LK, Parker MW. Treatment of endodontic urgent care cases. *Dent Clin North Am* 1986;30:549–572.
4. Dummett CO Jr. Dental management of traumatic injuries to the primary dentition. *J Calif Dent Assoc* 2000;28:838–845.
5. Roberts G, Scully C, Shotts R. ABC of oral health: dental emergencies. *BMJ* 2000;321:559–562.

Luxation Injuries (Avulsion)

Matthew Spencer

Clinical Presentation

Clinical presentation of a luxation injury depends on the category of injury, but all such injuries involve tooth or jaw pain after trauma. In extrusive luxation, the involved tooth is loose, shows gingival bleeding at the base, and is taller than the adjacent teeth. With intrusive luxation, the tooth is not loose, gingival bleeding may be seen, and the tooth appears to be shortened. Sometimes the tooth has been impacted so deeply that it is not visible. Lateral luxation results in a loose tooth that is displaced horizontally. It is often accompanied by a gingival laceration or an alveolar root fracture, or both. In complete luxation, there is gingival bleeding and the tooth is completely removed from the socket.[1-3]

Pathophysiology

Avulsion or luxation injuries of the teeth result when a tooth is displaced or loosened from its socket and account for approximately 17% of all dentoalveolar trauma. There are four categories: (1) extrusive luxation, or partial avulsion, which occurs when the tooth is partially displaced in an outward direction; (2) intrusive luxation, which results when the tooth is displaced downward into the alveolar bone; (3) lateral luxation, or displacement of the tooth in a horizontal plane; and (4) complete luxation, in which the tooth is entirely extracted from the socket.[1-3] Luxation injuries are most commonly caused by blunt trauma, usually from a fall, motor vehicle collision, assault, or sports-related trauma.[1-3]

Clinical Complications

The most common complications of luxation injuries are pulp necrosis, root resorption, and marginal bone loss. Intrusive and complete luxations carry a worse prognosis. Two other complications, which occur less frequently, are calcification of the pulp chamber and transient apical breakdown.[1-3]

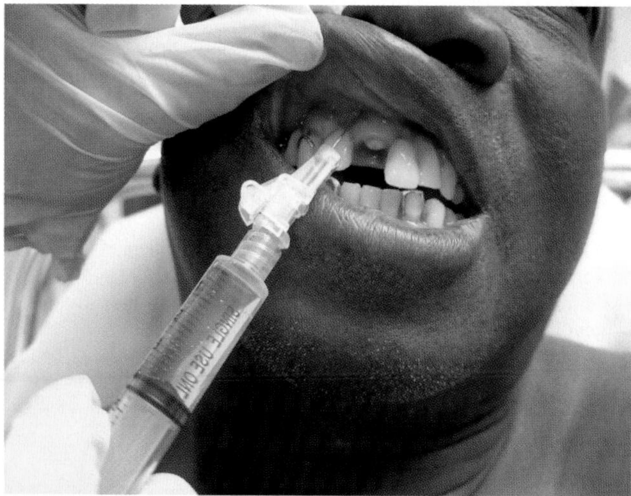

FIGURE 6–7 Avulsion of tooth no. 8 with partially retained root. (Courtesy of Mark Silverberg, MD.)

Management

Extrusive or lateral luxation injuries require manual reduction and nonrigid splinting for 1 to 3 weeks. In cases of intrusive luxation, the tooth often reerupts on its own over the course of a few months, but occasionally slow orthodontic extrusion is required. Complete luxation requires immediate reimplantation or storage in an appropriate transport medium and prompt medical attention. All luxation injuries should be treated as an open dental fracture with systemic antibiotics, and tetanus status should be updated if necessary. Penicillin or clindamycin is the first-line antibiotic of choice and should be prescribed until the patient can be seen by a dentist. If the injury occurs in a primary tooth, the tooth should be removed, because reimplantation may damage the developing permanent tooth.[4]

Outcome from tooth reimplantation in the setting of complete luxation is time dependent. The tooth should be reimplanted as soon as possible. Patients who telephone to the emergency department (ED) should be instructed to reimplant the tooth themselves or to place it in a proper transport medium and go directly to the hospital or dental office. Acceptable transport solutions include Hank's Balanced Salt Solution (Save-A-Tooth), milk, normal saline, saliva, and tap water. Soda, sports drinks, alcoholic beverages, or contact lens solution should not be used. If the tooth has been out of its socket for less than 20 minutes, it should be manipulated only by the crown and its root should be irrigated gently with normal saline. It should then be reimplanted into the socket, using firm pressure, with the convex surface facing out. If 20 to 60 minutes has elapsed, the tooth should be soaked for 30 minutes in Hank's solution and an additional 5 minutes in doxycycline (1 mg in 20 mL saline) before it is reimplanted. If the tooth has been out of the socket for longer than 60 minutes, it should be soaked in citric acid for 5 minutes, 2% stannous fluoride for 5 minutes, and then doxycycline for 5 minutes before reimplantation.[4]

REFERENCES

1. Dumsha TC. Luxation injuries. *Dent Clin North Am* 1995;39:79–91.
2. Dale RA. Dentoalveolar trauma. *Emerg Med Clin North Am* 2000;18:521–538.
3. Roberts G, Scully C, Shotts R. ABC of oral health: dental emergencies. *BMJ* 2000;321:559–562.
4. Trope M. Clinical management of the avulsed tooth. *Dent Clin North Am* 1995;39:93–112.

Alveolar Fracture

Matthew Spencer

Clinical Presentation

Patients presenting with alveolar fracture may report tooth or jaw pain after blunt or penetrating trauma. Alveolar fractures are often associated with tooth avulsion or other oral soft tissue injuries. They may involve a single tooth or multiple teeth, creating a segmental defect. They can be recognized clinically as one or multiple displaced or mobile teeth, or as movement of a group of teeth when checking the mobility of only a single tooth.[1–5] The diagnosis is primarily clinical and may be confirmed radiographically by intraoral periapical or occlusal films, or by extraoral Panorex films.[4,5] Computed tomographic scanning usually is not needed in the absence of associated facial injuries.

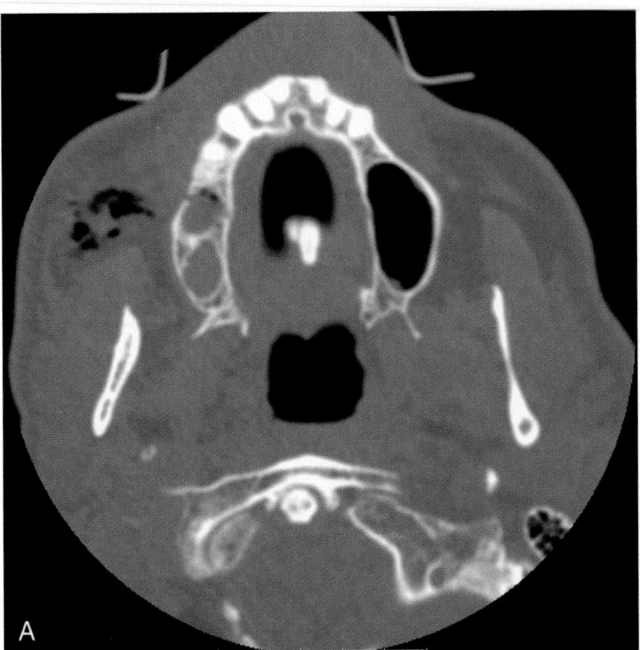

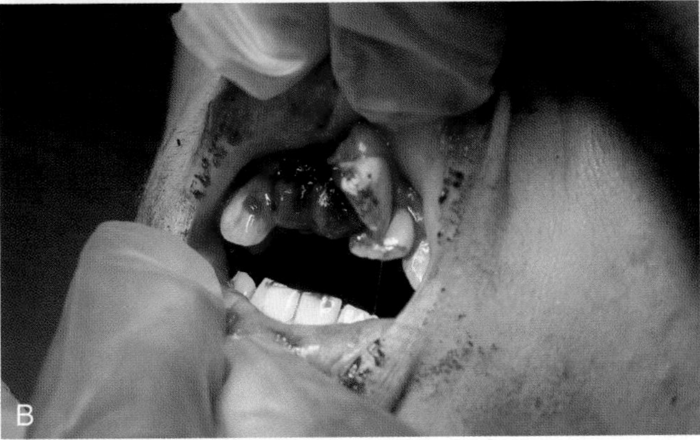

FIGURE 6–8 Alveolar ridge fracture seen on computed tomography **(A)** and clinically **(B)**. (**A,** Courtesy of Barry Hahn, MD. **B,** Courtesy of Anthony Morocco, MD.)

Pathophysiology

The alveolar ridge is that portion of the maxilla and mandible that contains the roots of the teeth. Fractures of the alveolar ridge usually involve the anterior teeth and account for 5% to 9% of injuries from dentoalveolar trauma.[1]

Clinical Complications

Pulp necrosis of the involved teeth occurs in 75% of patients, loss of marginal bone support in 13%, and root resorption in 11%.[1] The risk of all three complications is decreased if therapy is initiated within 1 hour after injury.[1]

Management

Treatment of alveolar fractures is the same for primary and permanent teeth and consists of manual reduction, splinting, antibiotics, and tetanus prophylaxis.[1,3,4] Manual reduction under local anesthesia and rigid to semirigid splinting by the emergency physician, dentist, or oral surgeon should be performed as soon as possible.[1–5] If the emergency department (ED) does not have the facilities for dental splinting, a consultant should be contacted and prompt referral arranged. Alveolar fractures are considered to be open fractures and should receive appropriate antibiotic coverage, usually penicillin, clindamycin, or metronidazole, within 6 hours after presentation.[4] On discharge from the ED, the patient should be referred to a dentist or oral surgeon within 24 hours.

REFERENCES

1. Dale RA. Dentoalveolar trauma. *Emerg Med Clin North Am* 2000;18:521–538.
2. Oikarinen KS. Clinical management of injuries to the maxilla, mandible, and alveolus. *Dent Clin North Am* 1995;39:113–131.
3. Flores MT, Andreasen JO, Bakland LK et al. Guidelines for the evaluation and management of traumatic dental injuries. *Dent Traumatol* 2001;17:1–4.
4. Padilla RR, Felsenfeld AL. Treatment and prevention of alveolar fractures and related injuries. *J Craniomaxillofac Trauma* 1997;3:22–27.
5. Bernstein L, Keyes KS. Dental and alveolar fractures. *Otolaryngol Clin North Am* 1972;5:273–281.

Tooth Wear from Bruxism

Matthew Spencer

Clinical Presentation

The most common symptom on presentation of patients with bruxism is erosion of the facets of the teeth, either incisal or occlusal. Patients may also report any or all of the following: jaw muscle stiffness or pain at night or on awakening, temporomandibular pain or clicking, tooth hypersensitivity or pain, and masseter muscle hypertrophy.[1–3]

Pathophysiology

Tooth wear may result from clenching or grinding of the teeth (bruxism), usually during sleep. The estimated incidence of bruxism varies widely, and most patients are unaware of their activity until someone else notices or their dentition is affected.[1–3] The cause of bruxism is unknown and controversial. It is thought to be essentially a sleep disorder and may relate to emotional stress or neurotransmitter imbalances in the brain.[1–3]

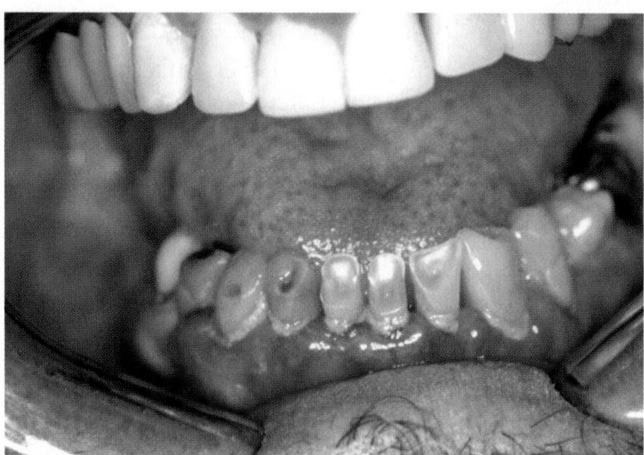

FIGURE 6–9 Severe damage to the lower teeth from chronic clinching and jaw grinding (bruxism). (Courtesy of Alfredo Aguirre, D.D.S., M.S.)

Clinical Complications

Complications include severe tooth wear resulting in changes in facial symmetry, food impaction, and thermal hypersensitivity. Hypermobility and fractures of the teeth may be encountered, as well as pulpitis and pulp necrosis.[2,3]

Management

Treatment for this disorder involves a combination of behavioral therapy, dental orthotics, and pharmaceutical therapy. The emergency physician suspecting the diagnosis may prescribe short-term, night-time use of benzodiazepines or other muscle relaxants. Dental follow-up is essential.[2,3]

REFERENCES

1. Lavigne GJ, Goulet JP, Zuconni M, Lobbezoo F. Sleep disorders and the dental patient. *Oral Surg Oral Med Oral Pathol* 1999;88:257–272.
2. Attanasio R. An overview of bruxism and its management. *Dent Clin North Am* 1997;41:229–239.
3. Attanasio R. Nocturnal bruxism and its clinical management. *Dent Clin North Am* 1991;35:245–252.

Gingival Hyperplasia

Matthew Spencer

Clinical Presentation

The clinical appearance of gingival hyperplasia resulting from phenytoin, cyclosporine, or calcium-channel blocker therapy is identical. It is commonly noticed 2 to 3 months after initiation of the therapy.[1] The overgrowth originates in the interdental papilla and then slowly spreads until the teeth are partially or completely covered.

Pathophysiology

Gingival enlargement and overgrowth is most often related to chronic phenytoin, cyclosporine, or calcium-channel blocker therapy. However, not all patients taking these medications become afflicted. In fact, only 50% of those taking phenytoin, 8% to 70% of those taking cyclosporine, and 15% to 21% of those taking nifedipine develop such complications.[1]

There are many hypotheses as to the exact cause of gingival hyperplasia, but none has been confirmed experimentally. Increased fibroblast proliferation and collagen secretion is the most commonly accepted theory. It is believed that these medications directly induce stimulation of fibroblasts to secrete the collagen in susceptible individuals.[1,2]

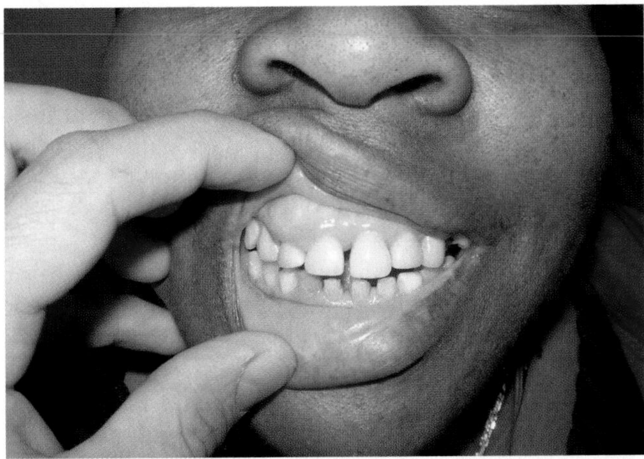

FIGURE 6–10 Gingival hypertrophy, secondary to chronic Dilantin therapy, is evident along the right upper gum line. (Courtesy of Mark Silverberg, MD.)

Clinical Complications

Patients usually complain only of altered cosmesis, but masticatory function may occasionally be impaired.

Management

Good oral hygiene may decrease a patient's risk of developing gingival hyperplasia, but there are no known medications that effectively treat it. In the emergency department (ED), these patients should be encouraged to use good oral hygiene and then referred to a dentist in 1 to 2 weeks or as needed. If severe impairment is present, the medication must be discontinued, or a dentist or oral surgeon may be called to perform a gingivectomy or an excisional flap.[1]

REFERENCES

1. Dongari A, McDonnell HT, Langlais RP. Drug-induced gingival overgrowth. *Oral Surg Oral Med Oral Pathol* 1993;76:543–548.
2. Keith DA. Side effects of diphenylhydantoin: a review. *J Oral Surg* 1978;36:206–209.

Tooth Discoloration

Matthew Spencer

Clinical Presentation

Patients generally complain of discoloration of the teeth that results in an unappealing cosmetic problem. Usually it is a change that has developed slowly over time, sometimes after trauma. Patients do not commonly present to the emergency department (ED) with this complaint, but it is often inadvertently found on examination, and it is frequently treated by dental practitioners.[1–3]

Pathophysiology

Tooth discoloration is any abnormal coloration or staining of the teeth. Tooth discoloration is classified by location as intrinsic or extrinsic, with extrinsic tooth discoloration further divided into metallic and nonmetallic subclasses.[1] Intrinsic discoloration may result when a chromogen is incorporated into the substance of the enamel or dentin, resulting in abnormal tooth color.[1–3] Common causes for tooth discoloration include congenital metabolic abnormalities, systemic disease, and chromogen introduction during tooth development. Etiologic examples include alkaptonuria, congenital erythropoietic porphyria, congenital hyperbilirubinemia, amelogenesis imperfecta, dentinogenesis imperfecta, tetracycline staining, fluorosis, enamel hypoplasia, and trauma resulting in accumulation of hemoglobin.[1–3] Extrinsic discoloration results from incorporation of a chromogen onto the external surfaces of the teeth, or incorporation into the pellicle. Staining can result directly from the color of the chromogen or indirectly from a localized chemical reaction on the surface of the tooth. Metallic discolorations may be caused by indirect staining from iron, copper, potassium permanganate, silver nitrate, or stannous fluoride. Nonmetallic staining is usually a result of direct staining from products such as tea, coffee, wine, other beverages; tobacco; or mouth rinses containing chlorhexidine and quaternary ammonium.[2]

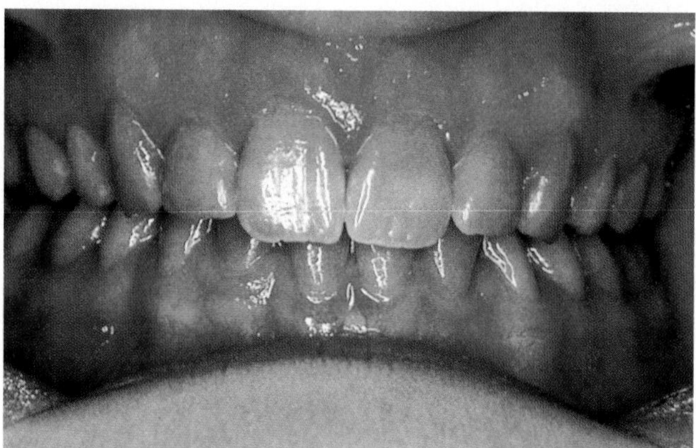

FIGURE 6–11 Tetracycline staining. This patient received systemic tetracycline during the period when her tooth buds were forming, resulting in discoloration of the permanent teeth. (From Benjamin, with permission.)

Diagnosis

The diagnosis is made entirely by clinical examination of the teeth.

Clinical Complications

There are no serious clinical complications from tooth discoloration alone. However, some causes of intrinsic discoloration are associated with systemic disorders that involve serious systemic signs and symptoms.[1–3]

Management

Treatment depends on the type of discoloration. Intrinsic staining generally is more difficult to treat than extrinsic staining. The mainstay of therapy is the use of abrasives and toothpastes to help reduce the accumulation of staining agents and eliminate some extrinsic stains. For the ED patient, recommendation of improved oral hygiene with brushing twice a day should be provided, as well as referral to a dental practitioner in a nonemergency time frame. More aggressive techniques of stain removal (e.g., hydrogen peroxide, vital bleaching, acid-etch bonding, crown placement) are usually necessary for intrinsic discoloration, as well as some extrinsic stains. These treatment modalities are beyond the realm of therapy provided by the emergency physician.[2,3]

REFERENCES

1. Watts A, Addy M. Tooth discoloration and staining: a review of the literature. *Br Dent J* 2001;190:309–316.
2. Nathoo SA. The chemistry and mechanisms of extrinsic and intrinsic discoloration. *J Am Dent Assoc* 1997;128:6S–10S.
3. Faunce F. Management of discolored teeth. *Dent Clin North Am* 1983;27:657–670.

Hutchinson's Teeth

Matthew Spencer

Clinical Presentation

In Hutchinson's teeth, the upper central incisors are small and have a rounded shape, with a taper from the gingival margin to the unusually thickened incisal surface, where a broad central notch can usually be found.[1-3] The increased space between the two central incisors and between the central and lateral incisors results in large gaps between these teeth. Such characteristic features are found in 11% to 45% of patients with congenital syphilis, but they are considered late findings because they are not present in the primary dentition.[3,4] Although rare today in developed countries due to perinatal testing for syphilis, Hutchinson's teeth are still often seen in the developing world.

Pathophysiology

Hutchinson's teeth are a characteristic deformity of the upper central incisors seen in the secondary dentition of patients with congenital syphilis. Hutchinson's teeth were first described by Sir Jonathan Hutchinson in 1857–1858. They have often been referred to as "barrel-like", "peg-shaped", or "screwdriver" teeth.[1-3] Syphilis is caused by infection with the spirochete *Treponema pallidum.* Congenital syphilis results from the vertical transplacental transmission of *T. pallidum* from mother to fetus. The spirochete causes Hutchinson's teeth by interfering with the development of the central upper incisors of the secondary dentition when the tooth buds are forming, during the 16th to 20th weeks of fetal life.[3] *T. pallidum* has a predilection for the middle of the three dental centers in the incisors. This leads to the teeth's characteristic barrel appearance with a central notch.

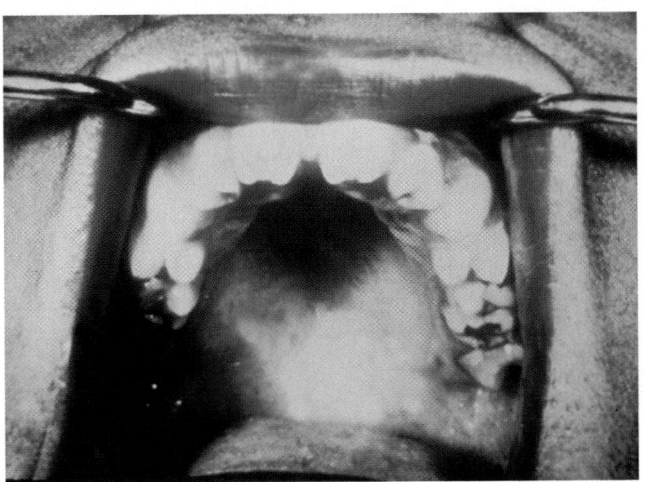

FIGURE 6–12 Hutchinson's teeth, showing "screwdriver" incisors. (From Sweet and Gibbs Atlas, with permission.)

Diagnosis

The diagnosis for this disorder is entirely clinical. Radiographs are not indicated.

Clinical Complications

The only complications are an increased tendency to dental wear and dental caries.

Management

Hutchinson's teeth are a late manifestation of congenital syphilis and are extremely rare in developed countries due to routine serologic testing of pregnant mothers for syphilis. Because they result from early fetal exposure and infection, even children who were diagnosed and treated for congenital syphilis at birth can develop Hutchinson's teeth.[2] If a child presents to the emergency department (ED) with a characteristic pattern of Hutchinson's teeth and no history of treatment for congenital syphilis, the emergency physician should look for other signs and symptoms of syphilis and obtain serologic testing on the mother and child. If either test is positive, that patient should be treated with penicillin, 100,000 to 150,000 U/kg per day in children or 50,000 U/kg per dose in adults divided every 8 to 12 hours for 10 to 14 days.[5] Two other adult regimens are procaine penicillin 50,000 U/kg per dose given once a day intramuscularly for 10 days, or benzathine penicillin 2.4 million units given once a week intramuscularly for 3 weeks.

REFERENCES

1. Hillson S, Grigson C, Bond S. Dental defects of congenital syphilis. *Am J Phys Anthropol* 1998;107:25–40.
2. Southby R. Hutchinson's teeth. *Aust Paediatr J* 1981;17:226.
3. Robinson RC. Congenital syphilis. *Arch Dermatol* 1969;99:599–610.
4. Bernfeld WK. Hutchinson's teeth and early treatment of congenital syphilis. *Br J Vener Dis* 1971;47:54–56.
5. Treadwell P. Sexually transmitted diseases in neonates and infants. *Semin Dermatol* 1994;13:256–261.

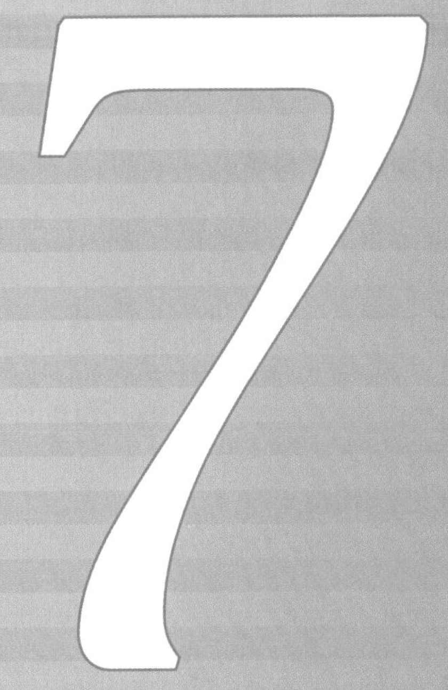

Cardiovascular

7-1

Acute Myocardial Infarction

Ralph Weiche

Clinical Presentation

Patients with acute myocardial infarction (AMI) present with chest discomfort, tightness, pressure, or a "squeezing sensation" located over the anterior chest. The chest pain may radiate to the jaw, neck, arms, back, or epigastrium. Associated symptoms may include dyspnea, nausea, anxiety, lightheadedness, syncope, or diaphoresis. Elderly patients, women, and patients with diabetes are more likely to have atypical presentations.

Pathophysiology

The term *acute myocardial infarction* refers to myocardial necrosis secondary to ischemia. Ischemia typically results from coronary artery atherosclerotic plaque rupture, with thrombus formation and consequent occlusion of the blood supply in a coronary vessel. Ischemia may also result from coronary artery vasospasm. In some patients, this vasospasm results from the use of sympathomimetic or serotonergic medications (e.g., cocaine, amphetamines).

Diagnosis

The diagnosis requires a high index of suspicion in patients with historical risk factors for coronary artery disease (smoking, age greater than 55 years, hypertension, diabetes, family history) and consistent symptoms. Patients may present with an absence of chest pain ("silent MI"), with an atypical history, or before visible changes in the electrocardiograph (ECG) or serum markers.

ECG manifestations of AMI include sinus tachycardia (ST)-segment elevation greater than 1 mm in two contiguous leads and new Q waves.[1] Myocardial ischemia may produce ST-segment depression or T-wave inversion. However, normal or nonspecific findings on ECG do not exclude the diagnosis of AMI, and ECG changes may be late findings.[1]

The anatomic localization of an AMI can be inferred by the distribution of ECG abnormalities: inferior wall (II, III, aVF), lateral wall (I, aVL, V4–V6), anteroseptal (V1–V3), anterolateral (V1–V6), right ventricular (RV4, RV5), and posterior wall (R/S ratio >1 in V1 and V2; upright T-waves in V1, V8, and V9).

Clinical Complications

Complications include systolic or diastolic dysfunction, decreased ejection fraction, cardiogenic shock, arrhythmias, valvular dysfunction (rupture of a papillary muscle or chordae tendineae), and septal or ventricular wall rupture.

Management

The management of AMI is complex, and as the state of the art evolves, so do the standards of care for AMI. Published guidelines should be reviewed for details.[1] The initial management of suspected AMI should include adequate intravenous (IV) access, oxygen, cardiac monitoring, and placement in a location with defibrillation and cardiac medications readily available.[1] All pa-

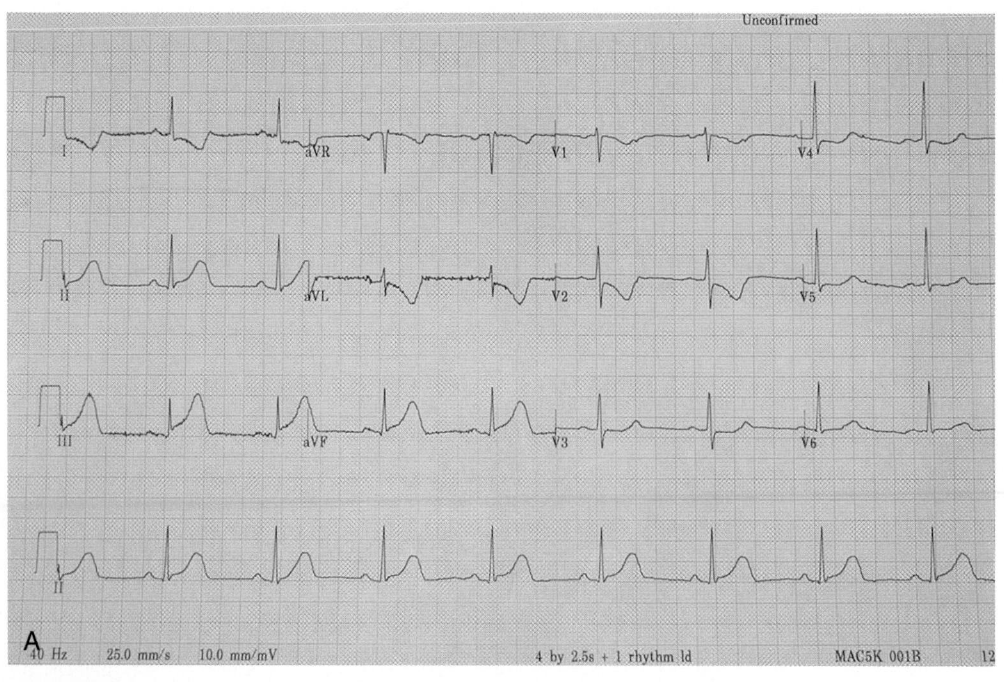

FIGURE 7–1 **A:** Inferior wall myocardial infarction. (Courtesy of Robert Hendrickson, MD.)

Acute Myocardial Infarction

Ralph Weiche

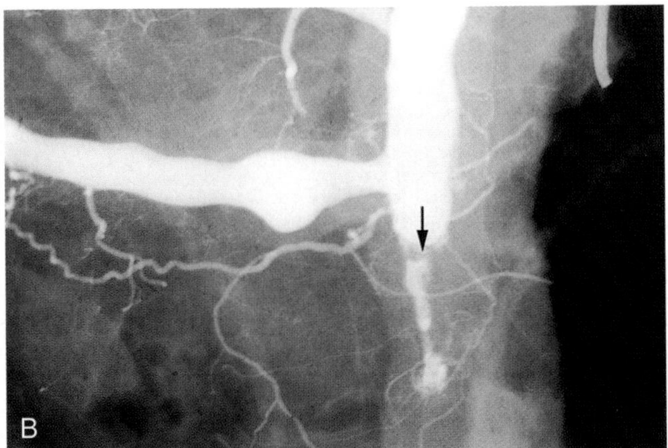

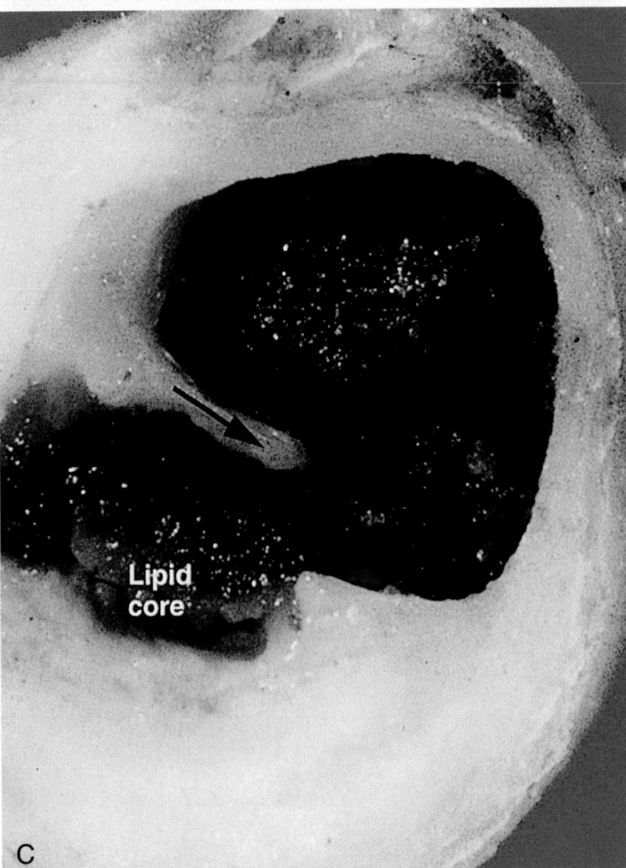

FIGURE 7–1, cont'd. **B:** The occluded artery *(arrow)* shows a thread of angiographic medium passing some distance into the thrombus, but there is no distal artery filling. **C:** The end of the torn plaque cap is visible *(arrow);* thrombus within the lipid core is in continuity with thrombus within the arterial lumen. (**B** and **C,** from Davies, with permission.)

tients should be treated with aspirin (unless allergic) and β-blockade (unless bradycardic, hypotensive, or intoxicated with sympathomimetics). Chest pain may be relieved with nitroglycerin or morphine sulfate. Patients should be evaluated with an ECG and laboratory values (myoglobin, creatine phosphokinase [CPK], troponin, or some combination of these). Reperfusion therapy with cardiac catheterization (if available) or fibrinolytics or both should proceed immediately on the diagnosis of AMI.[1] Patients with an AMI should be placed in an intensive care setting, and on-site consultation with a cardiologist should be obtained.

REFERENCES

1. Ryan TJ, Antman EM, Brooks NH, et al. 1999 update: ACC/AHA guidelines for the management of patients with acute myocardial infarction. *Circulation* 1999;100:1016–1030.

Unstable Angina

Todd McGrath

Clinical Presentation

Patients may present with substernal chest pain with or without radiation to the left arm, worsening pain similar to previous angina, resting chest pain, congestive heart failure (CHF), nausea, diaphoresis, and shortness of breath.[1] Patients may have the following risk factors: age older than 70 years, diabetes, cigarette smoking, peripheral vascular disease (PVD), coronary artery disease, and male gender.[1]

Pathophysiology

Unstable angina refers to chest pain of cardiac origin that is either increasing in intensity and frequency or occurring without inciting events (i.e., pain at rest).

The cause of unstable angina is ischemia of the cardiac myocytes, which results from thromboembolization within the coronary arteries, most commonly due to rupture of atherosclerotic plaques.[2]

Diagnosis

The diagnosis is made by recognition of the clinical history and confirmed with an electrocardiograph (ECG) and cardiac biomarkers. Sinus tachycardia (ST)-segment depression or elevation or the presence of T-wave changes is sufficient to confirm the diagnosis of unstable angina.[1] In patients with unchanged ECGs, biomarkers may reveal evidence of ischemia/unstable angina. Troponin T and I are highly specific for cardiac myocytes, and elevation of either of these isoenzymes is also highly specific for acute coronary syndrome.[1,2]

Clinical Complications

Patients with unstable angina are at increased risk for a myocardial infarction (MI) or sudden cardiac death.[1]

Management

Patients with unstable angina should be admitted to the hospital and given supplemental oxygen, aspirin (which reduces mortality and morbidity by 50% to 70%), nitrates, and β-blockers as well as antithrombotic treatment with unfractionated heparin or low-molecular-weight heparin (LMWH).[1,2] Clopidogrel may further reduce morbidity and mortality when added to aspirin.[1] The glycoprotein IIb/IIIa inhibitors may decrease the risks of recurrent angina and MI when used to treat unstable angina.[1]

REFERENCES

1. Cannon CP, Turpie AG. Unstable angina and non-ST-elevation myocardial infarction: initial antithrombotic therapy and early invasive strategy. *Circulation* 2003;107:2640–2645.
2. Parchure N, Brecker SJ. Management of acute coronary syndromes. *Curr Opin Crit Care* 2002;8:230–235.

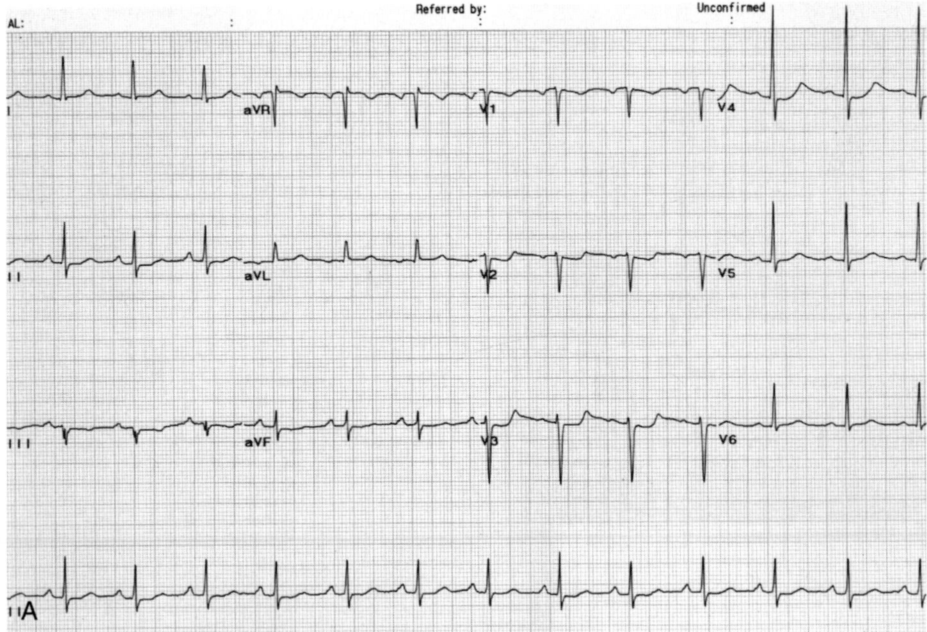

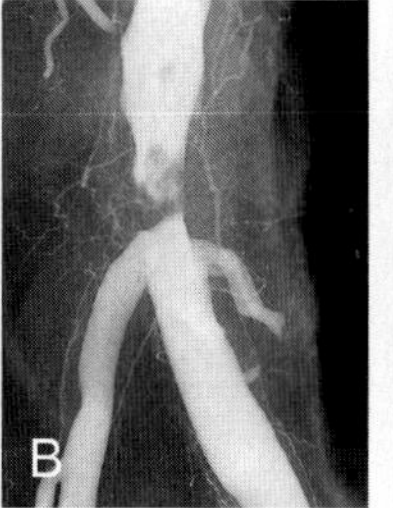

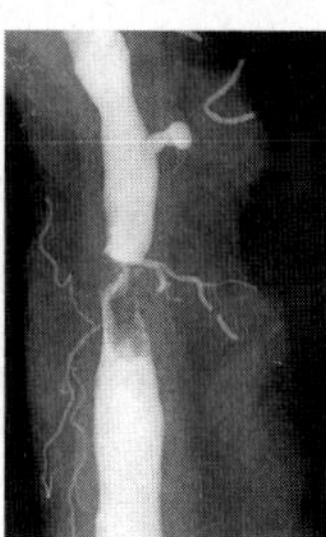

FIGURE 7–2 **A:** Sinus tachycardia (ST) segment depression in V2–V4, consistent with ischemia. (From Fowler, with permission.) **B:** Angiogram shows characteristic eccentric ragged stenosis with a small amount of attached intraluminal thrombus. (From Davies, with permission.)

Ventricular Aneurysm

Todd McGrath

Clinical Presentation

Ventricular aneurysms (VA) develop progressively over a 4- to 6-week period after infarction.[1] Patients may have signs of left-sided congestive heart failure (CHF) (including pulmonary edema, third heart sound [S_3] gallop, and jugular venous distention), thromboembolic phenomena secondary to mural thrombus formation, or ventricular arrhythmias.[1,3] VAs may be detected on electrocardiographs (ECGs) of asymptomatic patients (sinus tachycardia [ST] elevations in the area of the aneurysm).

Pathophysiology

VA is a complication of a myocardial infarction (MI) that results in gradual thinning of the ventricular wall in the area of infarction. The thin-walled area may paradoxically bulge outward during ventricular contraction.[1,2]

After an acute myocardial infarction (AMI), the ventricular wall remodels and gradually thins in the area of infarction.[1-3] Cardiac contractility, heart rate (tachycardia or bradycardia), and/or increased afterload after an MI may have roles in aneurysmal development.[1]

Diagnosis

The diagnosis of VA should be suspected based on the clinical history in a patient with a recent AMI (within 4 to 6 weeks); it is confirmed by echocardiography.[1]

Clinical Complications

Clinical complications of VAs are related to the paradoxic outward bulging of the ventricle during systole and loss of uniform ventricular contraction.[1] The patient may develop CHF secondary to poor left ventricular (LV) function. The aneurysm itself allows for the development of a thrombus within the ventricle that may cause thromboembolic phenomena. Finally, there is an increased risk for various potentially lethal ventricular arrhythmias.[1,2] Rupture of a VA is an uncommon event.[2]

Management

Prevention is the key to management early in the postinfarction period. Control of heart rate, contractility, and afterload reduction help in the prevention of VA and in the initial medical treatment of an aneurysm. Thrombolytic therapy at the time of infarction has also been shown to reduce the incidence of VA.[1] Patients presenting with VAs should receive immediate treatment of their presenting pathology (CHF, arrhythmias, embolic phenomena) and stabilization of airway, breathing, and circulation (ABCs) until definitive surgical correction of the aneurysm can be accomplished.[1,2]

REFERENCES

1. Bartel T, Vanheiden H, Schaar J, Mertzkirch W, Erbel R. Biomechanical modeling of hemodynamic factors determining bulging of ventricular aneurysms. *Ann Thorac Surg* 2002;74:1581–1588.
2. Das AK, Wilson GM, Furnary AP. Coincidence of true and false left ventricular aneurysm. *Ann Thorac Surg* 1997;64:831–834.
3. Tikiz H, Atak R, Balbay Y, Genc Y, Kutuk E. Left ventricular aneurysm formation after anterior myocardial infarction: clinical and angiographic determinants in 809 patients. *Int J Cardiol* 2002;82:7–16.

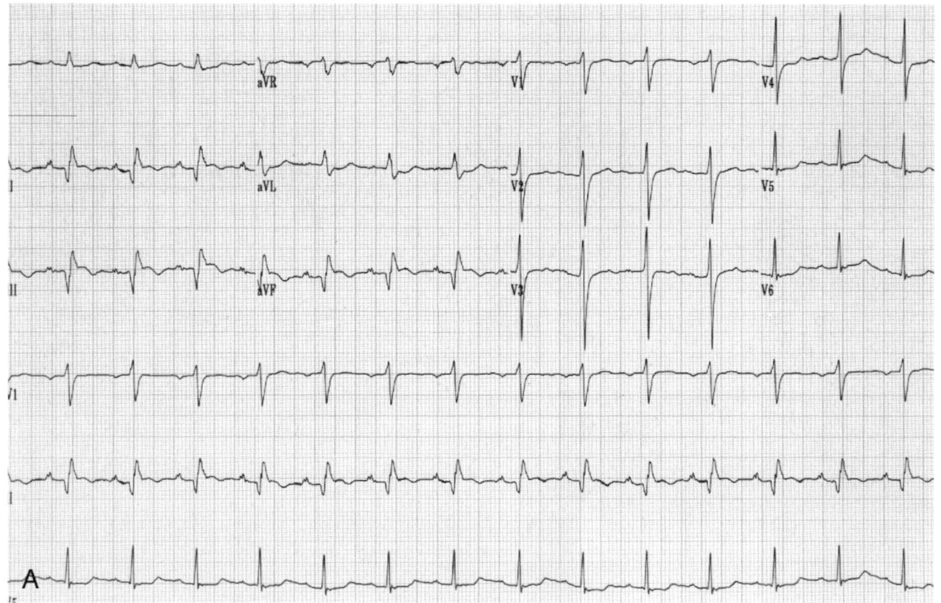

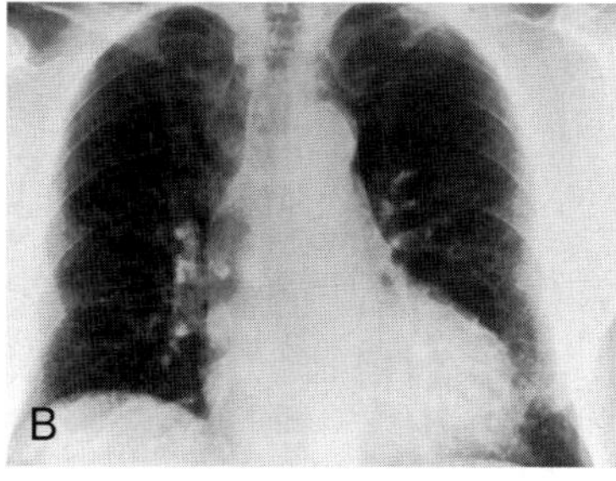

FIGURE 7–3 **A:** Persistent sinus tachycardia (ST) elevation consistent with ventricular aneurysm. (From Fowler, with permission.) **B:** Posterior chest radiograph of a patient with an aneurysm of the anterolateral wall of the left ventricle, which is enlarged. Note also the deformity of the left lower border of the cardiac silhouette. (From Kassner, with permission.)

Pericarditis

Lisa Freeman

Clinical Presentation

Patients most commonly present to the emergency department (ED) with chest pain that may be either sharp and pleuritic, or dull and pressure-like. The pain radiates to the back, left shoulder, neck, arm, or trapezial ridge and is classically worse when supine and relieved by sitting up and leaning forward. Cough, dyspnea, dysphagia, nausea, and fever may be present. The cardinal sign of pericarditis on examination is the pericardial friction rub. The rub is often intermittent, positional, and best heard at the lower left sternal border.[1]

Pathophysiology

Pericarditis refers to inflammation and infection or infiltration of the pericardium, with or without pericardial effusion. It has many infectious and noninfectious causes.[1]

Inflammation of the pericardium usually is secondary to disorders in or about the heart, but in some cases it is caused by systemic disorders or by metastatic disease. Whatever the cause of the pericarditis, there is an inflammatory reaction of the epicardial and pericardial surfaces. The most frequent type of pericarditis, which is not bacterial in origin, produces serous fluid mixed with a fibrinous exudate. Bacterial pericarditis leads to a collection of purulent effusion in the pericardial sac. The most important causes of pericarditis are idiopathic (most common), viral, bacterial, tuberculous, fungal, parasitic, and neoplastic causes, as well as uremia, postmyocardial infarction (MI) complications, connective tissue diseases, radiation, chest trauma, and drugs such as hydralazine and procainamide.[1]

Diagnosis

Diagnosis can be made with electrocardiograph (ECG) analysis. ECG changes occur in stages, and presenting patients may demonstrate any of the following. The first changes demonstrate diffuse sinus tachycardia (ST) elevation except in leads AVR and V1. The elevation is concave upward, and there are no reciprocal ST-T changes in other leads. This progresses to normalization of the ST segments and flattening of the T waves. The PR seg-

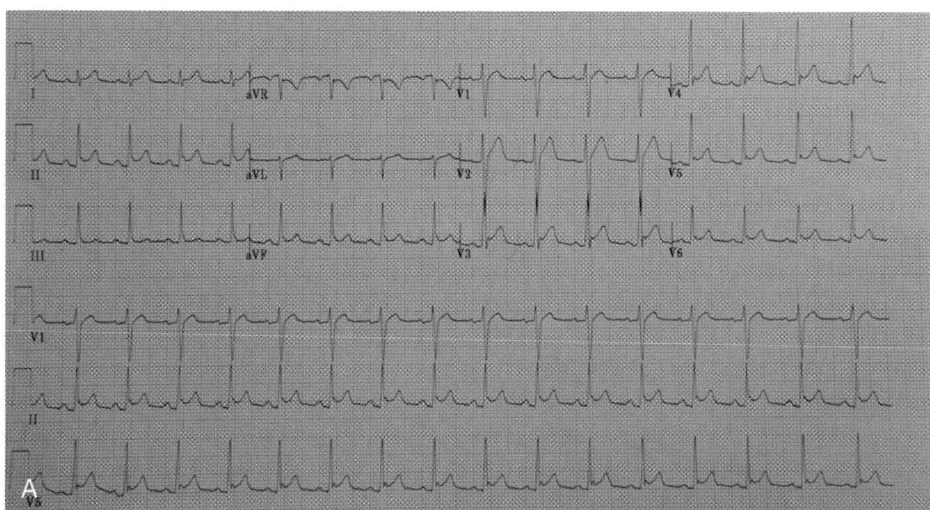

FIGURE 7–4 **A:** Electrocardiogram showing PR depression and diffuse sinus tachycardia (ST) elevation, as commonly seen in pericarditis. (Courtesy of Robert Hendrickson, MD.)

Pericarditis

Lisa Freeman

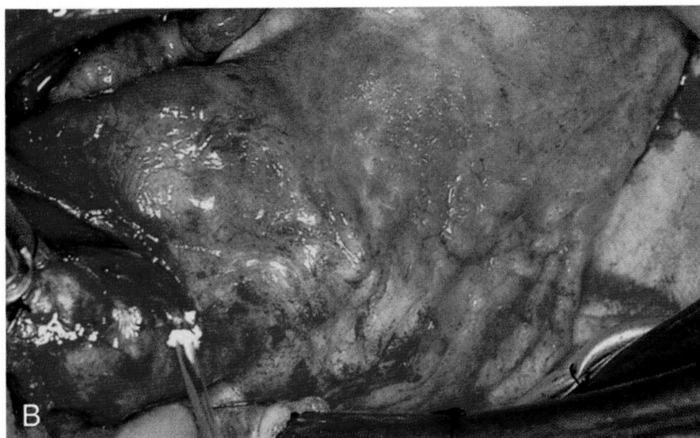

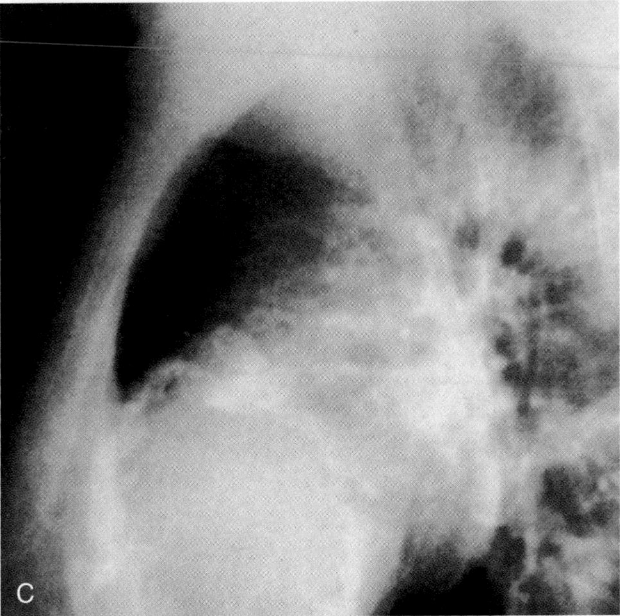

FIGURE 7–4 cont'd. B: Operative view of the heart showing the epicardial surface with a fine granular appearance. (From Hurst, with permission.) **C:** Lateral chest radiograph showing calcified pericardium surrounding the heart. (From Hurst, with permission.)

ment may become depressed. The T waves may then become inverted. Eventually, all the abnormal changes resolve and the ECG may return to baseline. Laboratory evaluation may reveal leukocytosis and an elevated erythrocyte sedimentation rate (ESR). The chest radiograph is usually normal but may show cardiomegaly if there is a sizable pericardial effusion. An echocardiogram can exclude pericardial effusion. Pericardiocentesis may be performed to examine any pericardial fluid that is present, especially if a bacterial infectious cause is suspected or tamponade is present.[1]

Clinical Complications

Pericarditis usually results in at least a small amount of excess pericardial fluid. In some cases, the fluid accumulation becomes large and leads to cardiac tamponade. Constrictive pericarditis may develop secondary to chronic inflammation, resulting in thickening and adherence of the pericardium to the heart.[1]

Management

Pericarditis without significant pericardial effusion needs no specific treatment other than pain control. Most patients can be discharged from the ED with antiinflammatory medication and follow-up within 48 hours. These patients should also be instructed to return to the ED if symptoms worsen. Pericarditis that may be secondary to a systemic illness usually requires hospital admission for diagnosis and management of the primary condition.[1]

REFERENCES

1. Spodick DH. Acute pericarditis: current concepts and practice. *JAMA* 2003;289:1150–1153.

Pericardial Effusion and Tamponade

Robert Chisholm

Clinical Presentation

The classic manifestation of acute pericardial tamponade is Beck's triad: hypotension, jugular venous distention, and muffled heart sounds. It may present insidiously, with a slowly developing effusion not exhibiting this triad. These patients may present with dyspnea and exercise intolerance.[1]

Pathophysiology

The most common cause of pericardial effusion with tamponade is malignancy. Other important causes are tuberculosis, uremia, hemorrhage (excessive anticoagulation), myxedema, systemic lupus erythematosus (SLE), radiation therapy, and chronic pericarditis.[1]

A pericardial effusion involves accumulation of fluid in the potential space between the fibrinous outer pericardium and the serous inner pericardium. This space normally contains about 20 mL of plasma-like fluid. Hemodynamic compromise can occur with an acute (minutes to hours) increase in a small amount of fluid (as little as 50 mL) or with a more lengthy (weeks to months) accumulation of fluid (up to 120 mL). However, if the intrapericardial pressure matches or exceeds ventricular diastolic pressures, systemic venous congestion occurs, cardiac output falls, and hypotension results.[1]

Diagnosis

Diagnosis is suggested by history and clinical examination. Examination may show the clinical findings of tamponade, such as jugulovenous distention, hypotension, distant heart sounds, pulsus paradoxus, and narrow pulse pressure. Chest radiography may show an enlarged heart if the effusion is chronic, and the electrocardiograph (ECG) may have low-voltage QRS complexes or electrical alternans suggestive of effusion. Emergency echocardiography should be performed for all suspected cases of pericardial tamponade. Ultrasonography shows fluid in the pericardial space and impaired cardiac motion. Inferior vena cava dilatation without inspiratory collapse is also seen and is highly suggestive of tamponade. If echocardiography is not immediately available but the patient is in critical condition and suspicion for tamponade exists, pericardiocentesis may be both diagnostic and therapeutic. Definitive intervention by a general or cardiothoracic surgeon is required.[1]

Clinical Complications

Pericardial tamponade, if not identified and treated, can lead to impaired cardiac output, hypotension, and death.[1]

Management

Patients with pericardial tamponade and hemodynamic instability should have immediate pericardiocentesis, followed by definitive surgical intervention and admission to the intensive care unit (ICU). Patients without hemodynamic instability should be treated with intravenous (IV) fluids, and urgent consultation with a thoracic surgeon should be obtained. Those with identified cardiac effusions with no tamponade physiology should be admitted to the cardiology inpatient unit or equivalent for telemetry monitoring and further evaluation. Pericardial effusions and tamponade in a nontrauma patient are suspicious for malignancy, and further workup is needed.[1]

REFERENCES

1. Spodick DH. Pathophysiology of cardiac tamponade. *Chest* 1998;113:1372–1378.

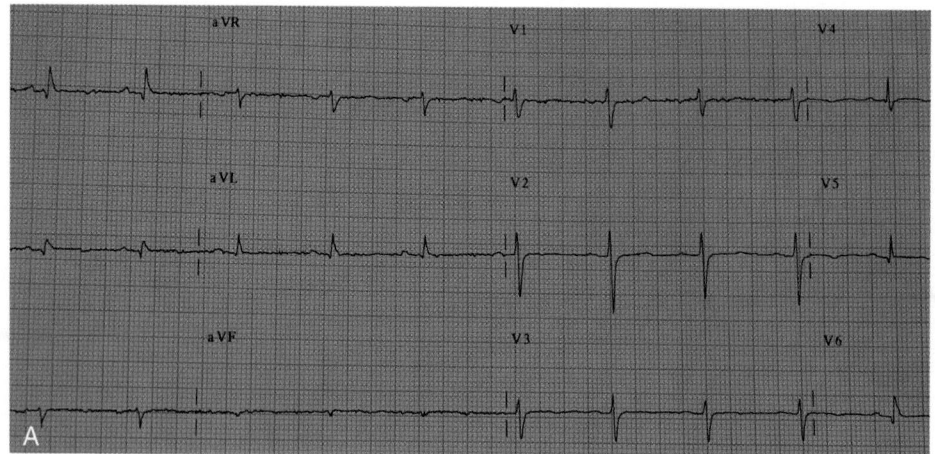

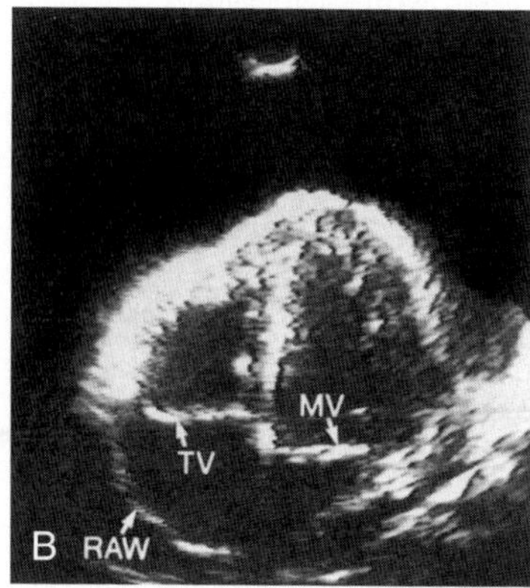

FIGURE 7–5 **A:** Electrocardiogram showing electrical alternans as seen in pericardial effusion. (Courtesy of John Fojtik, MD.) **B:** Apical four-chamber echocardiogram showing right atrial wall (RAW) collapsing inwardly, suggesting early tamponade. TV, tricuspid valve; MV, mitral valve. (From Hurst, with permission.)

Congestive Heart Failure

Robert Chisholm

Clinical Presentation

Patients with congestive heart failure (CHF) typically complain of shortness of breath and dyspnea on exertion, orthopnea, paroxysmal nocturnal dyspnea, a cough productive of pink frothy sputum, weakness, lightheadedness, abdominal pain, malaise, and nausea.

Pathophysiology

CHF may develop from a variety of causes, including valvular disease, ischemic cardiomyopathy (CM), dysrhythmia, hypertensive cardiomyopathy (HCM), constrictive heart disease, and dilated cardiomyopathy (DCM).[2] The end result is an imbalance in the myocardial Starling forces, from either inadequate filling or inadequate emptying.[1,2]

Diagnosis

The diagnosis is typically made clinically and confirmed with chest radiography, echocardiography, β-natriuretic peptide (BNP), or some kind of these. Examination may reveal tachypnea, jugular venous distention, peripheral edema, hypertension, pulmonary rales and rhonchi, a laterally displaced cardiac apical impulse, and S_3 or S_4 heart sounds. Chest radiography may reveal cardiomegaly; an increase in the prominence of the pulmonary vasculature, particularly in the apical areas ("cephalization"); and Kerley's lines. Electrocardiograph (ECG) may be used to determine the presence of myocardial ischemia. Laboratory analysis may reveal hepatic congestion or renal hypoperfusion. BNP is released from myocardial cells with stretching and is often elevated in CHF. BNP may be particularly helpful as a diagnostic test if the cause of dyspnea is in doubt (e.g., chronic obstructive pulmonary disease [COPD] versus CHF).

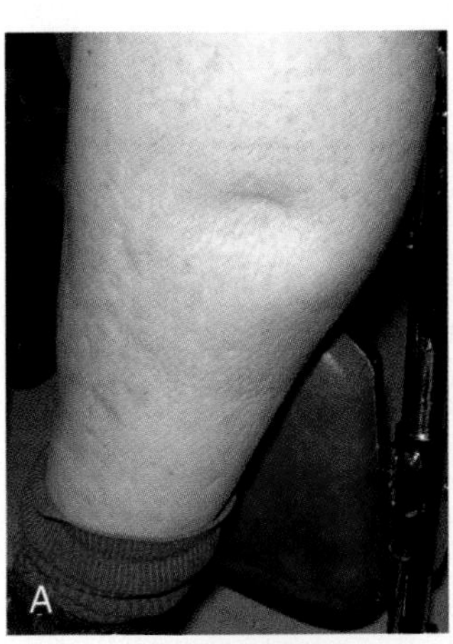

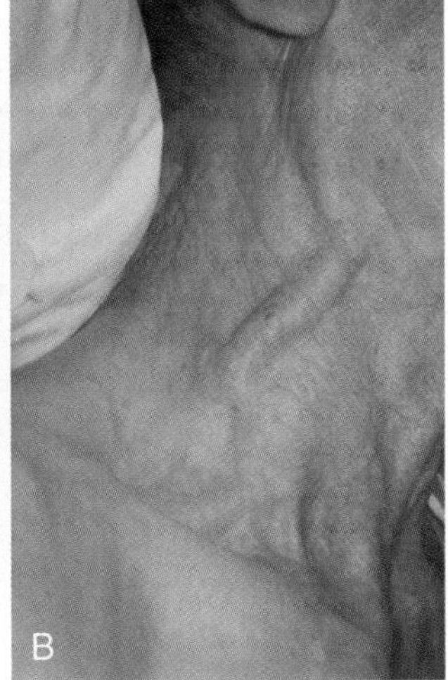

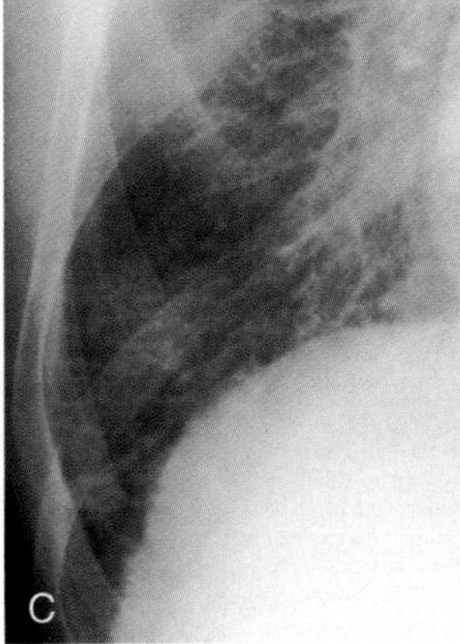

FIGURE 7–6 **A:** Pitting edema. (Courtesy of Mark Silverberg, MD.) **B:** Neck vein distention. (Courtesy of Michael Greenberg, MD.) **C:** Chest radiograph demonstrating pulmonary interstitial edema with Kerley's B lines. (From Hurst, with permission.)

Clinical Complications

Complications may include pulmonary edema, respiratory failure, end-organ hypoperfusion, shock, and death.

Management

Patients in extremis may require high-flow oxygen, large-bore intravenous (IV) access, endotracheal intubation, and inotropic support. In patients with mild to moderate symptoms, a determination of the cause of the heart failure is an initial priority, because it leads therapy. Initial steps may include administration of oxygen and elevation of the head of the bed.[2] Typical therapeutic strategies aim to decrease preload (nitrates, angiotensin-converting enzyme [ACE] inhibitors, diuretics, BNP), decrease afterload (ACE inhibitors, nitroprusside, BNP), increase inotropic support (dobutamine, dopamine), and decrease anxiety and myocardial oxygen demand (opioids).[1,2]

Patients with new-onset CHF should be admitted to the hospital on a telemetry ward for further evaluation. Patients with chronic heart failure with a clear inciting cause (e.g., increased water intake) and no suspicion of an acute event (e.g., myocardial infarction [MI], dissection, pulmonary embolism [PE]) who improve in the emergency department (ED) may be discharged to home with close follow-up.[1,2]

REFERENCES

1. Jessup M, Brozena S. Heart failure. *N Engl J Med* 2003;348:2007–2018.
2. Millane T, Jackson G, Gibbs CR, Lip GY. ABC of heart failure: acute and chronic management strategies. *BMJ* 2000;320:559–562.

Dilated Cardiomyopathy

Lisa Freeman

Clinical Presentation

Patients may present with symptoms of left-sided congestive heart failure (CHF) that have developed gradually. Shortness of breath, chest pain, fatigue, and weakness may be present. Physical examination often reveals S_3 and S_4 murmurs that reflect atrioventricular (AV) valve regurgitation, pulmonary rales, and signs of systemic shock. The blood pressure may be normal or low, and there is often tachycardia if CHF has developed. If right-sided heart failure develops, patients have jugular venous distention, ascites, and peripheral edema. Some patients have minimal or no symptoms, whereas others have progressive deterioration leading to death in 1 to 5 years.[1]

Pathophysiology

Dilated cardiomyopathy (DCM) refers to cardiac enlargement and impaired contraction of the left ventricular (LV) or of both ventricles. The causes are variable and include cardiovascular disease, alcohol- or drug-related, familial, viral, immune, and idiopathic causes. The estimated incidence is 5 to 8 cases per 100,000 population per year and is increasing.[1]

DCM is the most common form of cardiomyopathy (CM), accounting for 60% of all cases. It is characterized by ventricular dilatation and contractile dysfunction. The coronary arteries are often normal, and chest pain in these patients is thought to be caused by subendocardial ischemia. Excessive ethanol intake is a major cause of DCM, accounting for one third of cases. Ethanol may have a direct toxic effect on the myocardial cells, or secondary nutritional effects (e.g., lack of thiamine) in alcoholic patients may be contributory. Genetics is also thought to play a factor, because 20% of patients have a first-degree relative with DCM.[1]

Diagnosis

Identification of the reversible causes of DCM (ethanol, cobalt, mercury, lead, antiretroviral drugs, thiamine deficiency, hypothyroidism, acromegaly, thyrotoxicosis, hypocalcemia, hypophosphatemia, toxoplasmosis, and sarcoidosis) is particularly important during the first presentation.[1]

The goal of emergency department (ED) care is to exclude potentially reversible causes in a patient who has a clinical presentation suspicious for DCM. These include hypophosphatemia, hypocalcemia, ethanol, mercury, lead, antiretroviral agents, thiamine deficiency, toxoplasmosis, sarcoidosis and hyperthyroidism, and hypothyroidism.[1] Chest radiography usually reveals generalized cardiomegaly and pulmonary vascular redistribution. Interstitial and alveolar pulmonary edema are less common on initial presentation. Electrocardiograph (ECG) reveals sinus tachycardia when heart failure is present. Poor R-wave progression is seen, as is an interventricular conduction delay. Virtually any dysrhythmia may be seen, although atrial fibrillation (AF) is common, especially in patients with alcohol-induced DCM. Echocardiography makes the definitive diagnosis. It also is useful to assess the degree of LV dysfunction and to exclude valvular or pericardial disease. Myocardial biopsy may be needed if a reversible cause is suspected.

Clinical Complications

Intracavitary thrombi are common and may lead to systemic emboli. Pulmonary embolism (PE) is also a known complication. Prominent causes of death in patients with DCM include fulminant heart failure and dysrhythmias.

Dilated Cardiomyopathy

Lisa Freeman

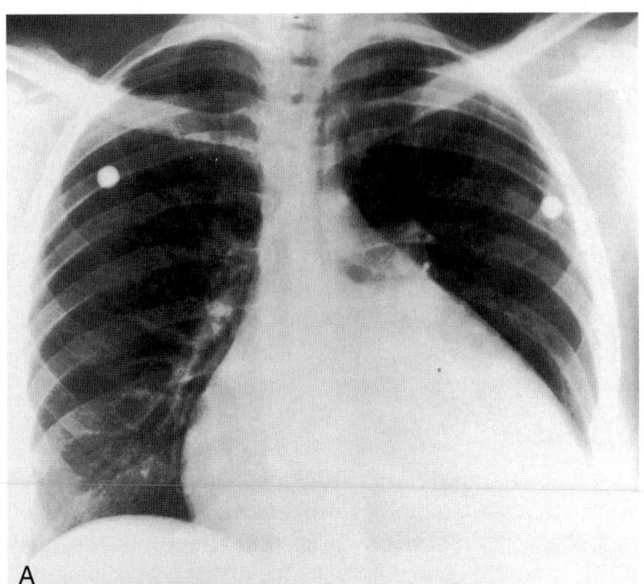

FIGURE 7–7 **A:** Chest radiograph in a patient with cardiomyopathy, demonstrating cardiomegaly with biventricular enlargement and pulmonary venous hypertension. (From Kassner, with permission.) **B:** Cross-sectional echocardiogram in the long-axis view recorded during systole in a patient with dilated cardiomyopathy. The systolic dimension of the left ventricle was 7.4 cm, and the diastolic dimension was 8.6 cm. (From Becker, with permission.)

Management

The basic management for idiopathic DCM is the same for CHF. Useful therapeutic agents include vasodilators (angiotensin-converting enzyme [ACE] inhibitors, nitrites, hydralazine), diuretics, digoxin, and carvedilol. Patients with DCM due to alcohol abuse will benefit from abstaining from alcohol, because the early manifestations may reverse.

REFERENCES

1. Dec GW, Fuster V. Medical progress: idiopathic dilated cardiomyopathy. *N Engl J Med* 1994;331:1564–1575.

Hypertrophic Cardiomyopathy

Robert Chisholm

Clinical Presentation

Hypertrophic cardiomyopathy (HCM) is the most common genetic cardiovascular disease (0.2% of the population). Patients may present with a variety of problems, including dyspnea, syncope, presyncope, angina, palpitations, congestive heart failure (CHF), and sudden death.[1,2] Patients may develop sudden cardiac death from ventricular outflow obstruction or arrhythmias. Patients are typically young and previously asymptomatic, and sudden cardiac death may occur after physical exertion.

Examination may reveal cardiac arrhythmias, signs of CHF, a systolic ejection crescendo–decrescendo murmur that is heard best between the apex and left sternal border (and increases with Valsalva maneuvers), and the holosystolic murmur of mitral regurgitation.[1]

There are no specific laboratory studies. The electrocardiograph (ECG) is abnormal in 90% of people with HCM, but there are no abnormalities that are specific for the disease. Chest radiography may be normal or show cardiomegaly. In severe HCM, radiographic findings of CHF may be present. Patients who are considered to be at risk for adverse events related to HCM should undergo Holter monitoring for surveillance of ventricular tachycardia and exercise testing to gauge the presence and severity of exercise-induced hypotension.[1]

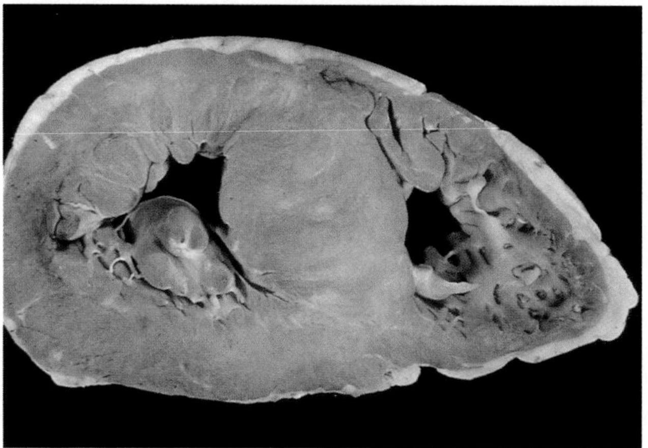

FIGURE 7–8 Cross-section through a heart with hypertropic cardiomyopathy and asymmetry of the affected interventricular septum. (From Becker, with permission.)

Pathophysiology

HCM is a genetic disorder that is characterized by the inappropriate, asymmetric hypertrophy of the left ventricular (LV).[1]

Patients with HCM may have asymmetric septal hypertrophy. In addition to obstruction from the hypertrophy, patients may have further obstruction of the left ventricular outflow tract from systolic anterior motion of the mitral valve. Greater ventricular contractile force leads to higher ejection velocity, which translates to increased displacement of the mitral valve, resulting in further narrowing of the outflow tract.[1]

Diagnosis

The ECG is abnormal in 90% of patients, showing left ventricular hypertrophy (LVH) with Q waves in the anterior and lateral leads.[1] Echocardiography is the diagnostic study of choice for suspected HCM. The diagnosis is suggested by the finding of a hypertrophied but nondilated left ventricle in the absence of illness capable of producing the hypertrophy.[1]

Clinical Complications

The most common complications are CHF, arrhythmia, atrial fibrillation (AF) with embolic stroke, and sudden death.[1,2]

Management

Patients presenting to the emergency department (ED) with new-onset heart failure, chest pain, or syncope should be admitted for further workup. β-blockers may be used for heart failure or AF, because they decrease heart rate, increase diastolic filling time, and decrease the LV outflow tract obstruction.[2] Any child or young person who presents with cardiac arrhythmia or syncopal/presyncopal complaints may be at risk for sudden cardiac death. If the diagnosis is suggested in a child or adult with new-onset symptomology, an echocardiogram and cardiology consultation are warranted.[2]

REFERENCES

1. Maron BJ. Hypertrophic cardiomyopathy: a systemic review. *JAMA* 2002;287:1308–1320.
2. Spirito P, Seidman CE, McKenna WJ, Maron BJ. The management of hypertrophic cardiomyopathy. *N Engl J Med* 1997;336: 775–785.

High-Output Cardiac Failure

Jennifer Larson

Clinical Presentation

The characteristic physical findings are all related to the hyperdynamic state and include relative tachycardia, bounding pulses with a quick upstroke, wide pulse pressure, venous hum (usually over deep internal jugular veins and occasionally over the femoral veins), systolic bruit over the carotids, S_3 gallop, and midsystolic murmur. Patients with chronic high-output heart failure typically present with signs and symptoms of low-output (or "congestive") heart failure, with systemic congestion and pulmonary edema. Acute presentations correlate with the underlying cause. Some specific causes have obvious physical findings, such as congenital fistulas (cutaneous hemangiomas or hemorrhagic telangiectasia) or hyperthyroidism (exophthalmos and a fine tremor). Laboratory data and radiologic studies are directed toward suspected causes. Chest radiography confirms pulmonary edema if there is associated congestive heart failure (CHF) in the chronic setting. If the cause is unknown, evaluation of hemoglobin/hematocrit, thyroid studies, thiamine concentration, aminotransferase levels, and a coagulation profile may be prudent.

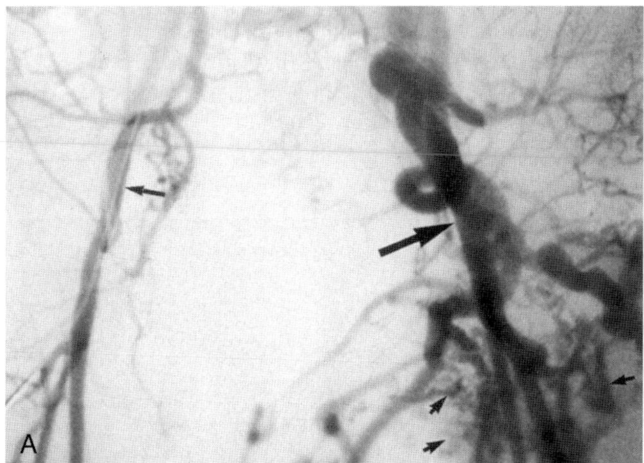

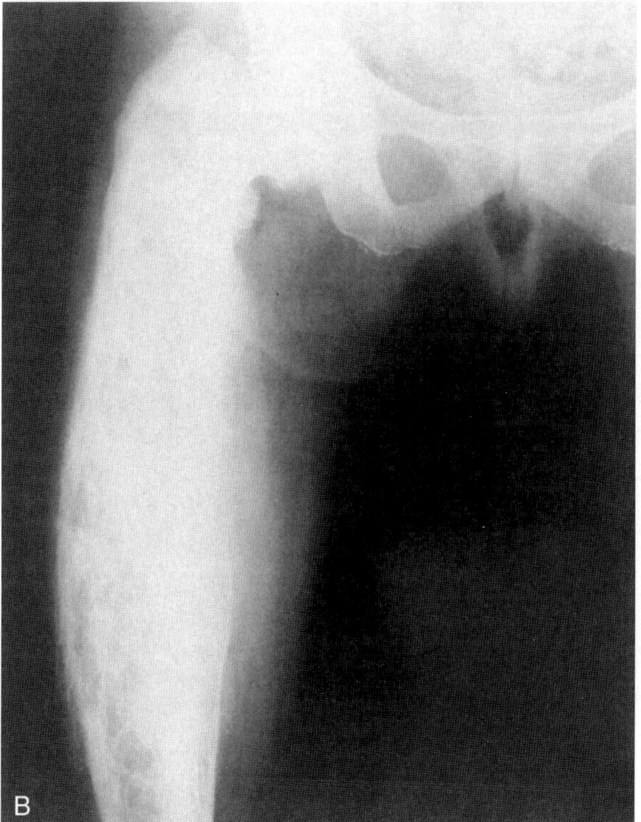

FIGURE 7–9 **A:** Arteriovenous communication. (From Hurst, with permission.) **B:** Paget's disease. (From Kassner, with permission.)

Pathophysiology

High-output cardiac failure is defined as heart failure in the presence of elevated cardiac output and low systemic vascular resistance.[1]

Several physiologic conditions may cause an increase in cardiac output (pregnancy, fever, exercise); however, heart failure usually does not occur in these cases unless there is an underlying cardiac pathology. Disorders associated with the development of high-output cardiac failure include hyperthyroidism, anemia, "wet" beriberi (thiamine deficiency), renal disease, hepatic disease, systemic arteriovenous fistulas, polycythemia vera, and carcinoid syndrome.

Diagnosis

Diagnosis depends on the primary condition.

Clinical Complications

Complications include acute coronary ischemia from high cardiac output, typically seen with underlying atherosclerotic disease, and CHF from the chronic high-output state.

Management

Management is best aimed at treatment of the underlying cause (e.g., hyperthyroidism, anemia, atrioventricular (AV) fistula, hemangioma, Paget's disease). If the patient is clinically stable in the emergency department (ED), close follow-up with outpatient workup and treatment of the primary condition is acceptable. The patient may require admission for treatment of CHF and, in the setting of low systemic vascular resistance, may require vasopressor therapy.

REFERENCES

1. Braverman AC, Steiner MA, Picus D, White H. High-output congestive heart failure following transjugular intrahepatic portal-systemic shunting. *Chest* 1995;107:1467–1469.

Abdominal Aortic Aneurysm

Lisa Freeman

Clinical Presentation

The majority of abdominal aortic aneurysms (AAA) are asymptomatic, and patients who present to the emergency department (ED) usually do so when the AAA expands or is leaking (bleeding). The pain is often nonspecific in location and character, and it is necessary to have a high index of suspicion to make a diagnosis. AAAs may also mimic other conditions that cause trunk pain, such as renal colic and mechanical low back pain. A ruptured AAA can cause signs of rapid blood loss, including syncope, hypotension, and tachycardia, as well as a pulsatile abdominal mass and abdominal tenderness.[2–4]

Pathophysiology

An AAA is defined as a focal dilatation of the abdominal aorta that results in a diameter at least 50% larger than the expected normal diameter.[1] The exact diameter of a normal aorta is variable, depending on gender, body habitus, and age, but typically ranges from 17 to 24 mm. A diameter of 30 mm is generally accepted as aneurysmal dilatation. AAAs are rare before the age of 50 years, but they are found in 2% to 5% of patients older than 65 years of age. At least 15,000 patients die from ruptured AAAs each year in the United States.[1]

Several biochemical aberrations can occur that lead to the loss of elastin and collagen in the aortic wall. These

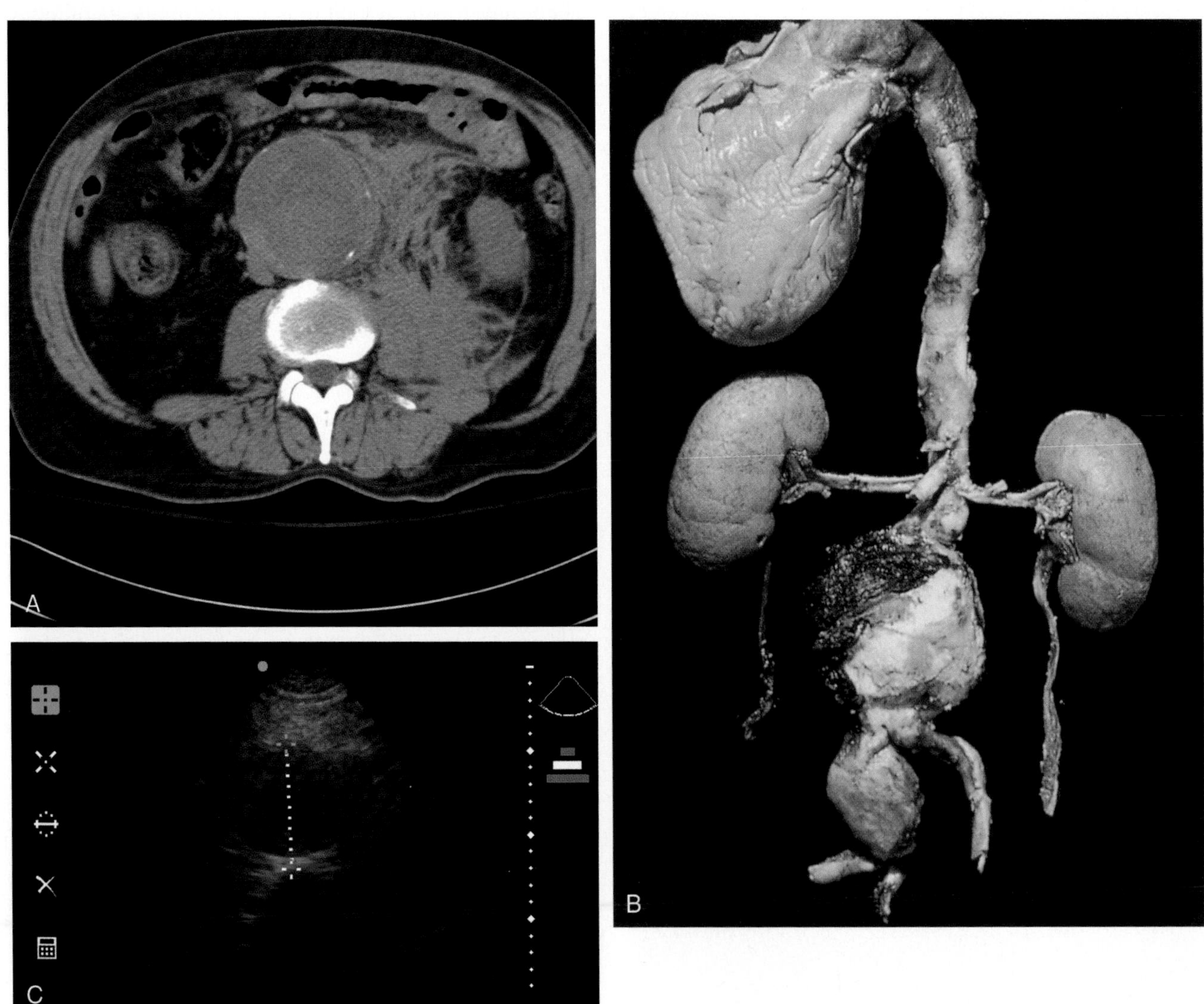

FIGURE 7–10 **A:** An 8.3 cm infrarenal abdominal aortic aneurysm (AAA) with peritoneal blood. (Courtesy of Robert Hendrickson, MD.) **B:** Artherosclerotic AAA located distal to the renal arteries. There is an additional aneurysm in the right common iliac artery. The atherosclerosis of the aorta is associated with obstructive atherosclerotic coronary artery disease. (From Hurst, with permission.) **C:** Transverse view of infrarenal AAA. (Courtesy of Al Sabbaj, MD.)

structural changes result in degeneration and aneurysmal dilatation. The risk of rupture increases with aneurysm size and significantly increases after the aneurysm reaches 5 cm or greater. Intraperitoneal rupture usually is rapidly fatal. Retroperitoneal rupture may be contained, giving the patient time to present to the ED for treatment. Risk factors for AAA include advanced age, gender (males carry higher risk), hypertension, and smoking. Conditions such as chronic obstructive pulmonary disease (COPD), coronary artery disease, peripheral vascular disease (PVD), or a predisposed family history also contribute to the risk of developing AAA.[1–4]

Diagnosis

The diagnostic approach taken depends on the stability of the patient and the index of suspicion. An unstable patient with a convincing presentation should receive immediate attention to their airway, breathing, and circulation (ABCs), followed by intravenous (IV) access and emergency surgical consultation. Blood products should also be available. Surgical consultation should not be delayed for any diagnostic study, because the only treatment of a ruptured AAA is immediate surgery.[2–4] Palpation of a pulsatile mass in the epigastrium should be attempted. However, palpation cannot be used to rule out a diagnosis of AAA, because the physical examination is only 68% sensitive in detecting an enlarged aorta (up to 82% sensitive for AAAs larger than 5 cm).[3]

Ultrasonography can be done at the bedside to attempt visualization of an enlarged aorta for rapid confirmation of the diagnosis. Bedside ultrasound should not be used to identify peritoneal blood (focused abdominal sonography for trauma [FAST] examination), because most bleeding is retroperitoneal, and the lack of peritoneal blood cannot be used to rule out AAA. Stable patients should undergo computed tomography (CT) with IV contrast, which is almost 100% sensitive in detecting AAA.[2] All patients with a symptomatic AAA should have a complete blood count, typing and cross-matching for 6 units of packed red blood cells (PRBCs), coagulation studies, and creatinine administration.[2–4]

Clinical Complications

The most feared complication of AAA is rupture with exsanguination. Other complications, such as obstruction of surrounding structures (e.g., ureters) and thrombosis of the AAA, are very rare. Patients with repaired AAAs are at risk for development of aortoenteric fistulas or graft failure.[2–4]

Management

Patients should have immediate assessment of their ABCs, placement of two large-bore IV access tubes, use of a cardiac monitor, and administration of oxygen. Patients with significant shock require IV fluids and unmatched blood products. Ruptured AAA requires immediate surgical intervention. Intubation may also be required.[1–4]

REFERENCES

1. Shames ML, Thompson RW. Abdominal aortic aneurysms: surgical treatment. *Cardiol Clin* 2002;20:563–578.
2. Clinical policy: critical issues for the initial evaluation and management of patients presenting with a chief complaint of nontraumatic acute abdominal pain. *Ann Emerg Med* 2000;36:406–415.
3. Fink HA, Lederle FA, Roth CS, Bowles CA, Nelson DB, Haas MA. The accuracy of physical examination to detect abdominal aortic aneurysm. *Arch Intern Med* 2000;160:833–836.
4. Lederle FA, Simel DL. The rational clinical examination: does this patient have abdominal aortic aneurysm? *JAMA* 1999;281:77–82.

Aortic Dissection

Samuel Kim

Clinical Presentation

Patients with aortic dissection commonly present to the emergency department (ED) with complaints of chest pain or back pain or both. The pain is usually abrupt in onset (85%) and is classically described as a "tearing" or "ripping" pain (51%). The location of the pain is most commonly the chest (73%), followed by the back (53%) and then the abdomen (30%).[2] Depending on the extent of the dissection, perfusion of branch arteries of the aorta may be affected, resulting in a myriad of possible ischemic presentations. Neurologic findings occur in 18% to 30% of cases, caused by stroke/cerebral ischemia, decreased spinal cord perfusion, or compression of peripheral nerves. Renal ischemia with resultant renal failure may occur. Mesenteric artery involvement may also cause mesenteric ischemia with acute abdominal pain. Pulse pressure and blood pressure differentials between the upper extremities may be seen (38%) and are the most specific physical examination finding. Lower-extremity perfusion may also be compromised, with symptomatic ischemia seen in 15% to 20% of cases. Involvement of the ascending aorta may cause compromise of coronary artery perfusion with resultant ischemia. Acute aortic valve insufficiency and pericardial effusion with tamponade may occur, with resultant hypotension and shock. The electrocardiograph (ECG) is often nonspecific and varies depending on coronary artery involvement. Chest radiography shows mediastinal widening in up to 50% of cases but is normal in up to 12% of cases.[2] Other findings may include changes in the position of the aorta, double aortic shadow, enlargement of the aortic knob, displacement of aortic calcifications, left pleural effusion, and disparity in the sizes of the ascending and descending aorta.

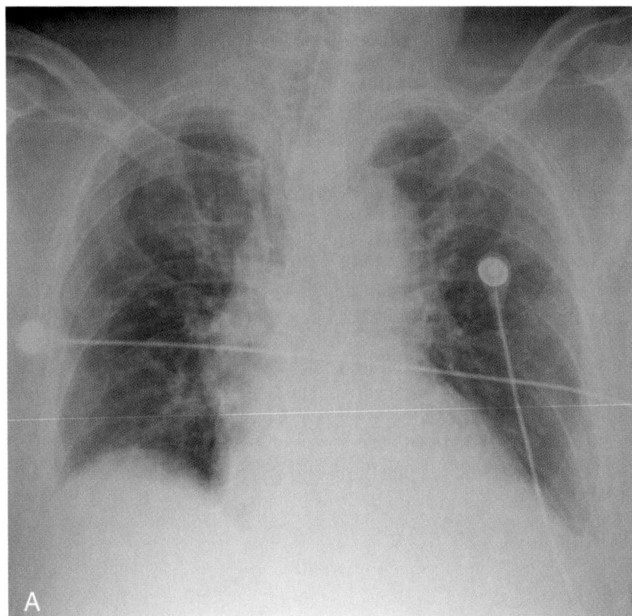

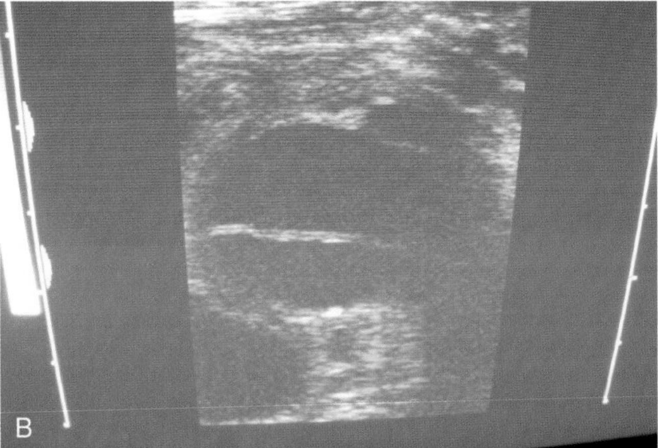

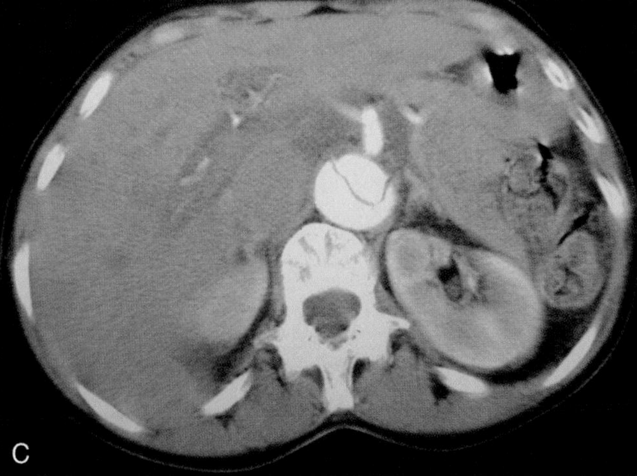

FIGURE 7–11 **A:** Chest radiograph showing widened mediastinum and displacement of trachea and esophagus. (Courtesy of Robert Hendrickson, MD.) **B:** Ultrasonogram showing a false lumen filled with clot. (Courtesy of Mark Silverberg, MD.) **C:** Computed tomogram showing aortic dissection with false lumen. (Courtesy of Colleen Campbell, MD.)

Aortic Dissection

Samuel Kim

Pathophysiology

Aortic dissection refers to separation of the layers of the aortic wall, usually caused by a tear in the intima. Aortic dissections are classified by two different schematics, the Stanford and DeBakey systems. Under the Stanford classification, dissections involving the ascending aorta are type A, and type B dissections involve only the descending aorta. Under the DeBakey classification, type I dissections include the ascending aorta, aortic arch, and descending aorta, whereas type II dissections involve only the ascending aorta and type III involve only the descending aorta.[1]

Aortic dissection may result from an initial intimal tear followed by cleavage of the intimal and medial layers and subsequent extension. Much more rarely, cleavage of the intimal and medial layers is caused by an initial intramural hematoma that expands and then ruptures through the intima. Usually, the intima tears around areas with the greatest pressure gradients and fluctuations, most commonly in the ascending aorta and the first portion of the descending aorta.[2] The ratio of type A to type B dissections is approximately 2:1. There is a male-to-female ratio of approximately 2:1, and the peak incidence is in the sixth and seventh decades of life.[3] Other risk factors include long-standing untreated hypertension, aortic dilatation, aneurysm, coarctation, aortic arteritis, aortic arch hypoplasia, chromosomal aberrations (Turner's and Noonan's syndromes), and connective tissue diseases (Marfan's and Ehlers-Danlos syndromes). Iatrogenic trauma has also been implicated. Cocaine users and pregnant women have been cited as higher-risk population groups.[3]

Diagnosis

All patients in whom aortic dissection is suspected should be imaged with transesophageal echocardiography (TEE), magnetic resonance imaging (MRI), computed tomography (CT), or angiography. Any modality except transthoracic echocardiography (TTE) may be used to rule out aortic dissection if the clinical suspicion is low. If the pretest probability is moderate to high, a second test should be ordered if the first test is negative.[4] The selection of the second test should be made with time delays in mind, because time to diagnosis and treatment significantly affects survival. TEE and MRI are the most sensitive and specific studies, with TEE having a sensitivity of 95% to 100% and a specificity of 70% to 95%, and MRI having a sensitivity of 95% and a specificity of 100%. CT has a sensitivity of 83% to 90% and a specificity of 90% to 100%.[4]

Clinical Complications

Aortic dissection may result in rupture, with type A dissections being most prone to rupture. The mortality rate after rupture is 1% per hour after onset of symptoms.[4] Aortic dissection may also result in stroke, shock, hypotension, acute renal failure, neurologic deficits, symptomatic limb ischemia, and mesenteric ischemia.

Management

Patients with aortic dissection should receive rapid control of hypertension and tachycardia with intravenous (IV) antihypertensive medications, regardless of dissection type. A combination of a β-blocker and a vasodilator (e.g., nitroprusside) usually is used,[3] although single therapy with labetalol or esmolol also may be used. Patients with probable aortic dissection should have immediate consultation with an appropriate surgeon or cardiologist or both. Definitive treatment is based on the type of dissection. Type A dissections are treated by surgery unless comorbid conditions preclude surgery as an option, and type B dissections are managed medically. All aortic dissections require intensive care unit (ICU) admission.[1–4]

REFERENCES

1. Pretre R, Von Segesser L. Aortic dissection. *Lancet* 1997;349:1461–1464.
2. Hagan PG, Nienaber CA, Isselbacher EM, et al. The International Registry of Acute Aortic Dissection (IRAD): new insights into an old disease. *JAMA* 2000;283:897–903.
3. Sarasin FP, Louis-Simonet M, Gaspoz JM, Junod A. Detecting acute thoracic aortic dissection in the emergency department: time constraints and choice of the optimal diagnostic test. *Ann Emerg Med* 1996;28:278–288.
4. Khan I, Nair C. Clinical, diagnostic, and management perspectives of aortic dissection. *Chest* 2002;122:311–328.

Thoracic Aortic Aneurysm

Robert Hendrickson

Clinical Presentation

Patients with a rupture of a thoracic aortic aneurysm (TAA) typically develop rapid exsanguination and rarely survive to hospitalization. If they survive to the emergency department (ED), these patients have hypovolemic shock and evidence of exsanguination (widened mediastinum and hemothorax) on chest radiography. Occasionally, patients present with chest pain that is attributable to rapid expansion of the aneurysm and impending rupture.[1]

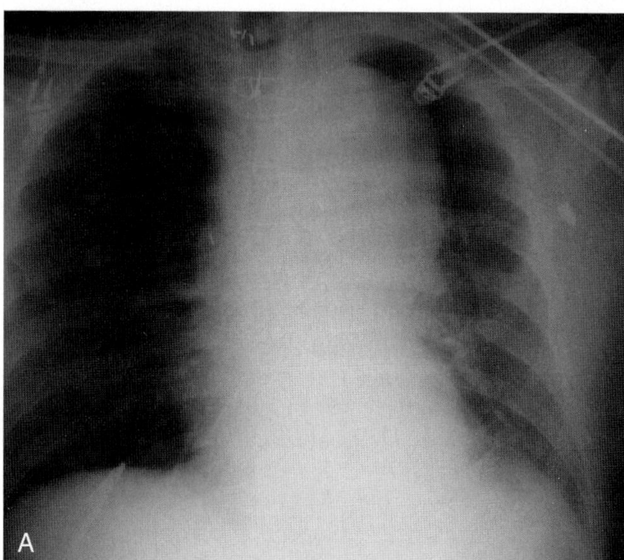

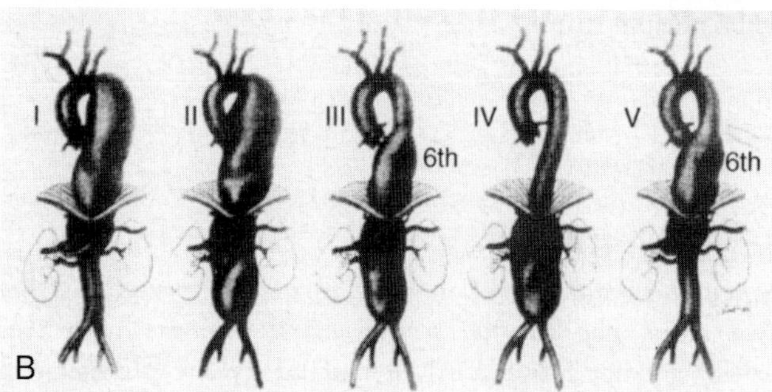

FIGURE 7–12 **A:** Thoracic aneurysm. (Courtesy of Donald Sallee, MD.) **B:** Thoracoabdominal aortic aneurysm classification: I, between left subclavian and renal arteries; II, between left subclavian and bifurcation; III, between 6th rib and bifurcation; IV, between the 12th rib and the bifurcation; V, between the 6th rib and the renal arteries. (From Safi HJ, Winnerkvist A, Miller CC 3rd, et al. Effect of extended cross-clamp time during thoracoabdominal aneurysm repair. *Ann Thorac Surg* 1998;66:1204–1209, with permission.)

Patients with unruptured TAAs may present with symptoms that are related to compression of thoracic structures, such as hoarseness, dysphagia, dyspnea, chest pain, or superior vena cava syndrome.[2] TAA may also be detected on routine chest radiography as a widened inferior mediastinum and enlarged aortic shadow. An enlarged aorta may be evident on abdominal examination if the aneurysm extends to the abdomen.

Pathophysiology

TAA refers to aneurysmal dilatation of the ascending (50%), arch (10%), or descending (40%) portion of the aorta within the thorax.[1] Aneurysms may be primarily thoracic or thoracoabdominal.[1]

Aneurysmal dilatation may be related to atherosclerosis, trauma, medial degeneration (Marfan syndrome), aortitis (syphilis), mycotic infections, and vasculitis (Takayasu's arteritis).[1,2] Dilatation of the proximal aorta may also occur with bicuspid valves and after surgical repair of aortic dissection.[2]

Diagnosis

Diagnosis of an unruptured TAA typically is made on chest radiography and should be confirmed with a thoracic computed tomography (CT) to differentiate aneurysmal dilatation from anatomic tortuosity of the aorta.

Clinical Complications

The primary complication is rupture. Rupture occurs in up to 50% of patients with TAA and has a mortality rate of 90%.[2] Survival rates are approximately 57% at 1 year, 35% at 3 years, and 19% at 5 years.[2]

Management

Patients with a ruptured TAA or impending rupture require oxygen, large-bore fluid and blood infusions, emergency surgical consultation, and rapid transport to the operating theater. Patients without rupture who have radiographic signs of aortic dilatation should be further evaluated with a thoracic CT and close follow-up with a thoracic surgeon. Control of hypertension and smoking cessation may also be helpful.[2]

REFERENCES

1. Fann JI. Descending thoracic and thoracoabdominal aortic aneurysms. *Coron Artery Dis* 2002;13:93–102.
2. Moon MR, Sundt TM 3rd. Aortic arch aneurysms. *Coron Artery Dis* 2002;13:85–92.

Septal Wall Rupture

Todd McGrath

Clinical Presentation

Patients with septal wall rupture (SWR) present with chest pain, shortness of breath, and signs of cardiogenic shock. This condition is typically seen either within the first 24 hours of an acute myocardial infarction (AMI) or 3 to 5 days after myocardial infarction (MI). Patients may have a new, harsh systolic murmur at the left sternal border.[1]

Pathophysiology

SWR occurs when the intraventricular septum ruptures, creating a left-to-right shunting of blood flow within the heart after an AMI.

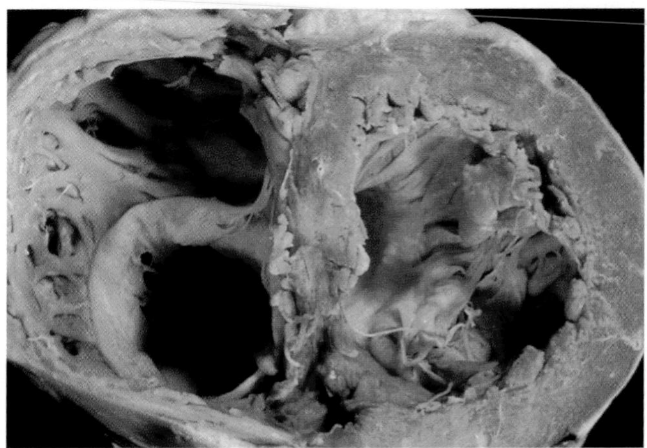

FIGURE 7-13 Rupture of ventricular septum. (From Hurst, with permission.)

SWR involves necrosis of the intraventricular septum associated with an AMI. If the rupture occurs in the first 24 hours, it is usually associated with an intramural hematoma within the septum. Delayed rupture is typically related to coagulation necrosis of the septum.[1] SWR complicates between 1% and 3% of infarctions, although reperfusion therapy lowers this rate to approximately 0.2%.[1,2]

Diagnosis

The diagnosis of SWR is made by use of bedside echocardiography in patients presenting with consistent symptoms.[1]

Clinical Complications

Complications of SWR include left-to-right shunting, biventricular heart failure, and cardiogenic shock.[1]

Management

Initial management of SWR involves medical stabilization with attention to hypotension using inotropic agents and vasopressors.[1] The use of an intraaortic balloon pump may be necessary for stabilization.[1,2] Definitive treatment requires surgical repair of the defect.[1]

REFERENCES

1. Birnbaum Y, Fishbein MC, Blanche C, Siegel RJ. Ventricular septal rupture after acute myocardial infarction. *N Engl J Med* 2002;347:1426–1432.
2. Deja MA, Szostek J, Wildenka K, et al. Post infarction ventricular septal defect: can we do better? *Eur J Cardiothorac Surg* 2000;18: 194–201.

7-14

Papillary Muscle Rupture

Todd McGrath

Clinical Presentation

Patients with papillary muscle rupture (PMR) present with an acute myocardial infarction (AMI) or recent history of myocardial infarction (MI) (more commonly after an inferior MI) and mitral regurgitation. Severely affected patients may present with cardiovascular collapse and pulmonary edema.[1]

Pathophysiology

There are three papillary muscles (anterior, inferior, and posterior) that may infarct and necrose in association with an AMI. Theories suggest that postinfarction ischemia, infarct extension, and physical strain after MI may lead to PMR, secondary to local necrosis. This is usually seen within 5 days after the initial infarction; it is more common in patients who present late in the course of their infarction and in more physically active post-MI patients.[1] The kinetic energy of a sudden deceleration can shear the papillary muscle in trauma patients.[2]

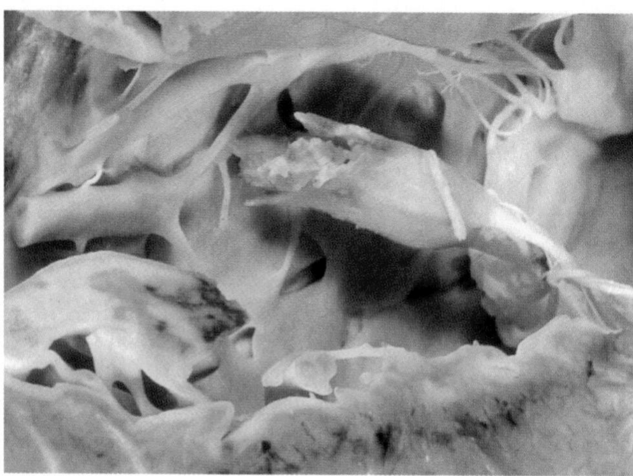

FIGURE 7–14 Rupture of the posteromedial papillary muscle. (From Hurst, with permission.)

Diagnosis

PMR should be suspected in any patient with a recent history of AMI who presents with pulmonary edema and a murmur consistent with mitral regurgitation. The definitive diagnosis is made by transesophageal echocardiography.[1,2]

Clinical Complications

Complications are related to the sudden loss of mitral valve competence. Patients typically develop pulmonary edema and cardiovascular collapse secondary to sudden valvular insufficiency.[1,2]

Management

The initial management includes use of inotropic agents and afterload reduction with a vasodilator to treat any cardiovascular collapse. Patients may also require standard AMI therapy. The definitive treatment involves surgical repair of the papillary muscle and mitral valve, which carries a mortality rate of 45.8%.[1,2]

REFERENCES

1. Figueras J, Calvo F, Cortadellas J, Soler-Soler J. Comparison of patients with and without papillary muscle rupture during acute myocardial infarction. *Am J Cardiol* 1997;80:625–627.
2. Simmers TA, Meijburg HW, de la Riviere AB. Traumatic papillary muscle rupture. *Ann Thorac Surg* 2001;72:257–259.

Aortic Regurgitation

Robert Chisholm

Clinical Presentation

The hallmark of aortic regurgitation (AR) is a high-pitched decrescendo diastolic murmur at the left sternal border, heard best with the patient leaning forward in expiration. Patients may present to the emergency department (ED) with complaints related to either acute or chronic AR, and symptoms vary depending on the time course of disease.

AR occurs as an acute manifestation in 20% of patients. Symptoms include dyspnea (50% of patients), weakness, hypotension, angina, paroxysmal nocturnal dyspnea, orthopnea, diaphoresis, palpitations, and abdominal pain. Critically ill patients may develop signs of congestive heart failure (CHF) or shock (or both), which include hypotension, tachycardia, cyanosis, pulmonary edema, and peripheral vasoconstriction.

Chronic AR eventually leads to heart failure and its associated signs and symptoms. A variety of physical signs have been identified in patients with chronic AR: Austin Flint murmur (low-pitched, rumbling, late diastolic apical murmur), Hill sign (lower extremity systolic blood pressure greater than upper extremity systolic blood pressure), Corrigan pulse ("water-hammer pulse"; rapid rise and fall of arterial pulse by palpation of radial artery), Duroziez sign (to-fro murmur auscultated by compressing the femoral artery with the stethoscope), and Quincke sign (capillary pulsations of the nail beds).[1]

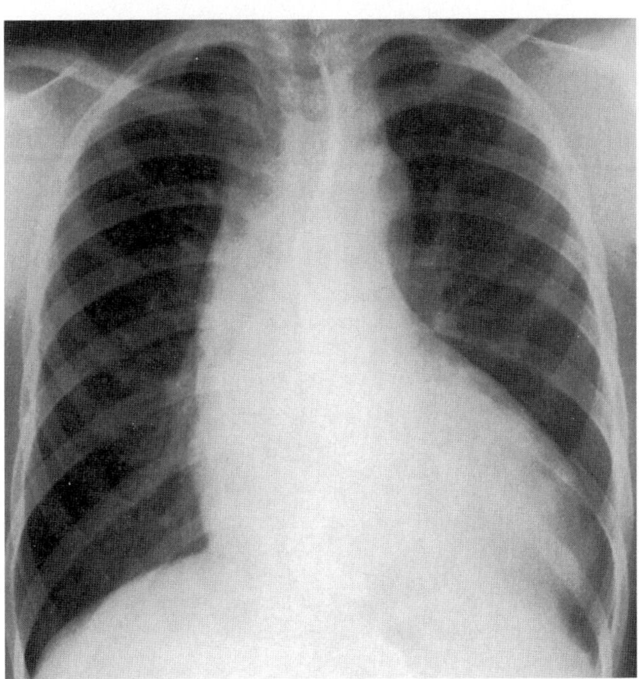

FIGURE 7–15 Barium opacifies the esophagus on the chest films of a patient with aortic regurgitation, and reveals marked enlargement of the left ventricle, with dilation of the aorta beginning in the root and extending through the distal arch. (From Hurst, with permission.)

Pathophysiology

Regurgitation is caused by disease of the aortic valve, aorta, or trauma. The diastolic retrograde blood flow into the ventricle causes left ventricular (LV) volume overload. The severity of disease depends on the degree of valvular incompetence. Causes of AR include infective endocarditis, aortic dissection, trauma, rheumatic heart disease (RHD), syphilis, connective tissue diseases such as Marfan syndrome, bicuspid aortic valve, and autoimmune diseases such as Reiter's syndrome, and systemic lupus erythematosus (SLE).[1]

Diagnosis

The diagnosis can be made with a thorough history and physical examination and confirmed with echocardiography.[1] Chest radiography in acute AR may be normal or may show an increased pulmonary venous pattern representing pulmonary edema. Chronic AR may illustrate marked cardiac enlargement with a prominent aortic arch and a normal pulmonary venous pattern. The electrocardiograph (ECG) may depict left-axis deviation in chronic AR.[1]

Clinical Complications

Acute AR may lead to LV overload, dysfunction, shock, and death. Chronic AR is a more indolent process, which also eventually produces symptoms related to ventricular dysfunction and heart failure.[1]

Management

Acute AR is an emergency and mandates cardiac intensive care unit (ICU) admission and prompt cardiology or cardiothoracic surgery consultation. Positive inotropes help support forward flow and blood pressure, and vasodilators decrease afterload.[1]

REFERENCES

1. Babu AN, Kymes SM, Carpenter Fryer SM. Eponyms and the diagnosis of aortic regurgitation: what says the evidence. *Ann Intern Med* 2003;138:736–742.

Aortic Stenosis

Lisa Freeman

Clinical Presentation

The onset of symptoms occurs late in the course of disease and only after significant stenosis occurs. Presenting symptoms are an indication for valve replacement and can include exercise-induced syncope, dyspnea, and angina-type chest pain. Eventually, symptoms may occur at rest, and congestive heart failure (CHF) and atrial fibrillation (AF) may develop. On physical examination, the blood pressure may be normal or low with a narrow pulse pressure. There is often a split S_2, and an S_3 or S_4 present. The classic murmur is a harsh systolic ejection crescendo–decrescendo murmur that radiates to the neck.[2]

Pathophysiology

Aortic stenosis is a chronic valvular disease that can lead to CHF and death if untreated. The most common causes are congenital (bicuspid valve), rheumatic heart disease (RHD), and degenerative heart disease (calcific aortic stenosis).[1]

Because of the stenotic aortic valve, blood flow into the aorta is restricted. The resultant left ventricular hypertrophy (LVH) leads to low cardiac output and significant reduction in coronary blood flow. This predisposes the patient to development of lethal arrthymias.[1,2]

Diagnosis

Initial diagnosis made by physical examination is confirmed via echocardiogram. A normal aortic valve has an area of 2.5 cm^2 without a gradient between the ventricle and the aorta. A valve with an area of less than 0.8 cm^2 or a gradient greater than 50 mm Hg defines critical aortic stenosis.[1] Electrocardiograph (ECG) may reveal evidence of LVH or a bundle branch block. Chest radiography may be normal at the onset of symptoms, but will eventually reflect LVH or CHF.[1,2]

Clinical Complications

After the onset of symptoms, prognosis is poor. Survival is only 2 to 3 years,[2] and sudden death from an arrhythmia occurs in 25% of patients. CHF and AF may also occur.[1,2]

Management

Other than supportive care in an acute case, there is no efficacious therapy for aortic stenosis. Aortic valve replacement is the only effective intervention, and patients with aortic stenosis should receive endocarditis prophylaxis before any indicated procedure.[2]

REFERENCES

1. Shipton B, Wahba H. Valvular heart disease: review and update. *Am Fam Physician* 2001;63:2201–2208.
2. Carabello BA. Aortic stenosis. *N Engl J Med* 2002;346:677–682.

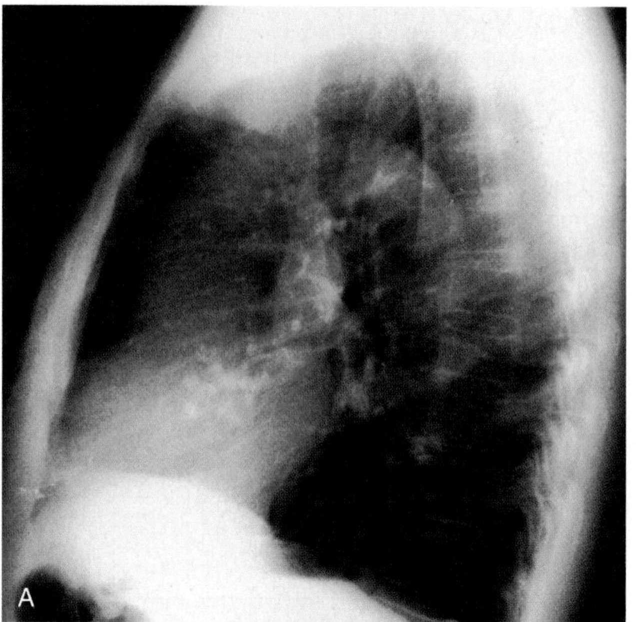

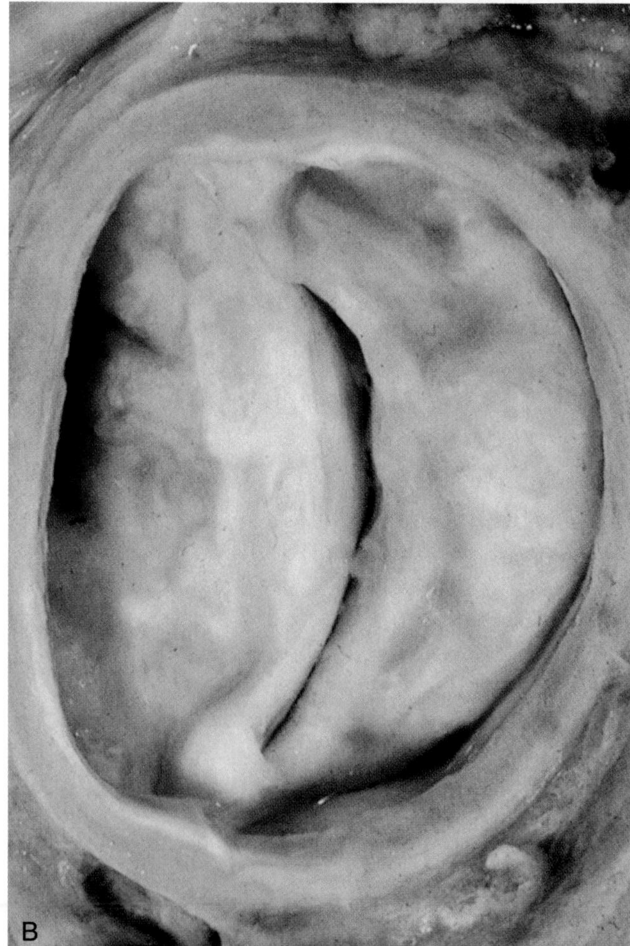

FIGURE 7–16 A: Chest radiograph showing calcific aortic stenosis. Note normal-sized heart with a slightly enlarged ascending aorta. (From Hurst, with permission.) **B:** Isolated calcific stenosis in association with a congenitally bicuspid aortic valve. (From Becker, with permission.)

Phlegmasia Cerulea and Alba Dolens

Jennifer Larson

Clinical Presentation

Patients with phlegmasia cerulea dolens (PCD) present with a clinical triad of extremity edema, severe pain, and cyanosis.[1] The pain is constant and progresses distally. Secondary manifestations, such as blebs and bullae due to massive fluid sequestration, may occur. Between 50% and 60% of PCD cases are preceded by phlegmasia alba dolens (PAD), which manifests as extremity edema with pain but no cyanosis.[1] Alba is a descriptive term for the blanching seen. Lower extremities are the site of disease in the majority of patient presentations, and the left extremity is affected more commonly than the right.[1]

Pathophysiology

PCD and PAD are acute massive venous thromboses that obstruct venous drainage of an extremity. PCD is associated with ischemia of the limb, whereas PAD is not.[1]

PCD is caused by thrombosis of major deep venous channels, as well as collateral veins, leading to decreased venous drainage, fluid sequestration, and edema.[1] Elevations in tissue pressure from edema and decrease in perfusion pressure due to hypovolemia may lead to ischemia of the limb and gangrene of the skin, subcutaneous tissue, and muscles. PAD spares the collateral veins, allowing for some venous drainage.[1]

Risk factors for PCD and PAD include malignancy, hypercoagulable state, surgery, trauma, and third trimester of pregnancy. However, up to 10% of patients have no known risk factor.[1]

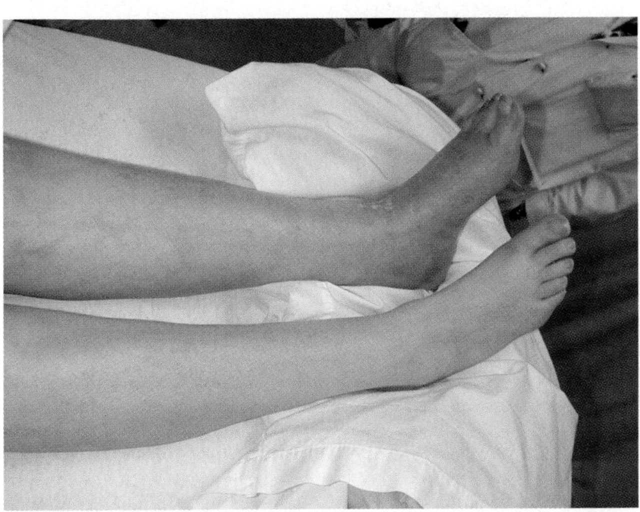

FIGURE 7–17 Phlegmasia cerulea dolens. (Courtesy of William S. Schroder, MD.)

Diagnosis

The diagnosis is made by recognition of the typical clinical features and identification of a deep venous thrombosis (DVT) by ultrasonography, venography, or magnetic resonance imaging (MRI).

Clinical Complications

Complications include gangrene, hypotension, arterial insufficiency, amputation, and death.[1] Other complications include postphlebitic syndrome and rethrombosis after thrombectomy.[1]

Management

All patients with PCD or PAD require hospital admission. For PAD and mild forms of PCD, medical therapy is the initial treatment. This includes steep limb elevation, anticoagulation with intravenous (IV) heparin, and fluid resuscitation, followed by long-term anticoagulation with warfarin and compression stockings. For all other forms of PCD, surgical thrombectomy with concomitant anticoagulation is the course of action with or without fasciotomy. Thrombolysis with tissue plasminogen activator (tPA) is an alternative therapy and may be combined with anticoagulation.[1]

REFERENCES

1. Perkins JM, Magee TR, Galland RB. Phlegmasia caerulea dolens and venous gangrene. *Br J Surg* 1996;83:19–23.

Deep Venous Thrombosis

Paul Prator

Clinical Presentation

Presenting symptoms in patients with deep venous thrombosis (DVT) may include the gradual onset of unilateral lower extremity pain, tenderness, warmth or erythema, swelling (circumferential difference between extremities greater than 1 to 2 cm), a Homan sign (pain in the calf with dorsiflexion of the foot), a painful pale extremity (phlegmasia alba dolens; PAD), a painful cyanotic extremity (phlegmasia cerulea dolens; PCD), or a low-grade fever.[1]

Pathophysiology

Venous stasis, endothelial injury, and hypercoagulable states predispose to the development of DVT. Ultimately, fatal thrombi may form at many sites in the venous system; however, approximately 80% of symptomatic DVT occur at or proximal to the popliteal veins.[1] Risk factors include hypercoagulable states (malignancies, contraceptive use, sepsis, protein C/S deficiencies), inflammatory disease (systemic lupus erythematosus [SLE], inflammatory bowel disease), trauma (burns/surgery), intravenous (IV) access (central venous catheters, pacemakers), tobacco use, obesity, immobilization (casting, travel, bed rest, stroke, paralysis, congestive heart failure [CHF]/acute myocardial infarction [AMI]), or a past history of thromboembolism.[1]

Diagnosis

The diagnosis may be considered clinically but must be confirmed with laboratory or radiographic testing. The initial diagnostic test usually is compression/color-flow duplex Doppler ultrasonography. However, ultrasound cannot reliably detect pelvic or calf DVT. Contrast venography is a highly sensitive option; however, it requires specialized equipment, is invasive, and may result in serious side effects. Magnetic resonance imaging (MRI) may become increasingly useful as a highly sensitive tool in detecting DVT. MRI has the advantage of detecting other pathologic conditions that may be responsible for the presenting complaints (cysts, hematomas, enlarged lymph nodes, pelvic masses), but it is expensive, is not readily available, and cannot be used in patients with indwelling metallic hardware.[1,2]

The D-dimer laboratory assay is a sensitive test often used concurrently with imaging studies for the detection of DVT; the strength of this test lies in its ability to exclude the diagnosis of DVT. Other causes of an elevated D-dimer concentration include infection, recent surgery, malignancies, trauma, and cardiovascular disease. The combination of a low D-dimer and a normal duplex Doppler ultrasound study has a negative predictive value of approximately 99% for a proximal DVT.[2]

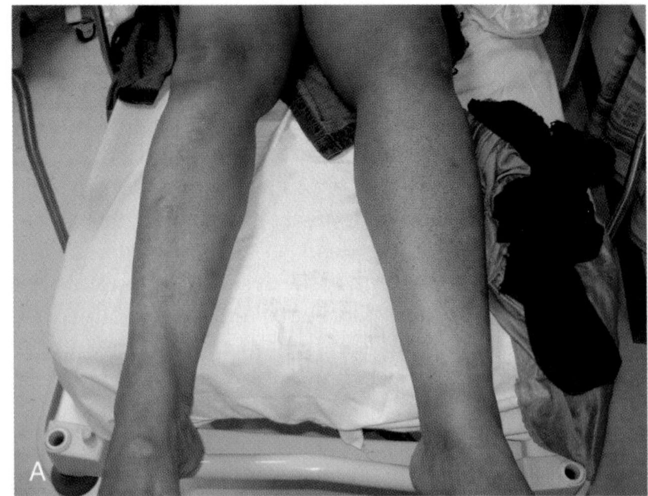

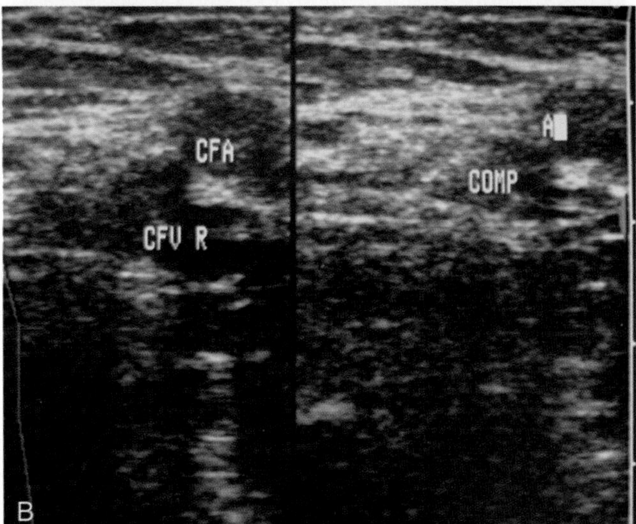

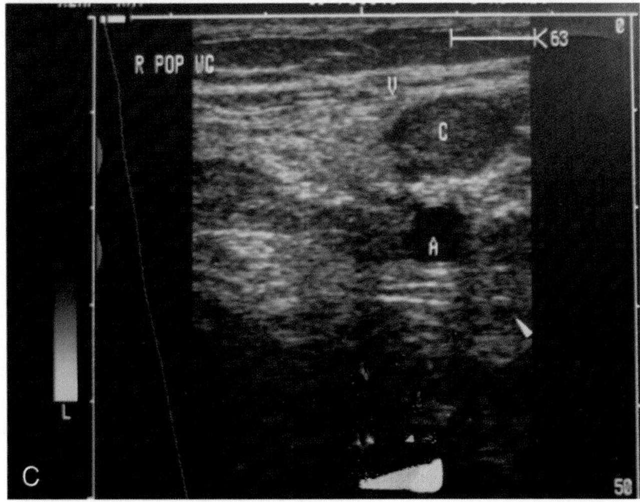

FIGURE 7–18 **A:** Lower extremity erythema and edema as typical of deep venous thrombosis. (Courtesy of Mark Silverberg, MD.) **B:** Ultrasonogram showing incompressible vein. (Courtesy of John Fojtik, MD.) **C:** Ultrasonogram showing visible clot. (Courtesy of John Fojtik, MD.)

Deep Venous Thrombosis

Paul Prator

Clinical Complications

The major complication of DVT is pulmonary embolism (PE). Chronic venous insufficiency, limb ischemia (secondary to acute or complete venous obstruction), and postphlebitic syndromes are other potentially serious manifestations of DVT.[1,2]

Management

Prompt anticoagulation is the mainstay of treatment for proven proximal DVT. Current therapies use unfractionated heparin versus fractionated heparin or low-molecular-weight heparin (LMWH). LMWHs have the added advantages of simplified administration, longer half-life, lower incidence of bleeding complications and heparin-induced thrombocytopenia, a more predictable anticoagulant effect, and no need to monitor serial activated partial-thromboplastin times (aPTT).[2] Oral anticoagulation with warfarin is often started concurrently with heparin therapy, and a course of 3 to 6 months is recommended. The daily warfarin dose is adjusted to achieve an international normalized ratio (INR) between 2.0 and 3.0.[2] In patients in whom anticoagulation is contraindicated, placement of a vena cava filter (Greenfield filter) may be considered.[1,2]

REFERENCES

1. Hirsh J, Hoak J. Management of deep venous thrombosis and pulmonary embolism: a statement for healthcare professionals from the Council on Thrombosis, American Heart Association. *Circulation* 1996;93:2212–2245.
2. Ginsberg JS. Drug therapy: management of venous thromboembolism. *N Engl J Med* 1996;335:1816–1828.

Acute Arterial Occlusion

Robert Hendrickson

Clinical Presentation

Patients may present to the emergency department (ED) with acute onset of pain in an extremity that is associated with numbness and change in skin color ("blue toe"). Occlusion most commonly occurs in the lower extremity.[1,2]

Pathophysiology

Acute arterial occlusion occurs when a thrombus or embolus acutely occludes a terminal artery and produces ischemia.

Acute arterial occlusion may result from an embolus, a thrombus, or a vascular dissection. Emboli from cardiac valvular vegetations, from aortic aneurysms, or from within the heart (e.g., from atrial fibrillation [AF]) may occlude the upper or lower extremities. Thrombi may form on the endothelium of a vessel containing atherosclerotic plaques. Finally, proximal occlusion may occur as a result of an aortic or femoral dissection or thrombosis of an abdominal aortic aneurysm (AAA). Gradual onset of vascular occlusion, as occurs with atherosclerosis or fibrosis, does not produce acute arterial occlusion, because the artery has time to develop effective collateral circulation.[1,2]

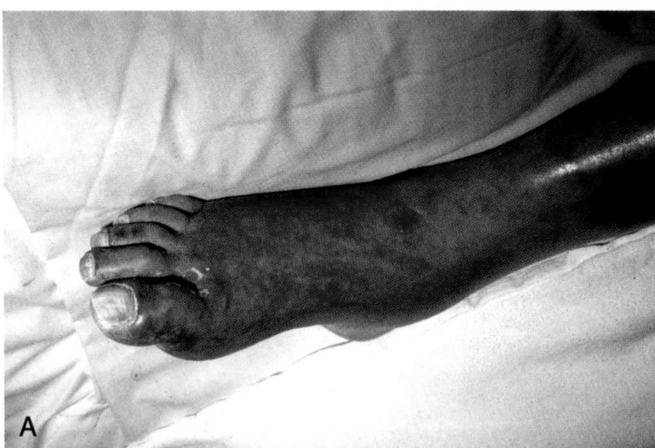

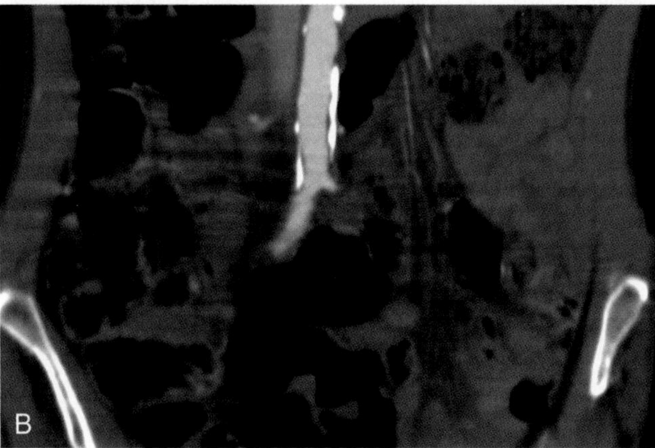

FIGURE 7–19 **A:** Mottled skin on foot in acute arterial occlusion. (Courtesy of William B. Schroder, MD.) **B:** Left femoral artery thrombosis. (Courtesy of Robert Hendrickson, MD.)

Diagnosis

The diagnosis of acute arterial occlusion may be made clinically by noting an extremity that is pale, cool, paresthetic, and with diminished or absent pulses. Care should be taken to rule out other causes of ischemia, including compartmental syndrome, trauma, aortic dissection, and thrombosis of an AAA. AF or a cardiac murmur should increase the suspicion of emboli, and truncal pain and older age should increase the suspicion of dissection. The diagnosis usually can be confirmed with contrast computed tomography (CT) or arteriography. A metabolic panel and an arterial blood gas determination may reveal acidosis and hyperlactatemia, which are often associated with partial vascular occlusion and limb ischemia.[1,2]

Clinical Complications

Arterial occlusion may lead to ischemia, necrosis, amputation, systemic acidosis, and infection of the involved limb.[1,2]

Management

Patients should be immediately evaluated for other causes of ischemia, including compartmental syndrome, aortic dissection, and thrombosis of an AAA. Surgical and interventional radiology consultation should be obtained as soon as possible. Thrombectomy/embolectomy may be accomplished via intraarterial urokinase or surgical intervention.[1] Both interventions have similar rates of amputation-free survival.[1] Urokinase has a higher rate of intracranial hemorrhage,[1] but it may be more appropriate if a delay in revascularization is unacceptable.[2] Surgical thrombectomy should be used in patients with contraindications to fibrinolytics or intravenous (IV) dye allergies.[2]

REFERENCES

1. Ouriel K, Veith FJ, Sasahara AA. A comparison of recombinant urokinase with vascular surgery as initial treatment for acute arterial occlusion of the legs. *N Engl J Med* 1998;338:1105–1111.
2. Ouriel K. Thrombolytic therapy for acute arterial occlusion. *J Am Coll Surg* 2002;194:S32–S39.

Peripheral Vascular Disease (Arteriosclerosis Obliterans)

Robert Chisholm

Clinical Presentation

The early sign of peripheral vascular disease (PVD) is typically claudication, which is pain that is reproducible on walking a specific distance. Claudication occurs at a specific activity level and is relieved after a short rest.[1] The location of pain may reflect the arteries involved—calf claudication (femoral-popliteal) or thigh and buttock pain (aortoiliac). As the condition advances, intermittent claudication can lead to rest claudication. Occasionally, PVD manifests as an acute extremity ischemic event from an embolus or thrombus in an atherosclerotic plaque.

Pathophysiology

PVD results from atherosclerosis, a gradual process of arterial occlusion by enlarging cholesterol plaques. Many factors contribute to the development of cholesterol atheromas, including genetic factors, hypertension, diabetes, diet, and smoking.

Diagnosis

The diagnosis can be made with a thorough history and physical examination. Patients with PVD may have thin and atrophic skin, loss of hair, rubor, and distal ulcerations of the affected extremity. The ankle-brachial index (ABI) can be helpful to determine hypoperfusion. The systolic pressure at the ankle is divided by the systolic pressure in the arm, both measured in the supine position. Results are classified as incompressible (greater than 1.3; for example, calcified vessels), normal (0.9 to 1.3), suggestive of PVD (0.4 to 0.9), or critical stenosis (less than 0.4).[1]

An assessment of limb pallor with the patient supine may also be helpful in quantitating the degree of disease. Pallor manifesting while the limb is held level indicates severe disease, whereas pallor with 60-degree elevation indicates less advanced, but significant disease.

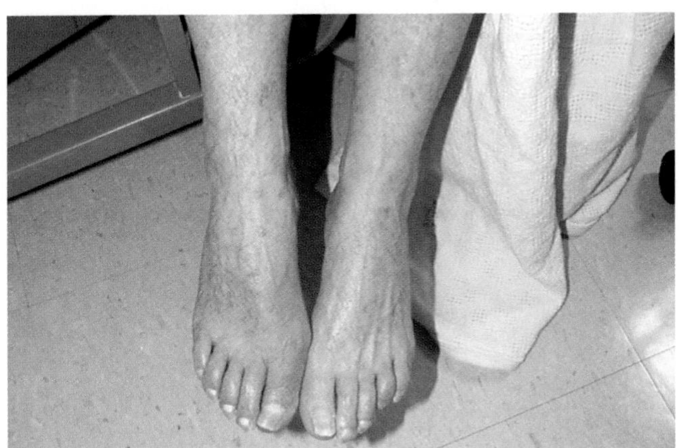

FIGURE 7–20 Left foot is noticeably pale, indicative of reduced blood flow. (Courtesy of William B. Schroder, MD.)

Clinical Complications

Acute limb ischemia can lead to irreversible tissue damage, gangrene, and limb loss (less than 1%). Patients with PVD are at higher risk for other atherosclerotic diseases, including myocardial infarction (MI) and cerebrovascular accident (CVA) (5% to 10% per year).[2]

Management

Chronic claudication is not an emergency but is best treated with lifestyle modification (exercise, cessation of smoking); treatment of diabetes, hyperlipidemia, and hypertension; angiotensin-converting enzyme (ACE) inhibitors; antiplatelet therapy (aspirin, ticlopidine, or clopidogrel); and referral back to the primary physician for monitoring and surgical referral, if needed.[1,2] Acute limb ischemia is a true emergency and must be approached with the end goal of reperfusion in mind. The patient should be resuscitated and given oxygen, pain medication, and intravenous (IV) access. Laboratory evaluation may reveal acidosis and hyperlactatemia secondary to limb ischemia. Empiric treatment with anticoagulants should be considered, and emergency general or vascular surgery consultation should be obtained.

REFERENCES

1. Hiatt WR. Medical treatment of peripheral arterial disease and claudication. *N Engl J Med* 2001;344:1608–1621.
2. Burns P, Gough S, Bradbury AW. Management of peripheral arterial disease in primary care. *BMJ* 2003;326:584–588.

Venous Stasis Ulcer

Samuel Kim

Clinical Presentation

Patients with venous stasis ulcers often present with complaints of a recurrent ulcer in the same location that does not heal. These ulcers are typically painless, but may be painful for some patients. Patients may report symptoms suggestive of venous insufficiency, including aching pain and swelling of the legs that is worse at the end of the day. These symptoms typically are relieved with rest and elevation of the legs. The most common location for venous stasis ulcers is on the lower extremities near the medial malleolus.[1] These ulcers are usually irregular in shape, with a shallow ulcer bed and a thin layer of overlying granulation tissue.[1] Frank necrosis and exposure of deeper underlying tissue (e.g., tendons) usually are not seen, but, if present, these findings suggest other possible causes of ulceration. Additional findings usually associated with venous ulcers include hemosiderin deposition (due to exudated erythrocytes), which results in reddish-brown discoloration; dependent edema of lower extremities; varicose veins; and eczematous skin changes overlying these areas.[1]

Pathophysiology

Venous stasis ulcers are limb lesions that occur secondary to chronically elevated venous pressures caused by venous insufficiency.

The exact mechanism by which elevated venous pressures result in ulceration is unknown. There are several theories: (1) elevated venous pressures result in exudation of fibrinogen through capillary walls and subse-

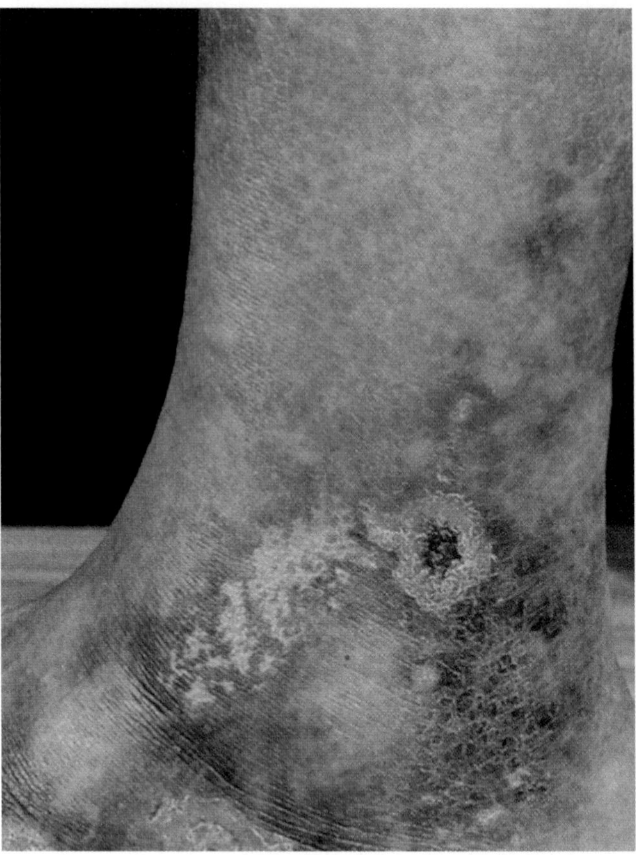

FIGURE 7–21 Typical appearance of postphlebitic skin changes and brawny edema associated with chronic deep venous valvular insufficiency. (From Hurst, with permission.)

Venous Stasis Ulcer

Samuel Kim

quent deposition of fibrin around capillaries; (2) leukocytes adhere to venous endothelium, activating and releasing proteolytic enzymes; (3) exudation into surrounding tissue traps growth factors, preventing them from aiding in repair processes.[2] A number of specific risk factors have been identified for venous stasis ulcers, including obesity, prior history of lower extremity injury, family history of varicose veins, occupational activities that include long hours of standing or sitting, previous surgery, and history of deep venous thrombosis (DVT).

Diagnosis

A properly completed patient history and physical examination are essential in making a diagnosis of venous stasis ulcer. However, adjunct studies may be necessary to rule out other possible causes of ulceration, because the most common alternative causes are peripheral vascular disease (PVD) and peripheral neuropathy. Color duplex ultrasonography is useful in evaluating venous system disease, because it can provide information on both arterial and venous system flow and may be used to evaluate for DVT in a patient with leg swelling. An ankle-brachial index (ABI) may be measured to evaluate the presence of PVD (ABI greater than 0.7). Nylon monofilament testing may be useful to help rule out neuropathy. Blood glucose testing may be used to evaluate for occult diabetes. In patients with suspected osteomyelitis, radiographs, bone scans, and bone biopsies may be necessary.

Clinical Complications

Venous stasis ulcers may progress to deeper ulceration and secondary infections, leading to cellulitis, myositis, and other soft tissue infections. This condition may also result in osteomyelitis and, in cases with significant arterial disease, to gangrene as well.

Management

The mainstay of therapy for venous ulcers remains elevation and compression. Both inelastic compression dressings (e.g., Unna boot) and elastic compression bandages may be used. Noncompressive therapy should be used if there is significant arterial disease or significant congestive heart failure (CHF). Usually, venous ulcers can be managed on an outpatient basis unless significant secondary infection or deep ulceration is evident.[2] Vascular surgical consultation should be arranged, because these wounds require long-term care and evaluation for malignancy, as well as plastic surgery if the wound fails to heal.[2]

REFERENCES

1. de Araujo T, Valencia I, Federman DG, Kirsner RS. Managing the patient with venous ulcers. *Ann Intern Med* 2003;138:326–334.
2. Phillips, TJ. Current approaches to venous ulcers and compression. *Dermatol Surg* 2001;27:611–621.

Gangrene

Jennifer Larson

Clinical Presentation

Venous gangrene is rare; the exact incidence is not known. Gangrene is part of a spectrum of presentations of tissue ischemia. Gangrene is always preceded by phlegmasia cerulea dolens (PCD), because 40% to 60% of PCD cases progress to gangrene.[1] PCD is an acute massive venous thrombosis associated with limb ischemia. Gangrene occurs when limb ischemia progresses toward necrosis of the limb. PCD manifests as extremity edema, severe pain, and cyanosis. When this condition progresses to gangrene, it can be described as either "wet" or "dry." Wet gangrene is characterized by swelling and a moist appearance and is often associated with blebs and bullae caused by massive fluid sequestration. Dry gangrene is characterized by swelling associated with a hard, dry texture and often has a clear demarcation between viable and necrotic tissue. Gangrene moves distally to proximally and occurs within the first 48 hours after ischemia. Superficial gangrene is seen in 10% to 20% of cases; arterial pulses are present. Deep gangrene is a pulseless state.[1]

Pathophysiology

Gangrene is characterized by cyanotic, anesthetic tissue, associated with or progressing toward necrosis, that is caused by obstruction of the venous drainage of an extremity.

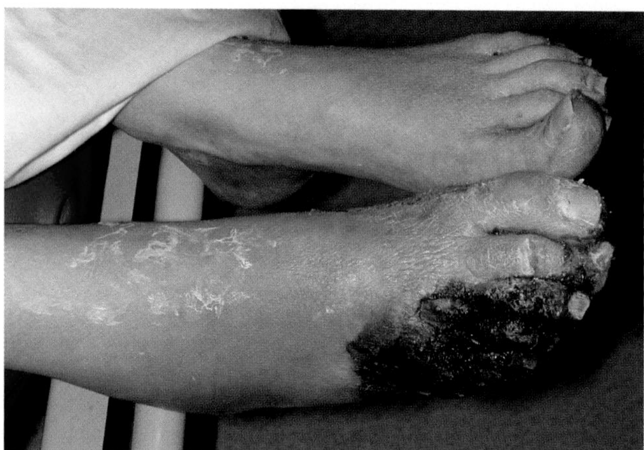

FIGURE 7–22 Gangrene of the lower extremity. (Courtesy of Robert Hendrickson, MD.)

Venous gangrene is caused by total thrombotic occlusion of venous drainage, including the microvascular collateral veins. With total obstruction, tissue pressures become elevated and lead to decreased perfusion pressure, which then results in ischemia. Limb ischemia can involve the skin, subcutaneous tissues, muscles, or a combination of these.

Risk factors are generally the same as those for deep venous thrombosis (DVT) and include malignancy (20% to 40%); hypercoagulable state; surgery; trauma; peripartum status (third trimester and postpartum); inflammatory conditions such as ulcerative colitis, pneumonitis, and gastroenteritis; and prolonged immobility. Up to 10% of patients have no known risk factors.[1]

Diagnosis

The diagnosis is based on high clinical suspicion and the presence of classic presenting signs and symptoms, with confirmation of a DVT by continuous-wave or duplex Doppler ultrasonography, or by the gold standard, contrast venography.

Clinical Complications

Complications include arterial insufficiency (present in 80% to 90% of cases), hypotension (due to massive fluid sequestration, as well as possible sepsis), amputation of the affected limb or some part thereof (20% to 50%), and death (20% to 40%).[1] Postphlebitic syndrome and rethrombosis are common.

Management

Patients with venous gangrene require hospital admission. Initial management involves correction of hypotension by intravenous (IV) administration of fluids to improve tissue perfusion. Definitive treatment (thrombolysis and thrombectomy) remains controversial, and success rates are dismal. Amputation often is the only chance of survival.

REFERENCES

1. Perkins JM, Magee TR, Galland RB. Phlegmasia caerulea dolens and venous gangrene. *Br J Surg* 1996;83:19–23.

Rheumatic Heart Disease

Ralph Weiche

Clinical Presentation

Acute rheumatic fever occurs most frequently in children between 4 and 9 years of age after pharyngitis with group A β-hemolytic *Streptococcus* species (i.e., *Streptococcus pyogenes*). The onset of the disease usually is characterized by an acute febrile illness occurring several weeks after the sore throat has resolved, with some combination of migratory arthritis predominantly involving the large joints, carditis, valvulitis, central nervous system effects (i.e., Sydenham's chorea), and a rash.[1,2]

Pathophysiology

Rheumatic heart disease (RHD) encompasses carditis occurring during acute rheumatic fever and the residual chronic valvular deformities. Acute rheumatic fever is an inflammatory condition that occurs as a delayed sequela of group A β-hemolytic streptococcal pharyngitis in children.[1,2]

Rheumatic fever is thought to result from an autoimmune response in children and adolescents after group A β-hemolytic streptococcal pharyngitis. Some strains of group A *Streptococcus* have antigenic domains similar to those of antigens in components of the human heart.[1,2]

Diagnosis

The revised Jones criteria are used to establish the diagnosis of acute rheumatic fever.[2] The diagnosis requires that two major, or one major and two minor criteria, be satisfied, in addition to evidence of recent streptococcal infection. The five major criteria are carditis, polyarthritis, chorea, erythema marginatum, and subcutaneous nodules. The minor criteria are fever, arthralgias, and previous rheumatic fever or heart disease. A preceding streptococcal infection may be evidenced by either increased antistreptolysin O antibodies, a positive throat culture for group A β-hemolytic streptococci, or recent scarlet fever.[1,2]

Clinical Complications

RHD is the most serious sequela of acute rheumatic fever. Patients with chronic RHD may develop valve stenosis with varying degrees of regurgitation, atrial dilation, arrhythmias, and ventricular dysfunction. RHD usually occurs 10 to 20 years after rheumatic fever and is the major cause of acquired valvular disease in the world. The most common valvular abnormalities are mitral stenosis, mitral regurgitation, aortic stenosis, and aortic regurgitation.[1,2]

Management

Management of acute rheumatic fever involves antibiotic treatment of group A streptococcal pharyngitis, suppressing inflammation from the autoimmune response (high-dose aspirin, corticosteroids), and providing supportive treatment for congestive heart failure (CHF). Treatment of valvular abnormalities of RHD may require treatment for CHF as well as surgical correction.[1]

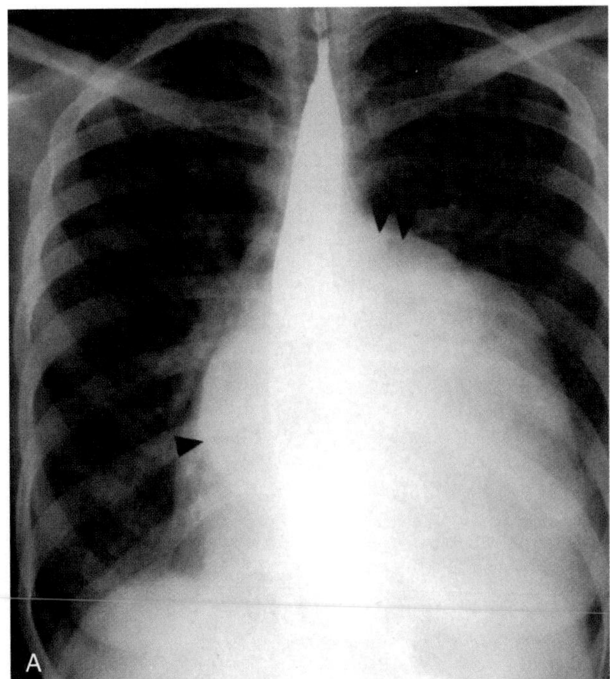

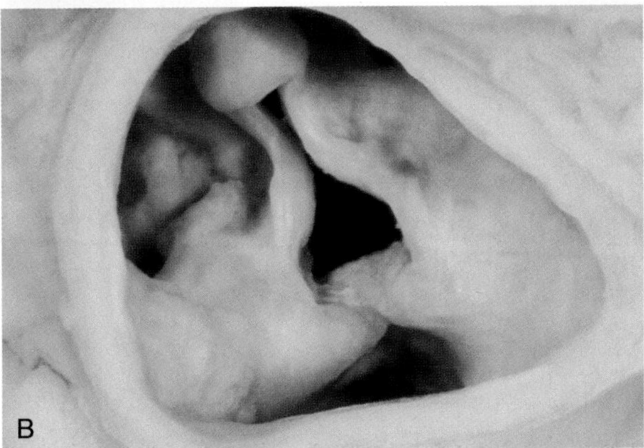

FIGURE 7–23 A: Chest radiograph of the barium-filled esophagus of a patient with rheumatic mitral regurgitation; cardiomegaly is present, with the left ventricle extending toward the lateral chest wall. The enlarged left atrium can be seen as a double density *(single arrow)*, and the pulmonary artery segment *(double arrows)* is prominent. (From Hurst, with permission.) **B:** Rheumatic aortic valve with commissural fusion and leaflet fibrosis; the pathology suggests stenosis and regurgitation as a functional consequence. (From Becker, with permission.)

REFERENCES

1. Stollerman GH. Rheumatic fever. *Lancet* 1997;349:935–942.
2. Veasy GL, Hill HR. Immunologic and clinical correlations in rheumatic fever and rheumatic heart disease. *Pediatr Infect Dis J* 1997;16:400–407.

Bacterial Endocarditis

Gail Rudnitsky

Clinical Presentation

The clinical presentation of endocarditis is variable, although fever is usually present. Patients with bacterial endocarditis may be severely ill, or they may have nonspecific symptoms such as weakness, anorexia, malaise, and low-grade fevers lasting weeks to months. The patient may present with a new murmur or in fulminate congestive heart failure (CHF). Extracardiac immunologic manifestations of the disease, such as Roth's spots, Osler's nodes, glomerulonephritis, and positive rheumatoid factors, are more likely to occur with the subacute form of the disease.[1]

Pathophysiology

The hallmark of endocarditis is a vegetation on one of the valves of the heart. This is an inflammatory lesion consisting of a collection of platelets, fibrin, microorganisms, and inflammatory cells. Patients with congenital heart defects, mitral valve prolapse, acquired valvular defects such as rheumatic fever, and artificial heart

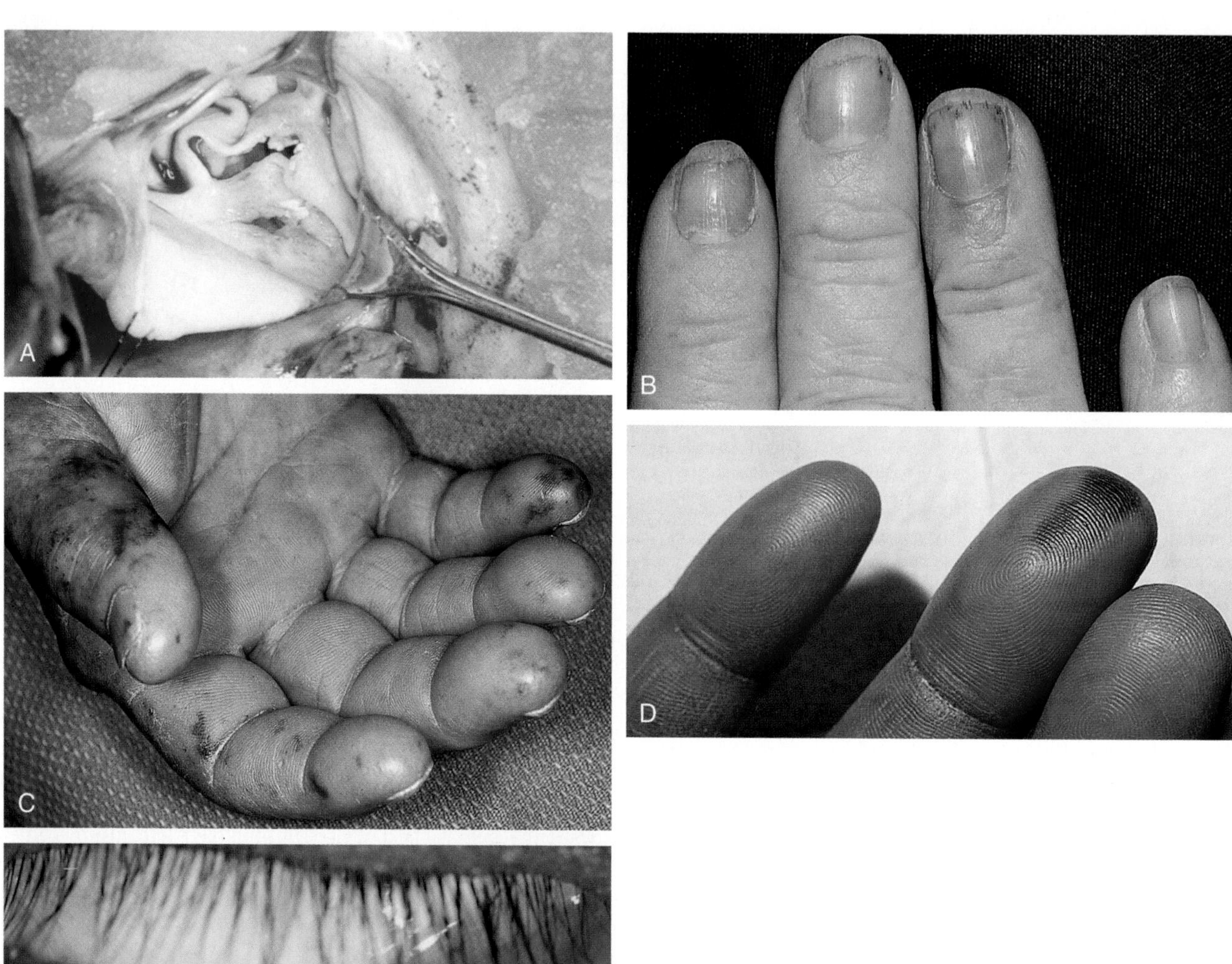

FIGURE 7–24 **A:** Operative view of a severely damaged aortic valve, secondary to bacterial endocarditis. (From Hurst, with permission.) **B:** Splinter hemorrhages. (From Sontheimer, with permission.) **C:** Janeway lesions. **D:** Ostler node. **E:** Petechiae. (**C** through **E,** from Ostler, with permission.)

Bacterial Endocarditis

Gail Rudnitsky

valves are predisposed to develop bacterial endocarditis. Other risk factors include poor dental hygiene, hemodialysis, intravenous (IV) drug abuse, diabetes mellitus, and possibly human immunodeficiency virus (HIV) infection. Although any organism can cause endocarditis, staphylococci and streptococci are the two most common organisms, with staphylococci being more common in patients with artificial valves, and *Streptococcus viridans* occurring most commonly in native valve endocarditis.[1–3]

Diagnosis

All patients with suspected endocarditis should have blood cultures and an electrocardiograph (ECG) performed on admission. Patients with new heart blocks should be admitted to a monitored setting. Because it is noninvasive and highly specific (98%), transthoracic echocardiography (TTE) should be performed on all patients with suspected bacterial endocarditis. However, because TTE misses up to 20% of vegetations in adults with bacterial endocarditis, transesophageal echocardiography (TEE) (sensitivity, 76% to 100%; specificity, 94%) should be performed for patients with suspected bacterial endocarditis.

Clinical Complications

CHF and stroke are the two most serious complications of infective endocarditis. CHF results from disruption of the valve by the organisms and from the inflammatory process. Extension beyond the valve can cause disturbances of the conduction system, pericarditis, or fistula formation. Pieces of vegetation can break off and embolize to the brain or other organs. Patients can also develop mycotic aneurysms, which may lead to hemorrhagic strokes.[1,2]

Management

Treatment consists of prolonged administration of the appropriate antibiotics. Treatment is usually begun in the hospital but may be continued on an outpatient basis. Empiric treatment for suspected bacterial endocarditis consists of vancomycin and gentamycin. Once culture results are available, more directed therapy can be started. Patients with CHF, perivalvular invasive disease, or artificial valves may require surgical therapy.[2,3]

REFERENCES

1. Mylonakis E, Calderwood SB. Infective endocarditis in adults. *N Engl J Med* 2001;345:1318–1330.
2. Bayer AS, Bolger AF, Taubert KA, et al. Diagnosis and management of infective endocarditis and its complications. *Circulation* 1998;98:2936–2948.
3. Giessel BE, Koenig CJ, Blake RL Jr. Management of bacterial endocarditis. *Am Fam Physician* 2000;61:1725–1732,1739.

Patent Ductus Arteriosus

Michael Greenberg

Clinical Presentation

Patients with patent ductus arteriosus (PDA) present with a wide variety of age-dependent and severity-dependent symptoms, ranging from no symptoms at all to frank congestive heart failure (CHF) and cardiorespiratory arrest. Most present with increasing fatigue, difficulty breathing, or palpitations. PDA is a form of acyanotic congenital heart disease.[1]

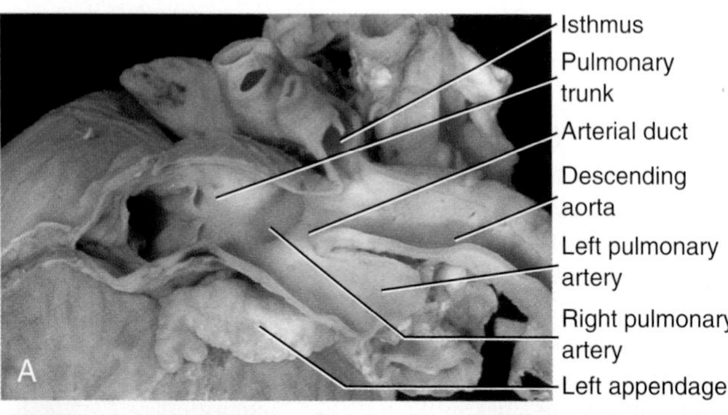

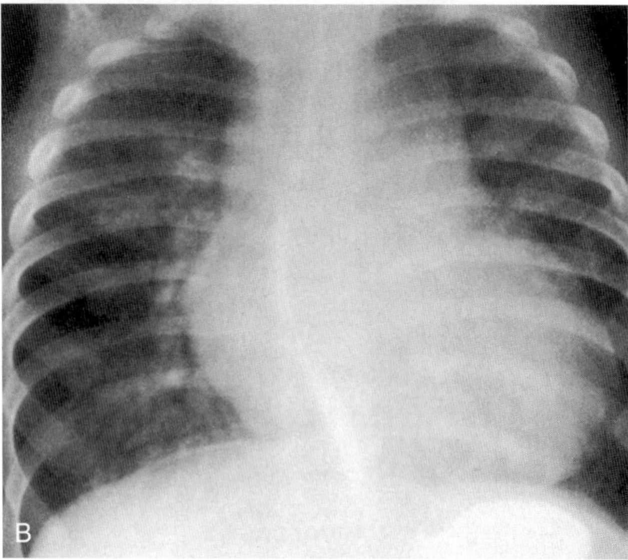

FIGURE 7–25 **A:** Heart with persistent patency of the arterial duct sectioned to replicate the view obtained by the echocardiographer from the suprasternal window. (From Hurst, with permission.) **B:** Chest radiograph of a 1-month-old infant with a large patent ductus arteriosus; moderate cardiac enlargement with increased pulmonary flow is seen. (From Hurst, with permission.)

Pathophysiology

The descending aorta is connected to the left pulmonary artery via the ductus arteriosis. During fetal life, the ductus allows pulmonary arterial blood to go directly to the descending aorta, as opposed to the fetal lungs, for oxygenation. The ductus arteriosis normally closes spontaneously after birth, but in some cases this does not occur. Consequently, a continuous flow of blood is allowed to enter the aorta from the pulmonary artery, creating a left-to-right shunt. This PDA is involved in approximately 1 of every 10 cases of congenital heart disease. PDA is more common after pregnancies that involve perinatal hypoxia, in infants who are born at altitude, in premature infants, and in those born to mothers infected with rubella.[1]

Most PDAs do not close spontaneously, and a small PDA may be tolerated for life without symptoms. However, approximately 30% of patients with more than minimal PDAs that are not repaired die of CHF, endocarditis, or pulmonary hypertension by the age of 40 years. The remainder of untreated patients usually die by the age of 60 years.[1]

Diagnosis

Patients manifest "bounding" arterial pulses, wide pulse pressures, and so-called "machinery" heart murmurs, heard best in the left second intercostal space on the anterior chest wall.[1] Advanced imaging techniques, including two-dimensional echocardiography and Doppler flow studies, are used to confirm the diagnosis, and cardiac catheterization and angiography are used to define the severity of the lesion.[1]

Clinical Complications

Complications of untreated PDA include infective endocarditis, pulmonary hypertension, CHF, and death.

Management

Patients with symptomatic PDAs should be evaluated by a cardiothoracic surgeon. Surgical resolution of this lesion is routine and usually can be completed without the use of cardiopulmonary bypass. The perioperative mortality rate is less than 1%.[1]

REFERENCES

1. Brickner ME, Hillis LD, Lange RA. Congenital heart disease in adults: first of two parts. *N Engl J Med* 2000;342:256–263.

Aortic Coarctation

Robert Hendrickson

Clinical Presentation

Most cases of aortic coarctation (AC) first manifest in infants, although some patients first develop symptoms during adulthood.[1] Infants present with systolic hypertension or weak pulses with poor perfusion in the lower extremities. Adult patients may present with symptoms related to hypertension of the upper extremities (headache, epistaxis, heart failure, lightheadedness, alteration of mental status), underperfusion of the lower extremities (claudication), or complications of the coarctation, including infectious endocarditis, premature coronary artery disease, and aortic dissection.[1]

Patients may have elevations of systolic blood pressure and wide pulse pressures in the upper extremities compared with the lower extremities (systolic pressure gradient greater than 30 mm Hg). A harsh systolic murmur may be heard over the left sternal border and possibly in the back (due to collateral flow through intercostal and axillary branches).[1] The femoral pulse may be delayed and less prominent than the neck and arm pulses. Electrocardiograph (ECG) may reveal ventricular hypertrophy. Chest radiography may reveal notching of the posterior third through eighth ribs caused by collateral blood vessel engorgement and, occasionally, a visible indentation of the aortic shadow.[1]

Pathophysiology

AC is an idiopathic disorder. A thin ridge of tissue extends into the aortic lumen and is typically located just distal to the attachment of the left subclavian artery. This ridge partially obstructs blood flow, increases systolic pressure in the upper extremities (head and heart), and decreases systolic pressure distally.

Diagnosis

The diagnosis should be considered in patients who have a typical history, or systolic pressure differences between the upper and lower extremities, or both. The diagnosis may be confirmed with additional studies, including magnetic resonance imaging (MRI), aortography, and echocardiography. Selection of the workup depends on the age and condition of the patient.

Clinical Complications

Complications include aortic dissection, heart failure, hypertension, intracranial edema or hemorrhage (due to hypertension), claudication, and infectious endocarditis.[1]

Management

Patients who have symptoms that are consistent with coarctation should have a cardiothoracic surgery consultation and further testing. Long-term management options include medical blood pressure control and surgical repair or balloon dilatation of the coarctation.[2]

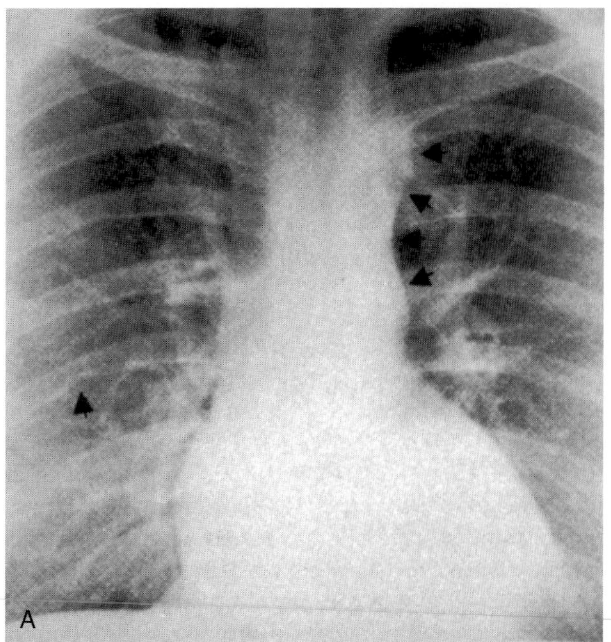

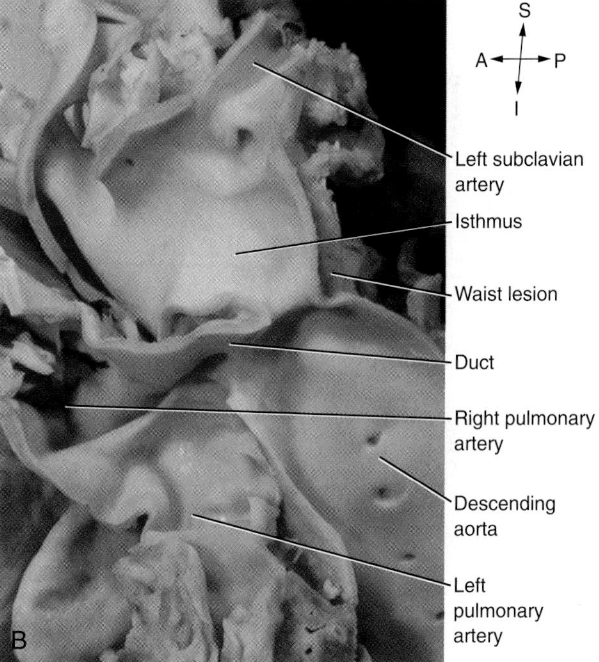

FIGURE 7–26 **A:** The x-ray shows a large notch in the seventh posterior rib, which is the premier differential diagnostic finding, with coarctation of the aorta. Left ventricular contour *(arrows)* is normal. **B:** Coarctation with open arterial duct due to waist lesion in immediate preductal position. (**A** and **B** Reprinted from Hurst with permission.)

REFERENCES

1. Brickner ME, Hillis LD, Lange RA. Congenital heart disease in adults: first of two parts. *N Engl J Med* 2000;342:256–263.
2. McCrindle BW. Coarctation of the aorta. *Curr Opin Cardiol* 1999;14: 448–452.

Ventricular Septal Defect

Samuel Kim

Clinical Presentation

Patients with ventricular septal defects (VSDs) vary in their presentation, depending on the size and the precise anatomic location of the defect. Small VSDs are often asymptomatic and may spontaneously close over time without treatment.[1] Infants with moderate to large VSDs may present to the emergency department (ED) with growth restriction, fatigue during feedings, diaphoresis, irritability, tachycardia, and tachypnea. Infants in whom symptoms progress typically present with congestive heart failure (CHF) at 6 to 8 weeks of age.

Pathophysiology

VSDs are the most common congenital heart malformations and consist of a defect in the septal wall that divides the ventricles.

VSD is the most common congenital heart defect.[2] It may be associated with chromosomal abnormalities, most notably Down syndrome. Shortly after birth, blood flow through a VSD is from the left to the right ventricle. This leads to an increase in pulmonary artery blood flow and pressure and to left and right ventricular hypertrophy. This hypertrophy and hypertension result in CHF. If uncorrected, right ventricular pressures may become greater than the left ventricular (LV) pressure, leading to a right-to-left shunt and cyanotic heart disease, known as Eisenmenger's complex.

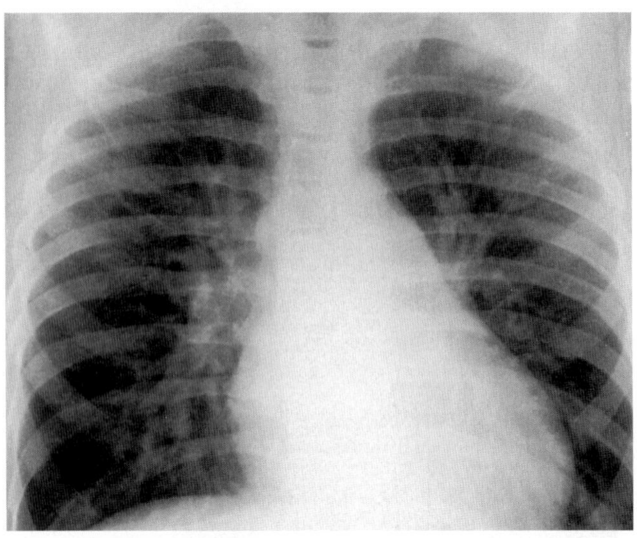

FIGURE 7–27 Moderate-sized ventricular septal defect with a pulmonary/systemic blood flow ratio of 2.5. (From Chatterjee, with permission.)

Diagnosis

The physical examination findings associated with VSD may include nasal flaring, respiratory retractions, tachypnea, and a palpable thrill. Rales and lower-extremity edema occur only rarely in infants. Patients with a VSD have a holosystolic murmur, best heard at the left parasternal border, and the character of the murmur depends on the location and size of the defect.[2] The diagnosis of VSD is confirmed by the use of echocardiography. Electrocardiograph (ECG) may reveal left atrial enlargement and biventricular hypertrophy. Chest radiographs may show increased pulmonary vascular markings and enlargement of the left atrium, LV, and right ventricle.

Clinical Complications

VSDs may progress to CHF, Eisenmenger's complex, or conduction abnormalities. Patients with a VSD should receive antibiotic prophylaxis for bacterial endocarditis before potentially high-risk procedures such as major surgery, dental procedures, and incision and drainage. VSDs may also present a pathway for the occurrence of paradoxic emboli.

Management

Patients with CHF need urgent pediatric cardiology consultation and probably intensive care unit (ICU) admission. Treatment usually includes digoxin and diuretics.[1] Patients in whom a new murmur suspicious of VSD is detected who have no evidence of hemodynamic compromise may not require hospitalization. However, prompt referral to a pediatric cardiologist is needed.

REFERENCES

1. Burton DA, Cabalka AK. Cardiac evaluation of infants. *Pediatr Clin North Am* 1994;41:991–1013.
2. Flynn PA, Engle MA, Ehlers KH. Cardiac issues in the pediatric emergency room. *Pediatr Clin North Am* 1992;39:955–986.

Atrial Septal Defect

Michael Greenberg

Clinical Presentation

Patients with atrial septal defect (ASD) present with a wide variety of age-dependent and severity-dependent manifestations of ASD ranging from no symptoms at all to frank congestive heart failure (CHF) and cardiorespiratory arrest. Most present with increasing fatigue, difficulty breathing, or palpitations. ASD is a form of acyanotic congenital heart disease.[1]

Pathophysiology

Approximately 30% of congenital heart disease in adults involves ASD, and ASD is decidedly more common in females (3:1). ASDs cause intraatrial shunting of blood. The direction and amount of blood flow depends on the size of the ASD. Small defects may have no clinically important hemodynamic manifestations. Larger ASDs may be associated with substantial and serious manifestations. In most cases, left-to-right shunting develops, causing increased blood flow to the lungs and dilation of the right ventricle, both atria, and the pulmonary arteries. As the condition persists, the direction of flow may change, depending on various factors. Some patients with unrepaired ASD have survived for long periods. However, those with large shunts often succumb in the fourth decade of life to right-sided heart failure and arrhythmias.

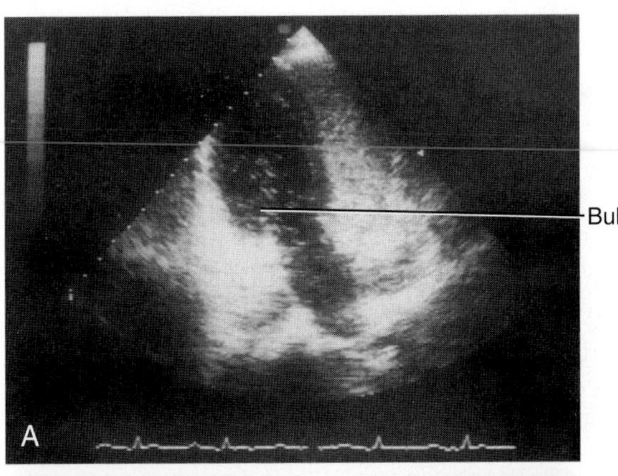

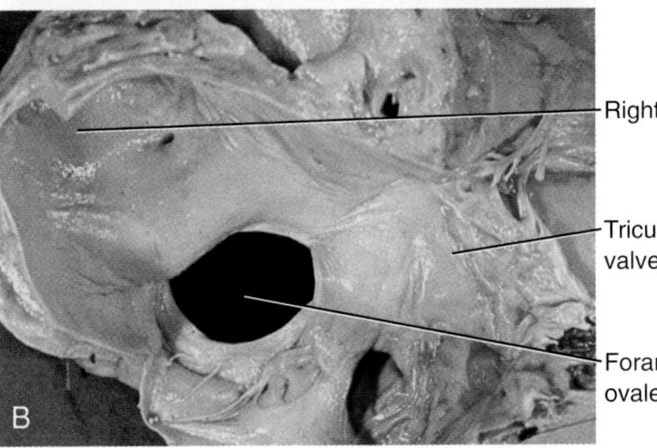

FIGURE 7–28 **A:** Contrast echocardiogram demonstrating bubbles in both atria in this patient with a patent foramen ovale who had a brainstem infarction. (From Hurst, with permission.) **B:** Pathologic specimen showing a patent foramen ovale. (From Perkin, with permission.)

Diagnosis

Patients may initially be asymptomatic for many years. However, over time, the right side of the heart dilates and manifestations of right-sided heart failure become obvious. Patients with sizable ASDs demonstrate systolic ejection murmurs, heard best in the second intercostal space. The electrocardiograph (ECG) may show right-axis deviation with incomplete right bundle block. The chest radiograph shows prominent pulmonary artery shadows and an apparently enhanced peripheral vascular pattern. Advanced imaging techniques including two-dimensional echocardiography and Doppler flow studies are used to confirm the diagnosis, and cardiac catheterization and angiography are used to define the severity of the lesion.[1]

Clinical Complications

Complications of untreated ASD include infective endocarditis, right-sided heart failure, multiple arrhythmias, and death.

Management

Patients with symptomatic ASDs should be stabilized and evaluated by a cardiothoracic surgeon as soon as possible.[1]

REFERENCES

1. Brickner ME, Hillis LD, Lange RA. Congenital heart disease in adults: first of two parts. *N Engl J Med* 2000;342:256–263.

Atrial Myxoma

Samuel Kim

Clinical Presentation

Atrial myxomas may manifest with symptoms of cardiac obstruction, including cardiac failure (67%), constitutional symptoms (34%), and systemic emboli of tumor fragments (29%).[1] Atrial myxomas cause obstructive symptoms by a ball-valve mechanism and may mimic mitral stenosis. Obstruction may vary with body position, a finding that is strongly suggestive of atrial myxoma. Constitutional symptoms include myalgias, muscle weakness, arthralgia, fever, weight loss, and fatigue. Embolic phenomena are greatly varied, but more than two thirds of emboli travel to the cerebral circulation.[1] There is a 2:1 female-to-male ratio, and most cases occur between the third and sixth decades.[1] Physical examination may reveal cardiac auscultatory findings. Usually, an apical presystolic or diastolic murmur is heard, similar to mitral stenosis, but it may be positional in nature. The most specific auscultatory finding, termed a "tumor plop," is a low-frequency sound heard after the second heart sound. Electrocardiograph (ECG) findings, when present, are usually nonspecific. The most common ECG finding is left atrial enlargement, which is present in 62% of patients.[1] Laboratory findings are also not very specific; they include anemia (usually microcytic, hemolytic), elevated erythrocyte sedimentation rate (ESR), and elevated C-reactive protein. Chest radiographs are usually nonspecific and may show signs of pulmonary congestion and left atrial enlargement. Rarely, a heavily calcified myxoma may be visible on

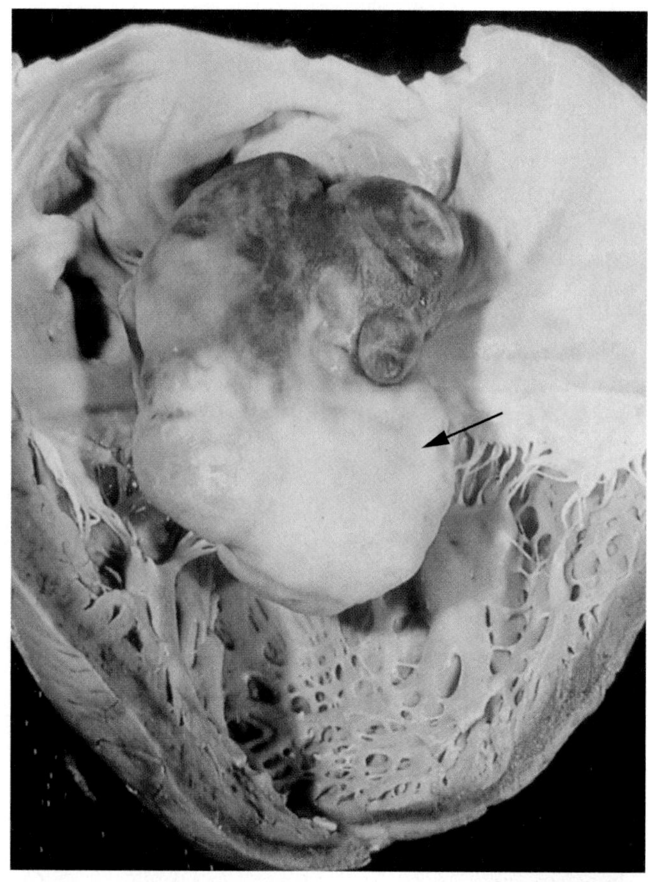

FIGURE 7–29 Atrial myxoma. (From Becker, with permission.)

Atrial Myxoma

Samuel Kim

plain films. Myxomas are usually diagnosed by cardiac echocardiography.

Pathophysiology

Atrial myxomas are tumors, usually pedunculated, that are found most commonly within the left atrium. Atrial myxoma is the most common benign tumor of the heart.

Atrial myxomas are benign neoplasms of endocardial origin.

Diagnosis

The most common modality for diagnosis is cardiac echocardiography. Transthoracic echocardiography (TTE) has a sensitivity of approximately 95%, and transesophageal echocardiography (TEE) has a sensitivity that approaches 100%. Computed tomography (CT) and magnetic resonance imaging (MRI), may also be used as diagnostic modalities. These modalities provide some advantages over echocardiography in that they can better characterize the attachment site, tumor stalk presence, and size. Echocardiography usually is sufficient to make the decision for operation. Once atrial myxoma is suspected, cardiac catheterization is usually performed concomitantly to rule out coronary artery disease in patients older than 40 years of age. Also, confirmation by pathology of the surgical specimen must be done to rule out other cardiac neoplasms.[1]

Clinical Complications

Atrial myxomas can lead to embolic phenomena, especially cerebrovascular accidents (CVA), and sudden death. They can also lead to cardiac failure.

Management

Atrial myxoma is treated by surgical excision. All patients with a suspected atrial myxoma need urgent cardiothoracic consultation for resection. Often, this diagnosis is made not in the emergency department (ED) but on cardiac echocardiography done after admission. Disposition should be based on hemodynamic stability, except in the rare cases in which atrial myxoma is diagnosed in the ED. Intensive care unit (ICU) admission should be considered, given the high rate of embolic and sudden death complications.[1]

REFERENCES

1. Pinede L, Duhaut P, Loire R. Clinical presentation of left atrial cardiac myxoma: a series of 112 consecutive cases. *Medicine (Baltimore)* 2001;80:159–172.

Supraventricular Tachycardia

Brandt Delhamer

Clinical Presentation

The symptomatic patient with a supraventricular tachycardia (SVT) may present with acute episodes known as paroxysmal supraventricular tachycardia (PSVT). These patients may complain of lightheadedness, palpitations, or dizziness. Chest pain or pressure and dyspnea are less common complaints. Except in patients with underlying coronary artery disease, SVT is rarely associated with myocardial ischemia.[1]

Pathophysiology

SVTs include all arrhythmias that result from electrical activity originating above the bifurcation of the bundle of His. However, the term SVT is more commonly used to describe reentrant rhythms specifically, and it generally does not include atrial fibrillation/flutter, multifocal atrial tachycardia, or sinus tachycardia.[1]

Several varieties of reentrant SVT exist. atrioventricular (AV) nodal reentrant tachycardia (AVNRT) and AV

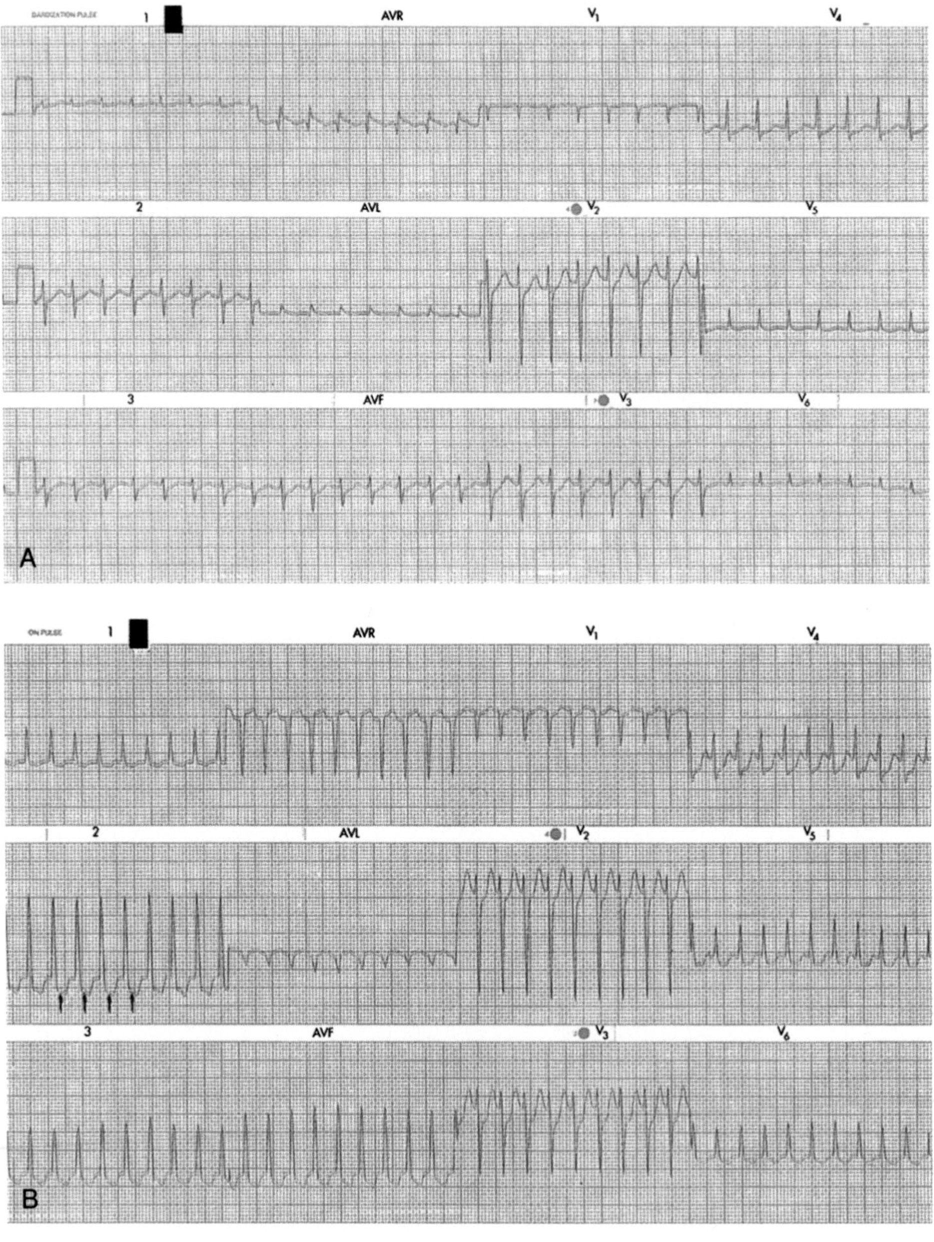

FIGURE 7–30 **A:** Regular, narrow-complex tachycardia consistent with atrioventricular (AV) nodal re-entry tachycardia. **B:** Regular, narrow-complex tachycardia consistent with AV re-entry tachycardia. (From Hurst, with permission.)

Supraventricular Tachycardia

Brandt Delhamer

reentrant tachycardia (AVRT) are the most common, accounting for 60% and 20% of patients, respectively.[1]

In AVNRT, the QRS complex is narrow and the P wave is buried within the QRS complex. In a minority of cases (10%), a retrograde P wave is visible before the QRS complex. Rates of 160 to 200 beats/minute are common and may be sustained for extended periods. Reentry within the AV node is usually initiated when an ectopic atrial impulse encounters the AV node during the partially refractory period.[1]

AVRT occurs when two parallel tracks with different conduction velocities are present between the atria and ventricles. The two tracks form a circuit—the normal AV node and the bypass tract—through which a sustained electrical loop may occur. Orthodromic conduction describes the condition in which the electrical impulse first travels down the AV node and reenters up through the bypass tract. Antidromic conduction refers to the opposite conduction pattern. Orthodromic conduction produces a narrow-complex QRS, whereas antidromic conduction produces a wide QRS complex. Both antidromic and orthodromic conduction typically form a retrograde P wave that appears after the QRS complex.[1]

Reentrant SVT may occur in the normal heart, but it is also seen in patients with myocardial infarction (MI), Wolff-Parkinson-White (WPW) syndrome, acute pericarditis, mitral valve prolapse, or rheumatic heart disease (RHD).

Diagnosis

The diagnostic test for SVT is the 12-lead electrocardiograph (ECG). Narrow-complex (orthodromic) or wide-complex (antidromic) tachycardia with a P wave that is retrograde or buried in the QRS complex is a finding consistent with the diagnosis.[1]

Clinical Complications

SVT may lead to heart failure with resultant pulmonary edema in patients with preexisting left ventricular (LV) pathology, because the decrease in diastolic filling cannot be tolerated in combination with reduced cardiac output. In patients with preexisting coronary artery disease, the rapid heart rate may cause cardiac ischemia with the concomitant sensation of chest pain and dyspnea.[1]

Management

Patients with SVT who are hemodynamically unstable should receive immediate synchronized cardioversion with 100 J, intravenous (IV) access, and resuscitation. IV adenosine may be attempted if it does not delay cardioversion. In stable patients, a 12-lead ECG should be obtained to confirm the diagnosis.

For reentry SVT, the goal is to impede conduction through the AV node, thus eliminating the reentry mechanism. The least invasive method of decreasing AV nodal conduction is to increase vagal tone. To achieve this, the patient may be instructed to bear down or the physician may massage the carotid bodies.[1] Carotid massage should be avoided in patients with carotid bruits, because they may be at higher risk of embolization and cerebrovascular accident (CVA).

After vagal maneuvers, adenosine may be administered into a large peripheral or central vein. Adenosine is an ultra-short-acting drug that does not cause hypotension and has no sustained antiarrhythmic effect. Calcium-channel antagonists or β-channel antagonists may also be used to convert SVT.

REFERENCES

1. Ganz LI, Friedman PL. Medical progress: supraventricular tachycardia. *N Engl J Med* 1995;332:162–173.

Ventricular Tachyarrhythmias

Phillip Woodward

Clinical Presentation

The presentation of ventricular tachyarrhythmias (VTs) ranges from pulseless apnea or syncope (unstable VT) to nonspecific symptoms or palpitations (stable VT). Patients may report a brief prodrome of chest discomfort, shortness of breath, diaphoresis, or lightheadedness, followed by a loss of consciousness. The stable patient may present with the same symptoms but is able to maintain adequate circulation.[1,2]

Pathophysiology

VT may be caused by scarring from an acute myocardial infarction (AMI) (most common),[1] myocarditis, drugs, electrolyte abnormalities, sarcoidosis, Chagas' disease, or prolonged QT syndrome.[2] VT develops when an alteration of the conduction system, from any of these causes, increases the susceptibility of the myocardium to reentry circuits. VTs can be divided into monomorphic and polymorphic forms. Monomorphic forms are commonly associated with ischemic heart disease and cardiomyopathies and result from a reentrant circuit through a fixed tract. Polymorphic tachycardia is associated with congenital or acquired long QT syndrome and results from a continuously moving reentrant circuit.

Diagnosis

The diagnosis is made by the recognition of a regular wide-complex tachycardia on a rhythm strip. VT may be differentiated from supraventricular tachycardia with aberrancy by historical factors (i.e., history of myocardial infarction [MI] and older age imply VT) and by electrocardiograph (ECG) findings (fusion beats, capture beats, and atrioventricular [AV] dissociation imply VT).[2]

Management

Patients with ventricular fibrillation (VF) or pulseless VT require up to three immediate defibrillation attempts (200, 300, and 360 J) before airway management. Epinephrine (every 3 to 5 minutes) or vasopressin (one-time dose) should be administered to pulseless patients. Patients with persistent VF or pulseless VT should be given amiodarone or lidocaine alternating with defibrillation attempts.[2] In patients with stable or intermittent monomorphic VT, pharmacotherapy is based on the patient's presumed cardiac function. Patients with a normal ejection fraction (EF) may receive intravenous (IV) procainamide. In patients with suspected poor EF, amiodarone or lidocaine may be used.[2]

Stable polymorphic VT may be secondary to prolongation of the QT interval from an underlying cause that is potentially correctable (i.e., drugs, electrolytes). Patients with persistent polymorphic VT require synchronized cardioversion. Intermittent polymorphic VT may be treated with agents aimed at decreasing the QT interval, such as magnesium, overdrive pacing, or isoproterenol. It may also be treated with phenytoin or lidocaine.[2]

REFERENCES

1. Saliba WI, Natale A. Ventricular tachycardia syndromes. *Med Clin North Am* 2001;85:267–304.
2. Atkins DL, Dorian P, Gonzalez ER, et al. Treatment of tachyarrhythmias. *Ann Emerg Med* 2001;37[4 Suppl]:S91–S109.

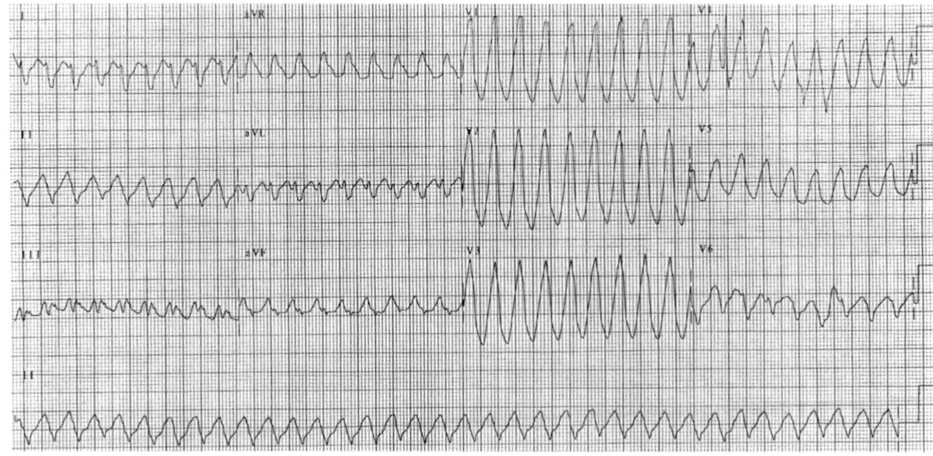

FIGURE 7–31 Ventricular tachycardia. (Courtesy of Jerrica Chen, MD.)

Atrial Fibrillation

Ralph Weiche

Clinical Presentation

Patients with atrial fibrillation (AF) may be asymptomatic, or they may present with symptoms related to rapid ventricular rate (palpitations, 26%; chest pain, 34%; lightheadedness, 19%), decreased cardiac output (dyspnea, 52%; heart failure, fatigue), or thromboembolic events (cerebrovascular accident [CVA], distal arterial embolus).[1]

Pathophysiology

AF is the chaotic depolarization of the atria caused by multiple atrial reentrant circuits.[1,2] The uncoordinated, rapid depolarization may lead to decreases in ventricular filling and, if it is transmitted to the ventricle, to a rapid ventricular rate.[2] AF can be associated with underlying heart disease, particularly conditions that dilate or increase pressure in the atria (rheumatic heart disease [RHD], hypertrophic cardiomyopathy [CM], dilated cardiomyopathy [DCM], pulmonary embolism [PE], hypertension). "Lone AF" may occur without structural heart disease; in some cases, it is reversible (e.g., thyrotoxicosis, the postsurgical state, fever, certain medications). AF is not commonly associated with coronary heart disease unless there are associated factors such as congestive heart failure (CHF) or hypertension.

Diagnosis

The diagnosis may be made by observation of a chaotic atrial rhythm without P waves and a narrow, irregularly irregular ventricular rhythm on electrocardiograph (ECG). It is important to diagnose the reversible causes of AF early in the hospital or emergency department (ED) course. These causes include thyrotoxicosis, fever, alcohol, and sympathomimetic drugs.[1,2]

Clinical Complications

The morbidity of AF is primarily the result of CHF and stroke. Patients younger than 60 years of age who have AF but no apparent heart disease (lone AF) have a better prognosis. The coexistence of cardiovascular disease and chronic AF worsens the prognosis.[1]

Management

Hypotension secondary to rapid AF should be treated with immediate cardioversion.[1] In normotensive patients with rapid rates, the first priority is rate control via blockade of the atrioventricular (AV) node, using calcium-channel blockers or β-blockers.[2] In patients with irregular, wide tachycardia, the diagnosis of ventricular tachycardia or AF with aberrant conduction (e.g., Wolff-Parkinson-White [WPW] syndrome) should be considered and treatment initiated with an agent that does not block the AV node (e.g., procainamide).

If AF has persisted for less than 72 hours, consideration may be given to chemical cardioversion (procainamide, amiodarone, ibutilide). If the onset of AF was more than 72 hours earlier, or if the time of onset is questionable, anticoagulation should be considered because of the increased risk of atrial thrombus and embolization.[2]

REFERENCES

1. Narayan SM, Cain ME, Smith JM. Atrial fibrillation. *Lancet* 1997; 350:943–950.
2. Falk RH. Medical progress: atrial fibrillation. *N Engl J Med* 2001;344:1067–1078.

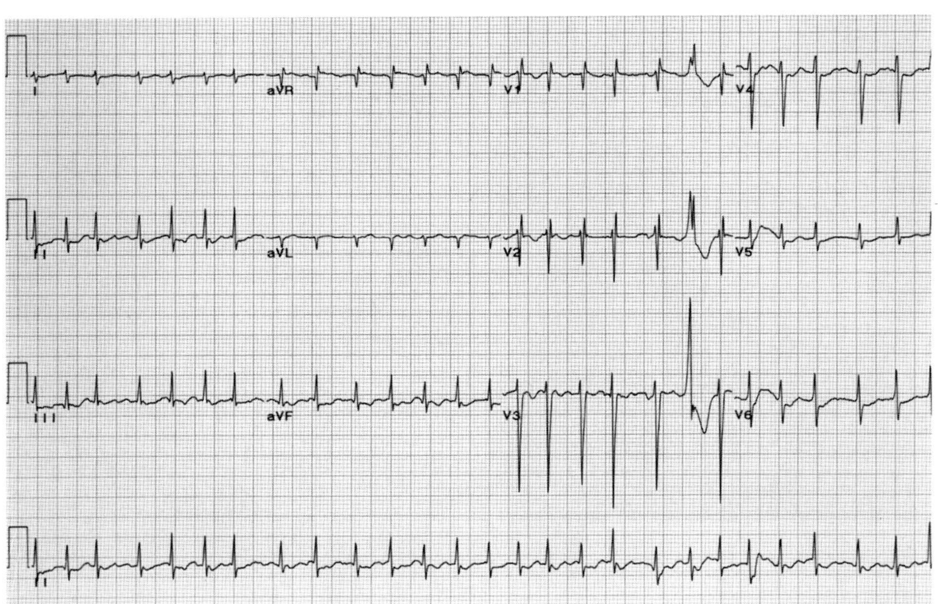

FIGURE 7–32 Typical electrocardiogram for atrial fibrillation. (From Fowler, with permission.)

Atrial Flutter

Gail Rudnitsky

Clinical Presentation

Patients with atrial flutter may be asymptomatic, or they may present with palpations. If hemodynamic compromise is present, patients may present with chest pain, heart failure, shortness of breath, syncope, or fatigue.[1,2]

Pathophysiology

Atrial flutter results from a single reentry circuit within the right atrium. The atrial rate is usually 300 beats/minute and regular, although it may range from 250 to 350 beats/minute. Ventricular conduction is usually 2:1. Associated comorbid conditions may include hypertension, coronary artery disease, valvular heart disease, sick sinus syndrome, and chronic obstructive pulmonary disease (COPD).[1,2]

Diagnosis

Diagnosis is made by observation of the characteristic sawtooth flutter waves on the electrocardiograph (ECG). A regular rate of 150 is characteristic of 2:1 conduction. Carotid sinus massage or administration of adenosine may slow the rate enough to make visible the characteristic flutter waves. Caution should be taken with adenosine, because it may promote 1:1 conduction.[1,2]

Clinical Complications

Clinical complications of atrial flutter involve the effects of hypoperfusion or embolization and include congestive heart failure (CHF), myocardial infarction (MI), and stroke. The incidence of embolization with atrial flutter is unknown; however, this rhythm is often associated with other diseases that are also related to thromboembolic disease (e.g., valvular heart disease, hypertension, CHF).[1,2]

Management

Unstable patients should undergo prompt DC cardioversion (25 to 50J). Stable patients may also be cardioverted, but anticoagulation should be considered if atrial flutter has been present for longer than 48 hours. Electrical cardioversion converts 90% of patients to sinus rhythm. Alternatively, a class III drug such as ibutilide, dofetilide, or sotalol can be used to chemically convert the rhythm. These drugs may result in torsades de pointes. Alternative drugs to consider are procainamide and amiodarone. Class I drugs such as procainamide may lower the flutter rate, resulting in 1:1 conduction and a much faster ventricular rate. Class IC drugs may also result in QRS widening and ventricular tachycardia. Before cardioversion, the ventricular rate may be controlled by drugs that prolong the refractory period of the atrioventricular (AV) node, such as β-blockers, calcium-channel blockers, or amiodarone.[1,2]

REFERENCES

1. Atkins DL, Dorian P, Gonzalez ER, et al. Treatment of tachyarrhythmias. *Ann Emerg Med* 2001;37[4 Suppl]:S91–S109.
2. Wellens HJ. Contemporary management of atrial flutter. *Circulation* 2002;106:649–652.

Atrial Flutter

Gail Rudnitsky

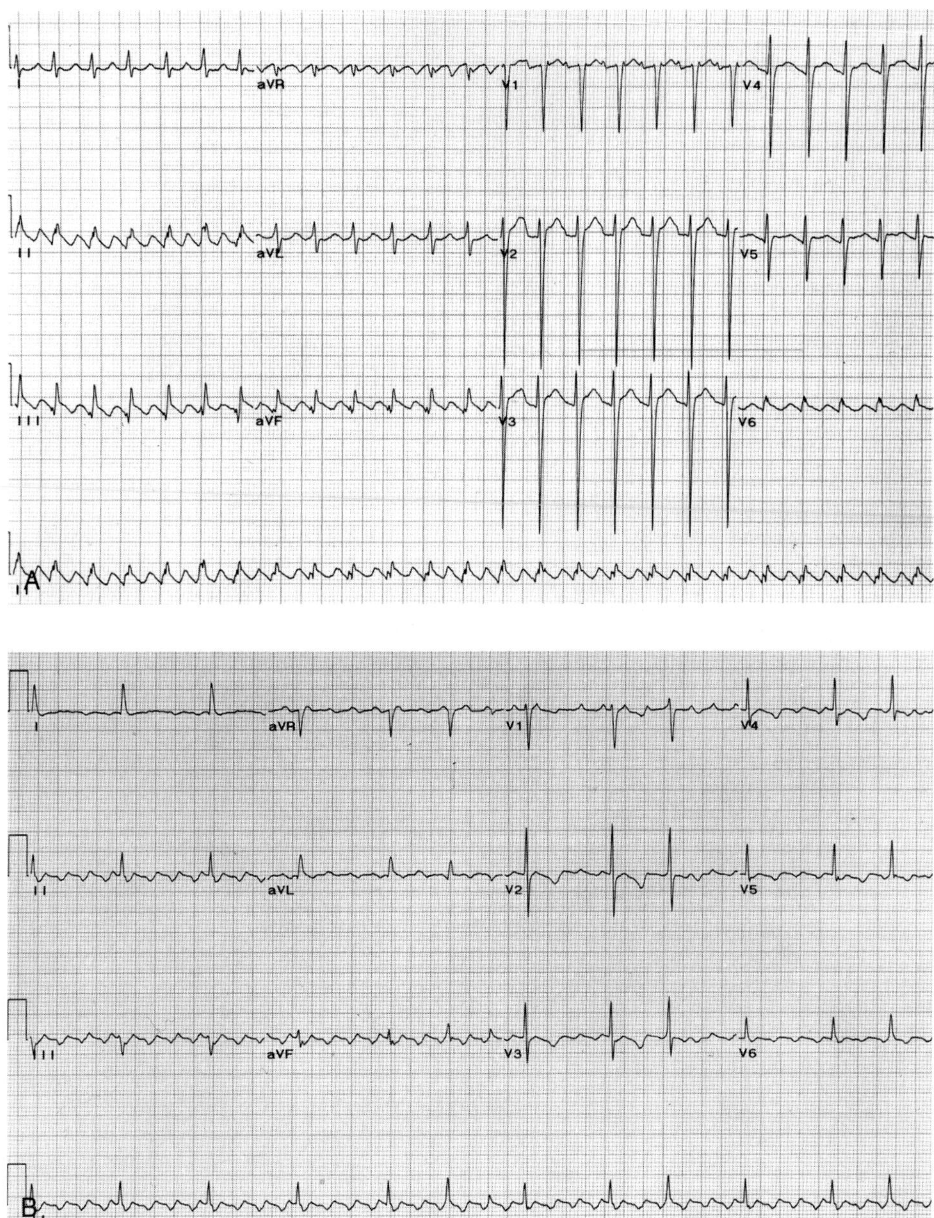

FIGURE 7–33 **A:** Atrial flutter with 2:1 block. (From Fowler, with permission.) **B:** Atrial flutter with variable ventricular response. (From Fowler, with permission.)

Wolff-Parkinson-White Syndrome

Michael Greenberg

Clinical Presentation

The most common presenting symptoms for Wolff-Parkinson-White (WPW) syndrome is palpitations. Additional presenting symptoms may include dizziness, syncope, shortness of breath, and chest pain. Some patients with WPW syndrome remain asymptomatic.[1-3]

Pathophysiology

WPW syndrome is the most common ventricular preexcitation syndrome. It derives from the presence of accessory cardiac conduction pathways within the myocardium.[2] These accessory pathways have electrophysiologic properties that are different from normal. The accessory pathways conduct at greater speed when compared with the normal pathways. Atrioventricular (AV) nodal tissue slows impulse conduction, whereas the speed of conduction in the accessory pathways is accelerated. This accounts for the electrocardiograph (ECG) findings associated with WPW syndrome: short PR interval and the so-called delta wave.[1-3]

Diagnosis

The diagnosis of WPW syndrome requires symptoms of recurrent tachyarrhythmias in conjunction with ECG findings that are consistent with preexcitation. The primary ECG findings are (1) a shortened PR interval, (2) a QRS duration greater than 0.12 seconds, and (3) the presence of a delta wave (a slowly rising onset of the QRS complex). Paroxysmal atrial tachycardia is the most common arrhythmia associated with WPW syndrome.[1-3]

Clinical Complications

Complications include arrhythmias, syncope, and cardiac arrest.

Management

Treatment depends on the specific arrhythmias and symptoms manifested by the patient. Patients with WPW syndrome who survive cardiac arrest should undergo radiofrequency ablation of the accessory pathways. Patients with atrial fibrillation (AF) and adverse hemodynamic effects should be immediately cardioverted. AV blocking agents (digoxin, verapamil, adenosine, β-blockers, diltiazem) should not be used, but patients with supraventricular tachycardia (SVT) may be treated with adenosine. Asymptomatic patients may require no treatment at all.[1-3] Patients first identified in the emergency department (ED) should be admitted for monitoring and further evaluation.

REFERENCES

1. Al-Khatib SM, Pritchett EL. Clinical features of Wolff-Parkinson-White syndrome. *Am Heart J* 1999;138:403–413.
2. Ganz LI, Friedman PL. Supraventricular tachycardia. *N Engl J Med* 1995;332:162–173.
3. Trohman RG. Supraventricular tachycardia: implications for the intensivist. *Crit Care Med* 2000;28[10 Suppl]:N129–N135.

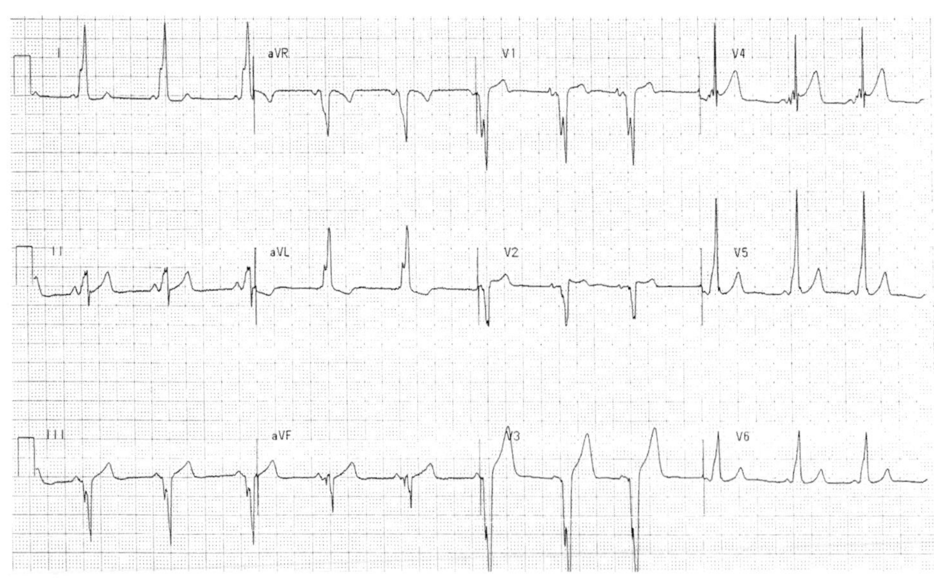

FIGURE 7–34 Short PR interval and delta waves consistent with Wolff-Parkinson-White syndrome. (Courtesy of Kristen Curtis, MD.)

Multifocal Atrial Tachycardia

Robert G. Hendrickson

Clinical Presentation

Patients with multifocal atrial tachycardia (MAT) may present with signs and symptoms of tachycardia (palpitations, anxiety), increased myocardial demand (chest pain, lightheadedness, syncope), or the underlying disorder (dyspnea, tachypnea, wheezing, hypoxemia). MAT is typically a transient rhythm that is present during exacerbation of cardiopulmonary disease. Patients are typically older (mean age, 72 years) and have underlying disorders, including chronic obstructive pulmonary disease (COPD) (55%), congestive heart failure (CHF) (28%), hypokalemia (23%), hypomagnesemia, or hypoxemia (43%).[1] However, MAT may rarely be seen in children or young adults without underlying disorders.[1]

Pathophysiology

MAT is defined as an atrial rate greater than 100 beats/minute with at least three morphologically distinct P waves, irregular PP intervals (and PR intervals), and an isoelectric baseline (no evidence of atrial fibrillation/flutter).[1] MAT may develop when early-triggered atrial beats are caused by delayed afterdepolarizations (DAD).[1] DAD are membrane depolarizations that occur in phase 4 of the action potential. If the DAD reaches the threshold value, an early, ectopic atrial beat is triggered, followed by activation of the atrioventricular (AV) node and a normal, narrow ventricular beat. Factors that increase the risk of MAT are the same as those that lead to excess intracellular calcium and DADs: catecholamines, theophylline, acidemia, hypoxemia, hypokalemia, and hypomagnesemia.[1]

Diagnosis

MAT may be diagnosed by recognition of a tachycardic rhythm with more than two distinct morphologies of P waves, with alteration of the PR and PP intervals, with narrow-complex QRS (or baseline QRS morphology) in the setting of hypoxemia, COPD, CHF, or electrolyte disturbance.

Clinical Complications

Complications include deterioration into atrial fibrillation/flutter, increased myocardial demand (myocardial infarction ([MI], cerebrovascular accident [CVA], hypotension), and decompensation of the triggering event (hypoxemia, hypokalemia, COPD, CHF).

Management

The treatment of MAT begins with management of the underlying condition—hypoxemia, COPD, CHF, pulmonary embolism (PE), acidosis, hypokalemia, or hypomagnesemia. Several treatment modalities may worsen the MAT until hypoxemia is resolved (theophylline, β-adrenergic agonists, digoxin).[1] If MAT remains after treatment of the underlying condition or puts the patient at risk of increased myocardial oxygen demand, then suppression of atrial beats with medications may be indicated. Metoprolol may be used to decrease the rate, but it is contraindicated in patients with significant bronchospasm or CHF.[1] Magnesium may also be used to control rate and correct hypomagnesemia. If metoprolol and magnesium fail to control the rate or are contraindicated, verapamil may be given.[1]

REFERENCES

1. McCord J, Borzak S. Multifocal atrial tachycardia. *Chest* 1998;113: 203–209.

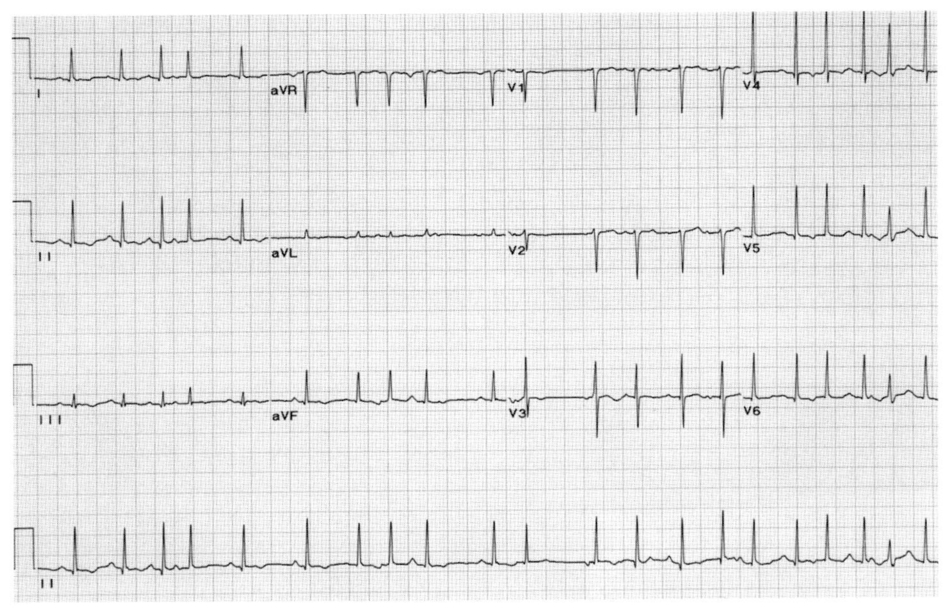

FIGURE 7-35 Varying P-wave morphologies and PR intervals consistent with multifocal atrial tachycardia. (From Fowler, with permission.)

7–36

Sinus Tachycardia

Ralph Weiche

Clinical Presentation

Sinus tachycardia (ST) is often asymptomatic, although the patient may complain of palpitations or symptoms consistent with the cause (e.g., agitation or tremor with sympathomimetic drugs).

Pathophysiology

ST has been defined as a sinus rhythm with a rate exceeding 100 beats/minute. However, the heart rate naturally varies with age. The heart rate may be 150 beats/minute in infants and gradually slows over the next 6 years. The resting sinus rate in adults is approximately 65 to 85 beats/minute.

ST is most often a normal physiologic response to exercise or a number of other factors. The more common factors that can induce ST include hyperthyroidism, fever, hypovolemia, sepsis, anemia, hypotension, shock, pulmonary embolism (PE), acute coronary ischemia and myocardial infarction (MI), congestive heart failure (CHF), chronic pulmonary disease, pheochromocytoma, or drugs.

Diagnosis

ST can be diagnosed by a rhythm strip, or preferably a 12-lead electrocardiograph (ECG), that demonstrates a normal QRS complex with a rate greater than 100 beats/minute. The P waves in a sinus tachycardia have a normal morphology. The PR interval tends to decrease with increasing heart rate.

Clinical Complications

ST rarely causes complications. Patients with organic heart disease and ST may develop CHF or ischemia. In these patients, ST results in a shortened ventricular filling time, decreased cardiac output, increased myocardial oxygen consumption, and reduced coronary blood flow.

Management

No therapy is required for a physiologic ST. However, ST may often be an indicator of significant disease, and attention should be focused on identification and treatment of the underlying cause. Initial therapy may include treatment of the potential underlying disorder (e.g., opioids for pain, acetaminophen for fever, resuscitation for dehydration). ST resulting from an acute myocardial infarction (AMI) increases myocardial oxygen consumption, may increase the size of ischemic injury and infarction, and is associated with increased morbidity and mortality. In this setting, ST should be treated with β-blockers. The disposition of the patient depends on the underlying cause of the ST.

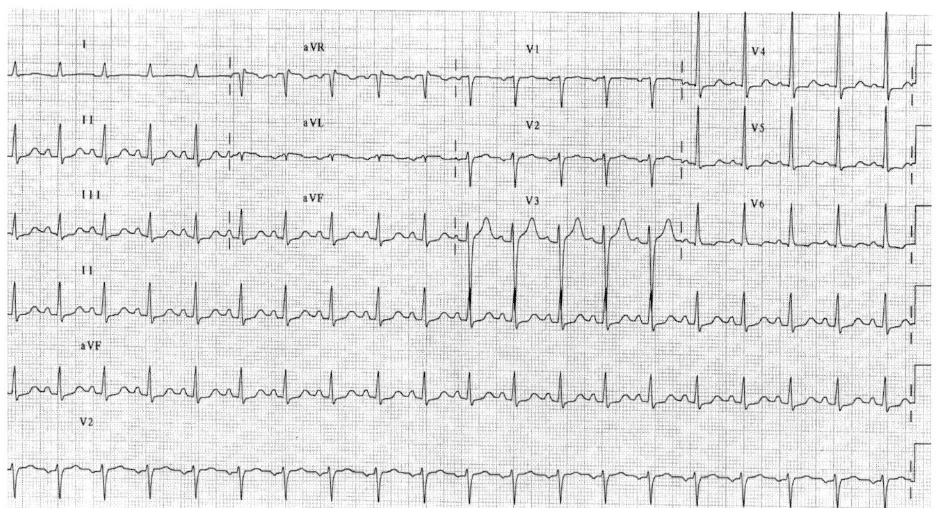

FIGURE 7–36 Sinus tachycardia. (Courtesy of Mark Silverberg, MD.)

Torsades de Pointes

Lisa Freeman

Clinical Presentation

The patient may present in cardiac arrest or with palpitations, syncope, chest pain, or shortness of breath. Heart rates may vary but are typically between 200 and 240 beats/minute.

Pathophysiology

Torsades de pointes ("twisting of the points") is a form of atypical ventricular tachycardia in which the QRS axis essentially "swings" from a positive to a negative direction in a single lead.

Torsades usually occurs in patients with serious heart disease who have a prolonged and uneven ventricular repolarization and a prolonged QT interval. Prolongation of the QT interval may be congenital, or it may be acquired secondary to hypokalemia, hypocalcemia, hypomagnesemia, or various drugs.[1] Drugs that are known to prolong the QT interval include quinidine, procainamide, phenothiazines, amiodarone, butyrophenones, and tricyclic antidepressants.[2]

Diagnosis

The diagnosis is based on the characteristic undulating axis on the electrocardiograph (ECG). Episodes of torsades usually occur in short runs of 5 to 15 seconds at a rate of 200 to 240 beats/minute. Torsades should be suspected in patients with intermittent palpitations or syncope who have a prolonged QT interval on ECG.

Clinical Complications

Torsades de pointes can degenerate into a pulseless ventricular tachycardia, ventricular fibrillation (VF), asystole, and death.

Management

The termination of life-threatening, nonterminating torsades or ventricular tachycardia requires immediate unsynchronized cardioversion. To decrease the incidence of intermittent torsades, temporary overdrive pacing is the safest and most effective method. Magnesium sulfate may abolish bursts of torsades, but recurrences are not uncommon. Hypokalemia and hypocalcemia should also be corrected urgently.

REFERENCES

1. Viskin S. Long QT syndromes and torsades de pointes. *Lancet* 1999;354:1625–1633.
2. Nelson LS. Toxicologic myocardial sensitization. *J Toxicol Clin Toxicol* 2002;40:867–879.

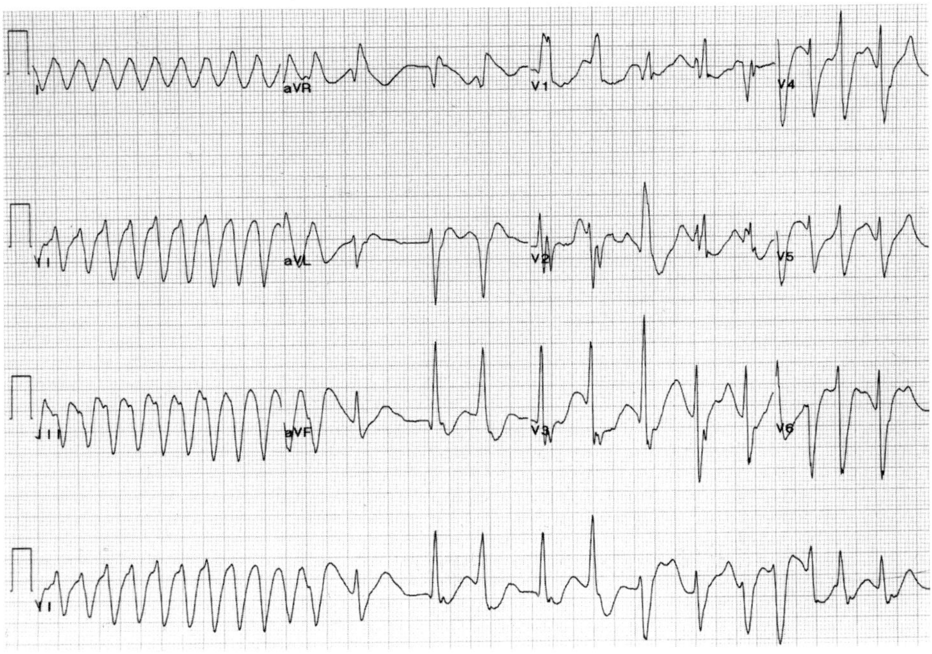

FIGURE 7–37 Electrocardiogram demonstrating two bouts of torsades de pointes, the second consisting of seven cycles. The ventricular rhythm between these episodes is uncertain but may represent junctional rhythm with premature ventricular systoles. (From Fowler, with permission.)

Atrioventricular Blocks

Todd McGrath

Clinical Presentation

Patients with an atrioventricular (AV) block may be asymptomatic, or they may present with increasing exercise intolerance or syncope.[1]

Pathophysiology

The cause of AV block is most commonly coronary artery disease that leads to chronic fibrotic changes of the cardiac conduction system.[1] AV blocks may also have pharmacologic causes (e.g., calcium-channel or β-blockers, cardiac glycosides).

Diagnosis

The diagnosis of AV block is made by electrocardiograph (ECG). AV blocks are further divided into a classification of degrees. First-degree AV block involves simply a prolongation of the PR segment to greater than 200 msec. Second-degree AV blocks are those in which the impulse is not completely conducted after every atrial beat and the ventricular beat is occasionally dropped. Second-degree AV blocks are further divided into type I, in which the PR interval progressively lengthens until a beat is dropped (commonly called Wenckebach's block); and type II, in which the PR interval is constant until a beat is dropped abruptly. Finally, third-degree AV blocks are those in which there is complete AV dissociation and the atria and ventricles beat independently of each other.[1]

Clinical Complications

The clinical complications of AV blocks are those related to decreased heart rate with subsequent decrease in cardiac output, hypotension, and syncope.[1]

Management

The management of AV blocks depends on the degree and type of block and the clinical status of the patient. First-degree AV blocks require no immediate intervention. Second-degree type I blocks also require no immediate intervention in an asymptomatic patient, but they do respond to atropine or cardiac pacing if indicated.[1,2] Second-degree type II blocks and third-degree blocks require emergency cardiac pacing (transcutaneous as a bridge to transvenous) for definitive treatment, because they are likely to progress to third-degree AV block. Atropine is contraindicated in patients with type II second-degree blocks.[2]

REFERENCES

1. Bourke JP. Atrioventricular block and problems with atrioventricular conduction. *Clin Geriatr Med* 2002;18:229–251.
2. Barold SS. 2:1 Atrioventricular block: order from chaos. *Am J Emerg Med* 2001;19:214–217.

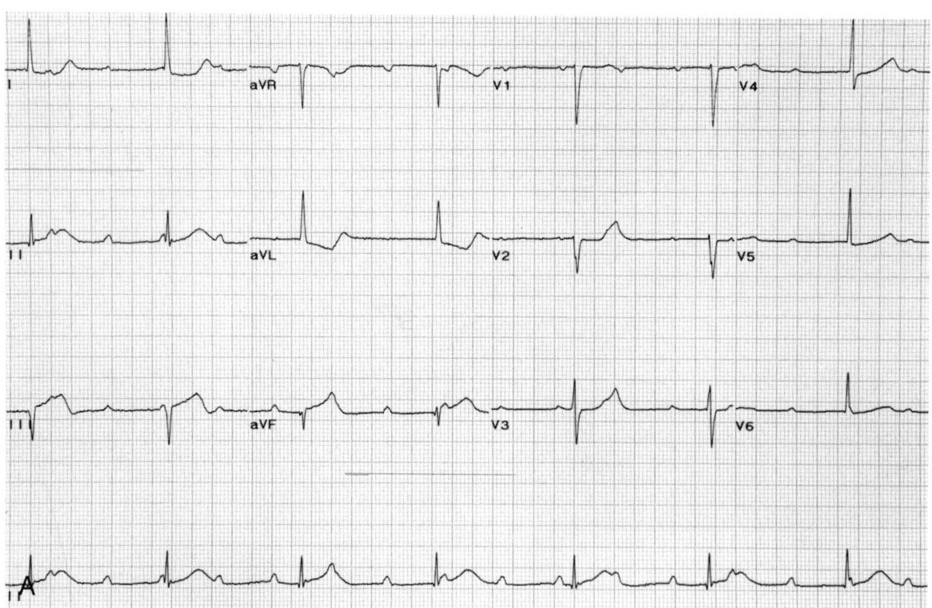

FIGURE 7–38 A: Complete atrioventricular (AV) block.

Atrioventricular Blocks

Todd McGrath

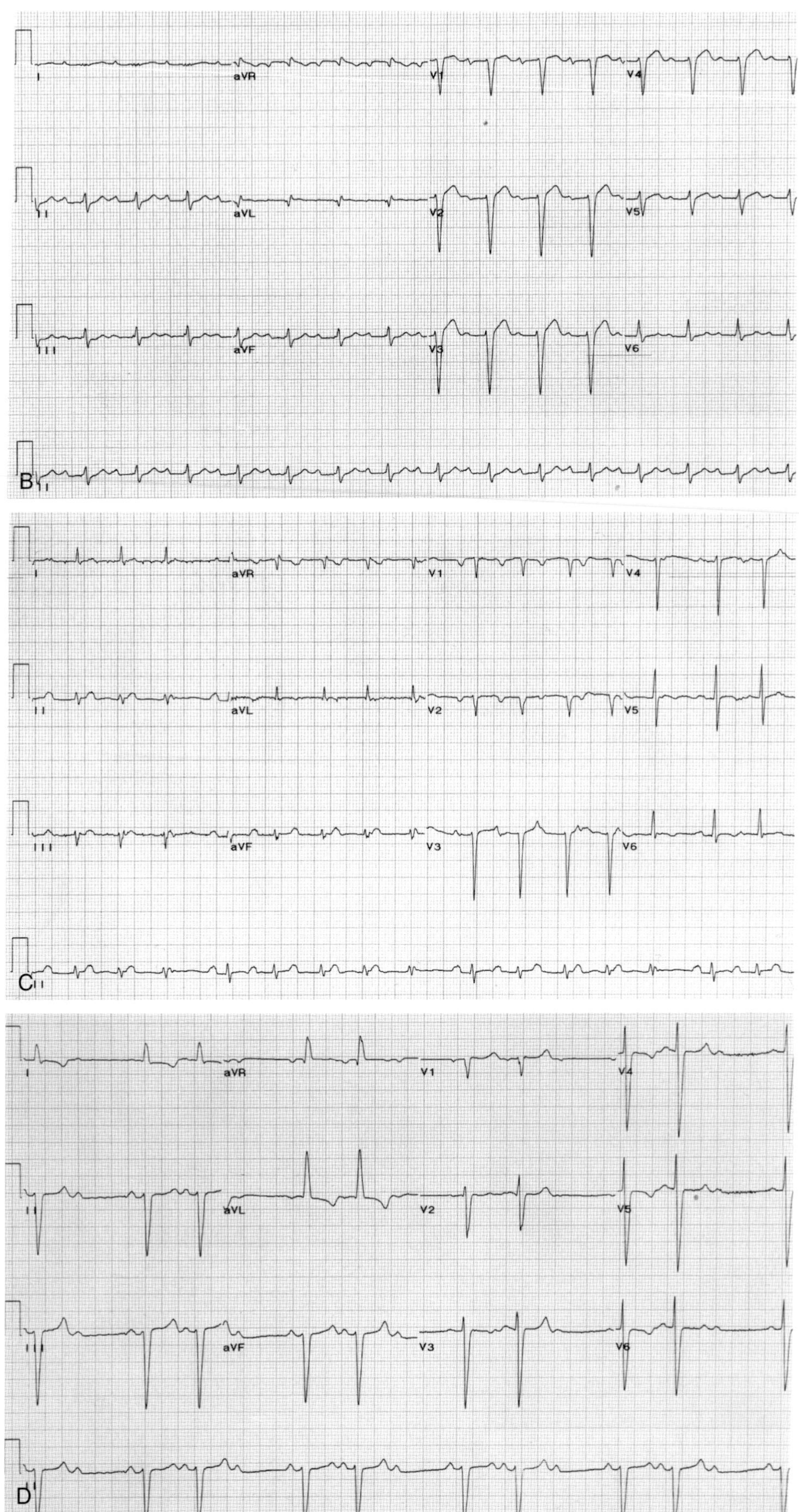

FIGURE 7–38, cont'd. B: First-degree AV block. **C:** Mobitz type 1 second-degree AV block. **D:** Mobitz type 2 second-degree AV block. (**A** through **D** from Fowler with permission.)

Sinus Bradycardia

Ralph Weiche

Clinical Presentation

Sinus bradycardia (SB) is usually asymptomatic. However, symptoms related to the slow heart rate may include dizziness, presyncope, syncope, and worsening of angina or congestive heart failure (CHF). The sick sinoatrial (SA) node often does not respond appropriately to exercise, and fatigue or dyspnea on exertion may be the presenting complaint.

Pathophysiology

SB is an incidental finding in otherwise healthy individuals, particularly in young or sleeping patients. There is no prognostic significance to SB in otherwise healthy patients. Other causes include vagal response, sinus node dysfunction, drugs, acute myocardial infarction (AMI), and increased intracranial pressure. Vasovagal response may be associated with a profound bradycardia caused by direct parasympathetic action on the SA node. The vagal response can be stimulated by pressure on the carotid sinus, vomiting, a Valsalva maneuver when straining to stool, or cold water on the face. SB may be the result of SA-node dysfunction and the sick sinus syndrome, which can be caused by any of a number of disorders affecting the SA node. Many classes of drugs can depress the SA node and slow the heart rate, including parasympathomimetic agents, α- and β-adrenergic blockers, digitalis, calcium-channel blockers, amiodarone and other antiarrhythmic drugs, cimetidine, and lithium. SB can occur in patients with AMI, particularly infarctions affecting the inferior wall. Increased vagal activity and ischemia of the SA node are responsible for the slowing of the heart rate. SB also may be a reperfusion arrhythmia after thrombolysis. Increased intracranial pressure should be considered if SB occurs in a patient with neurologic dysfunction. Other causes of SB are hypothyroidism, hypothermia, hypoxia, and some infections.

Diagnosis

SB is diagnosed by demonstration on electrocardiograph (ECG) of a sinus rhythm with a resting heart rate of 60 beats/minute or less.

Clinical Complications

Symptomatic bradycardia can lead to hypoperfusion, shock, CHF, myocardial ischemia or infarction, or death, and it can precipitate other fatal dysrrhythmias.

Management

Asymptomatic patients with SB may not require any intervention. The underlying cause should be considered and addressed. In patients with SB secondary to use of digitalis, β-blockers, or calcium-channel blockers, discontinuation of the drug and monitored observation may be all that is necessary. Symptomatic patients require intravenous (IV) access, supplemental oxygen, and cardiac monitoring. Atropine and drug-specific medications may be used to treat the bradycardia if hypotension is present. Refractory symptomatic bradycardia may require transcutaneous or transvenous pacing. Patients in unstable condition may require intensive care unit (ICU) admission.

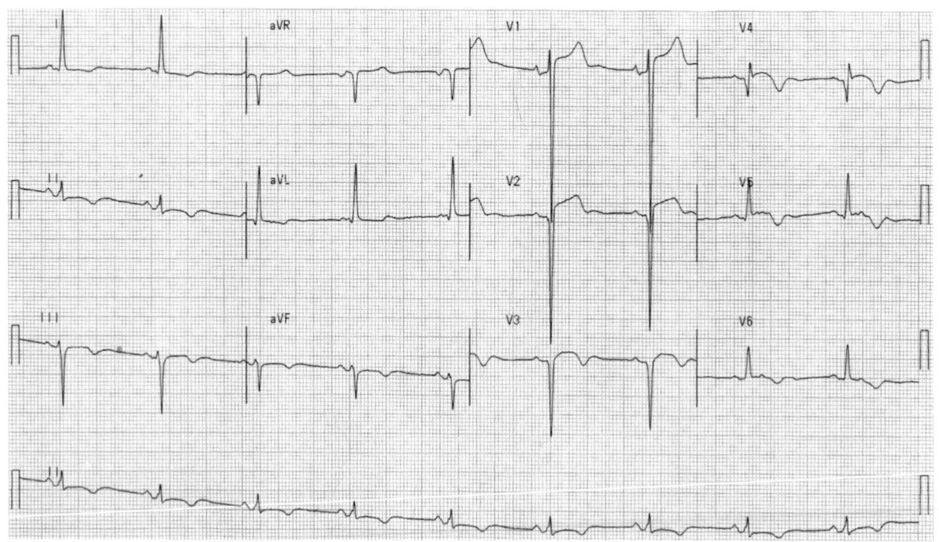

FIGURE 7–39 Sinus bradycardia. (Courtesy of Mark Silverberg, MD.)

Pacemaker Failure

Brandt Delhamer

Clinical Presentation

The patient may be asymptomatic or may have symptoms ranging from syncope or near-syncope to orthostatic dizziness, lightheadedness, dyspnea, or palpitations.

Pathophysiology

Pacemaker failure refers to an implanted pacemaker's inability to sense, to produce pacemaker spikes, or to conduct electrical complexes.[1]

The causes of pacemaker failure include failure to pace (e.g., lead disconnection, break, or displacement; exit block), failure to sense, and failure of the pacing generator (e.g., battery depletion).[1] Of these, the most common cause for failure is lead displacement; for example, ventricular wires may migrate to the pulmonary outflow tract or atrial wires to the atria or superior vena cava). Exit block is the failure of the heart to capture a normally firing pacer stimulus due to changes in the adjacent myocardium from infarct or ischemia, class III antiarrhythmics, or electrolyte abnormalities. Failure to sense is often caused by local fibrosis at the tip of the pacing wire.

Diagnosis

The diagnosis of pacemaker failure usually depends on the interpretation of an electrocardiograph (ECG), combined with an understanding of the device in question. Normal posteroanterior and lateral radiographs may show displaced or fractured leads.

If the pacemaker is not sensing, the ECG shows an entirely paced rhythm, despite intrinsic electrical activity (e.g., a pacer spike shortly after an intrinsic QRS). If the pacemaker is failing to fire or to capture, the ECG shows no pacemaker activity. If the intrinsic heart rate is more rapid than the set pacemaker rate, a magnet may be applied to the pacemaker to disconnect the sensing mode. This should result in an entirely paced rhythm if the pacemaker is outputting normally. Oversensing, or sensing of a non-QRS signal as a QRS complex (e.g., sensing body movement as a QRS), may also result in failure to pace. If the pacemaker is failing to capture, pacemaker spikes are visible on the ECG, but they do not produce a QRS complex.[1,2]

Clinical Complications

Complications include bradycardia, syncope, hypotension, and death.[1]

Management

Patients with symptomatic bradycardia or hypotension may be treated with transcutaneous pacing. Chest radiographs should be obtained and the catheter tip positions identified. The pulse generator should also be evaluated for possible lead disconnection. A 12-lead ECG should be obtained, and the relationship between the pacer spikes and the complexes should be determined.

REFERENCES

1. Harper RJ, Brady WJ, Perron AD, Mangrum M. The paced electrocardiogram: issues for the emergency physician. *Am J Emerg Med* 2001;19:551–560.
2. Sarko JA, Tiffany BR. Cardiac pacemakers: evaluation and management of malfunctions. *Am J Emerg Med* 2000;18:435–440.

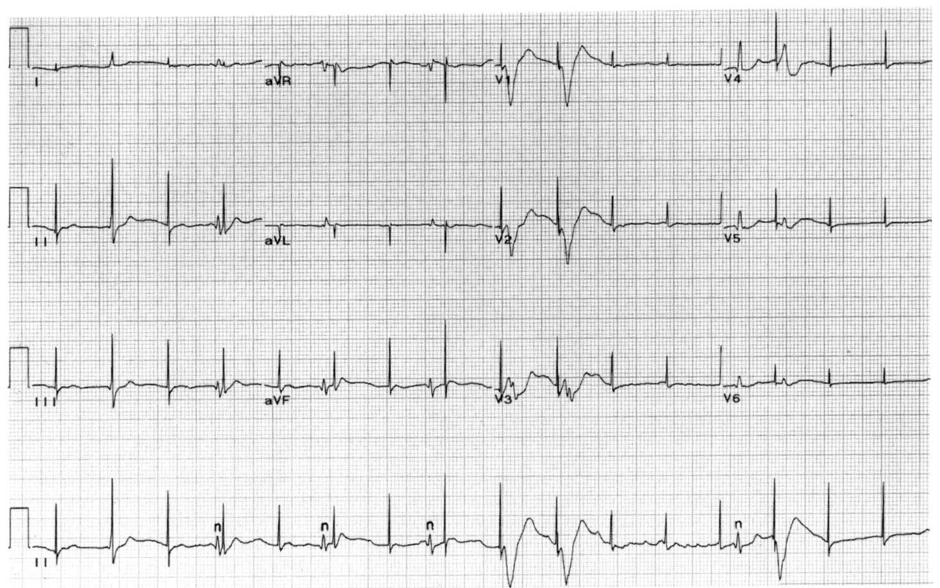

FIGURE 7–40 Electronic pacing record shows failure to sense and failure to capture in this patient with an overdose of verapamil. Electronic pacing spikes are occurring at the rate of 100 per minute. Some pacing spikes closely follow the native QRS complexes (n), indicating failure to sense. There are only three paced beats in the record; the remainder of the time there is failure to capture. (From Fowler, with permission.)

Mitral Valve Prolapse

Cara Marie Cenera and Michael Greenberg

Clinical Presentation

Most patients are asymptomatic; however, in approximately 5% of all cases, mitral valve prolapse (MVP) is associated with musculoskeletal disorders including Marfan's syndrome, Ehlers-Danlos syndrome, pectus excavatum, and severe scoliosis.[1] Symptomatic patients may present with palpitations, chest pain, or symptoms of mitral regurgitation. Rare symptoms include various arrhythmias, such as paroxysmal reentry supraventricular tachycardia and ventricular tachycardia.[2]

Pathophysiology

MVP involves the displacement of one or both of the mitral valve leaflets into the left atrium during systole.[1,2]

MVP probably involves an inherited autosomal dominant connective tissue disorder and results from myxomatous degeneration of the supporting structure of the mitral valve leaflets.[1,2] Secondary MVP may result from elongated chordae tendinae or atypical left ventricular (LV) wall motion, or both.[2]

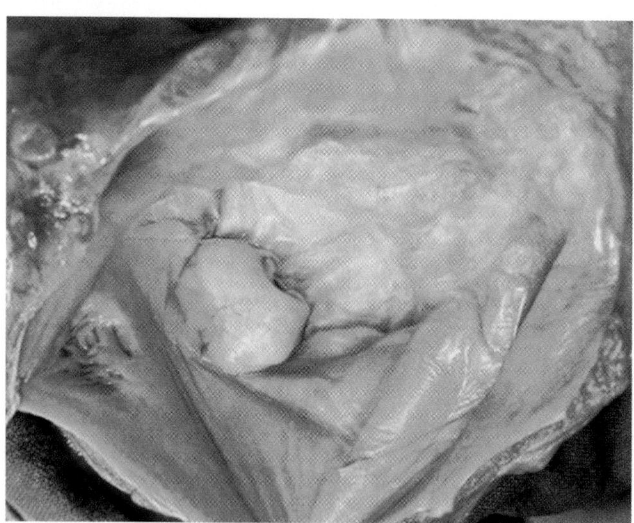

FIGURE 7–41 Prolapsed mitral valve observed from the left ventricle. (From Perkin, with permission.)

Diagnosis

On auscultation, a midsystolic to late systolic click, with or without a late systolic murmur, may be appreciated.[1] The electrocardiograph (ECG) is typically normal but in some cases demonstrates sinus tachycardia (ST) depression/T-wave inversion in the inferior leads.[2] Echocardiography is the gold standard diagnostic technique for MVP and typically demonstrates posterior displacement of the mitral leaflets.[1,2]

Clinical Complications

Clinical complications are related to abnormal friction of the valves (accounting for 11% to 29% of all cases of infective endocarditis) and arrhythmias (e.g., sinus tachycardia, atrial fibrillation [AF], ventricular tachycardia).[1] In addition, 10% of patients with MVP also develop mitral regurgitation. Any connection between MVP and cerebral ischemic events is controversial.[2]

Management

Patients with mitral regurgitation or a murmur, or both, should be treated with antibiotic prophylaxis to prevent infective endocarditis. β-adrenergic blockers should be used to relieve the palpitations or chest pain.[2] Severe MVP may require surgical intervention.[1]

REFERENCES

1. Jacobs W, Chamoun A, Stouffer GA. Mitral valve prolapse: a review of the literature. *Am J Med Sci* 2001;321:401–410.
2. Hanson EW, Neerhut RK, Lynch C. Mitral valve prolapse. *Anesthesiology* 1996;85:178–195.

Situs Inversus and Dextrocardia

Lisa Freeman

Clinical Presentation

Patients with undiagnosed situs inversus may present as a diagnostic and therapeutic challenge, because they may have unusual signs and symptoms.[1] One source for clinical confusion is the fact that, although the viscera are anatomically transposed, their nerve supply is not. As an example of the potential clinical confusion that can occur, symptoms are often referable to the right lower quadrant in appendicitis, but in biliary tract disease, the pain is usually where the gall bladder is located, in the left upper quadrant.[1,2]

Pathophysiology

Situs inversus refers to a perfect mirror image of the normal physiologic positions of the visceral organs, with preservation of their anteroposterior relationships.[1] Transpositions may be complete or incomplete, and there are multiple variations. In dextrocardia, the heart is on the right side of the chest. Dextrocardia may coexist with situs inversus.[2]

Conditions known to be associated with situs inversus include polysplenia, asplenia, annular pancreas, horseshoe kidney, and diaphragmatic hernia.[1] Consequently, the potential for an untraditional presentation of referred pain in virtually any chest or abdominal problem does exist. Most anatomic and scientific evidence supports the contention that the central nervous system does not share in the transposition. The presence of polysplenia may be associated with occult splenic rupture and uncontrolled hemorrhage if not identified. The heart usually functions normally, even in cases of dextrocardia, unless there are significant other associated cardiac malformations. If dextrocardia is present without situs inversus, cardiac abnormalities often coexist. Kartagener's syndrome is a condition that includes situs inversus, bronchiectasis, and sinusitis.[1]

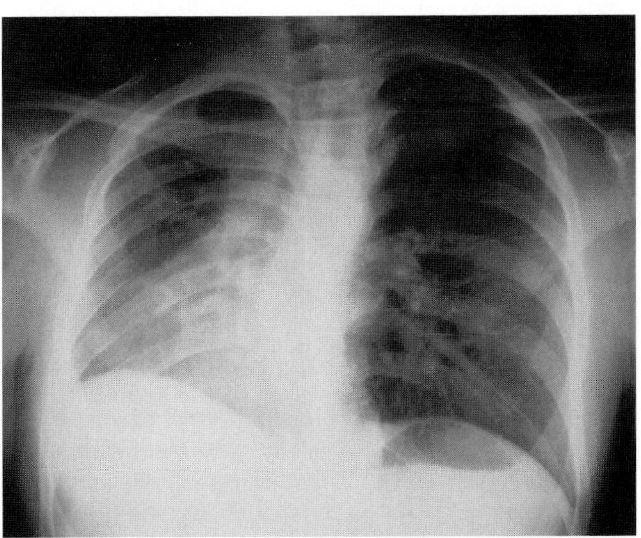

FIGURE 7–42 Dextrocardia. Note cardiac shadow on right and gastric bubble on left. (Courtesy of Mark Silverberg, MD.)

Diagnosis

The initial diagnosis of these conditions rests on careful physical examination. In dextrocardia, the physical examination may reveal heart sounds and an apical impulse in the right chest rather than the left. In situs inversus, the liver may be palpated on the left and the spleen on the right. Often, the diagnosis of these conditions is fortuitous on plain radiography, where left-right confusion is initially assumed.[1] The chest radiograph reveals a right-sided cardiac apex, a lower left hemidiaphragm, and a right-sided stomach bubble. In cases of dextrocardia, the electrocardiograph (ECG) may show inverted P- and T-waves in lead I, with a negative QRS deflection and a reverse pattern between aVR and aVL.[2]

Clinical Complications

Delayed or missed diagnoses are important complications of situs inversus, because the failure to recognize these conditions may place the patient at future risk for problems such as missed appendicitis.[1,2]

REFERENCES

1. Janchar T, Milzman D, Clement M. Situs inversus: emergency evaluations of atypical presentations. *Am J Emerg Med* 2000;18: 349–350.
2. Goldman L, Bennett JC: *Cecil textbook of medicine,* 21st. ed. Philadelphia: WB Saunders, 2000.

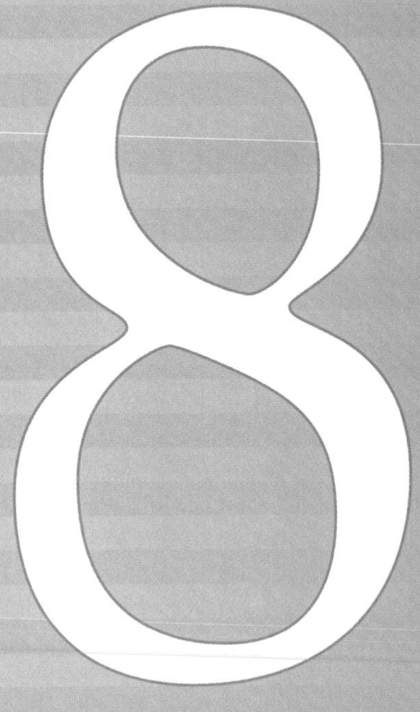

Respiratory

Asthma

Robert Hendrickson

Clinical Presentation

Patients with mild asthma exacerbations may present with cough, dyspnea, or pleuritic chest pain. Less commonly, patients present in extremis with symptoms developing from hypercarbia and hypoxemia, including altered mental status, anxiety, and respiratory arrest.

Physical examination findings vary with the severity of hypoxemia and airway obstruction. Mild signs may include tachycardia, tachypnea, and expiratory wheezing. As airway obstruction worsens, wheezing may be evident during both inspiration and expiration. With severe obstruction, air movement through the bronchi may be too decreased to detect wheezing at all. In these severe cases, pulsus paradoxus may occasionally be seen.[1]

Pathophysiology

Asthma is a reversible pulmonary obstructive airway disorder caused by bronchoconstriction, pulmonary mucosal edema, and mucosal hypersecretion.

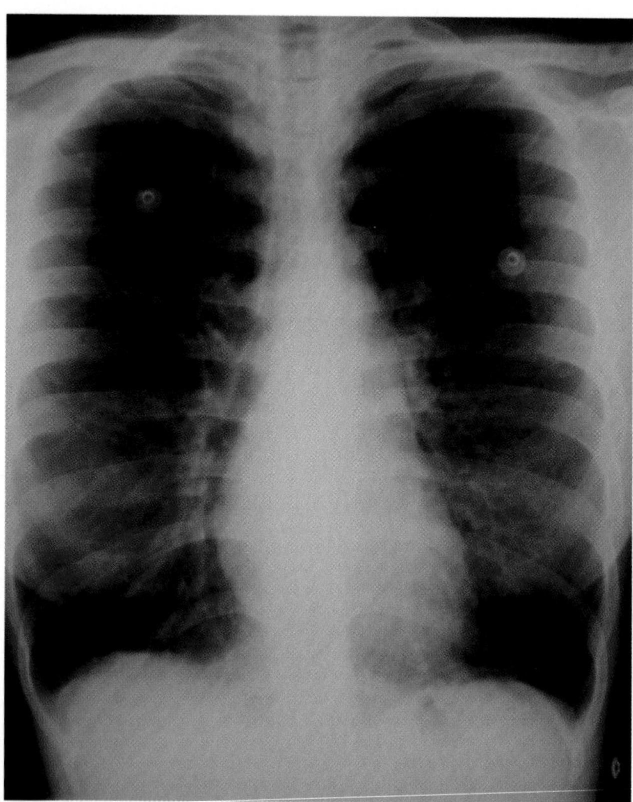

FIGURE 8–1 Radiographs of an adult with asthma, demonstrating hyperinflated lungs. (Courtesy of Anthony Morocco, MD.)

Asthma exacerbations usually are triggered by viral infections, exposure to antigens (e.g., dog, cat, pollen), changes in weather (e.g., cold, humid), or exposure to irritants (e.g., ammonia, perfume). Other, less common triggers include gastroesophageal reflux, exercise, anxiety, nonsteroidal antiinflammatory drugs (NSAIDs), and menses.[2]

Asthmatic patients have an increased response to triggers compared with nonasthmatics. When an asthmatic encounters a trigger, the bronchiolar smooth muscle contracts, lessening the diameter of the airway. In addition, several inflammatory mediators, including histamine and leukotrienes, are released and cause mucosal edema and increased mucous secretion, which further decreases the airway lumen. Exposure to triggers may also increase vagal tone, particularly in children, causing bronchoconstriction.

Diagnosis

The diagnosis of mild asthma is made clinically from the typical history and physical examination. Occasionally, peak flow testing diagnoses an atypical asthma exacerbation, such as cough-variant asthma. In moderate or severe cases, pulse oximetry and peak flow testing may help predict the need for admission and help track improvements with therapy.[3]

Blood tests are of little value in the diagnosis. Chest radiography may reveal flattening of the diaphragm that is consistent with air trapping. In addition, chest radiography may be used to rule out pneumonia, heart failure, or pneumothorax, which sometimes mimic asthma. Arterial blood gas (ABG) analysis may be helpful to diagnose hypercarbia if the patient has an alteration of mental status, but it is not necessary to obtain as a "baseline" measurement.[1] ABG results should not be the primary reason for deciding to initiate mechanical ventilation. Intubation and mechanical ventilation do little to improve the pulmonary dynamics of asthma and may increase the risk of barotrauma and air trapping. The decision to intubate should be based on the need to protect the airway (secondary to alterations of mental status, hypercarbia, and so on) or to improve severe hypoxemia.

Clinical Complications

Severe hypoxemia may result in myocardial infarction, cerebrovascular accident, hypoxic encephalopathy, respiratory failure, and death. Positive-pressure ventilation of an asthmatic patient may lead to hyperinflation, self-controlled positive end-expiratory pressure (auto-PEEP), hypotension, and barotrauma.

Asthma

Robert Hendrickson

Management

An initial assessment of the need for an emergency airway and the adequacy of breathing should be rapidly performed, because it leads the initial management. The treatment of asthma is aimed at relieving bronchospasm and decreasing bronchiolar edema.

Patients *in extremis* in whom inhalational therapy is not practical (e.g., altered mental status, weak respiratory excursion) may receive subcutaneous β-adrenergic agonists or an intravenous terbutaline infusion in addition to inhaled/nebulized β-agonists. In addition, systemic corticosteroids and oxygen should be provided. Patients with mild to moderate asthma exacerbations may receive nebulized or inhaled β-agonists (albuterol or terbutaline) repeated hourly or given as a continuous infusion. The addition of an anticholinergic (vagolytic) inhaled agent (e.g., ipratropium bromide) may improve bronchodilatation.

Patients with moderate or severe asthma may be treated with corticosteroids, such a prednisone, 1 mg/kg orally; dexamethasone, 0.1 mg/kg intravenously; or Solu-Medrol (methylprednisolone) 2 mg/kg IV. Patients with an inflammatory condition as a trigger for their asthma (e.g., upper respiratory tract infection) should be treated with corticosteroids. The methylxanthines, theophylline and aminophylline, are still used occasionally to treat chronic asthma, but they have little role in acute asthma therapy. Magnesium has been used to treat acute asthma exacerbation with mixed results and remains controversial.

Patients with a complete response to therapy (peak expiratory flow [PEF] greater than 70%), may be discharged with a short course of oral corticosteroids and β-agonist therapy. Patients with incomplete response to therapy (PEF 50% to 70% with continued mild wheezing) may require admission to the hospital or discharge with close follow-up. Nonresponders (PEF less than 50%) require further therapy and hospitalization.

REFERENCES

1. Marik PE, Varon J, Fromm R. The management of acute severe asthma. *J Emerg Med* 2002;23:257–268.
2. Lemanske RF, Busse WW. Asthma. *JAMA* 1997;278:1855–1873.
3. Emond SD, Camargo CA, Nowak RM. 1997 National Asthma Education and Prevention Program guidelines: a practical summary for emergency physicians. *Ann Emerg Med* 1998;31:579–589.

Chronic Obstructive Pulmonary Disease

Jennifer Larson

Clinical Presentation

Patients with chronic obstructive pulmonary disease (COPD) may present with acute exacerbations beyond their baseline chronic airway obstruction and may have increased cough, sputum production, or dyspnea.[1] Precipitating factors include infection (viral or bacterial) and bronchospasm.

Pathophysiology

COPD is characterized by decreased airway diameter secondary to loss of lung parenchyma, chronic inflammation, and hyperplasia of mucous-secreting cells.[2] Risk factors include tobacco abuse, cystic fibrosis, α_1-antitrypsin deficiency, and bronchiectasis.[1,2]

Diagnosis

The diagnosis is based on the history and physical examination. Obstruction may be confirmed with peak flow and pulmonary function testing. On physical examination, there may be hyperresonance of the chest with wheezing and coarse rhonchi, or a decrease in air movement and lung sounds. Patients may exhibit accessory muscle use, pursed lips, or the tripod sitting position. Radiography may reveal hyperinflation with diminished pulmonary vasculature (emphysema) or increased bronchovascular markings (chronic bronchitis).[1,2]

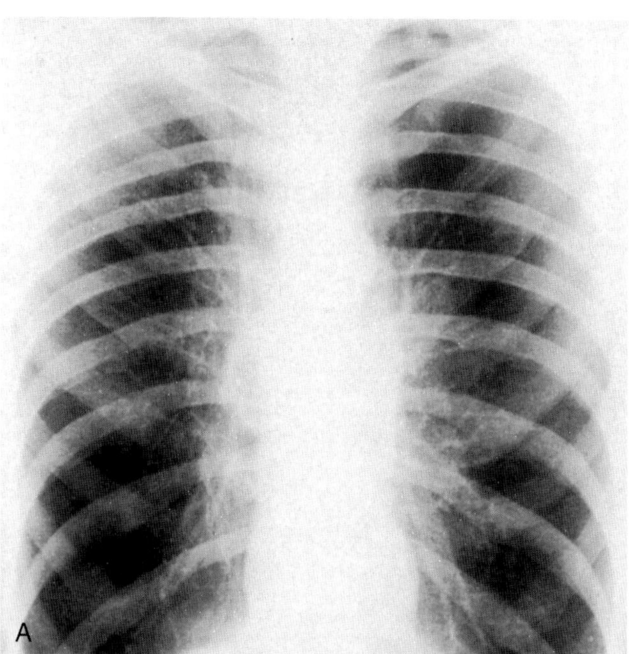

FIGURE 8–2 **A:** Chest radiograph showing overaeration of lungs, centralized flow pattern, and small heart size. (From Hurst, with permission.)

Clinical Complications

Respiratory failure is the most significant complication. Pneumothorax due to bleb formation may occur. Other complications include infection, cor pulmonale, pulmonary hypertension, malnutrition, adrenal crisis (with chronic steroid use), secondary polycythemia, and bullous lung disease.[1,2]

Management

Patients with hypoxemia may be treated with supplemental oxygen to keep the blood oxygen saturation higher than 88% to 90%. Overaggressive oxygen therapy may lead to elevations in the carbon dioxide concentration, with subsequent narcosis and need for intubation. Patients with depressed mental status may require endotracheal intubation. Arterial blood gas (ABG) analysis helps to determine the extent of respiratory acidosis (pH less than 7.30 or carbon dioxide tension [$P\text{CO}_2$] higher than baseline), and peak flow measurements determine the degree of airway obstruction. Emergency department (ED) management includes inhaled β-agonists and anticholinergics, corticosteroids, antibiotics (if bacterial infection appears to be the exacerbating factor), continuous positive airway pressure (CPAP) or bilevel positive airway pressure (BiPAP), and intubation for respiratory failure. Patients who return to their baseline status with immediate therapies in the ED may be discharged home; however, they most likely will require a short steroid burst and close follow-up with their primary physician. Patients with poor responses to therapy require admission.[1,2]

REFERENCES

1. Mannino DM. COPD: epidemiology, prevalence, morbidity and mortality, and disease heterogeneity. *Chest* 2002;121[5 Suppl]: 121S–126S.
2. Singh JM, Palda VA, Stanbrook MB, Chapman KR. Corticosteroid therapy for patients with acute exacerbations of chronic obstructive pulmonary disease: a systematic review. *Arch Intern Med* 2002;162:2527–2536.

Chronic Obstructive Pulmonary Disease

Jennifer Larson

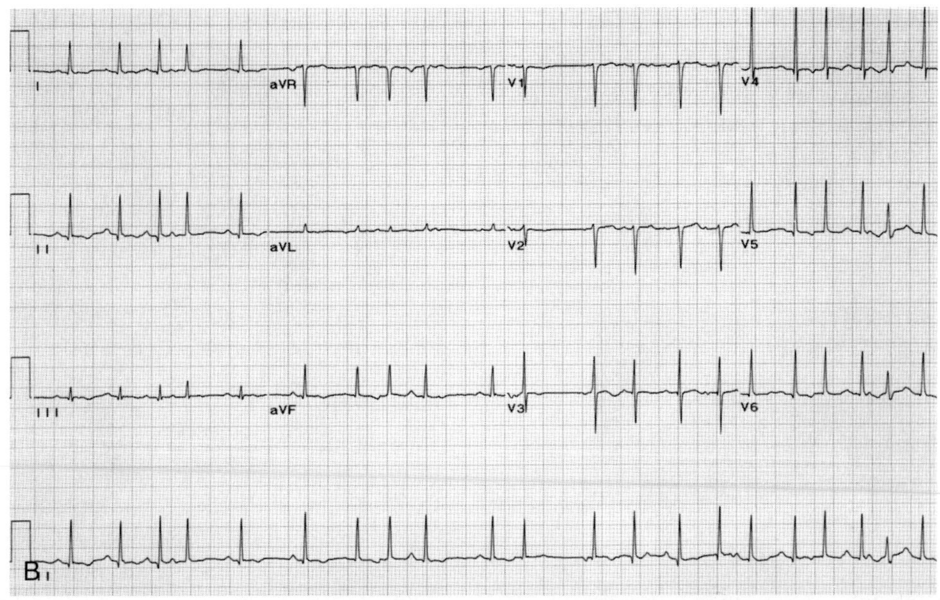

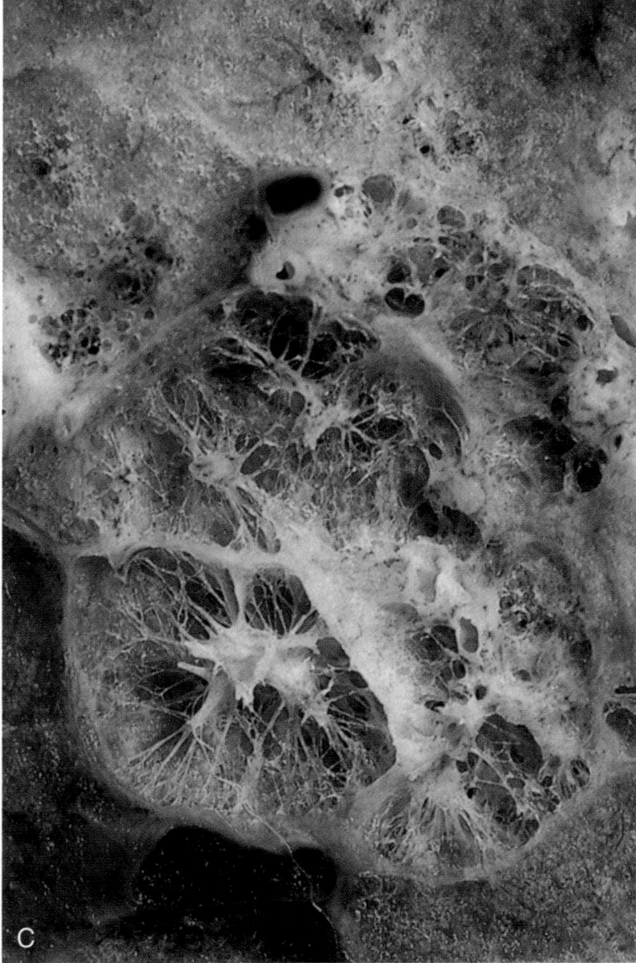

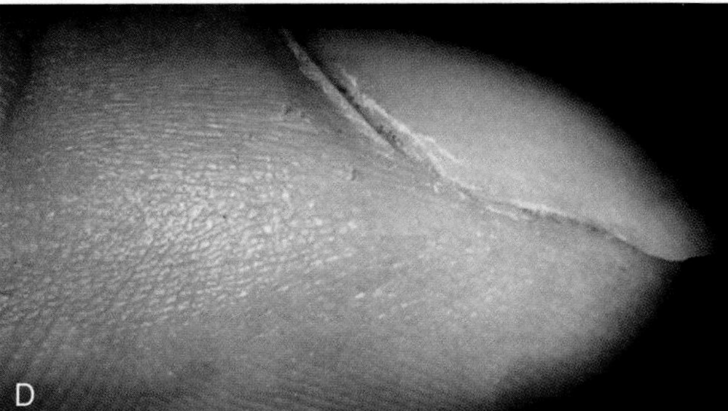

FIGURE 8–2, cont'd. B: Multifocal atrial tachycardia, commonly seen in patients with chronic obstructive pulmonary disease. (From Fowler, with permission.) **C:** Gross aspect of lung with pulmonary emphysema. Note the centrally dilated air spaces. (From Hurst, with permission.) **D:** Finger clubbing. (From Habif, with permission.)

Pulmonary Embolism

Michael Greenberg

Clinical Presentation

The classic presentation of pulmonary embolism (PE) involves dyspnea, pleuritic chest pain, tachypnea, and tachycardia of relatively acute onset. However, patients may present with a wide variety of symptoms, ranging from asymptomatic or subtle to cardiorespiratory arrest. Patients with risk factors for or clinical evidence of venous thrombosis are at special risk.[1-3]

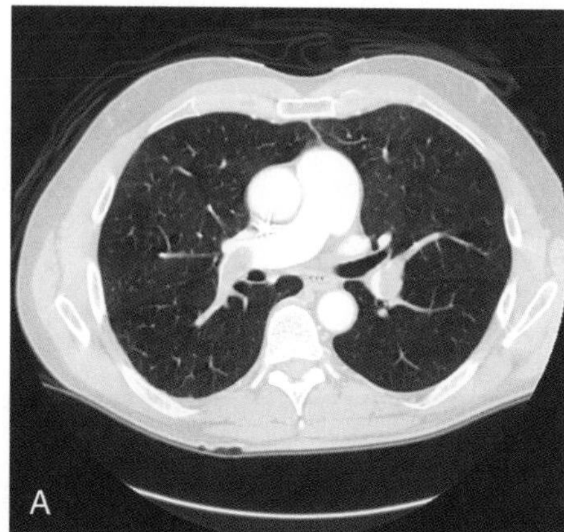

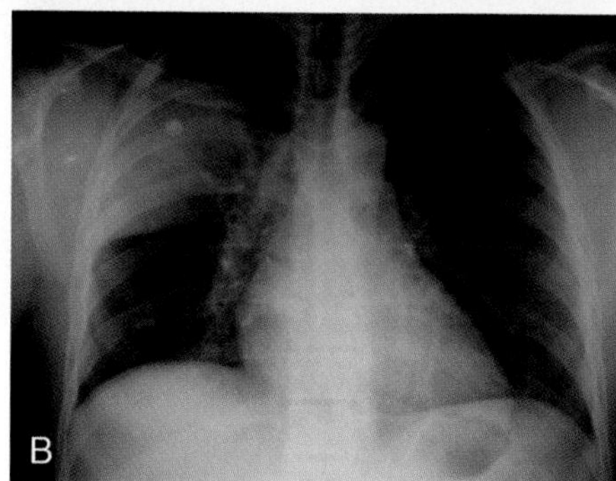

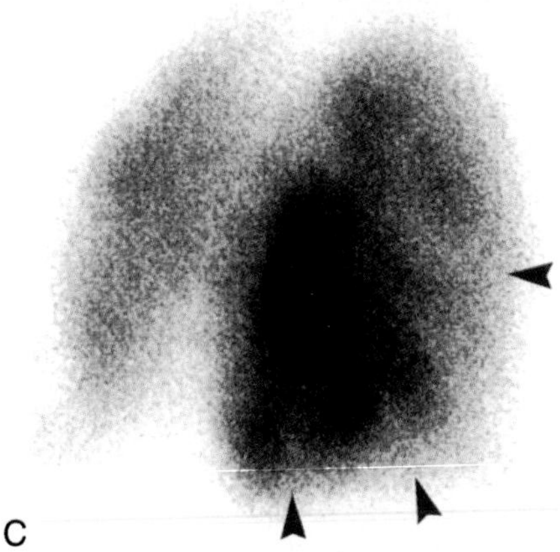

FIGURE 8–3 **A:** Computed tomogram showing pulmonary embolism. (Courtesy of Robert Hendrickson, MD.) **B:** Chest radiograph showing pulmonary infarct. (Courtesy of Donald Sallee, MD.) **C:** Right posterior view of a perfusion scan showing multiple subsegmental defects *(arrows)*. (**C,** from Hurst, with permission.)

Pathophysiology

As many as 600,000 cases of PE occur annually in the United States, with up to 200,000 fatal events each year.[1] Risk factors for venous thromboembolism include age greater than 40 years, previous history of venous thromboembolism, surgery with more than 30 minutes of anesthesia, prolonged immobilization, congestive heart failure (CHF), malignancy, lower-extremity and pelvic fractures, obesity, pregnancy or recent delivery, estrogen-containing medications, inflammatory bowel disease, and various genetic disorders.[1]

Diagnosis

The diagnosis of PE is "confounded by a clinical presentation that may be subtle, atypical, or obscured by another coexisting disease."[1] Multiple and varied diagnostic tests exist, allowing assessments of probability for PE as "low" (10% or less), "intermediate" (about 30%), or "high" (70% or greater).[1] Diagnostic tests that may be used include D-dimer testing, ventilation-perfusion scanning, computed tomography (CT), and pulmonary angiography. Pulmonary angiography remains the gold standard for diagnosing PE.[1] The physical examination in conjunction with the electrocardiogram (ECG), chest radiograph, chest CT, and echocardiogram may show evidence of dysfunction of the right ventricle, which constitutes an important indicator of high risk as well as poor outcome.[1,2] Measurements of troponin levels, pro-B-type natriuretic peptide, and B-type natriuretic peptide may also assist in evaluating right ventricular function. The ECG may show the classic "S1Q3T3" pattern.

Clinical Complications

Complications include ventricular dysfunction, respiratory failure, multiorgan failure, and death.

Management

Heparin anticoagulation is the mainstay of immediate therapy, with the initiation of longer-term anticoagulation as an essential component of care.[1] Vena cava filters may be considered to reduce the chance of additional emboli getting to the lungs. Thrombolysis may be considered for use in some cases but is currently controversial. Surgical or catheter-assisted embolectomy may be considered for selected patients.[1]

REFERENCES

1. Fedullo PF, Tapson VF. Clinical practice: the evaluation of suspected pulmonary embolism. *N Engl J Med* 2003;349:1247–1256.
2. Goldhaber SZ, Elliott CG. Acute pulmonary embolism. Part II: risk stratification, treatment, and prevention. *Circulation* 2003;108: 2834–2838.
3. Guidelines on diagnosis and management of acute pulmonary embolism. Task Force on Pulmonary Embolism, European Society of Cardiology. *Eur Heart J* 2000;21:1301–1336.

Spontaneous Pneumothorax

Swapan Dubey

Clinical Presentation

Patients with spontaneous pneumothorax (SP) usually present with acute pleuritic chest pain, dyspnea (proportional to the size of the pneumothorax), and cough. With a small pneumothorax, signs may include decreased breath sounds, decreased tactile fremitus, and ipsilateral hyperresonance. In the case of a large spontaneous pneumothorax, tachycardia, tachypnea, and hypoxemia may be evident.

Pathophysiology

Primary SP occurs without identifiable external precipitating factors in patients without obvious underlying lung disease. Secondary SP occurs as a complication of an underlying lung disease.[1] In primary SP, disruption of the alveolar-pleural barrier is thought to occur when a subpleural bulla (or bleb), typically located at the lung apex, ruptures into the pleural space.[1] Factors associated with primary SP include cigarette smoking and changes in ambient atmospheric pressure. Physical exertion does not appear to be a precipitating factor, whereas familial patterns, mitral valve prolapse, and Marfan's syndrome are associated with SP.

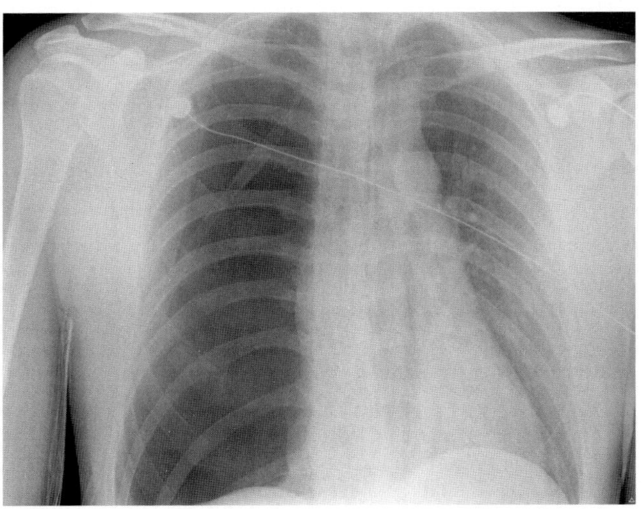

FIGURE 8–4 A 100% right-sided spontaneous pneumothorax. (Courtesy of Robert Hendrickson, MD.)

Catamenial pneumothorax is a rare condition in which recurrent SPs occur in association with menses (typically within 72 hours of onset). Although it has been termed thoracic endometriosis syndrome, the exact cause of catamenial pneumothorax remains uncertain. One possibility is that this condition results from passage of intraabdominal air through diaphragmatic defects.[1]

Diagnosis

Suspicion based on the clinical presentation and physical examination are crucial in identifying SP. Chest radiography may reveal a visceral pleural line with absence of lung markings distal to the line. Formulas used to estimate size are unreliable. Associated electrocardiogram (ECG) changes may include axis deviation, decreased QRS voltage, and T-wave inversions.[1]

Clinical Complications

Approximately 3% of SPs become tension pneumothoraces, with possible associated hypoxemia, cyanosis, hypotension, and death. Reinflation pulmonary edema has been reported after correction of large SPs.[1]

Management

Supportive measures that should be initiated include intravenous (IV) access and supplemental oxygen. Treatment with oxygen by a nonrebreather mask may increase the rate of absorption of the pneumothorax. The ultimate goal of the management of an SP is evacuating the pleural space and minimizing the possibility of recurrence.[1] Decisions in the management of a pneumothorax must take into account several factors, including size of the pneumothorax, severity of signs, presence of underlying pulmonary disease, comorbidities, patient reliability, and availability for follow-up monitoring. Needle aspiration of pneumothorax has been advocated by some, with a variable degree of success. Tube thoracostomy is the most common approach to the treatment of pneumothorax.[1]

REFERENCES

1. Weissberg D, Rafaely Y. Pneumothorax: experience with 1,199 patients. *Chest* 2000;117:1279–1285.

Severe Acute Respiratory Syndrome

Michael Greenberg

Clinical Presentation

Severe acute respiratory syndrome (SARS) begins with a prodrome, often with fever, chills and rigors, headache, malaise, and myalgias. After 3 to 7 days, a lower respiratory tract illness develops, in most cases with a dry, nonproductive cough or dyspnea, sometimes with hypoxemia. Diarrhea has been described in a large percentage of SARS patients.[1–4]

Pathophysiology

SARS is an emerging infectious disease that was first identified in China in November, 2002. It is caused by a unique coronavirus, SARS-CoV. The SARS-CoV genome has been sequenced, and it does not appear to be related to any previously known coronaviruses of humans or animals.[2] It is likely that SARS-CoV started out as an animal virus that transformed to be able to accommodate human-to-human transmission. Within the first 10 days, the histology reflects diffuse alveolar damage with a mixture of inflammatory cells, edema, and hyaline membrane formation. Desquamation of pneumatocytes is a consistent finding.[2]

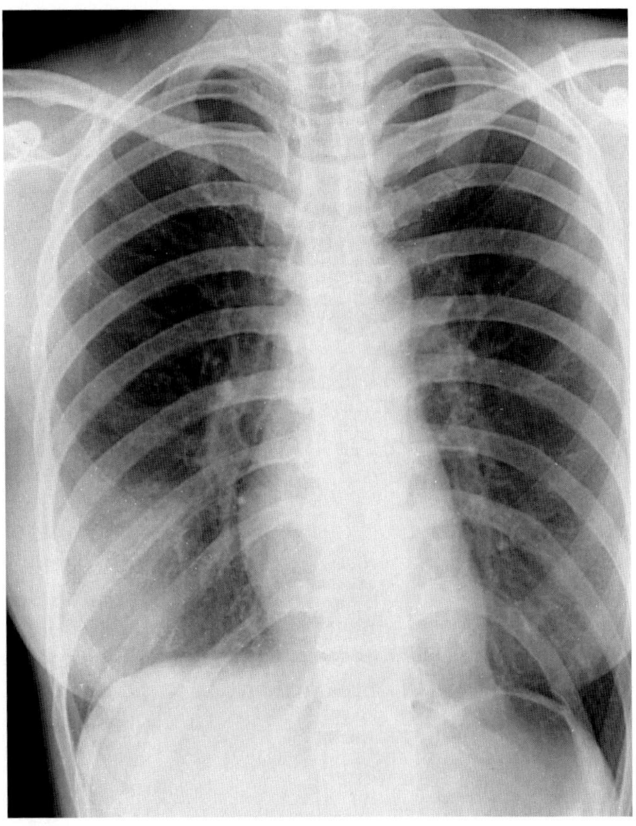

FIGURE 8–5 Severe acute respiratory syndrome. (From Rainer TH, Cameron PA, Smit D, et al. Evaluation of WHO criteria for identifying patients with severe acute respiratory syndrome out of the hospital: prospective observational study. *BMJ* 2003;326:1354–1358, with permission.)

Diagnosis

The diagnosis requires an elevated index of suspicion in conjunction with findings on examination. Chest radiographs demonstrate either focal or generalized infiltrates in most cases, with no cavitation, lymphadenopathy, or pleural effusion.[4] Lymphopenia, thrombocytopenia, and elevated lactate dehydrogenase (LDH) levels are common. The diagnosis may be confirmed by detection of serum antibody to SARS-CoV by enzyme-linked immunosorbent assay (ELISA), polymerase chain reaction (PCR), or other techniques. The differential diagnosis includes adult respiratory distress syndrome (ARDS), cytomegalovirus pneumonitis, acute interstitial pneumonitis, bronchiolitis obliterans–organizing pneumonia (BOOP), and alveolar proteinosis.

Clinical Complications

Complications include progressive pneumonia, spontaneous pneumothorax, spontaneous pneumomediastinum, and death.[1–4]

Management

In many cases, management requires admission to an intensive care unit (ICU) with mechanical ventilatory support. Some have advocated the use of ribavirin and corticosteroids. However, a number of cases have progressed to irreversibility despite all efforts. The optimal treatment for SARS has yet to be derived.

REFERENCES

1. Hui D, Wong P, Wang C. SARS: Clinical features and diagnosis. *Respirology* 2003;8[Suppl]:S20–S24.
2. Nicholls J, Dong X, Jiang, G, et al. SARS: Clinical virology and pathogenesis. *Respirology* 2003;8[Suppl]:S6–S8.
3. Yeung M, Xu R. SARS: epidemiology. *Respirology* 2003;8[Suppl]: S9–S14.
4. OOI G, Daqing M. SARS: radiological features. *Respirology* 2003;8[Suppl]:S15–S19.

Hospital-Acquired Pneumonia

Robert Hendrickson

Hospital-acquired pneumonia (HAP) is defined as a pulmonary infection that develops at least 48 hours after admission to the hospital. The emergency physician may see HAP in patients who recently were discharged from a health care facility, particularly an intensive care unit (ICU).[1-3]

Clinical Presentation

Patients may present to the emergency department (ED) with fever, cough, pleuritic chest pain, or some combination of these. Fever and leukocytosis, with or without a leftward differential shift, may be evident but are nonspecific and not essential to the diagnosis.[1]

Pathophysiology

HAP differs from community-acquired pneumonia (CAP) in that the pathogens that produce the disease are variable. In addition to the more typical staphylococcal and streptococcal infections, HAP may be produced by enteric gram-negative bacilli or by resistant organisms (e.g., *Klebsiella, Pseudomonas, Acinetobacter*).[1] These organisms are present in hospitals and are thought to gain access to the pulmonary tree by microaspiration.

Diagnosis

The diagnosis of HAP is made in patients with respiratory symptoms and a pulmonary infiltrate who recently were discharged from a health care facility. It is important to consider alternative causes of pulmonary infiltrate in these patients, including pulmonary embolus and pulmonary edema.[2] The reliability of other methods (e.g., computed tomography [CT], invasive microbiologic techniques) used to diagnose pneumonia in patients with clinical HAP is questionable.[2]

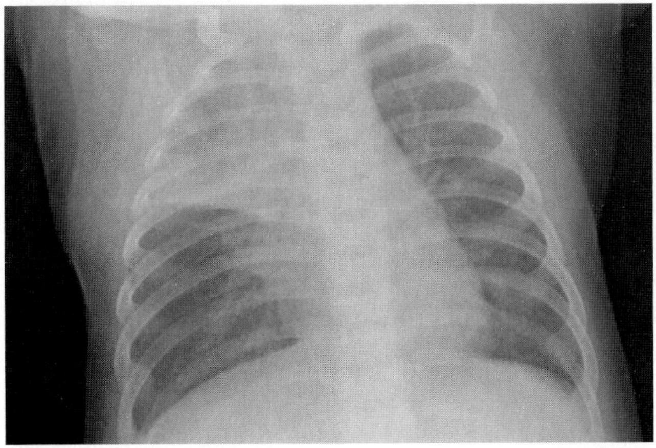

FIGURE 8–6 Right upper lobe pneumonia developed during an inpatient stay after admission for croup. (Courtesy of Jay Itzkowitz, MD.)

Clinical Complications

Complications of nosocomial pneumonia include sepsis, hypoxemia, adult respiratory distress syndrome (ARDS), and death.[1-3]

Management

Risk stratification and empiric antibiotic therapy are the essential factors when deciding on treatment. Patients with mild to moderate symptoms may be treated with a third-generation cephalosporin (ceftriaxone or cefotaxime) or a β-lactam penicillin (ampicillin/sulbactam or piperacillin/tazobactam). Patients with mild to moderate symptoms and risk factors for anaerobes (witnessed aspiration, trauma, coma, diabetes mellitus, high-dose steroids, preceding antibiotics, prolonged ICU stay) may be treated with combination therapy using a cephalosporin and a β-lactam (e.g., ceftriaxone and ampicillin/sulbactam) or a cephalosporin with clindamycin. Patients with severe disease who are mechanically ventilated should be treated with ciprofloxacin, an aminoglycoside, and either ticarcillin/clavulanate, aztreonam, imipenem, or vancomycin.[3]

REFERENCES

1. Fiel S. Guidelines and critical pathways for severe hospital-acquired pneumonia. *Chest* 2001;119:412S–418S.
2. Cunha BA. Nosocomial pneumonia: diagnostic and therapeutic considerations. *Med Clin North Am* 2001;85:79–114.
3. American Thoracic Society. Hospital-acquired pneumonia in adults: diagnosis, assessment of severity, initial antimicrobial therapy, and preventative strategies. *Am J Respir Crit Care Med* 1996;153: 1711–1725.

Community-Acquired Pneumonia

Swapan Dubey

Clinical Presentation

Common presenting symptoms include fever, myalgias, cough, and pleuritic chest pain. Severe symptoms may develop, including respiratory distress and hypoxemia. Physical examination findings may include fever, elevation of the respiratory rate, and localized rhonchi, rales, or wheezes.[1]

Pathophysiology

Community-acquired pneumonia (CAP) is an infection of the lung parenchyma that develops in patients who have not recently been hospitalized and are not at risk for aspiration. It is the sixth leading cause of death overall and the leading cause of death from infectious causes in the United States.

Lung parenchymal infection is thought to develop from microaspiration of oral flora or inhalation of infectious agents. The most common organisms are *Streptococcus pneumoniae* (20% to 60%), *Haemophilus influenzae* (3% to 10%), *Mycoplasma pneumoniae* (1% to 3%), *Chlamydia pneumoniae* (5% to 17%), *Legionella pneumophila* (2% to 8%), and oral anaerobes (6% to 10%).[1] *Pneumocystis carinii* can cause pneumonia in patients with acquired immunodeficiency syndrome (AIDS).

Diagnosis

CAP may be diagnosed clinically by history and physical examination. Chest radiography may reveal an infiltrate in one or more lobes. Blood cultures and sputum Gram staining may be helpful for inpatient care but should not delay the administration of empiric antibiotics.

Clinical Complications

CAP may progress to hypoxemia, respiratory failure, bacteremia (especially with pneumococcus), and sepsis. The mortality rate in admitted patients approaches 20%; among outpatients, it is less than 5%.[1]

Management

The mainstay of treatment of CAP is antibiotic therapy. Recommendations for specific antibiotics are continuously evolving due to an expanding spectrum of pathogens, antibiotic resistance, and new generations of antibiotics. The American Thoracic Society based its 2001 recommendations on site of care (outpatient, inpatient, or intensive care unit [ICU]) and the presence of cardiopulmonary disease and modifying risk factors (CPD/MRF).

Mildly symptomatic, young patients without evidence of hypoxemia may be treated in the outpatient setting. Those without CPD/MRF may be treated with a

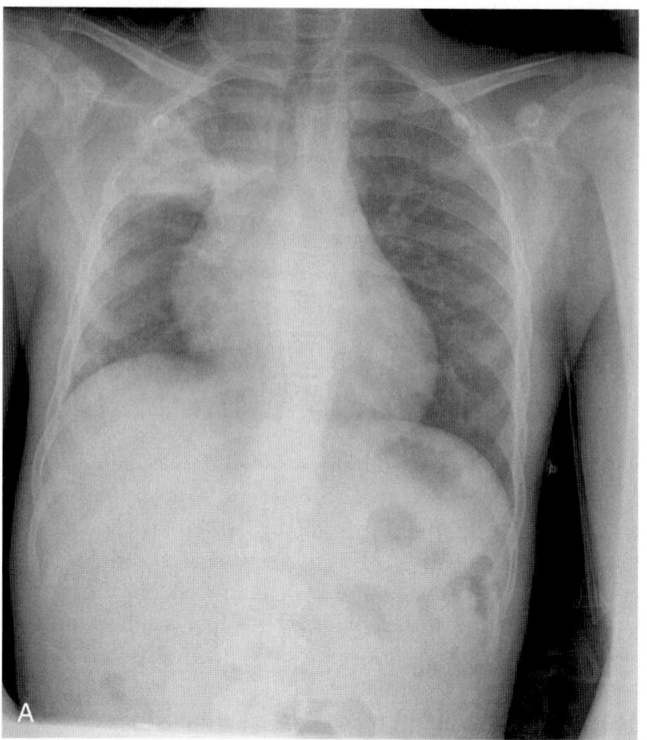

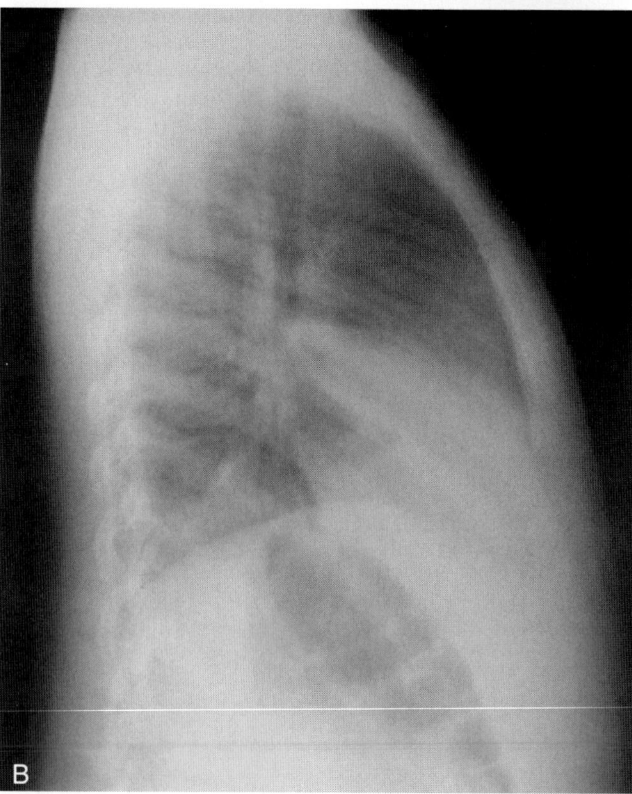

FIGURE 8–7 **A:** Right upper lobe pneumonia. (Courtesy of Robert Hendrickson, MD.) **B:** Right middle lobe pneumonia. (Courtesy of Christy Salvaggio, MD.)

Community-Acquired Pneumonia

Swapan Dubey

macrolide (azithromycin, clarithromycin) or doxycycline. Those patients with CPD/MRF should be treated with an antipneumococcal quinolone (gatifloxacin, gemifloxacin, levofloxacin, moxifloxacin, sparfloxacin) alone, or with the combination of a β-lactam (ceftriaxone, cefpodoxime, cefuroxime, high-dose amoxicillin, or amoxicillin/clavulanate) and a macrolide.[2]

Patients with advanced age, more severe symptoms, or hypoxemia may be treated as inpatients. Those without CPD/MRF may be treated with azithromycin monotherapy. Those with CPD/MRF may require the combination of a β-lactam and a macrolide or an antipneumococcal quinolone alone.[2]

Patients who require intensive care may be treated with a β-lactam plus a macrolide or a quinolone. Patients with bronchiectasis, malnutrition, chronic corticosteroid use, or recent antibiotic use require an antipseudomonal β-lactam (cefepime, imipenem, meropenem, piperacillin/tazobactam) with either an intravenous antipseudomonal quinolone (ciprofloxacin) or an intravenous aminoglycoside (gentamicin, tobramycin, amikacin) and a macrolide (azithromycin).[2,3]

REFERENCES

1. Halm EA, Teirstein AS. Management of community-acquired pneumonia. *N Engl J Med* 2002;347:2039–2045.
2. American Thoracic Society: Guidelines for the management of adults with community-acquired pneumonia. *Am J Respir Crit Care Med* 2001;163:1730–1754.
3. Bernstein JM. Treatment of community-acquired pneumonia-IDSA guidelines. Infectious Diseases Society of America. *Chest* 1999;115:9S–13S.

Aspiration Pneumonia

Swapan Dubey

Clinical Presentation

Symptoms may vary with regard to the volume, pH, and content of the aspirate. Common symptoms include cough, fever, myalgias, respiratory distress, and pleuritic chest pain. Severe symptoms may develop, including respiratory distress and hypoxemia.[1] Physical examination findings may include tachypnea, hypoxia, hypotension, and localized rhonchi, rales, or wheezes.[1] Fever has been noted in 50% of patients within 36 hours after aspiration.

Pathophysiology

Aspiration pneumonia is inflammation of the lung caused by aspiration of the contents of the nasopharynx or oropharynx.[1] The cause of this inflammation may be chemical, bacterial, mechanical, or a combination of all three.

Aspiration pneumonia is almost always a mixed-flora infection composed of anaerobic and microaerophilic bacteria. Organisms commonly involved are *Peptostreptococcus, Fusobacterium, Bacteroides melaninogenicus,* aerobic streptococci, and mixed aerobes or anaerobes present in the mouth.[1]

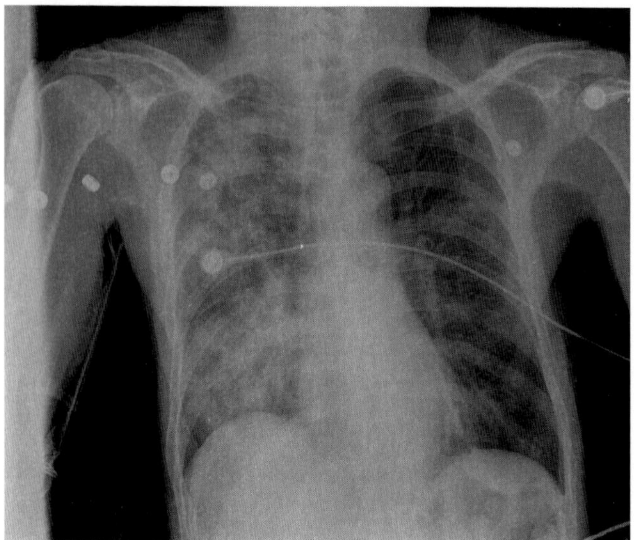

FIGURE 8–8 Multilobar aspiration pneumonia. (Courtesy of Alex Lapidus, MD.)

Diagnosis

The diagnosis of aspiration begins with a high index of suspicion. Patients at high risk of aspiration include those with seizure disorders, repeated vomiting, alcohol dependence, or excessive sedation.[1] Aspiration pneumonia should be considered in patients with these disorders who have developed respiratory distress, cough, or hypoxemia. Chest radiography may be initially normal because pulmonary inflammation and edema has not yet developed. Later in the course, the chest radiograph may demonstrate infiltrates in the inferior segment of the right upper lobe or in the apical segment of the lower lobe. Nonspecific laboratory findings may include leukocytosis with left shift, hypoxemia, and occasionally hypercapnia or hypoxemia.

Clinical Complications

Aspiration pneumonia can lead to progressive hypoxemia, mechanical ventilation, overwhelming infection, and pulmonary abscesses.[1]

Management

The treatment of patients with witnessed aspiration includes maintaining an adequate airway, suctioning particulate matter from the oropharynx, and providing supplemental oxygen to maintain the arterial partial pressure of oxygen (Pao_2). Empiric antibiotic therapy for witnessed aspiration is not well studied in the absence of a confirmed infectious process. Patients with confirmed infection requiring antibiotics should receive antibiotics with known activity against anaerobes, in addition to standard community-acquired pneumonia (CAP) therapy. Prophylactic corticosteroids are not generally necessary for patients with aspiration pneumonia.

Patients usually present to the emergency department (ED) with fever and respiratory symptoms and risk factors for aspiration. In this case, patients should be treated with antibiotics to cover CAP, as well as antibiotics that treat anaerobic infections.

REFERENCES

1. Marik PE. Aspiration pneumonitis and aspiration pneumonia. *N Engl J Med* 2001;344:665–671.

Acute Bronchitis

Swapan Dubey

Clinical Presentation

The predominant feature of acute bronchitis is cough, which is usually productive. Systemic symptoms such as fever, myalgias, headache, or rhinitis are variably present. If there is bronchospasm, the patient may have dyspnea, wheezing, or an unproductive cough.

Pathophysiology

Acute bronchitis is an infection of the conducting airways of the lungs. This produces inflammation, which leads to the production of exudate and, occasionally, bronchospasm. Most cases of acute bronchitis are caused by viruses, such as rhinovirus, influenza, respiratory syncytial virus, and adenovirus. Bacterial causes include *Bordetella pertussis, M. pneumoniae,* and *C. pneumoniae.*

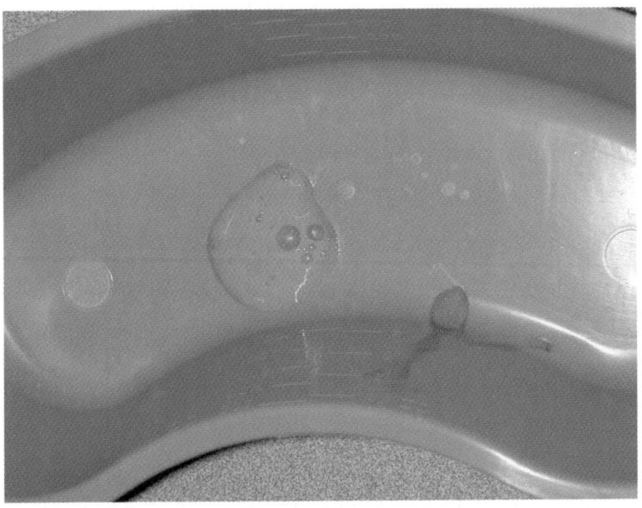

FIGURE 8–9 Green sputum is typical of bronchitis. (Courtesy of Robert Hendrickson, MD.)

Diagnosis

The diagnosis of acute bronchitis may be made clinically, because no confirmatory diagnostic tests are available. Patients typically present with a history of cough for less than 1 week. The physical examination is usually normal and without hypoxia. Wheezing may be present with associated bronchospasm. Chest radiography is indicated only to exclude pneumonia in patients who have fever, clinical toxicity, or pathologic findings on lung examination. Of note, the color of the sputum cannot be used to differentiate a bacterial from a viral infection. Blood and sputum studies are of limited utility and generally are not indicated.

Clinical Complications

Acute bronchitis usually resolves without sequelae, with or without intervention. The cough, however, may persist for several weeks.

Management

The routine use of antibiotics for acute bronchitis is controversial. Although antibiotics may decrease symptom duration by up to one-half day,[1] they are also associated with significant side effects (relative risk, 1.48).[1] Furthermore, because of concerns about worsening bacterial antibiotic resistance and limited efficacy, some guidelines have discouraged their use.[1] Clearly, a large clinical benefit from antibiotic therapy is unlikely and, in most cases, does not outweigh the risk of adverse reactions to the drugs. In patients with obstructive airway symptoms, wheezing, or a lower than expected peak flow, β2-agonists may be effective in decreasing cough.

REFERENCES

1. Edmonds ML. Evidence-based emergency medicine: antibiotic treatment for acute bronchitis. *Ann Emerg Med* 2002;40:110–112.

Chemical Pneumonitis

Mark Su

Clinical Presentation

Patients with chemical pneumonitis present with varying degrees of respiratory distress after some type of known or unknown exposure. Patients may exhibit any combination of respiratory symptoms, including tachypnea, cough, rales, rhonchi, wheezing, hypoxemia, cyanosis, and hemoptysis.

Pathophysiology

Mechanisms of pulmonary toxicity vary, based on the causative agent. All agents capable of causing chemical pneumonitis have three common mechanisms of pathogenesis: alveolar mucous membrane damage, systemic absorption, and asphyxiation.[1] Local alveolar damage may be caused by membrane irritation, capillary leakage, or burns from aerosolized caustics.

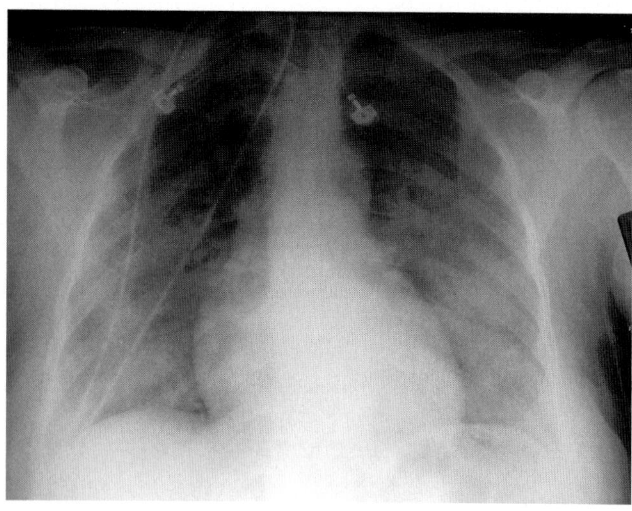

FIGURE 8–10 Pneumonitis from inhalation of trichloroethylene. (Courtesy of Robert Hendrickson, MD.)

Diagnosis

The history is of critical importance in diagnosis of chemically induced pneumonitis. Plain chest radiographs may be helpful in confirming the diagnosis. Depending on the degree of injury and the time since exposure, the chest film may reveal perihilar densities, unilateral or bilateral consolidation, well-defined nodules, interstitial pneumonitis, pneumatoceles, or fulminant acute lung injury (ALI).[2]

Clinical Complications

A critical acute complication is ALI, previously referred to as noncardiogenic pulmonary edema, or adult respiratory distress syndrome (ARDS). Secondary bacterial infections may occur. Long-term complications may include bronchiectasis, bronchiolitis obliterans, and permanent lung scarring and parenchymal destruction.[1]

Management

Uncomplicated chemical pneumonitis may be managed acutely with good supportive care. However, some inciting agents, including chlorine gas, phosgene, and nitrogen dioxide, are associated with delayed presentation of ALI and require monitoring for at least 24 hours. Intensive ventilatory support may also be required.[1] Specific therapy, such as nebulized sodium bicarbonate for chlorine gas inhalation, is rarely indicated.[3]

REFERENCES

1. White CS, Templeton PA. Chemical pneumonitis. *Radiol Clin North Am* 1992;30:1231–1243.
2. Kim KI, Kim CW, Lee MK, et al. Imaging of occupational lung disease. *Radiographics* 2001;21:1371–1391.
3. Chisolm CD, Singletary EM, Okerberg CV, et al. Inhaled sodium bicarbonate therapy for chlorine inhalational injuries. *Ann Emerg Med* 1989;18;466.

Aspirated Foreign Body

Michael Greenberg

Clinical Presentation

Aspirated foreign body (AFB) is primarily a pediatric problem. However, adults may also aspirate various foreign bodies. Patients may present with a variety of symptoms, including coughing, stridor, respiratory distress, choking, wheezing, chest pain, hemoptysis, fever, and cyanosis.[1-3]

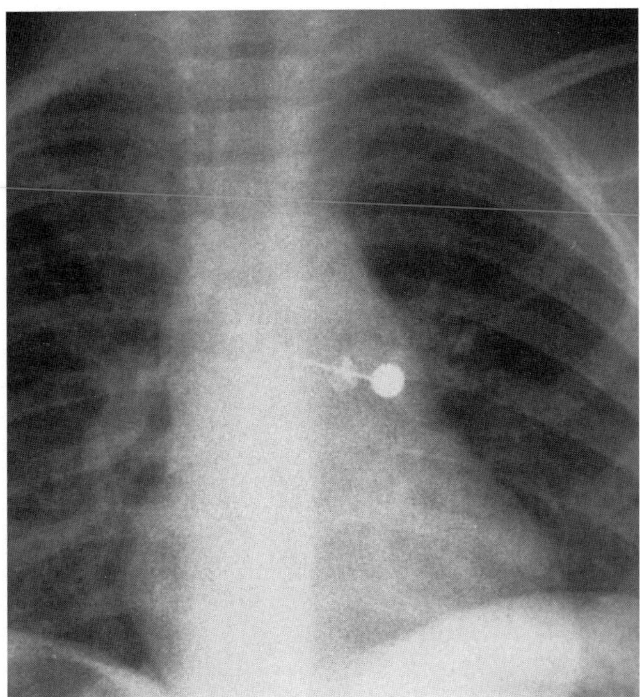

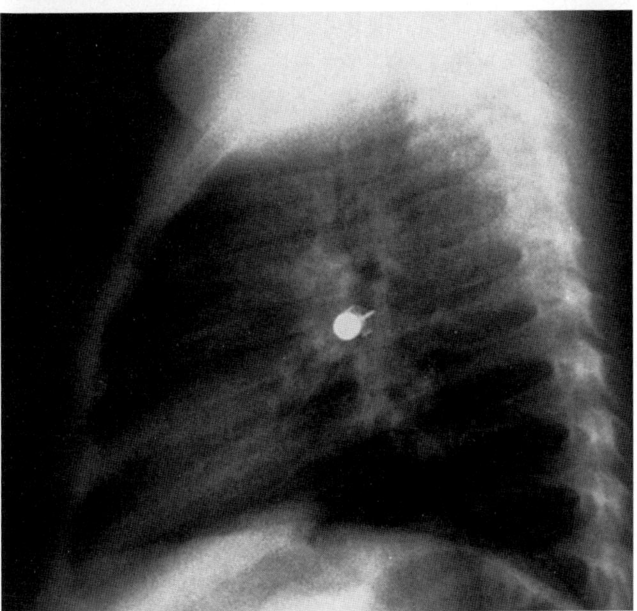

FIGURE 8–11 Two-view chest radiograph demonstrating an aspirated radiopaque foreign body (an earring) located in the left bronchus. (From Fleisher et al., with permission.)

Pathophysiology

Choking on food is the sixth most common cause of accidental deaths in children. Approximately 80% of pediatric AFBs are food materials, commonly peanuts or other nuts. Approximately 10% of AFBs are metallic.[1] Adults who are edentulous or mentally or neurologically impaired may be more prone to foreign body aspiration. AFBs are most commonly located in the right mainstem bronchus in children older than 3 years of age. In children younger than 3 years, the distribution between right and left is approximately equal.[2]

Diagnosis

AFB should be suspected based on history and physical examination. A chest radiograph should always be obtained, with the understanding that most AFBs are not radiopaque. Inspiratory and expiratory views are necessary in some cases, because air trapping may be the only radiographic indication of a nonradiopaque object. AFB bronchoscopy often is required to make the definitive diagnosis and should be pursued if the clinical suspicion is high, even in the face of negative findings on chest radiography. C-arm fluoroscopy may be helpful, especially for AFBs that are in the periphery of the respiratory tree.[1]

Clinical Complications

Complications include atelectasis, pneumonia, sepsis, and death.

Management

The mainstay of treatment is removal by bronchoscopy in most cases. If the clinical suspicion for AFB is high, or if the diagnosis cannot be clearly ruled out clinically, prompt on-site evaluation by an otolaryngologist prepared to perform bronchoscopy is essential.

REFERENCES

1. Deskin R, Young G, Hoffman R. Management of pediatric aspirated foreign bodies. *Laryngoscope* 1997;107:540–543.
2. Van Looij MA, Rood PP, Hoeve LJ, Borgstein JA. Aspirated foreign bodies in children: why are they more commonly found on the left? *Clin Otolaryngol* 2003;28:364–367.
3. Tan HK, Brown K, McGill T, Kenna MA, Lund DP, Healy GB. Airway foreign bodies (FB): a 10-year review. *Int J Pediatr Otorhinolaryngol* 2000;56:91–99.

Lung Abscess

Robert Hendrickson

Clinical Presentation

Patients with lung abscess present with fever (78%), productive cough (57%), chest pain (29%), malaise (21%), weight loss (15%), or hemoptysis (9%).[1] Abscesses typically occur in patients older than 60 years of age and in those with comorbid conditions such as chronic obstructive pulmonary disease (COPD), cancer, or immunocompromise.[1,2] Patients with acutely or chronically altered consciousness are also at higher risk for abscess formation due to aspiration.

Pathophysiology

Infection may develop secondary to aspiration of gastric or oral contents, but it may also occur through hematogenous spread (e.g., endocarditis) or alveolar spread (e.g., community-acquired pneumonia). Anaerobic organisms are typically found in community-acquired lung abscesses and in those caused by aspiration; they are associated with a low mortality rate.[2] Aerobes (e.g., *Klebsiella pneumoniae, Staphylococcus aureus, Pseudomonas aeruginosa*) may also be isolated, particularly in hospital-acquired cases. Aerobes are associated with high mortality rates (more than 50%).[1,2]

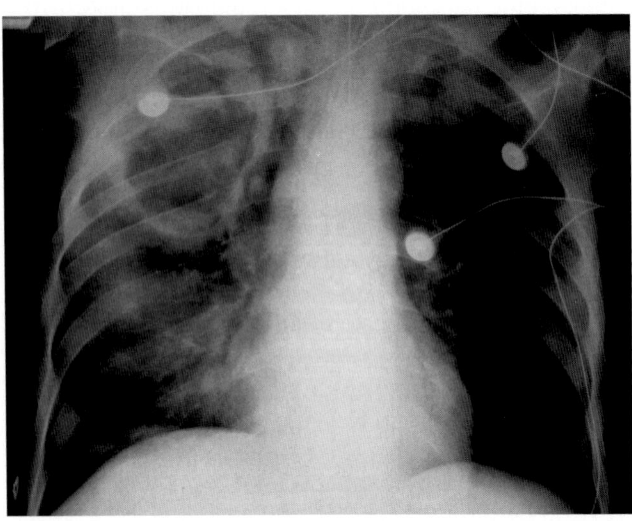

FIGURE 8-12 Right upper lobe lung abscess. (Courtesy of Mark Silverberg, MD.)

Diagnosis

The diagnosis is made from the clinical history and chest radiography. Occasionally, computed tomography (CT) scanning is helpful in detecting abscesses. A well-circumscribed capsule with an air–fluid level may be evident on chest radiography, typically in the right lower or right upper lobe.[1] Laboratory evaluation may reveal a leukocytosis.[1]

Clinical Complications

Complications include empyema, hemorrhage, adult respiratory distress syndrome (ARDS), sepsis, and death (15% to 20%).[1] Patients at higher risk of death include those with predisposing conditions and those with large abscesses.[1,2]

Management

Patients should be admitted to the hospital for intravenous (IV) antibiotics (e.g., clindamycin and cefoxitin). Percutaneous drainage and lobectomy are therapeutic options if conservative therapy fails (fewer than 10% of cases).[1]

REFERENCES

1. Hirshberg B, Sklair-Levi M. Nir-Paz R, Ben-Sira L, Krivoruk V, Kramer MR. Factors predicting mortality of patients with lung abscess. *Chest* 1999;115:746–750.
2. Mwandumba HC, Beeching NJ. Pyogenic lung infections: factors for predicting clinical outcome of lung abscess and thoracic empyema. *Curr Opin Pulm Med* 2000;6:234–239.

Sarcoidosis

Lisa Freeman

Clinical Presentation

Sarcoidosis is a multiorgan systemic granulomatous disease with a variable clinical picture. The lungs are the primary organ of pathology and are affected in more than 90% of patients. Dyspnea, dry cough, and chest pain occur in up to 50% of patients. Constitutional signs and symptoms, including fever, malaise, lymphadenopathy, and fatigue, are seen in one third of the patients. Clinically significant cardiac involvement is uncommon (approximately 5% of patients) and ranges from benign arrhythmias to high-grade heart block and sudden death.[1] Skin involvement usually manifests as erythema nodosum and lupus pernio. Other findings include uveitis, hypercalcemia, and arthralgias. Deforming arthritis is rare.[1]

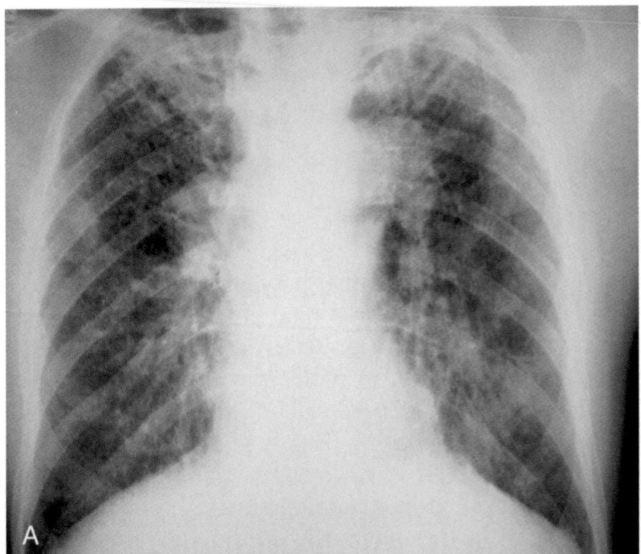

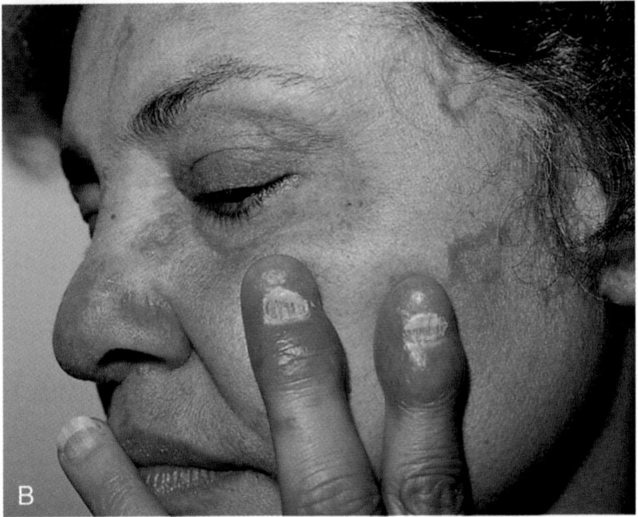

FIGURE 8–13 **A:** Sarcoidosis. Note prominent hilar adenopathy and the reticular/nodular pattern of the lung parenchyma. (Courtesy of Mark Silverberg, MD.) **B:** Annular lesions of the face with mild lupus pernio of the nose and severe involvement of the fingers and nails with sarcoidosis. (From Ostler, with permission.)

Pathophysiology

Sarcoidosis is a systemic granulomatous disease that affects mainly the lung and lymphatic system.[1] Symptoms are caused by local inflammatory reactions associated with noncaseating granulomas. Black women between the ages of 20 and 40 years seem to be the most commonly affected group, although the disease is seen in people of both sexes and all ages and races.[1]

The cause of sarcoidosis is unknown, but genetic, environmental, and immunologic factors have been postulated.[1] The myriad of clinical problems seen in sarcoidosis are caused by the presence of noncaseating granulomas and subsequent fibrosis of the affected organs.

Diagnosis

Sarcoidosis is often first suspected in a previously undiagnosed patient by the presence of bilateral hilar adenopathy on a chest radiograph. Radiographic changes progress from hilar adenopathy to interstitial lung disease and scarring. Suspicious chest radiographic findings should be followed with computed tomography (CT) of the chest and subsequent biopsy for confirmation.

Patients may also present to the emergency department (ED) with worsening respiratory symptoms secondary to worsening of sarcoidosis or secondary to an additional respiratory stress (e.g., pneumonia, upper respiratory tract infection), known as a "flare". Sarcoidosis is usually self-limited, and most patients have complete resolution of symptoms within 1 to 2 years. Approximately 10% progress to worsening fibrotic disease.

Clinical Complications

Complications include respiratory and cardiac decompensation, as well as metabolic complications such as hyponatremia, hypercalcemia, and renal insufficiency.

Management

Treatment of sarcoidosis includes corticosteroids, nonsteroidal antiinflammatory drugs (NSAIDs) (for arthralgias and erythema nodosum), methotrexate, azathioprine, cyclophosphamide, and chloroquine. Patients in the ED who have worsening respiratory symptoms should be evaluated for infectious causes (e.g., pneumonia, upper respiratory tract infection). Treatment with increased corticosteroids, followed by a taper, may be effective in decreasing respiratory symptoms in the acute setting.

REFERENCES

1. Statement on sarcoidosis. *Am J Respir Crit Care Med* 1999;160:736–755.

Tuberculosis

Lisa Freeman

Clinical Presentation

Patients with primary tuberculosis (TB) may report cough, fever, night sweats, and weight loss. Patients with reactivation of TB have a history of previous infection that has been latent. Reactivation of the latent infection may lead to pulmonary symptoms similar to those of primary TB, but with chest radiography findings localized in the upper lobes, as well as pleural effusion and hilar lymphadenopathy. Miliary TB is a systemic dissemination of TB that appears as multiple small nodules on chest radiography. Reactivation TB may also occur distant from the lungs (i.e., extrapulmonary TB) and may affect the liver, spleen, brain, adrenals, bones, vertebrae (Pott's disease), pericardium, peritoneum, or pleura. Reactivation of TB most commonly occurs in patients who are young, elderly, or immunosuppressed.

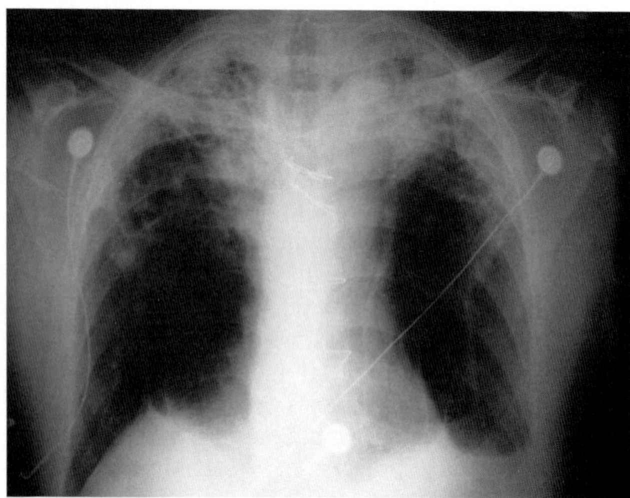

FIGURE 8–14 Chest radiograph demonstrating pulmonary tuberculosis. (Courtesy of Mark Silverberg, MD.)

Pathophysiology

Mycobacterium tuberculosis is a fastidious, acid-fast bacillus that is spread via aerosolization of respiratory droplets. There is initially no host reaction while the organisms multiply in the lungs. Over 4 to 6 weeks, the immune system responds and may be able to contain the infection in granulomas (i.e., tubercles), resulting in no further disease, or a progressive primary infection may occur, with development of a pleural effusion and lymphadenitis. Organisms that survive are contained by the immune system in tubercles that may caseate (necrose) or calcify (e.g., Ghon's complex). In most cases, the organisms remain in the tubercles, but some may enter the thoracic duct, spreading systemically and remaining dormant. TB can remain dormant for years after the initial infection and then reactivate, most frequently in the lung apex.

Diagnosis

Patients with typical symptoms (e.g., fever, night sweats, cough, weight loss) and potential exposure to TB should be placed in respiratory isolation for the protection of the emergency department (ED) staff. Chest radiography findings may include upper lobe necrotic granulomas with pleural effusion and hilar adenopathy. Findings may be atypical in patients with AIDS, and chest radiography may be normal in patients with extrapulmonary TB (mainly immunosuppressed or immunocompromised patients). Patients with positive radiographic findings should be admitted to an isolation room, and sputum specimens for acid-fast staining should be obtained for confirmation of the diagnosis. Consideration should be given to treating for community-acquired pneumonia, pending the results of the sputum tests. A protein purified derivative (PPD) skin test may be placed,[1] but it must be read in 48 to 72 hours. Routine laboratory analysis is generally unhelpful but may occasionally reveal hyponatremia or anemia.

Patients may also present to the ED with a positive PPD skin test. A positive PPD result means that the patient has been exposed to TB but is not necessarily symptomatic or infectious. PPD tests are positive if the area of induration is greater than 5 mm (in patients with HIV, immunosuppression, or abnormal chest radiograph); greater than 10 mm (in foreign-born patients, IV drug users, homeless patients, health care workers, and children younger than 4 years old); or greater than 15 mm (in all other patients).[2] A chest radiograph is indicated for patients with a new positive PPD. Patients who have positive PPD tests and findings on chest radiography may require admission to an isolation room, treatment, and sputum tests. If the chest radiograph is normal, outpatient therapy may be arranged, because the patient is not infectious.

Clinical Complications

Complications include multiorgan failure, drug resistance, and death.

Management

A healthy patient with a positive PPD result and a normal chest radiograph require a 6-month course of isoniazid (INH) or rifampin.[2,3] Patients with active disease require a multidrug regimen that may include INH, rifampin, ethambutol, and pyrazinamide.[3] Patients with known or suspected TB should be admitted to the hospital if they are actively coughing or have radiographic findings of TB, if the diagnosis is uncertain, if they cannot comply with therapy, or if evidence of multisystem disease is present. The patient should be treated in a negative-pressure ventilation room to avoid spread of the disease to staff and other patients.[3] High-efficiency particulate air (HEPA) masks are required for all staff while in respiratory contact with the patient.[4]

REFERENCES

1. Horsburgh CR Jr, Feldman S, Ridzon R. Practice guidelines for the treatment of tuberculosis. *Clin Infect Dis* 2000;31:633–639.
2. Jasmer RM, Nahid P, Hopewell PC. Clinical practice: latent tuberculosis infection. *N Engl J Med* 2002;347:1860–1866.
3. Treatment of tuberculosis. American Thoracic Society, CDC, and Infectious Diseases Society of America. *MMWR Morb Mortal Wkly Rep* 2003;52(RR-11): 1–77.
4. Small PM, Fujiwara PI. Management of tuberculosis in the United States. *N Engl J Med* 2001;345(3):189–200.

Pleural Effusion

Lisa Freeman

Clinical Presentation

The patient with pleural effusion may present with symptoms ranging from asymptomatic to marked respiratory distress. Often, the symptoms associated with a pleural effusion are caused by the underlying disease. A history of congestive heart failure (CHF), malignancy, liver disease, or kidney failure should be sought. The patient may present with a variety of complaints, including shortness of breath, chest pain, or shoulder pain. Physical examination may be normal in a patient with a small effusion. Larger effusions may cause decreased breath sounds, dullness to percussion, or a pleural friction rub. Stigmata of underlying illnesses should be sought.[1]

Pathophysiology

Pleural effusion is defined as the presence of an abnormally large amount of fluid in the space between the visceral and the parietal pleura. Depending on the content of this fluid, the effusion is a transudate or an exudate; the two types have different causes and different management strategies. A pleural effusion associated with a pulmonary infection is called a parapneumonic infection. The most common causes of pleural effusions in developed countries are CHF, malignancy, bacterial pneumonia, and pulmonary embolism (PE). In developing countries, the most common cause is tuberculosis (TB).[1]

Normally the pleural space has less than 30 mL of fluid, which functions primarily as a lubricant. Fluid balance is determined by the action of colloid and hydrostatic forces. A pleural effusion develops when the influx of fluid into the pleural space exceeds the efflux. A transudate is basically an ultrafiltrate of plasma, and the pleural surface is not involved in the primary pathologic process. Common causes of transudates include CHF, cirrhosis, pulmonary embolism, nephrotic syndrome, sarcoidosis, hypoalbuminemia, and trauma. An exudate is the result of a pathologic process involving the pleural surface or a disruption of lymphatic reabsorption. The most common causes of exudates are infectious, including pneumonia, parasitic or fungal infection, neoplastic disease, pancreatitis, connective tissue disease, or subdiaphragmatic abscess.[1]

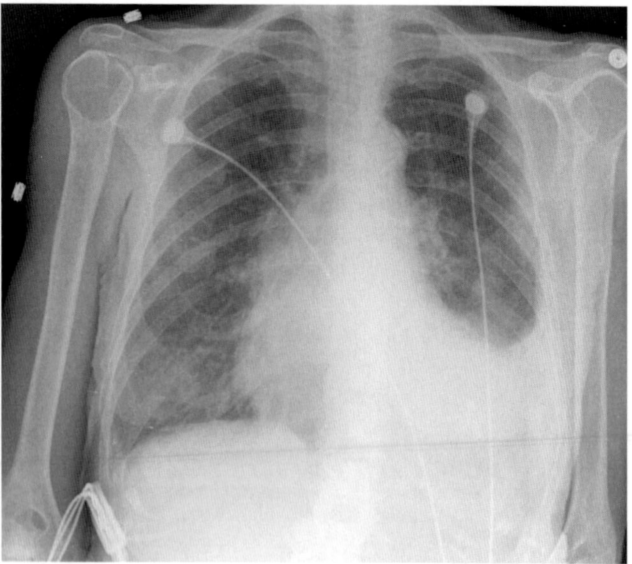

FIGURE 8–15 Left-sided pleural effusion. (Courtesy of Robert Hendrickson, MD.)

Diagnosis

A pleural effusion may be incidentally discovered on chest radiography, or radiography may be used to verify a suspected effusion. Blunting of the costophrenic angle is the most sensitive radiographic sign. This finding indicates the presence of at least 250 mL of fluid. Smaller effusions may be detected on lateral decubitus films. Laboratory studies may include complete blood count, blood chemistry measurements, arterial blood gas (ABG) analysis, coagulation studies, total protein determination, and measurement of the lactate dehydrogenase (LDH) concentration. The decision to perform thoracentesis in the emergency department (ED) should be individualized for each patient. Patients with large effusions causing respiratory compromise should undergo urgent thoracentesis in the ED. Most other patients with effusions can have thoracentesis deferred to the admitting or referral physician. If thoracentesis is performed, the fluid should be sent for white blood cell count, red blood cell count, LDH, protein, Gram strain, culture, amylase, and cytology if malignancy is suspected.[1]

In an exudate, the ratio of pleural fluid protein to serum protein is greater than 0.5, and the ratio of pleural fluid LDH to serum LDH is greater than 0.6. The presence of more than 100,000 red blood cells suggests malignancy, infarction, or trauma. The presence of more than 10,000 white blood cells suggests parapneumonic effusion, pancreatitis, collagen vascular disease, malignancy, or TB.

Clinical Complications

The most urgent complication of a pleural effusion is respiratory compromise.

Management

Patients with pleural effusions should be admitted to the hospital if there is respiratory or hemodynamic compromise, if the primary disease process requires admission, or if a parapneumonic effusion or empyema is suspected.[1]

REFERENCES

1. Light RW. Clinical practice: pleural effusion. *N Engl J Med* 2002;346: 1971–1977.

Empyema

Samuel Kim

Clinical Presentation

Patients with empyema present with variable symptoms that may range from nondescript chest pain with shortness of breath to frank sepsis. The classic presentation is that of dyspnea, fever, and pleuritic chest pain.

Pathophysiology

Empyema usually occurs after an episode of pneumonia. It may also occur as a result of fluid accumulation and secondary infection after surgery or trauma, or in association with malignancy. Anaerobic bacteria are responsible for most cases of empyema (76%).[1]

Diagnosis

Physical examination findings are essentially the same as for pleural effusions, including decreased breath sounds on the side of the affected lung and consolidation on percussion. Empyema is difficult to distinguish radiologically from a simple effusion on normal chest radiographs. Empyema may eventually become loculated as a late manifestation. Features suggestive of a loculated empyema include an irregular contour to the fluid/parenchyma interface and lack of a shift of fluid on lateral decubitus films. Empyema may be further characterized by ultrasonography and computed tomography (CT), both of which may be used to determine whether the empyema is loculated. Chest radiography may be used as an initial investigation, but ultrasonography, CT, or both are usually necessary to determine the presence of loculation. Analysis and culture of the pleural fluid is necessary for definitive diagnosis.[1]

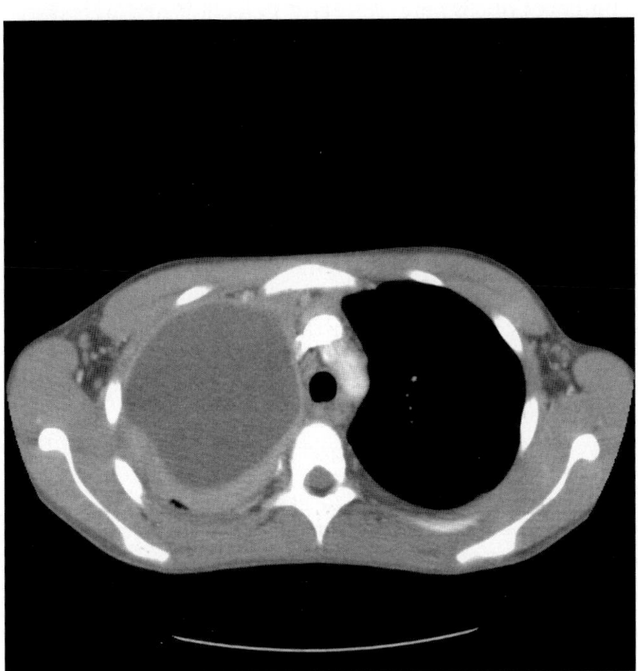

FIGURE 8–16 Loculated empyema. (Courtesy of John McManus, MD.)

Clinical Complications

Large fluid collections may compromise lung expansion, with resultant ventilation/perfusion mismatch and hypoxemia. A loculated empyema can cause adherence of the lung parenchyma to the chest wall. A chest tube or a thoracentesis into such an empyema may result in lung perforation or pneumothorax, or both.

Management

Empyema, when early in its course and not loculated, may be drained via simple thoracentesis. If it is loculated, decortication by a cardiothoracic surgeon may be needed. The fibrinous peel around the lung and around the abscess cavity may be removed laparoscopically. This procedure is known as a video-assisted thoracic surgery (VATS) procedure. Most patients who are diagnosed with empyema require hospital admission for definitive therapy.[1]

REFERENCES

1. Peek GJ, Morcos S, Cooper G. The pleural cavity. *BMJ* 2000;320: 1318–1321.

Pulmonary Fibrosis

Mark Su

Clinical Presentation

Patients with pulmonary fibrosis (PF) present with a history of progressive dyspnea on exertion for months to years and a nonproductive, paroxysmal cough. On physical examination, they have fine inspiratory crackles and may have digital clubbing.[1-4]

Pathophysiology

The pathogenesis of PF involves a combination of genetic and environmental factors. Inherited abnormalities of surface proteins, specifically a mutation in the surfactant protein C gene, have been implicated.[1] Although the most common cause is idiopathic, there are many identified environmental causes, such as infections, autoimmune disorders, and medications. Occupations that reportedly increase risk include farming, hair dressing, raising birds, stone cutting and polishing, and others involving exposure to animal and vegetable dust.[2]

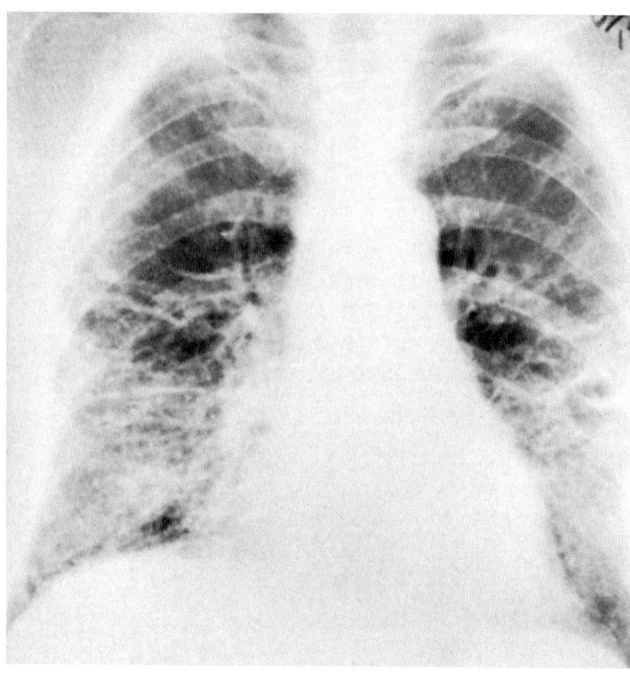

FIGURE 8–17 End-stage pulmonary fibrosis. (From George, with permission.)

Diagnosis

Imaging studies such as chest radiographs and high-resolution computed tomography (CT) are useful in making the diagnosis. High-resolution chest CT allows the correct diagnosis to be made in 60% to 80% of patients.[1] The performance of a surgical lung biopsy should be undertaken only if clinical findings in combination with chest CT results are not diagnostic. Plain radiographs usually demonstrate an interstitial reticular pattern.[1-4]

Clinical Complications

Complications include persistent cough and reduced exercise tolerance. Patients with idiopathic PF also have an increased risk of lung cancer, accounting for approximately 10% of all deaths related to this condition.[4]

Management

The goals of therapy are early detection and aggressive intervention, removal of the patient from exposure to possible causes, and palliation of complications. Although corticosteroid therapy is commonly used and is believed to be effective in up to 20% of patients, properly designed studies have not yet been performed.[1] Interferon-γ and nonsteroidal antiinflammatory drugs (NSAIDs) are currently being studied as potential therapies.[1,3] Disposition of patients presenting to the emergency department (ED) with this condition is based on the severity of clinical signs and symptoms (e.g., degree of hypoxia) and underlying comorbid conditions.[1]

REFERENCES

1. Green FH. Overview of pulmonary fibrosis. *Chest* 2002;122[6 Suppl]:334S–339S.
2. Baumgartner KB, Samet JM, Coultas DB, et. al. Occupational and environmental risk factors for idiopathic pulmonary fibrosis: a multicenter case-control study. *Am J Epidemiol* 2000;152:307–315.
3. American Thoracic Society. Idiopathic pulmonary fibrosis: diagnosis and treatment. International consensus statement: American Thoracic Society (ATS) and the European Respiratory Society (ERS). *Am J Respir Crit Care Med* 2000;161:646–664.
4. Collard HR, King TE Jr. Demystifying idiopathic interstitial pneumonia. *Arch Intern Med* 2003;163:17–29.

Lung Cancer

Lisa Freeman

Clinical Presentation

Signs and symptoms related to lung cancer include those related to the primary tumor, those related to localized spread, those related to metastatic disease, and those related to paraneoplastic syndromes. Most patients (73%) present with symptoms that are not directly related to the primary tumor, and many present with nonspecific symptoms such as anorexia, weight loss, and fatigue.

Pathophysiology

More than 90% of patients with lung cancer are symptomatic at presentation, from either the primary tumor, metastatic disease, or paraneoplastic syndromes.[1]

Occlusion of the distal bronchi by tumor or compression by enlarged lymph nodes can cause postobstructive pneumonia or wheezing or both. Tumor involvement of the airway may produce hemoptysis. Localized spread involving the recurrent laryngeal nerve leads to hoarseness, whereas phrenic nerve involvement causes paralysis of the hemidiaphragm, resulting in difficulty breathing deeply. Horner's syndrome occurs when the sympathetic chain is involved; it is marked by unilateral enophthalmos, ptosis, miosis, and ipsilateral anhydrosis.[1] Lung cancer can also invade locally to involve the heart and pericardium (15%). Distant metastases are commonly seen in the liver, various bones, adrenals, and central nervous system (CNS). Paraneoplastic syndromes are not directly related to the physical effects of the primary or metastatic tumor. Their exact pathogenesis is not fully understood, but they are thought to be caused by production of biologically active substances or possibly by an immune-mediated response.[1]

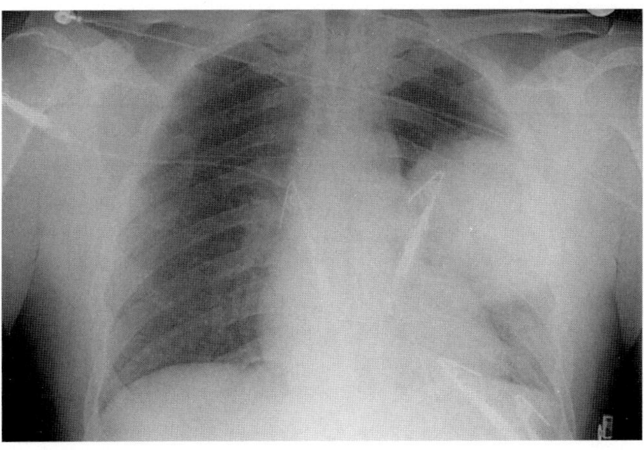

FIGURE 8–18 Left-sided pulmonary neoplasm. (Courtesy of Mark Silverberg, MD.)

Diagnosis

The chest radiograph is key in making at least a presumptive diagnosis of lung cancer. If the chest radiograph is normal or nondiagnostic in a patient whom the physician suspects may have lung cancer, computed tomography (CT) of the chest is warranted. Physical examination depends on the extent of disease. There may be neurologic findings related to intrathoracic spread of the tumor (recurrent laryngeal nerve or phrenic nerve paralysis or Horner's syndrome) or to CNS metastasis. There also may be signs and symptoms resulting from superior vena cava (SVC) obstruction, such as swelling of the face and upper extremities and plethora.

Clinical Complications

Complications of lung cancer may result from local invasion that causes bleeding and obstruction of the airways. The SVC may become obstructed or compromised, resulting in SVC syndrome. Various endocrine, neurologic, and systemic abnormalities caused by paraneoplastic syndromes may require more extensive diagnostic evaluations for identification.

REFERENCES

1. Beckles MA, Spiro SG, Colice GL, Rudd RM. Initial evaluation of the patient with lung cancer: symptoms, signs, laboratory tests, and paraneoplastic syndromes. *Chest* 2003;123[1 Suppl]:97S–104S.

Pancoast Tumor

Swapan Dubey

Clinical Presentation

Pancoast tumors involve the apex of the lung and invade the first and second ribs posteriorly. They typically involve the lower brachial plexus nerve roots (C8 and T1), producing pain that radiates down the inner arm and forearm. If the stellate ganglion is involved, Horner's syndrome may result. Horner's syndrome consists of unilateral ptosis (drooping of the eyelid), miosis (papillary dilatation), and anhydrosis (absence of sweating).[1]

Pathophysiology

A Pancoast tumor, also known as a superior sulcus tumor, occurs in the apex of the lung and invades chest wall structures.[1]

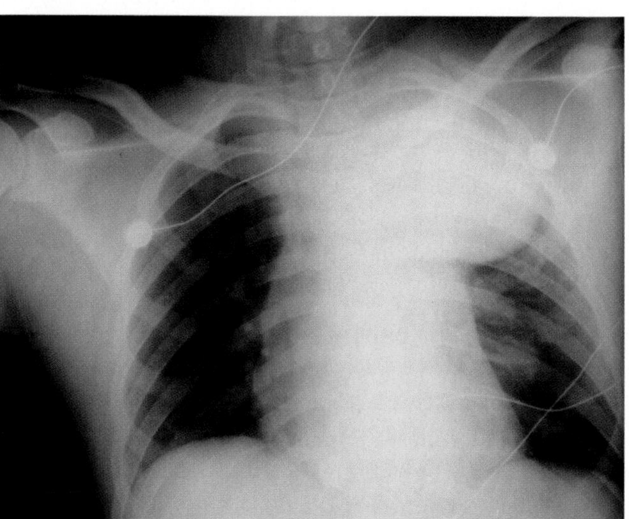

FIGURE 8–19 Left upper lobe Pancoast tumor. (Courtesy of Michael Lucchesi, MD.)

The tumor is a cancerous primary lung lesion, usually of squamous cell histology. The characteristic symptoms are caused by local invasion of contiguous structures, such as the upper ribs, subclavian vessels, chest wall, brachial plexus, and sympathetic chain.[1]

Diagnosis

The diagnosis may be suspected in patients with symptoms consistent with lower brachial plexus injury, Horner's syndrome, or lung cancer (weight loss, hemoptysis, dyspnea, cough). The diagnosis may be confirmed with chest radiography. Computed tomography (CT) of the chest can identify the extent of the tumor and nodal enlargement, as well as involvement of contiguous structures.[1]

Clinical Complications

Pancoast tumors may metastasize to other portions of the lung, as well as the liver, adrenals, and brain. Average survival time is 22 months, with a 5-year survival rate of approximately 27%.[1]

Management

Pancoast tumors usually are treated with radiation therapy followed by surgical resection.[1] Symptomatic patients who are first diagnosed in the emergency department (ED) usually require hospital admission.

REFERENCES

1. Detterbeck FC, Jones DR, Kernstine KH, Naunheim KS, American College of Physicians. Lung cancer: special treatment issues. *Chest* 2003;123[1 Suppl]:244S–258S.

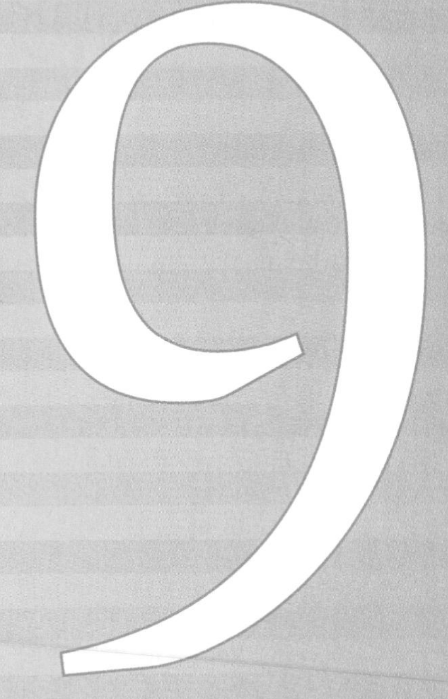

9 Gastrointestinal

9-1

Thermal Esophageal Injury

Michael Greenberg

Clinical Presentation

Patients with thermal esophageal injury (TEI) present with odynophagia, dysphagia, and retrosternal chest pain minutes to hours after swallowing excessively hot fluid.[1-3]

Pathophysiology

In some reports, histologic examination of the mucosa of the esophagus was "characterized by superficial mummified layers of necrotic anucleated nonviable squamous epithelium firmly adherent to the viable underlying squamous epithelial cells."[1] This is consistent with TEI resulting from direct contact with hot fluid to the mucosa.

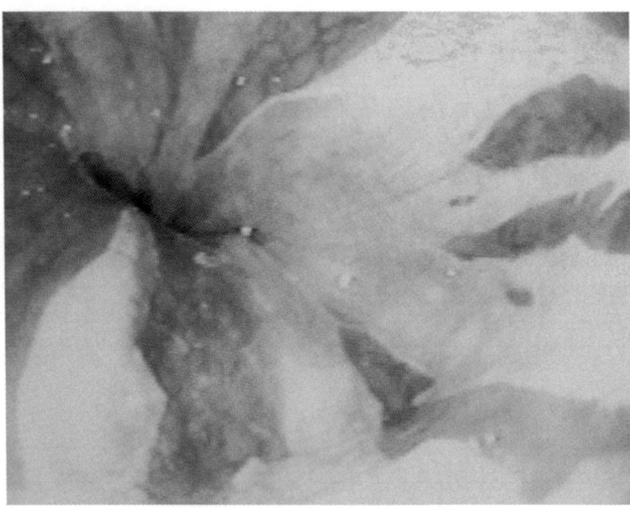

FIGURE 9-1 Local thermal injury of esophagus from hot fluid creates "candy cane" appearance of esophagus. (Reprinted from Cohen ME, Kegel JG. Candy cocaine esophagus. *Chest* 2002;121:1701-1703, with permission.)

Diagnosis

At endoscopy, a characteristic pattern of alternating white and pink bands or stripes is seen that reflects the passage of the hot fluid through the esophagus. This has been termed "candy-cane esophagus."[1,2]

Clinical Complications

Complications include esophageal perforation, esophagitis, infection, and stricture formation.[3]

Management

Concomitant disease must be ruled out, especially in patients who complain of chest pain. Referral for immediate endoscopy is essential if TEI is suspected. Steroid administration and prophylactic antibiotics are controversial and should be considered in consultation with the ear, nose, and throat (ENT) surgeon who will be caring for the patient.

REFERENCES

1. Dutta SK, Chung KY, Bhagavan BS. Thermal injury of the esophagus. *N Engl J Med* 1998;339:480-481.
2. Cohen ME, Kegel JE. Candy cocaine esophagus. *Chest* 2002;121: 1701-1703.
3. Javors BR, Panzer DE, Goldman IS. Acute thermal injury of the esophagus. *Dysphagia* 1996;11:72-74.

Gastroesophageal Reflux Disease

Derek Halvorson

Clinical Presentation

Gastroesophageal reflux disease (GERD) manifests as "heartburn"; patients describe a burning sensation in the epigastrium and lower substernal chest region. The sensation may progress into the throat or radiate into the back. Patients may complain of a sour taste in the mouth, persistent cough, wheezing, or hoarseness. Less commonly, patients may report dysphagia or a foreign body (FB) sensation in the throat. Symptoms may be more common at night (while lying supine) or after eating, especially after a large meal.[1]

Pathophysiology

GERD is a condition in which gastric acid secretion irritates and inflames the esophagus due to backward flow of gastric content.[1] GERD is caused by the movement of gastric contents cephalad, into the esophagus, as a result of transient laxity of the lower esophageal sphincter (LES). Symptoms may be precipitated by exercise, bending forward, lying down, or ingestion of certain foods (peppermint, alcohol, onions, or fat).

Diagnosis

The diagnosis is made by recognition of the typical history and elimination of more serious causes of the symptomatology. A 2-week treatment trial with a proton pump inhibitor (PPI) may provide symptomatic relief and sensitivity and specificity equivalent to the more invasive gold standard, esophageal monitoring.[1]

Outpatient endoscopy may be useful for patients with treatment failure, symptoms of complications (Barrett's esophagus, strictures, esophagitis), dysphagia, bleeding, chest pain, choking, weight loss, or persistent symptoms.[1,2]

Management

The treatment for GERD requires long-term modification of lifestyle and other medication interventions. Patients should be instructed to avoid large meals and not to lie down for 3 to 4 hours after eating. Patients should avoid caffeinated beverages, peppermint, fatty foods, onions, chocolate, spicy foods, citrus foods, alcohol, and tomato-based products. Lifestyle changes include discontinuation of smoking, weight loss, and elevation for the head of the bed. If there is no concern for other possible causes or complications (perforation, gastrointestinal [GI] bleeding, ulceration, or cardiac, pulmonary, or vascular symptoms), the patient can be referred to a primary care physician for follow-up and consideration for further testing such as a 24-hour pH monitoring, endoscopy, or motility studies as needed.[1,2]

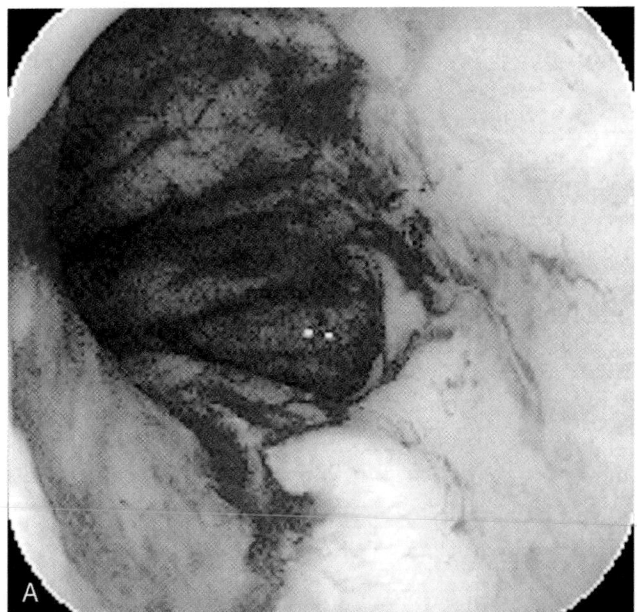

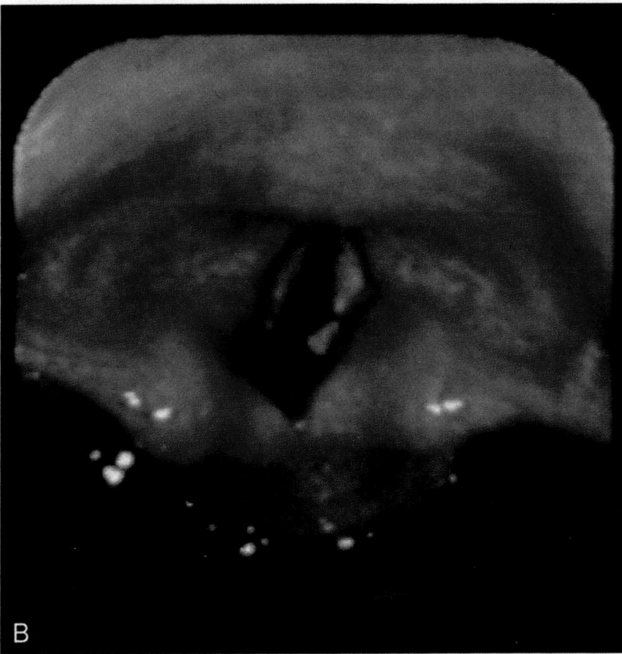

FIGURE 9–2 **A:** Endoscopic view of an oozing distal esophageal ulcer. (From Yamada, with permission.) **B:** Edema and erythema of the vocal cords and posterior glottis (reflux laryngitis). (From Yamada, with permission.)

REFERENCES

1. Dent J, Jones R, Kahrilas P, Talley NJ. Management of gastro-oesophageal reflux disease in general practice. *BMJ* 2001;322:344–347.
2. DeVault KR, Castell DO. Updated guidelines for the diagnosis and treatment of gastroesophageal reflux disease. *Am J Gastroenterol* 1999;94:1434–1442.

Esophageal Foreign Body

Derek Halvorson

Clinical Presentation

Most esophageal foreign bodies (FBs) occur in children younger than 4 years of age. Children may ingest a variety of small objects.[1] Prisoners and psychiatric patients may ingest potentially harmful objects for a variety of reasons. In adults, the most commonly seen esophageal FBs are food-related boluses that are accidentally or purposefully ingested.

Children with a history of FB ingestions may be brought to the emergency department (ED) by a parent or a sibling, and they are often asymptomatic (7% to 35%).[2] Adults more commonly have symptoms on presentation, and they often report anorexia, salivation, chest pain, dysphagia, or vomiting. Other complaints may include wheezing (often new-onset), persistent cough, stridor, choking, and recurrent pneumonia.

Pathophysiology

Esophogeal foreign body ingestions are found at one of three anatomic narrowings: (1) the cricopharyngeus muscle at the thoracic inlet, (2) the level of the aortic arch, and (3) the lower esophageal sphincter (LES).[2] Most objects, once they reach the LES, pass without incident through the intestinal tract. Large objects (greater than 5 cm long or 2 cm wide) and sharp objects may be exceptions to this rule. In children, esophageal FBs are most commonly found at the cricopharyngeus muscle (approximately 75% of children and 25% of adults). Conversely, retained esophageal FBs in adults are more commonly found at the LES (approximately 70% of adults and 10% of children).

Diagnosis

Clinical suspicion should be confirmed with an anteroposterior (AP) and lateral chest and abdominal radiograph, as well as a lateral neck radiograph. Coins in infants and children appear circular on the AP film and flat on the lateral film because of the flat coronal orientation of the esophagus within the mediastinum. In the airway, however, coins may appear either flat or "on edge" on the AP radiographs. Patients who have swallowed food boluses should similarly undergo plain radiography to look for imbedded bones. An esophagogram with barium or Gastrografin is indicated for radiolucent ingested objects. Computed tomography (CT) of the esophagus is reliable for identifying FBs in the esophagus and is superior to plain films for identifying fish or chicken bones (successful in up to 83% of patients with negative plain radiographs).

Clinical Complications

Retained esophageal FBs can cause a wide range of complications, the severity of which is often related to the duration of the entrapment. Complications include mucosal scratches or abrasions, esophageal stricture, retropharyngeal abscess, and esophageal perforation leading to fistula formation, mediastinitis, pneumomediastinum, pneumothorax, vascular injuries, and pericarditis or pericardial tamponade. Small disk batteries pose a substantial threat, because esophageal necrosis and perforation can occur within 6 hours.

Management

Management depends on the location and type of object as well as the clinical circumstances. Any evidence of airway compromise (e.g., stridor, wheezing, dyspnea) should be managed first by securing the airway if respiratory failure is imminent, followed by urgent consultation for endoscopic removal. If there is evidence for complete esophageal obstruction (i.e., drooling), the patient should be kept in the sitting position with a suction catheter to aid with oral secretions.

Uncomplicated retained FBs can be removed by other techniques. Single, smooth, and blunt radiopaque items that have been retained for less than 72 hours can be removed with the use of a Foley catheter. This procedure is most commonly performed on objects retained high in the thoracic inlet and is often done under fluoroscopic guidance. Removal is successful more than 90% of the time, but the patient may be at risk for aspiration.[1,2] If the FB is at the distal esophagus, is smooth and not caustic, and has been retained for less than 24 hours, a period of observation and oral feeding is reasonable. However, FBs should not be allowed to remain in the esophagus.[1]

Retained button batteries in the esophagus are a serious threat and require urgent transfer and removal to prevent burns (within 4 hours) and perforation (within 6 hours). Batteries located less than 15 mm beyond the gastroesophageal junction may be observed, with repeat radiography in 1 week if the battery does not pass. If the battery is more than 15 mm past the gastroesophageal junction, repeat radiography within 48 hours is recommended. Endoscopic removal is indicated if the battery is still in the stomach after 48 hours.[3]

REFERENCES

1. McGahren ED. Esophageal foreign bodies. *Pediatr Rev* 1999;20: 129–133.
2. Chen MK, Beierle EA. Gastrointestinal foreign bodies. *Pediatr Ann* 2001;30:736–742.
3. Litovitz T, Schmitz BF. Ingestion of cylindrical and button batteries: an analysis of 2382 cases. *Pediatrics* 1992;89:747–757.

Esophageal Foreign Body

Derek Halvorson

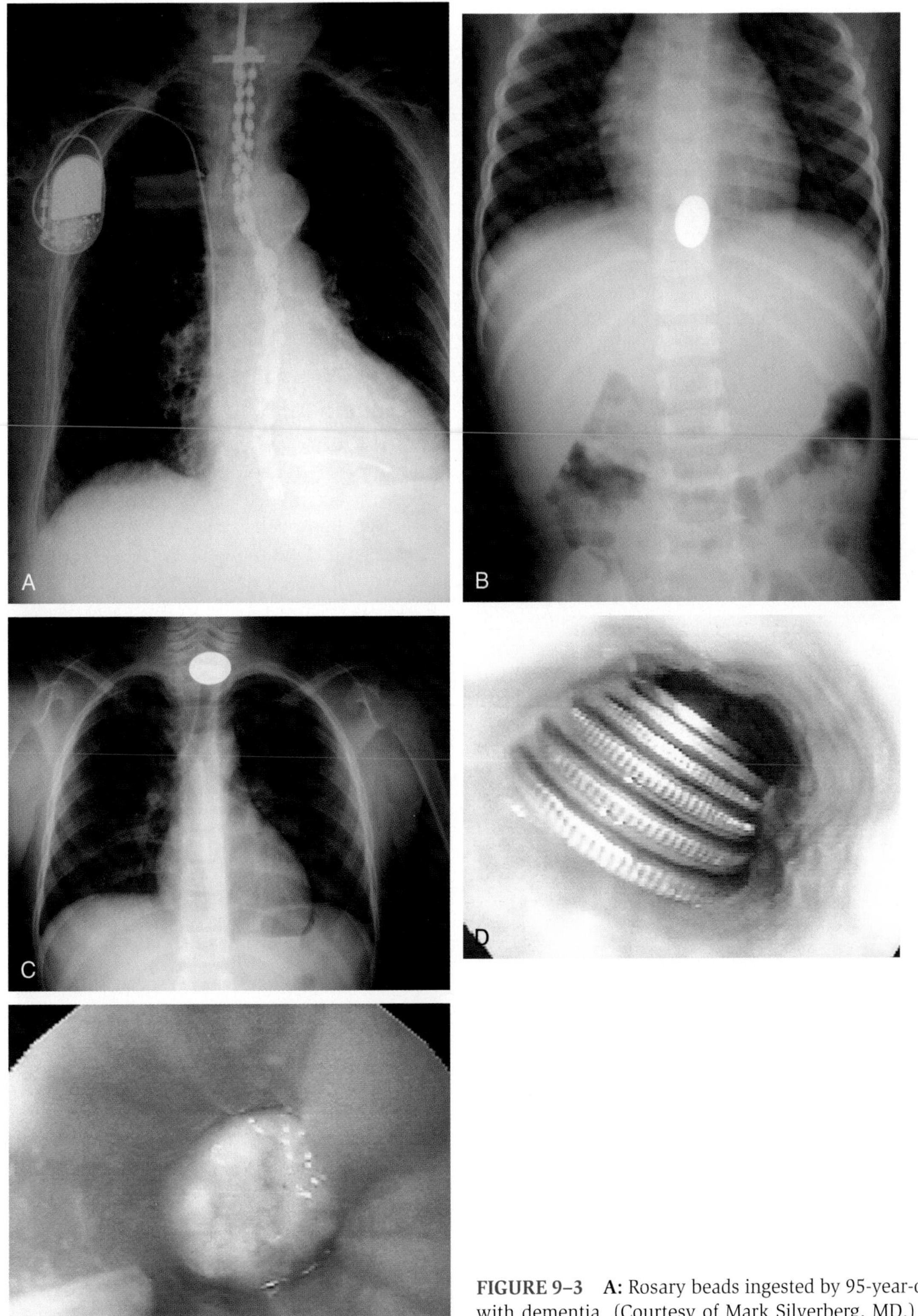

FIGURE 9–3 **A:** Rosary beads ingested by 95-year-old woman with dementia. (Courtesy of Mark Silverberg, MD.) **B:** Coin at the lower esophageal sphincter. (Courtesy of Robert Hendrickson, MD.) **C:** Coin in the thoracic inlet. (Courtesy of Donald Sallee, MD.) **D:** Change in the amount of $1.30 in the esophagus. (From Yamada, with permission.) **E:** Food impaction in the distal esophagus. (From Yamada, with permission.)

Barrett's Esophagus

John Curtis

Clinical Presentation

Barrett's esophagus, although associated with both reflux of gastric contents into the esophagus and the eventual development of esophageal adenocarcinoma, is typically an asymptomatic clinical entity that is found during endoscopy for symptomatic gastroesophageal reflux disease (GERD).[1-3]

Pathophysiology

The chronic reflux of gastric contents causes damage to the esophageal epithelium. During the healing process, the mucosa takes on the characteristics of specialized intestinal cells. This abnormal mucosa is at increased risk for neoplastic transformation; esophageal adenocarcinoma develops at the rate of 0.5% per patient-year.

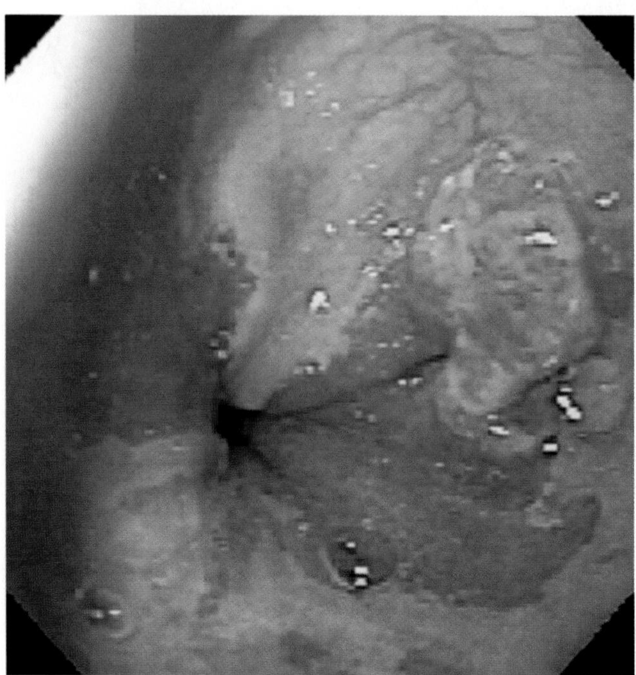

FIGURE 9–4 Barrett's esophagus with an early adenocarcinoma identified on surveillance endoscopy. (From Yamada, with permission.)

Diagnosis

Diagnosis is made by endoscopy. The typical whitish squamous epithelium is seen to be replaced by beefy red columnar epithelium, more typical of intestinal columnar epithelium.[1] Biopsy confirms the intestinal morphology of the epithelium and allows for detection of the dysplasia associated with neoplastic transformation.

Clinical Complications

Adenocarcinoma may complicate untreated Barrett's esophagus.

Management

Antireflux therapy with proton pump inhibitors (PPIs) or histamine H_2 receptor blockers does not effectively reduce the incidence of carcinoma. Antireflux surgery, however, has been shown to cause regression.[2] For patients with documented Barrett's esophagus, surveillance and therapy are determined by the findings on endoscopy. For those without dysplasia, routine endoscopy is recommended every 3 to 5 years. For those with low-grade dysplasia, repeat endoscopy at 6 and 12 months should be followed by annual evaluations to screen for progression.[1-3] High-grade dysplasia is treated with esophagectomy or intensive surveillance in suitable candidates. In those patients who are deemed to be poor surgical candidates, endoscopic ablation is a potential option.[3]

REFERENCES

1. Spechler SJ. Managing Barrett's oesophagus. *BMJ* 2003; 326:892–894.
2. Gurski RR, Peters JH, Hagen JA, DeMeester SR, Bremner CG, Chandrasoma PT, DeMeester TR. Barrett's esophagus can and does regress after antireflux surgery: a study of prevalence and predictive features. J Am Coll Surg 2003;196:706–712, discussion 712–713.
3. Spechler SJ. Barrett's esophagus. *N Engl J Med* 2002;346:836–842.

Esophageal Stricture

Gregory Schneider

Clinical Presentation

Patients with esophageal stricture complain of difficulty swallowing solids, which may progress to difficulty swallowing liquids. Patients may also complain of painful swallowing.[1]

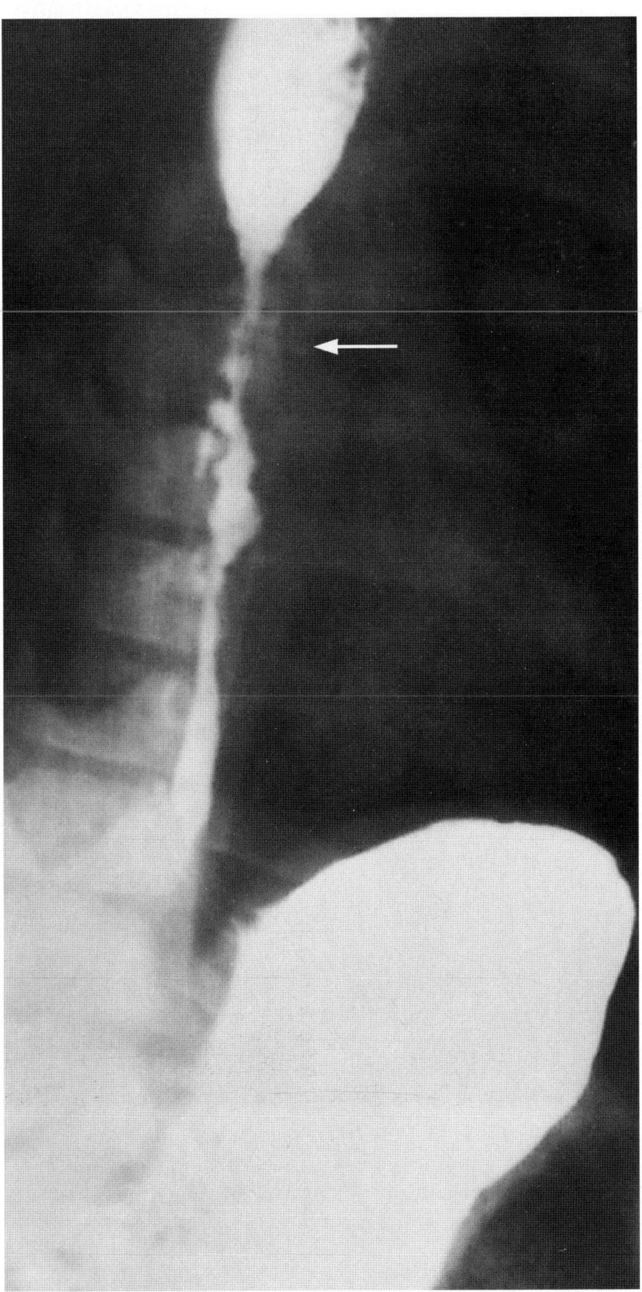

FIGURE 9–5 Esophageal stricture caused by caustic injury to the esophagus. (From Yamada, with permission.)

Pathophysiology

More than 90% of esophageal strictures arise as a complication of long-term gastroesophageal reflux disease (GERD). Stricture formation is preceded by ulcerative esophagitis, leading to full-thickness esophageal inflammation and eventually to scar tissue and contraction. Strictures may also result from ingestion of caustic substances, from extrinsic compression by tumors or anatomic prominences (enlarged thyroid, cardiac or aortic compression), or from surgery. Strictures may also be congenital.[1,2]

Diagnosis

History is the key to suspecting esophageal stricture. Patients typically have a history of dysphagia and long-term GERD. Barium swallow esophagography should be performed to look for a narrowing of the esophagus. Once an esophageal stricture is identified, patients must be referred to a gastroenterologist for endoscopy and biopsy to rule out a malignancy. Antacid therapy should also begin once a stricture is diagnosed.[1,2]

Clinical Complications

Malignant transformation may occur secondary to GERD. Barrett's esophagus is a well-known complication of GERD and progresses to cancer in 5% to 10% of patients.[1,2]

Management

Endoscopy and biopsy are required in every new case. Once malignancy is ruled out, the patient usually undergoes a series of esophageal dilations. This treatment has been shown to effectively and safely manage esophageal strictures. If it is performed properly, the percentage of esophageal rupture is less than 1%.[1,2]

REFERENCES

1. Henderson RD. Management of the patient with benign esophageal stricture. *Surg Clin North Am* 1983;63:885–903.
2. Broor SL, Raju GS, Bose PP, et al. Long term results of endoscopic dilatation for corrosive oesophageal strictures. *Gut* 1993;34: 1498–1501.

Esophageal Diverticula

Christopher Keane

Clinical Presentation

Dysphagia is the most common symptom of esophageal diverticula. Large diverticula can become filled with food, causing regurgitation and aspiration. Patients also complain of chest pain or upper gastrointestinal (GI) bleeding.[1–3]

Pathophysiology

An esophageal diverticulum is an outpouching of the esophagus. A true diverticulum contains all layers of the intestinal tract wall. A false diverticulum (pseudodiverticulum) occurs when the mucosa and submucosa herniate through a defect in the muscular wall. Most esophageal diverticula are thought to be caused by an underlying motility disorder. However, structural lesions, incomplete relaxation of the upper or lower esophageal sphincter, or stricture may also play a role. Symptoms may be related to the location of the diverticulum. Zenker's diverticula are located in the hypopharynx. Midesophageal diverticula are rare. Diverticula occurring in the lower esophagus (6 to 10 cm from the lower esophageal sphincter [LES]) are called epiphrenic diverticula.[1] Rarely, esophageal intraluminal diverticulosis occurs, in which numerous, 1- to 4-mm, saccular outpouchings form in the wall.[1]

Diagnosis

The physical examination findings usually are normal. In Zenker's diverticulum, patients may present with a neck mass or halitosis. Patients may also have signs of aspiration pneumonia. Barium swallow esophagography is the radiographic test of choice. Endoscopy, esophageal manometry (indispensable for detection of any motor alterations, which are often at the root of the pathogenesis for the diverticulum), and 24-hour pH monitoring are all used to diagnose this condition. Laboratory testing is generally not helpful.[1–3]

Clinical Complications

Recurrent aspiration pneumonia can complicate large esophageal diverticula. Carcinoma, fistulization, and perforation are uncommon complications.[2]

Management

Asymptomatic patients can benefit from surveillance. Patients with pulmonary aspiration may require surgery.[3]

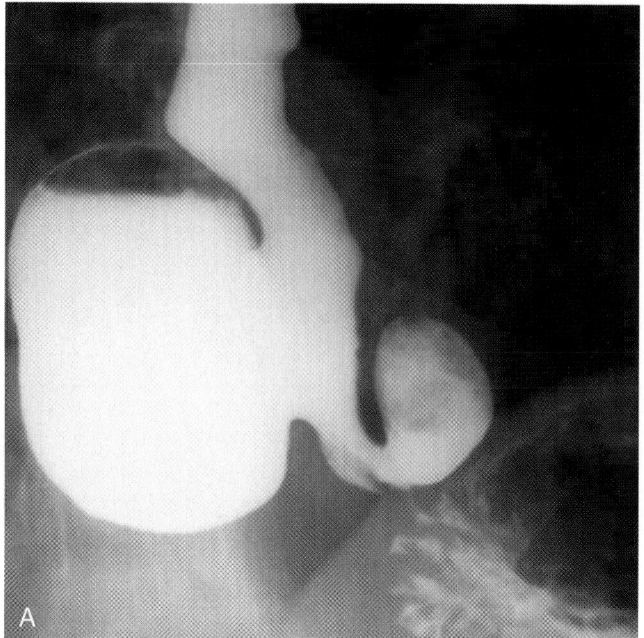

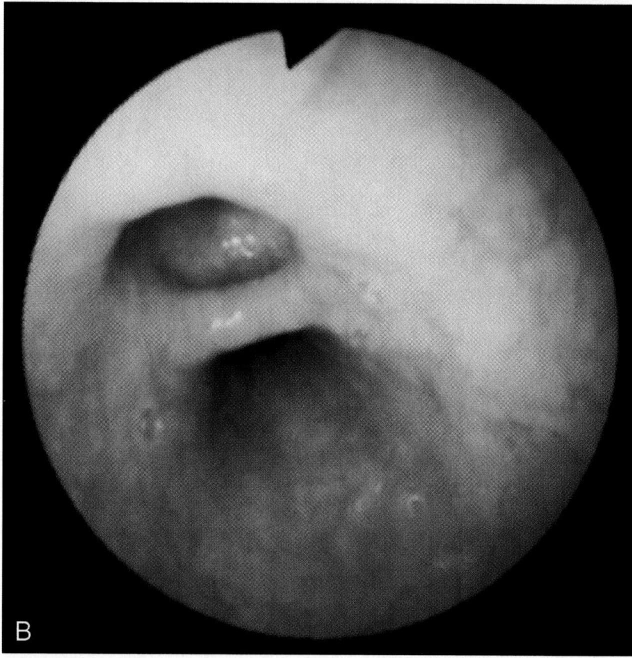

FIGURE 9–6 A: Barium esophagogram demonstrating an esophageal epiphrenic diverticulum. (From Yamada, with permission.) **B:** Midesophageal diverticulum. The lumen is in the center of the field. (From Yamada, with permission.)

REFERENCES

1. Dado G, Bresadola V, Terrosu G, Bresadola F. Diverticula of the midthoracic esophagus: pathogenesis and surgical treatment. *Surg Endosc* 2002;16:871.
2. Lopez A, Rodriguez P, Santana N, Freixinet J. Esophagobronchial fistula caused by traction esophageal diverticulum. *Eur J Cardiothorac Surg* 2003;23:128–130.
3. Ipek T, Eyuboglu E. Laparoscopic resection of an esophageal epiphrenic diverticulum. *Acta Chir Belg* 2002;102:270–273.

Achalasia

Cameron Symonds and Jonathan Glauser

Clinical Presentation

Patients with achalasia present with dysphagia, chest pain, regurgitation, weight loss, and coughing. Dysphagia occurs with both solids and liquids, differentiating the process from obstructive strictures and tumors. Swallowing may be improved by standing or by raising the arms above the head. The chest pain is characterized by retrosternal burning pain and is precipitated by eating. Regurgitation can lead to nocturnal cough, aspiration, and respiratory distress. Patients with advanced disease commonly have significant weight loss. Age at onset typically ranges from 25 to 60 years.

Pathophysiology

Achalasia is a primary motility disorder of the esophagus characterized by a lack of esophageal peristalsis and a hypertonic lower esophageal sphincter (LES). There is an absence of inhibitory ganglion cells throughout the esophageal wall, resulting in unopposed acetylcholine stimulation of the LES and resultant hypertonicity. Persistently elevated pressures lead to mechanical dilation of the esophageal wall and decreased peristalsis.

Diagnosis

Barium esophagography is the initial study of choice. Classically, the contrast medium is retained in the atonic esophagus and the nonskeletal muscular distal esophagus is dilated. The dilatation tapers abruptly at the LES, creating a "bird-beak" appearance on the film. A chest radiograph may demonstrate a double mediastinal stripe and a retrocardiac air–fluid level. Endoscopy may rule out malignancy, stricture, or coexistent pathology such as candidal infection. Esophageal manometry is useful if radiographs are equivocal.[1]

Clinical Complications

Chronic irritation of the esophageal mucosa can cause esophagitis, metaplasia, or squamous cell carcinoma of the esophagus. Nocturnal cough and aspiration may occur.

Management

Therapy is palliative and is directed at relieving obstructive symptoms. Calcium-channel blockers and nitrates can improve LES relaxation and offer mild symptomatic relief early in the course of the disease. Endoscopically guided injections of botulinum toxin into the hypertonic LES produce transient focal neuromuscular paralysis. Symptoms recur in most patients by 1 year. Mechanical dilation or myotomy of the LES has been successful in more than 50% of cases.[2]

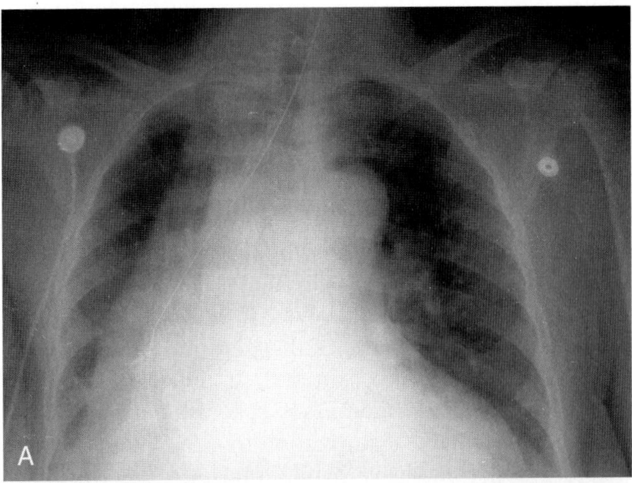

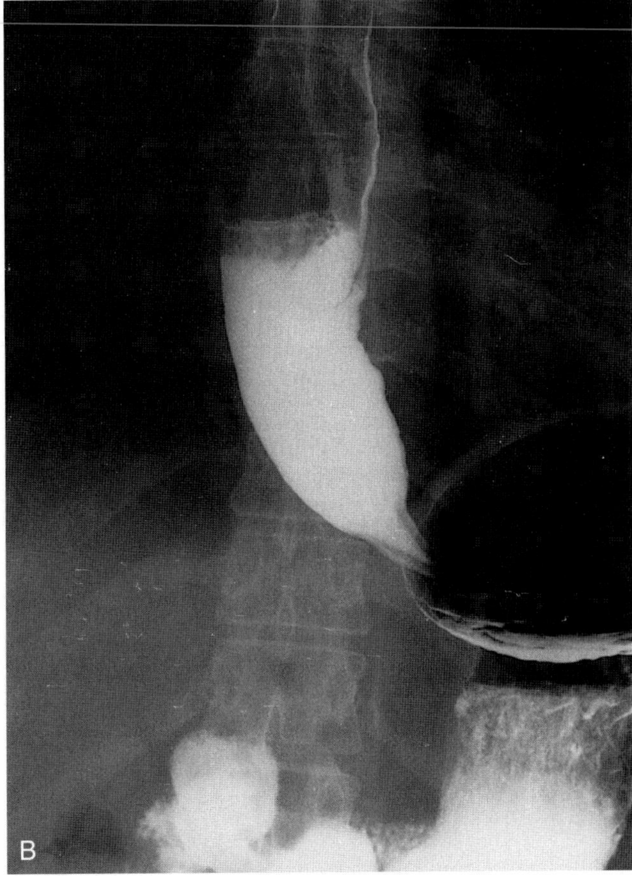

FIGURE 9–7 **A:** Radiographic findings consistent with achalasia. (Courtesy of Mark Silverberg, MD.) **B:** Barium esophagogram showing achalasia. (From Yamada, with permission.)

REFERENCES

1. Ferguson MK. Achalasia: current evaluation and therapy. *Ann Thorac Surg* 1991;52:336–342.
2. Patti MG, Fisichella PM, Perretta S, et al. Impact of minimally invasive surgery on the treatment of esophageal achalasia: a decade of change. *J Am Coll Surg* 2003;196:698–703.

Candidal Esophagitis

Jason Kitchen

Clinical Presentation

Patients with candidal esophagitis present with dysphagia, odynophagia, and retrosternal pain. Occasionally, they may have only constitutional symptoms such as fever.[1]

Pathophysiology

Candida albicans is the species implicated in most patients with candidal esophagitis. Little is known about host and yeast factors involved in the pathogenesis of esophageal candidiasis, but they are most likely to be similar to those involved in oral candidiasis (defects in either T-helper or T-suppressor cell function, accompanied by increased transformation of *Candida blastoconidia* to the more invasive hyphal phase).[1]

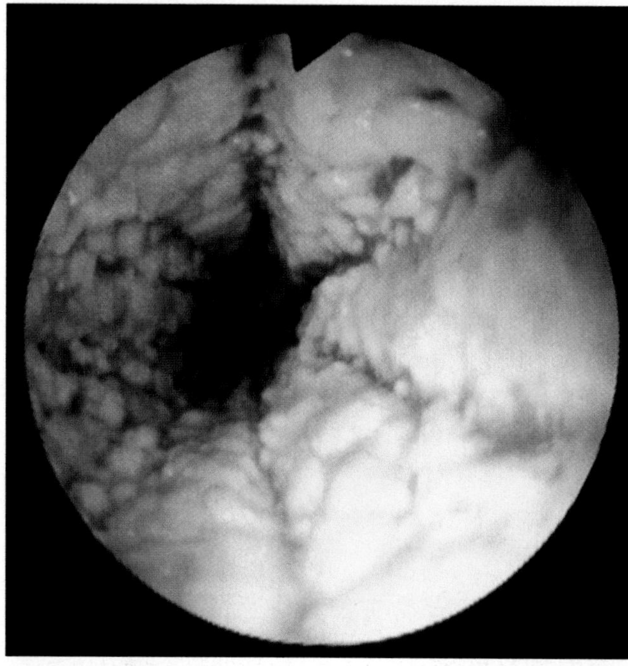

FIGURE 9–8 Severe candidiasis of the esophagus in a patient with acquired immunodeficiency syndrome. (From Yamada, with permission.)

Diagnosis

Endoscopy provides the most rapid diagnosis and the one with the highest sensitivity. The characteristic endoscopic appearance is yellow-white plaques on an erythematous background, with varying degrees of ulceration. However, erythema in the absence of plaques may be the only finding. Biopsy is the only definitive method of diagnosis. In patients with acquired immunodeficiency syndrome (AIDS), it is not uncommon to identify more than one agent causing esophagitis.[1]

Clinical Complications

Candidal esophagitis occurs late in the natural history of human immunodeficiency (HIV) infection, and usually at a low CD4-positive T-cell count. Cases refractory to antifungal therapy are indicative of worsening immunosuppression on course to a nonfunctional immune system. Treatment success is limited, and recurrence is common. Treatment that focuses more on the dysfunctional immune system in these patients (e.g., highly active antiretroviral therapy) may yield better results.[2]

Management

Oral and intravenous fluconazole are the drugs of choice. Intravenous amphotericin B is used primarily for azole-refractory cases. In uncomplicated cases, an oral course of therapy may be started, and patients may be discharged with arrangements for close follow-up. In complicated or refractory cases, the patient should be admitted for further evaluation and intravenous therapy.[1]

REFERENCES

1. Vazquez JA, Sobel JD. Mucosal candidiasis. *Infect Dis Clin North Am* 2002;16:793–820.
2. Zingman BS. Resolution of refractory AIDS-related mucosal candidiasis after initiation of didanosine plus saquinavir. *N Engl J Med* 1996;334:1674–1675.

Mallory-Weiss Syndrome

George S. Kim

Clinical Presentation

Patients with Mallory-Weiss syndrome (MWS) present with acute upper gastrointestinal (GI) bleeding after forceful emesis; 10% of patients present with melena alone.[1] Most patients are between 30 and 50 years of age. Emesis may initially involve gastric contents with subsequent episodes of vomiting, resulting in hematemesis. In 90% of cases, bleeding ceases spontaneously.[1]

Pathophysiology

MWS involves partial-thickness tearing of the gastric/esophageal mucosa at the gastroesophageal junction, resulting in upper GI bleeding. MWS accounts for 5% to 15% of upper GI bleeds. MWS tears are caused by a sudden increase of abdominal pressure that causes tears at the gastroesophageal junction.[1,2] MWS tears are associated with episodes of vomiting and retching, but heavy lifting, straining, seizures, trauma, colonic lavage, and cardiopulmonary resuscitation have been implicated as well.[1] Most MWS tears occur within 2 cm of the cardiac side of the gastroesophageal junction on the lesser curvature of the stomach.[1]

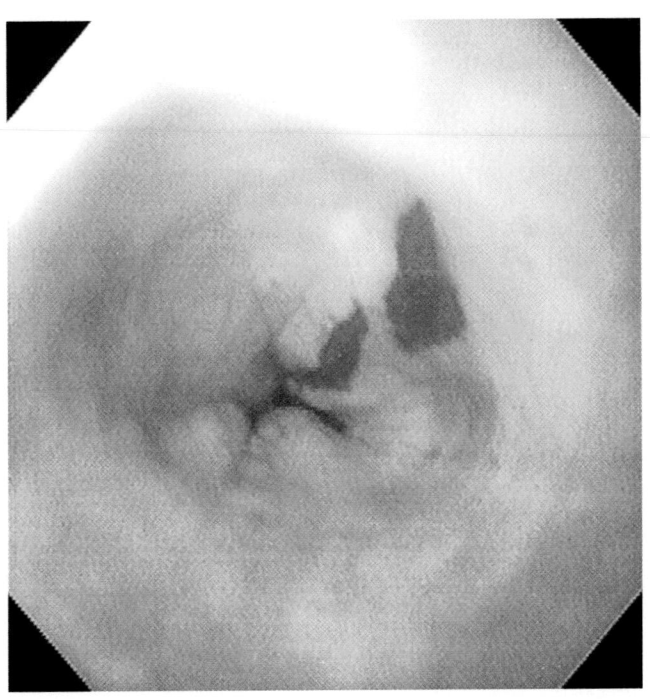

FIGURE 9–9 Endoscopic view of a Mallory-Weiss tear. (From Yamada, with permission.)

Diagnosis

Diagnosis is made by clinical history. Definitive diagnosis is made by endoscopy.

Clinical Complications

Severe GI bleeding that does not resolve with conservative management occurs in 5% to 35% of patients.[1,2]

Management

Treatment in most cases involves supportive care, fluid resuscitation, H_2 receptor blockers, and antiemetics.[2] Cases involving severe bleeding require more invasive techniques, such as balloon tamponade or endoscopy for ligation, injection therapy, or electrocoagulation.[3] Vasopressin therapy and angiographic embolization also have been employed.[2,3]

REFERENCES

1. Younes Z, Johnson DA. The spectrum of spontaneous and iatrogenic esophageal injury: perforations, Mallory-Weiss tears, and hematomas. *J Clin Gastroenterol* 1999;29:306–317.
2. Terada R, Ito S, Akama F, et al. Mallory-Weiss syndrome with severe bleeding: treatment by endoscopic ligation. *Am J Emerg Med* 2000;18:812–815.
3. Huang SP, Wang HP, Lee YC, et al. Endoscopic hemoclip placement and epinephrine injection for Mallory-Weiss syndrome with active bleeding. *Gastrointest Endosc* 2002;55:842–846.

Boerhaave's Syndrome

Marco Garza

Clinical Presentation

Presentations of Boerhaave's Syndrome (BS) range from sepsis and shock to mild pain and vomiting.[1] Patients may complain of lower thoracic pain that is progressive and is exacerbated by swallowing or neck flexion. Leakage of air and fluid into the surrounding mediastinal structures may lead to subcutaneous emphysema or a change in the patient's voice.

Pathophysiology

Boerhaave's syndrome (BS) occurs predominantly in men (70%) between the ages of 40 and 60 years old.[2] Esophageal perforation may result if the upper esophageal sphincter fails to open during emesis and pressure builds in the lower esophagus. Impaired sphincter relaxation may be associated with alcohol, general anesthesia, sedatives, or repeated vomiting. Rupture usually occurs in the distal esophagus (90%), and risk may increase with preexisting esophageal disease. Tears in the mucosa and media vary in length from less than 1 to more than 8 cm. Because the esophagus lacks a serosal layer, rupture of the media exposes the mediastinum to gastric contents. The ensuing inflammation and infection of the mediastinum is the cause of morbidity and mortality associated with esophageal rupture.

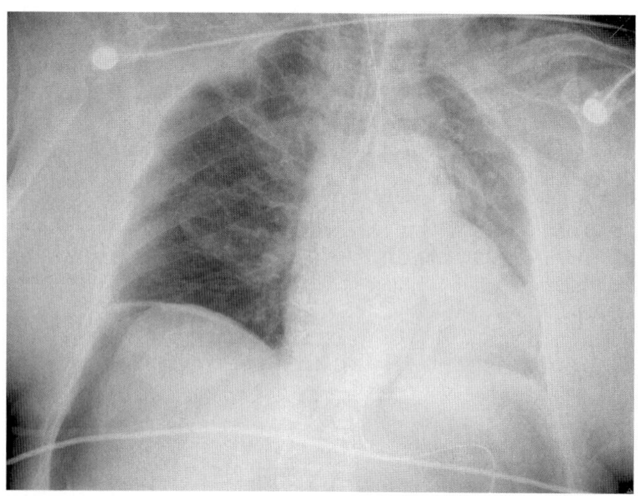

FIGURE 9–10 Perforated distal esophagus leading to pneumoperitoneum, pneumomediastinum, and subcutaneous air. (Courtesy of Robert Hendrickson, MD.)

Diagnosis

The diagnosis is often delayed, and BS can be confused with perforated peptic ulcer, myocardial infarction, pancreatitis, dissecting aortic aneurysm, or pneumonia.[2] Chest radiographs may be normal, or they may reveal subcutaneous emphysema, pneumomediastinum, pleural effusions, or a widened mediastinum. Noncontrast chest computed tomography (CT) may reveal small amounts of mediastinal air in the surrounding esophagus, small pleural effusions, and direct communication of the esophagus with the mediastinum.[1] The gold standard of diagnostic testing is the contrast esophagogram. A water-soluble contrast agent should be used first, because water-soluble agents are rapidly absorbed and do not cause a significant inflammatory response in the mediastinum.

Clinical Complications

Complications include mediastinitis, sepsis, multiorgan failure, and death. The mortality rate ranges from 5% to 14%, depending on the rapidity of the diagnosis.[1]

Management

Patients with sepsis or shock require airway management, intravenous fluids, vasopressors, antibiotics, and admission to an intensive care unit (ICU). Broad-spectrum antibiotics may be used, although the mediastinitis is generally chemical and not infectious. H_2 receptor blockers or proton pump blockers may also be used. On-site emergency surgical consultation is essential.

REFERENCES

1. Younes Z, Johnson DA. The spectrum of spontaneous and iatrogenic esophageal injury: perforations, Mallory-Weiss tears, and hematomas. *J Clin Gastroenterol* 1999;29:306–317.
2. Reeder LB, DeFilippi VJ, Ferguson MK. Current results of therapy for esophageal perforation. *Am J Surg* 1995;169:615–617.

Peptic Ulcer Disease

Derek Halvorson

Clinical Presentation

Patients with peptic ulcer disease (PUD) may present with epigastric pain, belching, bloating, and distention (40% to 70%). The pain may begin after meals (1 to 3 hours after eating in 60% to 90%); it may be improved with eating or with antacids, or it may radiate and follow a daily pattern. Vomiting may represent gastric outlet obstruction resulting from stricture due to chronic inflammation at the pylorus. Sudden, severe pain and abdominal distention or peritoneal signs may represent acute perforation. Hematemesis, melena, and hypotension may occur with significant bleeding. Physical examination findings may be subtle and consist of mild to moderate epigastric tenderness. Patients with acute perforation or bleeding may develop hypotension, melena, hematemesis, or peritoneal signs.

Pathophysiology

PUD results from a breakdown of the normal mucosal barrier of the stomach and intestine by high concentrations of acid and pepsin. The two main causes for this breakdown are *Helicobacter pylori* infection and use of nonsteroidal antiinflammatory drugs (NSAIDs).[1] Other causes include severe physiologic stress (e.g., burns), central nervous system trauma, surgery, and rare hypersecretory states such as Zollinger-Ellison syndrome. Chronic medical conditions such as renal or hepatic failure, pulmonary diseases, radiation, or chemotherapy may also lead to the destruction of mucosal protection. Factors that may potentiate PUD include smoking, alcohol use, steroid use, psychological stress, and bisphosphonates. *H. pylori* infections are the most common cause of PUD (90% of duodenal ulcers and 70% to 75% gastric ulcers). They produce PUD via inflammatory, mucoprotective, and hormonal influences.[1] NSAID use causes a suppression of protective gastric prostaglandins that leads to a weakening of the mucosal protective barrier.[2]

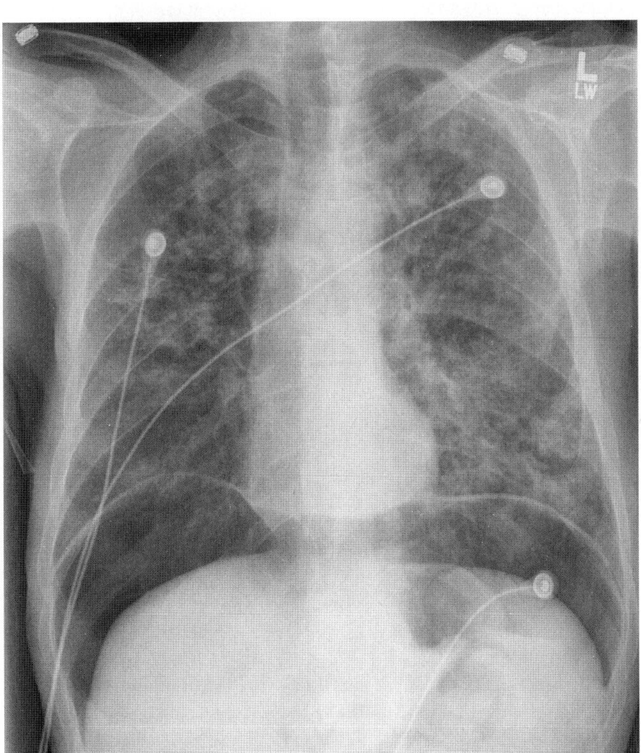

FIGURE 9–11 Perforated peptic ulcer with air under the diaphragm. (Courtesy of Robert Hendrickson, MD.)

Diagnosis

The diagnosis is suspected by the clinical history and physical examination findings and confirmed by contrast radiography or endoscopy.

Clinical Complications

Complications include bleeding, perforation, and obstruction.

Management

Patients who present with symptoms consistent with PUD should have consideration of other, non-PUD diseases (e.g., acute coronary syndrome, pancreatitis, abdominal aortic aneurysm, aortic dissection) and PUD-related complications (e.g., gastrointestinal [GI] bleeding, perforation). A stool guaiac test should be performed, and use of a nasogastric tube (NGT) should be considered if there is a history of hematemesis. Patients should be instructed to cease NSAID use and smoking. Treatment for PUD should be instituted early and may include use of proton pump inhibitors (PPIs), H_2 receptor antagonists, or sucralfate.[2] Patients should be referred to their primary care physician for further management and possible *H. pylori* testing and treatment.

REFERENCES

1. Chan FK, Leung WK. Peptic-ulcer disease. *Lancet* 2002;360: 933–941.
2. Soll AH. Consensus conference. Medical treatment of peptic ulcer disease: practice guidelines. Practice Parameters Committee of the American College of Gastroenterology. *JAMA* 1996;275:622–629.

9–12

Bezoars

Robert Hendrickson

Bezoars are masses of food (phytobezoars), medication (pharmacobezoars), hair (trichobezoars), or other ingested items that conglomerate in the stomach or intestine.[1]

Clinical Presentation

Patients with bezoars may present with a painless epigastric mass, weight loss, anemia, or obstruction of the bowels. Patients at highest risk are children with pica and adults with previous gastric surgery or psychiatric disorders, including trichotillomania (urge to pull one's hair) or trichophagia (urge to eat one's hair).[1] Bezoars may be found in patients who chronically ingest fibrous materials (e.g., pistachio nut shells, sunflower seeds). Lactobezoars, or bezoars of formula or milk, may be seen in neonates.[1]

Diagnosis

The diagnosis may be suspected clinically and is confirmed with visualization of a large density filling the stomach on radiography or computed tomography (CT) scan.[1]

Clinical Complications

Complications include acute obstruction of the gastric outlet or bowel and chronic obstruction of the stomach leading to malnutrition, anemia, and weight loss.[1]

Management

Small bezoars may be removed via endoscopy, whereas larger bezoars may require operative removal. Chemical dissolution has been attempted in the past with inconsistent results.[1]

REFERENCES

1. Phillips MR, Zaheer S, Drugas GT. Gastric trichobezoar: case report and literature review. *Mayo Clin Proc* 1998;73:653–656.

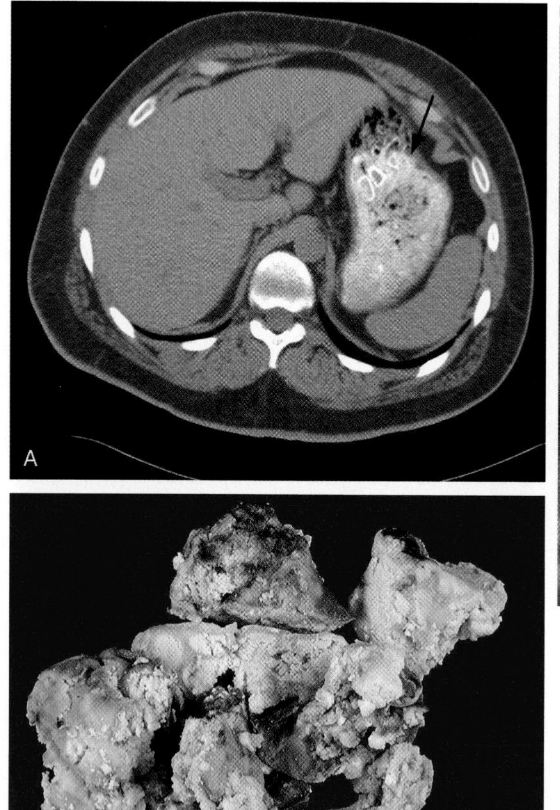

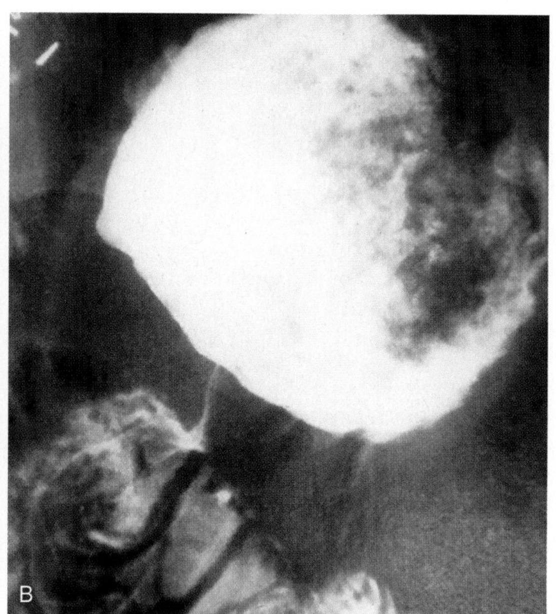

FIGURE 9–12 **A:** Computed tomogram showing a bezoar in a patient who eats his hair (trichotillomania). (Courtesy of Robert Hendrickson, MD.) **B:** Gastric phytobezoar demonstrated by barium examination. (From Yamada, with permission.) **C:** Pharmacobezoar. (From Schwartz, with permission. Massive verapamil pharmacobezoar resulting in esophageal perforation. *Int J Med Toxicol* 2004;7:4.)

Upper Gastrointestinal Bleeding

Swapan Dubey

Clinical Presentation

The clinical presentation of patients with upper gastrointestinal bleeding (UGIB) ranges from massive hematemesis to an asymptomatic positive random stool sample.

Pathophysiology

UGIB is defined as any bleeding that occurs proximal to the ligament of Treitz in the distal duodenum. The majority of UGIB results as a consequence of peptic ulcer disease (PUD) (caused by *H. pylori* or use of nonsteroidal antiinflammatory drugs [NSAIDs] or alcohol). Mallory-Weiss tears, esophageal varices, and gastritis are less common causes of UGIB.[1,2]

Diagnosis

The diagnosis can be made by inspection of the patient's emesis or by placing a nasogastric tube (NGT) and detecting frank blood, blood-stained fluid, or "coffee grounds." The return of a clear aspirate, however, may simply indicate bleeding has stopped, is intermittent, or cannot be detected due to pyloric spasm.

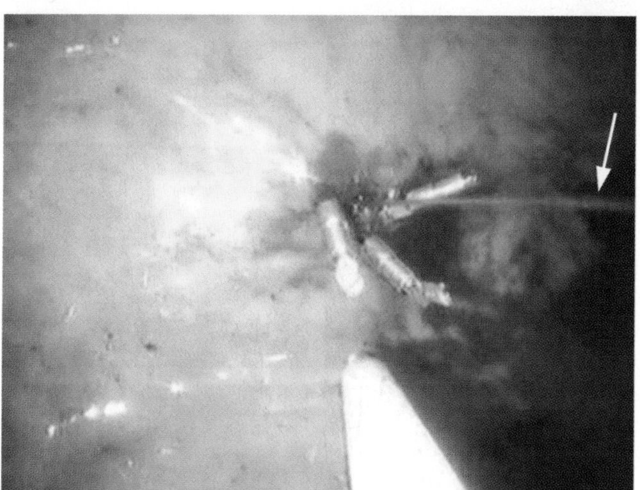

FIGURE 9–13 Spurting blood from an erosive lesion. These lesions are dilated aberrant vessels that can erode through the mucosal surface to cause recurrent vigorous bleeding. (From Yamada, with permission.)

Clinical Complications

Complications of UGIB include hemodynamic instability, surgical morbidity, and infection by blood-borne pathogens from transfusions.

Management

Maintenance of a patent airway and restoration of intravascular volume are the goals of preliminary management. Initial crystalloid infusion, up to 30 mL/kg, may be followed by transfusion of O-negative or cross-matched blood as needed. Patients with active bleeding require emergency consultation for esophagogastroduodenoscopy (EGD). Those without active bleeding may be monitored, observed, and possibly scheduled for an EGD.[1] Interventions during EGD include submucosal injection of epinephrine, sclerotherapy, and band ligation. If these measures fail to stop the bleeding, angiography with embolization or surgery may be necessary. For those patients with presumed variceal bleeding, medical management may be initiated while awaiting definitive care. Octreotide may be used to lower portal venous pressures, and a Sengstaken-Blakemore tube may be placed as a temporizing measure (see "Variceal Bleeding").[1]

REFERENCES

1. Dallal HJ, Palmer KR. ABC of the upper gastrointestinal tract: upper gastrointestinal haemorrhage. *BMJ* 2001;323:1115–1117.
2. McGuirk TD, Coyle WJ. Upper gastrointestinal tract bleeding. *Emerg Med Clin North Am* 1996;14:523–545.

Lower Gastrointestinal Bleeding

Swapan Dubey

Clinical Presentation

Lower gastrointestinal bleeding (LGIB) may manifest as hematochezia (red blood per rectum), as melena (tarry, black stool), or as an occult finding on routine physical examination.[1,2]

Pathophysiology

LGIB is defined as any bleeding that occurs within the gastrointestinal (GI) tract distal to the ligament of Treitz. Common causes of LGIB are diverticulosis, angiodysplasia, colitis, anorectal causes, upper gastrointestinal bleeding (UGIB), neoplasms, and inflammatory bowel disease.[1,2]

Diagnosis

Patients with LGIB should have a nasogastric tube (NGT) placed to exclude a lesion proximal to the pylorus. Historical and physical features may help determine the location of bleeding. Red blood streaks or blood found only on toilet paper may imply an anal source. Bright red or maroon stool (hematochezia) may imply a distal source of bleeding (in about 90% of cases).[1] Melena results from the oxidation of hematin and is typically associated with lesions of the upper GI tract but may have a lower GI tract focus. Anoscopy may reveal a bleeding internal hemorrhoid, but in up to 25% of cases melena is associated with a second, more proximal source of bleeding.[1]

Clinical Complications

Complications include cardiac ischemia and cerebral hypoperfusion resulting from blood loss.

Management

Initial resuscitation of the unstable patient may include airway management and resuscitation with crystalloid and blood products. Evaluation of the hemoglobin/hematocrit, platelet count, and a coagulation profile should be performed. Patients with massive LGIB should have surgical consultation and may require angiography for localization and therapeutic embolization. Colonoscopy may be performed for patients with less severe or intermittent bleeding. In addition, red blood cell (RBC) scans may be used for identification of continued bleeding and general localization of bleeding.[2]

REFERENCES

1. Peter DJ, Dougherty JM. Evaluation of the patient with gastrointestinal bleeding: an evidence based approach. *Emerg Med Clin North Am* 1999;17:239–261.
2. Zuccaro G Jr. Management of the adult patient with acute lower gastrointestinal bleeding. *Am J Gastroenterol* 1998;93:1202–1208.

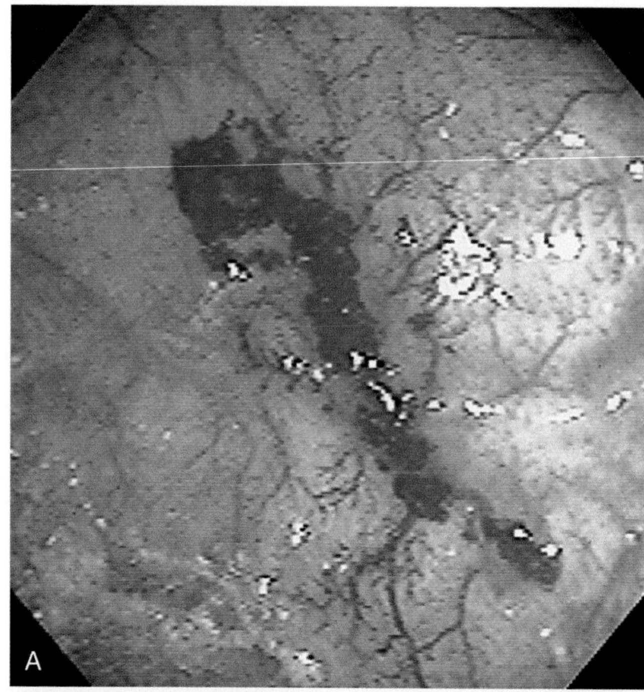

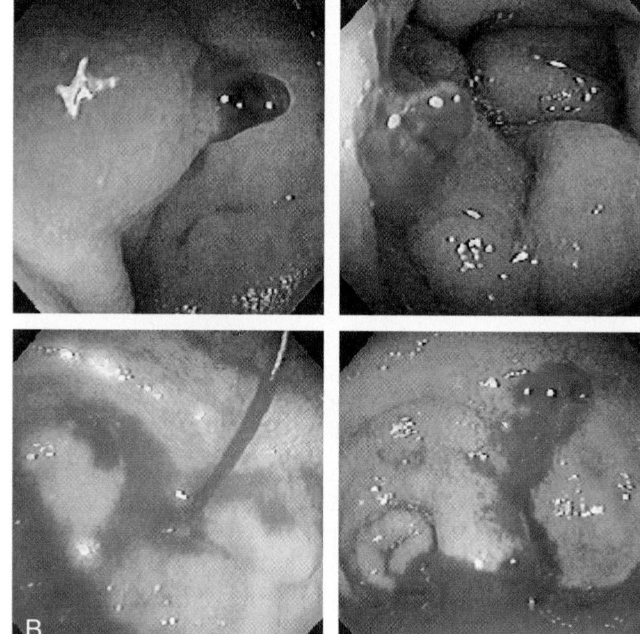

FIGURE 9–14 **A:** Vascular malformation. (From Yamada, with permission.) **B:** Active bleeding from angiodysplasia. (From Yamada, with permission.)

Black Stool

Robert Hendrickson

The emergency physician may be confronted by a patient whose chief complaint is black stools, or black stool may be discovered during care of a patient with other complaints. Melena is the maroon or black stool produced by bleeding in the upper GI tract. It is typically thick and tarry and produces a positive bedside occult blood test. Ingestion of iron supplements, antacids, and bismuth-containing products (e.g., Pepto-Bismol) may turn stool dark, but in all of these cases the bedside occult blood test is negative.[1]

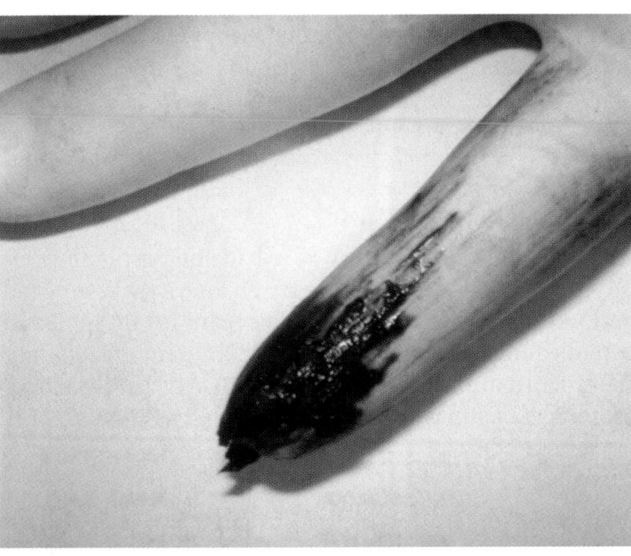

FIGURE 9–15 Black, tarry stool as seen on digital rectal examination. (Copyright James R. Roberts, MD.)

REFERENCES

1. Rockey DC. Occult gastrointestinal bleeding. *N Engl J Med* 1999; 341:38–46.

Ingested Foreign Bodies

Maria Halluska

Clinical Presentation

Patients with ingested foreign bodies (FBs) may present with anxiety, difficulty swallowing, drooling, violent retching, and pain localized anywhere from the mouth and throat to the neck or substernal or epigastric area. Pediatric patients present with refusal to eat, vomiting, gagging, choking, stridor, drooling, and pain.[1,2]

Pathophysiology

Although ingested FBs may become lodged anywhere in the digestive tract, they are most often found within one of several physiologic areas of relative constriction. In the pediatric patient, these areas are all located within the esophagus and include the cricopharyngeal narrowing (C6), the thoracic inlet (T1), the aortic arch (T4), the tracheal bifurcation (T6), and the hiatal narrowing (T10–11). In children most ingested FBs lodge in the proximal third of the esophagus, whereas in adults most ingested FBs lodge at the lower esophageal sphincter (LES). Risk factors in adult patients include dentures, esophageal abnormalities, alcohol consumption, prisoner status, a psychiatric disorder, and mental retardation.[1,2] Ingested FBs are also common in incarcerated persons.

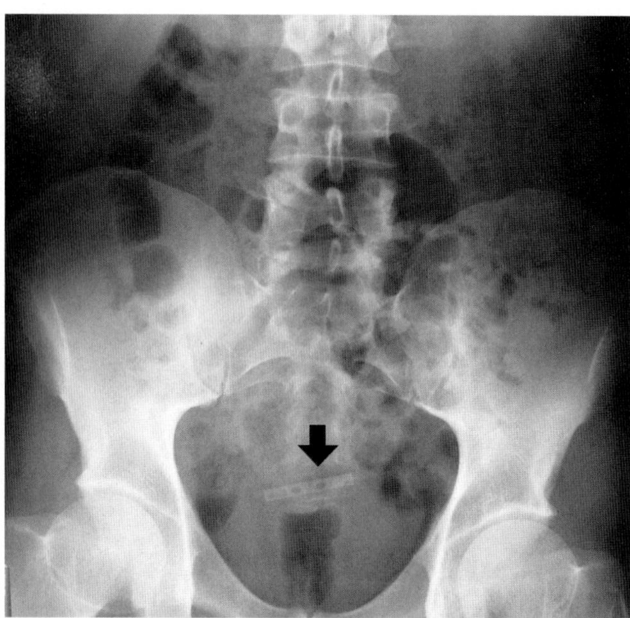

FIGURE 9–16 Swallowed taped razor blade in small intestine. (Courtesy of Mark Silverberg, MD.)

Diagnosis

A history of ingested FB, the time of ingestion, the item ingested, and a careful examination are key to proper diagnosis. In the instance of radiopaque FBs, plain radiographic films of the neck and chest help localization of the item and planning of the removal strategy. If the ingested FB is not localized by these techniques, more invasive measures may need to be undertaken, including direct or indirect laryngoscopy, contrast plain films, computed tomography (CT), endoscopy, or some combination of these. Most FB ingestions result in spontaneous passage; however, 10% to 20% of cases require some medical intervention, with 1% needing surgical intervention.[1,2]

Clinical Complications

Complications include airway occlusion, aspiration injury, mechanical and chemical erosion, stricture, and perforation. Luminal perforations can result in lethal complications (mediastinitis, cardiac tamponade, abscess formation, and aortoesophageal or tracheoesophageal fistulas).[1,2]

Management

Most ingested FBs can ultimately be managed conservatively, but airway patency is the first priority. Patients who have ingested sharp objects usually require imaging, endoscopy, and/or surgery for removal. Early consultation for these services is essential. Patients at risk for perforation require water-soluble contrast imaging to rule out this complication, and those at risk for aspiration should receive nasogastric tube (NGT) removal of any material proximal to the obstructing object. Those patients who are symptomatic and those with high-risk ingestions need esophagoscopy and observation for signs of complications.

REFERENCES

1. Wahbeh G, Wyllie R, Kay M. Foreign body ingestion in infants and children: location, location, location. *Clin Pediatr (Phila)* 2002;41:633–640.
2. Passey JC, Meher R, Agarwal S, Gupta B. Unusual complication of ingestion of a foreign body. *J Laryngol Otol* 2003;117:566–567.

Small Bowel Obstruction

Lalena Yarris

Clinical Presentation

The most common symptoms of small bowel obstruction (SBO) are abdominal pain, abdominal distention, nausea and vomiting, and an inability to pass flatus or stool. Proximal obstruction is more likely to cause early nausea and vomiting and causes less abdominal distention than distal obstruction does. Although obstipation is classically associated with SBO, a partial obstruction may allow passage of flatus or stool, including diarrhea. Because it takes 12 to 24 hours for the colon to empty, even a complete obstruction can manifest with diarrhea early in the clinical course.[1]

Pathophysiology

The stomach, small bowel, biliary tract, and pancreas collectively secrete 8 to 10 L of fluid daily. Intestinal obstruction prevents the passage of this fluid to the colon, where it can be reabsorbed. As the fluid collects proximally, intraluminal pressure develops, which accounts for the clinical symptoms associated with SBO. As the pressure builds, the intestine is at risk for development of edema and eventually ischemia.[1]

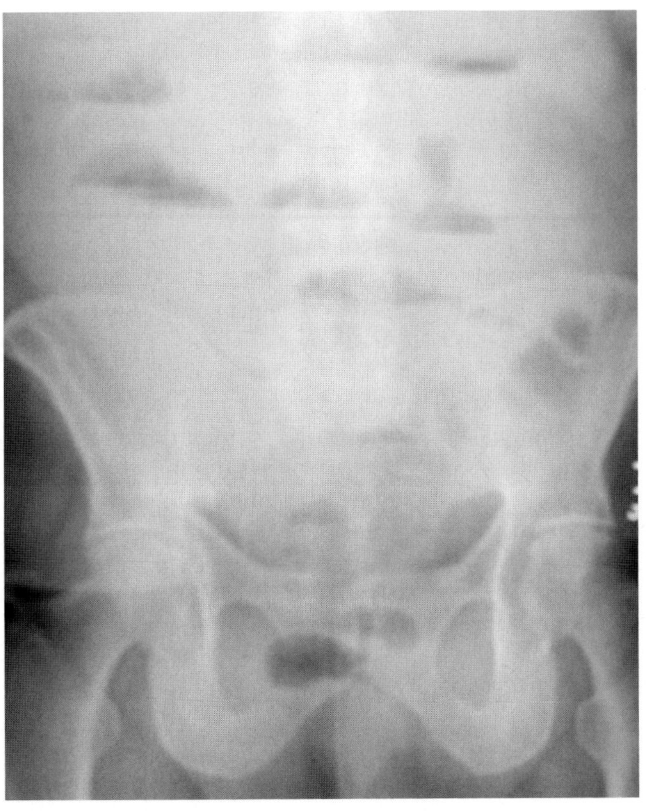

FIGURE 9–17 Multiple air–fluid levels in a patient with small bowel obstruction. (Courtesy of Robert Hendrickson, MD.)

Diagnosis

The diagnosis is primarily clinical, but laboratory studies may help in determining the severity of the process. Fever, tachycardia, elevated white blood cell (WBC) count, electrolyte or metabolic abnormalities, and peritoneal signs are suggestive of infection or bowel ischemia. Physical examination usually is significant for abdominal distention and tympany to percussion.

The most appropriate early imaging study is an abdominal series of plain radiographic films. Findings may include intestinal dilatation proximal to the obstruction and a paucity of bowel gas distally, as well as air–fluid levels.[2] Computed tomography (CT) scanning may demonstrate small bowel dilatation and air–fluid levels. The sensitivity and specificity of CT scanning for intestinal obstruction are 93% and 100%, respectively.[3]

Clinical Complications

Complications include hypovolemia, electrolyte abnormalities, acid–base disturbances, strangulation, bowel necrosis, sepsis, and death.

Management

Early surgical consultation is important in suspected intestinal obstruction. Patients with SBO should receive early fluid resuscitation, placement of a nasogastric tube (NGT), and admission to the hospital. Symptomatic treatment with antiemetics and narcotic analgesia is appropriate. Although some cases of intestinal obstruction resolve on their own, 50% to 70% require surgery. The overall mortality rate approaches 2%.[2]

REFERENCES

1. Miller G, Boman J, Shrier I, Gordon PH. Etiology of small bowel obstruction. *Am J Surg* 2000;180:33–36.
2. Maglinte DD, Heitkamp DE, Howard TJ, Kelvin FM, Lappas JC. Current concepts in imaging of small bowel obstruction. *Radiol Clin North Am* 2003;41:263–283.
3. Ogata M, Imai S, Hosotani R, et al. Abdominal ultrasonography for the diagnosis of strangulation in small bowel obstruction. *Br J Surg* 1994;81:421–424.

Large Bowel Obstruction

Lalena Yarris

Clinical Presentation

Patients with colonic obstruction usually present with abdominal distention and crampy, abdominal pain. Nausea and vomiting typically occur after the onset of pain. Obstipation may result if the large bowel obstruction (LBO) is complete. Patients with an incompetent ileocecal valve may present with symptoms suggestive of a small bowel obstruction (SBO). In most patients with a competent ileocecal valve, there is a "closed loop" between the valve and the obstruction. Because there is a finite area of colon and luminal space between these two points, obstruction may lead to massive distention and an increased risk of bowel perforation or bowel wall ischemia.[1]

Pathophysiology

LBO refers to a bowel obstruction that prevents the free passage of fluid and intestinal contents through the colon. The three most common causes for LBO are colorectal cancer (59%), volvulus (17%), and scarring associated with diverticulitis (12%).[1] Obstruction of the colon leads to distention of the proximal section of colon, resulting in increased intraluminal pressure. If the intraluminal pressure exceeds the venous pressure, the intestinal wall becomes edematous and no longer absorbs fluids. Intraluminal and interstitial fluid accumulates until the wall pressure exceeds the arterial pressure, and the bowel segment becomes ischemic.[1]

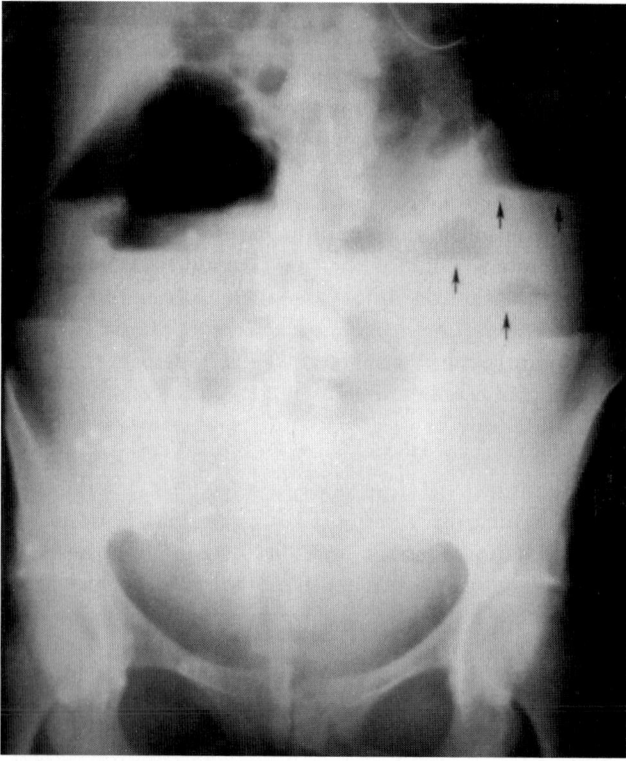

FIGURE 9–18 An upright abdominal radiograph reveals multiple air–fluid levels *(arrows)* in the dilated left hemicolon, with no gas distally. (From Yamada, with permission.)

Diagnosis

Patients with a history and physical examination suggestive of LBO require plain radiographic films of the abdomen. The abdominal series usually contains an upright and supine abdomen radiograph, as well as an upright chest or left lateral decubitus view to identify free air under the diaphragm. Radiographic findings in LBO include colonic distention with air–fluid levels within the colon. The large bowel is often distended proximal to the obstruction and decompressed distally. Cecal distention of greater than 12 cm often requires surgical intervention. Distended colon often can be differentiated from small bowel by the presence of haustra and the absence of plicae circulares. However, with ileocecal incompetence or if the bowel is very distended, it may be very difficult to differentiate between the two with plain films. A barium or Gastrografin enema often can confirm the diagnosis of colonic obstruction and identify the point of obstruction.[1] Colonoscopy may be performed in Ogilvie's syndrome (isolated paralytic ileus of the colon without mechanical obstruction) and volvulus. Computed tomography (CT) may also be helpful in identifying mass lesions and determining the point of transition in obstruction.

Clinical Complications

Complications of LBO include perforation, peritonitis, and sepsis. All of these complications can be life-threatening, and the mortality rate associated with a cecal perforation approaches 30%.[1]

Management

Early management of colonic obstruction is symptomatic and supportive. The administration of analgesics and antiemetics is appropriate, and patients should be given nothing by mouth. Nasogastric decompression and fluid resuscitation should be initiated, and emergency, on-site surgical consultation should be obtained. Findings that may necessitate emergency laparotomy include cecal distention greater than 12 cm, peritoneal free air, evidence of peritonitis, and sepsis. All patients with obstruction require admission to the hospital.[1]

REFERENCES

1. Lopez-Kostner F, Hool GR, Lavery IC. Management and causes of acute large bowel obstruction. *Surg Clin North Am* 1997;77: 1265–1290.

Ileus

Lalena Yarris

Clinical Presentation

Patients with a paralytic ileus present with abdominal distention, vomiting, and sometimes obstipation. The constant pain of colicky exacerbations associated with small bowel obstruction (SBO) is often absent, but frequently abdominal discomfort is associated with the distention. Quiet or absent bowel sounds are classically described, but this is an inconsistent physical finding associated with adynamic ileus. Laboratory studies are often normal. Plain abdominal radiographs may show dilated loops of small bowel with air–fluid levels. It can be difficult to distinguish ileus from mechanical obstruction. However, distention of the entire length of the colon is more common in paralytic ileus.[1,2]

Pathophysiology

Ileus is defined as a mechanical, dynamic, or adynamic obstruction of the bowel. In practice, the term usually refers to the latter of these forms of obstruction. Adynamic, or paralytic, ileus is a functional bowel obstruction secondary to bowel paralysis. Adynamic ileus is a common cause of bowel obstruction and may result from a variety of peritoneal insults, ranging from intraabdominal processes to surgery. Mechanical ileus involves obstruction of the bowel due to mechanical causes. Dynamic, or spastic, ileus is an uncommon condition resulting from extreme and prolonged contraction of the intestine associated with conditions such as heavy metal poisoning, uremia, porphyria, and extensive intestinal ulcerations.[1,2]

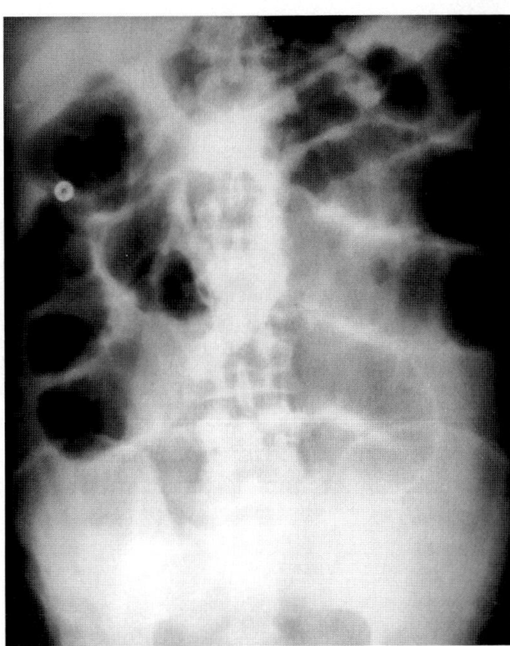

FIGURE 9–19 Plain radiograph shows a large amount of gas distending the ileum, suggesting a perforated viscus. (From Yamada, with permission.)

The bowel paralysis causing an adynamic ileus is thought to be the result of autonomic, pharmacologic, and hormonal factors.[1] Cases of refractory adynamic ileus are most likely to be caused by an imbalance of sympathetic and parasympathetic tone in the colon.[2] Adynamic ileus is commonly seen after abdominal surgery, but it may also occur with retroperitoneal hematomas, ureteral calculi, pyelonephritis, pancreatitis, bowel ischemia, electrolyte disturbances, and thoracic disorders such as lower-lobe pneumonia, rib fractures, and myocardial infarction. The degree of ileus depends on the severity and duration of the insult. Substances associated with peritoneal injury include hydrochloric acid, colonic contents, pancreatic enzymes, blood, and urine.[1,2]

Diagnosis

The diagnosis of ileus usually is based on the history and physical examination. Imaging studies such as plain abdominal radiographs, contrast enemas, and computed tomography (CT) scans may be used at times to exclude mechanical obstruction.[1,2]

Clinical Complications

Paralytic ileus is often self-limited and in most cases resolves in less than 4 days. If a postsurgical ileus does not resolve within this time period, other causes of ileus, including mechanical obstruction, intraabdominal abscess, or another source of infection, should be considered. A complication of ileus, especially in the case of "pseudo-obstruction" or Ogilvie's syndrome, is a failure to resolve, with the development of a chronic ileus.[1,2]

Management

Chronic ileus can be life-threatening and has been difficult to treat, with colonoscopic and surgical intervention being the mainstays of therapy. More recently, intravenous neostigmine has been shown to promptly resolve some cases of pseudo-obstruction within minutes, eliminating the need for more aggressive measures.[2] Paralytic ileus occurs secondary to another disorder, and treatment is symptomatic (i.e., by addressing the primary process). Patients should receive analgesics and antiemetics if needed, should receive nothing by mouth, and should be given intravenous fluids. Nasogastric suction is appropriate. In most cases, the ileus is self-limited and the prognosis good. Patients need inpatient admission to either a surgical or a medical service, depending on the primary process and the patient's comorbid conditions.[1,2]

REFERENCES

1. Lopez-Kostner F, Hool GR, Lavery IC. Management and causes of acute large bowel obstruction. *Surg Clin North Am* 1997;77: 1265–1290.
2. Ponec RJ, Saunders MD, Kimmey MB. Neostigmine for the treatment of acute colonic pseudo-obstruction. *N Engl J Med* 1999;341: 137–141.

Volvulus

Lalena Yarris

Clinical Presentation

The clinical presentation of volvulus varies somewhat, according to the site of torsion. The symptoms of sigmoid volvulus resemble those of a distal colonic obstruction and include abdominal pain and distention, nausea, constipation, and, occasionally, vomiting. The pain is usually continuous and severe, with a superimposed colicky exacerbation of the pain with peristalsis. In some patients, particularly children, the volvulus resolves spontaneously and then recurs, producing intermittent symptoms and making the diagnosis challenging.[1] Cecal volvulus manifests with symptoms more similar to those of small bowel obstruction (SBO), including abdominal pain, nausea, vomiting, obstipation, and some degree of distention. As with sigmoid volvulus, the pain is often severe and constant, with peristaltic exacerbations.[1,2]

Pathophysiology

Volvulus occurs when a portion of the gastrointestinal (GI) tract rotates upon itself, a condition that often leads to obstruction with compromise of the blood supply. The two most common sites of volvulus are the cecum and the sigmoid colon. Rarely, colonic volvulus is seen at the transverse colon or splenic flexure.[1,2] Patients may be predisposed to colonic volvulus by certain anatomic features. Redundant sigmoid colon with a narrow mesenteric attachment is considered a risk factor for sigmoid torsion, and increased cecal mobility for cecal torsion.[2] There is also assumed to be some stretching and elongation of the colon with age, and in more than 50% of cases the first incidence of volvulus occurs after the age of 65 years.[1] There is also an increased incidence of sigmoid volvulus among patients in nursing homes and other institutions, for reasons that are not clearly understood.[2]

Diagnosis

Volvulus should be suspected based on the history and physical examination and may be confirmed with imaging studies. Plain radiographic films of the abdomen can confirm the diagnosis of sigmoid volvulus in approximately 60% of patients.[1] The classic radiographic appearance includes a massively dilated sigmoid colon with loss of haustra and a "kidney bean" or "bent inner tube" appearance. Obstructive findings, such as dilated bowel proximal to the volvulus with air-fluid levels, may also be seen. Similar findings may be observed in

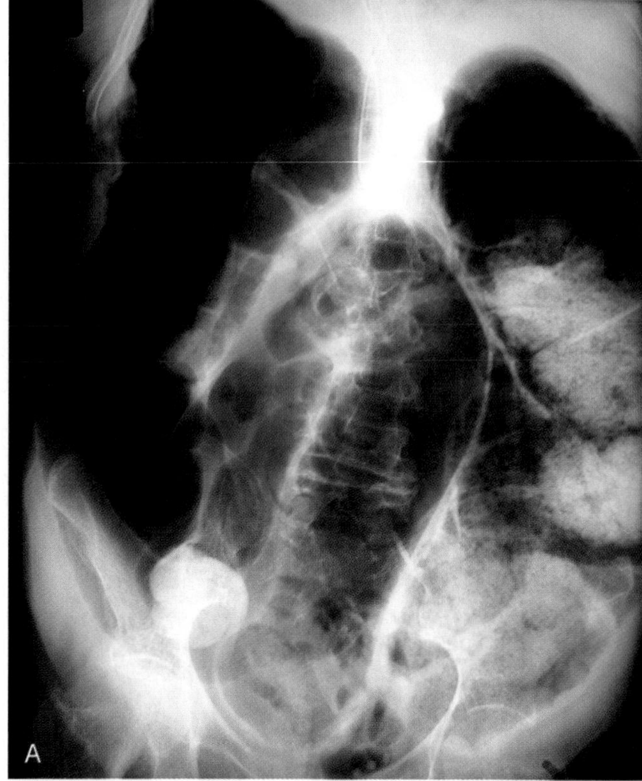

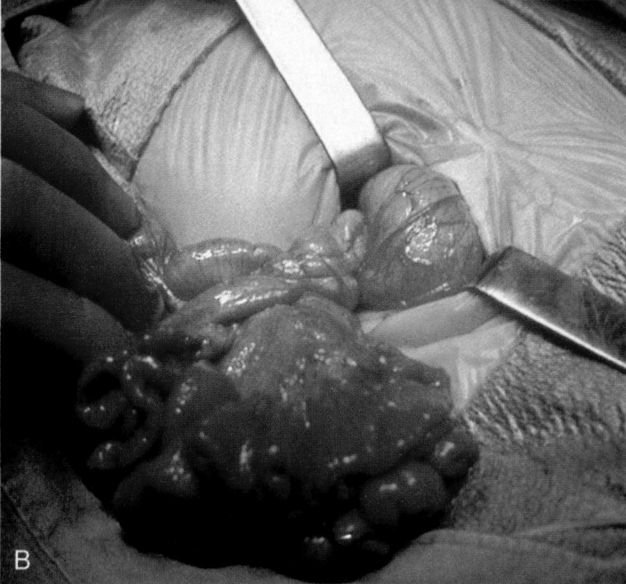

FIGURE 9–20 **A:** Sigmoid volvulus. (Courtesy of Mark Silverberg, MD.) **B:** Volvulus. There is complete twisting of the small bowel around the axis of its mesentery. (From Yamada, with permission.)

cecal volvulus, but a barium or water-soluble contrast enema is more likely to be diagnostic. Characteristic findings include a funnel-like narrowing that often resembles a bird's beak or ace of spades at the location of the volvulus. Contrast enema should be reserved for cases that are unclear and in which gangrene is not suspected, because gangrene raises the risk of perforation. Computed tomography (CT) may also be helpful if the diagnosis is unclear and a contrast enema is difficult to obtain or deemed unsafe. In sigmoid volvulus, sigmoidoscopy often has both a diagnostic and a therapeutic role, but colonoscopy is rarely helpful in cecal volvulus and risks colonic perforation.[1]

Clinical Complications

A life-threatening complication of colonic volvulus is intestinal gangrene with peritonitis and sepsis. Although gangrene is relatively uncommon, it can develop rapidly in patients with an uncorrected volvulus. Close observation and repeat examinations are advised, as is early surgical consultation.[1]

Management

Patients with volvulus should receive early symptomatic treatment, including intravenous fluids, nothing by mouth, analgesic, antiemetics, and nasogastric decompression. In sigmoid volvulus, detorsion of the volvulus can be achieved with sigmoidoscopy and placement of a rectal tube for decompression, although in most instances this procedure is not done by the emergency physician. Success rates as high as 55% to 75% have been reported with this technique, but recurrence rates approach 60% in the ensuing hours to weeks.[1,2] Definitive treatment after detorsion includes a variety of surgical approaches in a nonemergency setting that allows ample time for bowel preparation. Cecal volvulus, in contrast, is always treated surgically, with cecopexy or cecal resection. In addition to early surgical consultation, patients with volvulus require hospital admission for observation and surgical treatment.[1]

REFERENCES

1. Mangiante EC, Croce MA, Fabian TC, Moore OF 3rd, Britt LG. Sigmoid volvulus: a four-decade experience. *Am Surg* 1989;55: 41–44.
2. Lopez-Kostner F, Hool GR, Lavery IC. Management and causes of acute large-bowel obstruction. *Surg Clin North Am* 1997;77: 1265–1290.

Abdominal Hernia

Cameron Symonds and Jonathan Glauser

Clinical Presentation

Many abdominal hernias are asymptomatic. There may be a noticeable bulge. Pain may be acute with incarceration. Symptoms may be worsened by cough, exercise, or Valsalva maneuvers. Nausea, vomiting, and clinical toxicity may represent bowel obstruction. Femoral and obturator hernias commonly manifest as bowel obstruction rather than a noticeable bulge. Infants may present with irritability.

An abdominal hernia occurs with any viscus that protrudes through the borders of its native cavity. Hernias affect 10% of the population. Inguinal hernias are defined by a defect in the transversalis fascia. Most are indirect, resulting from failure of obliteration of the processus vaginalis in infancy. Direct hernias are protrusions through the transversalis fascia and are acquired. Umbilical hernias occur through the umbilical fibromuscular ring, which usually is obliterated by 2 years of age. These hernias are congenital and typically are repaired if they persist in children older than 2 to 4 years of age. A femoral hernia is a protrusion below the inguinal ligament. It is uncommon and occurs more frequently in females. Hernias may occur at incision sites (incisional), through the linea alba of the rectus sheath (ventral), or at the obturator foramen (obturator). Rarely, spigelian hernias occur through the spigelian fascia, located at the lateral border of the rectus at the semilunar line. Richter's hernia occurs when the antimesenteric border of the bowel passes through any of the described fascial defects.

Hernia can be classified into three types, independent of location: reducible, incarcerated, and strangulated. In a reducible hernia, the contents of the hernia return to the original cavity either spontaneously or manually. An incarcerated hernia occurs when the hernia is irreducible, usually due to bowel edema. Strangulated hernias develop as the bowel edema of an incarcerated hernia progresses until building pressure occludes the vascular supply.[1]

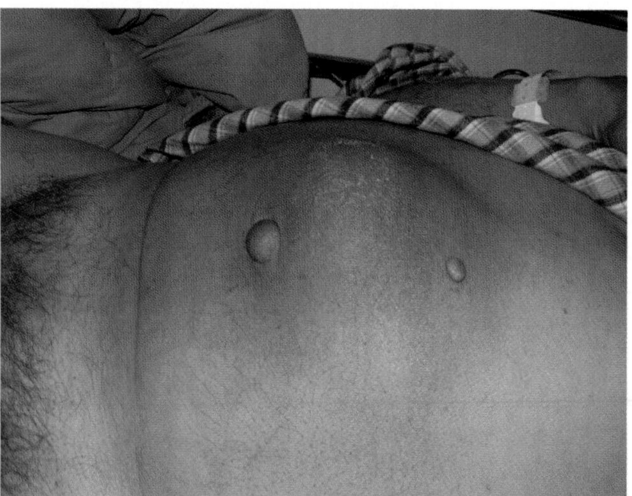

FIGURE 9–21 This abdominal wall hernia became painful and incarcerated, necessitating surgical reduction. (Courtesy of Mark Silverberg, MD.)

Pathophysiology

Increased intraabdominal pressure may force a viscus through various weak points in the abdominal wall. Associated conditions include repeated coughing, ascites, peritoneal dialysis, ventriculoperitoneal shunts, peritoneal masses or organomegaly, obstipation, and muscular effort. Other predisposing conditions include prematurity, collagen disorders, neonatal intraventricular hemorrhage, and myelomeningocele.

Diagnosis

The diagnosis of a hernia is usually made when the patient, parent, or physician observes a bulge. Plain radiographic films are useful only in detecting bowel obstruction or perforation.[2] Computed tomography (CT) is useful for localizing intraabdominal hernias and for delineating bowel wall integrity, perforation, gangrene, and abscess formation.[3] Ultrasonography may be useful to differentiate hernias from other pathologies such as adenopathies, abscesses, and masses.

Clinical Complications

Complications include bowel incarceration, strangulation, and obstruction. Strangulation of the bowel, common with Richter's hernias, may lead to bowel perforation, gangrene, abscess formation, peritonitis, and sepsis.

Management

Gentle attempts at manual reduction in the emergency department (ED) may be appropriate. However, with signs of obstruction, prostration, fever, or peritonitis, the hernia should not be reduced, and prompt surgical consultation should be obtained for operative reduction with possible bowel resection. Most patients who have reducible hernias with viable bowel can be referred for elective surgical repair. Any incarcerated or strangulated hernia requires immediate surgical intervention.

REFERENCES

1. Bobrow RS. The hernia. *J Am Board Fam Pract* 1999;12:95–96.
2. Toms AP, Dixon AK, Murphy JM, Jamieson NV. Illustrated review of new imaging techniques in the diagnosis of abdominal wall hernias. *Br J Surg* 1999;86:1243–1249.
3. Hojer AM, Rygaard H, Jess P. CT in the diagnosis of abdominal wall hernias: a preliminary study. *Eur Radiol* 1997;7:1416–1418.

Abdominal Abscess

William J. Meurer

Clinical Presentation

Patients with abdominal abscess frequently present with abdominal pain, fever, and tachycardia in light of a recent history of abdominal or pelvic surgery. Violation of the peritoneal cavity by surgery or trauma and inflammatory bowel disease (IBD) are important risk factors.[1–3]

Pathophysiology

Incidence rates as high as 24% after laparoscopic appendectomy, 4.2% after open appendectomy,[1] and 10% to 30% in patients with Crohn's disease (CD) have been reported.[2]

Diagnosis

The essential laboratory workup includes a complete blood count, urinalysis, electrolyte levels, and renal function analysis. Blood cultures may be indicated in the septic patient. Abdominal computed tomography (CT) with oral and intravenous contrast is the imaging test of choice. Unless viscus perforation is suspected, there is little utility in obtaining plain abdominal radiographic films.[1–3]

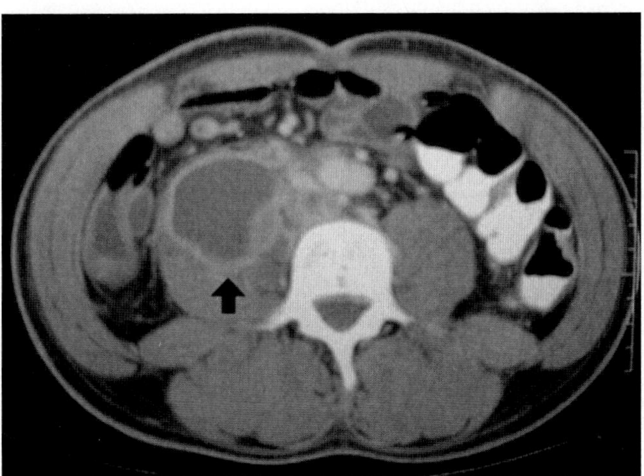

FIGURE 9–22 Computed tomogram showing abdominal abscess. (Courtesy of Mark Silverberg, MD.)

Clinical Complications

Sepsis and multiple organ dysfunction syndrome (MODS) are the major complications.[1–3]

Management

Fluid resuscitation and broad-spectrum antibiotics should be promptly initiated in the ED. A recent prospective, randomized study demonstrated that ertapenem and piperacillin/tazobactam are equivalent in efficacy and safety.[3] Urgent surgical consultation should be obtained, and patients with intraabdominal abscesses should be admitted.[2,3]

REFERENCES

1. Krisher SL, Browne A, Dibbins A, Tkacz N, Curci M. Intra-abdominal abscess after laparoscopic appendectomy for perforated appendicitis. *Arch Surg* 2001;136:438–441.
2. Jawhari A, Kamm MA, Ong C, Forbes A, Bartram CI, Hawley PR. Intra-abdominal and pelvic abscess in Crohn's disease: results of noninvasive and surgical management. *Br J Surg* 1998;85:367–371.
3. Solomkin JS, Yellin AE, Rotstein OD, et al. Ertapenem versus piperacillin/tazobactam in the treatment of complicated intraabdominal infections: results of a double-blind, randomized comparative phase III trial. *Ann Surg* 2003;237:235–245.

Acute Appendicitis

Michael Greenberg

Clinical Presentation

Although the classic presentation for acute appendicitis (AA) involves the onset of periumbilical pain that migrates to the right lower quadrant in association with fever, anorexia, nausea, and vomiting, substantial variations in presentation may be the rule rather than the exception. Clinical presentations can be complex and confusing in the very young, the elderly, immunocompromised individuals, and pregnant women.[1-3]

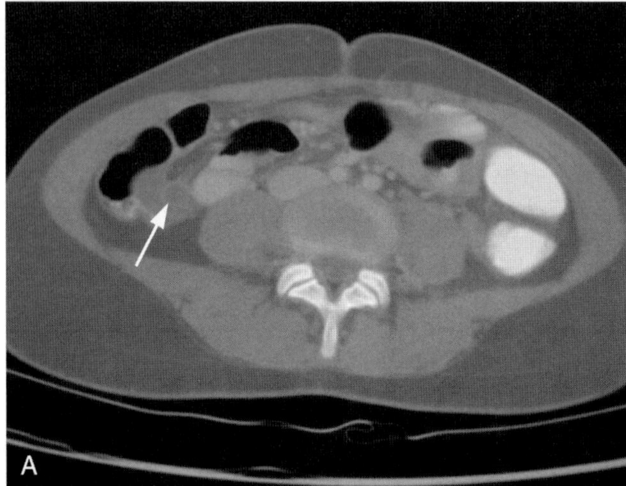

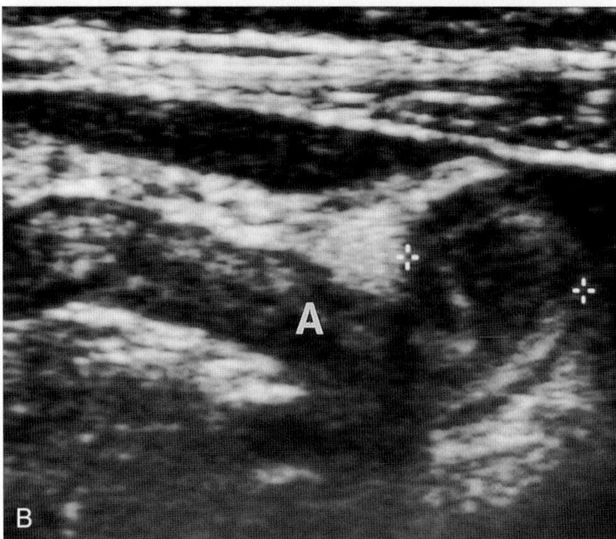

FIGURE 9-23 **A:** Dilated appendix ("bull's-eye sign"). (Courtesy of Robert Hendrickson, MD.) **B:** The distended appendix (A) has a dilated tip *(cursors)*. (From Yamada, with permission.)

Pathophysiology

AA is the most common cause for acute abdominal pain in the United States. The lifetime risk has been estimated to range from 5% to 20%.[1-3]

Diagnosis

History and physical examination are the mainstay for diagnosis. Approximately 95% of patients with right lower quadrant pain and tenderness who present as described can be expected to have AA. If the diagnosis is in doubt or the findings are equivocal, abdominal computed tomography (CT) may help to establish the diagnosis. CT is superior to ultrasonography in this regard.[1-3]

Clinical Complications

Complications include failure to diagnosis the problem, appendiceal rupture, intraabdominal abscess formation, postoperative wound infection, prolonged ileus, pneumonia, and systemic sepsis.

Management

The definitive treatment for AA is surgical removal of the appendix. Most surgeons advocate intravenous hydration and antibiotic coverage before operation, and the emergency physician may be in the best position to facilitate preoperative preparation of the patient. If the diagnosis is suspected, timely on-site surgical consultation is essential. If the diagnosis is in doubt, prudence dictates that patients with lower right-sided abdominal pain, fever, nausea, and vomiting should be observed in the hospital for a period adequate to determine the diagnosis.[3]

REFERENCES

1. Even-Bendahan G, Lazar I, Erez I, et al. Role of imaging in the diagnosis of acute appendicitis in children. *Clin Pediatr (Phila)* 2003;42:23–27.
2. Paulson EK, Kalady MF, Pappas TN. Clinical practice: suspected appendicitis. *N Engl J Med* 2003;348:236–242.
3. Margenthaler JA, Longo WE, Virgo KS, et al. Risk factors for adverse outcomes after the surgical treatment of appendicitis in adults. *Ann Surg* 2003;238:59–66.

Crohn's Disease

Robert Hendrickson

Clinical Presentation

Patients may present with an exacerbation of known Crohn's disease (CD), extraintestinal or fistulous complications, or undiagnosed disease. During exacerbations, patients typically develop fever, abdominal pain, weight loss, and diarrhea with or without blood in the stool.[1] Pain typically occurs in the right lower quadrant secondary to ileitis; however, patients may have pain in any location within the gastrointestinal (GI) tract. Bowel inflammation may lead to bowel obstruction, periintestinal abscesses, or fistulization.

Pathophysiology

CD is an idiopathic disorder with some genetic predisposition that most likely is caused by a transmural inflammatory response to bowel bacterial proteins.[2,3] The presence of intestinal bacterial proteins leads to an increase in intestinal type 1 helper (Th1) T cells, release of interferon-γ and interleukin-2 (IL-2), and a resultant inflammatory cascade.[2] The inflammation may include all layers of the bowel wall and may produce fistulas as well as periintestinal abscesses. The inflammatory regions may occur anywhere in the GI tract and are not necessarily contiguous.

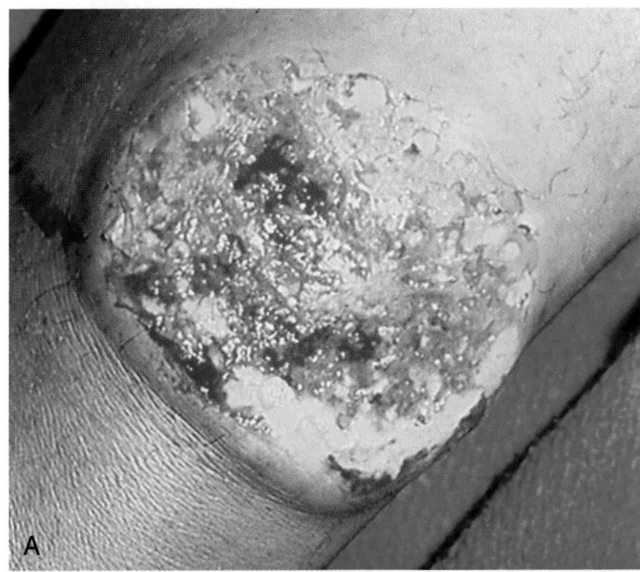

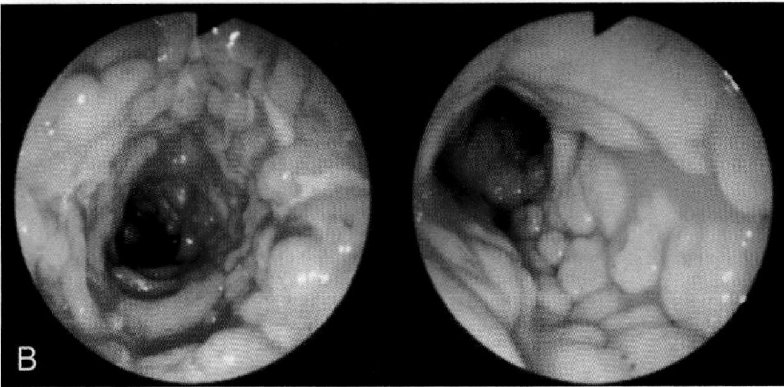

FIGURE 9–24 **A:** Pyoderma gangrenosum of a patient with Crohn's disease. (From Yamada, with permission.) **B:** Active phase of Crohn's disease shows cobblestoning, caused by interconnecting ulcerations *(left)*. An area of cobblestoning after therapy is shown on the right. (From Yamada, with permission.)

Clinical Complications

Extraintestinal complications include arthritis (nondeforming monoarthritis), sacroiliitis, cholelithiasis, iritis, uveitis, and erythema nodosum. Transmural bowel inflammation may lead to large bowel obstruction (LBO) or small bowel obstruction (SBO), intraabdominal abscesses, and fistulization from the GI tract to the bladder, abdominal wall, vagina, or another abdominal organ.

Management

Patients may require resuscitation and should initially be evaluated for fistulas, obstruction, perforation, and abscess formation. Those with significant dehydration, vomiting, anemia, complications, or pain require admission to the hospital for bowel rest, intravenous corticosteroids, surgical consultation (if indicated), and antibiotics (ciprofloxacin and metronidazole).[1]

Patients with mild exacerbations of CD may be considered for discharge on oral steroids and an increase in their chronic medications, with close follow-up by their primary provider. Patients with significant disease are typically treated with 5-acetylsalicylate (5-ASA) compounds, including sulfasalazine, mesalamine, olsalazine, or balsalazide. Patients with no response to these drugs may be treated with an immunomodulatory agent (e.g., azathioprine, mercaptopurine, cyclosporine, methotrexate), or an anti–tumor necrosis factor (TNF) infusion (infliximab).[2,3]

Patients without a diagnosis of CD who have consistent symptoms (abdominal pain, fever, diarrhea) should have other infectious causes excluded. Computed tomography (CT) of the abdomen may reveal inflammatory bowel wall changes anywhere in the GI tract, but typically at the ileum. Laboratory evaluation may reveal a leukocytosis.[1–3]

REFERENCES

1. Regueiro MD. Update in medical treatment of Crohn's disease. *J Clin Gastroenterol* 2000;31:282–291.
2. Podolsky DK. Inflammatory bowel disease. *N Engl J Med* 2002;347: 417–429.
3. Rampton DS. Management of Crohn's disease. *BMJ* 1999;319: 1480–1485.

Ulcerative Colitis

Robert Hendrickson

Clinical Presentation

Patients may present to the emergency department (ED) with exacerbations of known ulcerative colitis (UC), extraintestinal complications, or undiagnosed disease. Patients with severe exacerbations of UC may present with abdominal pain, profuse bloody diarrhea, fever, or evidence of dehydration.[1] Toxic megacolon may occur if the colonic muscularis layer becomes inflamed, leading to dilatation of the colon with constipation and, potentially, bowel perforation with resulting peritonitis and sepsis.

Extraintestinal manifestations of UC include episcleritis, uveitis, erythema nodosum, pyoderma gangrenosum, and migratory monoarticular arthritis. Sclerosing cholangitis may also occur in UC and typically produces asymptomatic elevations of liver enzymes; it may also cause fever, pain, and jaundice. Patients with UC are at increased risk for thromboembolic events.

Pathophysiology

UC is an idiopathic disorder that most likely is caused by a mucosal inflammatory response to colonic bacterial proteins.[2] The presence of intestinal bacterial proteins lead to an increase in T-helper type 2 cells, production of interleukin 5 and transforming growth factor-β, and an inflammatory cascade.[2] The colitis begins in the distal aspect of the colon, primarily affects the mucosa and submucosa, and may progress proximally in a contiguous manner, but it does not affect the small bowel.[1]

Clinical Complications

Complications include fulminant colitis, toxic megacolon, intestinal perforation, sepsis, uveitis, pyoderma gangrenosum, erythema nodosum, sclerosing cholangitis, liver failure, and colon cancer.

Management

Patients with fulminant colitis, toxic megacolon, or intestinal perforation require rapid resuscitation, nasogastric suction, intravenous antibiotics (ampicillin/cephalosporin and gentamycin and metronidazole), surgical consultation, and admission to the hospital. Laboratory evaluation may reveal increased white blood cells, an elevated erythrocyte sedimentation rate, and acute or chronic anemia. Patients without bowel perforation may be treated with intravenous corticosteroids.

Patients with mild to moderate symptomatic UC may be treated with a 5-acetylsalicylate (5-ASA) compound (e.g., sulfasalazine, mesalamine, olsalazine, balsalazide), either topically (e.g., enema) or orally.[2] Patients with no response to 5-ASA compounds may be treated with corticosteroids until the exacerbation resolves (usually 7 to 10 days).[2] Patients may also be treated with immunomodulatory agents such as azathioprine, mercaptopurine, cyclosporine, methotrexate, or the anti-tumor necrosis factor (TNF) agent, infliximab.

Patients who have symptoms suggestive of UC but are without a diagnosis of UC should have infectious causes (e.g., *Clostridium difficile, Salmonella* spp., *Shigella* spp.) and hemorrhagic causes (e.g., arteriovenous malformation, diverticula) of their symptoms excluded. Consultation with a gastroenterologist should be obtained to confirm the diagnosis with proctoscopy or colonoscopy.

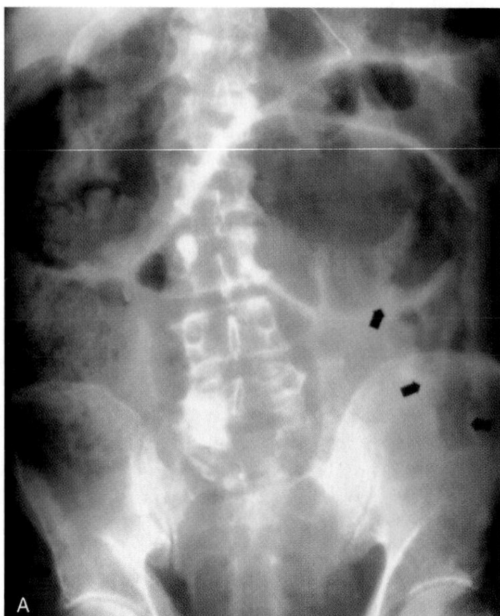

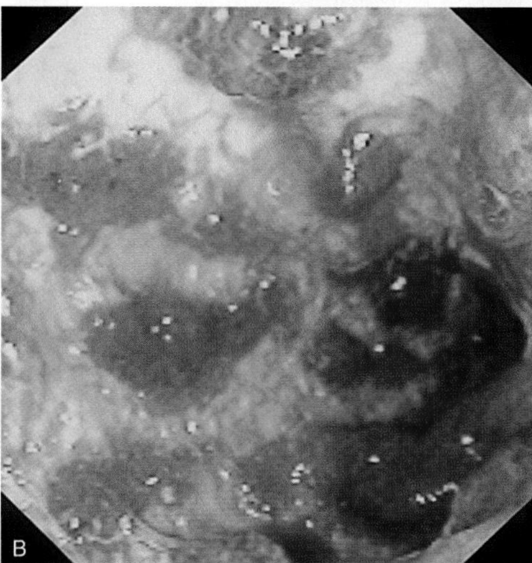

FIGURE 9–25 **A:** Radiograph of the abdomen shows distended colon with absence of normal haustra. The mucosal surface is nodular *(arrows)*. (From Yamada with permission.) **B:** Severely active ulcerative colitis. At least half of the surface area is denuded by ulcers, and there are intervening areas of edematous granular mucosa. (From Yamada, with permission.)

REFERENCES

1. Ghosh S, Shand A, Ferguson A. Ulcerative colitis. *BMJ* 2000;320:1119–1123.
2. Podolsky DK. Inflammatory bowel disease. *N Engl J Med* 2002;347:417–429.

Diverticulosis

Jason Sundseth

Clinical Presentation

Diverticulosis is common in elderly patients in western societies (65% prevalence at age 85 years). Symptoms are unusual (only 10% to 20% of people with diverticulosis) and may include intermittent lower abdominal pain and bloating that may be exacerbated by a meal and relieved with either flatus or a bowel movement. Bloating, diarrhea, constipation, or the passage of mucus can accompany the pain.[1]

Pathophysiology

Diverticulosis refers to saclike protrusions of the colonic mucosa. Diverticulosis may develop secondary to age-related alterations of collagen deposition, disordered colonic motility, or chronically elevated intraluminal pressure.[1] Diverticula occur in areas where the mesenteric vessels penetrate the colon, leaving an area of colonic wall weakness. Elevations of intraluminal pressure and contraction of colonic muscle may lead to herniation of the mucosa and submucosa through these weak areas (pseudodiverticula). True diverticula, which are very rare, occur when all layers are herniated.[1]

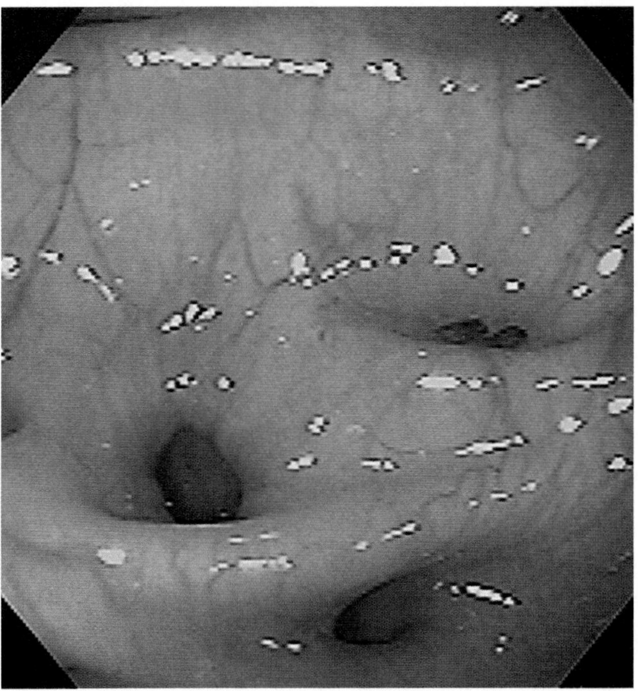

FIGURE 9–26 Multiple diverticular orifices. (From Yamada, with permission.)

Diagnosis

The diagnosis may be made by recognizing the typical history and physical examination findings (patients older than 40 years of age with lower abdominal pain and intermittent diarrhea, constipation, increased flatulence, or some combination of these symptoms). The diagnosis may be confirmed with computed tomography (CT), barium enema, or colonoscopy.[1]

Clinical Complications

Clinical complications include diverticulitis (10% to 25% of patients with colonic diverticula) and diverticular hemorrhage.[1]

Management

Symptomatic treatment includes relaxation of the painful muscle spasm. Application of heat or administering anticholinergics can reduce contractions.[1] Sedatives can decrease anxiety, which also helps to decrease contractions. A high-fiber diet, bulk laxatives, and stool softeners should be initiated to decrease intraluminal pressures.[1]

REFERENCES

1. Stollman NH, Raskin JB. Diverticular diseases of the colon. *J Clin Gastroenterol* 1999;29:241–252.

Diverticulitis

Jason Sundseth

Clinical Presentation

Patients may present with persistent left lower quadrant abdominal pain with diarrhea or constipation or both, low-grade fever, anorexia, and nausea. Dysuria and urinary frequency may reflect bladder or ureter irritation from the inflamed sigmoid colon. Patients of Asian descent may present with right-sided symptoms due to a predominance of diverticula in the ascending colon.[1]

Pathophysiology

Diverticula of the colon may become obstructed by stool in the diverticular neck. This fecalith abrades the mucosa and compromises the blood supply of the sac, leading to inflammation. The obstruction leads to a decrease in venous outflow, translocation of bacterial flora, localized ischemia, and diverticular perforation. Microperforations can be localized and contained by the pericolic fat and mesentery. Larger perforations may result in more extensive abscesses, fistulas, and even bacterial peritonitis.[1]

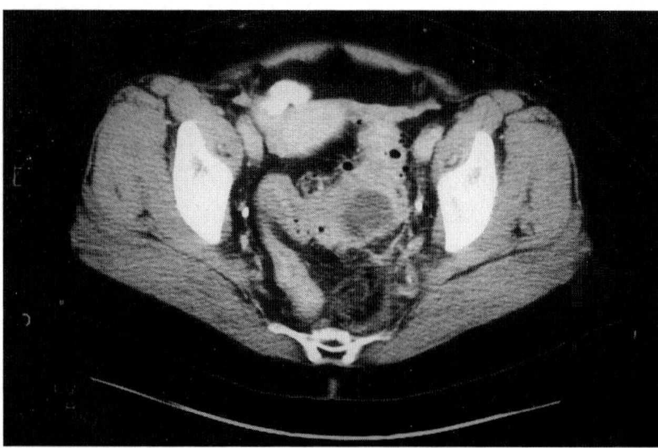

FIGURE 9–27 Computed tomogram with oral and intravenous contrast. The central, low-density region within the mass, the pockets of surrounding gas, and inflammatory changes in pericolic tissues are consistent with diverticular disease. (From Yamada, with permission.)

Diagnosis

The diagnosis may be suspected in patients with the typical history and physical examination. Plain radiography shows pneumoperitoneum in as many as 11% of patients with acute diverticulitis.[1] Small or large bowel dilatation or ileus, bowel obstruction, or soft tissue densities suggesting abscesses are found in up to 30% to 50% of patients.[1] CT with oral, rectal, and intravenous contrast may be used to determine or confirm the diagnosis and allows for the evaluation of extraluminal disease. Endoscopy is generally avoided because of the risk of perforation. Laboratory studies may reveal leukocytosis.

Clinical Complications

Complications include peritonitis, fistula formation, peritonitis, sepsis, and intestinal obstruction.

Management

Patients with mild symptoms, no comorbidities, and a confirmed diagnosis may be treated at home with a clear liquid diet, oral analgesia, and a broad-spectrum oral antibiotic (amoxicillin/clavulanate or a quinolone and metronidazole). If there is high fever, severe pain, or significant comorbid illness or the diagnosis is in doubt, the patient should be admitted to the hospital for strict bowel rest and intravenous administration of fluids, analgesics, and antibiotics (ampicillin-sulbactam or ticarcillin-clavulanate), starting in the emergency department (ED). Treatment for peritonitis or perforation requires immediate surgical consultation.[1]

REFERENCES

1. Stollman NH, Raskin JB. Diverticular disease of the colon. *J Clin Gastroenterol* 1999;29:241–252.

Hirschsprung's Disease

William J. Meurer

Clinical Presentation

Hirschsprung's disease (HD) almost invariably manifests in the neonatal period or in early infancy; however, it can manifest at any age and has been reported far into adulthood. Common clinical features are constipation, obstipation, and irritability. Fullness or mass in the left lower quadrant may be palpable, reflecting impaction of fecal material proximal to the aganglionic segment.[1,2]

Pathophysiology

The incidence is approximately 1 in 5,000, with a 4:1 male to female ratio.[1] Congenital absence of the ganglion cells of the myenteric plexus in the colon prevents proper bowel motility, and stool accumulates proximal to the affected area. The anus is almost always involved.[1]

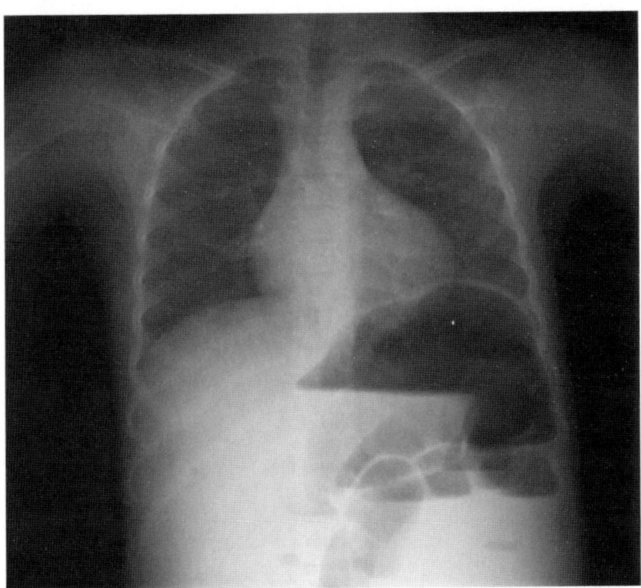

FIGURE 9–28 This child with Hirschsprung's disease has multiple air–fluid levels, consistent with obstruction. (Courtesy of Mark Silverberg, MD.)

Diagnosis

With a clinical history of constipation in the neonate, an abdominal plain film is reasonable. In older children, an abdominal radiograph should be obtained based on history and clinical suspicion. If a partial or full obstruction is seen, a water-soluble contrast enema should be obtained; this has sensitivity and specificity equivalent to barium enema and is preferred, given the complications of barium enema if a perforation is present.[2] Children who are febrile or toxic-appearing should have additional laboratory testing, including complete blood count, electrolyte measurements, and blood cultures. Pediatric surgery consultation is essential. Rectal biopsy confirms the diagnosis.[2]

Clinical Complications

Enterocolitis and toxic megacolon are the most feared and immediately lethal complications of HD. If the diagnosis is delayed, chronic constipation and failure to thrive may complicate the course of the disease.[2]

Management

Definitive therapy consists of excision of the affected area of bowel. Fluid resuscitation and broad-spectrum antibiotics for bowel flora coverage are indicated for the febrile or ill-appearing child. Patients with enterocolitis and toxic megacolon warrant admission to an intensive care unit (ICU). Patients with complete obstruction who are clinically stable warrant floor admission. If the obstruction is partial, discharge with symptomatic treatments, including enemas and stool softeners, and close follow-up with a surgeon may be appropriate.[2]

REFERENCES

1. Russell MD, Russell CA, Niebuhr E. An epidemiological study of Hirschsprung's disease and additional anomalies. *Acta Paediatr* 1994;83:68–71.
2. O'Donovan AN, Habra G, Somers S, Malone DE, Rees A, Winthrop AL. Diagnosis of Hirschsprung's disease. *AJR Am J Roentgenol* 1996;167:517–520.

Intestinal Perforation

John Curtis

Clinical Presentation

A perforated appendix, a stab wound, or iatrogenic rupture of the intestine secondary to endoscopic retrograde cholangiopancreatography (ERCP) or colonoscopy are clearly distinct clinical scenarios. Nausea, vomiting, pain, and the development of fever and diffuse peritonitis are some of the common symptoms and signs of perforation. The small bowel is the most commonly injured organ in penetrating trauma (including 80% of abdominal gunshot wounds) and the third most commonly injured organ in blunt trauma.[1]

Pathophysiology

Nontraumatic intestinal perforation can be caused by increased intraluminal pressure, local erosion of bowel wall, or an ingested object. The incidence of traumatic perforation is rising in both blunt and penetrating trauma, perhaps because of the increasing use of firearms, use of seatbelts, and the increasing speed of travel.[1] Colonic perforation has been shown to complicate 0.196% of colonoscopies and 0.088% of sigmoidoscopies.[2]

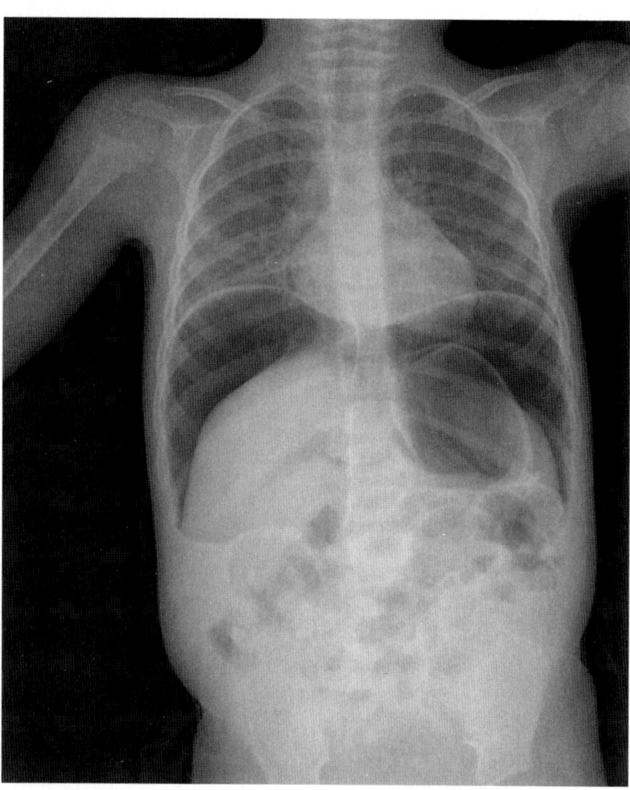

FIGURE 9–29 Free air under diaphragm secondary to intestinal perforation. (Courtesy of Robert Hendrickson, MD.)

Diagnosis

The diagnosis of perforation is suggested by free air on abdominal or chest radiography. Diagnostic peritoneal lavage yielding greater than 100,000 red blood cells (RBCs) or 500 white blood cells (WBCs) is nonspecific. Computed tomography (CT), preferably with oral contrast, is much more sensitive and specific for perforation, but it may be misleading in blunt trauma.[1]

Clinical Complications

Hemorrhage as well as spillage of intestinal contents can complicate perforations and leads to sepsis and multisystem organ failure in more than 70% of patients with perforation.[3] Surgical intervention can lead to multiple complications, including short-gut syndrome.

Management

Broad-spectrum antibiotic coverage should be started early. A typical regimen would include a third-generation cephalosporin and metronidazole. The treatment for perforation is primarily surgical and includes resection of the damaged bowel, with diversion and eventual reanastomosis.[1–3]

REFERENCES

1. Espinoza R, Rodriguez A. Traumatic and nontraumatic perforation of hollow viscera. *Surg Clin North Am* 1997;77:1291–1304.
2. Gatto NM, Frucht H, Sundararajan V, Jacobson JS, Grann VR, Neugut AI. Risk of perforation after colonoscopy and sigmoidoscopy: a population-based study. *J Natl Cancer Inst* 2003;95:230–236.
3. Barie PS, Hydo LJ, Fischer E. Development of multiple organ dysfunction syndrome in critically ill patients with perforated viscus: Predictive value of APACHE severity scoring. *Arch Surg* 1996;131:37–43.

Ischemic Colitis

John Curtis

Clinical Presentation

In 50% of patients with ischemic colitis, in whom the damage is limited to the mucosa and submucosa, the key symptoms and signs are abdominal pain (75%), bloody diarrhea, and abdominal distention. In the 10% of patients who experience full-thickness necrosis, perforation of the gangrenous segment and spillage of colonic bacteria into the peritoneal space and bloodstream cause rapidly progressive peritonitis, sepsis, and multisystem organ failure.[1–3]

Pathophysiology

In occlusive ischemic colitis, blood flow to a segment of the colon is interrupted by emboli, thrombi, mesenteric arteritis, dissection, or the vascular changes of diabetes or atherosclerosis. Vasoconstricting drugs, including cocaine and decongestants, can cause arterial insufficiency as well.[1] Venous occlusion also occurs in portal hypertension and in hypercoagulable states.[2] Nonocclusive ischemia is caused by low-flow states, including shock of any cause.

Diagnosis

The diagnosis is primarily clinical. Serum markers such as lactate, creatine phosphokinase (CPK), and lactate dehydrogenase (LDH) are relatively nonspecific. Radiographic evidence includes pneumatosis coli, thumbprinting on plain films, portal venous air, and bowel wall edema on computed tomography (CT). The definitive diagnosis of ischemic colitis is made by endoscopic evaluation of the affected segment.[1–3]

Clinical Complications

Chronic pain may complicate this disease after it is resolved acutely. Ischemia that enters the muscular layers can heal with scarring, resulting in strictures that may lead to obstruction.[1–3]

Management

The emergency management of ischemic colitis involves vigorous resuscitation with intravenous fluids and broad-spectrum antibiotics. Peritoneal signs mandate prompt surgical treatment, with resection of the involved bowel segment and a temporary diverting colostomy. Underlying causes should be sought and treated. This may include the discontinuation of vasoconstricting drugs, evaluation of hypercoagulable states, and screening for cardiac sources of embolism, which are present in up to 43% of patients with segmental nongangrenous ischemic colitis.[3]

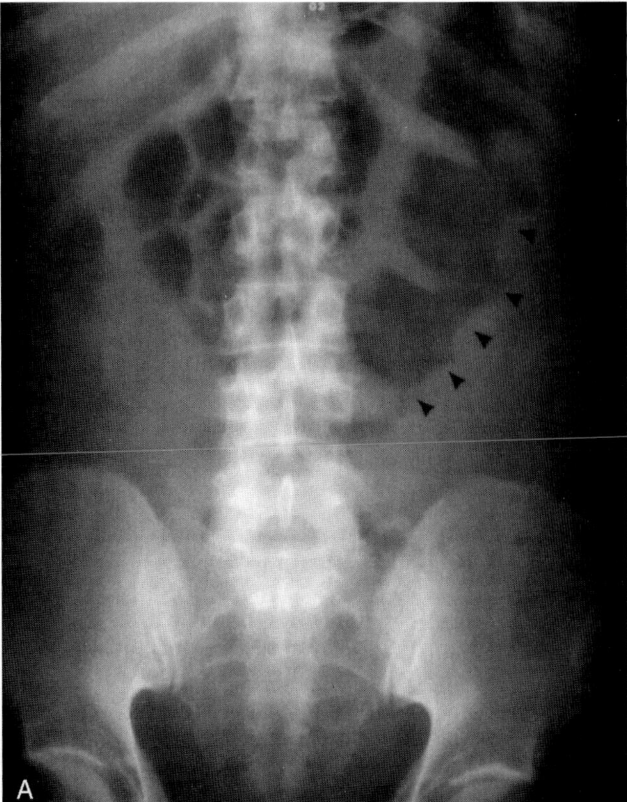

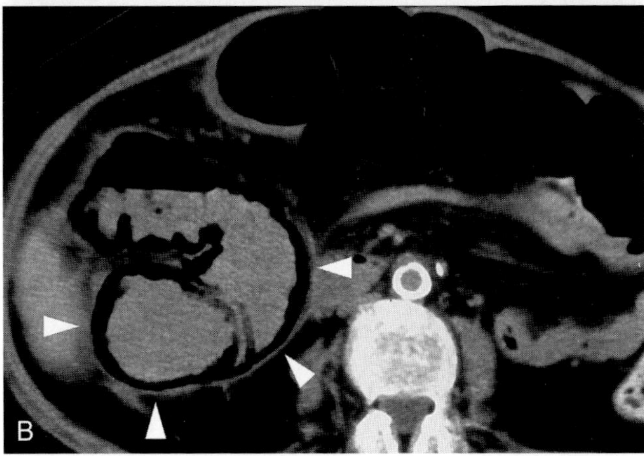

FIGURE 9–30 **A:** Mesenteric ischemia (ileus). On the first plain radiograph of the abdomen, the right colon and transverse colon are distended with gas and demonstrate a scalloped margin *(arrowheads)* and thickened, edematous haustra (From Yamada, with permission.) **B:** Severe ischemic colitis in a patient with septic shock. Transverse computed tomography scan section shows extensive pneumatosis in the colonic wall *(arrowheads)*. (From Yamada, with permission.)

REFERENCES

1. Toursarkissian B, Thompson RW. Ischemic colitis [Review]. *Surg Clin North Am* 1997;77:461–477.
2. Yee NS, Guerry D 4th, Lichtenstein GR. Ischemic colitis associated with factor V Leiden mutation. *Ann Intern Med* 2000;132:595–596.
3. Hourmand-Ollivier I, Bouin M, Saloux E, et al. Cardiac sources of embolism should be routinely screened in ischemic colitis. *Am J Gastroenterol* 2003;98:1573–1577.

Meckel's Diverticulum

Jesse Walck

Clinical Presentation

Patients with Meckel's diverticulum (MD) usually present with painless rectal bleeding. Bleeding is more common in children, who may present with bright red blood per rectum or maroon, tarry stools.

Pathophysiology

MD is an embryologic remnant of the omphalomesenteric duct in the gastrointestinal (GI) tract. MD is the most common congenital GI anomaly and is found in approximately 2% of the population. During embryologic development of the gut, the omphalomesenteric or vitelline duct temporarily connects the embryologic midgut and the future umbilicus. Normally, this duct is obliterated during subsequent development, but it may persist as a fibrous tract, a patent fistula, an enterocyst, or, most commonly, a diverticulum. If the remnant remains as a proximal diverticulum from the midgut, it is referred to as an MD.[1] MDs are typically located 40 to 65 cm proximal to the ileocecal valve. The size of the diverticulum is variable and can range from a small bump to several centimeters in length.[1–3]

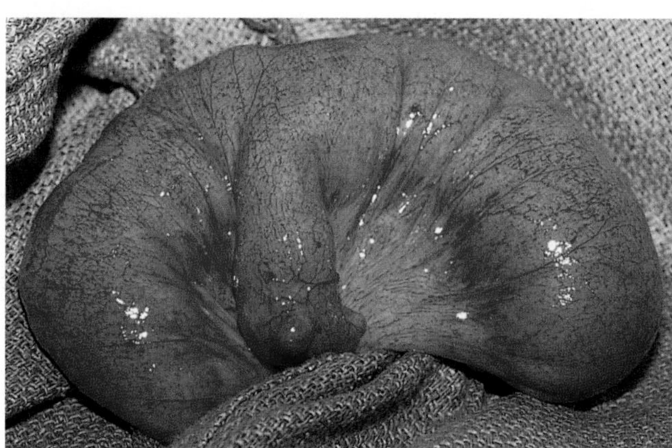

FIGURE 9–31 Meckel's diverticulum. These true diverticula contain all layers of the intestinal wall. (From Yamada, with permission.)

Diagnosis

A radionuclide scan is the diagnostic study of choice for MD; it shows uptake by the heterotopic gastric mucosa with a reported accuracy of 90% in pediatric patients. Computed tomography (CT) and ultrasonography usually are not diagnostic. Because symptoms other than painless rectal bleeding are less specific, an MD often is diagnosed only at laparotomy.[1–3]

Clinical Complications

Bleeding is the most common complication. It occurs in 50% of symptomatic patients and results from ulceration of ileal mucosa adjacent to the heterotopic gastric mucosa. Other complications include obstruction, intussusception, and fibrous bands, which can cause intestinal obstruction or volvulus.[1–3]

Management

Symptomatic patients should receive supportive care followed by timely surgical resection. The treatment of asymptomatic MD found on laparotomy remains controversial. One study supported diverticulectomy for an MD discovered incidentally, suggesting that its associated risk is less than the lifetime risk of complications from an MD.[2]

REFERENCES

1. Weinstein EC, Cain JC, Remine WH. Meckel's diverticulum: 55 years of clinical and surgical experience. *JAMA* 1962;182:251–253.
2. Cullen JJ, Kelly KA, Moir CR, Hodge DO, Zinmeister AR, Melton LJ 3rd. Surgical management of Meckel's diverticulum: an epidemiologic, population-based study. *Ann Surg* 1994;220:564–569.
3. Yahchouchy EK, Marano AF, Etienne JC, Fingerhut AL. Meckel's diverticulum. *J Am Coll Surg* 2001;192:658–662.

Carcinoid Syndrome

Cameron Symonds and Jonathan Glauser

Clinical Presentation

Patients with carcinoid syndrome (CS) may present with flushing, telangiectasia of the face and neck, diarrhea, bronchospasm, abdominal cramping, and fatigue. Cutaneous flushing typically involves the head and neck and may last minutes to hours. Symptoms may be provoked by exertion or by consumption of food or alcohol and may include tachycardia and hypotension.[1]

Pathophysiology

CS is caused by the hormonal action of various amines and peptides (e.g., serotonin, bradykinin, histamine) secreted by carcinoid tumors. It is characterized by paroxysmal vasomotor disturbances, diarrhea, and bronchospasm.[1] Carcinoid tumors occur in the appendix (40%), small bowel (20%), rectum (15%), bronchi (12%), and, less frequently, other parts of the gastrointestinal (GI) tract. Chemicals that can generate symptoms of CS include serotonin, chromogranin-A, neurokinin-A, bradykinin, tachykinin, and other hormones.[1]

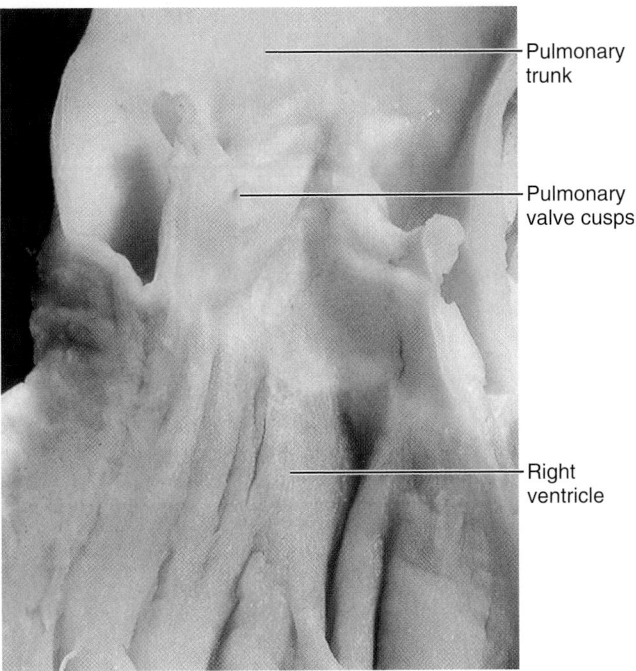

FIGURE 9–32 Pulmonary valve stenosis resulting from carcinoid syndrome. The pulmonary valve shows marked thickening. (From Hurst, with permission.)

Diagnosis

Laboratory testing is for elevated 24-hour urine 5-hydroxyindoleacetic acid (5-HIAA), a serotonin metabolite. Some common foods (bananas, pineapples) and medications (acetaminophen, caffeine) falsely elevate 5-HIAA levels. Iodine 131–labeled metaiodobenzylguanidine (MIBG) and octreotide scanning are the primary imaging modalities for localizing carcinoids. Other radiologic tests include computed tomography (CT) of the abdomen, barium examinations, angiography, and venous blood sampling with radioimmunoassay of tumor products.[1]

Clinical Complications

Complications include hypotension, increased platelet aggregation leading to disseminated intravascular coagulation, deep venous thromboses, stroke, and bronchospasm. Between 50% and 60% of patients develop carcinoid heart, with endocardial fibrosis and right-sided heart failure.[2] Chronic diarrhea and malabsorption may lead to nutritional deficiencies. Decreased tryptophan from serotonin synthesis can lead to niacin deficiency or pellagra.[2]

Management

Somatostatin analogues (e.g., octreotide, lanreotide) and interferon-α provide symptomatic relief from the flushing and other endocrine manifestations of the syndrome. H_2 receptor blockers, antidiarrheal medications, and albuterol all may reduce the visceral and peripheral effects of the hormones. Nutritional support and niacin supplementation can prevent malnutrition and pellagra.[1] Definitive treatment is surgical resection if the tumor is localized.[1-3]

REFERENCES

1. Anderson AS, Krauss D, Lang R. Cardiovascular complications of malignant carcinoid disease. *Am Heart J* 1997;134:693–702.
2. Boushey RP, Dackiw AP. Carcinoid tumors. *Curr Treat Options Oncol* 2002;3:319–326.
3. Soga J, Yakuwa Y, Osaka M. Carcinoid syndrome: a statistical evaluation of 748 reported cases. *J Exp Clin Cancer Res* 1999;18;133–141.

Peutz-Jeghers Syndrome

Gregory Schneider

Clinical Presentation

Patients with Peutz-Jeghers syndrome (PJS) may present with complaints consistent with bowel obstruction, abdominal pain, gastrointestinal (GI) bleeding, or actual extrusion of a polyp.[1]

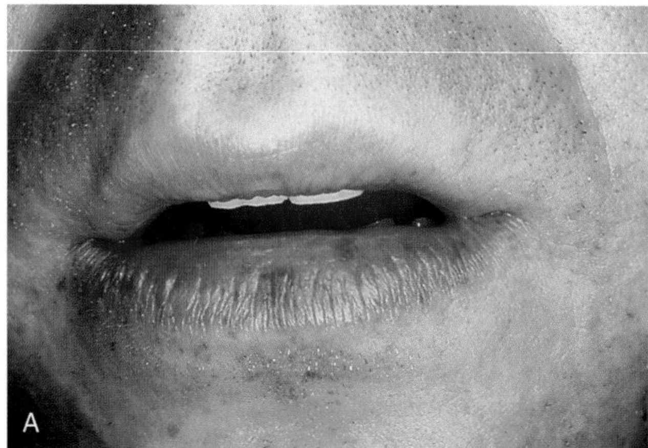

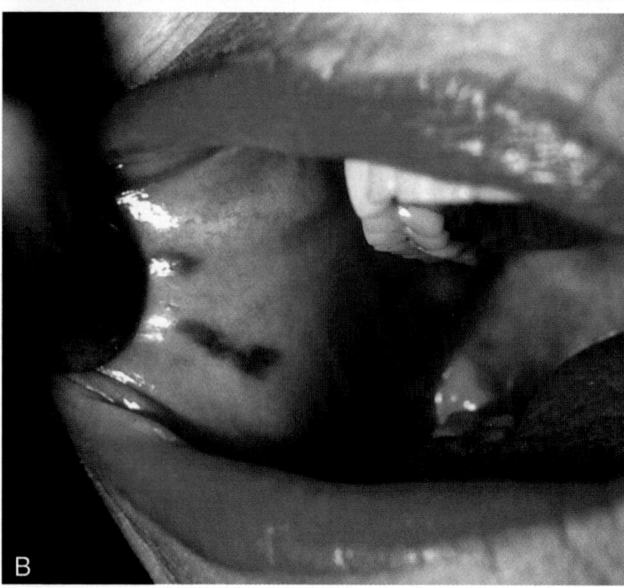

FIGURE 9–33 **A:** Peutz-Jeghers syndrome. Note pigmented macules on the lips that cross the vermilion border. (Courtesy of Jeffrey P. Callen, MD.) (From Yamada, with permission.) **B:** Peutz-Jeghers syndrome. The buccal and perioral pigment spots are characteristic of this syndrome. (From Yamada, with permission.)

Pathophysiology

PJS is an autosomal dominant inherited condition with variable penetrance.[1,2] The mechanism by which this abnormality manifests is poorly understood, but PJS is thought to be a cancer susceptibility syndrome. Multiple hamartomatous polyps form throughout the GI system, including stomach, colon, and rectum, with the greatest prevalence in the small intestine.[2]

Diagnosis

The diagnosis rests on a careful history and physical examination. Patients often have a history of previous GI surgery. Pigmented macules are present primarily around the mouth, eyes, nostrils, perianal area, and buccal mucosa. Family history may reveal a parent with a similar pigmented pattern and a history of multiple GI surgeries. Genetic testing confirms the diagnosis.[2]

Clinical Complications

Recurrent intussusception and GI bleeding are common, and an increased susceptibility to various cancers at a young age has been described.[1,2]

Management

Treatment of acute surgical problems in patients with PJS should not differ from that in normal patients, but there is a significantly increased likelihood of intussusception and obstruction. In long-term management, the goal is to remove all polyps. Genetic testing should be suggested for all first-degree relatives of PJS patients.[2]

REFERENCES

1. Utsunomiya J, Gocho H, Miyanaga T, Hamaguchi E, Kashimure A. Peutz-Jeghers syndrome: its natural course and management. *Johns Hopkins Med J* 1975;136:71–82.
2. McGarrity TJ, Kulin HE, Zaino RJ. Peutz-Jeghers syndrome. *Am J Gastroenterol* 2000;95:596–604.

Gallstone Ileus

Swapan Dubey

Clinical Presentation

Patients with gallstone ileus (GSI) often present with undifferentiated acute abdominal pain, but they may have signs and symptoms of intestinal obstruction, including nausea, vomiting, obstipation, inability to pass flatus, and abdominal pain. Symptoms of biliary colic are present in 50% to 66% of cases.[1–3] Symptoms may be vague and mild, and patients may not present until several days after initial onset.[1,2]

Pathophysiology

GSI may be preceded by an episode of acute cholecystitis. A biliary-enteric fistula may result from gallbladder inflammation, adhesions, and gangrene with perforation into the adjacent viscus, or from pressure necrosis from an impacted gallstone. Fistulas usually are located in the duodenum. Less frequent sites are the stomach, colon, and small bowel. The stone traverses the small bowel and increases in size due to intestinal sediment. Stones may become impacted in the distal ileum at the ileocecal valve.[1,2] Symptoms may be intermittent as stones lodge temporarily distally along the colon. Once the stone becomes lodged, classic symptoms of bowel obstruction predominate.

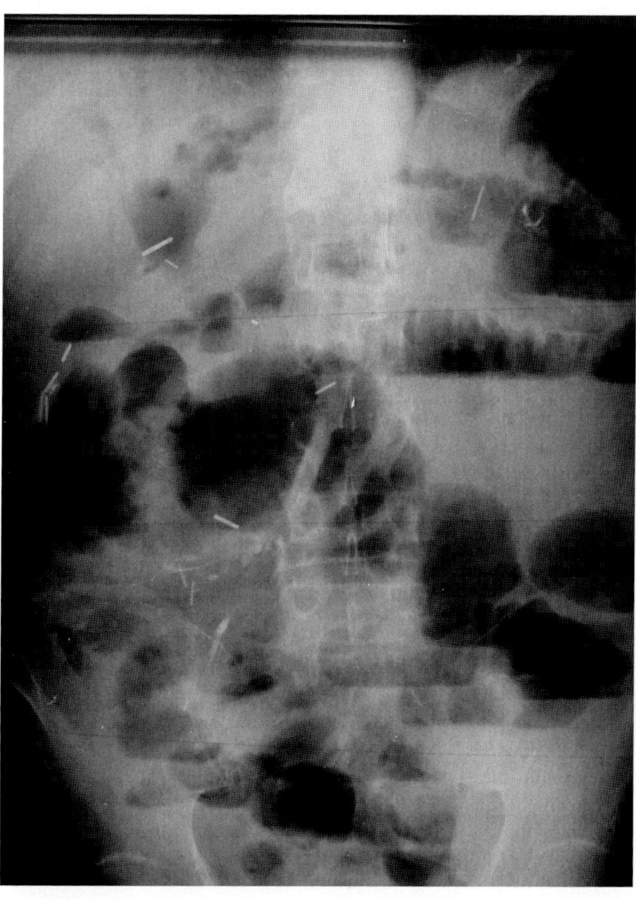

FIGURE 9–34 Small bowel obstruction and pneumobilia in a patient with gallstone ileus. (Courtesy of John Fojtik, MD.)

Diagnosis

A correct, preoperative diagnosis is made in only 50% of cases of GSI, with an average delay of 3 to 4.5 days between admission and surgical intervention.[1–3] Plain abdominal radiographs continue to have a role for patients with suspected bowel obstruction. The classic triad of GSI on abdominal films consists of small bowel obstruction (SBO), pneumobilia, and an ectopic gallstone. This triad is found in one third of cases of GSI, and two of the three signs are present in an additional 40% to 50%. Computed tomography (CT) findings may include pneumobilia and signs of liver inflammation, including free perihepatic fluid, and perihepatic fat-stranding.[1–3]

Clinical Complications

GSI is an uncommon complication of gallbladder disease. It frequently occurs in elderly patients who have comorbid diseases, and the diagnosis often is delayed. The mortality rate is reported to be 15% to 18%.[1–3]

Management

Emergency department (ED) management includes nasogastric tube (NGT) placement, bowel rest, fluid resuscitation, and, if indicated, administration of broad-spectrum antibiotics appropriate for peritonitis. Careful attention should be given to addressing exacerbations of underlying disease. Emergency surgical consultation is essential.

REFERENCES

1. Abou-Saif A, Al-Kawas FH. Complications of gallstone disease: Mirizzi syndrome, cholecystocholedochal fistula, and gallstone ileus. *Am J Gastroenterol* 2002;97:249–254.
2. Lyburn ID, Harris AC, Torreggiani WC et al. Gall-stone ileus: imaging features. *Hosp Med* 2002;63:434–435.
3. Reisner RM, Cohen JR. Gallstone ileus: a review of 1001 reported cases. *Am Surg* 1994;60:441–446.

Cholelithiasis

Lalena Yarris

Clinical Presentation

Most gallstones are asymptomatic. When biliary symptoms do develop, the patient usually presents with vague midepigastric or right upper quadrant (RUQ) tenderness that may radiate into the back or right shoulder region and is sometimes accompanied by nausea and vomiting. The term biliary "colic" is a misnomer, because biliary pain usually is constant, lasting up to 4 hours.[1] Although classically described as occurring after a fatty meal, biliary pain may occur at any time and may awaken the patient at night.

Biliary colic is caused by pressure as the gallbladder contracts against an impacted ductal stone. Since colic is not associated with inflammation or infection, fever, leukocytosis, or peritoneal signs should raise the suspicion of a complication of cholelithiasis, such as acute cholecystitis.

Pathophysiology

Gallstone disease is a common entity with life-threatening complications. Up to 10% of adults have gallstones. In adults older than 50 years of age, the prevalence rises to 25% in women and 15% in men. Emergency physicians should be familiar with the clinical course of gallstones, both to avoid being misled by the incidental finding of cholelithiasis and to correctly identify acute complications of chronic disease. The gallbladder is a thin-walled, contractile organ attached to the underside of the liver that serves to store and concentrate bile. Bile is composed of cholesterol, bile acids, and phospholipids, and the relative concentrations of each must be maintained within a fairly narrow range to prevent the precipitation of cholesterol crystals and the formation of gallstones. Mixed cholesterol stones account for approximately 75% of all stones in populations of western nations. Most of the remaining stones are pigment stones.[1]

Diagnosis

The diagnosis must be suspected based on a typical clinical history of RUQ abdominal pain. Laboratory studies are generally unremarkable in uncomplicated cholelithiasis. Acute cholecystitis is associated with a leukocytosis with a left shift, mildly elevated bilirubin, and mild increases in the transaminases, alkaline phosphatase, and amylase. Significantly elevated amylase should prompt consideration of pancreatitis.

The preferred imaging modality for cholelithiasis is ultrasonography. It is noninvasive and can detect the presence or absence of gallstones with a high degree of sensitivity and specificity (96% and 88%, respectively).[2] In addition, acute cholecystitis may be suggested by the findings of gallbladder wall thickening, a sonographic Murphy's sign, or pericholecystic fluid. Abdominal radiographs are generally not helpful, because only 10% of gallstones are radiopaque. However, they may be helpful in evaluating for pneumoperitoneum in the ill patient who presents with a complication of cholecystitis, or if there is a clinical suspicion for other intraabdominal processes.

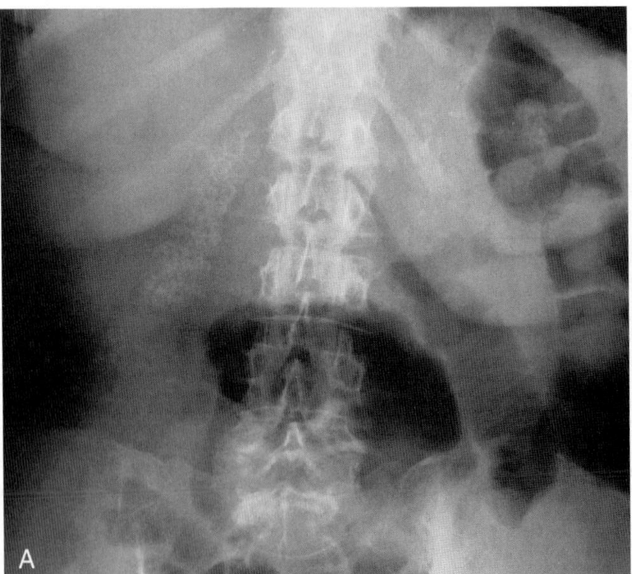

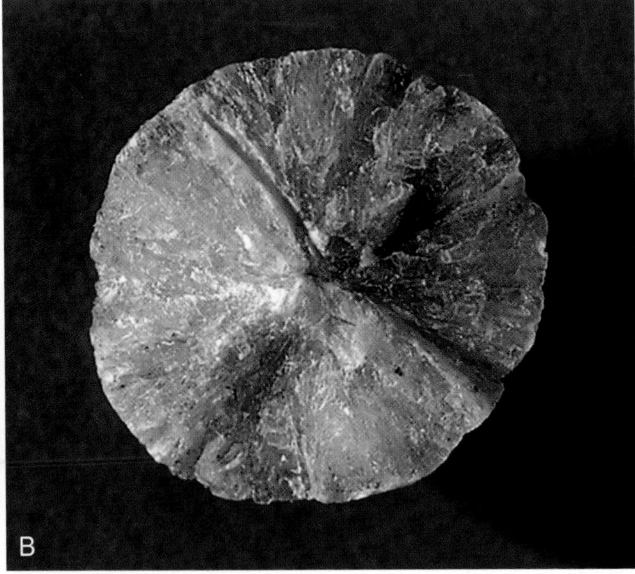

FIGURE 9–35 **A:** This patient has multiple gallstones. Note the hollow center of each stone. (Courtesy of Mark Silverberg, MD.) **B:** Pure, usually solitary, cholesterol gallstone (cholesterol solitaire). (From Yamada, with permission.)

Cholelithiasis

Lalena Yarris

Clinical Complications

Complications of cholelithiasis include acute cholecystitis, common bile duct stones, ascending cholangitis, pancreatitis, and gallstone ileus.

Management

Appropriate emergency department (ED) management of cholelithiasis depends on the symptoms. If gallstones are identified as an incidental finding and the patient is asymptomatic, there is no need for further evaluation or referral. Because of the low rate of symptom development, prophylactic cholecystectomy is rarely indicated. Management of biliary colic should include hydration, analgesia, and antiemetics. If the patient can be made comfortable and appears well, an extensive workup is not needed; outpatient ultrasonography and follow-up is appropriate. If the patient cannot be made comfortable or cannot tolerate oral fluids due to nausea or vomiting, inpatient admission may be necessary. In the ill-appearing patient, management should include laboratory studies, appropriate imaging studies, and consideration of early surgical or gastroenterology consultation. If the patient is febrile and acute cholecystitis is suspected, blood cultures and antibiotics are indicated. Therapy should be directed toward coverage of typical biliary pathogens, including enteric gram-negative bacteria, gram-positive species, and anaerobes in the elderly.

REFERENCES

1. Beckingham IJ. Gallstone disease. *Br Med J* 2001;322:91–94.
2. Kendall JL, Shimp RJ. Performance and interpretation of focused right upper quadrant ultrasound by emergency physicians. *J Emerg Med* 2001;21:7–13.

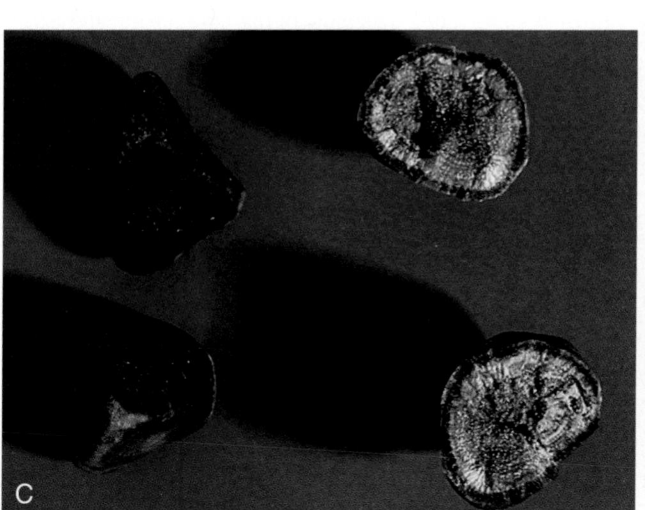

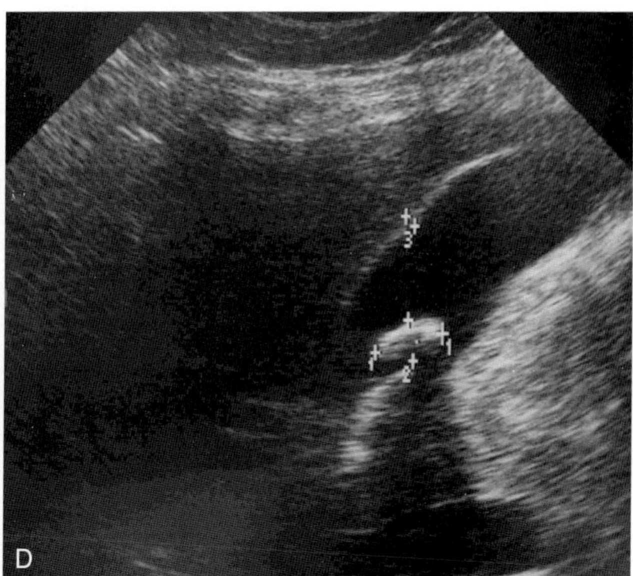

FIGURE 9–35, cont'd. C: Mixed cholesterol gallstones, which usually are multiple and faceted. The fractured surface shows a pigment center and concentric "growth" rings. (From Yamada, with permission.) **D:** Hyperdensity with acoustic shadowing, indicative of a 1.6 × 0.9 cm gallstone. (Courtesy of John Fojtik, MD.)

Acute Cholecystitis

Lisa Freeman

Clinical Presentation

Patients with acute cholecystitis typically present with constant pain below the right costal margin or epigastrium that radiates to the back. There may be a history of previous episodes of intermittent, colicky pain in the same area of the abdomen, occurring after intake of fatty foods. Nausea, vomiting, and fever may also be present. Physical examination may reveal tenderness in the right upper quadrant (RUQ), Murphy's sign (inspiratory arrest with palpation of the RUQ, secondary to pain), and localized peritoneal signs (guarding and rebound tenderness).

Pathophysiology

Acute calculous cholecystitis starts with persistent obstruction of the gallbladder outlet by a stone impacted in the neck of the gallbladder, Hartmann's pouch, or the cystic duct. As a result, the pressure inside the gallbladder rises, causing rapid distention of the gallbladder, decreased blood supply, ischemia of the gallbladder wall, release of inflammatory mediators, and, possibly, bacterial invasion. Acalculous cholecystitis occurs in critically ill patients (sepsis, trauma, burns, AIDS) and may manifest as sepsis of unknown origin. The pathogenesis of acalculous cholecystitis is thought to be related to biliary

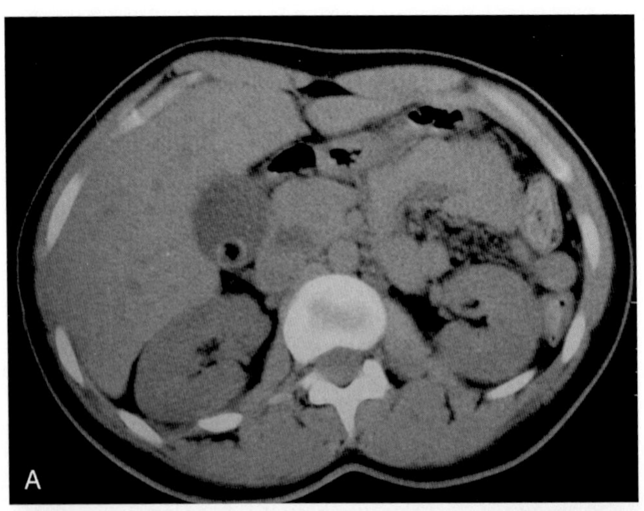

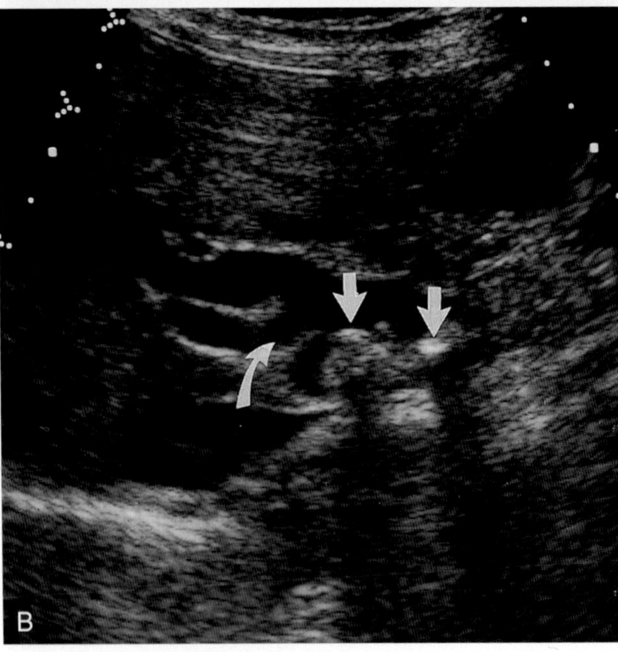

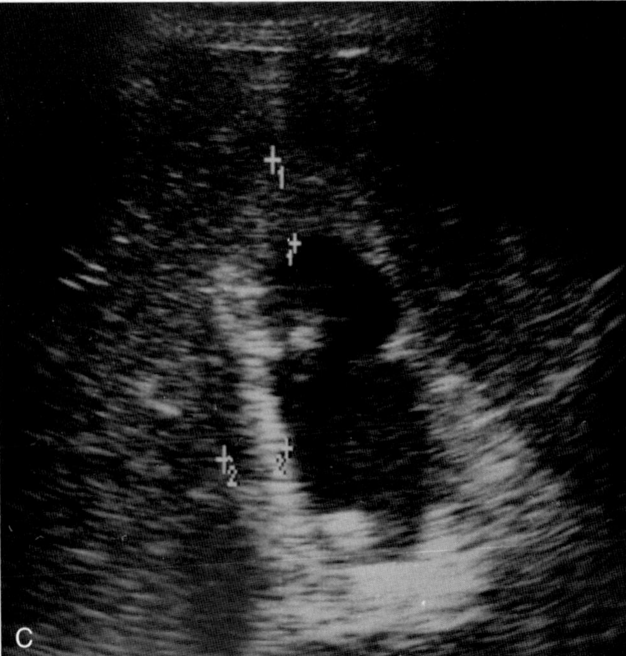

FIGURE 9–36 **A:** A single large gallstone with a typical hollow center. (Courtesy of Mark Silverberg, MD.) **B:** Common bile duct stone. Long-axis view of the intrahepatic and extrahepatic bile ducts reveals two echogenic common duct stones *(arrows)*. (From Yamada, with permission.) **C:** Gallstones and the presence of a thickened gallbladder wall, pericholecystic fluid, and a sonographic Murphy's sign are all indicative of cholecystitis. (Courtesy of John Fojtik, MD.)

Acute Cholecystitis

Lisa Freeman

stasis and mucosal ischemia that results in inflammation and infection.

Diagnosis

The diagnosis of acute cholecystitis is made by historical and physical examination findings and is confirmed by laboratory and radiologic studies. Leukocytosis with neutrophilia or bandemia (left shift) may occur. Elevation of total bilirubin, alkaline phosphatase, and transaminases may occur and suggest choledocholithiasis with obstruction of the common bile duct. Ultrasonographic study of the RUQ can detect signs of cholecystitis with a sensitivity of 88% and a specificity of 80%.[1] Typical sonographic findings include thickening of the gallbladder wall (greater than 4 mm), a sonographic Murphy's sign, and the presence of inflammatory fluid around the gallbladder. Hepatobiliary scintigraphy (HIDA scan) is used to evaluate biliary excretion of the intravenous nuclear isotope to determine the patency of the cystic duct. In a positive scan, there is nonvisualization of the gallbladder with normal excretion of the nuclear isotope into the biliary ducts and duodenum; this confirms obstruction of the cystic duct. HIDA scanning is up to 95% sensitive and 90% specific for the detection of acute cholecystitis.[2] Endoscopic retrograde cholangiopancreatography (ERCP) may be used for patients with elevated transaminases, amylase, or lipase to exclude choledocholithiasis and gallstone pancreatitis.[3]

Clinical Complications

Complications include gallbladder perforation, ascending cholangitis, and sepsis.

Management

All patients with acute cholecystitis require hospital admission, bowel rest, intravenous fluids, antiemetics, narcotic analgesics, and intravenous antibiotics. Recommended antibiotics include fourth-generation extended-spectrum penicillins such as piperacillin-tazobactam and ticarcillin-clavulanate.[3]

REFERENCES

1. Trowbridge RL, Rutkowski NK, Shojania KG. Does this patient have acute cholecystitis? *JAMA* 2003;289:80–86.
2. Kalloo AN, Kantsevoy SV. Gallstones and biliary disease. *Prim Care* 2001;28:591–606.
3. Indar AA, Beckingham IJ. Acute cholecystitis. *BMJ* 2002;325: 639–643.

Acute Pancreatitis

Lisa Freeman

Clinical Presentation

Patients with acute pancreatitis may complain of mild to severe epigastric pain that radiates to the back or flank. The pain is constant and dull and is typically worse when supine. A drinking binge or heavy meal may trigger the pain. Nausea and vomiting is present in 75% to 90% of patients.[1] Respiratory complaints such as chest pain or dyspnea may be present as well, reflecting the possible presence of a pleural effusion, atelectasis, or infiltrate. On physical examination, there is tenderness in the epigastrium or in the left upper quadrant, or both, and abdominal distention may be observed. The patient may have fever, tachycardia, dehydration, hypotension, and altered mental status.

Pathophysiology

Pancreatitis is inflammation of the pancreas, which typically results from obstruction of the exocrine pancreatic ducts. Up to 80% of cases are caused by alcohol abuse or biliary tract obstruction. About 20% to 30% of patients with acute pancreatitis develop necrosis, organ failure, or both.[1] Obstruction may be the result of a biliary stone, thickening of pancreatic secretions, or damage to exocrine duct linings (e.g., alcohol, endoscopic retrograde cholangiopancreatography [ERCP]). Obstruction of the ducts leads to interstitial release of amylase, lipase, and proteases, which can cause destruction of the gland. The exocrine and endocrine functions of the gland may be impaired for weeks.[1] There are many causes of acute pancreatitis[2]:

- Biliary tract disease (80%)
- Alcohol abuse
- Pancreatic duct obstruction
- Ischemia
- Drugs (angiotensin-converting enzyme inhibitors, thiazides, estrogens)
- Infectious (mumps, Epstein-Barr virus, coxsackievirus, cytomegalovirus)
- Postoperative status
- Post-ERCP status (5%)
- Metabolic disease (hyperlipidemia)
- Penetrating peptic ulcer
- Idiopathic (10%)

Diagnosis

The diagnosis of pancreatitis is made by history and physical examination and confirmed with laboratory and radiologic studies. The diagnosis requires a high index of suspicion and is misdiagnosed as much as 43% of the time.[1] Amylase and lipase concentrations may vary during pancreatitis, depending on the severity of the disease. Amylase concentrations begin to rise by 2 to 12 hours after symptom onset, peaking at 12 to 72 hours and returning to normal in 1 week. Lipase concentration increases within 4 to 8 hours after symptom onset, peaks at 24 hours, and normalizes in 1 to 2 weeks. Amylase is somewhat sensitive (75% to 92%), but not specific (20% to 60%) for diagnosis of pancreatitis. Lipase is somewhat more sensitive (86% to 100%) and specific (50% to 99%).

Serum testing may reveal elevations in liver transaminases, dehydration, hypokalemia, hypocalcemia, and hypomagnesemia. Chest radiographs should be obtained to evaluate respiratory complications. Plain films of the abdomen may be used to exclude other significant causes of pain, including obstruction and perforation. Computed tomography (CT) is the imaging modality of choice and may be obtained if the diagnosis is unclear or if the patient is severely ill. CT reveals diffuse or segmental enlargement of the pancreas with an irregular contour and obliteration of the peripancreatic fat, necrosis, or pseudocyst. Ultrasound studies may be obtained to exclude gallstones and biliary duct obstruction.

Several classification schemes exist to predict the severity of disease and the prognosis. Ranson's criteria are the most widely known:

- Age > 55 years
- White blood cells (WBCs) > 16,000 cells/hpf
- Glucose > 200 mg/dL
- Lactate dehydrogenase (LDH) > 350 IU/L
- Aspartate aminotransferase (SGOT) > 250 IU/dL

The criteria are expanded after the first 48 hours. The prognosis of the disease is correlated with the number of criteria met. Amylase and lipase are not used as prognostic criteria.

Clinical Complications

Multiple significant complications of acute pancreatitis are possible. These include hypovolemia, pancreatic necrosis or abscess, pseudocyst, acute respiratory distress syndrome, renal failure, ileus, shock, and sepsis.

Management

Management of airway, breathing, and circulation (the ABCs) is crucial, especially in severe cases, with emphasis on fluid resuscitation. Nasogastric suction is necessary only for intractable nausea and vomiting. Oral intake should be restricted until nausea and vomiting have subsided. Opioid analgesics and antiemetics should be provided as necessary. Morphine should be avoided as an analgesic, because it can cause spasm of the sphincter of Oddi. Although such spasm has not been proven to change the outcome in patients with acute pancreatitis, there are many other opioid options, including hydromorphone and meperidine. The use of antibiotics is controversial and should be reserved for cases of necrotizing pancreatitis. Most patients should be admitted. Patients may be discharged if they have mild disease, have adequate pain control, and are tolerating oral intake and biliary duct obstruction has been excluded.

REFERENCES

1. Munoz A, Katerndahl DA. Diagnosis and management of acute pancreatitis. *Am Fam Physician* 2000;62:164–174.
2. Beckingham IJ, Bornman PC. Acute pancreatitis. *BMJ* 2001;322: 595–598.

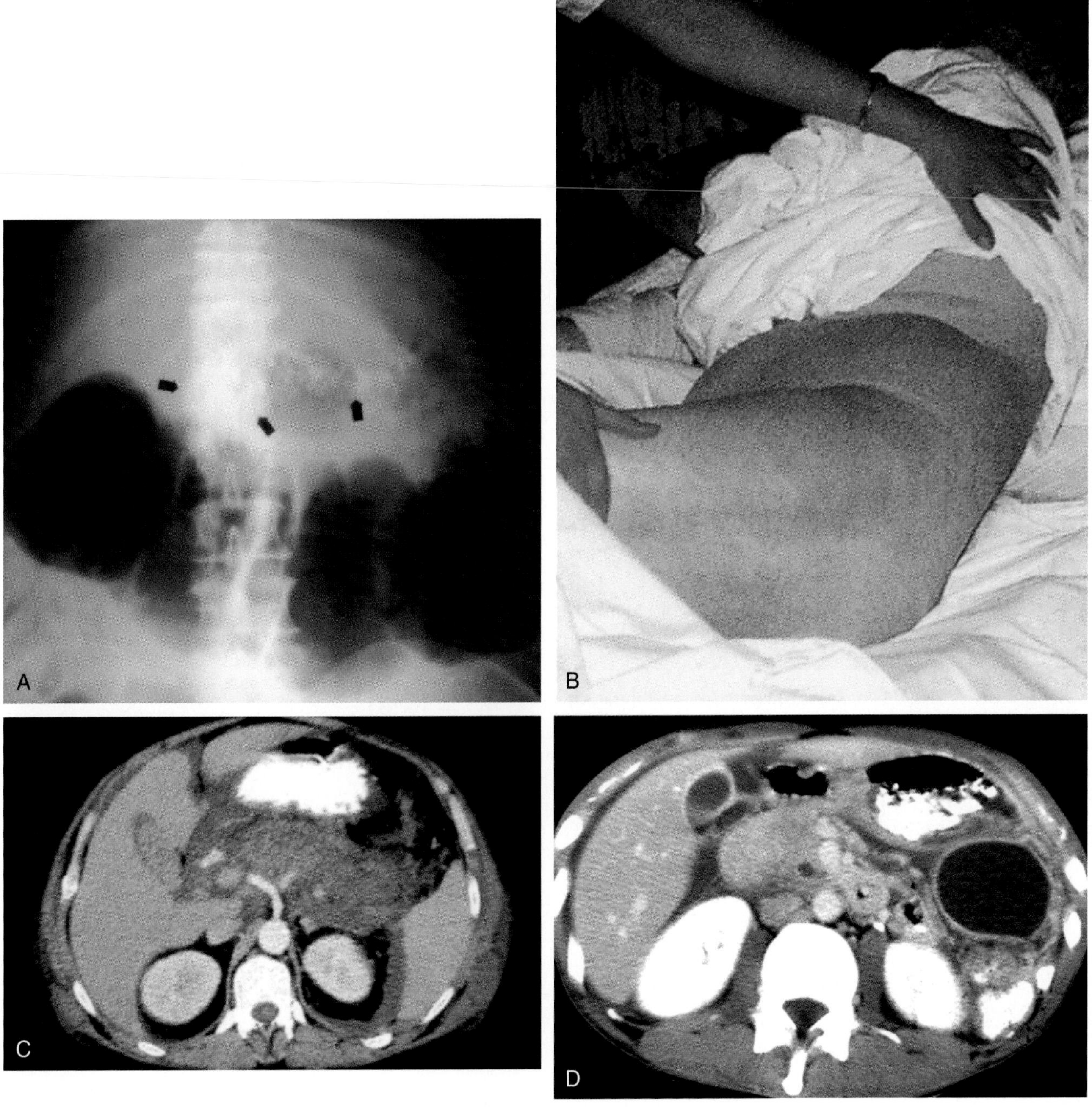

FIGURE 9–37 **A:** Localized colonic ileus caused by pancreatitis. (From Yamada, with permission.) **B:** Grey Turner's sign. (From Yamada, with permission.) **C:** Contrast-enhanced computed tomographic scan of the pancreas. There is absence of contrast enhancement, which suggests complete necrosis of the pancreas. (From Yamada, with permission.) **D:** A pseudocyst is seen near the tail of the pancreas. (From Yamada, with permission.)

Peliosis Hepatis

Michael Greenberg

Clinical Presentation

With the increase in the use of anabolic steroids to enhance athletic performance by young men, it is probable that patients with peliosis hepatis, a complication of steroid use, will be seen in the emergency department (ED). At times, the vascular lakes that characterize this condition rupture and result in intraabdominal hemorrhage. These patients may present in severe hypovolemic shock in the face of minimal or absent abdominal trauma. In addition, blood-filled lacunae may expand and then compress normal liver tissue, resulting in jaundice as well as frank liver failure.

Pathophysiology

Peliosis hepatis is a condition that affects the liver and is characterized by the development of many variably sized, blood-filled lacunae. This condition is most commonly associated with the chronic use of anabolic steroids as well as progestational and estrogenic steroids.[1] The drug danazol has also been reported to produce this lesion.[2] The pathophysiology of this condition involves marked dilatation of the vascular hepatic sinuses. The lesions tend to be widely distributed throughout the liver and "consist of blood-filled, ecstatic veins and some extremely dilated sinusoids."[3]

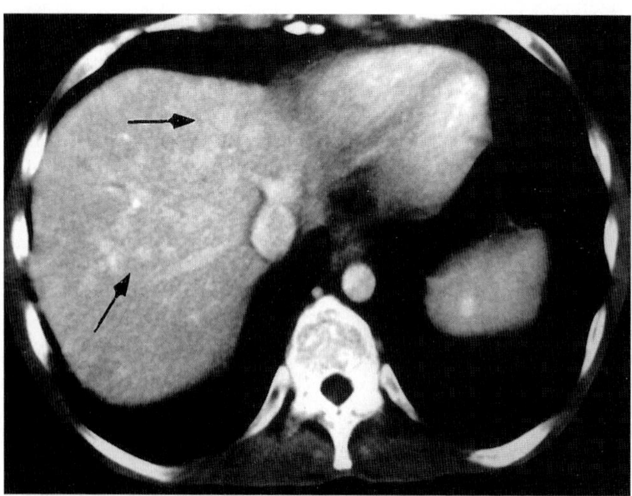

FIGURE 9–38 Peliosis hepatis. A computed tomographic image demonstrates multiple peliotic lesions, two of which are indicated by arrows. (From Yamada, with permission.)

Diagnosis

This condition should be considered in any patient who has been chronically taking anabolic steroids and presents to the ED with atraumatic right upper quadrant (RUQ) pain, unexplained jaundice, hypovolemic shock, or any combination of these findings. This condition may be diagnosed effectively by the use of abdominal ultrasonography.[1,3]

Clinical Complications

If peliosis hepatis remains undiagnosed, patients may die of unrecognized intraabdominal hemorrhage.

Management

Patients who are taking anabolic steroids should be monitored by the use of periodic abdominal ultrasonographic studies, and steroids should be cut back or discontinued if the condition develops. Patients with known peliosis hepatis must be counseled to avoid contact sports and to guard against any abdominal or RUQ trauma.[1,3]

REFERENCES

1. Bagatell CJ, Bremner WJ. Androgens in men: uses and abuses. *N Engl J Med* 1996;334:707–714.
2. Nesher G, Dollberg L, Zimran A, Hershko C. Hepatosplenic peliosis after danazol and glucocorticoids for ITP. *N Engl J Med* 1985;312:242–243.
3. Walter E, Mockel J. Images in clinical medicine: peliosis hepatis. *N Engl J Med* 1996;337:1603.

Budd-Chiari Syndrome

Gregory Schneider

Clinical Presentation

The Budd-Chiari syndrome (BCS) is characterized by right upper quadrant (RUQ) abdominal pain, ascites, liver enlargement, renal insufficiency or failure, and jaundice. The chronic form manifests with ascites that develop over several months. Jaundice is absent.[1]

Pathophysiology

Thrombosis of the hepatic veins in BCS is typically secondary to paroxysmal nocturnal hematuria; antiphospholipid syndrome; deficiency in antithrombin, protein C, or protein S; or presence of factor V Leiden.[1] Most cases are associated with myeloproliferative disease. Thrombosis of the hepatic veins leads to liver congestion with painful hepatomegaly. The degree of subsequent liver failure is variable.[2]

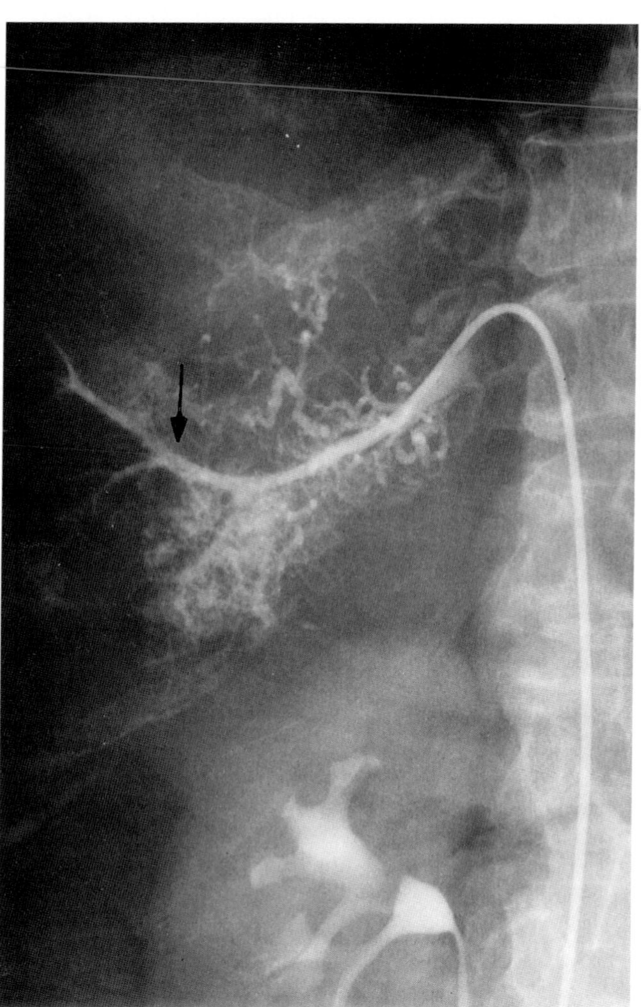

FIGURE 9–39 Budd-Chiari syndrome. The angiogram demonstrates the spiderweb pattern that is characteristic of the syndrome. (From Yamada, with permission.)

Diagnosis

BCS is suspected if ascites, liver enlargement, and upper abdominal pain are present, if liver disease is documented in a patient with a known thrombogenic disorder, or if chronic liver disease remains unexplained after other common causes have been excluded. Diagnosis is made by Doppler sonographic documentation of absent flow in hepatic veins or the presence of large intrahepatic collateral vessels, which develop to help decompress the liver in chronic cases. Magnetic resonance imaging may be helpful if ultrasonography is inconclusive.[1]

Clinical Complications

Liver failure is the most serious complication. Fibrosis may develop, leading to nodular regeneration and cirrhosis. Other complications include gastrointestinal (GI) bleeding and hepatocellular carcinoma.[1,2]

Management

Treatment depends on the acuteness of the patient's condition. Focal obstruction may be helped by dilation and stent placement to achieve vascular patency. Shunts may be used to decompress the liver. Portacaval and mesocaval shunts effectively relieve hepatic engorgement. Radiologically placed transjugular intrahepatic portasystemic shunts have recently gained favor because of their less invasive nature and the fact that their location does not complicate liver transplantation. Liver transplantation is considered in fulminant hepatic failure and if shunting procedures have failed.[1,2]

REFERENCES

1. Valla DC. Hepatic vein thrombosis (Budd-Chiari syndrome). *Semin Liver Dis* 2002;22:5–14.
2. Olzinski AT, Sanyal AJ. Treating Budd-Chiari Syndrome: making rational choices from a myriad of options. *J Clin Gastroenterol* 2000;30:155–161.

Cirrhosis/Portal Hypertension

Robert Hendrickson

Clinical Presentation

Patients with portal hypertension (PH) may present to the emergency department (ED) with a variety of complications, including variceal gastrointestinal (GI) bleeding, spontaneous bacterial peritonitis (SBP), ascites, and hepatic encephalopathy. Variceal bleeding may be brisk and may result in rapid exsanguination, tachycardia, hypotension, hematemesis, and alteration of mental status. Ascites may produce abdominal distention or dyspnea (from inhibition of diaphragmatic movement). SBP is an infection of the ascitic peritoneal fluid and may manifest as abdominal pain with or without a fever. Hepatic encephalopathy occurs when the cirrhotic liver cannot metabolize substances, including ammonia; it may manifest with an alteration of mental status and asterixis.

Patients with cirrhosis and PH may have several clinical signs: varices of the esophagus, hemorrhoids, jaundice, spider angiomata, gynecomastia, splenomegaly, caput medusae, and palmar erythema.

Pathophysiology

Cirrhosis of the liver refers to the fibrotic alteration of the liver parenchyma that leads to liver contraction and an increase in pressure of the portal venous system (PH). Cirrhosis usually is caused by excessive alcohol use or by viral hepatitis (hepatitis B or C), but it may also be caused by autoimmune disease, medications, biliary cirrhosis, or various metabolic disorders.[1,2] Chronic inflammation from alcohol, hepatitis, metabolic disorders, or medications leads to a cycle of fibrous scarring and hepatocellular regeneration that results in a nodular, shrunken liver with limited ability to produce proteins or metabolize chemicals. There is also an elevation of the portal venous pressure.

Diagnosis

PH and cirrhosis may be identified with a thorough history and physical examination.

Clinical Complications

Complications include variceal bleeding, ascites, SBP, hypoalbuminemia, hepatorenal syndrome, hepatic encephalopathy, and coagulopathy.

Management

A patient with variceal bleeding should be rapidly evaluated and treated with oxygen, large-bore intravenous access and infusion of fluids, packed red blood cells (RBCs), and fresh-frozen plasma, if necessary. Rapid consultation with an endoscopist is necessary. The patient may be treated with a splanchnic vasoconstrictor (octreotide, somatostatin, terlipressin) while awaiting endoscopic sclerotherapy.[2] Balloon tamponade may be used to temporarily tamponade the bleeding while awaiting more definitive therapy.[1]

Patients with ascites may initially be treated with bed rest, sodium and fluid restriction, and a diuretic for symptomatic relief.[1] These patients occasionally require therapeutic sterile paracentesis for symptomatic relief, particularly from dyspnea.[1] Patients with suspected SBP also require paracentesis for diagnostic purposes, as well as antibiotics (e.g., cefotaxime).[1]

Patients with hepatic encephalopathy require admission to the hospital and therapy to decrease intestinal ammonia (lactulose, neomycin or metronidazole), increase ammonia breakdown (ornithine aspartate), and a low-protein diet.[2] Patients with PH may be taking several chronic medications, including β-blockers (propranolol) and nitrates (isosorbide dinitrate).[2]

REFERENCES

1. Menon KV, Kamath PS. Managing the complications of cirrhosis. *Mayo Clin Proc* 2000;75:501–509.
2. D'Amico G, Pagliaro L, Bosch J. Pharmacological treatment of portal hypertension: an evidence-based approach. *Semin Liver Dis* 1999;19:475–505.

Cirrhosis/Portal Hypertension

Robert Hendrickson

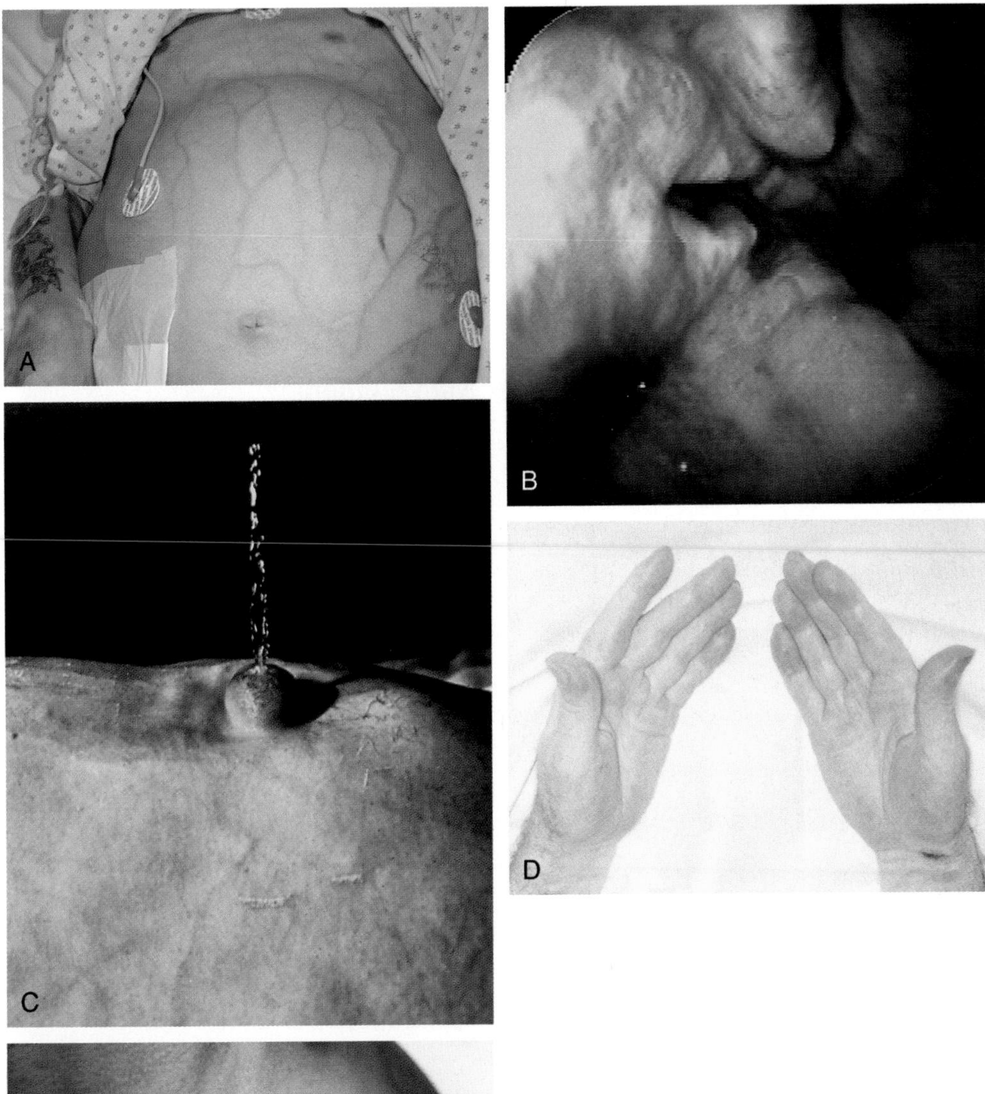

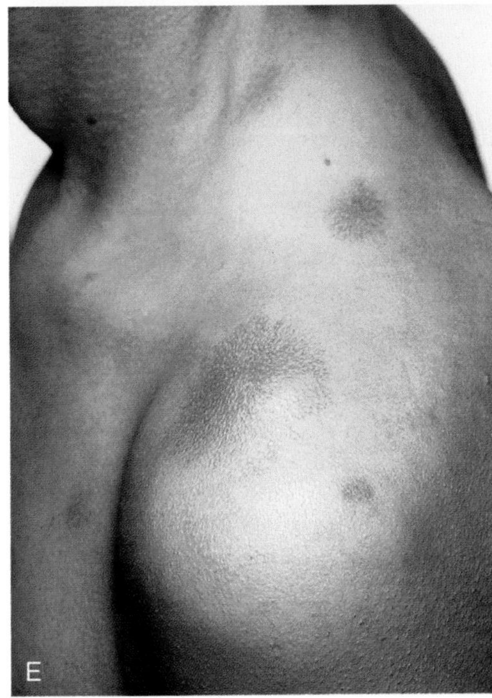

FIGURE 9–40 **A:** Caput medusae. (Courtesy of Rafi Israeli, MD.) **B:** Endoscopic view of moderate-sized esophageal varices with multiple red marks. (From Yamada, with permission.) **C:** Ruptured umbilical hernia, one of the most feared complications of ascites. (Courtesy of Telfer B. Reynolds, MD.) (Reprinted from Yamada with permission.) **D:** Palmar erythema of severe liver disease. (Courtesy of Telfer B. Reynolds, MD.) (From Yamada, with permission.) **E:** Cutaneous spider angiomas of cirrhosis on the upper torso. (Courtesy of Telfer B. Reynolds, MD.) (From Yamada, with permission.)

Hepatorenal Syndrome

Michael Greenberg

Clinical Presentation

Patients with hepatorenal syndrome (HRS) present with renal failure in the face of late-stage cirrhotic liver disease.

Pathophysiology

HRS is a common complication of cirrhotic liver disease associated with renal failure. HRS is defined by vascular constriction of the renal circulation, the specific mechanism of which is unclear. It is probable that portal hypertension causes essentially systemic vascular "underfilling," which activates homeostatic mechanisms that result in widespread systemic (and renal) vasoconstriction.[1] Renal perfusion is markedly decreased, and HRS develops. HRS may be precipitated by gastrointestinal (GI) bleeding, systemic infections, or paracentesis in which large volumes of fluid are removed.[1]

TABLE 9–41 Major Criteria for a Diagnosis of Hepatorenal Syndrome*

1. Chronic or acute liver disease with advanced hepatic failure and portal hypertension
2. Low glomerular filtration rate, as indicated by serum creatinine >225 μM or creatinine clearance <40 mL/min
3. Absence of shock, ongoing bacterial infection, or recent treatment with nephrotoxic drugs; absence of excessive fluid losses (including gastrointestinal bleeding)
4. No sustained improvement in renal function after expansion with 1.5 L isotonic saline
5. Proteinuria <0.5 g/day, and no ultrasonographic evidence of renal tract disease

*Additional criteria NOT required for diagnosis but commonly present include urine volume <500 mL/day, urine sodium <10 mM, urine osmolality >plasma osmolality, urine red blood cells <50 per high-power field, and serum sodium <130 mM.
From Dagher L, Moore K. The hepatorenal syndrome. *Gut* 2001;49:729-737, with permission.

Diagnosis

See Table 9–41. HRS must be suspected in any patient with late-stage cirrhosis and evidence of renal failure.

Clinical Complications

HRS carries a grave prognosis.

Management

Patients with HRS require meticulous supportive care, with special attention to fluid and electrolyte issues.[1] The treatment of choice for HRS is liver transplantation.[1] Early involvement of liver transplantation teams is appropriate. Measures aimed at preventing HRS are appropriate in the setting of spontaneous bacterial peritonitis or alcoholic hepatitis (or both).[1] In spontaneous bacterial peritonitis, the intravenous administration of albumin plus antibiotics greatly decreases the risk for HRS.[1] In patients with alcoholic liver disease, the administration of pentoxifylline may decrease the incidence of HRS. Pentoxifylline probably acts to inhibit the production of tumor necrosis factor (TNF), vascular endothelial factor, and other tissue factors that may be associated with the development of HRS.[1]

REFERENCES

1. Gines P, Guevara M, Arroyo V, Rodes J. Hepatorenal syndrome. *Lancet* 2003;362:1819–1827.

Rectal Foreign Bodies

Jason Sundseth

Clinical Presentation

Patients usually present with rectal pain, bleeding, abdominal pain, or complaining of the presence of a rectal foreign body (FB).[1] Patient history may be unreliable due to embarrassment.[1] Elderly patients may present after attempting fecal disimpaction or a prostatic massage. Identifying whether the FB is a result of assault is important, because this cause typically results in a higher incidence of injury.

Pathophysiology

Rectal FBs are objects that have been placed into the rectum and cannot be retrieved by the patient. Rectal FBs usually are inserted. However, they may result from incomplete passage of a swallowed FB.[1] The FBs are termed high-lying or low-lying, depending on their location in relation to the rectosigmoid junction. Edema and muscular spasms can result from the obstruction and may worsen with delays in presentation. Lacerations and perforation are possible but are uncommon.[1]

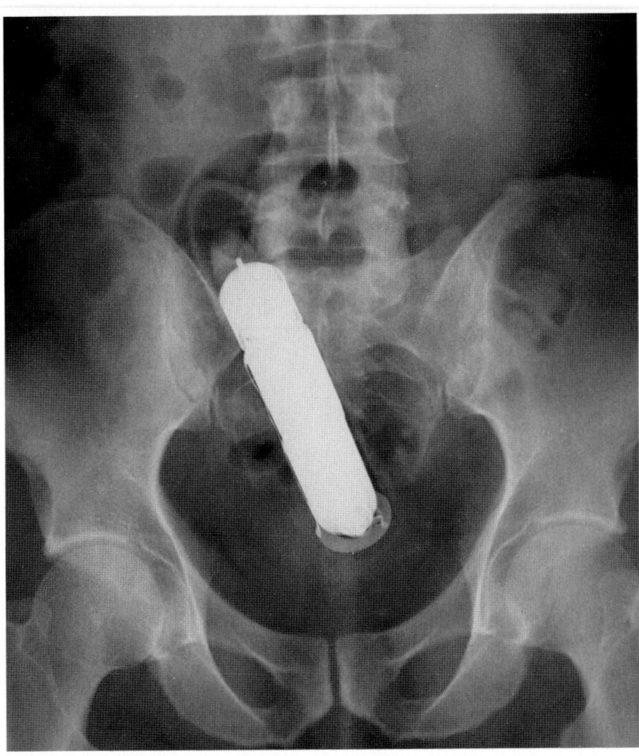

FIGURE 9–42 Vibrator in rectum. (Courtesy of Robert Hendrickson, MD.)

Diagnosis

Laboratory studies may include a hematocrit and white blood cell (WBC) count to evaluate the extent of rectal bleeding or the presence of infection. Radiographic studies include a flat plate of the abdomen and pelvis to evaluate the object's size, location, and orientation. An upright chest or lateral abdominal film may help identify free air if perforation is suspected.[1,2]

Clinical Complications

Rectal lacerations, perforations, and infection with abscess formation and sepsis may complicate this problem.[1,2]

Management

Removal of the object may be attempted in the emergency department (ED) for low-lying objects that are easily palpated on rectal examination. Rectal examination should not be performed before review of the radiographs for location, orientation, and the nature of the object. The presence of blood indicates laceration or perforation and warrants a surgery consultation. Attempts may be made with visualization through an anoscope or proctoscope and removal with forceps or snares.[2] Adequate sedation and analgesia are vital for easier removal. Abdominal manipulation can be performed for high-lying objects in an attempt to move them into a low-lying position for removal. If the object appears difficult or dangerous to remove, consultation with a surgeon for removal under general anesthesia would be prudent.[1,2]

REFERENCES

1. Ooi BS, Ho YH, Eu KW, Nyam D, Leong A, Seow-Choen F. Management of anorectal foreign bodies: a cause of obscure anal pain. *Aust N Z J Surg* 1998;68:852–855.
2. Cohen JS, Sackier JM. Management of colorectal foreign bodies. *J R Coll Surg Edinb* 1996;41:312–315.

Anorectal Abscesses

Derek Halvorson

Clinical Presentation

Patients with perianal abscesses, which comprise 60% of all anorectal abscesses (ARAs), usually present with dull perianal discomfort that is typically worse with increased perineal pressure (e.g., sitting, coughing, defecating). Physical examination may reveal an erythematous, warm, tender area with well-defined fluctuance near the anal orifice. No induration or fluctuance is noted on the digital rectal examination (DRE), and fever and leukocytosis are rare.[1]

Patients with perirectal abscesses have fewer, and more diffuse, external anal signs. These patients are more likely to have fever, leukocytosis, and fluctuance above the anal verge on DRE. Ischiorectal abscesses extend from the external anal sphincter to the ischiorectal space. Pain is noted in the region of the buttock and typically is throbbing and constant. External findings may be absent or may include more diffuse tenderness; fluctuance may be noted on DRE just above the dentate line. Intersphincteric abscesses extend between the internal and external sphincter and rarely cause outward skin changes. A tender mass may be noted within the anal canal or distal rectum. Supralevator and deep space abscesses cause rectal pain, fever, and leukocytosis and may produce urinary retention. DRE may reveal a tender, fluctuant mass in the anal canal or distal rectum.[1]

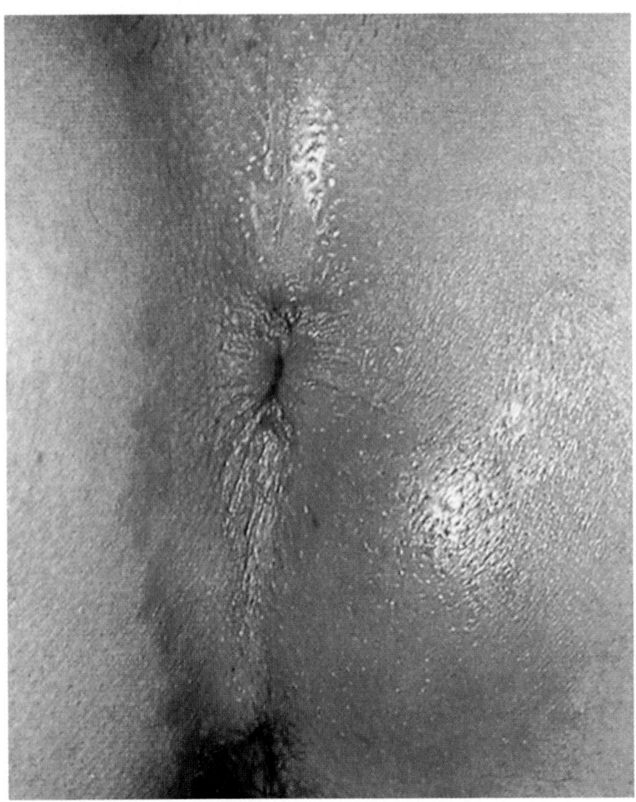

FIGURE 9–43 A right ischiorectal abscess in the left posterior quadrant. (From Yamada, with permission.)

Pathophysiology

ARAs are soft tissue infections that involve one or more of the anorectal tissue planes, including perianal, ischiorectal, intersphincteric, supralevator, horseshoe, and deep-space infections.[1] ARAs are caused by the obstruction of anal crypts.[1,2] Anal crypts are glands that drain at the level of the dentate line to lubricate the anal canal for defecation.[2] If the crypts are obstructed, bacteria proliferate, resulting in suppuration and abscess formation. The most common bacteria involved are *Escherichia coli*, enterococci, staphylococci, and streptococci.[1]

Diagnosis

The diagnosis is made by history and physical examination, including a DRE. Computed tomography may aid in localizing the abscess to help guide the surgical approach.

Management

The definitive management of anorectal abscess is surgical drainage. Small, superficial abscesses may be drained in the emergency department (ED) under local anesthesia, with packing placement for 24 hours and daily sitz baths.[1] All other cases require surgical consultation and drainage, often under general anesthesia. All patients require surgical referral within 48 hours because of the potential for fistula formation. Antibiotics are reserved for high-risk individuals, including those with immunosuppression, diabetes, or valvular heart disease.

REFERENCES

1. Janicke DM, Pundt MR. Anorectal disorders. *Emerg Med Clin North Am* 1996;14:757–788.
2. Saclarides TJ, Brand MI. Evolving trends in the treatment of anorectal diseases. *Dis Colon Rectum* 1999;42:1245–1252.

Hemorrhoids

Jason Sundseth

Clinical Presentation

Patients with internal hemorrhoids typically present with painless rectal bleeding that typically consists of blood-streaked stool occurring with or after defecation.[1] Patients with external hemorrhoids may present with signs of inflammation or thrombosis (dull, aching pain with pruritus and swelling).

Pathophysiology

Hemorrhoids are classified according to their location and degree of severity. External hemorrhoids originate below the dentate line, are innervated by the inferior rectal nerve, receive their blood supply from the inferior hemorrhoidal plexus, and are covered by modified squamous epithelium. Internal hemorrhoids originate above the dentate line, lack sensory innervation, receive their blood supply from the superior hemorrhoidal plexus, and are covered by transitional or columnar epithelium.[2] The most common explanation of hemorrhoidal pathophysiology theorizes that these veins become engorged secondary to loss of support structures of the rectal connective tissue. The dilated, engorged veins cause surrounding inflammation as well as thrombosis, ulceration, and bleeding.

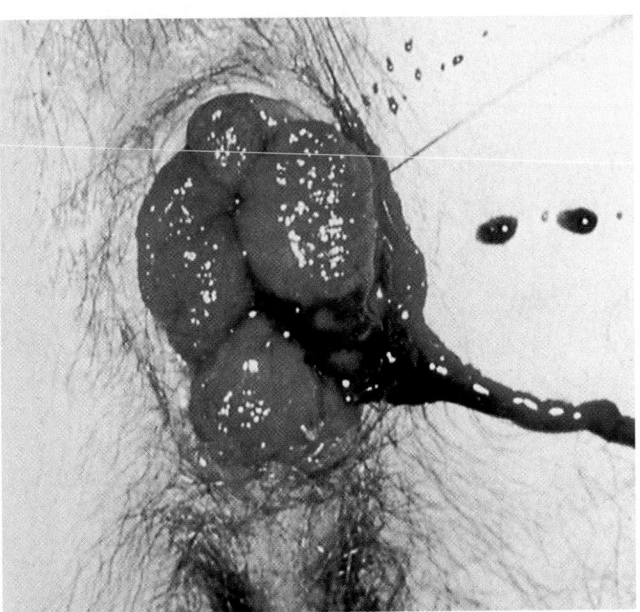

FIGURE 9–44 Third-degree internal hemorrhoids. Spontaneous bleeding is apparent. (From Yamada, with permission.)

Diagnosis

The diagnosis is made by visual inspection, digital rectal exam, and anoscopy.[1] Hemorrhoids are typically located at the 5-, 9-, or 12-o'clock position. Potential physical findings include skin tags from old hemorrhoids, an inflamed hemorrhoid (red, soft, tender mass), and a thrombosed hemorrhoid (bluish, tender, hard mass).[2] Anoscopy is required to diagnose internal hemorrhoids.

Clinical Complications

Complications include thrombosis, ulceration, infection, abscess, anemia, and incontinence. The recurrence rate is 10% to 50%.

Management

Thrombosed external hemorrhoids may be excised surgically in the emergency department (ED) if the patient presents during the first 2 to 3 days of symptoms, or if medical therapy has failed.[2] Patients with less severe disease may be treated initially with simple outpatient methods (the mnemonic "WASH" may be helpful): **w**arm water (sitz bath); oral **a**nalgesia (e.g., nonsteroidal antiinflammatory drugs [NSAIDs]) or topical anesthetics/steroid creams; **s**tool softeners; and a **h**igh-fiber diet.

The treatment of internal hemorrhoids is based on their severity. Hemorrhoids may protrude into the anal cavity but without prolapse (grade 1), prolapse but spontaneously reduce (grade 2), require manual reduction (grade 3), or be irreducible (grade 4). Patients with grade 3 or 4 internal hemorrhoids should be referred to a surgeon, because surgical therapy or office treatment may be appropriate.[1] Grade 1 or 2 internal hemorrhoids may be treated medically with the "WASH" treatments described earlier.

REFERENCES

1. Alonso-Coello P, Castillejo MM. Office evaluation and treatment of hemorrhoids. *J Fam Pract* 2003;52:366–374.
2. Janicke DM, Pundt MR. Anorectal disorders. *Emerg Med Clin North Am* 1996;14:757–788.

Inguinal Hernia

George S. Kim

Clinical Presentation

Many inguinal hernias are asymptomatic. Patients present complaining of a mass in the groin that becomes more swollen with Valsalva maneuvers or standing. Patients with incarcerated hernias may also complain of pain and swelling in the groin region. Incarcerated hernias can also manifest as bowel obstruction. Low-grade fever and vomiting may also be present.[1]

Pathophysiology

Inguinal hernias can be divided into two types, indirect and direct. Indirect inguinal hernias are caused by a congenital patent process vaginalis, which allows passage of abdominal contents through the internal inguinal ring and into the scrotum. Direct inguinal hernias result from a weakness of the transversalis fascia. This typically occurs in Hesselbach's triangle above the inguinal ligament. The overall incidence of inguinal hernias is 3% to 5%; approximately two thirds are indirect and one third direct.

The incidence is higher in men, and there is a bimodal distribution, with peaks at age 1 year and at an average age of 40 years. Inguinal hernias occur more commonly on the right. In children, the incidence is 1% to 2%, with 10% of hernias developing the complication of incarceration.[1,2]

Diagnosis

Diagnosis is made by physical examination findings of a palpable mass in the groin or scrotum. On occasion, the abdominal wall defect can be palpated. Bowel sounds may be auscultated in the scrotal sac. Hernias can also be detected on ultrasonography or computed tomography (CT).

Clinical Complications

The most serious complications of inguinal hernias are incarceration and strangulation, both of which are surgical emergencies. Incarceration occurs when the herniated portion of bowel can no longer be reduced through the abdominal defect. Strangulation occurs when the incarcerated portion of herniated bowel shows evidence of ischemia. Approximately 5% of hernias diagnosed in the emergency department (ED) require emergency surgical exploration for incarceration or strangulation. Between 10% and 15% of incarcerated hernias show evidence of strangulation.

Management

Reduction of the hernia should be attempted, with sedation as necessary.[1,2] Hernias that are reducible may be treated conservatively with analgesia and outpatient surgical follow-up. Hernias that cannot be reduced require fluid resuscitation, antibiotics, analgesia, and immediate surgical consultation.[1,2]

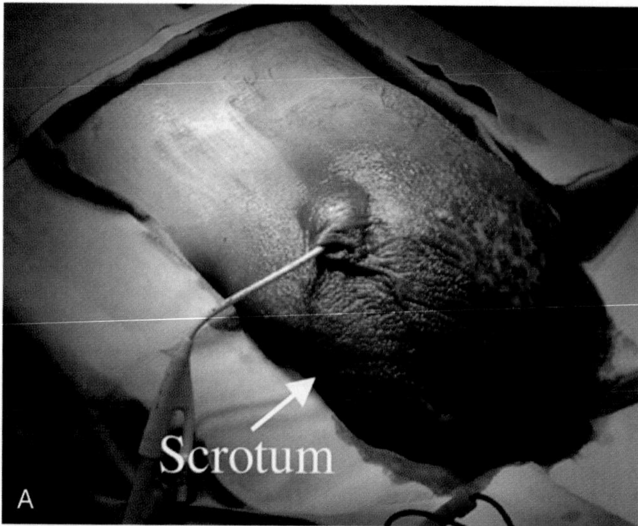

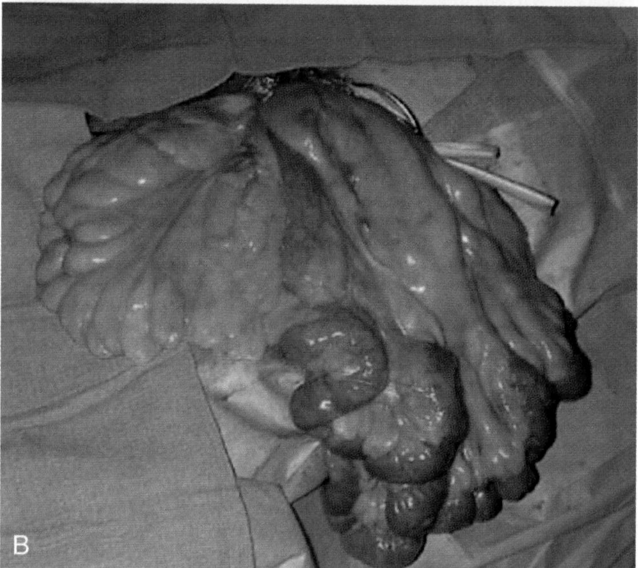

FIGURE 9–45 Giant inguinal hernia. **A:** Large bilateral inguinal hernia. (From Yamada, with permission.) **B:** At operation, most of the small and large intestinal contents were present in the hernia sac in the scrotum. Repair was performed with polypropylene mesh. (From Yamada, with permission.)

REFERENCES

1. Kulah B, Kulacoglu IH, Oruc MT, et al. Presentation and outcome of incarcerated external hernias in adults. *Am J Surg* 2001;181: 101–104.
2. D'Agostino J. Common abdominal emergencies in children. *Emerg Med Clin North Am* 2002;20:139–153.

Femoral Hernias

Cameron Symonds and Jonathan Glauser

Clinical Presentation

Patients with femoral hernias complain of a painful bulge localized to the medial thigh and groin that typically is worsened by activity or straining. Nausea and vomiting may represent bowel obstruction from the entrapped hernia. Femoral hernias may be mistaken for inguinal lymphadenopathy or abscess.[1]

Pathophysiology

Conditions creating excessive pressures that may be associated with hernias include repeated coughing, ascites, increased peritoneal fluid from biliary atresia, peritoneal dialysis, ventriculoperitoneal shunts, peritoneal masses or organomegaly; obstipation, and muscular effort.[1] Femoral hernias are predisposed to incarceration and strangulation because of the small diameter of the femoral canal.[1]

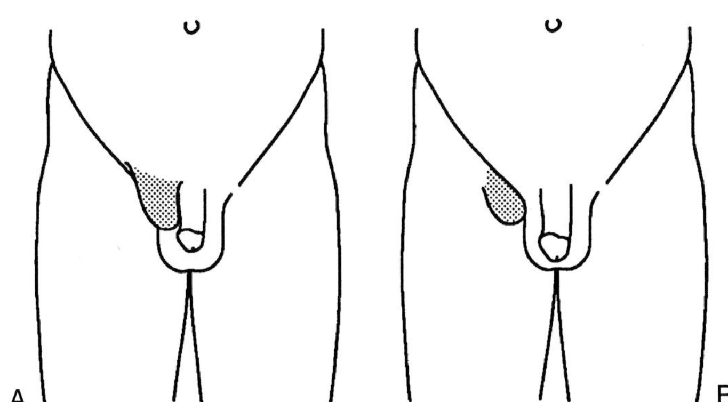

FIGURE 9–46 In contrast to inguinal hernias **(A)**, femoral hernias **(B)** occur below the inguinal ligament. (From Greenfield, with permission.)

Diagnosis

The diagnosis of a femoral hernia usually is made because the patient, parent, or physician observes a bulge. Femoral hernias are particularly difficult to diagnose because of their small size, female preponderance, and late presentation. A bulge is often palpable below the inguinal ligament; however, the hernia sac can dissect superiorly and mimic an inguinal hernia. Ultrasonography can differentiate hernia from other inguinal pathologies, including adenopathy and abscess. Computed tomography can define viscera in the femoral canal, identify bowel obstruction, and delineate other inguinal pathologies.

Clinical Complications

Complications include delayed diagnosis, incarceration, strangulation, and bowel obstruction.[2]

Management

Acutely, a clinical determination of the bowel integrity must be made. If the entrapped viscus is considered viable, gentle attempts at manual reduction can be made in the emergency department (ED). If the patient exhibits signs of obstruction, prostration, fever, or peritonitis, the hernia should not be reduced and prompt surgical consultation should be obtained. If the hernia is reducible, urgent surgical repair of the femoral defect is recommended, because of the predilection for strangulation.[2]

REFERENCES

1. Bobrow RS. The hernia. *J Am Board Fam Pract* 1999;12:95–96.
2. Naude GP, Ocon S, Bongard F. Femoral hernia: the dire consequences of a missed diagnosis. *Am J Emerg Med* 1997;15:680–682.

Rectal Prolapse

Colleen Campbell

Clinical Presentation

Patients with rectal prolapse (RP) present with complaints of pruritus and a mass at the anus, along with bloody mucus noted on toilet paper with wiping. Because this condition is progressive, patients may initially notice the mass only with straining. Most patients have a history of fecal incontinence and chronic constipation. On examination, a erythematous, friable, edematous mucosa may be visible externally. Patients often have other symptoms of pelvic floor damage, including stress incontinence and vaginal prolapse.[1,2]

Pathophysiology

RP (procidentia) occurs when all layers of the rectal wall protrude through the anal canal as a result of intussusception of the rectosigmoid below the level of the rectal sphincter. RP typically occurs in elderly women as a result of chronic straining secondary to constipation. Pudendal nerve damage or damage to the levator ani related to childbirth contributes to underlying pelvic floor weakness.[1] Women are affected with RP 10 times more commonly than men, and most of those women are parous. Women most commonly seek treatment for this disorder during the sixth decade of life.[2]

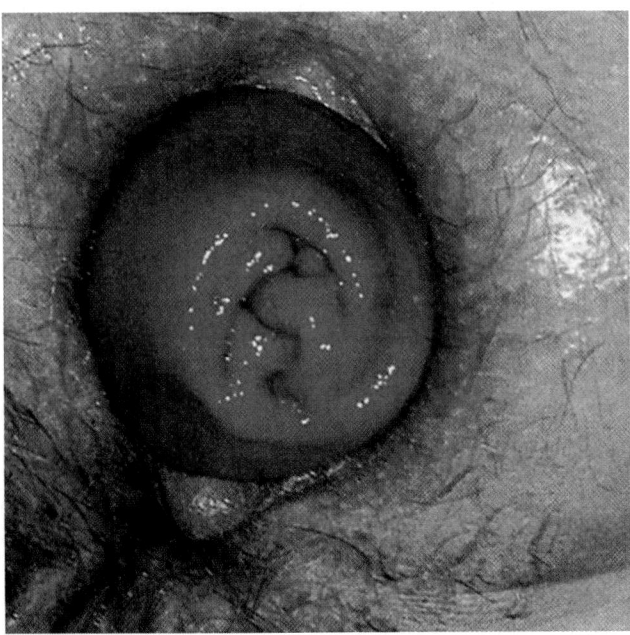

FIGURE 9–47 Complete rectal prolapse. (From Yamada, with permission.)

Diagnosis

The diagnosis of rectal prolapse is based on clinical history and physical examination. Examination should be done while the patient is straining and is most revealing if done while the patient is upright. Concentric mucosal folds visibly differentiate this condition from a thrombosed hemorrhoid. Manometry uniformly reveals low anal sphincter pressures. Defecography can be used to confirm the diagnosis.[1–3]

Clinical Complications

Complications include rectal bleeding, nerve damage to the pudendal nerves, and fecal incontinence. There is progressive impairment of internal sphincter function as a result of mucosal extrusion that leads to incontinence.[3]

Management

RP can usually be reduced with gentle manual pressure. Sugar has been used as an osmotic agent to reduce swelling and to aid manual reduction in some cases. Abdominal rectopexy is the procedure of choice for complete RP, but a perineal approach is an alternative.[2] Abdominal rectopexy may be done laparoscopically or by an open procedure.

REFERENCES

1. Felt-Bersma RJ, Cuesta MA. Rectal prolapse, rectal intussusception, rectocele, and solitary rectal ulcer syndrome. *Gastroenterol Clin North Am* 2001;30:199–222.
2. Peters WA 3rd, Smith MR, Drescher CW. Rectal prolapse in women with other defects of pelvic floor support. *Am J Obstet Gynecol* 2001;184:1488–1494.
3. Nagle D. Rectal prolapse and fecal incontinence. *Prim Care* 1999;26: 101–111.

Osler-Weber-Rendu Syndrome

Colleen Campbell

Clinical Presentation

Patients with Osler-Weber-Rendu syndrome (OWRS) usually (85%) present in their second decade with recurrent epistaxis.[1-3] Affected women have menorrhagia. Recurrent gastrointestinal (GI) bleeding becomes more common, beginning in the fifth decade, due to arteriovenous malformations and aneurysms. Because the bleeding is usually painless, patients often present with symptoms of anemia, such as dyspnea on exertion and fatigue. On examination, small telangiectases are found on mucosal surfaces as well as on the nose, hands, feet, and chest.[1] These are usually very small, pinpoint macules or papules that are violaceous in color and are most often found on the face and lips.[1-3]

Pathophysiology

OWRS is an autosomal dominant inherited disorder that is characterized by hemorrhagic telangiectases affecting the skin, lung, GI tract, and central nervous system. OWRS is thought to result from a genetic defect in the gene that encodes for endoglin. This protein is essential in angiogenesis and maintenance of vascular integrity.[2] The telangiectases may not become apparent until adulthood. The GI tract is diffusely affected, with lesions being found in the stomach, duodenum, small bowel, or colon. Virtually every organ system in the body may be involved. Bleeding is intermittent and progressive.

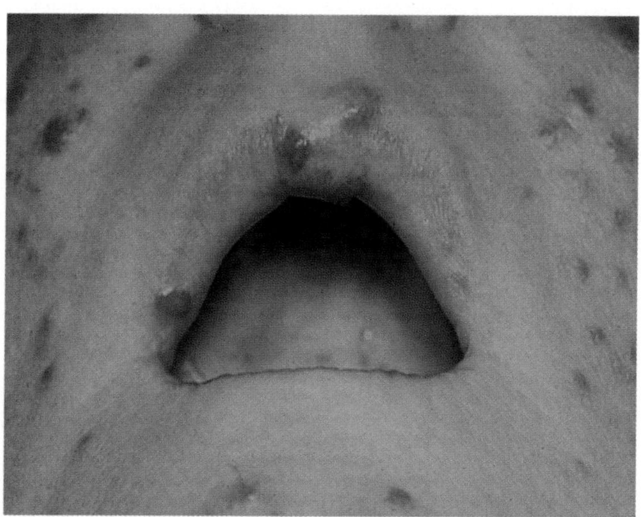

FIGURE 9–48 Osler-Weber-Rendu syndrome. Similar-appearing lesions occur throughout the gastrointestinal tract, especially in the gastroduodenal region. (From Yamada, with permission.)

Diagnosis

Diagnosis of the disease is suggested based on history and physical examination. A complete blood panel, blood chemistry analysis, and coagulation tests are indicated to evaluate for anemia and to rule out other causes of bleeding. Laparoscopy or biopsy may be necessary to evaluate solid organ involvement. Endoscopy is necessary to identify the source of GI bleeding and to characterize the nature of the lesions.

Clinical Complications

Chronic anemia is the most common complication resulting from recurrent bleeding. Mortality is increased in OWRS due to bleeding episodes.

Management

Large-bore intravenous access, along with rapid saline infusion, may be necessary for acute symptomatic anemia secondary to bleeding. Blood transfusions have significantly reduced the mortality rate.[3] Iron supplementation becomes important given the chronic nature of blood loss. Surgical resection is rarely indicated because of the diffuse nature of the disease. Interventional angiography may be successful in controlling bleeding. Estrogen and progesterone supplements have been used with some success to control menorrhagia.[2]

REFERENCES

1. Boh EE, al-Smadi RM. Cutaneous manifestations of gastrointestinal diseases. *Dermatol Clin* 2002;20:533–546.
2. Ward SK, Roenigk HH, Gordon KB. Dermatologic manifestations of gastrointestinal disorders. *Gastroenterol Clin North Am* 1998;27:615–636.
3. Fuchizaki U, Miyamori H, Kitagawa S, Kaneko S, Kobayashi K. Hereditary hemorrhagic telangiectasia (Rendu-Osler-Weber disease). *Lancet* 2003;362:1490–1494.

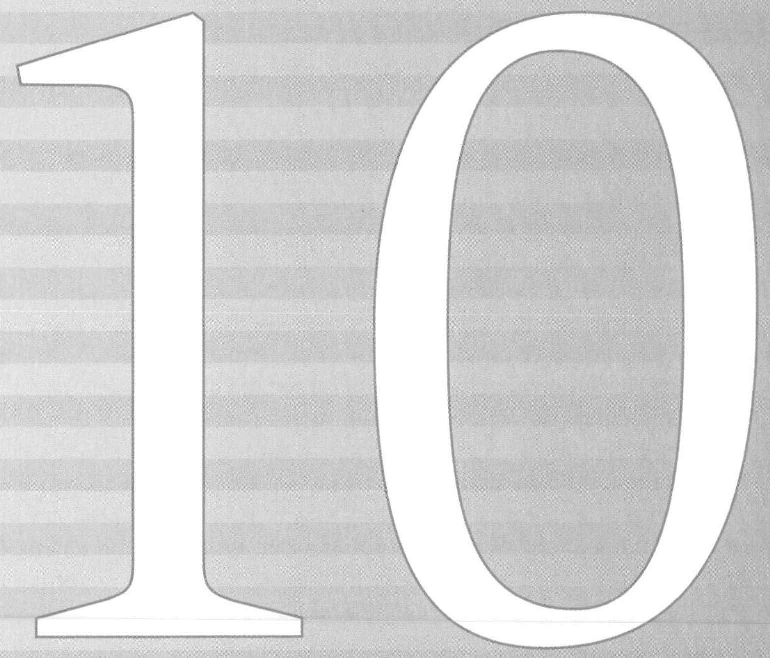

Genitourinary/Renal

10–1

Penile Fracture

Colleen Campbell

Clinical Presentation

Penile fracture is rupture of the tunica albuginea that results from a rapid, blunt force to an erect penis. This force is usually a bending or impaction motion induced by vaginal intercourse or aggressive masturbation. Patients give a history of a "popping" or "cracking" sound followed by pain and rapid detumescence.[1] On physical examination, the penile shaft is ecchymotic and swollen, with deviation most often away from the side of injury. This is often referred to as the "eggplant" deformity or "aubergine sign." The fracture site may be directly palpable where the hematoma forms; this is referred to as the "rolling sign." Most often the fracture is proximal and ventral in coital injuries. The incidence of penile fracture is relatively rare, but it is thought to be underreported.

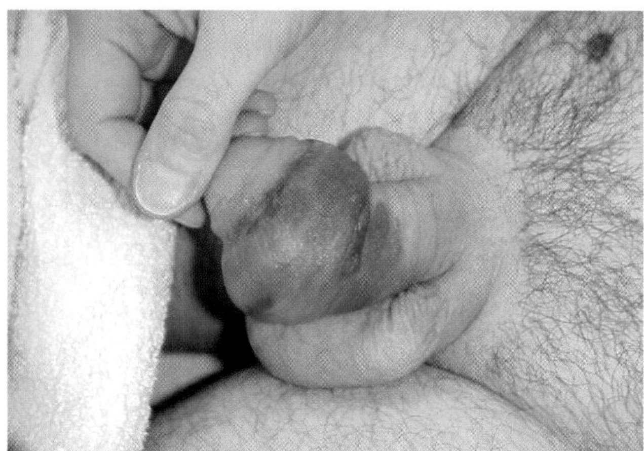

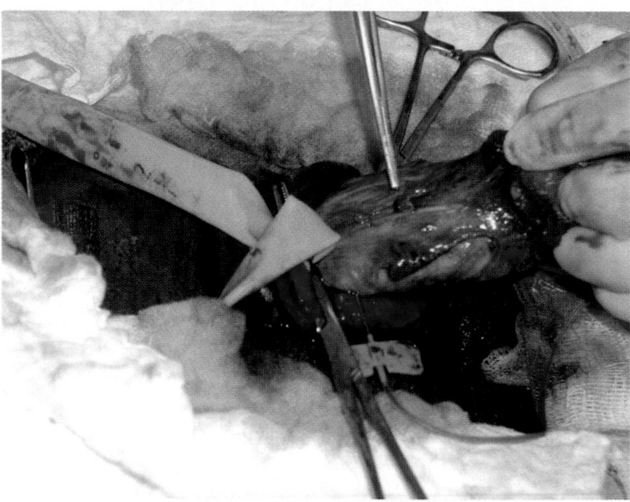

FIGURE 10–1 **A:** Penile fracture. Note swelling, deformity, and ecchymosis. (Courtesy of Donald Sallee, MD.) **B:** Operative repair of penile fracture. Note tissue disruption with local hemorrhage. (Courtesy of Sam N. Chawla, MD and Laura Spivak, MD.)

Diagnosis

The diagnosis is largely clinical, but it may be aided by cavernosography, urethrography, ultrasonography, or magnetic resonance imaging (MRI).[1] Retrograde urethrography is necessary in all patients who are unable to void, in those with blood at the urethral meatus, and in those with frank hematuria.

Clinical Complications

The rate of complications with conservative management in some series has been as high 40%, compared with 11% among operatively treated patients.[2] The most common complications are unacceptable penile curvature, painful erections, penile abscess formation secondary to missed urethral injuries, and late penile plaque formation akin to Peyronie's disease.[2] Less frequently, impotence, penile aneurysm, skin necrosis, fistulas, and high-flow priapism occur as a result of this injury.

Management

Penile fracture requires immediate urologic consultation for urgent surgical repair. This treatment includes evacuation of hematoma and suture repair of the ruptured tunica albuginea. The urethra is most often stented with the catheter to aid in restoration of anatomy and maintenance of the repair. Antiandrogens such as diethylstilbestrol, amyl nitrate, and benzodiazepines are used to prevent erection during convalescence. Some authors advocate conservative management consisting of Foley catheterization, penile splinting and pressure dressings, nonsteroidal antiinflammatory drugs (NSAIDs), fibrinolytics, and antibiotics. This is recommended only in milder cases with normal findings on cavernosography.[2]

REFERENCES

1. Beysel M, Tekin A, Gurdal M, Yucebas E, Sengor F. Evaluation and treatment of penile fractures: accuracy of clinical diagnosis and the value of corpus cavernosography. *Urology* 2002;60:492–496.
2. Eke N. Fracture of the penis. *Br J Surg* 2002;89:555–565.

Penile Amputation

Colleen Campbell

Pathophysiology

Penile amputation is an uncommon traumatic injury.[1] Automutilation has been reported in psychotic (schizophrenic) men with sexual fears and in intoxicated men.[2] Traumatic amputations may result from industrial or motor vehicle accidents.[1] Circumcision performed by laypersons may result in accidental amputation.[1–3]

Diagnosis

Diagnosis of penile amputation is based on history and physical examination. Retrograde urethrography is useful in evaluating the extent of urethral injury. A complete blood count (CBC) and a basic chemistry panel are useful in the evaluation of the hypovolemia and acidosis that occur in association with amputation.[1–3]

Clinical Complications

Amputation of the penis has devastating social and physical ramifications for the patient. Urethral strictures and voiding problems are common. Loss of sexual function and necrosis occur. Replantation complications include skin loss, fistula formation, urethral contracture or stricture, necrosis, and loss of sensation and sexual function.[1,3] These complications are significantly reduced with the use of microsurgical anastomosis of the dorsal penile artery and vein, as well as nerves.

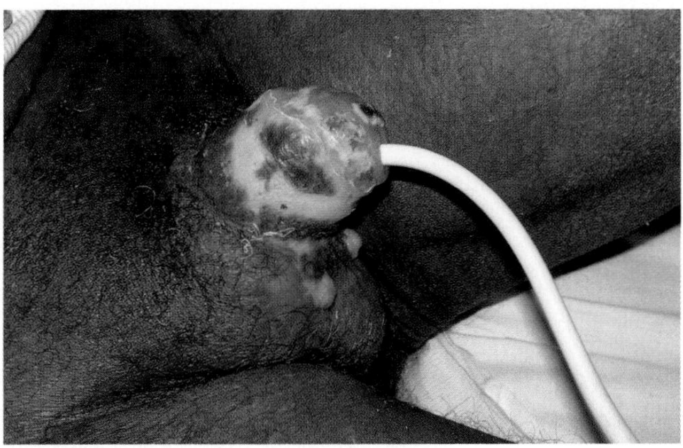

FIGURE 10–2 Traumatic penile amputation. (Courtesy of Mark Silverberg, MD.)

Management

Penile amputations are often associated with other injuries, making a secondary survey and workup of associated injuries or drug overdose mandatory. Treatment of hypovolemia and shock are the primary goals, because substantial bleeding is possible. Emergency suprapubic catheterization is necessary if the urethra is involved. The amputated penis should be wrapped in a moist, saline-soaked, sterile dressing and placed in a plastic bag. Cooling should be maintained by placing the plastic bag in ice water slush. Care should be taken to avoid cold injury by avoiding direct penile contact with ice. Tetanus prophylaxis and antibiotics covering skin and urethral flora should be initiated in the emergency department (ED). Emergency referral to a urology specialist is indicated in any penile amputation case. Viable reconstruction has been initiated as late as 16 hours after the amputation.[1] The treatment of choice for proximal amputation is microvascular replantation and repair of the dorsal artery, vein, and nerve.[1–3]

REFERENCES

1. Jezior JR, Brady JD, Schlossberg SM. Management of penile amputation injuries. *World J Surg* 2001;25:1602–1609.
2. Ignajatovic I, Potic B, Paunkovic L, Ravangard Y. Automutilation of the penis performed by the kitchen knife. *Int Urol Nephrol* 2002;34:113–115.
3. Darewicz B, Galek L, Darewicz J, Kudelski J, Malczyk E. Successful microsurgical replantation of an amputated penis. *Int Urol Nephrol* 2001;33:385–386.

10-3

Male Genital Degloving Injury

Michael Greenberg

Clinical Presentation

Patients with male genital degloving injury (MGDI) present after forceful trauma affecting the male genitals. MGDI is an uncommon injury that is frequently work-related.[1-3]

Pathophysiology

Mechanical injury involving farm workers is the mechanism of injury in most cases of MGDI. The redundant skin of the scrotum and penis are entrapped when a pants leg becomes entangled in a piece of moving machinery with rotating parts. Finical and Arnold[1] pointed out that the penile and scrotal skin is often avulsed in one piece, leaving a proximally based flap, and that the "loose skin of the penis usually tears behind the coronal sulcus, leaving the glans intact and pulling the skin off the penis down to the base."

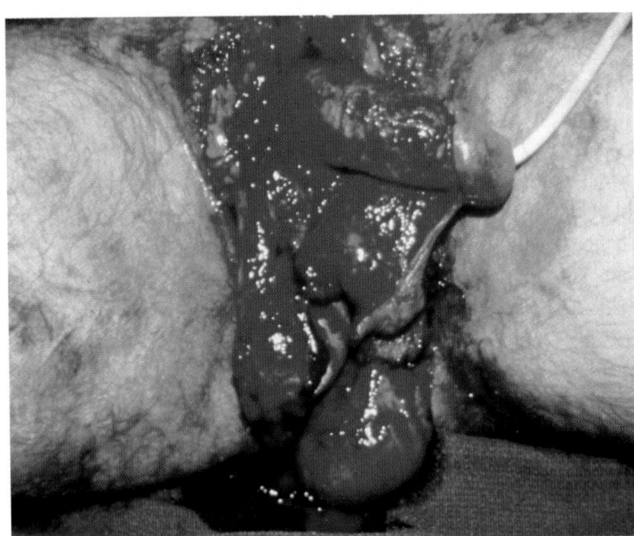

FIGURE 10–3 Genital degloving injury. (Courtesy of Lewis J. Kaplan, MD.)

Diagnosis

The diagnosis is usually apparent on physical examination; however, these injuries cannot be fully assessed unless the patient is completely unclothed.

Clinical Complications

Complications include chronic genital deformity with the potential for permanent urologic dysfunction, sexual dysfunction, or both, as well as concomitant posttraumatic stress disorder.

Management

Advanced trauma life support (ATLS) protocols should be adhered to, and the injured areas should be covered with sterile dressings soaked in sterile saline solution. Immediate on-site consultation with urology and/or plastic surgery specialists should be obtained. There should be no hesitation to transfer hemodynamically stable patients in order to obtain maximally experienced plastic surgical and urologic treatment. Prevention is the optimum treatment for these injuries.[1-3]

REFERENCES

1. Finical SJ, Arnold PG. Care of the degloved penis and scrotum: a 25-year experience. *Plastic Recon Surg* 1999;104:2074–2078.
2. Georgiou P, Liakopoulos P, Gamatasi E, Komninakis E. Degloving injury of the penis from pig bite. *Plastic Recon Surg* 2001;108:805–806.
3. Gencosmanoglu R, Bilkay U, Alper M, Gurler T, Cagdas A. Late results of split-grafted penoscrotal avulsion injuries. *J Trauma* 1995;39:1201–1203.

Penetrating Genital Trauma (Male)

Colleen Campbell

Clinical Presentation

Penetrating penile injuries are uncommon. Only 5% of all urologic injuries occurring during the Vietnam War were penile injuries.[1] Patients often present with signs and symptoms of hypovolemia. After proper attention to the standard ABCs (airway, breathing, and circulation), secondary survey of the trauma victim (after mandatory removal of all clothing) reveals the injury. Blood at the urethral meatus indicates a urethral injury. Bruising or swelling of the scrotum may be present with associated testicular injury. Careful examination of all related areas, including the abdomen, thighs, and rectum, is necessary to identify otherwise occult entry or exit wounds.

Diagnosis

The history and physical examination are the mainstays of diagnosis. Further evaluation includes retrograde urethrography to evaluate the extent of urethral injury. In one series, urethral damage was found in 22% of patients who sustained penetrating penile trauma.[2] Blast effect alone can cause testicular injury.[2] Testicular ultrasonography or nuclear scanning is necessary in patients with a suspected testicular injury. In one series, 72% of patients with penetrating trauma to the genitourinary tract had associated injuries, most commonly to the thigh.[2] Evaluation of the abdomen and extremities is necessary, because major vascular injury is commonly associated with gunshot wounds to this region. Plain radiography, computed tomography (CT), and angiography are often necessary to rule out such injuries. Proctoscopy may also be used to evaluate associated rectal injury.

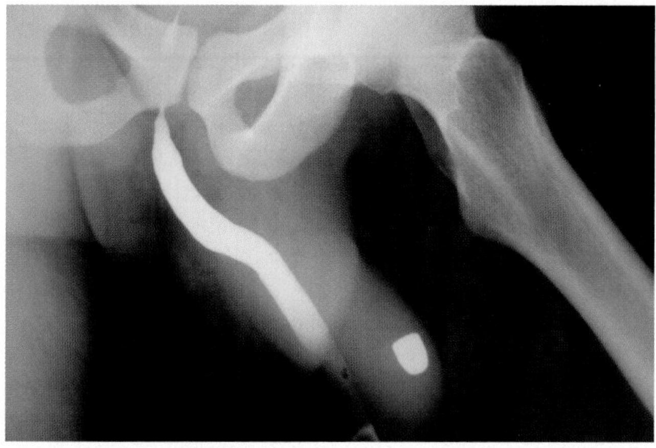

FIGURE 10–4 Gunshot wound of the penis with retained bullet fragment. (Courtesy of Mark Silverberg, MD.)

Clinical Complications

Hypovolemia and shock are the most life-threatening complications associated with genital gunshot wounds. Infection is the most common complication. Gangrene, urethral stricture, and fistula formation may result after penile gunshot wounds. Penile shortening, buildup of granulation tissue, and sexual dysfunction have also been documented.[3]

Management

Emergency urology and trauma team referral are warranted as soon as the injury is discovered. Tetanus and antibiotic prophylaxis should be initiated in the emergency department (ED). Skin and urethral flora should be covered as usual, with a cephalosporin or quinolone. Operative irrigation and débridement of the wounds may be necessary, especially if secondary missiles (e.g., clothing particles) are suspected to remain in the wound.[2] Primary closure or reconstructive repair is performed at the discretion of the urologist.

REFERENCES

1. Cline KJ, Mata JA, Venable DD, Eastham JA. Penetrating trauma to the male external genitalia. *J Trauma* 1998;44:492–494.
2. Mydlo JH, Harris CF, Brown JG. Blunt, penetrating, and ischemic injuries to the penis. *J Urol* 2002;168:1433–1435.
3. Selikowitz, SM. Penetrating high velocity genitourinary injuries: statistics, mechanisms, and renal wounds. *Urology* 1977;9:371–376.

Scrotal Hematoma

Timothy Lum

Clinical Presentation

Patients with scrotal hematoma (SH) present after blunt or penetrating trauma to the lower torso or genitalia.[1] If the SH is secondary to a pelvic fracture, the patient may also have blood at the urethral meatus and a high-riding, boggy prostate with or without pelvic instability.[1]

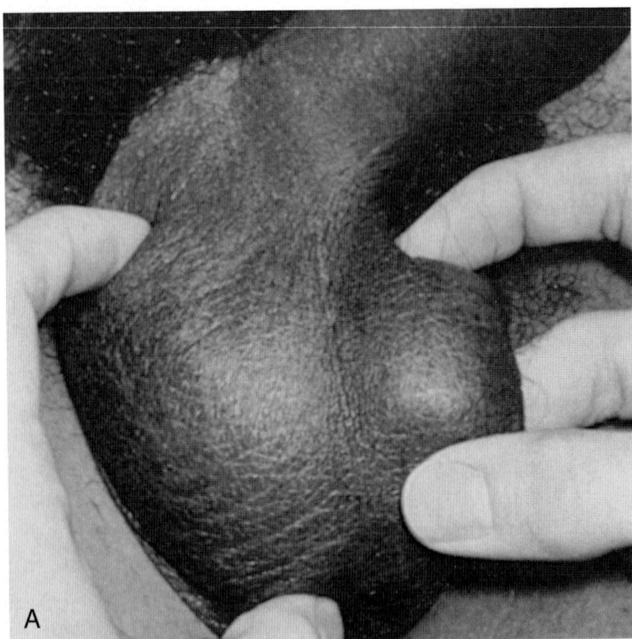

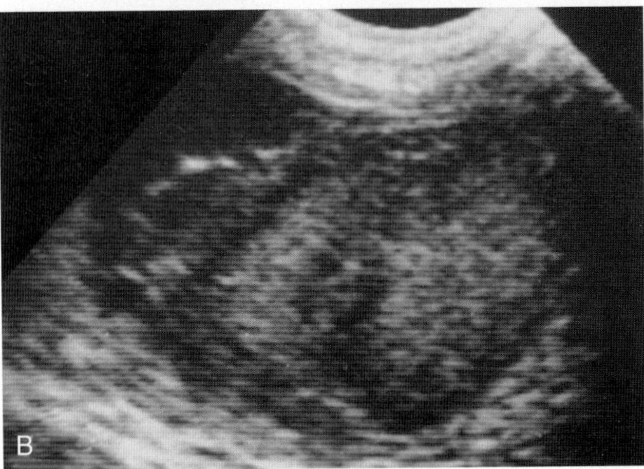

FIGURE 10–5 **A:** Testicular swelling and tenderness after a kick to the scrotum. **B:** Sonographic examination showed a central, linear, sonolucent area reflecting testicular rupture, which requires surgical repair. (From Fleisher *Textbook*, with permission.)

Pathophysiology

SHs can arise by many mechanisms. They may occur after direct genital trauma, or they may be the result of a pelvic fracture, with blood tracking downward through the fascial planes and settling in the scrotum. Some of these pelvic fractures may be associated with urethral disruption. If the SH is caused by direct scrotal trauma, testicular rupture should be a concern. Urologic procedures such as orchiectomy or hydrocelectomy can also lead to SH formation. Large volumes of blood can accumulate in the scrotum because of the distensibility of the scrotal skin, which has little to no ability to tamponade bleeding.[2]

Diagnosis

The diagnosis of SH can be made based on history and physical examination. Scrotal examination reveals an erythematous, edematous scrotum with blood discoloring the scrotal wall.[1,2] However, pelvic radiography, urinalysis, and ultrasonography of the testicles with color flow Doppler are helpful to rule out concomitant injuries.[2]

Clinical Complications

Prolonged scrotal pain, infection, and hematocele formation have been reported to complicate SHs.[1,2]

Management

Advanced trauma life support (ATLS) protocols should be followed until the patient is stabilized. Urology consultation and possible surgical exploration are mandated if the scrotal injury is associated with a significant hematocele, gross hematuria, blood at the urethral meatus, testicular hematoma, or testicular rupture.[1,2] SHs, especially those that develop postoperatively, may require drainage by a urologist and further exposure of the scrotal contents.[2] A drain may be inserted, and the patient is administered antibiotics until it is removed.[1] SHs or injuries not resulting in testicular hematoma or rupture can be treated with ice to reduce swelling and control pain, elevation to promote venolymphatic drainage, and oral analgesics.[2]

REFERENCES

1. Dreitlein DA, Suner S, Basler J. Genitourinary trauma. *Emerg Medicine Clin North Am* 2001;19:569–590.
2. Edelsberg JS, Surh YS. The acute scrotum. *Emerg Med Clin North Am* 1988;6:521–546.

Penile Zipper Injury

Christian M. Sloane

Clinical Presentation

The patient with penile zipper injury presents guarding the affected area and is usually anxious and in pain. There may be little or copious amounts of bleeding. The age group most commonly affected is 2 to 6 years. The tissue may be caught in one of two ways—in the movable zipper part itself, or between the teeth of the zipper.[1]

Pathophysiology

Typically, the loose skin of the foreskin or volar aspect of the penis becomes entrapped. This can occur during either closure or opening of the zipper; there is no clear predominance of either mechanism.

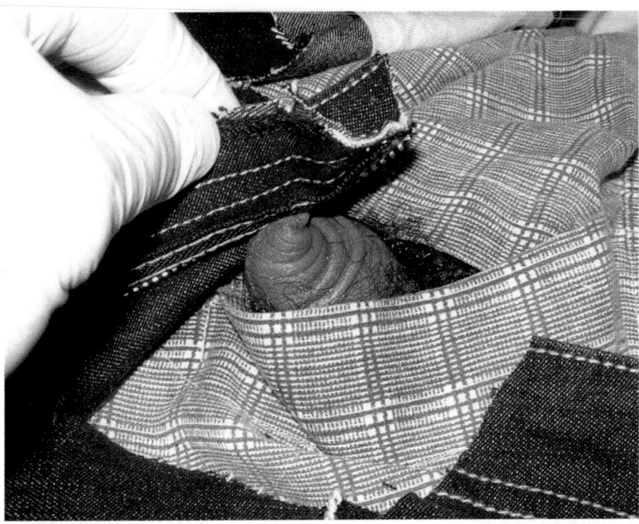

FIGURE 10–6 Foreskin entrapped in zipper. (Courtesy of Mark Silverberg, MD.)

Diagnosis

Diagnosis is straightforward and is made by visual inspection.

Clinical Complications

Injury to the urethra is possible if a significant laceration is present, and a urologic evaluation is warranted. Infection and hemorrhage are possible.

Management

For tissue caught in the teeth of the zipper, cutting transversely beneath the location of entrapment and pulling the teeth apart usually releases the area. For tissue caught in the moving part of the zipper, release can be more difficult, and anesthesia or sedation may be necessary. Gentle manipulation of the zipper after anesthesia and the addition of mineral oil are the simplest treatments and are often successful. If not, cutting the median bar (diamond or bridge) of the zipper in half will cause the interlocking teeth of the zipper to fall apart, freeing the skin. A bone cutter or wire clippers may be required to break the bar.[1,2]

REFERENCES

1. Wyatt JP, Scobie WG. The management of penile zip entrapment in children. *Injury* 1994;25:59–60.
2. Lundquist ST, Stack LB. Diseases of the foreskin, penis and urethra. *Emerg Med Clin North Am* 2001;19:529–546.

Constricting Penile Ring

David Flores and Colleen Campbell

Clinical Presentation

The presentation of a patient with a constricting penile ring is usually obvious upon physical examination. Patients may give a history of preceding use of a vacuum suction device. The penis appears engorged, may have purple discoloration, and may be cool to the touch. Priapism is evident.

Pathophysiology

Penile rings are constrictive bands that are placed around the shaft of the penis to maintain erection or to prevent premature ejaculation. The penile ring was first described in the Far East. A myriad of devices have been used, including bullrings, wedding rings, hammerheads, plumbing devices, and marketed products such as Electro-flex rings® and the Stormy Leather® penis ring.[1,2] Patients often present after trying to use a constricting penile ring in conjunction with a vacuum device to achieve a more satisfactory erection. Once the venous flow is constricted, the penis remains erect. Ensuing edema may then cause the ring to become entrapped onto the penis.

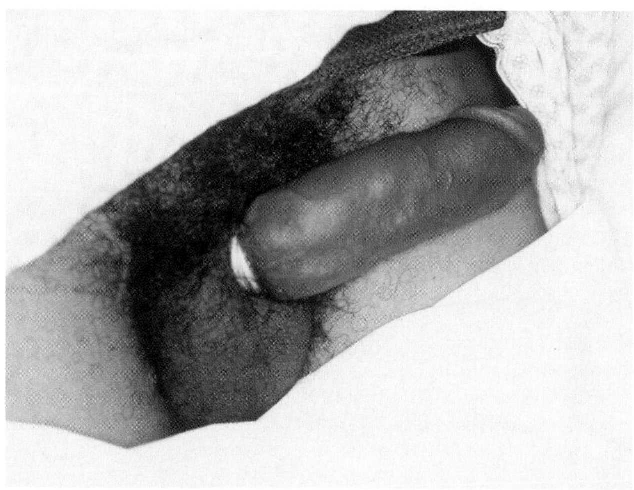

FIGURE 10–7 Constricting penile ring. (Copyright James R. Roberts, MD.)

Diagnosis

The diagnosis of a constricting penile ring is based on the history and physical examination.

Clinical Complications

Patients frequently complain of painful ejaculations while the ring is in place. Priapism can lead to fibrosis and permanent cell death within 6 hours. Neurovascular damage can also occur as a result of the constricting force of the ring. Petechiae may develop at the ring site. Penile tip necrosis or permanent erectile dysfunction may result. Peyronie's disease can also result from chronic use of penile rings in conjunction with vacuum erection devices.[1,2]

Management

Removal of the constricting device is necessary as quickly as possible to prevent irreversible neurovascular damage. Devices that are useful to this end include metal ring cutters and metal saws. The string method, in which umbilical tape is placed under the ring and the penis is wrapped distally, after which the proximal portion of the umbilical ring is gradually pulled, has been successful at times.[1,2]

REFERENCES

1. Levine LA, Dimitriou RJ. Vacuum constriction and external erection devices in erectile dysfunction. *Urol Clin North Am* 2001;28: 335–341.
2. Perabo FGE, Steiner G, Albers P, Muller SC. Treatment of penile strangulation caused by constricting devices. *Urology* 2002;59:137.

Priapism

Colleen Campbell

Clinical Presentation

Patients with priapism present with a painful erection. Patients may present after trauma with a painless erection resulting from an arterial high-flow state caused by injury to the cavernosal artery.

Pathophysiology

Priapism is the prolonged engorgement of the penis not related to sexual desire or stimulation. Most cases of priapism are caused by a low-flow state. The most common causes are sickle cell disease, drug-induced priapism, and malignancy-associated priapism. Sickled red blood cells (RBCs) may gather in sinusoidal spaces during physiologic erection, resulting in subsequent priapism; this is the most common type of priapism in children.[1] Local injection of papaverine, crack cocaine use, and ingestion of sildenafil, trazodone, or chlorpromazine have all been associated with increased incidence of priapism.[1] High-flow priapism is less acute in onset and results in fewer complications. It occurs when arterial inflow exceeds the capacity of the venous system, and it usually is painless. Most commonly, it is caused by trauma to the perineum in a straddle mechanism of injury.

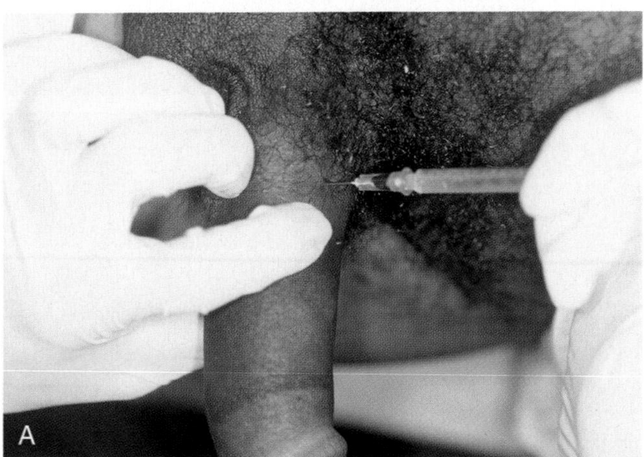

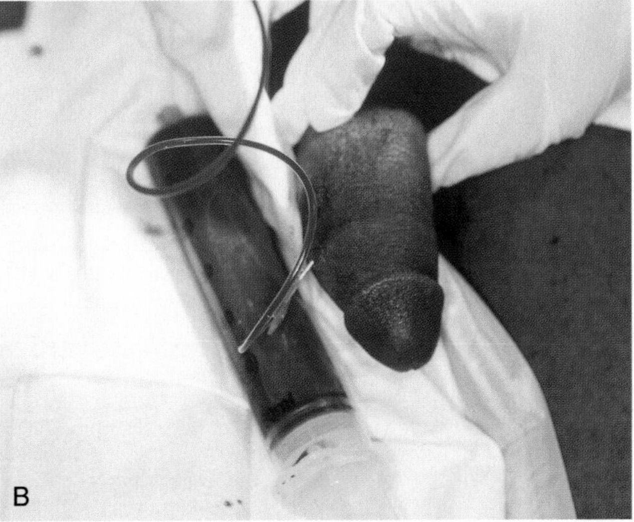

FIGURE 10–8 Local anesthetic penile block **(A)** preceding corpora irrigation **(B)** to relieve priapism. (Copyright James R. Roberts, MD.)

Diagnosis

Diagnosis is mostly clinical by history and physical examination. An intracavernous blood gas analysis may be obtained to differentiate high-flow priapism from low-flow or ischemic priapism. Penile technetium scans may also be used to assess blood flow states. On physical examination, the entire corpora cavernosa (or, rarely, only a segment of the cavernosa) is engorged.[2] The corpus spongiosum usually is not involved.

Clinical Complications

Erectile dysfunction is common after priapism and can be expected in as many as 70% of cases treated conservatively.[2]

Management

Pain relief is essential in the treatment of priapism. Algorithms for treatment start with less invasive measures, followed quickly by more invasive treatments. In patients with sickle cell disease, hydration and red blood cells (RBCs) exchange transfusions have been attempted without conclusive differences in outcome.[1] Hydroxyurea (a DNA synthesis inhibitor), hydralazine, and etilefrine (an α-adrenergic agonist) have also been used for their vasodilatory properties in the prevention of sickle cell–induced priapism.[1] Intracavernous injection of an α-agonist (phenylephrine, ephedrine, epinephrine) may be effective if priapism is treated within the first 12 hours after onset. A trial of corporal irrigation may be attempted for 20 minutes, before proceeding to a surgical shunt procedure. An intracavernous pressure monitor reading indicating pressure less than 40 mm Hg indicates successful treatment.[3]

REFERENCES

1. Powars DR, Johnson CS. Priapism. *Hematol Oncol Clin North Am* 1996;10:1363–1372.
2. Pautler SE, Brock GB. Priapism: from Priapus to the present time. *Urol Clin North Am* 2001;28:391–403.
3. Hatzichristou D, Salpiggidis G, Hatzimouratidis R, et al. Management strategy for arterial priapism: therapeutic dilemmas. *J Urol* 2002;168:2074–2077.

Phimosis

Colleen Campbell

Clinical Presentation

Phimosis occurs only in uncircumcised males. Physiologic phimosis occurs in all newborn males, because epithelial adhesion attaches the prepuce to the glans at birth.[1] By 5 years of age, 90% of boys are able to retract the foreskin.[1] Patients with phimosis are unable to retract the foreskin over the glans and may also present with symptoms and signs of balanoposthitis, urinary retention, or dyspareunia.

Pathophysiology

Phimosis results when a previously mobile penile foreskin cannot be retracted over the glans (after puberty). Phimosis may be caused by underlying infection of the glans or prepuce or by scarring from previous injury.[1,2]

Clinical Complications

Phimosis commonly results in balanoposthitis. Urinary retention may also result.[1,2]

Management

Temporary treatment includes application of nonsteroidal creams or steroidal creams to reduce inflammation. The distal foreskin may be opened with the use of a hemostat to dilate the stenotic meatus. Dorsal slit incision of the prepuce or circumcision constitutes definitive therapy.[1,2]

REFERENCES

1. Lundquist, ST, Stack LB. Diseases of the foreskin, penis and urethra. *Emerg Med Clin North Am* 2001;19:529–546.
2. Atilla MK, Dundaroz R, et al. A nonsurgical approach to the treatment of phimosis: local nonsteroidal anti-inflammatory ointment application. *J Urol* 1997;158:196–197(abst).

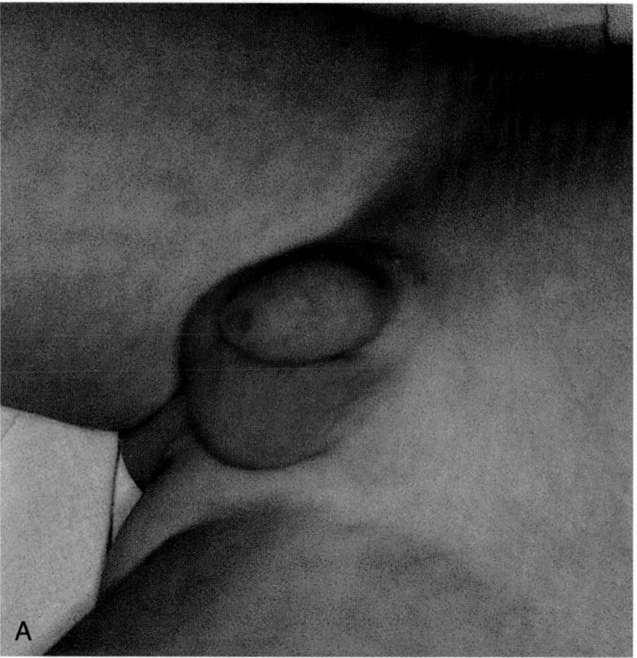

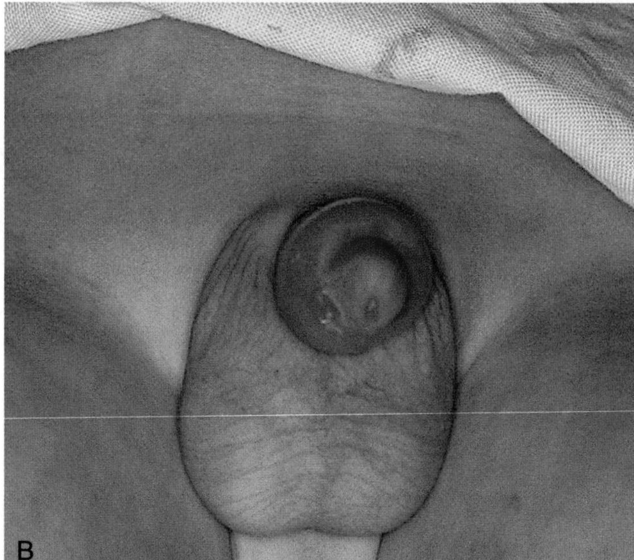

FIGURE 10–9 The parents of this boy with physiologic phimosis **(A)** retracted his foreskin, causing paraphimosis **(B)**. (From Fleisher *Atlas,* with permission.)

Balanitis

Colleen Campbell

Clinical Presentation

Balanitis is more common in uncircumcised diabetic men and in male children.[1] The patient may present with itching, swelling, or penile discomfort. The glans and foreskin may be erythematous, swollen, and malodorous. Discharge may be visible at the sulcus of the glans and prepuce. If a discharge from the urethra is present, a different diagnosis should be sought, because the urethra should not be involved in balanitis.

Pathophysiology

Balanitis is inflammation of the glans penis. Balanoposthitis involves inflammation of the prepuce as well. Balanitis may be caused by an acute or chronic infection or irritation of the glans. Poor personal hygiene is a major contributing factor. The most common infectious organisms are candidal species.[2] Other infectious causes are anaerobic bacteria including group B streptococci, *Gardnerella,* and sexually transmitted infections such as herpes simplex virus (HSV), human papillomavirus (HPV), syphilis, trichomoniasis, and amoebiasis. Noninfectious causes include local friction, irritation, or trauma; contact dermatitis, and dermatologic disorders such as psoriasis, lichen planus, and erythema multiforme exudativum.[1]

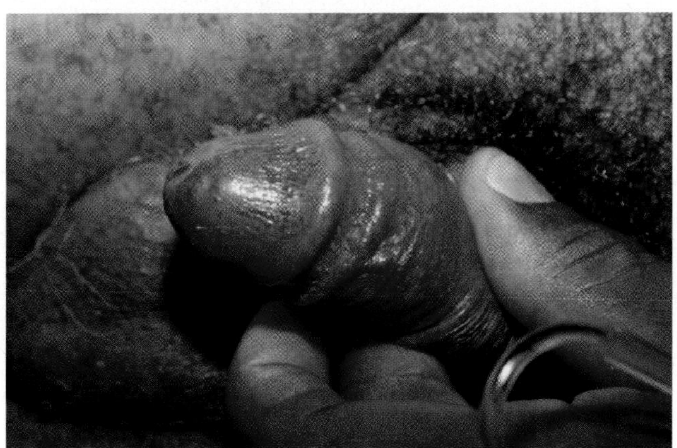

FIGURE 10–10 Monilial balanitis. (Copyright James R. Roberts, MD.)

Clinical Complications

Complications are rare. However, chronic balanoposthitis may develop in those patients with continued poor hygiene, especially if the patient is a diabetic. This can eventually lead to phimosis or paraphimosis.

Management

Frequent cleansing with a mild soap, followed by adequate drying, is the mainstay of treatment. Candidal infections are treated with antifungal creams such as nystatin or clotrimazole. Anaerobic infections, *Gardnerella,* and *Trichomonas* should be treated with oral metronidazole. If a specific bacterial or viral source is found, appropriate oral antibiotics or antiviral agents should be initiated. If the infection is refractory to medical treatment, referral to a urologist for biopsy is indicated.

REFERENCES

1. Waugh, MA. Sexually transmitted diseases: balanitis. *Dermatol Clin* 1998;16:757–762.
2. Lundquist ST, Stack LB. Genitourinary emergencies: diseases of the foreskin, penis, and urethra. *Emerg Med Clin North Am* 2001;19: 529–546.

Pearly Penile Papules

R. Zachary McDonald and Colleen Campbell

Clinical Presentation

Patients with pearly penile papules (PPPs) usually present concerned that they may have genital warts, because these entities are often mistaken for one another.

Pathophysiology

PPPs are benign, dome-shaped, asymptomatic angiofibromas that occur circumferentially around the coronal sulcus of the penis. The estimated incidence of PPP is 8% to 30%. The majority of cases occur in uncircumcised men, with all races being equally susceptible.[1] PPP are not related to human papillomavirus (HPV) and are different in their arrangement in rows and their singular dome shape.[1] Warts are not as linear or as clearly defined, and they usually form in clusters on the skin. Although the exact cause of PPP is unknown, uncircumcised men develop the papules more frequently than do those who are circumcised.

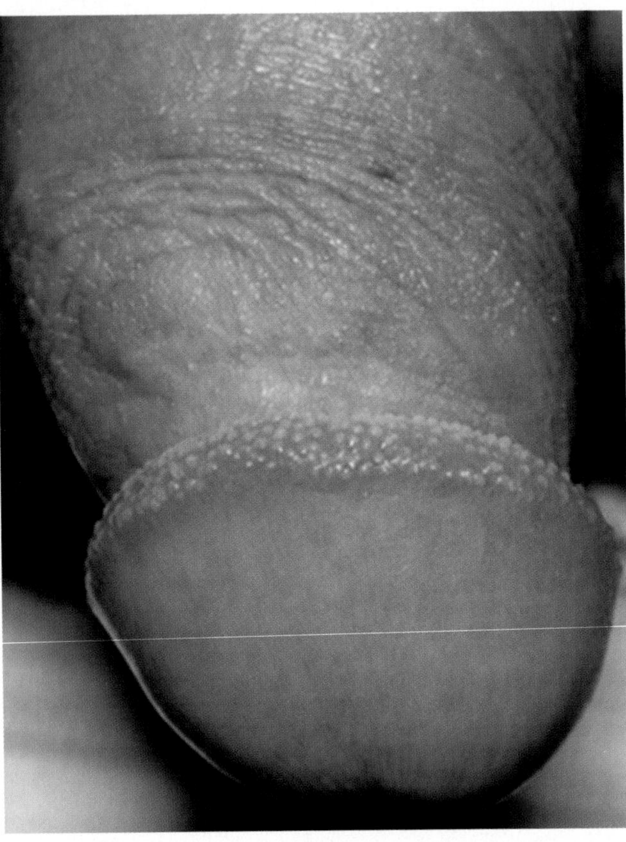

FIGURE 10–11 Pearly penile papules. Shiny papules are present around the corona of the glans penis. (From Goodheart, with permission.)

Diagnosis

The diagnosis is based on clinical history and physical examination. Patients have pale/white or skin-colored, 1- to 2-mm dome-shaped spots that typically are located in rows around the corona and sulcus of the glans penis. To confirm the presence of PPPs and to rule out other potentially serious diseases such as carcinoma, it may be necessary to obtain a tissue diagnosis via biopsy. Microscopic examination reveals a number of thin-walled, ectatic vessels in the dermis, as well as fibroblastic proliferation. Papule cells may appear either star-shaped or multinucleated.

Clinical Complications

PPP can cause a substantial amount of anxiety in patients, unless appropriate reassurance is forthcoming. Infection may be a complication if patients pick at or manipulate the lesions.

Management

Because of the harmless nature of PPP, most patients do not elect complex treatment. However, if patients insist on lesion removal, several modalities may be used, including podophyllin application, circumcision, electrodesiccation and curettage, cryotherapy, and carbon dioxide laser.[2]

REFERENCES

1. Hogewoning CJ, Bleeker MC, van den Brule AJ, et al. Pearly penile papules: still no reason for uneasiness. *J Am Acad Dermatol* 2003;49:50–54.
2. Lane JE, Peterson CM, Ratz JL. Treatment of pearly penile papules with CO_2 laser. *Dermatol Surg* 2002;28:617–618.

Testicular Torsion

Colleen Campbell

Clinical Presentation

Testicular torsion (TT) manifests as the sudden onset of unilateral, nonpositional testicular pain and tenderness. This may occur during athletic events or during sleep. Often, patients describe a history of previous episodes of similar symptoms lasting for short periods. Nausea and vomiting are present in 50% of cases.[1]

Pathophysiology

TT is most commonly caused by a congenitally loose fixation of the tunica vaginalis to the posterior scrotal wall; this is referred to as the "bell clapper deformity."[1] This defect is usually found bilaterally. The higher the degree of abnormal rotation, the more rapid the development of ischemia of the testicle. There is a bimodal incidence of this disease, with peaks occurring during infancy and adolescence, but it can occur at any age.[2]

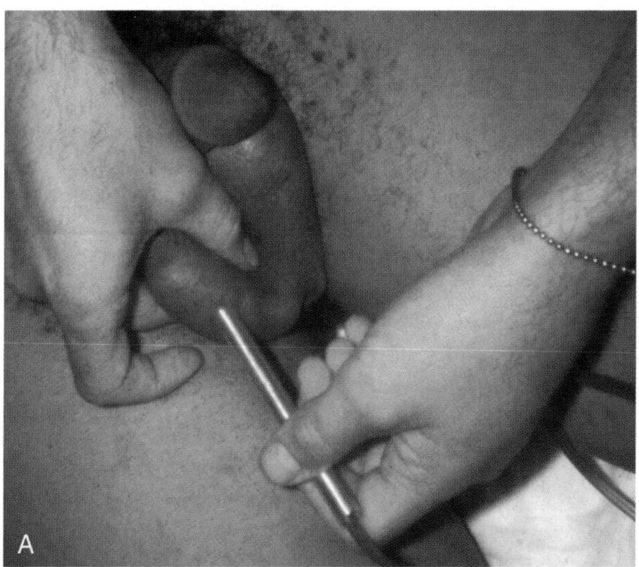

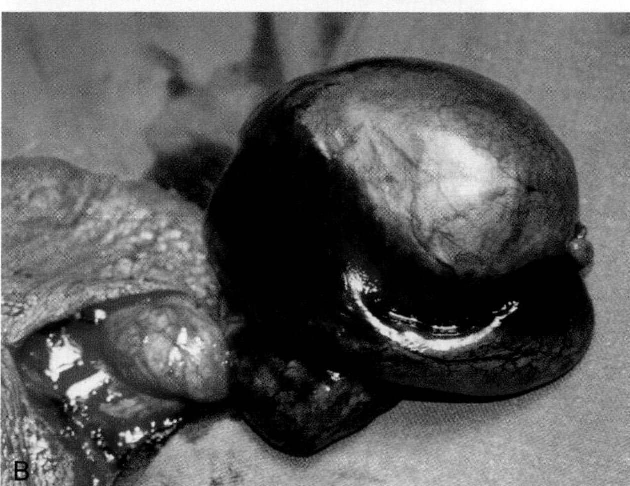

FIGURE 10–12 **A:** Probe placement for Doppler ultrasonography of testicle. (Copyright James R. Roberts, MD.) **B:** Gangrene of the right testicle in a boy 16 years of age who had a 720-degree torsion of the spermatic cord. (From Glenn, with permission.)

Diagnosis

TT is a urologic emergency, and an immediate consultation with a genitourinary specialist should be obtained if the diagnosis is suspected. Neither consultation nor surgery should be delayed to await diagnostic test results if torsion is strongly suspected. Confirmatory studies, when used, include Doppler ultrasonography and testicular radionuclide scanning. Doppler ultrasonography shows decreased flow in the affected testicle, with a sensitivity of 85% to 90%.[3] Technetium scintigraphy has a specificity and a sensitivity of at least 95% but may be more time-consuming to obtain.[1] There are no specific laboratory studies that aid in the diagnosis of TT, but it should be mentioned that the urinalysis is normal in 80% of patients with TT.[1] On physical examination, the affected testicle may be found to have an abnormal horizontal lie, with the testicle most often rotated medially. One sign of torsion is the absence of the cremasteric reflex on the affected side. This sign has been found to be more reliable in children than in adults.[2]

Clinical Complications

Tubular necrosis in the involved testicle is evident after 2 hours of torsion, so time to detorsion is of the essence.[1] There is almost complete testicular atrophy within 8 hours after the onset of ischemia. Clinical complications of TT are decreased fertility and testicular loss if the torsion is not corrected quickly enough. More extreme degrees of testicular rotation adversely affect the degree of testicular ischemia and chances of salvage.

Management

Manual detorsion may be attempted by rotating the involved testicle in the direction of external rotation (i.e., clockwise for the left testicle and counterclockwise for the right when standing at the patient's feet). This motion has been compared to opening the pages of a book. Definitive treatment involves operative scrotal exploration and detorsion of the testicle, followed by orchiopexy. This is usually done bilaterally, because the congenital defect commonly exists on both sides.

REFERENCES

1. Cummings JM, Boullier JA, Sekhon D, Bose K. Adult testicular torsion. *J Urol* 2002;167:2109–2110.
2. Kass EJ, Lundak B. The acute scrotum. *Pediatr Clin North Am* 1997;44:1251–1266.
3. Paltiel HJ, Connolly LP, Atala A, Paltiel AD, Zurakowski D, Treves ST. Acute scrotal symptoms in boys with an indeterminate clinical presentation: comparison of color Doppler sonography and scintigraphy. *Radiology* 1998;207:223–231.

Testicular Cancer

Colleen Campbell

Clinical Presentation

Patients with testicular cancer (TC) may present with a painless scrotal or testicular mass that does not transilluminate. Patients may also have a diffusely painful scrotum and may appear to have symptoms consistent with epididymitis. Signs of metastatic disease include lower-extremity swelling, back pain, or pulmonary symptoms.

Pathophysiology

TC is the most common malignancy in men between the ages of 15 and 34 years.[1] More than 95% are germ-cell tumors. Seminomas and testicular lymphomas are more common in older men.[2] Cryptorchidism is an important risk factor for disease: 20% of tumors occur in the contralateral testicle in cryptorchidism.[1] TC is 20 to 50 times more common in immunosuppressed persons.[2] White males and first-degree relatives of patients with TC are at increased risk for the disease. Seminomas are often diagnosed in older men with a history of undescended testicles.

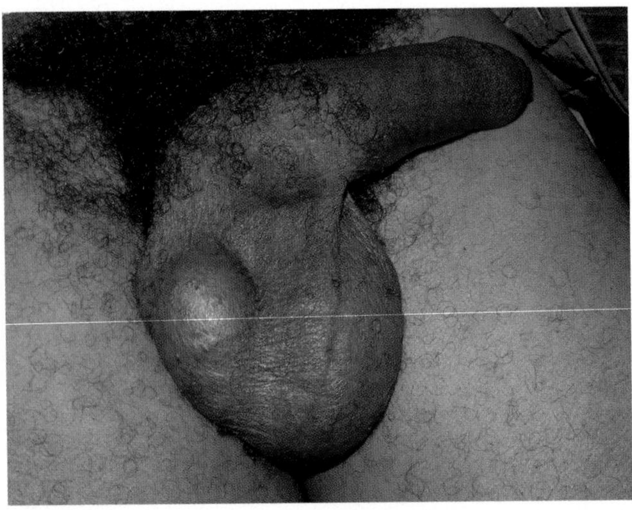

FIGURE 10–13 Left-sided testicular mass. (Courtesy of Mark Silverberg, MD.)

Diagnosis

The suspicion of TC is initiated on palpation of a testicular mass or testicular swelling. Tumor markers that may be used to signal the presence of a testicular malignancy include α-fetoprotein (AFP), β-human chorionic gonadotropin (β-hCG), lactic acid dehydrogenase (LDH), and placental alkaline phosphatase (pAP). Chest radiography and computed tomography (CT) of the abdomen and pelvis are necessary for staging, which is important in making prognostic predictions.

Clinical Complications

Complications of TC and its treatment are largely related to infertility. The overall mortality rate is low, and most recurrences happen within the first year after therapy.[2]

Management

Expedient referral to a urologist is indicated for all non-illuminating scrotal masses, because the doubling time for tumors is short (10 to 30 days).[1] Any patient with a recurrent or resistant epididymitis should also be referred, because this is a diagnosis commonly confused with TC. Inguinal orchiectomy is the treatment of choice for TC; it is combined with radiation therapy for early-stage disease. Seminomas, which are the most common form of TC, are very sensitive to radiation. Later-stage malignancies and non-seminomas should be treated with platinum-based chemotherapy as well. The overall survival rate is greater than 90%.[3]

REFERENCES

1. Kinkade S. Testicular cancer. *Am Fam Physician* 1999;59:2539–2544, 2549–2550.
2. Epperson WJ, Frank WL. Male genital cancers. *Prim Care* 1998;25:459–472.
3. Shelley MD, Burgon K, Mason MD. Treatment of testicular germ-cell cancer: a Cochrane evidence-based systematic review. *Cancer Treat Rev* 2002;28:237–253.

Epididymitis

Michael Greenberg

Clinical Presentation

Patients with epididymitis present with gradual onset of scrotal pain. Urethral discharge is a presenting complaint in 50% of patients.

Pathophysiology

Inflammation of the epididymis usually begins in the vas deferens and descends to the epididymis. In infants and in men older than 35 years of age, infection is usually caused by coliform bacteria. Unusual pathogens, such as tuberculosis, cryptococcus, and brucella, may be found in immunocompromised individuals. Reactive epididymitis may result from inflammatory conditions such as Henoch-Schönlein purpura, or from drugs such as amiodarone.[1-3]

Diagnosis

Dysuria, urgency, and frequency are characteristic of epididymitis. Scrotal swelling, edema, and erythema develop as the disease progresses. Prehn's sign is the relief of scrotal pain with elevation of the involved testicle, but it is not a reliable way to differentiate epididymitis from torsion. If three of the following criteria are present, the diagnosis of epididymitis is likely: gradual onset of pain, dysuria, urethral discharge or recent instrumentations, history of genitourinary abnormality or trauma, fever greater than 101°F, tenderness localized to the epididymis, urine sediment with greater than 10 white blood cells (WBCs) per high-power field (hpf) or greater than 10 red blood cells (RBCs)/hpf.

Fifty percent of patients have pyuria on urinalysis. Urine culture should be ordered along with the initial urinalysis. The WBC count is elevated on the complete blood count in 30% to 50% of patients with epididymitis, but this is a nonspecific finding. Perfusion studies are recommended if fewer than two of clinical criteria listed are present or if the diagnosis is unclear.

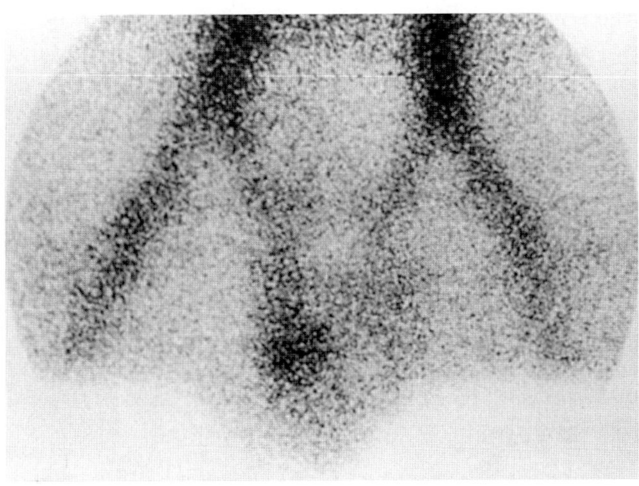

FIGURE 10–14 Epididymitis: testicular scan (technetium 99m). Diffuse photon-dense area in scrotum reflects uptake of radionuclide into the inflamed epididymis. (From Fleisher *Atlas,* with permission.)

Clinical Complications

Complications of epididymitis include chronic pain and infertility. In many cases, testicular atrophy results from thrombosis of the testicular artery.[1-3]

Management

Treatment of epididymitis involves pain relief and treatment of infection. Empiric antibiotic therapy against gonorrhea and chlamydia is recommended pending culture results. Treatment regimens involve doxycycline after initial treatment with ceftriaxone. Alternative therapies include ciprofloxacin or ofloxacin. For men older than 35 years of age and for homosexual men, treatment against enterobacteria is initiated with a fluoroquinolone for 14 to 21 days. Trimethoprim-sulfamethoxazole (TMP-SMX) may be used for children and older men. Patients should refer their partners for evaluation and treatment. Patients need urologic referral if symptoms have not improved within 72 hours after treatment initiation. Bed rest and pain control are the mainstays of treatment for sterile epididymitis.[1-3]

REFERENCES

1. Galejs LE. Diagnosis and treatment of the acute scrotum. *Am Fam Physician* 1999;59:817–824.
2. Burgher SW. Acute scrotal pain. *Emerg Med Clin North Am* 1998;16:781–809.
3. Can heavy lifting cause epididymitis? *J Occup Environ Med* 1997;39:609–610.

10–15

Varicocele

Colleen Campbell

Clinical Presentation

Most varicoceles are asymptomatic, but patients may notice a gradual decrease in testicular size on the affected side. A "bag of worms" is the classic description of the appearance of the spermatic cord region. The left side is affected more frequently than the right.[1] Bilateral varicoceles do occur but are less common.

Pathophysiology

A varicocele is a dilatation of the testicular vein and pampiniform plexus of the testis. Varicoceles are relatively common, with an incidence as high as 15% and a peak incidence during adolescence.[1] The scrotal veins are believed to dilate abnormally more often on the left because of the increased length of the spermatic vein on the left and also because of the increased angle of drainage of the left internal spermatic vein into the left renal vein (and subsequently to the inferior vena cava), which causes increased blood pooling in the pampiniform plexus of the left testicle. Loss of testicular volume occurs because of alteration in blood flow of the testis and increased temperature of the affected testicle.

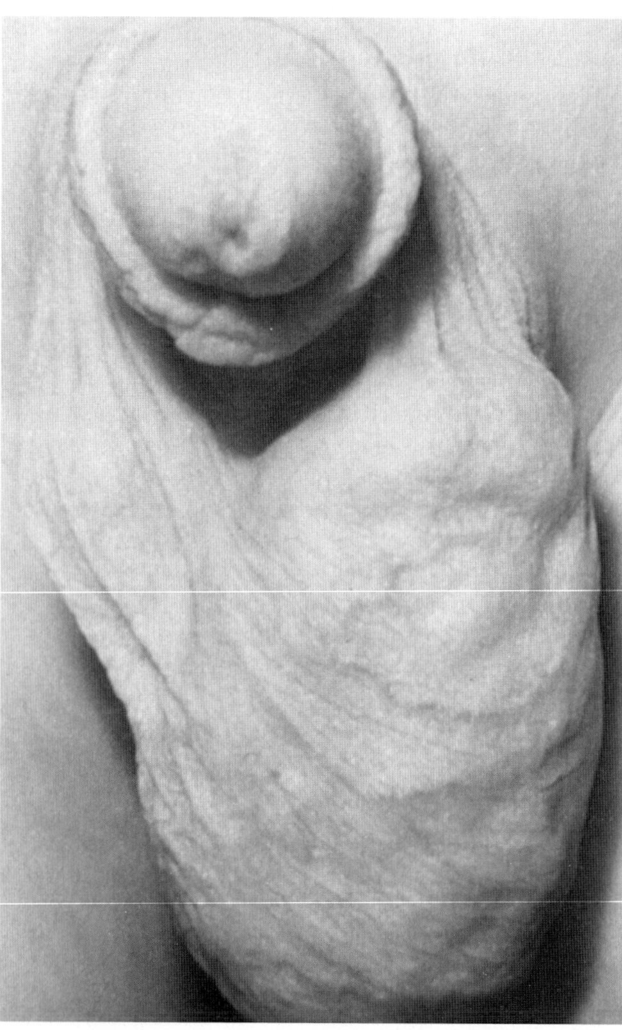

FIGURE 10–15 Varicocele: abnormal dilation of cremasteric and pampiniform venous plexuses surrounding the spermatic cord, giving the scrotum the appearance of a "bag of worms." (From Fleisher *Textbook*, with permission.)

Diagnosis

Varicoceles are detected on routine examination of the genitalia. The physical examination should be performed while the patient is standing and again while he is supine. Grade 1 varicoceles may be palpable on examination only during Valsalva maneuvers, whereas grade 2 and 3 lesions are easily palpated at any time. Ultrasonography, venography, magnetic resonance imaging (MRI), and scintography have all been used to diagnose varicoceles but have uncertain clinical utility.

Clinical Complications

Loss of testicular volume and decreased fertility are the most common complications of varicocele formation. The larger the varicocele, the more likely it is that fertility will be impaired. Eighty percent of patients with a varicocele do not have impaired fertility, but varicoceles are implicated in 70% to 80% of men with secondary infertility.[2,3]

Management

Patients should be referred in a timely manner to a urologist for definitive treatment. Treatment options include interventional radiology with transvenous occlusion or surgical correction. Interventional radiology is unsuccessful in venous occlusion at least 15% of the time.[1] Repair should be undertaken as soon as possible so as to prevent infertility.[3]

REFERENCES

1. Kass EJ. Adolescent varicocele. *Pediatr Clin North Am* 2001;48:1559–1569.
2. Fretz PC, Sandlow JI. Varicocele: current concepts in pathophysiology, diagnosis and treatment. *Urol Clin North Am* 2002;29:921–937.
3. Penson DF, Paltiel AD, Krumholz HM, Palter S. The cost-effectiveness of treatment for varicocele related infertility. *J Urol* 2002;168:2490–2494.

Hydrocele

Colleen Campbell

Clinical Presentation

Almost all hydroceles are reported in males, usually in infancy. Hydroceles in females have been reported within the canal of Nuck, the inguinal portion of the patent processus vaginalis.[1] Children present with a history of painless scrotal swelling that becomes more pronounced with exercise or when crying. Parents may note an increase in size of the mass during waking hours when the child is upright. Physical examination should include scrotal transillumination. In cases of hydrocele, the scrotum can be transilluminated, because light passes readily through the fluid-filled scrotum. The appearance of the scrotum is smooth, with no tenderness on palpation.

Pathophysiology

A hydrocele is a collection of peritoneal fluid that accumulates within the scrotum as a result of the congenital defect of a patent processus vaginalis. Hydroceles are considered sequelae of congenital anomalies, and most are apparent at birth. A communicating hydrocele results when there is a narrowing of the processus vaginalis without complete closure at the internal inguinal ring. A noncommunicating hydrocele results when the incomplete closure is more distal than the internal ring. Because the processus vaginalis usually fuses between 7 and 9 months of gestational age, hydroceles are more common in premature infants.[2] Hydroceles occur more frequently on the right side, but they may occur bilaterally.[2] In adults, hydroceles sometimes develop secondary to other disease processes, such as infection, testicular torsion (TT), or hypoalbuminemia.

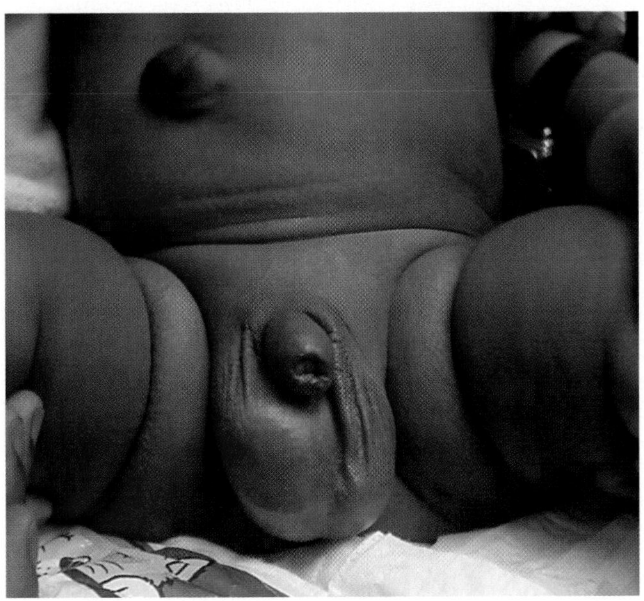

FIGURE 10–16 Right-sided hydrocele. (Courtesy of Christy Salvaggio, MD.)

Diagnosis

Hydroceles are usually apparent on physical examination with the demonstration of a soft, cystic mass palpable within the scrotum. However, if the mass is continuous with the inguinal canal, a hernia is the more likely diagnosis. Because incarcerated hernias also can transilluminate on physical examination, herniography is occasionally required to confirm the presence of a hydrocele. If the diagnosis is still in question, radiopaque contrast media can be injected into the peritoneal cavity and sequential radiographs taken of the inguinal region. A hydrocele is then diagnosed if contrast material enters the scrotum.[2]

Clinical Complications

A communicating hydrocele may result in an inguinal hernia if the patent processus vaginalis enlarges to the extent that bowel is able to slip into the scrotum. This bowel can become incarcerated and necrotic if blood flow becomes compromised.

Management

Infants with uncomplicated hydroceles are usually simply observed for 1 to 2 years, because most inguinal defects spontaneously resolve.[3] Surgical repair may be required if the hydrocele persists for a longer period.

REFERENCES

1. Wei, BP, Castles L, Stewart KA. Hydrocele of the canal of Nuck. *Aust N Z J Surg* 2002;72:603–605.
2. Kapur P, Caty MG, Glick PL. Pediatric hernias and hydroceles. *Pediatr Clin North Am* 1998;45:773–789.
3. Kass EJ, Lundak B. Pediatric urology: the acute scrotum. *Pediatr Clin North Am* 1997;44:1251–1266.

Orchitis

Mark Silverberg

Clinical Presentation

Bilateral testicular pain and swelling are frequently present in patients with orchitis, often in association with edema and erythema of the scrotum. Because orchitis is frequently a complication of epididymitis, it may also be accompanied by dysuria and penile discharge, but these associated findings are not specific for orchitis. Orchitis may result from infection with the mumps virus, most often affecting postpubertal boys 4 to 6 days after onset of parotid gland swelling.[1] Mumps orchitis is unilateral in as many as 70% of patients.[1]

Pathophysiology

Orchitis is inflammation or infection of the testicle, often resulting from direct extension from the epididymitis to the testicle.[2] Infection of only one testicle is uncommon but can result from hematogenous spread of bacteria. The most common cause of unilateral orchitis is mumps infection, but coxsackie A virus has also been implicated.[1] *Escherichia coli, Klebsiella,* and *Pseudomonas* are the most common bacterial infections of the testicle.[3] *Staphylococcus* and *Streptococcus* species have also been isolated. Pyogenic bacterial orchitis is usually a result of direct extension from epididymitis. Granulomatous orchitis usually occurs in immunocompromised hosts and may be a result of syphilis, mycobacterial, or fungal infection. Orchitis can also occur as a sequela of testicular trauma.

Diagnosis

See Tables 10–17A and B. Urinalysis often shows pyuria (greater than 10 white blood cells [WBCs]/hpf [high-power field] or greater than 10 red blood cells [RBCs]/hpf). Urethral swabs and blood cultures should be sent to help identify the infecting organism.[3] It is critical to remember that unilateral testicular pain, without pyuria, represents torsion until proven otherwise. All of these cases require prompt, on-site urology consultation, without exception.

Clinical Complications

Complications of orchitis include chronic pain, scarring, and infertility. Approximately one third of patients affected with mumps orchitis have decreased fertility as a

TABLE 10–17A Differential Diagnosis of Orchitis

Nonpainful scrotal swelling
Henoch-Schönlein purpura
Hydrocele
Idiopathic scrotal edema
Kawasaki disease
Nephrotic syndrome
Testicular neoplasm
Testicular torsion (early)
Reducible inguinal hernia
Varicocele
Painful swelling of the scrotum
Epididymitis
Fournier's gangrene
Incarcerated hernia
Orchitis
Renal colic
Scrotal abscess
Testicular torsion
Torsion of the appendix testis
Trauma

(From ref. 2, with permission.)

Mark Silverberg

TABLE 10–17B Comparison of Epididymitis, Orchitis, and Torsion of the Testicle

Factor	Epididymitis	Orchitis	Torsion
Age	Adolescent	Postpubertal	Prepubertal/adolescent
Common cause	Viral, chemicals, sexually transmitted disease	Viral (mumps)	Bell clapper deformity
Bilaterality	Unusual	20–60%	Almost never
Dysuria	Often +	Usually −	Usually −
Fever	+/−	+	Usually −
Nausea/vomiting	+/−	+/−	+/−
Onset	Gradual	1–2 d	Sudden
Localized pain	Epididymis (early)	Entire testicle	Testis, abdomen, flank
Urinalysis	+/−White blood cells (WBCs)	+/−WBCs	Usually no WBCs
Cremaster reflex	Usually present	Usually present	Usually absent
Doppler	Increased flow	Increased flow	Decreased flow

(From ref. 2, with permission.)

result of this infection.[1] A reactive hydrocele may also develop in response to infection.

Management

Management of orchitis is similar to that of epididymitis. Bacterial causes should be treated with a quinolone antibiotic or as culture sensitivities indicate.[4] Viral infections require good supportive care, including scrotal support, bed rest, analgesia, and appropriate follow-up.

REFERENCES

1. Marcozzi D, Suner S. Genitourinary emergencies: the nontraumatic, acute scrotum. *Emerg Med Clin North Am* 2001;19:547–568.
2. Kass EJ, Lundak B. Pediatric urology: the acute scrotum. *Pediatr Clin North Am* 1997;44:1251–1266.
3. Burgher SW. The difficult diagnosis: acute scrotal pain. *Emerg Med Clin North Am* 1998;16:781–809.
4. Galejs LE. Diagnosis and treatment of the acute scrotum. *Am Fam Physician* 1999;59:817–824.

Bladder and Urethral Foreign Bodies

Colleen Campbell

Clinical Presentation

Patients with bladder or urethral foreign bodies (FBs) may present with urinary frequency, dysuria, or hematuria in conjunction with poor urinary stream or hesitancy. Patients may have minimal bladder discomfort, or they may be asymptomatic for years. Patients with urethral FBs may have urinary obstruction or severe pain. Patients may not be forthcoming with vital history of urethral instrumentation due to embarrassment.

Pathophysiology

A wide variety of bladder FBs have been reported, including dollar bills, plants and wood, animal parts, thermometers, bullets, and buttons.[1–3] Most bladder FBs are sharp, lacerating, or wire-like objects.[1] FBs must migrate 20 to 25 cm against the flow of urine, through the bulbous urethra, to enter the bladder.[1] Objects have also been reported to migrate through the intraabdominal or pelvic route, including orthopedic pins, intrauterine devices, pessaries, chicken bones from the gastrointestinal tract, and cardioverter-pacemakers originally placed in the rectus muscles.[1–3] Live organisms that may burrow into the urethra include leeches and the ureophilic parasitic Amazon fish, candiru.[1]

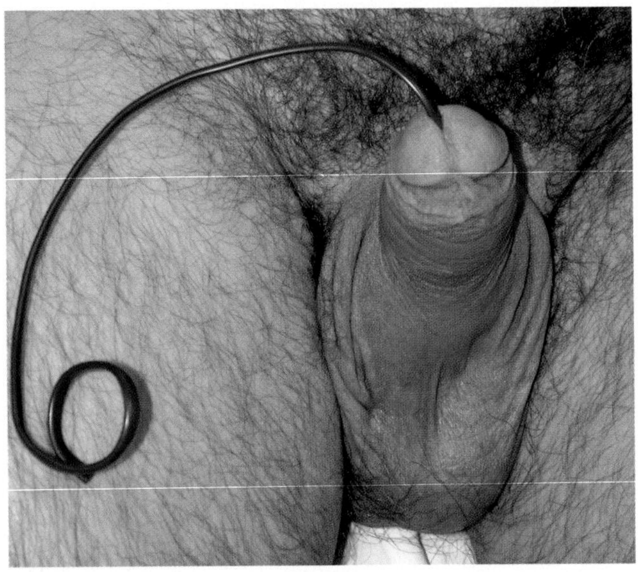

FIGURE 10–18 Telephone cord was knotted and placed in the urethra. (Courtesy of Lowan Stewart, MD.)

Diagnosis

Patients may hesitate to give an accurate history. Plain radiographs often are used to diagnose the FB, but ultrasonography may be useful in differentiating specific locations of bladder FBs.[2] For urethral FBs, plain films may identify radiolucent objects, but organic compounds will be missed on radiography. A voiding cystourethrogram may aid in diagnosis. Urinalysis may show evidence of infection.[1,3]

Clinical Complications

The most common complications of bladder FBs are infection and injury to the genitourinary tract. Patients may also have urinary obstruction requiring suprapubic catheterization. Injury of the bladder is surprisingly rare, given the vast array of FBs reported. Bladder injury is more common in the case of a gunshot wound to the bladder or bullet migration into the bladder. Urethral FB complications include ascending infections, septicemia, urethral diverticula, periurethral phlegmon, and urethral tears.

Management

All cases of bladder FB require prompt referral to a urology specialist for removal. Concomitant infection requires treatment with appropriate antibiotics. Most bladder FBs can be removed with cystoscopy using forceps or magnetic retrievers. Ultrasound-guided cystoscopy was used successfully in the removal of a test tube.[2] Fogarty catheters also have been used successfully.[3] Laparotomy may be required in the case of very large FBs.

When dealing with urethral FBs, the foreign body should be pushed into the bladder, where it can be more easily removed. Occasionally, an external urethrostomy is required, especially in the case of accompanying periurethral abscess.[1–4]

REFERENCES

1. van Ophoven A, deKernion JB. Clinical management of foreign bodies of the genitourinary tract. *J Urol* 2000;164:274–287.
2. Wang SM, Shih FY, Ma MH, Chen SC, Huang GT. Manual removal of urinary bladder foreign body under ultrasound localization. *Am J Emerg Med* 1998;16:329–330.
3. Phillips JL. Fogarty catheter extraction of unusual urethral foreign bodies. *J Urol* 1996;155:1374–1375.
4. Lundquist ST, Stack LB. Diseases of the foreskin, penis, and urethra. *Emerg Med Clin North Am* 2001;19:526–546.

Rhabdomyolysis

Matthew Spencer

Clinical Presentation

Patients with rhabdomyolysis are often asymptomatic but may present with diffuse myalgias. Patients may report a change in the color of their urine to tea-colored or "port-wine" colored.[1]

Pathophysiology

Rhabdomyolysis is a syndrome that results from breakdown of striated muscle fibers with the release of muscle constituents into the circulation. Rhabdomyolysis is often nontraumatic but may result from crush injuries, ischemic insult, or heat-related causes. Other causes of rhabdomyolysis include seizures, alcohol and drug abuse, and overexertion. Drugs associated with direct myotoxicity include 3-hydroxy-3-methylglutaryl coenzyme A (HMG-CoA) reductase inhibitors, cyclosporine, erythromycin, colchicines, zidovudine, and corticosteroids.[2] Indirect muscle damage is caused by alcohol, cocaine, amphetamines, 3,4-methylenedioxymethamphetamine (MDMA), and lysergic acid diethylamide (LSD).[2] Extracellular calcium leakage occurs with muscle injury. This leads to leakage of myoglobin, creatine kinase (CK), and urate into the circulation. Myoglobin, the most nephrotoxic byproduct of muscle breakdown, causes renal tubular obstruction when it precipitates.[3]

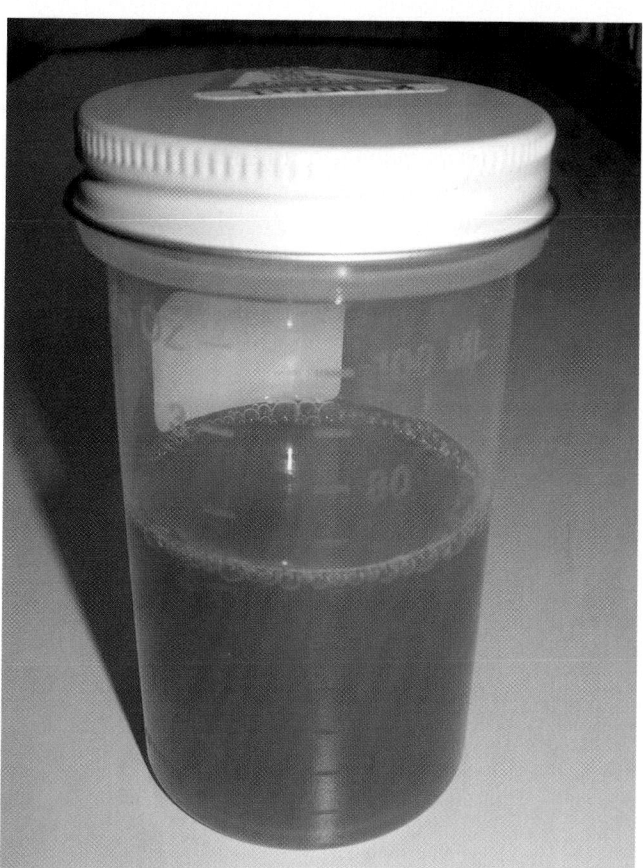

FIGURE 10–19 Urine specimen in rhabdomyolysis may have a brown to black color. (Courtesy of Mark Silverberg, MD.)

Diagnosis

Urine dipstick may be used as a screening examination. The dipstick turns blue in the presence of hemoglobin or myoglobin. Analysis of the corresponding spun urine is significant for the absence of red blood cells (RBCs). Uric acid crystals are often present on urinalysis as well.[1] The serum should be normal in color in the presence of myoglobin but discolored red or brown in the presence of hemoglobin.

Clinical Complications

The most life-threatening early complication is hyperkalemia, which can lead to cardiac arrhythmias or arrest. Hypocalcemia and hyperphosphatemia also occur early on.[2] Later in the disease course, acute renal failure (ARF) occurs in 15% of affected patients. Rhabdomyolysis is a leading cause of ARF.[1] Hepatic dysfunction occurs in 25% of patients with rhabdomyolysis.[2]

Management

Treatment of rhabdomyolysis is aimed at preserving renal function. Patients often require large amounts of fluids because of sequestration of fluids in necrotic muscle tissue.[2] Intravenous fluids should be directed to maintain a minimum urine output of 300 mL/hour until CK levels fall below 1000 μ/L. Sodium bicarbonate is recommended to alkalinize the urine to a pH greater than 6.5 if there is no evidence of oliguric renal failure.[3] This is done to enhance renal elimination of myoglobin casts. Mannitol is recommended by some authors.[1] Mannitol acts to draw fluid from the interstitial space as an osmotic diuretic to decrease myoglobin casts, and as a free-radical scavenger.[1] Hemodialysis is used aggressively to treat oliguric renal failure and severe hyperkalemia.

REFERENCES

1. Vanholder R, Sever MS, Erek E, Lameire N. Rhabdomyolysis. *J Am Soc Nephrol* 2000;11: 1553–1561.
2. Sauret JM, Marinides G, Wang GK. Rhabdomyolysis. *Am Fam Physician* 2002;65:907–912.
3. Lappalainen H, Tiula E, Uotila L, Manttari M. Elimination kinetics of myoglobin and creatine kinase in rhabdomyolysis: implications for follow-up. *Crit Care Med* 2002;30:2212–2215.

Hematuria

Mark Silverberg

Clinical Presentation

Gross hematuria may be evident on physical examination, but this may be a false diagnosis if the patient has ingested beets, rhubarb, or other substances containing red dyes that cannot be broken down enzymatically. Drugs that can change the color of urine include phenazopyridine, phenindione, and phenothiazine.[1] Most patients with hematuria are asymptomatic. Gross hematuria at the beginning of the urine stream suggests a urethral cause. Important historical elements include the presence of painful voiding, trauma, and a family history of renal or stone disease. Physical examination findings are usually absent or minimal. In the setting of hypertension, diabetes, and edema, glomerular causes of hematuria should be suspected. Lower-abdominal or flank tenderness may be present in the case of a urinary tract infection, nephrolithiasis, or an obstructing mass.

Pathophysiology

See Table 10–20. Hematuria is the presence of more than 3 red blood cells (RBCs)/hpf (high-power field) on microscopic analysis of centrifuged urine sediment.[1] Microscopic hematuria is thought to have a benign etiology in most cases. A single episode of transient microscopic hematuria was found in 39% of healthy young men, and up to 16% of the time it recurred once without any detectable disease process being present in these individuals.[1] Older patients with microscopic hematuria are at increased risk for malignancy, renal lithiasis, or intrinsic renal disease.[1] In older patients with persistent microscopic hematuria, the incidence of malignancy has been found to be approximately 5%; however, up to 20% of patients with gross hematuria have a neoplasm.[1] Hematuria may originate from glomerular causes, renal parenchymal disease, or extrarenal locations. Glomerular causes include primary and secondary glomerulonephritis. Classic primary disease processes leading to glomerulonephritis are diabetes and hypertension, and secondary causes include familial conditions such as Alport's syndrome and Fabry's disease. Vasculitic diseases and systemic lupus erythematosus (SLE) also occasionally result in hematuria. Renal parenchymal diseases that cause blood to appear in the urine include renal tumors, vascular disease (i.e., sickle cell disease and malignant hypertension), polycystic kidney disease, and medullary sponge kidney. Extrarenal causes include malignancy, nephrolithiasis, infection (i.e., cystitis, *Schistosoma haematobium*, or tuberculosis), and bleeding disorders (drug-induced or systemic), in addition to trauma (e.g., vigorous physical exercise).

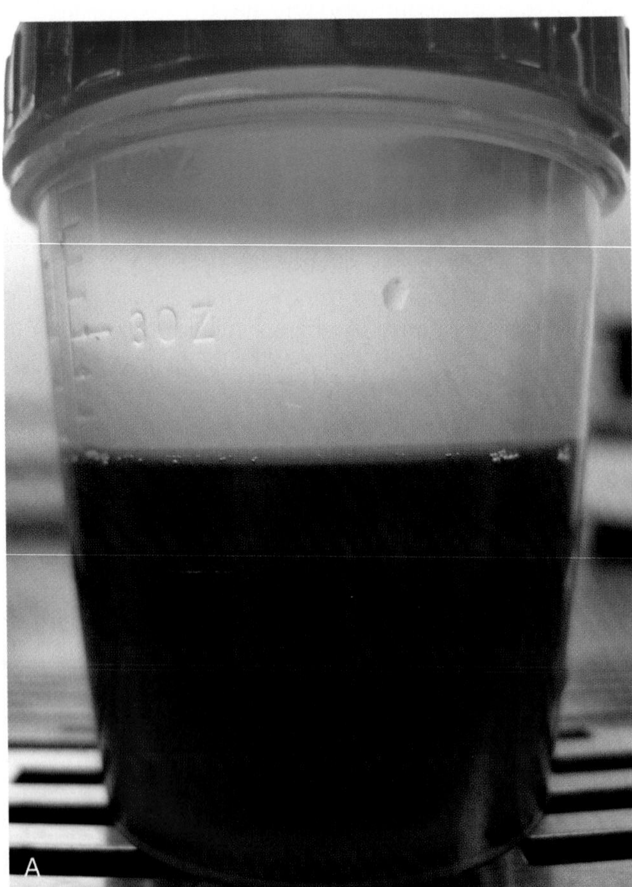

FIGURE 10–20 Gross hematuria. (Courtesy of Anthony Morocco, MD.)

TABLE 10–20 Most Common Causes of Hematuria by Age and Gender

Age (yr)	Cause
0–20	Acute glomerulonephritis
	Acute urinary tract infection (UTI)
	Congenital urinary tract anomalies with obstruction
20–40	Acute UTI
	Stones
	Bladder tumor
40–60	
Men	Bladder tumor
	Stones
	Acute UTI
Women	Acute UTI
	Stones
	Bladder tumor
60	
Men	Benign prostatic hyperplasia
	Bladder tumor
	Acute UTI
Women	Bladder tumor
	Acute UTI

From Gillenwater JY, Grayhack JT, Howards SS, Mitchell ME, eds. Adult and Pediatric Urology, Fourth Edition. Philadelphia: Lippincott Williams & Wilkins, 2001, with permission.

Hematuria

Mark Silverberg

Diagnosis

Microscopic hematuria is usually diagnosed by urine dipstick. A color change is noted when orthotolidine on the stick is oxidized by peroxide in the presence of hemoglobin or myoglobin.[2] This test can detect as few as 5 to 20 RBCs/mm^2 of urine.[3] Urine dipstick may be falsely positive in the presence of oxidizing agents or povidone-iodine, or falsely negative if left exposed to air or with vitamin C ingestion and excretion.[2] Microscopic urinalysis may help differentiate glomerular from nonglomerular causes of hematuria. Dysmorphic RBCs, cellular casts, and protein all point to the diagnosis of glomerular disease.[1] Blood clots or crystals in the urine favor nonglomerular causes. Because of the high incidence of benign microscopic hematuria, at least three samples on different days should be obtained. In the setting of traumatic gross hematuria, retrograde urethrography and computed tomography (CT) of the abdomen with intravenous contrast are indicated procedures to determine renal blood flow and the anatomic location and the extent of injury.

Clinical Complications

Hematuria can be benign with no significant clinical complications, or it can be a herald of a more serious underlying disease. Complications are diverse and are directly related to the underlying cause of hematuria as opposed to the symptom in itself.

Management

A first episode of asymptomatic hematuria requires follow-up with a primary physician for repeat urinalysis. In older patients with microscopic hematuria, referral to a urologist for further workup, including upper tract imaging, cystoscopy, and urine cytology, is warranted. Patients found to have RBC casts, dysmorphic RBCs, or proteinuria should be referred to a nephrologist. Patients with traumatic gross hematuria should have emergency urology consultation.

REFERENCES

1. Ahmed S, Lee, J. Asymptomatic urinary abnormalities: hematuria and proteinuria. *Med Clin North Am* 1997;81:641–652.
2. Grossfeld GD, Wolf JS Jr, Litwan MS, et al. Asymptomatic microscopic hematuria in adults: summary of the AUA Best Practice Policy Recommendations. *Am Fam Physician* 2001;63:1145–1154.
3. Feld LG, Waz WR, Perez LM, Joseph DB. Pediatric urology. Hematuria: an integrated and surgical approach. *Pediatr Clin North Am* 1997;44:1191–1210.

Urinary Tract Infections and Pyelonephritis

Colleen Campbell

Clinical Presentation

Some patients with urinary tract infection (UTI) are asymptomatic, whereas others present with dysuria, urinary frequency, hesitancy, hematuria, and lower abdominal discomfort. Flank pain, fever, chills, nausea, and malaise characterize pyelonephritis.

Pathophysiology

UTIs are the most common bacterial infections, with the incidence in females exceeding that in males. Infants, elderly individuals, pregnant women, diabetics, patients with spinal cord injury or multiple sclerosis, patients with human immunodeficiency virus (HIV) infection, and those patients who undergo routine or frequent urinary catheterization are susceptible to infection. *E. coli* causes more than 80% of uncomplicated infections.

Diagnosis

Urinalysis and culture are essential for accurate diagnosis. The finding of at least one organism per high-power field with pyuria is a sensitive indicator for infection. If many epithelial cells are also present, the specimen is considered contaminated and the results not reliable. Sterile catheterization should be performed to obtain urine in females only. The presence of greater than 100 colony-forming units (CFU) per milliliter in a patient with symptoms of UTI is considered diagnostic.[1] Traditionally, a culture revealing 100,000 bacteria per milliliter was considered the gold standard of diagnosis, although much lower colony counts have been found to be associated with infection.

Urinary leukocyte esterase and urinary nitrate cause colorimetric change on specially designed dipsticks. Leukocyte esterase is present when neutrophils release the substance in the urine in response to infection or inflammation. Nitrates are present when they are released in enzymatic reduction by gram-negative bacteria. If both are present in a symptomatic patient, the positive predictive value is approximately 67%.

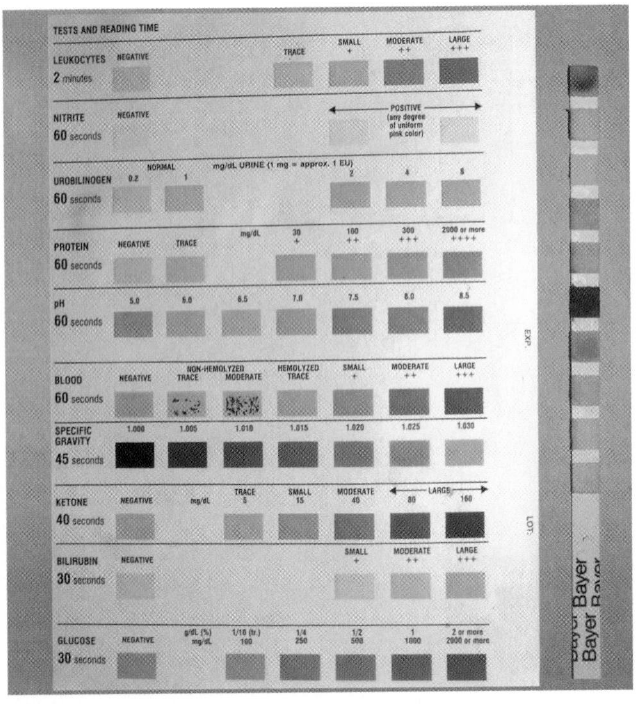

FIGURE 10–21 The urine of a patient with a urinary tract infection is usually positive for nitrite, leukocytes, and blood. (Courtesy of Lekha Shah, MD.)

Clinical Complications

UTIs in children are associated with higher complication rates. During pregnancy, UTI more often progresses to pyelonephritis.[1] There are increased risks of premature labor, fetal mortality, and low birth weight.

Management

In simple, uncomplicated lower tract UTIs, trimethoprim-sulfamethoxazole (TMP-SMX) may be used, but resistance to TMP-SMX has doubled in the last decade in some states.[2] Nitrofurantoin is also effective. Pregnant women may be treated with first- or second-generation cephalosporins. In upper tract UTIs, a 14-day course of therapy with quinolone is warranted. In any patient with systemic signs of toxicity, it is recommended that switch therapy be initiated with intravenous hydration plus aminoglycoside or a third-generation cephalosporin followed by parenteral quinolone therapy. Patients with complicated disease, or failure to improve within 24 hours, should be admitted for intravenous antibiotic therapy.

REFERENCES

1. Ronald A. The etiology of urinary tract infection: traditional and emerging pathogens. *Am J Med* 2002;113[Suppl 1A]:14S–19S.
2. Krieger JN. Urinary tract infections: what's new? *J Urol* 2002;168: 2351–2358.

Renal Stones

Colleen Campbell

Clinical Presentation

Patients with renal stones (RS) present with acute, severe, unilateral flank pain or lower abdominal pain, often with nausea and vomiting. In some, pain radiates to the vaginal or scrotal area.

Pathophysiology

Stone formation occurs in 2% to 3% of the population, with adult white men having a 12% lifetime risk.[1] Stone formation may be precipitated by dehydration, high dietary oxalate intake, or medications. Crixivan (indinavir) is the medication most commonly associated with stone formation, but acetazolamide and triamterene have also been implicated.[1]

Seventy-five percent of stones contain calcium complexed with phosphate or oxalate. Urea-splitting organisms such as *Proteus, Klebsiella,* and *Pseudomonas* predispose the patient to struvite stones (magnesium-ammonium-phosphate). Five percent of stones are composed of uric acid.[2]

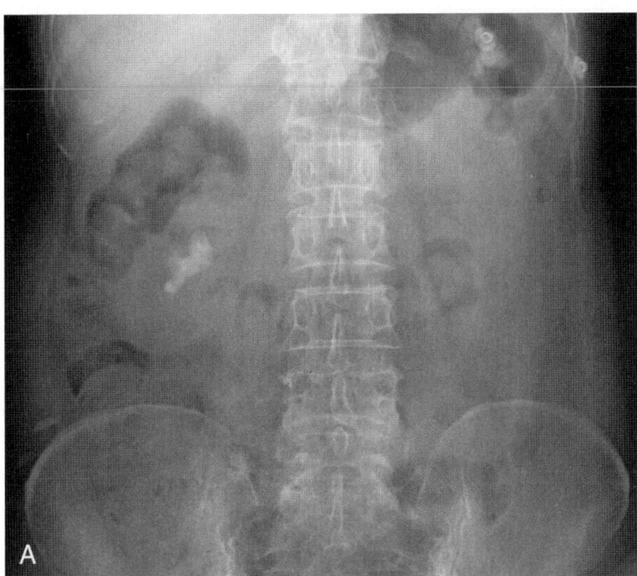

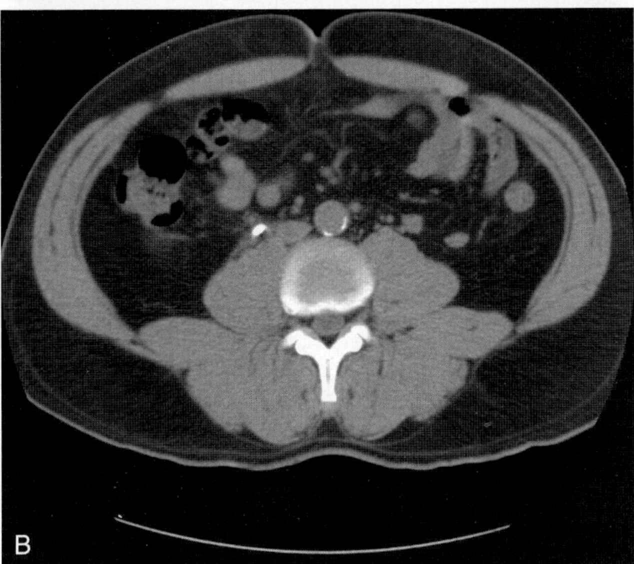

FIGURE 10–22 **A:** Staghorn kidney stone as seen on abdominal radiograph. (Courtesy of Roger D. Tillotson, MD.) **B:** Right ureteral stone as seen on abdominal computed tomogram. (Courtesy of Robert Hendrickson, MD.)

Diagnosis

Eighty percent of patients with stones have microscopic hematuria.[2] A lesser percentage have pyuria without bacturia due to ureteral inflammation.[1] Radiographic examination of the kidneys, ureter, and bladder (KUB) was traditionally used to screen for disease, but the sensitivity is low (45% to 60%).[3] Helical computed tomography (CT) has become the mainstay of diagnosis, with a sensitivity greater than 95% and a specificity of 92% to 100%.[3] Perinephric stranding, hydronephrosis, and an enlargement of the affected kidney are all common CT findings of stone disease.[3] Intravenous pyelography (IVP) is a more time-consuming study and has a lower sensitivity (64% to 87%).[2] Ultrasonography may detect hydronephrosis, but is only 19% sensitive for the detection of ureteral stones.[2]

Clinical Complications

Complications include sepsis, acute renal failure (ARF) secondary to bilateral obstruction, severe dehydration secondary to vomiting, and intractable pain.

Management

Initial management requires adequate analgesia. Randomized, prospective studies have shown equal efficacy of nonsteroidal antiinflammatory drugs (NSAIDs) and morphine.[1] NSAIDs may impair renal blood flow in patients with renal insufficiency, so narcotic analgesia is preferred for these patients. Ureteral stones greater than 10 mm usually require urologic intervention. Definitive treatment of stones includes extracorporeal shock-wave lithotripsy, ureteroscopic removal, or percutaneous nephrolithotomy. Ureteroscopy may require postoperative stenting, and this procedure may be complicated by stricture formation. Percutaneous nephrolithotomy usually is reserved for ureteral stones larger than 1 cm and renal stones larger than 2 cm.[1]

REFERENCES

1. Portis AJ, Sundaram CP. Diagnosis and initial management of kidney stones. *Am Fam Physician* 2001;63:1329–1338.
2. Shokeir AA. Renal colic: new concepts related to pathophysiology, diagnosis and treatment. *Curr Opin Urol* 2002;12:263–269.
3. Colistro R, Torreggiani WC, Lyburn ID. Unenhanced helical CT in the investigation of acute flank pain. *Clin Radiol* 2002;57:435–441.

Acute Urinary Retention

Mark Silverberg

Clinical Presentation

The patient population most commonly found to be in urinary retention consists of older men.[1] Even if complete obstruction causing retention is not present, impending obstruction may be preceded by such symptoms as urinary hesitancy, decreased force of flow or dribbling at the end of voiding, and overflow incontinence. The patient's urinary history is useful in differentiating infectious, drug-related, and obstructive causes of urinary retention. Dysuria, hematuria, and urgency with fever or chills point to an infectious origin. On physical examination, the patient may have a painful, distended bladder or suprapubic mass. Rectal examination can reveal a large, smooth prostate in the setting of benign prostate hypertrophy (BPH) or a firm, nodular prostate, signifying possible prostate cancer as a cause of urethral or bladder outlet impingement.

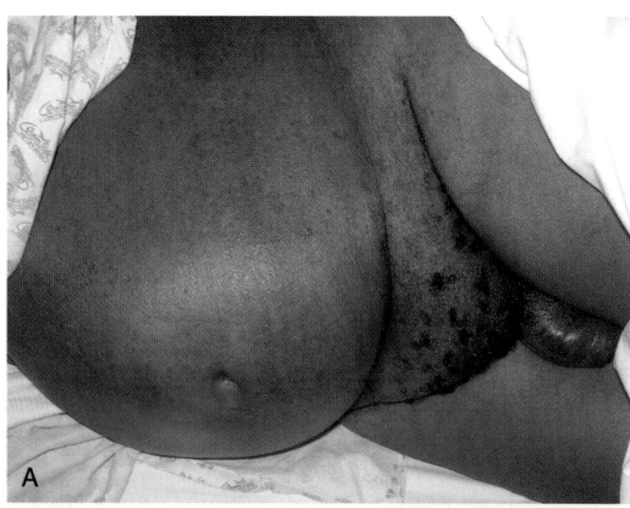

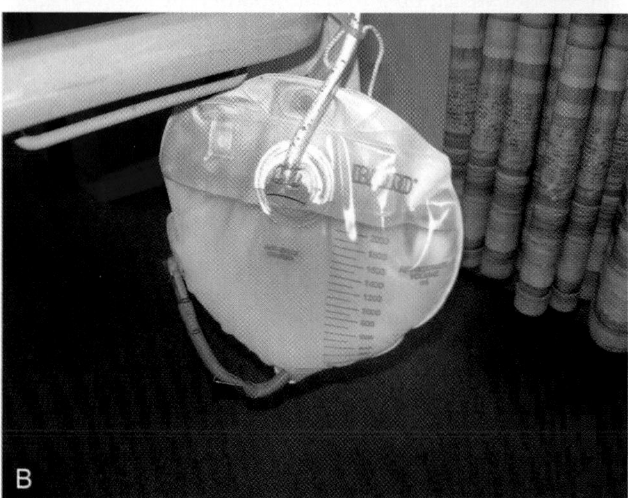

FIGURE 10–23 This patient with urinary retention **(A)** drained more than 2,000 mL of urine after a Foley catheter was inserted **(B)**. (Courtesy of Mark Silverberg, MD.)

Pathophysiology

BPH is the most common cause of urinary retention in men, whereas multiple sclerosis and diabetes are the most common causes among women.[2] Other obstructive causes include prostate cancer, urethral strictures, and bladder calculi or masses. Urethral obstruction may be caused by paraphimosis, phimosis, or sclerotic meatal stenosis. Infectious causes include prostatitis, cystitis, and herpes simplex virus (HSV) infection. Trauma to the genitourinary tract or strangulation of the penis (such as with a hair tourniquet) can also cause acute urinary retention. In men, the most common site of trauma is the membranous urethra (straddle injuries).[1] Anticholinergic medications cause retention by inhibiting detrusor muscle contraction, whereas sympathomimetics cause sphincter contraction. Many other pharmacologic agents have been implicated in retention, including monoamine oxidase inhibitors, calcium-channel blockers, and a host of other antihypertensive medications.[1] Upper motor neuron lesions can cause retention through dysfunction of the sacral micturition center, and lower motor neuron lesions often lead to bladder flaccidity. Disk herniation can manifest in this manner, with retention caused by lower motor neuron dysfunction. In women, urinary retention is the presenting symptom of multiple sclerosis in 10% of patients afflicted with this disease, and it is caused by local demyelination of micturition reflex neurons.[1] Diabetic neuropathy has also been found to cause acute urinary retention. Compressive pelvic masses, including fibroids, fecal impaction, abdominal aortic aneurysms, and a retroverted gravid uterus, are some of the less commonly described causes of urinary retention.[1]

Diagnosis

The cornerstone of diagnosis and treatment of urinary retention is bladder catheterization. A postvoid residual volume greater than 100 to 150 mL is considered diagnostic of obstruction. Urinalysis and culture should be obtained to diagnose infection, if suspected. Ultrasonography can be used to determine bladder volume, but it is unreliable. The gold standard of diagnosis remains urinary catheterization.

Clinical Complications

Complications of urinary retention include infection, postobstructive diuresis, hemorrhage, and autonomic dysreflexia. Ascending infection occurs in about 10% of patients with in-dwelling catheters.[3] If postobstructive diuresis develops after catheterization and urine output is greater than 200 mL/hour for 4 hours, then the patient should be admitted for observation and electrolyte monitoring. There has been no evidence to date to show that

Acute Urinary Retention

Mark Silverberg

gradual bladder decompression prevents this complication. Autonomic dysreflexia due to urinary retention can cause hypertension, vasoconstriction, and tachycardia in patients with spinal cord lesions above the T6 level.

Management

A 14F to 18F Foley catheter should be passed into the bladder as the first approach to relieve urinary retention. Suprapubic bladder drainage may be necessary in the setting of urethral trauma, or if transurethral catheterization cannot be performed. A spinal needle is inserted in the midline 2 cm above the pubic symphysis and aimed posteriorly, 30 degrees cephalad.[4] After aspiration of urine, a catheter is introduced using the Seldinger technique. Patients with chronic obstructive voiding symptoms should be observed, with intake and output monitored, for 4 to 6 hours for signs of postobstructive diuresis. α-Adrenergic blockade using prazosin three times a day or doxazosin each day has been shown to increase successful voiding after catheter removal.[1] Other medications used for this purpose, as well as to relieve bladder spasm, include baclofen, oxybutynin, bethanechol, dantrolene, and diazepam.[3] These medications act on the external sphincter or on the detrusor muscle. Prophylactic antibiotic use in catheterized patients is controversial, because patients usually develop asymptomatic bacterial infections and antibiotic use may lead to further bacterial resistance.[1–3]

REFERENCES

1. Curtis LA, Dolan TS, Cespedes RD. Acute urinary retention and urinary incontinence. *Emerg Clin North Am* 2001;19:591–619.
2. McConnell JD, Bruskewitz R, et al. The effect of finasteride on the risk of acute urinary retention and the need for surgical treatment among men with benign prostatic hyperplasia. *N Engl J Med* 1998;338:557–563.
3. Cravens DD, Zweig S. Urinary catheter management. *Am Fam Physician* 2000;61:369–376.

Acute Renal Failure

Colleen Campbell

Clinical Presentation

The cause of acute renal failure (ARF) may involve prerenal, postrenal (obstructive), or intrinsic causes. Patients with a prerenal cause have symptoms of volume depletion. Intrinsic failure can be asymptomatic. Patients with postrenal failure may complain of abdominal pain, inability to urinate, or incomplete voiding.

Pathophysiology

Prerenal causes account for 70% of cases of ARF, intrinsic renal failure for 11%, and postrenal or obstructive causes for 17%.[1] Prerenal failure results from hypoperfusion of the kidney. Angiotensin-converting enzyme (ACE) inhibitors and nonsteroidal antiinflammatory drugs (NSAIDs) have also been found to cause decreased renal perfusion.[2] Intrinsic renal failure results from tubular damage and necrosis within the kidney parenchyma and may be caused by surgery, sepsis, toxicants (including nephrotoxic medications), renal artery or vein thrombosis, or vasculitic syndromes such as hemolytic uremic syndrome or thrombotic thrombocytopenia purpura. Other causes of intrinsic renal failure include myoglobinuria and hemoglobinuria, glomerulonephritis, and interstitial nephritis. In postrenal or obstructive failure, the renal tubules or pelvis may be blocked.

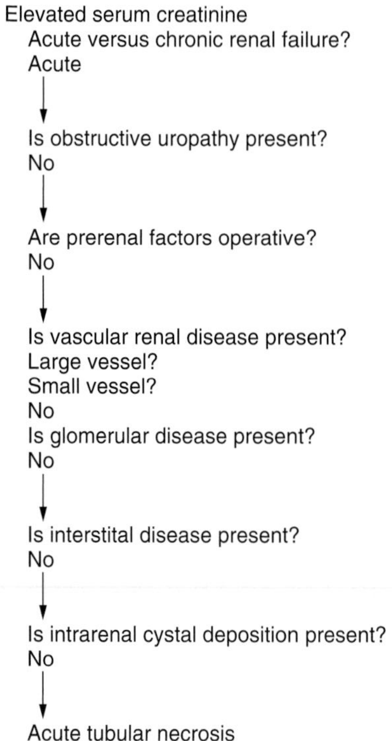

FIGURE 10–24 Schema for determining the cause of acute renal failure. (Modified with permission from Massry SG, Glassock RJ. *Textbook of nephrology,* 2nd ed. Baltimore: Williams & Wilkins, 1989.)

Diagnosis

See Table 10–24. The physical examination is generally unrevealing except in obstructive ARF, but it may be significant for new-onset hypertension. The bladder may be palpable or tender (or both) on abdominal examination if the patient is experiencing urinary retention. Decreased volume status may be discerned by evaluating skin turgor or finding flattened neck veins. If the baseline weight of the patient is known, the current weight may also provide useful information concerning hydration status. Laboratory values such as blood urea nitrogen (BUN), creatinine, and electrolyte levels are most important in determining ARF and its underlying cause. An increased creatinine level suggests ARF. If the ratio of BUN to creatinine is greater than 20:1, prerenal causes are the more likely culprit. Urine electrolyte measurements help differentiate prerenal from intrinsic causes, as do the urinalysis and urine osmolality. A highly concentrated urine with a specific gravity greater than 1.020 and hyaline casts suggest prerenal causes, as does a urine osmolality of greater than 500 mM. Intrinsic causes of renal failure are more likely to show a specific gravity of about 1.010, a serum osmolality of approximately 300 mM, and brown, granular casts. Urine may show muddy-brown casts in acute tubular necrosis or white blood cell (WBC) casts with interstitial nephritis. Red blood cell (RBC) casts are significant for glomerulonephritis. Hyaline casts are characteristic of prerenal ARF. Urine dipstick findings positive for blood may reveal myoglobinuria or hemoglobinuria if no RBCs are seen in the urinalysis. Calcium oxalate crystals may be found in nephrolithiasis. Renal ultrasonography may be performed to elucidate obstructive causes and kidney size.[1-3]

TABLE 10–24 Indications for Dialytic Therapy of Acute Renal Failure

Fluid overload (pulmonary edema)
Hyperkalemia (serum potassium >6.5 mEq/L)
Metabolic acidosis (pH >7.15)
Symptomatic severe hyponatremia (serum sodium >120 mEq/L)
Pericarditis
Encephalopathy (confusion, myoclonic jerks, seizures, coma)
Symptomatic uremia
Hypercatabolic state I (as assessed from clinical conditions, an increase in blood urea nitrogen >30 mg/dL per day or an increase in serum creatinine >2.0 mg/dL per day; an example of this condition is acute renal failure secondary to rhabdomyolysis)
Toxin removal (intoxication with ethylene glycol, salicylate, etc.)
Severe uremic bleeding

Modified with permission from Massry SG, Glassock RJ. *Textbook of nephrology,* 2nd ed. Baltimore: Williams & Wilkins, 1989.

Acute Renal Failure

Colleen Campbell

Clinical Complications

Complications of ARF include hyperkalemia, hypernatremia, metabolic acidosis, hyperphosphatemia, hypocalcemia, and hypermagnesemia. ARF can lead to uremic syndrome, which manifests as nausea, mental status changes, anemia, and bleeding, and can also cause pericarditis or pleuritis. The mortality rate of ARF is between 20% and 80%.[1] Among patients who survive to hospital discharge, 5% to 30% require long-term dialysis.[1]

Management

Treatment of prerenal failure requires restoration of renal perfusion. Intrinsic failure may be supported with dialysis. Prophylactic dialysis has not been shown to be beneficial in preventing complications or mortality related to ARF.[2] Loop diuretics have been advocated, based on theoretical advantages, but have failed to show clinical benefit in studies to date.[3] Dopamine has been advocated in low doses, as has atrial natriuretic peptide, because they cause dilation of the afferent arterioles.

REFERENCES

1. Brady HR, Singer GG. Acute renal failure. *Lancet* 1995;346:1533–1540.
2. Teschan PE, Baxter CR, O'Brien TF, Freyhof JN, Hall WH. Prophylactic hemodialysis in the treatment of acute renal failure. *J Am Soc Nephrol* 1998;9:2384–2397.
3. Mindell JA, Chertow GM: A practical approach to acute renal failure. *Med Clin North Am* 1997;81:731–748.

Chronic Renal Failure

Colleen Campbell

Clinical Presentation

Patients with chronic renal failure (CRF) may present with weakness, fatigue, decreased urine concentration, and poor appetite. Inability to concentrate urine occurs early in the disease; volume overload manifests later. Patients may present late with complaints including shortness of breath or chest pain resulting from pleural or pericardial effusions or volume overload.[1-4]

Pathophysiology

The most common causes of CRF are glomerular, including diabetic nephropathy and hypertensive nephrosclerosis, especially among African-Americans.[1] Reflux nephropathy is the most common cause in children.[1]

Diagnosis

Creatinine remains normal until the glomerular filtration rate (GFR) is reduced by 60% to 75%.[4] CRF is considered to be present whenever the creatinine concentration is greater than 1.5 mg/dL in a female patient or 2 mg/dL in a male.[4]

If the patient is still producing urine, the urinalysis shows broad, waxy casts, as opposed to the red blood cell (RBC) casts seen in acute renal failure (ARF).[1] An electrocardiogram should be obtained for all patients to screen for asymptomatic hyperkalemia. Ultrasonography most often shows bilateral renal atrophy in a patient with CRF. The skin may have a yellow tinge, known as "uremic frost," and may be pruritic due to local calcium deposition.[1]

Clinical Complications

Uremia and volume overload can lead to pericarditis, congestive heart failure, and pleural effusions.[1] Anemia is universal as the production of erythropoietin is decreased. The incidence of cardiovascular death is greatly increased in CRF patients because of accelerated coronary artery disease and an increased incidence of cardiac arrest.[1] Infection is the second leading cause of death; it is related to impaired humeral and cellular immunity, as well as increased exposure to blood-borne bacteria during dialysis.[1]

Management

The National Institutes of Health recommend that women with creatinine values greater than 1.5 or men with values greater than 2.0 be referred to a nephrologist.[4] Hyperkalemia must be aggressively treated. Indications for emergency dialysis include pulmonary edema, uncontrolled hypertension, hyperkalemia, severe refractory acidosis, hypermagnesemia or hyperphosphatemia, and pericarditis.[1]

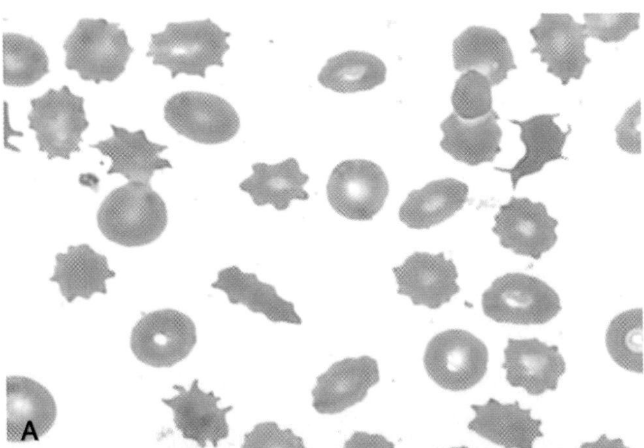

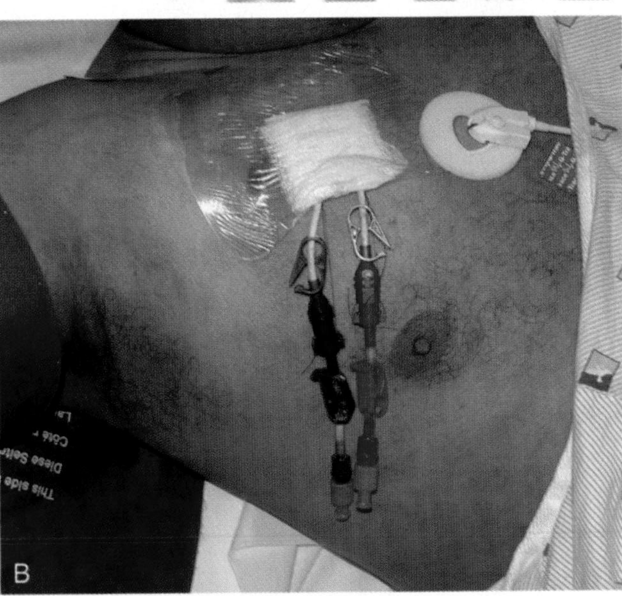

FIGURE 10-25 **A:** Peripheral blood smear showing burr cells characteristic of chronic renal failure. (From Anderson, with permission.) **B:** A Hickman catheter can be used for hemodialysis in patients with chronic renal failure. (Courtesy of Mark Silverberg, MD.)

REFERENCES

1. Dember LM. Critical care issues in the patient with chronic renal failure. *Crit Care Clin* 2002;18:421–440.
2. Mermel LA, Farr BM, Sherertz RJ, et al. Guidelines for the management of intravascular catheter-related infections. *Clin Infect Dis* 2001;32:1249–1272.
3. Eberst ME, Berkowitz LR. Hemostasis in renal disease: pathophysiology and management. *Am J Med* 1994;96:168–179.
4. Ifudu O, Dawood M, Iofel Y, Valcourt JS, Friedman EA. Delayed referral of black, Hispanic, and older patients with chronic renal failure. *Am J Kidney Dis* 1999;33:728–733.

Nephrotic Syndrome

Colleen Campbell

Clinical Presentation

Children with nephrotic syndrome (NS) present to the emergency department (ED) after parents notice increased abdominal girth or facial swelling.[1] Adults often present with hypertension with or without acute renal failure (ARF).

Pathophysiology

NS is a glomerular disorder characterized by proteinuria, hypoalbuminemia, edema, and hyperlipidemia. The peak age at onset in children is 2 to 3 years. Minimal change disease is the most common microscopic finding in children with nephrotic syndrome, whereas focal segmental glomerulosclerosis (FSGS) is common in adults.[1] Edema occurs when the albumin level drops to lower than 2.0 g/dL. Hypocalcemia commonly accompanies the hypoproteinemia but is rarely clinically evident.[2] Adults usually have a more progressive disease course (especially with FSGS) despite therapeutic measures and often progress to renal failure. This is especially true in the elderly.[3]

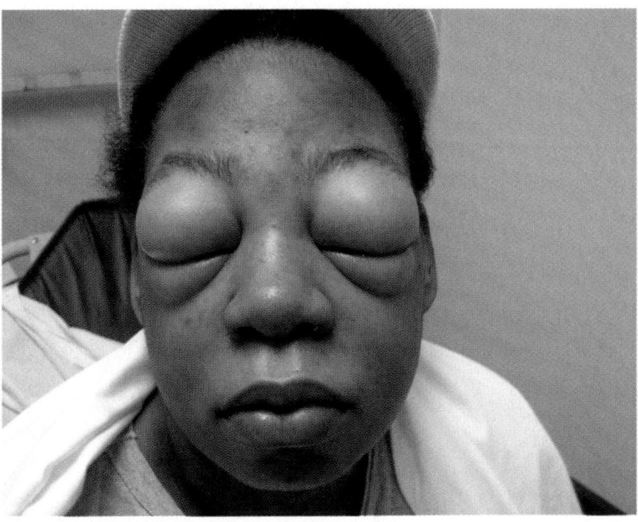

FIGURE 10–26 Severe eyelid edema in a patient with nephrotic syndrome. (Courtesy of Mark Silverberg, MD.)

Diagnosis

Diagnosis is based on the history and physical examination in conjunction with laboratory studies. Laboratory studies indicated include a complete blood count (CBC), chemistry panel, and urine protein and creatinine determinations. If the ratio of urine protein to creatinine is greater than 2, the patient is considered to have NS.[1] Pediatric patients who lose protein at a rate greater than or equal to 50 mg/kg in 24 hours are also considered to have NS.[2] Hypercholesterolemia greater than 200 mg/dL may be a clue to the diagnosis.[2]

Clinical Complications

Acute NS is associated with substantial mortality, probably secondary to sepsis, thromboembolic disease, atherosclerosis, and renal failure. Relapse is common (36% at 1 year), even with a long initial course of steroid therapy.[1] Other complications include testicular torsion (TT) secondary to scrotal edema and growth arrest in children.[1,2]

Management

Treatment of NS involves daily corticosteroid use, alkylating agents, and cyclosporine. Most patients respond within 3 weeks after initiation of steroid therapy. Patients who require high steroid doses may also need prolonged treatment with an alkylating agent such as chlorambucil or cyclophosphamide.[1] Cyclosporine is associated with a higher rate of renal toxicity in adults and a high rate of relapse on discontinuation.[1] Angiotensin-converting enzyme (ACE) inhibitors provide useful treatment of hypertension associated with NS, and daily aspirin is used to prevent thromboembolism.[2]

REFERENCES

1. Tune BM, Mendoza SA. Treatment of the idiopathic nephrotic syndrome: regimens and outcomes in children and adults. *J Am Soc Nephrol* 1997;8:824–832.
2. Roth KS, Amaker BH, Chan JC. Nephrotic syndrome: pathogenesis and management. *Pediatr Rev* 2002;23:237–248.
3. Dumoulin A, Hill GS, Montseny JJ, Meyrier A. Clinical and morphological prognostic factors in membranous nephropathy: significance of focal segmental glomerulosclerosis. *Am J Kidney Dis* 2003;41:38–48.

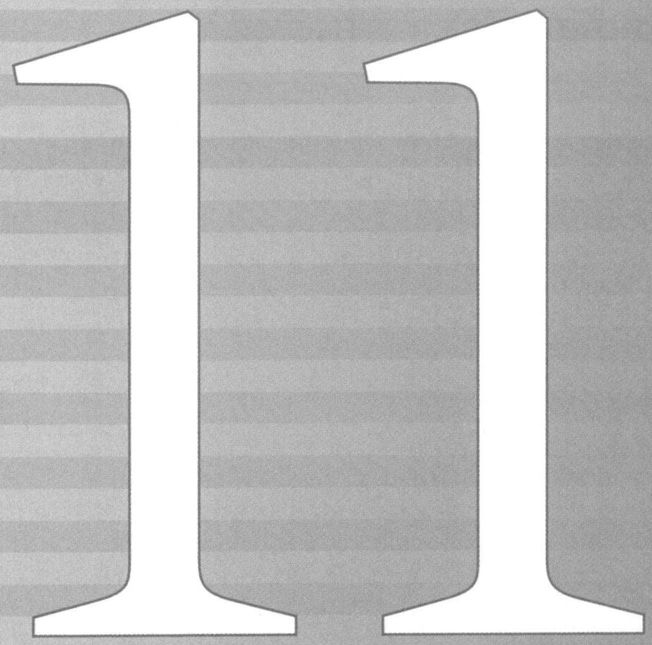

Gynecologic

Bartholin Gland Abscess

Anthony Morocco

Clinical Presentation

A Bartholin gland cyst manifests as a painless mass (1 to 3 cm) in the labia. Abscesses are larger (up to 8 cm or more), are more painful, and develop over 2 to 4 days. Patients complain of severe vulvar pain, dyspareunia, and difficulty sitting or walking. The abscess may spontaneously rupture and drain after several days.[1]

Pathophysiology

The Bartholin glands are paired structures located in the labia minora. Cysts or abscesses of these glands occur in 2% of women.[1] The glands are normally pea-sized and located at the 4- and 8-o'clock positions. They drain through ducts that exit between the hymenal ring and the labium. A Bartholin gland cyst results when the duct is blocked. An abscess occurs due to infection of a cyst.[1] The organisms most commonly found in these abscesses are *Bacteroides fragilis* and *Peptostreptococcus* spp. *Neisseria gonorrhoeae* is found in 10% to 15% of cases.[2]

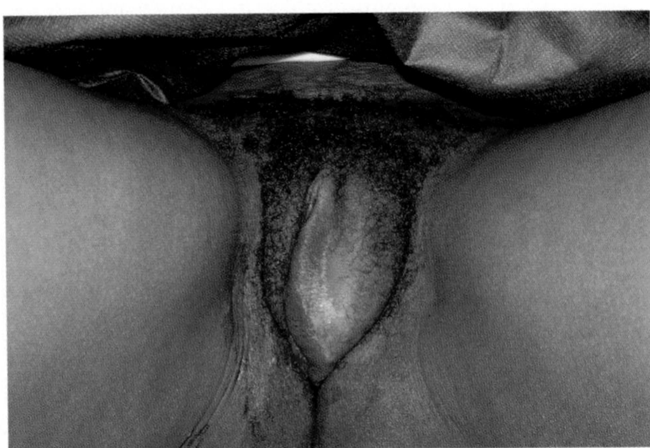

FIGURE 11–1 Left-sided Bartholin gland abscess. (Courtesy of Mark Silverberg, MD.)

Diagnosis

Differential diagnosis includes several types of cyst (e.g., sebaceous), hematoma, carcinoma, fibroma, lipoma, endometriosis, and inguinal hernia.[1]

Clinical Complications

Potential complications of the abscess or drainage procedure include dyspareunia, excessive bleeding, cellulitis, and sepsis.[1]

Management

In patients younger than 40 years of age, asymptomatic Bartholin gland cysts require only treatment for discomfort or cosmesis. Older patients should have the cyst removed and tested to rule out carcinoma. Ruptured cysts and abscesses should be treated with sitz baths. Early abscesses may also benefit from sitz baths, because drainage may be more successful if it is delayed until the abscess is "pointing." Simple lancing or needle aspiration of a cyst or abscess commonly results in recurrence of the lesion.[1] Appropriate emergency treatment involves drainage and placement of a drainage catheter. After local anesthesia, an incision is made into the abscess through the mucosal side (inside the labium). After the pus has been drained and any loculations broken up, the catheter is placed in the abscess cavity and its balloon is filled with water. The catheter should remain in place for 4 to 6 weeks to allow formation of a permanent fistula. The patient should be tested for gonorrhea and chlamydia.[2] Definitive treatment of recurrent Bartholin cyst or abscess by a gynecologist includes marsupialization, laser excision, or surgical excision.[1]

REFERENCES

1. Hill DA, Lense JJ. Office management of Bartholin gland cysts and abscesses. *Am Fam Physician* 1998;57:1611–1616, 1619–1620.
2. Zeger W, Holt K. Gynecologic infections. *Emerg Med Clin North Am* 2003;21:631–648.

Bacterial Vaginosis

Anthony Morocco

Clinical Presentation

Patients with bacterial vaginosis (BV) present with a thin, milky, malodorous, and homogeneous vaginal discharge. However, up to 50% of affected women are asymptomatic.[1,2]

Pathophysiology

BV is a common form of infectious vaginitis, with an incidence of 10% to 40%.[1] Despite its common occurrence, the precise cause remains unclear. The importance of sexual transmission is unknown, but BV is associated with multiple sex partners and frequent douching.[2] BV is most likely a polymicrobial anaerobic infection, with concurrent inhibition of the *Lactobacillus* organisms that normally inhabit the vagina. *Gardnerella vaginalis,* a gram-negative rod, plays a prominent role in BV, along with other anaerobes such as *Bacteroides, Peptococcus, Prevotella,* and *Mycoplasma hominis.*[2,3] *G. vaginalis* may also be part of the normal vaginal flora; men may harbor the organism in the urethra, but they do not develop symptoms.[3]

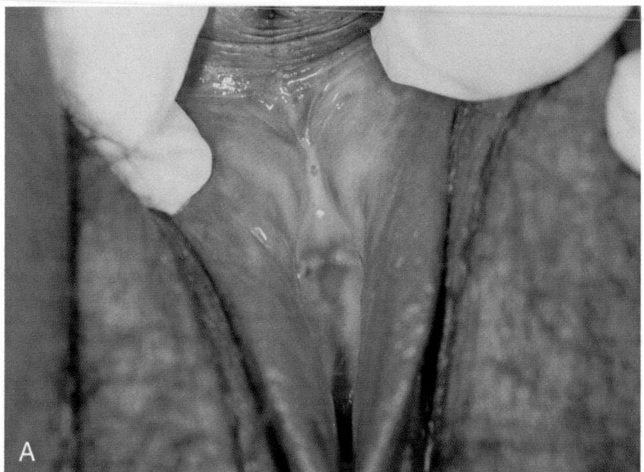

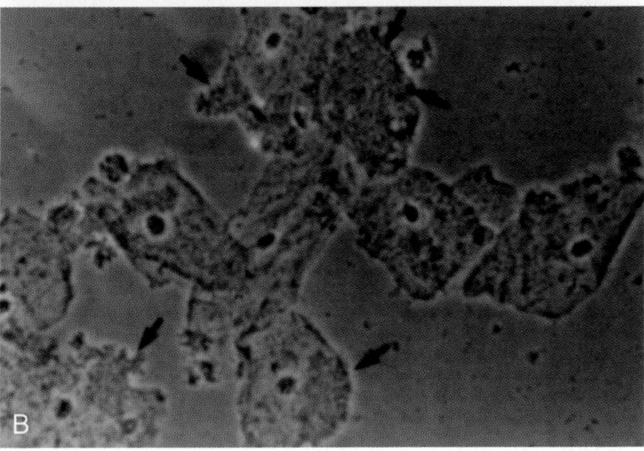

FIGURE 11–2 **A:** Thin, grey discharge, consistent with bacterial vaginosis. (From Sweet and Gibbs, with permission.) **B:** Bacteria lining endothelial cells (clue cells). (From Mandell, with permission.)

Diagnosis

The diagnosis is based on identification of three of the following four clinical criteria on examination of vaginal fluid: presence of clue cells (desquamated epithelial cells with adherent bacteria); pH greater than 4.5; positive "whiff test" (presence of amine odor with potassium hydroxide); and a thin, adherent vaginal discharge. Gram staining, DNA probes, and other commercial assays may assist in diagnosis.[1] Differential diagnosis includes infections such as *Trichomonas, Candida,* and *Chlamydia* and the presence of a vaginal foreign body.[3]

Clinical Complications

Complications occur primarily in pregnant patients and include postpartum endometritis, miscarriage, and preterm labor. BV can also lead to cervicitis and pelvic inflammatory disease, as well as postoperative infections after gynecologic procedures (e.g., hysterectomy, uterine curettage).[1,2]

Management

All symptomatic patients should be treated, as should asymptomatic pregnant patients.[2] Recommended antibiotic regimens for nonpregnant women include oral metronidazole 500 mg or intravaginal metronidazole gel. Less efficacious regimens include oral or intravaginal clindamycin and single-dose metronidazole therapy. Pregnant women should be treated with metronidazole or clindamycin. Treatment during pregnancy reduces the risk of obstetric complications.[1–3] Treatment of sex partners is not recommended.[2] Clinicians should consult current recommendations from the Centers for Disease Control and Prevention for doses and applicable duration of therapy.

REFERENCES

1. Zeger W, Holt K. Gynecologic infections. *Emerg Med Clin North Am* 2003;21:631–648.
2. Workowski KA, Levine WC. Sexually transmitted diseases treatment guidelines—2002. *MMWR Morb Mortal Wkly Rep* 2002;51(RR-6):1–80.
3. Fiumara NJ. Genital ulcer infections in the female patient and the vaginitides. *Dermatol Clin* 1997;15:233–245.

Vulvovaginal Candidiasis

Anthony Morocco

Clinical Presentation

Patients with vulvovaginal candidiasis (VVC) present with pruritus; a white, curd-like vaginal discharge; erythema of the vulva; vaginal pain; dyspareunia; and dysuria.[1]

Pathophysiology

VVC, also called monilial vaginitis, is a common infection of the female genital tract, affecting 75% of women at least once. Recurrent VVC is defined as four or more episodes per year.[1] VVC is most commonly caused by *Candida albicans*. Recurrent VVC is more likely to be caused by *Candida glabrata* or other non-*albicans* species (10% to 20% of cases).[1] Risk factors for infection include antibiotic use, pregnancy, immunocompromised state, diabetes, corticosteroids, and higher-dose estrogen-containing oral contraceptives.[2]

Diagnosis

Yeasts and pseudohyphae may be visualized on a saline preparation of vaginal fluid with 10% potassium hydroxide (KOH) added. *Candida* can also be cultured from vaginal fluid; however, this organism is part of the normal vaginal flora in 10% to 20% of women who are asymptomatic.[1]

Clinical Complications

Patients with severe infections may develop extensive areas of erythema, edema, excoriation, satellite lesions, and formation of fissures.[1]

Management

The topical azoles (e.g., clotrimazole, miconazole), used intravaginally, are 80% to 90% effective in relieving symptoms and eradicating the pathogen. Oral fluconazole is also effective. Longer courses of treatment may be needed for recurrent VVC, non-*albicans* infections, and severe cases. Recurrent VVC may also require long-term suppressive maintenance therapy. Treatment of sex partners is not generally recommended except in cases of recurrent infection or balanitis.[1]

REFERENCES

1. Workowski KA, Levine WC. Sexually transmitted diseases treatment guidelines—2002. *MMWR Morb Mortal Wkly Rep* 2002;51(RR-6):1–80.
2. Sobel JD, Faro S, Froce RW, et al. Vulvovaginal candidiasis: epidemiologic, diagnostic, and therapeutic considerations. *Am J Obstet Gynecol* 1998;178:203–211.

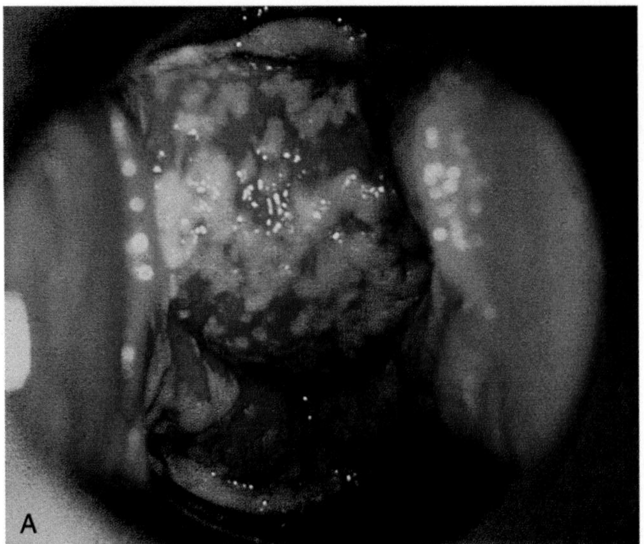

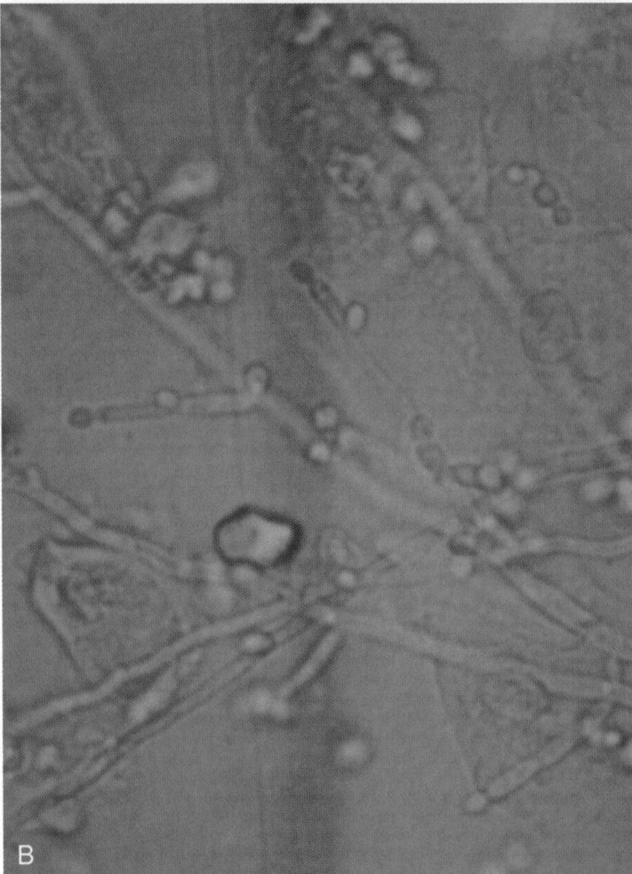

FIGURE 11–3 **A:** "Cheesy" white discharge consistent with candidal vaginitis. (From Sweet and Gibbs, with permission.) **B:** Hyphae as seen on wet mount preparation. (From Mandell, with permission.)

Uterine Prolapse

Anthony Morocco

Clinical Presentation

Patients with uterine prolapse may present with complaints of pelvic pressure, low back pain, dyspareunia, or a mass in the vagina. Symptoms and degree of prolapse worsen with increases in intraabdominal pressure.[1]

Pathophysiology

Prolapse of pelvic organs is caused by a weakening of the pelvic floor that normally supports these structures. The pelvic floor is made up of muscles (levator ani group and coccygeus) and endopelvic fascia. In addition, uterine prolapse results after weakening of the sacrouterine and cardinal ligaments. This may result from the trauma of childbirth or hysterectomy. Other potential causes include other trauma or surgical injury, chronic coughing, heavy labor, congenital abnormalities, and hormone-related tissue atrophy. Additional risk factors for uterine prolapse include asthma, chronic obstructive pulmonary disease, uterine or ovarian tumors, ascites, obesity, and spina bifida.[1]

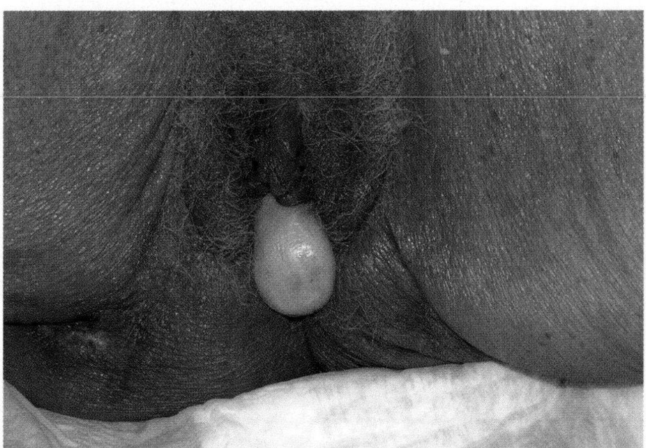

FIGURE 11–4 Grade IV uterine prolapse. (Courtesy of Mark Silverberg, MD.)

Diagnosis

Uterine prolapse extending outside the vagina is easily visible on gross inspection of the perineum. Pelvic examination allows assessment of the extent of prolapse within the vaginal vault. The degree of prolapse may be graded from I (mild) to IV (protrusion beyond the introitus).[1]

Clinical Complications

Cervical tissue may become macerated and bleed if it protrudes beyond the vaginal introitus for extended periods. Ischemic injuries do not occur.[1] Prolapse of other pelvic organs may also occur, resulting in cystocele, cystourethrocele, rectocele, ureterocele, urethral prolapse, or vaginal vault prolapse.[1]

Management

Patients should be referred to a gynecologist for possible surgical intervention. A vaginal pessary may be used for elderly patients and those with severe symptoms.[1]

REFERENCES

1. Harrison BP, Cespedes RD. Pelvic organ prolapse. *Emerg Med Clin North Am* 2001;19:781–797.

Ovarian Cysts and Masses

Jennifer Hendrickson

Clinical Presentation

Patients with ovarian cysts or masses usually present with lower abdominal pain. Unruptured cysts usually cause more chronic pelvic pain, pressure, or dyspareunia. Irregular menses may also occur. Cyst rupture is suspected with a history of acute onset of sharp pain and peritoneal signs.[1] Increasing abdominal girth, shortness of breath, or nausea and vomiting should raise suspicion of an ovarian malignancy.

Pathophysiology

Most ovarian cysts are the result of a normal follicle that either fails to rupture (follicular cyst) or fails to regress (corpus luteum cyst).[1] Numerous neoplastic processes can give rise to many types of ovarian tumors.

Diagnosis

Cysts may be suspected based on history and pelvic examination and confirmed with ultrasonography.[1] Transvaginal ultrasonography usually reveals characteristics of ovarian cysts that can raise or lower the suspicion of malignancy. For a woman of reproductive age, cyst size greater than 18 cm^3, presence of papillary excrescences, multiple loculations, or a mixed solid/cystic structure raise the concern for malignancy and require further gynecologic investigation.[2]

Clinical Complications

Ovarian cysts may undergo torsion, which is a surgical emergency. Cyst rupture can result in symptoms of acute abdomen, requiring surgical intervention. Certain cysts (teratomas, endometriomas) can cause dense pelvic adhesions and chronic pelvic pain with rupture. Ovarian malignancies are generally associated with high mortality rates.[2]

Management

If ectopic pregnancy, adnexal torsion, and tubo-ovarian abscess have been ruled out and the patient's pain has been controlled, outpatient follow-up with a gynecologist is appropriate. Pain may be controlled with nonsteroidal antiinflammatory drugs (NSAIDs) or opioids or both. Admission should be considered if there is a question of any emergency condition or if acute pain persists.[1,2]

REFERENCES

1. Lawrence LL. Unusual presentations in obstetrics and gynecology. *Emerg Med Clin North Am* 2003;21:649–665.
2. Crvenkovic G, Karlan BY, Platt LD. Current role of ultrasound in ovarian cancer screening. *Clin Obstet Gynecol* 1996;39:259–267.

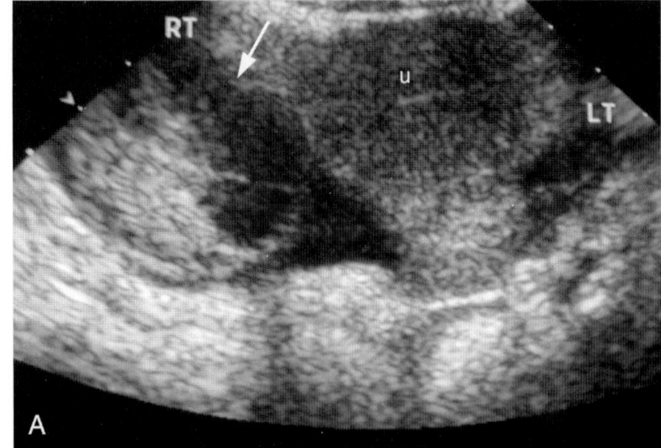

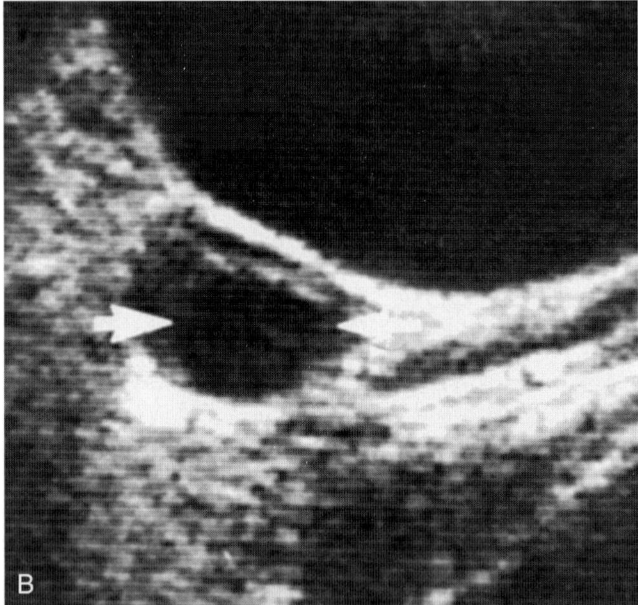

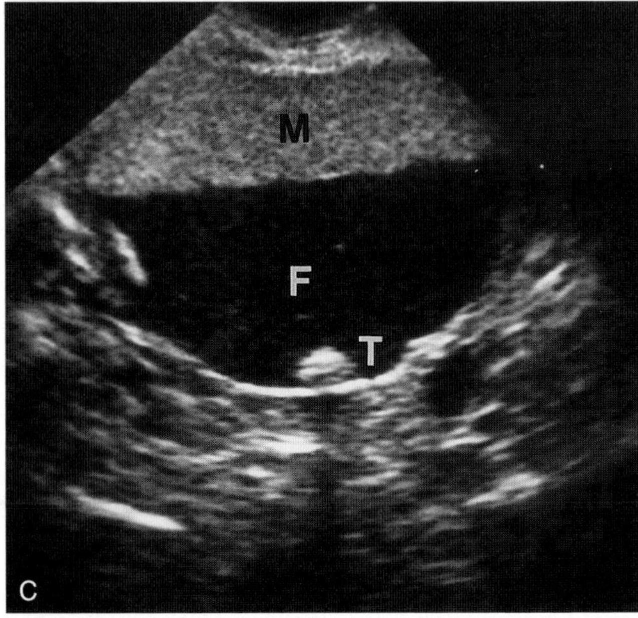

FIGURE 11–5 **A:** Complex right ovarian cyst. (Courtesy of Robert Hendrickson, MD.) **B:** Simple cystic structure consistent with a dominant follicle. (From Sauerbrei, with permission.) **C:** Teratoma. Note solid matter (M) with fluid (F) and tooth (T). (From Sauerbrei, with permission.)

Ovarian Torsion

Anthony Morocco

Clinical Presentation

Patients with ovarian torsion present with acute unilateral lower abdominal pain. Pain may be sharp, colicky, severe, and radiating to the back, flank, or groin. Nausea and vomiting also commonly occur (70% of patients). Physical examination reveals a tender abdomen and adnexal mass in 50% of affected patients. Thirty percent of patients in one series had no tenderness on pelvic examination.[1]

Pathophysiology

Ovarian torsion is an uncommon and frequently missed cause of lower abdominal pain in women. The term *adnexal torsion* is often used, because other structures (e.g., fallopian tubes) can also be affected. The average age at diagnosis is the late twenties, and 15% to 20% of cases occur in pregnant patients.[1] Enlargement of the ovary and prior pelvic surgery are risk factors for torsion. Ovarian enlargement may be caused by cysts, benign tumors, or malignancies. It is speculated that the ovary may enlarge asymmetrically, allowing twisting around the pedicle. Adnexal structures may also twist around postsurgical adhesions or other structural abnormalities.[1]

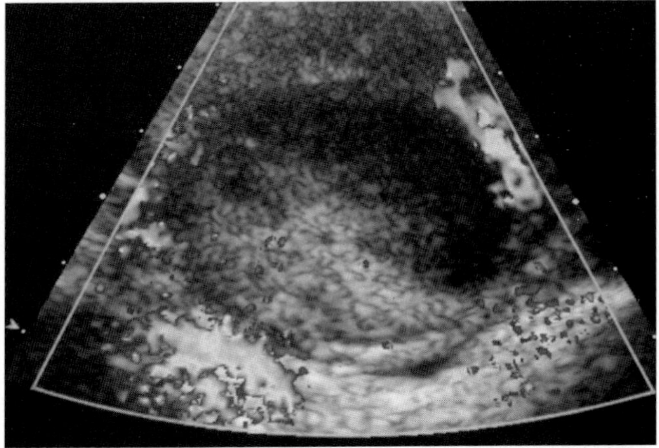

FIGURE 11-6 Ultrasound showing absence of blood flow to the ovary. (Courtesy of Robert Hendrickson, MD.)

Diagnosis

Diagnosis is difficult and is often missed in the emergency department (ED). The symptoms mimic those of other conditions, such as renal colic and ruptured ovarian cyst. These entities and others (e.g., appendicitis, ectopic pregnancy) should be ruled out. Ultrasonography with Doppler imaging should be used to assess the ovary for enlargement and blood flow, although its sensitivity for torsion is not 100%.[1]

Clinical Complications

Necrosis and loss of the ovary may occur. However, most women have no reduction of fertility with only one viable ovary.[1]

Management

Adnexal torsion requires prompt surgical intervention. Low ovarian salvage rates (10% or less) were previously reported, because ischemic-appearing ovaries are frequently removed. However, recent studies have shown that laparoscopic detorsion restores function in most cases, despite the poor appearance of the ovary.[1,2]

REFERENCES

1. Houry D, Abbott JT. Ovarian torsion: a fifteen-year review. *Ann Emerg Med* 2001;38:156–159.
2. Cohen SB, Wattiez A, Seidman DS, et al. Laparoscopic versus laparotomy for detorsion and sparing of the twisted ischemic adnexa. *JSLS* 2003;7:295–299.

Uterine Fibroids

Anthony Morocco

Clinical Presentation

Fibroids may result in abnormally heavy menstrual bleeding (menorrhagia), pelvic discomfort, or reproductive dysfunction. The pelvic discomfort includes pelvic pressure, acute or chronic pain, urinary difficulties, and constipation. On pelvic examination, an enlarged and irregular uterus may be palpated.[1]

Pathophysiology

Uterine fibroids, known as leiomyomas, are benign tumors that occur in as many as 77% of women. Clinically apparent fibroids occur in 25% of women (usually after 30 years of age), and they are the most common reason for hysterectomy. Black women are much more likely than white women to have fibroids.[1] The cause of fibroids is unclear, but they are both benign and hormone sensitive. Parity and oral contraceptive use decrease the likelihood of fibroids. Location of the tumor significantly affects the clinical symptoms; submucosal fibroids and those that intrude into the uterine cavity are more likely to cause menorrhagia. Most fibroid-related symptoms are caused by the size of the tumor, although the cause of menorrhagia is unclear.[1]

Diagnosis

Although an enlarged uterus can be detected on pelvic examination, diagnosis is confirmed by ultrasound imaging.

Clinical Complications

Anemia occurs with significant menstrual blood loss. A fibroid under the placenta increases the risk of abruption. Fibroids in the gravid uterus can result in premature labor.[1]

Management

No treatment is necessary unless symptoms occur. Pharmacologic treatment for fibroid-related bleeding usually begins with a trial of oral contraceptives or progestogen. The mainstays of pharmacologic therapy are the gonadotropin-releasing hormone (GnRH) agonists, which induce amenorrhea and decrease uterine size. These agents are generally used while awaiting surgery, because cessation of the drugs results in rapid reenlargement of the fibroids. Androgenic steroids such as danazol can decrease bleeding and uterine size. Hysterectomy may be performed to eliminate the fibroids and any chance of recurrence. Myomectomy involves removal of tumors with sparing of the uterus; it is commonly performed to preserve fertility. Small fibroids may be removed laparoscopically (or hysteroscopically if submucosal). The recurrence rate of fibroids detectable by ultrasonography is 50% at 5 years after myomectomy. Another procedure, myolysis, involves coagulation of the fibroid without removal. Endometrial ablation may be used for cases of menorrhagia. Uterine artery embolization is a possible alternative to surgery.[1]

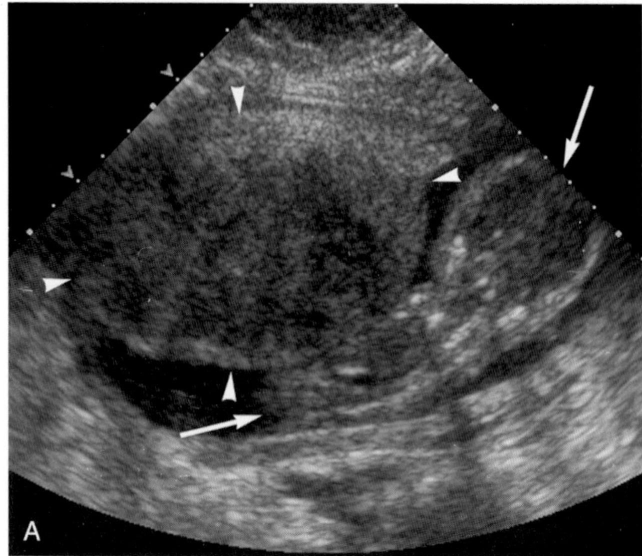

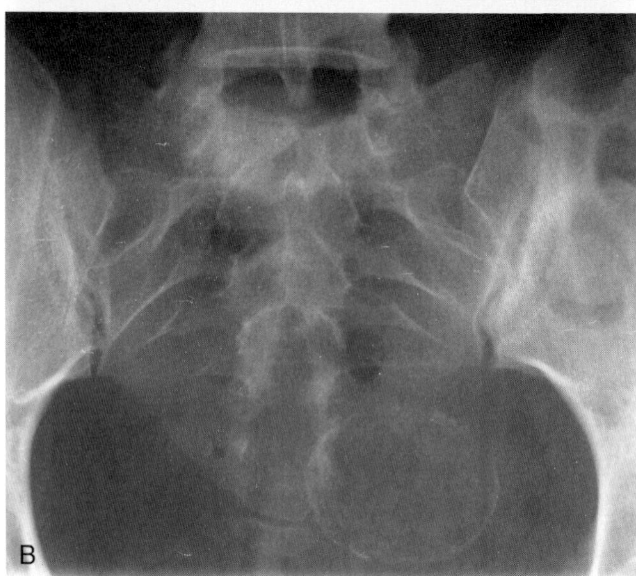

FIGURE 11–7 A: Uterine fibroid indenting the gestational sac. A large anterior fibroid *(arrowheads)* indents the gestational sac and presses against the fetus *(arrows)*. (From Doubilet and Benson, with permission.) **B:** Calcified fibroid visualized in the left lower pelvis. (Courtesy of Mark Silverberg, MD.)

REFERENCES

1. Stewart EA. Uterine fibroids. *Lancet* 2001;357:293–298.

Polycystic Ovary Syndrome

Anthony Morocco

Clinical Presentation

Patients may present for evaluation of one or more of the varied manifestations of polycystic ovary syndrome (PCOS). Seventy percent of affected women have irregular menstrual periods or amenorrhea. Seventy percent develop a male pattern of hirsutism, with hair growth on the upper lip, chin, periareolar area, chest, and other areas. Other abnormalities include upper body obesity, acne, and acanthosis nigricans.[1]

Pathophysiology

PCOS is an endocrine disorder that affects up to 6% of women of reproductive age.[1] The cause of PCOS is unclear. Patients exhibit insulin resistance and resulting hyperinsulinemia. Infertility results from a prolonged anovulatory state. Excess androgen production is responsible for the hirsutism.[1]

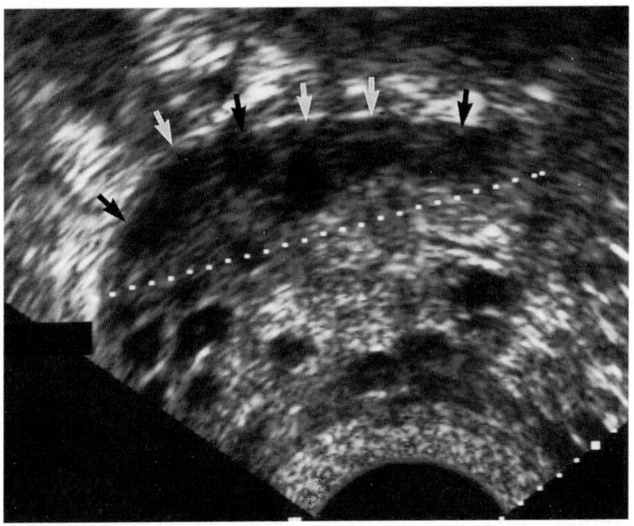

FIGURE 11–8 Transvaginal ultrasound scan showing multiple tiny follicles distributed in the periphery of an enlarged ovary *(arrows)*. (From Sauerbrei, with permission.)

Diagnosis

Diagnostic criteria for PCOS include menstrual irregularity, hyperandrogenism, and exclusion of other possible causes. Other causes of anovulatory states should be ruled out, including premature ovarian failure, pituitary adenoma, thyroid dysfunction, excessive physical exertion, eating disorders and excessive weight loss, and congenital adrenal hyperplasia. Ultrasound findings consistent with a diagnosis of PCOS are eight or more follicles smaller than 10 mm in the ovary. These follicles usually are located around the periphery, forming the appearance of a "pearl necklace." The ratio of leuteinizing hormone (LH) to follicle-stimulating hormone (FSH) is 3:1. Glucose and lipid levels may also be abnormal.[1,2]

Clinical Complications

A chronic anovulatory state with unopposed estrogen effect results in a threefold increase in the rate of endometrial cancer in patients with PCOS. The risk of breast cancer may also be increased. Diabetes and hyperlipidemia associated with PCOS increase the risk for cardiovascular disease.[1]

Management

Diet and exercise are useful, because weight reduction decreases androgen production and insulin resistance. Pharmacologic treatment includes oral contraceptives and antiandrogens for normalization of menstrual cycles and to treat acne and hirsutism. Treatment with ovulation-inducing agents may be used for patients who desire pregnancy. Metformin has been shown to improve insulin sensitivity, and it also normalizes menstrual periods and decreases androgen levels.[1]

REFERENCES

1. Hunter MH, Sterrett JJ. Polycystic ovary syndrome: it's not just infertility. *Am Fam Physician* 2000;62:1079–1088.
2. Taylor AE. Polycystic ovary syndrome. *Endocrinol Metab Clin North Am* 1998;27:877–902.

Endometriosis

Anthony Morocco

Clinical Presentation

Patients with endometriosis complain of pain that worsens during menses. The pain may involve the pelvis (dysmenorrhea, dyspareunia), low back, and rectum. Patients may also present for infertility evaluation. Clinical findings may include pelvic masses, adnexal or uterine tenderness, and a fixed and retroverted uterus.[1]

Pathophysiology

Endometriosis is a disorder that affects an estimated 5% to 10% of women. The diagnosis is most commonly made in women in their late twenties. Endometriosis is diagnosed in 20% of women undergoing laparoscopy for infertility workups and in 24% of women undergoing evaluation for chronic pelvic pain.[1] Endometriosis is caused by the presence of endometrial tissue at abnormal sites, including the ovaries and fallopian tubes. Location within the ovary causes the classic "chocolate cyst." The tissue responds to the fluctuation in hormones during the menstrual cycle with growth and bleeding, causing symptoms. The cause for this abnormal location is unknown. One theory blames retrograde menstruation, with endometrial cells refluxed into the pelvis, where they implant. The occasional occurrence of endometrial tissue in the lung or nose suggests an alternative origin.[1]

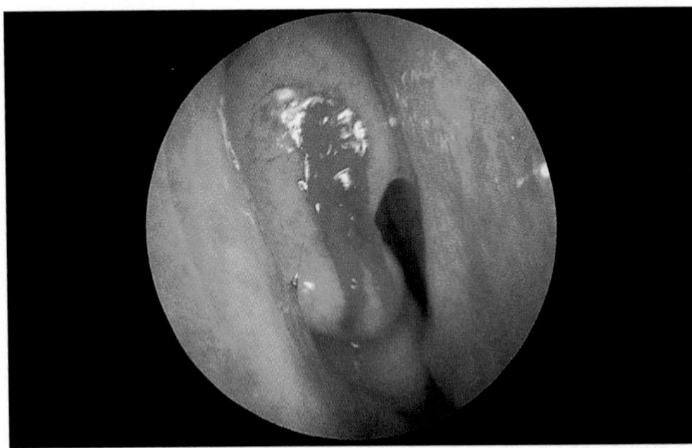

FIGURE 11-9 A small patch of ectopic endometriosis is seen in the head of the right inferior nasal turbinate. Menses were invariably preceded by a minor nosebleed by 1 day. (From Benjamin, with permission.)

Diagnosis

The new onset of dysmenorrhea and other pain during menses suggests the diagnosis. Laparoscopic visualization confirms the presence of lesions, although their extent can be difficult to assess. Staging systems can be used to classify the severity of disease.[1]

Clinical Complications

Complications include intraabdominal scarring and adhesions, rectal bleeding, bowel obstruction, urinary obstruction, and hemoptysis.[1]

Management

A trial of oral contraceptives or progestins may be useful in patients with mild symptoms; pain relief is achieved in 75% of cases. Gonadotropin-releasing hormone (GnRH) agonists such as leuprolide induce amenorrhea and effectively relieve pain in 90% of patients. Androgens such as danazol relieve symptoms but cause severe side effects. Because endometriosis-related infertility does not improve after these pharmacologic therapies, surgery may be required to remove adhesions and other obstructive lesions. Surgical treatment also frequently results in pain relief and lower recurrence rates than does pharmacologic treatment. Removal of pelvic organs (hysterectomy, oophorectomy) may be beneficial for intractable pain.[1]

REFERENCES

1. Wellbery C. Diagnosis and treatment of endometriosis. *Am Fam Physician* 1999;60:1753–1762, 1767–1768.

Breast Masses

Anthony Morocco

Clinical Presentation

Patients present with concerns about a recently discovered breast mass, or a mass may be discovered incidentally on any physical examination.

Pathophysiology

Breast masses may be related to normal physiologic processes, or they may be pathologic. Nodularity is a normal property of breast glandular tissue. The upper outer quadrant and inframammary ridge tend to be nodular, and the size of the tissue varies through the menstrual cycle. Dominant masses by definition do not vary with the menstrual cycle. These masses may be caused by cysts, fibroadenomas, fibrocystic changes, fat necrosis, or malignancy.[1]

Diagnosis/Treatment

Workup of a breast mass includes differentiation between cystic and solid structures. Fibrocystic change involves dilation of ducts and stromal edema. It is the most common cause of benign breast disease. Although fibrocystic changes and microcysts are common in young women, larger macrocysts are most common in premenopausal women older than 40 years of age. Macrocysts are uncommon in younger women and in postmenopausal women not receiving hormone replacement. Examination may reveal a well-demarcated, firm structure that may vary with the menstrual cycle. Consultation or referral to a breast surgeon for further workup is appropriate. The diagnosis of a cyst may be confirmed by ultrasonography or by needle aspiration of the fluid contents, which is also the treatment. Only cysts with bloody aspirate, remaining mass after aspiration, or multiple rapid recurrences require surgical biopsy.[1]

Women older than 40 years of age and those with risk factors for malignancy require an aggressive workup. Suspicious masses are hard, solitary, discrete, and adherent to adjacent to tissue. Consultation or referral to a breast surgeon should be made for suspicious masses. For women younger than age 40 years, equivocal findings on physical examination may first be evaluated by ultrasonography. Clinically benign-appearing masses may be excised or evaluated by imaging and needle aspiration. A concerning mass should be evaluated by fine-needle aspiration, needle biopsy, core cutting, or excisional biopsy. Needle biopsy can be guided ultrasonographically or mammographically (stereotaxis).[2] For women older than age 40 years, a mammogram is more often used as part of the initial workup for any breast mass, to evaluate the extent of the mass and to search for the presence of other lesions. A normal mammogram does not rule out breast cancer, because many cancers cannot be visualized on the mammogram. Histopathologic evaluation should be performed to rule out malignancy.[1]

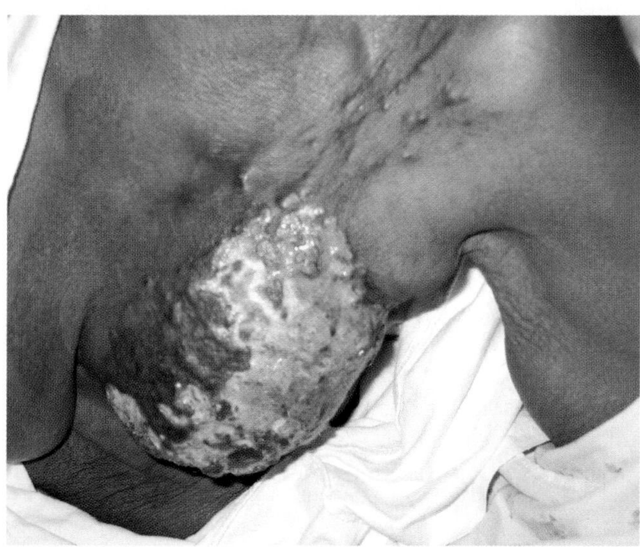

FIGURE 11–10 Extensive fungating cancerous lesion of the breast. (Courtesy of Michael S. Weingarten, MD.)

REFERENCES

1. Morrow M. The evaluation of common breast problems. *Am Fam Physician* 2000;61:2371–2378, 2385.
2. Newman LA, Sabel M. Advances in breast cancer detection and management. *Med Clin North Am* 2003;87:997–1028.

Breast Infections

Anthony Morocco

Clinical Presentation

Patients with mastitis present with low-grade fever, breast tenderness, local erythema and edema, and malaise. Nonlactating women may also complain of nipple discharge.[1]

Pathophysiology

Infections of the breast include mastitis and abscess. These conditions, including puerperal mastitis (also called "milk fever"), are most common in lactating women; they usually occur 2 to 3 weeks after delivery, with half of the infections occurring in the first 12 postpartum weeks. Infection in nonlactating women is much less common and may be related to duct ectasia. Other diseases such as carcinoma and fat necrosis can cause a breast mass and inflammation mimicking infection.[1] The most common site of lactational mastitis is in the upper outer quadrant. Lactational mastitis is blamed on milk stasis, which may be related to a number of factors, including erratic or interrupted feeding patterns, poor positioning during feeding, illness, damaged nipples, and hyperlactation. Stasis and inspissation results in an inflammatory response to milk components that infiltrate surrounding breast tissue. Secondary bacterial infection may then occur, usually involving *Staphylococcus aureus.* Nonlactational mastitis with subareolar abscesses is caused by duct ectasia, involving a complex process of ductal dilatation, inflammation, and secondary bacterial infection.[1]

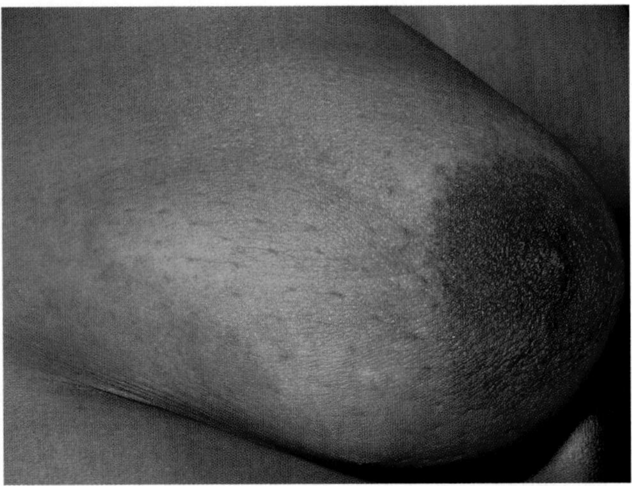

FIGURE 11–11 Inferiorly located abscess that drained 55 mL of pus. (Courtesy of Mark Silverberg, MD.)

Diagnosis

Abscesses can be difficult to diagnose because of an absence of palpable fluctuance and inability to palpate deeply due to patient discomfort. Ultrasonography may be useful in locating an abscess and guiding drainage procedures. Breast abscesses require surgical or gynecologic consultation for incision and drainage. Nonlactating women with suspected mastitis should be referred to a breast surgeon for biopsy to rule out inflammatory carcinoma.[1]

Clinical Complications

Untreated and improperly treated infections can result in abscess formation, sepsis, and recurrent mastitis. The incidence of recurrent mastitis within the same lactation period is 6% to 23%.[2] Subareolar abscesses can result in frequent recurrence and fistula formation.[1]

Management

Lactational mastitis should be treated with antibiotics (e.g., dicloxacillin, cephalexin) and pain medication. Patients should continue nursing with both breasts, or at least express milk on the affected side, because cessation of nursing can exacerbate the milk stasis that may be the underlying cause of the mastitis.[1] Abscesses should be treated with antibiotics started in the emergency department (ED), as well as prompt, on-site consultation for decompression by needle aspiration (with ultrasound guidance, if necessary), continuous catheter drainage, or incision and drainage in the operating room.[2]

REFERENCES

1. Marchant DJ. Inflammation of the breast. *Obstet Gynecol Clin North Am* 2002;29:89–102.
2. Dener C, Inan A. Breast abscesses in lactating women. *World J Surg* 2003;27:130–133.

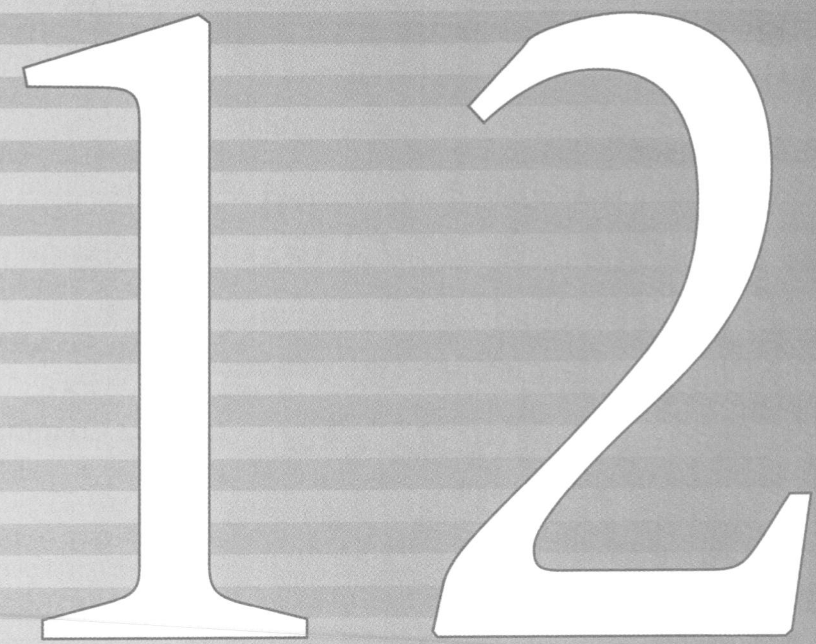

Sexually Transmitted Diseases

Urethritis

Dziwe Ntaba

Clinical Presentation

Patients with urethritis present with painful urination and a urethral discharge. Urethral itching is also common; however, many patients are relatively asymptomatic. Presenting symptoms may also include urinary frequency and urgency.

Pathophysiology

The most likely single etiologic agent causing acute urethritis is *Neisseria gonorrhoeae* (GCU). However, nongonococcal urethritis (NGU) is twice as common and is associated with greater morbidity than GCU. *Chlamydia* species are the predominate organisms involved in NGU; others include *Ureaplasma* spp., *Trichomonas* spp., and herpes simplex virus. Noninfectious causes of urethritis include Reiter's syndrome and Kawasaki disease. Traumatic urethritis is caused by an inflammatory reaction to the insertion of a foreign body, medical instrument, or urinary catheter.[1]

Diagnosis

A complete genitourinary examination is indicated. Suggestive findings include clear to yellow-brown discharge, meatal edema, and tenderness to palpation along the course of the urethra (in men). Consideration of possible joint or eye involvement is essential. Laboratory evaluation includes urinalysis, urethral swab for gonorrhea and chlamydia, cultures, and Gram staining. Ideally, swabs should be obtained at least 2 hours after voiding, to prevent bacterial washout. A complete absence of white blood cells on the urethral smear argues against urethritis.[1]

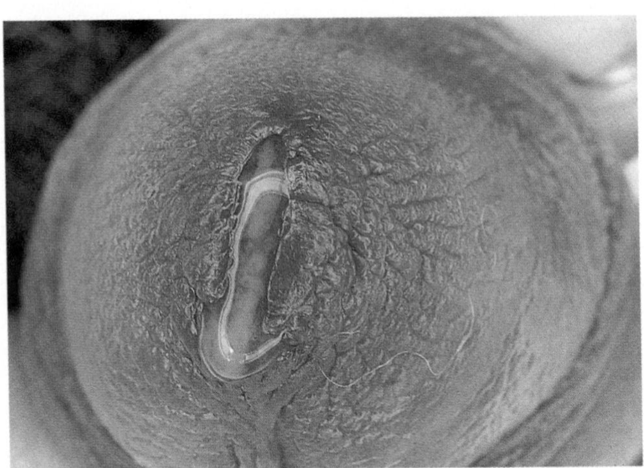

FIGURE 12–1 Gonococcal urethritis with purulent discharge. (From Ostler, with permission.)

Clinical Complications

Complications include pelvic inflammatory disease (PID) in women, prostatitis in men, disseminated gonococcal disease in both sexes, and epidemiologic spread within a community. Gonorrhea is highly infectious: a single episode of unprotected intercourse with an infected partner carries an 80% transmission risk to women, and 20% to men. The pharynx is involved in 40% of homosexual men and 7% of heterosexuals with GCU.[2] Notification of public health authorities, patient education regarding risks of reinfection, and referral of sexual partners are essential.

Management

Treatment for uncomplicated cases of urethritis is empirically geared toward coverage of both GCU and NGU, because coinfection is common. Single doses of ceftriaxone or of ciprofloxacin are recommended for GCU, although recent reports show a rise in quinolone-resistant *N. gonorrhea.* For NGU, azithromycin and doxycycline are equally efficacious.[2]

REFERENCES

1. Lundquist ST, Stack LB. Diseases of the foreskin, penis, and urethra. *Emerg Med Clin North Am* 2001;19:529–546.
2. Workowski KA, Levine WC. Sexually transmitted diseases treatment guidelines—2002. *MMWR Morb Mortal Wkly Rep* 2002;51(RR-6): 1–80.

Pelvic Inflammatory Disease

Anthony Morocco

Clinical Presentation

Patients with pelvic inflammatory disease (PID) present with a variety of symptoms, alone or in combination, including vaginal discharge, abdominal pain, dyspareunia, vaginal bleeding, dysuria, malaise, nausea, vomiting, and fever.

Pathophysiology

Various bacteria have been implicated in the pathogenesis of PID, including *N. gonorrhoeae, Chlamydia trachomatis, Haemophilus influenzae,* enteric bacteria (e.g., *Bacteroides fragilis*), *Streptococcus agalactiae,* cytomegalovirus (CMV), *Mycoplasma hominis,* and *Ureaplasma urealyticum.* Most cases of PID are probably caused by ascending infections of the lower genital tract.[1,2]

Diagnosis

The diagnosis can be difficult, and it is likely that many mild cases go unrecognized. Although most cases are diagnosed on clinical grounds, the gold standard for diagnosis is laparoscopy.[1] Physical findings include fever, tachycardia, abdominal tenderness, cervical motion tenderness, and bilateral adnexal tenderness. Guarding and rebound tenderness may be present on abdominal examination.[2] Minimal criteria for the clinical diagnosis include adnexal tenderness or cervical motion tenderness in a sexually active woman for which no other cause can be found. Supportive findings include oral temperature greater than 38.3°C, vaginal discharge, white blood cells on saline preparation of vaginal fluid, laboratory evidence of *N. gonorrhoeae* or *C. trachomatis* infection, elevation in C-reactive protein, and increased erythrocyte sedimentation rate (ESR). The positive predictive value of a clinical diagnosis ranges from 65% to 90%.[1]

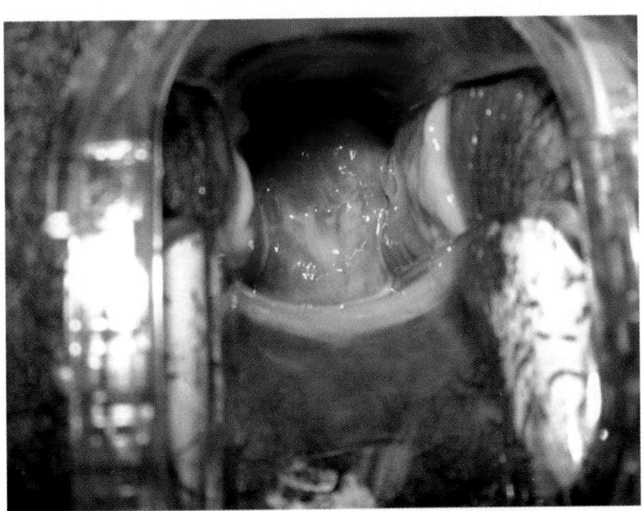

FIGURE 12–2 Mucopurulent cervicitis with inflammatory changes and copious discharge. (Courtesy of Rafi Israeli, MD.)

Clinical Complications

The most common complications are related to damage and scarring of the upper genital tract, which can result in infertility, future ectopic pregnancies, and chronic pelvic pain. Other complications include tubo-ovarian abscess (TOA) and Fitz-Hugh–Curtis syndrome.[2]

Management

The decision to treat PID on an inpatient rather than an outpatient basis is founded on factors such as pregnancy, failure of initial outpatient treatment, inability to follow oral antibiotic regimen, severe clinical illness, presence of TOA, and the potential presence of a serious alternative diagnosis (e.g., appendicitis).[1,2] Antimicrobial therapy should be broad-spectrum and directed at all the potential pathogens. Inpatient first-line therapy is cefoxitin or cefotetan, plus doxycycline or clindamycin, plus gentamicin. Outpatient therapy is ofloxacin or levofloxacin, or intramuscular ceftriaxone and oral doxycycline; either regimen may be given with or without metronidazole.[1] Clinicians should consult current recommendations of the Centers for Disease Control and Prevention (CDC) for dosages and applicable duration of therapy.

REFERENCES

1. Workowski KA, Levine WC. Sexually transmitted diseases treatment guidelines—2002. *MMWR Morb Mortal Wkly Rep* 2002;51(RR-6):1–80.
2. Zeger W, Holt K. Gynecologic infections. *Emerg Med Clin North Am* 2003;21:631–648.

Tubo-ovarian Abscess

Dziwe Ntaba

Clinical Presentation

Tubo-ovarian abscess (TOA) is a common complication of pelvic inflammatory disease (PID), with a clinical presentation similar to that of salpingitis (i.e., abdominal pain, fever, and gastrointestinal symptoms).

Pathophysiology

TOA is present in as many as 15% of women with PID and in approximately 33% of those requiring hospitalization for PID. TOA is less prevalent among postmenopausal women. The most common pathogens isolated from operative cultures are *Escherichia coli*, *Bacteroides*, and *Streptococcus*. *Neisseria* and *Chlamydia* species are less commonly isolated, but this may reflect selection bias among published case reports or among those cases requiring surgical intervention.[1]

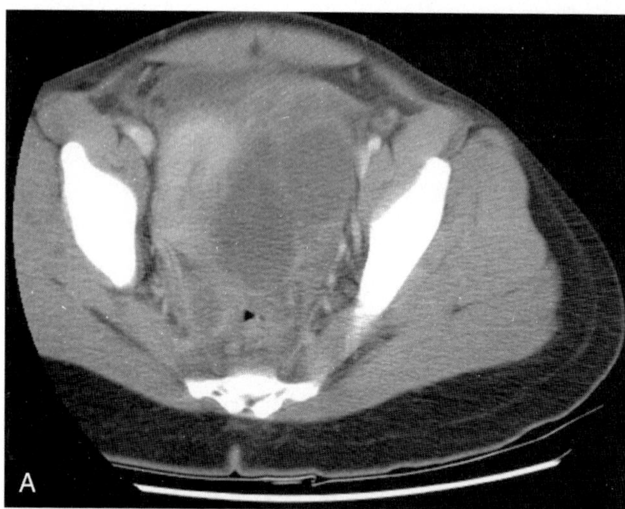

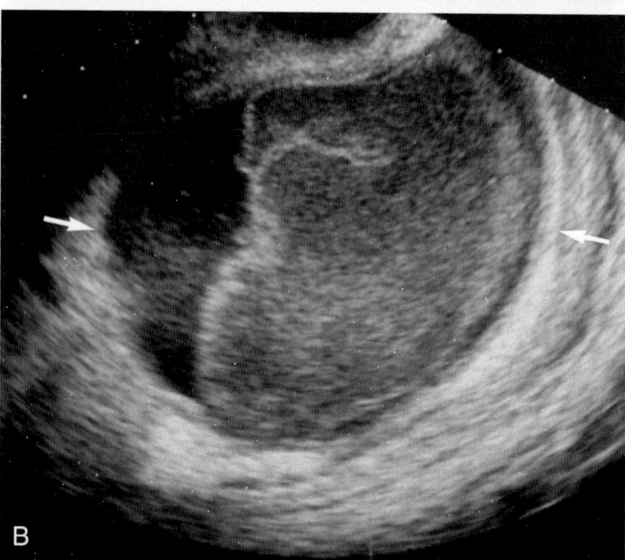

FIGURE 12–3 **A:** Contrast computed tomographic scan of tubo-ovarian abscess. (Courtesy of Jaimee O'Connor, MD.) **B:** Transvaginal sonographic image of the mass *(arrows)* shows predominantly cystic areas of the abscess. (From Doubilet, with permission.)

Diagnosis

Historical clues to the presence of TOA include one or more previous episodes of PID and the presence of an intrauterine device.[1] Physical examination usually reveals lower abdominal tenderness, cervical and adnexal tenderness, and the perception of adnexal fullness on pelvic examination. The diagnosis is confirmed by transvaginal sonography, which demonstrates a well-demarcated, tubular structure with thick, dense walls containing heterogeneous fluid–debris levels. If free fluid is seen, or if peritoneal signs are present on examination, computed tomography (CT) of the abdomen is indicated. Transabdominal ultrasonography may be confounded by bowel gas and body habitus.[2] Some authors recommend the routine use of ultrasonography in all patients admitted to the hospital with PID.[3] Laparoscopy is the diagnostic gold standard.

Clinical Complications

Complications include rupture and subsequent sepsis as well as septic shock. Posttreatment risks for ectopic pregnancy and infertility are substantial.

Management

Given the polymicrobial spectrum seen in TOA, triple therapy with ampicillin, gentamicin, and clindamycin has shown to be cost-effective. Surgery is required in all cases of TOA rupture, or failure of medical treatment.[2]

REFERENCES

1. El Khoury J, Stikkelbroeck MM, Goodman A, Rubin RH, Cosimi AB, Fishman JA. Postmenopausal tubo-ovarian abscess due to *Pseudomonas aeruginosa* in a renal transplant patient: a case report and review of the literature. *Transplantation* 2001;72:1241–1244.
2. Lee C, Henderson SO. Emergent surgical complications of genitourinary infections. *Emerg Med Clin North Am* 2003;21:1057–1074.
3. McNeely SG, Hendrix SL, Mazzoni MM, Kmak DC, Ransom SB. Medically sound, cost-effective treatment for pelvic inflammatory disease and tuboovarian abscess. *Am J Obstet Gynecol* 1998;178: 1272–1278.

Chancroid

Colleen Campbell

Clinical Presentation

Patients with chancroid may describe a history of preceding malaise for several days before the appearance of genital ulcers. Patients present with painful genital ulcers surrounded by erythema. Men usually present with one or more ulcers on the prepuce or frenulum, whereas women may present with ulceration involving the vulva, cervix, or perianal area.[1] Tender, unilateral lymphadenopathy is a common associated presenting complaint.

Pathophysiology

Chancroid, a sexually transmitted disease caused by *Haemophilus ducreyi,* is characterized by necrotizing genital ulcers. *H. ducreyi* is a fastidious, gram-negative organism.[1] Human immunodeficiency virus (HIV) infection is associated with a higher rate of chancroid infection. Men develop chancroid more commonly than women do. The ulcer begins as an erythematous papule about 4 days after exposure and progresses to ulceration after pustule rupture. There may be obvious bubo formation in the inguinal regions.

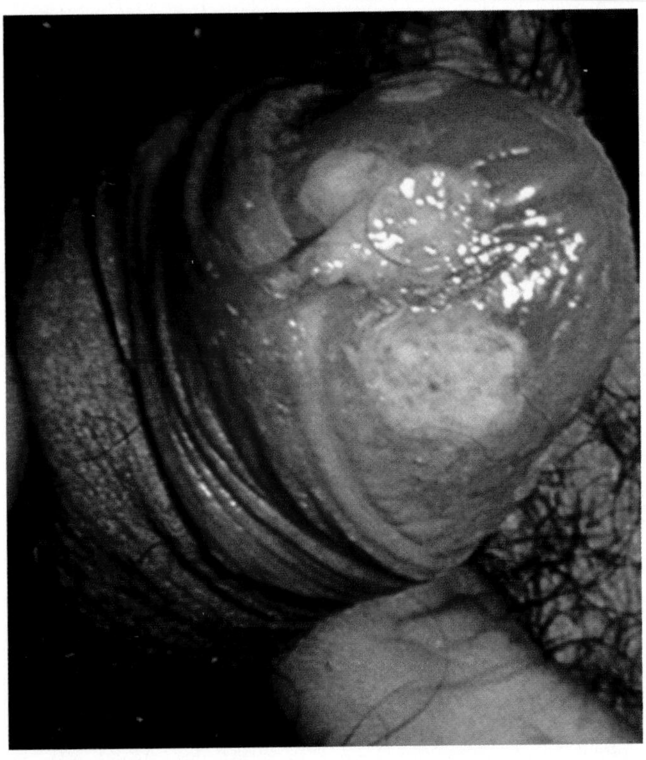

FIGURE 12–4 Chancroid in a patient with multiple painful ulcers on the glans penis. (From Goodheart, with permission.)

Diagnosis

The diagnosis of chancroid should be considered in all patients with painful genital ulcers characterized by irregular, inverted, and granulomatous borders. Physical examination, even when performed by experienced clinicians, is a relatively insensitive and nonspecific indicator of disease.[1] Multiplex polymerase chain reaction (M-PCR) tests exist and are a very sensitive means to differentiate chancroid from syphilis, but they are expensive and not widely available. Culture only approaches 75% sensitivity, because *H. ducreyi* is an extraordinarily fastidious microaerophilic organism.

Clinical Complications

Chancroid ulcers are associated with an increased rate of transmission. Phimosis may occur in men as a result of this disease.[1] Autoinoculation also occurs to other sites of the body. Balanitis and fistula formation are uncommon complications.[2]

Management

Effective treatment may be achieved by the use of ciprofloxacin, ceftriaxone, or erythromycin. The cure rate associated with these drugs is greater than 90%; ceftriaxone and erythromycin are a safer alternative during pregnancy.[1] Azithromycin and spectinomycin are other single-dose treatment regimens recommended by the World Health Organization (WHO) and the Centers for Disease Control and Prevention (CDC).[1] Prolonged courses of treatment may be necessary for patients with concomitant infection.[2] Healing of the ulcer can take up to 3 weeks. Notification and testing of sexual contacts is mandatory.

REFERENCES

1. Lewis DA. Chancroid: clinical manifestations, diagnosis, and management. *Sex Transm Infect* 2003;79:68–71.
2. Sehgal VN, Srivastava G. Chancroid: contemporary appraisal. *Int J Dermatol* 2003;42:182–190.

Condyloma Acuminata

Michael Greenberg

Clinical Presentation

Both male and female patients with condylomata acuminata (CA) present with genital and/or anorectal skin lesions, and they usually seek care when the lesions bleed, become painful or irritating, or somehow are cosmetically problematic.[1,2]

Pathophysiology

CA are external genital warts that are caused by infection with the human papillomavirus (HPV). Some 80 strains of HPV have been identified, and 30 of these cause genital infection. The incidence of CA ranges from 0.5% to 1% among sexually active young adults in the United States. There are reportedly up to 1 million new cases annually. Adolescents, young adults, and persons with multiple partners are at highest risk for infection. There is no evidence that condoms prevent the spread of HPV, and HPV may be spread by a variety of sexual activities beyond intercourse. The risk for cervical intraepithelial neoplasia in women infected with HPV is increased. Passive and active cigarette smoke exposure are strongly associated with HPV expression.[1,2]

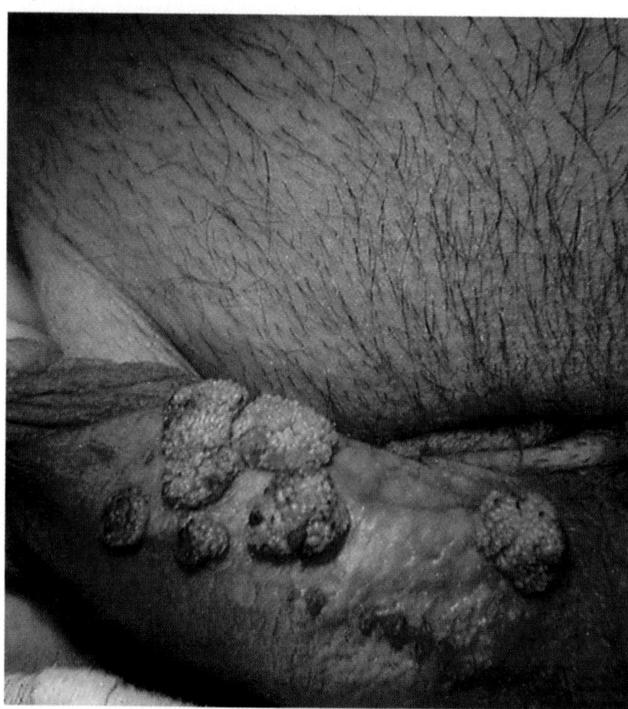

FIGURE 12–5 Condyloma acuminatum. Typical verrucous papules and nodules in the genital area. (From Yamada, with permission.)

Diagnosis

The diagnosis is based on the clinical appearance and location of the lesions. The lesions typically appear as mobile, grey-white, warty excrescences distributed as described earlier.

Clinical Complications

Complications include secondary infection and malignant transformation.

Management

Treatment is aimed at relief of symptoms and includes options such as the use of destructive chemicals (trichloroacetic acid, podophyllin, podofilox, 5-fluorouracil), immune modulators (α-interferon, imiquimod), and surgery (excision, carbon dioxide laser ablation). Imiquimod is a topical immune-response modifier that acts to upregulate the cells that are active in the normal immune response.[2]

REFERENCES

1. Van Den Eeden SK, Habel LA, Sherman KJ, McKnight B, Stergachis A, Daling JR. Risk factors for incident and recurrent condylomata acuminata among men: a population-based study. *Sex Transm Dis* 1998;25:278–284.
2. Fleisher AB Jr, Parrish CA, Glenn R, Feldman SR. Condylomata acuminata (genital warts): patient demographics and treating physicians. *Sex Transm Dis* 2001;28:643–647.

Lymphogranuloma Venereum

Anthony Morocco

Clinical Presentation

Lymphogranuloma venereum (LGV) begins as a painless papule, vesicle, or erosion on the labia, fourchette, or cervix in women, or on the corona, glans, or prepuce or intraurethrally in men. This primary lesion may be accompanied by systemic symptoms of fever, headache, nausea, and myalgias or arthralgias and usually resolves in a few days. The second stage, or the inguinal syndrome, occurs most commonly in men and begins with the formation of firm, tender, and immobile lymph nodes in the drainage area of the primary lesion. The enlarged nodes become elongated and form a groove ("sign of the groove") along Poupart's ligament. The overlying skin becomes dusky and breaks down; the draining sinuses that form may last for months. A genitoanorectal syndrome occurs as the third stage, most commonly in women and homosexual men. Patients develop enlarged perirectal and intestinal lymph nodes, anal discharge, proctocolitis, bloody diarrhea, abdominal pain, and perirectal abscesses.[1]

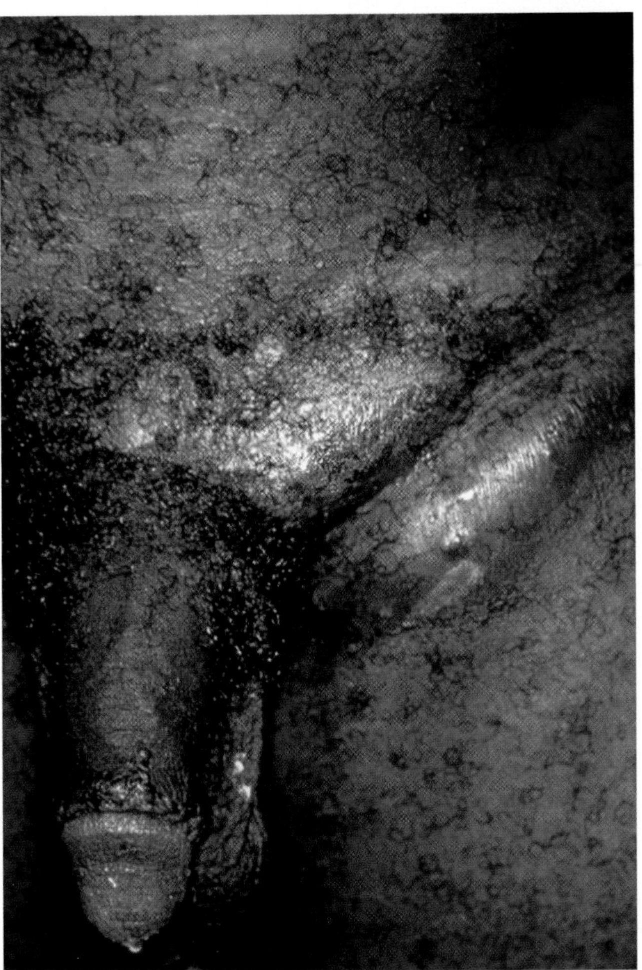

FIGURE 12–6 Lymphogranuloma venereum. Regional lymphadenitis (the "groove sign") is present. (From Goodheart, with permission.)

Pathophysiology

LGV is a sexually transmitted disease that is commonly found in southeast Asia, Africa, and Central and South America. LGV is uncommon in the United States, except among homosexual men.[1] LGV is caused by *Chlamydia trachomatis* serotypes L-1, L-2, and L-3.[1]

Diagnosis

The diagnosis usually is suspected based on clinical findings and verified by serology; a complement fixation titer greater than 1:64 represents a positive result.[2]

Clinical Complications

LGV can cause urethral obstruction, epithelialized fenestrations in the labia and clitoral prepuce, rectal strictures, rectovaginal and anal fistulas, intestinal obstruction, anal polyps, and elephantiasis of the genitals.[1]

Management

Incision and drainage or aspiration of buboes may be necessary. Doxycycline is the antibiotic of choice. Alternatively, erythromycin or azithromycin is also likely to be effective.[2]

REFERENCES

1. Fiumara NJ. Genital ulcer infections in the female patient and the vaginitides. *Dermatol Clin* 1997;15:233–246.
2. Workowski KA, Levine WC. Sexually transmitted diseases treatment guidelines—2002. *MMWR Morb Mortal Wkly Rep* 2002;51(RR-6): 1–80.

Granuloma Inguinale

Anthony Morocco

Clinical Presentation

Patients with granuloma inguinale first develop a "beefy red," easily bleeding, and moist papule on the labia majora or fourchette, or on the corona of the penis. Papules progress to nodules and ulcerate. Spread occurs along skin folds to the inguinal and perianal areas, with coalescence of lesions and elevation of borders.[1,2]

Pathophysiology

Granuloma inguinale, or donovanosis, is a chronic, granulomatous, sexually transmitted disease affecting fewer than 10 persons per year in the United States.[1,2] It is more commonly found in African-Americans, men, and homosexuals. The disease is endemic in several areas, including the Caribbean, India, Brazil, and Japan.[1] The gram-negative rod *Calymmatobacterium granulomatis* is the causative organism. The incubation period ranges from 8 days to 3 months.[1]

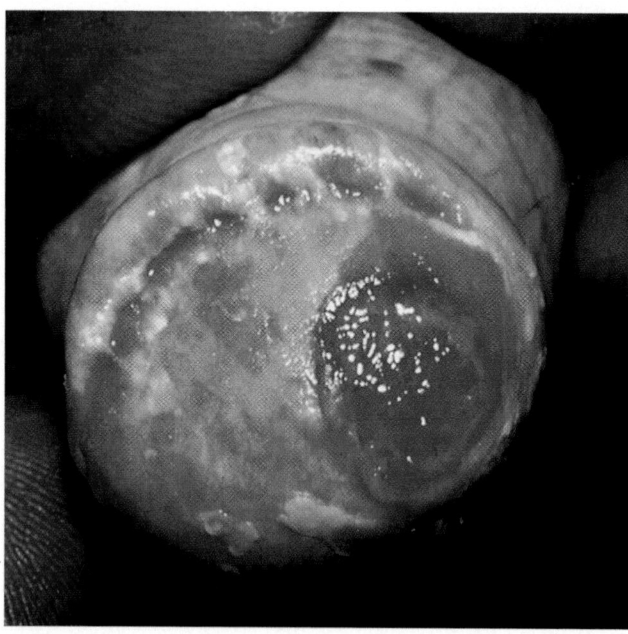

FIGURE 12–7 Granuloma inguinale, showing typical friable, beefy lesion. (Courtesy of William Henessy, MD.) (From Ostler, with permission.)

Diagnosis

Scrapings or a biopsy specimen should be stained and examined for the presence of organisms in large histiocytes (Donovan bodies) and plasma cells. Differential diagnosis includes syphilis, lymphogranuloma venereum, tuberculosis, squamous cell epithelioma, and pyogenic granuloma.[1]

Clinical Complications

Untreated lesions may develop squamous cell carcinoma.[1] Secondary bacterial infection of lesions also occurs. Relapse may occur 6 to 18 months after treatment.[2]

Management

Patients may be treated with doxycycline, trimethoprim-sulfamethoxazole, ciprofloxacin, erythromycin, or azithromycin. An aminoglycoside should be added if there is no improvement within a few days. Treatment should continue for at least 3 weeks, until lesions have healed. Any recent sexual partners should be examined and treated.[2]

REFERENCES

1. Fiumara NJ. Genital ulcer infections in the female patient and the vaginitides. *Dermatol Clin* 1997;15:233–246.
2. Workowski KA, Levine WC. Sexually transmitted diseases treatment guidelines—2002. *MMWR Morb Mortal Wkly Rep* 2002;51(RR-6): 1–80.

Gonococcal Arthritis

Robert Hendrickson

Clinical Presentation

Gonococcal arthritis (GA) typically manifests with the acute onset of monoarticular arthritis in a young adult, although polyarticular arthritis is possible. The joints most commonly affected are the knees, wrists, hands, and ankles.[1] Signs of mucosal gonococcal infection (vaginal, rectal, or urethral discharge; pelvic pain; sore throat; or dysuria) usually are not present.[2] Other signs of disseminated gonococcemia may be evident, including rash (painless and papular, pustular, or macular on an erythematous base) on the extremities (67%), fever, chills, and tenosynovitis of the wrists and ankles (67%).[1,2]

Pathophysiology

Gonococcal infection occurs at mucosal sites (cervix, urethra, pharynx, or rectum) and may be asymptomatic. Arthritis occurs during hematogenous dissemination of the bacteria.[1] Infection of the synovial tissue is followed by an inflammatory reaction within the joint.[2]

Diagnosis

The diagnosis should be suspected in all young, sexually active patients with monoarticular arthritis (GA is the cause in more than 50% of these presentations).[1,2] GA is more common in women, particularly within days after menses and shortly after or during pregnancy. Arthrocentesis with Gram staining, complete cell count, and culture of the synovial fluid should be performed to identify *Neisseria gonorrhoeae* and rule out other organisms. The synovial leukocyte count is typically 50,000 to 200,000, with greater than 90% polymorphonucleocytes (PMNs) in GA.[2]

Identification of *N. gonorrhoeae* is most likely at a mucosal site (cervix, urethra, pharynx, or rectum), even in asymptomatic patients.[1] Cultures should be grown on Thayer-Martin medium (chocolate agar with antibiotics). Gram stains and cultures of skin lesions, joint fluid, and blood generally are not diagnostic. Leukocytosis and an elevated erythrocyte sedimentation rate (ESR) may be present but are nonspecific. Other causes of arthritis should be considered, including Reiter's syndrome (urethritis, axial arthritis, and conjunctivitis secondary to chlamydia, seen more commonly in men), septic arthritis, bacterial endocarditis, rheumatic fever, hepatitis, and meningococcemia.

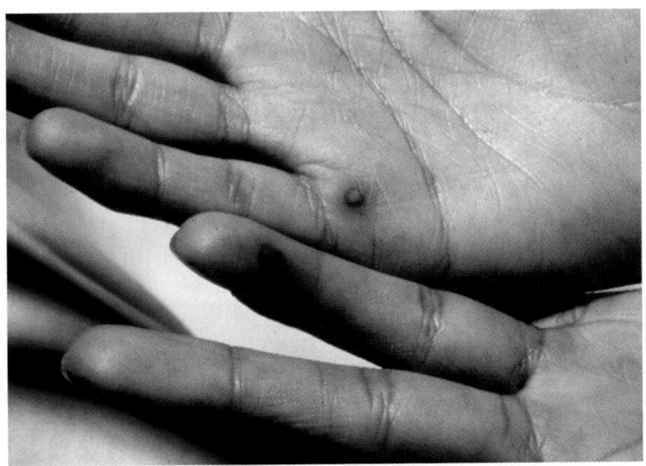

FIGURE 12–8 Disseminated gonococcemia. This is an example of septic vasculitis. Note the two palpable, purpuric, hemorrhagic vesicles. (From Goodheart, with permission.)

Clinical Complications

GA may rarely lead to joint destruction if left untreated. Disseminated gonococcemia may lead to meningitis, endocarditis, aortitis, myocarditis, or osteomyelitis.[1,2]

Management

Patients with suspected GA should have cervical or urethral swabs for identification of *N. gonorrhoeae* and may require arthrocentesis to rule out septic arthritis. Patients should be treated for gonorrhea, in the inpatient setting, with parenteral third-generation cephalosporins until 24 hours after symptoms improve (often 2-4 days).[1] All patients should also be treated for concomitant chlamydial infection (oral doxycycline), pending culture or PCR identification.[2]

REFERENCES

1. Scopelitis E, Martinez-Osuna P. Gonococcal arthritis. *Rheum Dis Clin North Am* 1993;19:363–377.
2. Cucurull E, Espinoza LR. Gonococcal arthritis. *Rheum Dis Clin North Am* 1998;24:305–322.

Syphilis

Christy Salvaggio

Clinical Presentation

Primary syphilis develops after direct contact with a chancre or other lesion of an infected individual. Because transmission is primarily sexual, lesions are most commonly genital and appear after an incubation period that can range from 10 days to as long as 3 months after exposure. The syphilitic chancre initially manifests as a red, firm papule, but it may be so small as to be easily overlooked. This papule erodes to a painless ulcer with a smooth, sharply demarcated border. The painless ulcer frequently goes undetected, especially in women, because the lesion is often located on the cervix. This single lesion of primary acquired syphilis contains infectious treponemes and is extremely contagious. Regional infected lymph nodes are typically enlarged and nontender. With or without treatment, the primary lesion of syphilis resolves within weeks; however, the hematogenous spread of treponemes results in secondary syphilis in approximately 25% of untreated cases.

Secondary syphilis is indicative of disseminated disease, and its onset is typically 6 to 12 weeks after infection. However, secondary disease may occur as long as 6 months after initial infection.[1] In most cases, the chancre of primary syphilis has resolved by the time secondary syphilis evolves. Constitutional symptoms associated with secondary syphilis are often nondescript, with vague flu-like symptoms of fever, malaise, myalgias, sore throat, and nontender, diffuse lymphadenopathy. Secondary syphilis generally involves multiorgan pathology, including gastrointestinal, renal, and rheumatologic disease; however, mucocutaneous lesions predominate.[1] The rash of secondary syphilis is classically a diffuse, coppery or dark-red rash with a symmetric distribution often involving the palms and soles. The rash is not painful or itchy, and patients are usually afebrile at the time the rash manifests. Both the severity of the rash and its appearance can be varied. Although maculopapular lesions are most common, the rash may be polymorphic, with macular, pustular, follicular, papular, and plaque-like lesions. Bullous or vesicular lesions are rare, whereas a superficial scaly component to the rash is common. Mucous membrane lesions are also common, contain many treponemes, and are highly contagious. Cutaneous lesions contain fewer treponemes but should also be treated as contagious. Relapses of the mucocutaneous lesions can occur for up to 4 years but are most common during the first year. The lesions seldom scar. Condylomata lata are highly infectious, wart-like lesions that appear on moist, intertriginous areas. They are especially common on perineal skin, on the vulva, and on the scrotum. Involvement of scalp hair follicles results in patchy alopecia that resolves after treatment.

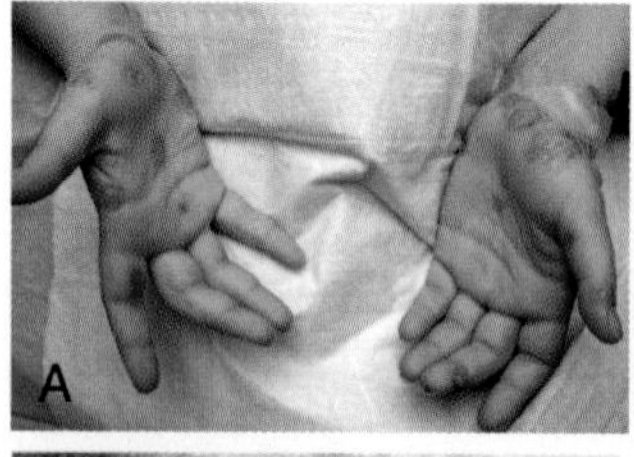

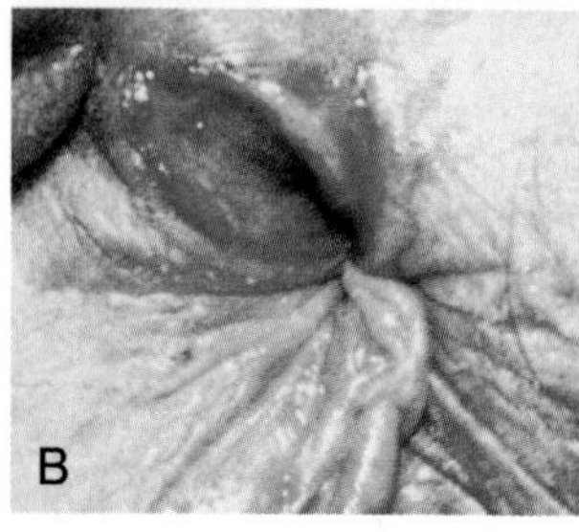

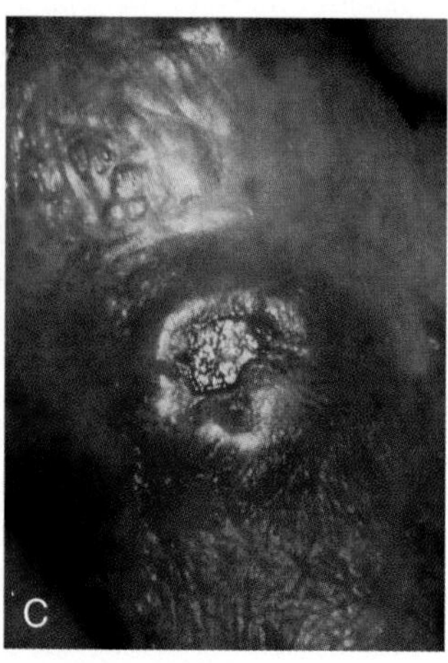

FIGURE 12–9 A: Palmer rash characteristic of secondary syphilis. (Courtesy of Ralph Weiche, MD.) **B:** Primary syphilitic chancre of the anus. Such lesions occur in people who engage in anoreceptive intercourse. Anorectal syphilitic chancres may be asymptomatic, or they may be painful, usually on defecation. (From Yamada, with permission.) **C:** Chancre of primary syphilis. (From Sweet and Gibbs, with permission.)

If left untreated, secondary syphilis eventually enters a latent stage, and the patient becomes asymptomatic; however, 30% of patients ultimately develop tertiary or latent disease.[2] Patients in the latent stage of disease who were infected within the last year have "early-latent" syphilis. All others have either "late-latent" syphilis or latent syphilis of unknown duration.

Tertiary syphilis may develop as long as 1 to 10 years after initial infection. Like secondary syphilis, tertiary syphilis produces multiorgan pathology with a predominance of cutaneous manifestations. Large, granulomatous lesions called "gummas" are pathognomonic of tertiary syphilis. Gummas represent an immune response to the treponemal infection, but, unlike the cutaneous lesions of primary and secondary syphilis, they do not contain live treponemes. Gummas occur on the skin, in bones, and, rarely, in other organs. They may contribute to the pathologic course of tertiary syphilis, because they can ulcerate and ultimately scar. Other problems associated with tertiary syphilis include aortitis (which potentially leads to aortic dissection, aortic aneurysm, or aortic regurgitation), central nervous system syphilis, general paresis, and tabes dorsalis. Tabes dorsalis results in sharp pain in the trunk and legs, incontinence, ocular palsies, paresthesias, Argyll-Robertson pupils (small, ir-

Syphilis

Christy Salvaggio

regular pupils that accommodate but do not react), absent deep tendon reflexes, and Charcot joints.[3]

Pathophysiology

Syphilis is a sexually transmitted infection caused by the spirochete, *Treponema pallidum.* Syphilis has primary, secondary, and tertiary (or latent) disease stages. Clinical presentation, patient infectivity, and treatment vary by disease stage. Similarly, congenital infections have unique clinical stages (see separate discussion of congenital syphilis elsewhere in this book). Humans are the only host, and this fragile spirochete cannot survive for long periods outside the human body. The highest incidence of infection occurs in young adults, and transmission is primarily via sexual contact, with rare transmissions occurring by other forms of close contact. Additionally, vertical transmission can occur during pregnancy, resulting in fetal infection and congenital syphilis (see separate discussion).[1]

Diagnosis

Motile spirochetes from tissue lesions or exudate can be identified by darkfield microscopy, which, in addition to direct fluorescent antibody tests, can be used to diagnose early disease. Generally, serologic testing is used to confirm or diagnose syphilis. Serology cannot be used to differentiate the clinical stage of syphilis, because patients are seroreactive at all stages. Two types of serologic tests are available, treponemal and nontreponemal tests. False-positive results occur with both test types; therefore, to confirm the diagnosis of syphilis, both a positive treponemal and a positive nontreponemal test are required.[4]

The fluorescent treponemal antibody absorbed (FTA-ABS) test and the *T. pallidum* particle agglutination (TP-PA) test are treponemal tests. Treponemal tests usually remain positive for life despite adequate treatment. The rapid plasma reagin serologic test (RPR) and the Venereal Disease Research Laboratory test (VDRL) are both nontreponemal tests. They do not directly test for antibodies to syphilis, but rather for cellular components. The RPR and VDRL tests are 70% reactive within 2 weeks of chancre appearance and 100% reactive in secondary or latent syphilis. After treatment, nontreponemal tests usually become nonreactive over time. A fourfold decrease in titers represents successful treatment, whereas a fourfold rise in titers represents a relapse or reinfection.[4]

Clinical Complications

Thirty percent of patients with untreated secondary syphilis go on to develop tertiary disease. Multisystem pathology associated with tertiary syphilis can include cardiovascular, ophthalmologic, and neurologic disease. Neurosyphilis is rare but can result from chronic meningeal inflammation.

Management

Parenteral penicillin remains the drug of choice for the treatment of syphilis. Tissue penetration of oral penicillin is inadequate. The recommended adult dose for treatment of primary, secondary, or latent syphilis is benzathine penicillin G, 2.4 million units given intramuscularly (IM) in a single dose. The pediatric dose is benzathine penicillin G, 50,000 units/kg IM, up to the adult dose of 2.4 million units in a single dose.[1] Tertiary syphilis must be treated with the same IM dose as primary syphilis, but the treatment repeated once a week for 3 weeks. Pediatric patients should also have evaluation of the cerebrospinal fluid for possible asymptomatic neurosyphilis. Syphilis involving the central nervous system (CNS) requires benzathine penicillin G, 4 million units IM or intravenously every 4 hours for 10 days. Cases of pediatric acquired syphilis require appropriate evaluation for sexual abuse. Treatment failures occur, and follow-up is mandatory, with repeat clinical examinations and serologic testing at least 6 months and 12 months after treatment. Penicillin-allergic patients without CNS disease should be treated with tetracycline (500 mg orally four times daily for 14 days) or doxycycline (100 mg orally twice daily for 14 days). Penicillin-allergic patients who are younger than 8 years of age, are pregnant, are infected with human immunodeficiency virus (HIV), or have CNS disease should undergo desensitization and then be treated with penicillin.[1]

The Jarisch-Herxheimer reaction is a febrile reaction seen within 24 hours after treatment for syphilis. Fever may be accompanied by other systemic complaints, including diffuse myalgias, headaches, hypotension, tachypnea, or some combination of these.[1] The Jarisch-Herxheimer reaction is seen in more than 50% of patients with primary or secondary disease, but it occurs less frequently in those with early latent disease.[2] During pregnancy, the Jarisch-Herxheimer reaction may result in contractions, premature delivery, or fetal demise, but fear of complications should not alter treatment.[1]

All sexual partners should seek medical care to determine their risk.[1] Empiric treatment is recommended for high-risk partners; others may be monitored with serologic testing. Testing for other sexually transmitted infections, including HIV, is imperative.

REFERENCES

1. Workowski KA, Levine WC. Sexually transmitted diseases treatment guidelines—2002. *MMWR Morb Mortal Wkly Rep* 2002;51(RR-6):1–80.
2. Ooi C, Dayan L. Syphilis: Diagnosis and management in general practice. *Aust Fam Physician* 2002;31:629–635.
3. Clyne B, Jerrard DA. Syphilis testing. *J Emerg Med* 2000;18:361–367.
4. Flores JL. Syphilis: a tale of twisted treponemes. *West J Med* 1995;163:552–559.

Condylomata Latum

Michael Greenberg

Clinical Presentation

Patients with condylomata latum present with grey-white or erythematous, painless, moist, flat, wart-like lesions of the genitalia, perineum, inner thighs, armpits, or breast folds. Concomitant findings consistent with secondary syphilis may be manifested, including fever, rash, anorexia, hair loss, lymphadenopathy, and weight loss.[1]

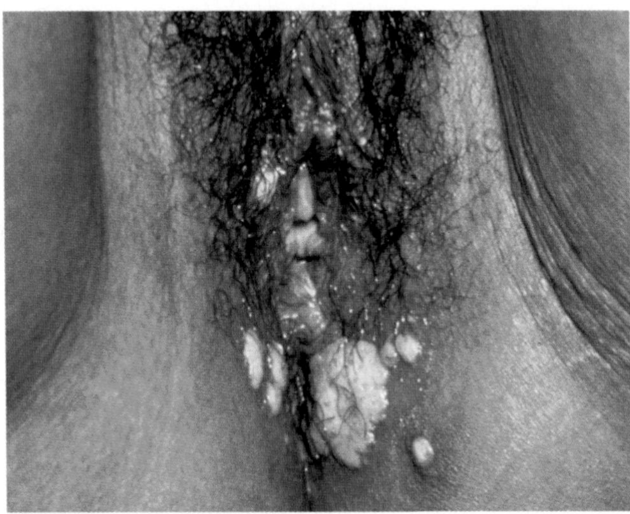

FIGURE 12–10 Secondary syphilis. Condylomata latum is noted. The moist, wart-like papule is highly infectious. (From Goodheart, with permission.)

Pathophysiology

Condylomata latum occur in cases of secondary syphilis. These lesions may develop from 2 to 8 weeks after the primary chancre.[1]

Diagnosis

The diagnosis may be suspected on clinical grounds but should be confirmed by specific laboratory tests. Nontreponemal tests such as the rapid plasma reagin (RPR), Venereal Disease Research Laboratory (VDRL), and automated reagin test (ART) may be useful in screening for syphilis. However, microscopic examination using darkfield techniques is the most specific means for diagnosing syphilis in the face of condylomata latum.[2]

Clinical Complications

Complications include disease progression to later stages of syphilis infection.

Management

Effective treatment for condylomata latum requires treatment of the underlying syphilis infection, in accord with current Centers for Disease Control and Prevention (CDC) guidelines and recommendations.

REFERENCES

1. Brown DL, Frank JE. Diagnosis and management of syphilis. *Am Fam Physician* 2003;68:283–290.
2. Larsen SA, Steiner BM, Rudolph AH. Laboratory diagnosis and interpretation of tests for syphilis. *Clin Microbiol Rev* 1995;8:1–21.

Trichomoniasis

Anthony Morocco

Clinical Presentation

Patients with trichomoniasis present with a frothy, malodorous, green-yellow vaginal discharge, with onset during or after menses. Local symptoms of discomfort include pruritus, labial tenderness, dysuria, dyspareunia, and dull, low abdominal pain. A strawberry appearance to the cervix or vulva may be seen; it is caused by punctate hemorrhages. Up to 50% of infected women are asymptomatic.[1,3] Infected men may complain of mild urethral discomfort and a slight discharge, but most have no symptoms.[1]

Pathophysiology

Trichomoniasis is a vaginal infection that is primarily sexually transmitted. Approximately 3 million cases occur annually in the United States, primarily in women aged 15 to 40 years.[1] The causative organism is *Trichomonas vaginalis,* a flagellated protozoan. The incubation period averages 7 days. Infection can occur by various alternative routes, including passage from mother to infant and bathing in a tub recently used by an infected individual.[1]

Diagnosis

Culture of the responsible organism is the most sensitive diagnostic test. The mobile trichomonads may be visualized on a saline wet-mount preparation, although the sensitivity for wet-mount analysis is only 60% to 70%.[2]

Clinical Complications

The organism may spread to cause infection in the Bartholin glands, urethra, bladder, and Skene's ducts.[1] Trichomoniasis also facilitates the spread of human immunodeficiency virus and is associated with preterm deliveries and low-birth-weight infants.[3]

Management

Patients should be treated with metronidazole for 7 days. Topical treatments such as metronidazole gel are not recommended because of their poor efficacy. Sexual contacts should also be treated.

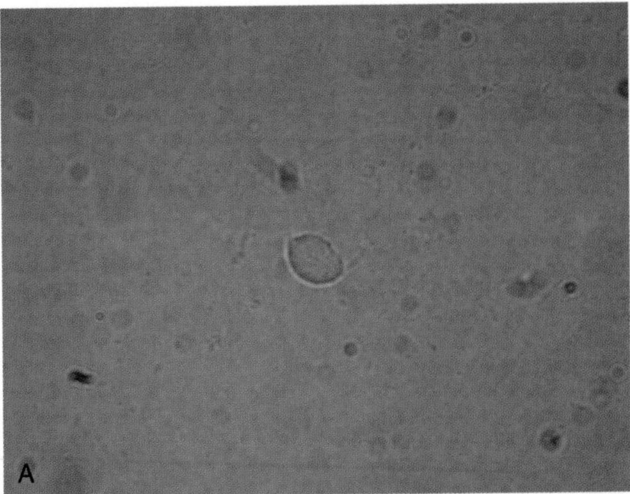

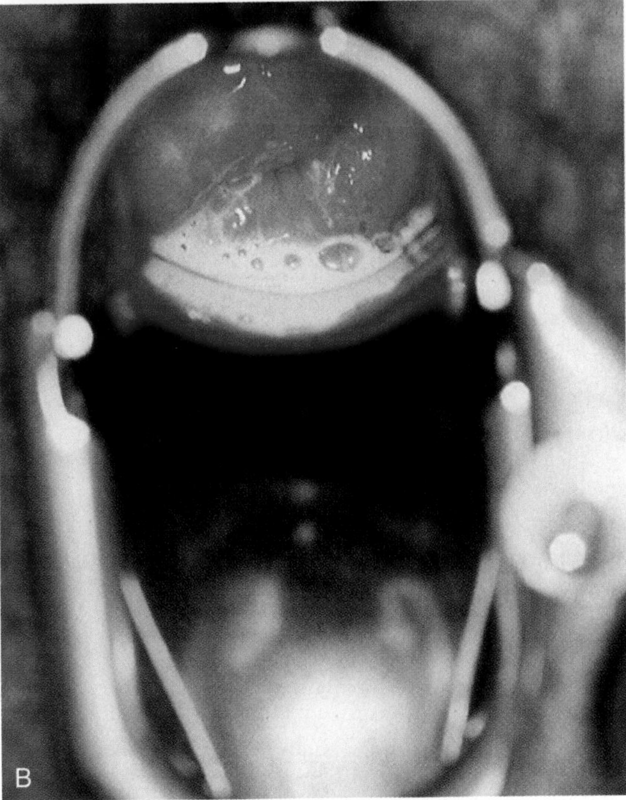

FIGURE 12–11 **A:** Trichomonad on microscopy. (Courtesy of Robert Hendrickson, MD.) **B:** Frothy vaginal discharge of trichomoniasis. (From Rein MF. In: Holmes KK et al, eds. *Sexually transmitted diseases.* New York: McGraw-Hill; 1984.)

REFERENCES

1. Fiumara NJ. Genital ulcer infections in the female patient and the vaginitides. *Dermatol Clin* 1997;15:233–245.
2. Workowski KA, Levine WC. Sexually transmitted diseases treatment guidelines—2002. *MMWR Morb Mortal Wkly Rep* 2002;51(RR-6): 1–80.
3. Zeger W, Holt K. Gynecologic infections. *Emerg Med Clin North Am* 2003;21:631–648.

Herpes Genitalis

Anthony Morocco

Clinical Presentation

Patients with herpes genitalis develop burning, painful, vesicular lesions on the vulva, vagina, or cervix. Lesions may also involve the urethra, buttocks, perineum, and upper thighs. Inguinal lymphadenopathy may be noted on examination. Vesicles rupture, leaving an erythematous ulcer that forms a crust. Time from initial symptoms to complete healing is 3 weeks. Dysuria is present in 80% of cases. With the first outbreak (primary genital herpes), systemic symptoms are present in 80% of cases and may include fever, malaise, myalgias, abdominal pain, and headache. The primary outbreak also results in more extensive and longer-lasting lesions. Recurrent attacks may be precipitated by stress, trauma, fever, menses, ultraviolet light, heat, cold, infection, or immunodeficiency.[1,2]

Pathophysiology

Genital herpes is a common sexually transmitted infection caused by the herpes simplex virus (HSV). It is the most common cause of genital ulcers.[1] Of the two subtypes, HSV-2 is the more common cause of genital infections. HSV-1, which commonly causes herpes labialis, is responsible for 15% to 30% of genital infections.[1] The viruses may be spread by oral or genital contact. The first outbreak occurs 3 days to 2 weeks after exposure. After primary infection, the virus becomes latent in the sacral sensory ganglia. Viral shedding occurs for 3 weeks after a primary outbreak, but for only 3 days after a recurrence. Viral shedding can occur even in the absence of lesions.[2]

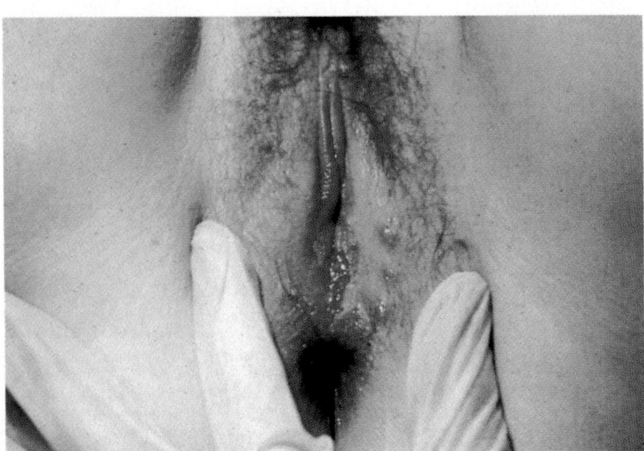

FIGURE 12–12 Primary genital herpes of the vulva. A woman with classic primary genital herpes shows the bilaterally distributed lesions. She complained of headache, malaise, and myalgias and had a low-grade fever. Primary herpes simplex virus (HSV) infection also involved the urethra and cervix in this woman, and HSV-2 was isolated from urethral swabs and urine. Clinically, one cannot distinguish primary genital herpes due to HSV-1 from that due to HSV-2; only laboratory assays can distinguish between the two viral subtypes. (From Mandell, with permission.)

Diagnosis

The diagnosis can generally be made by the appearance of the lesions and a history of recurrent outbreaks. Viral cultures and serology can confirm the diagnosis, and these tests have supplanted the Tzanck smear. Testing for syphilis should be considered in all cases.[1]

Clinical Complications

HSV infection can enhance the transmission of human immunodeficiency virus.[1] Primary HSV infection can result in urinary retention, neuralgia, and meningoencephalitis. Disseminated or severe infection occurs in neonates and in immunocompromised patients.[2]

Management

Treatment with the antiviral medications acyclovir, famciclovir, or valacyclovir within 24 hours after symptom onset may speed resolution.[3] These medications are also used prophylactically to prevent recurrences in those who have six or more episodes per year.[1,3]

REFERENCES

1. Zeger W, Holt K. Gynecologic infections. *Emerg Med Clin North Am* 2003;21:631–648.
2. Yeung-Yue KA, Brentjens MH, Lee PC, Tyring SK. Herpes simplex viruses 1 and 2. *Dermatol Clin* 2002;20:249–266.
3. Workowski KA, Levine WC. Sexually transmitted diseases treatment guidelines—2002. *MMWR Morb Mortal Wkly Rep* 2002;51(RR-6): 1–80.

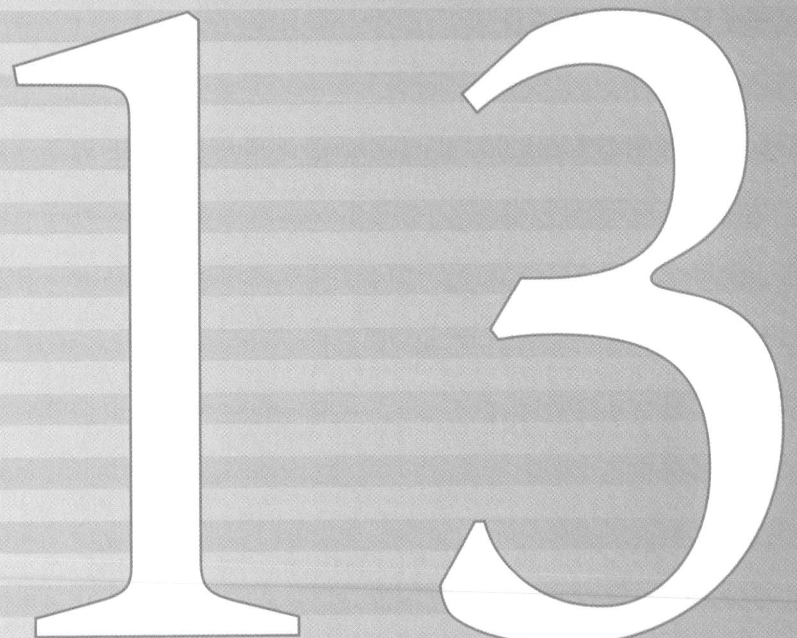

Obstetrics

13-1

Pelvic Ultrasonography

Anthony Morocco

Pelvic ultrasonography has become a valuable tool for the evaluation of lower abdominal pain and pregnancy-related pathology in the emergency department.

Pelvic sonograms may be performed by a transabdominal (TAS) or an endovaginal (EVS) approach. TAS allows a wider view of the pelvis and more superior structures, and it is less invasive. The advantages of EVS are greater resolution and better visualization of the uterus and adnexal structures, better visualization of a uterus that is retroverted or affected by large fibroids, no requirement for a full bladder, and better imaging in obese patients.[1]

Ultrasonography in the first trimester of pregnancy is useful for assessing fetal viability and ectopic pregnancy. A gestational sac can first be visualized by EVS at 4.5 weeks of gestational age and by TAS 7 to 10 days later. The true gestational sac is visualized as a double decidual sac, with an anechoic center surrounded by two echogenic concentric rings. At 5 to 6 weeks, the yolk sac is seen, followed by the fetal pole. Cardiac activity is visualized by EVS at 6 weeks of gestational age.[1]

Patients with bleeding or pain early in pregnancy can be evaluated for a number of findings, including fetal viability, location of pregnancy, retained products after incomplete abortion, and molar pregnancy. For ectopic pregnancy evaluation, evidence of an intrauterine pregnancy (IUP) should be present on EVS if the serum β-human chorionic gonadotropin (hCG) concentration is greater than approximately 1,500 to 2,000 mIU/mL. Findings consistent with ectopic pregnancy include lack of a definite IUP with this concentration of hCG and the presence of an adnexal mass, viable ectopic gestation, free fluid in the pelvis, and adnexal tenderness with probe pressure.[1]

Ultrasonography can diagnose a number of problems in the third trimester of pregnancy, including placenta previa, placental abruption, and traumatic injuries (e.g. abruption, uterine rupture).[1]

Several other diagnoses may be confirmed by pelvic ultrasound when evaluating lower abdominal pain. Tubo-ovarian abscess is diagnosed by visualization of a thickened, fluid-filled fallopian tube. Various types of cysts can be visualized in the ovaries, and free fluid in the pelvis may be indicative of cyst rupture. Color-flow Doppler ultrasonography may reveal an enlarged ovary with decreased blood flow in ovarian torsion.[1]

REFERENCES

1. Phelan MB, Valley VT, Mateer JR. Pelvic ultrasonography. *Emerg Med Clin North Am* 1997;15:789–824.

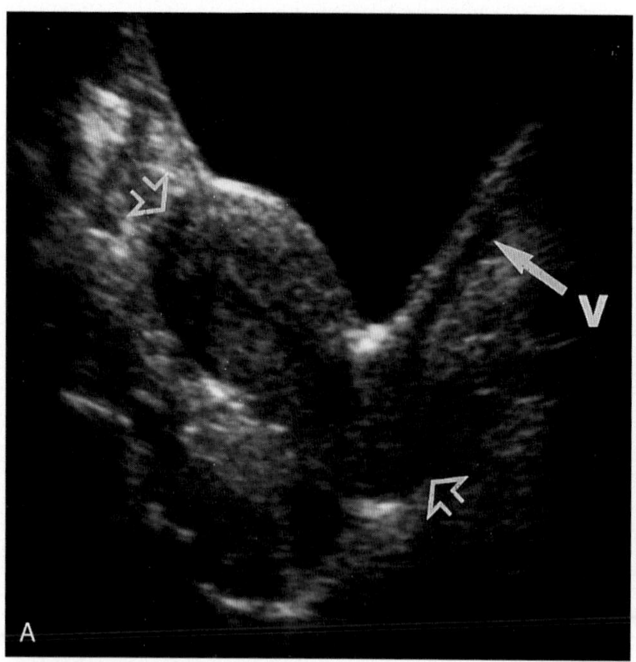

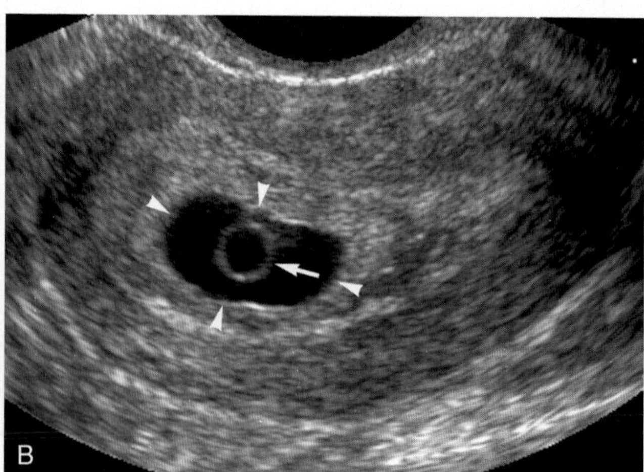

FIGURE 13–1 **A:** Normal sagittal pelvic ultrasonogram. (From Sauerbrei, with permission.) **B:** Gestational sac. (From Doubilet and Benson, with permission.)

Pelvic Ultrasonography

Anthony Morocco

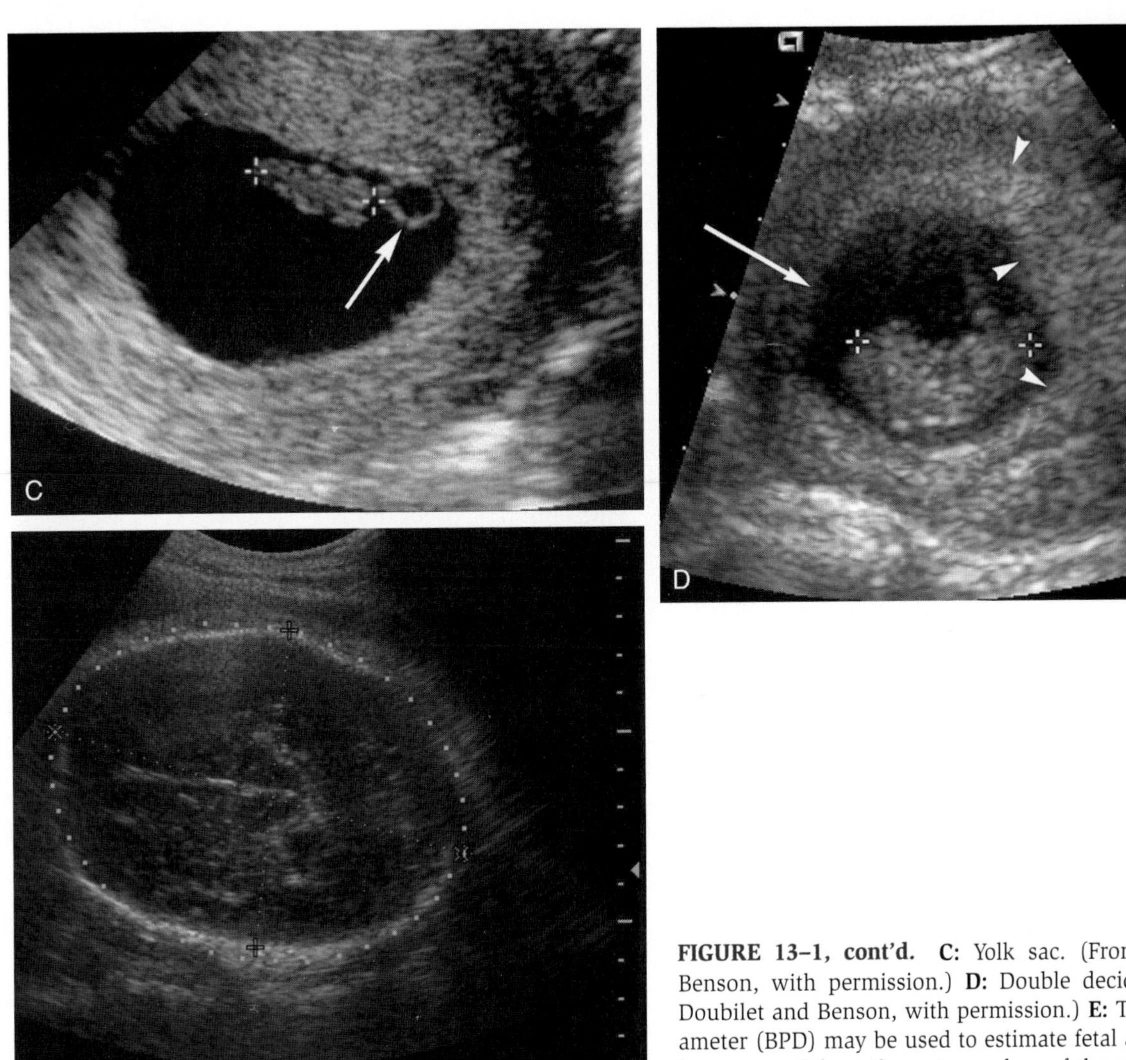

FIGURE 13–1, cont'd. C: Yolk sac. (From Doubilet and Benson, with permission.) **D:** Double decidual sac. (From Doubilet and Benson, with permission.) **E:** The biparietal diameter (BPD) may be used to estimate fetal age. BPD should be measured from the outer surface of the proximal calvaria to the inner surface of the distal calvaria in the thalamic scan plane. (Courtesy of Eric Adar, MD.)

Preeclampsia/Eclampsia

Jennifer Hendrickson

Clinical Presentation

Patients with preeclampsia typically present in the third trimester of pregnancy with hypertension and proteinuria, accompanied by any or all of the following: nondependent edema, epigastric or right upper quadrant pain, headache, and visual disturbances. **H**emolysis, **e**levated **l**iver enzymes, and **l**ow **p**latelet concentration are sometimes seen; these abnormalities are the hallmark of the HELLP syndrome, a subtype of preeclampsia. Rarely, a patient presents after or during an eclamptic seizure.[1]

Pathophysiology

Preeclampsia is a syndrome specific to pregnancy that is defined by hypertension (140/90 mm Hg or higher) and proteinuria (0.3 g or greater per 24 hours), with onset occurring after 20 weeks of gestation. Eclampsia is defined as the syndrome of new-onset seizures occurring in a patient who has been diagnosed with preeclampsia.[1] Preeclampsia is estimated to occur in 5% to 8% of pregnancies, with approximately 1% of those cases progressing to eclampsia.[2] The cause of preeclampsia is unknown; however, vascular changes occur that result in vasospasm and endothelial damage. This leads to hypertension, edema, and end-organ damage.[1] Risk factors for preeclampsia include primiparity, multiple gestations, prior preeclampsia, chronic hypertension, autoimmune disease, pregestational diabetes, nephropathy, obesity, age older than 35 years, and African-American race.[1]

Diagnosis

Because the presenting complaints for preeclamptics are often vague, the physician must have a high index of suspicion. Blood pressure assessment suggests the diagnosis, at which point a urine dipstick for protein can quickly be performed (1+ or greater is suspicious). Liver enzymes, complete blood count, and lactate dehydrogenase or peripheral blood smear are abnormal in patients exhibiting the HELLP variant. In those presenting with seizures, other causes should be ruled out, including arteriovenous malformations, ruptured aneurysm, and idiopathic seizure disorder.[1]

Clinical Complications

The hypertension, vasospasm, and endothelial damage that occur with preeclampsia can result in numerous adverse outcomes. Cerebral edema and herniation, intracranial hemorrhage, renal failure, subcapsular hepatic hematoma and capsule rupture, and pulmonary edema all contribute to maternal mortality. Fetal morbidity and mortality arise from placental abruption, premature delivery, and growth restriction.[1]

Management

The cure for preeclampsia is delivery; however, the mode and timing of delivery must be individualized. Obstetric consultation should be obtained as soon as possible, with transfer to a tertiary care facility for the preterm gestation. If gestation is less than 34 weeks, corticosteroids should be administered to promote lung maturity in the event of delivery. For the patient with eclampsia, control of blood pressure and seizure activity is paramount. Diastolic blood pressures greater than 105 to 110 mm Hg should be treated with parenteral antihypertensives; labetalol and hydralazine have both been extensively studied.[1] Prospective, randomized controlled trials have validated magnesium sulfate as the drug of choice for eclamptic seizures, and it can be given intravenously or intramuscularly.[2,3]

REFERENCES

1. ACOG Practice Bulletin. Diagnosis and management of preeclampsia and eclampsia. *Obstet Gynecol* 2002;99:159–167.
2. Witlin AG. Prevention and treatment of eclamptic convulsions. *Clin Obstet Gynecol* 1999;42:507–518.
3. Which anticonvulsant for women with eclampsia? Evidence from the Collaborative Eclampsia Trial. *Lancet* 1995;345:1455–1463.

Preeclampsia/Eclampsia

Jennifer Hendrickson

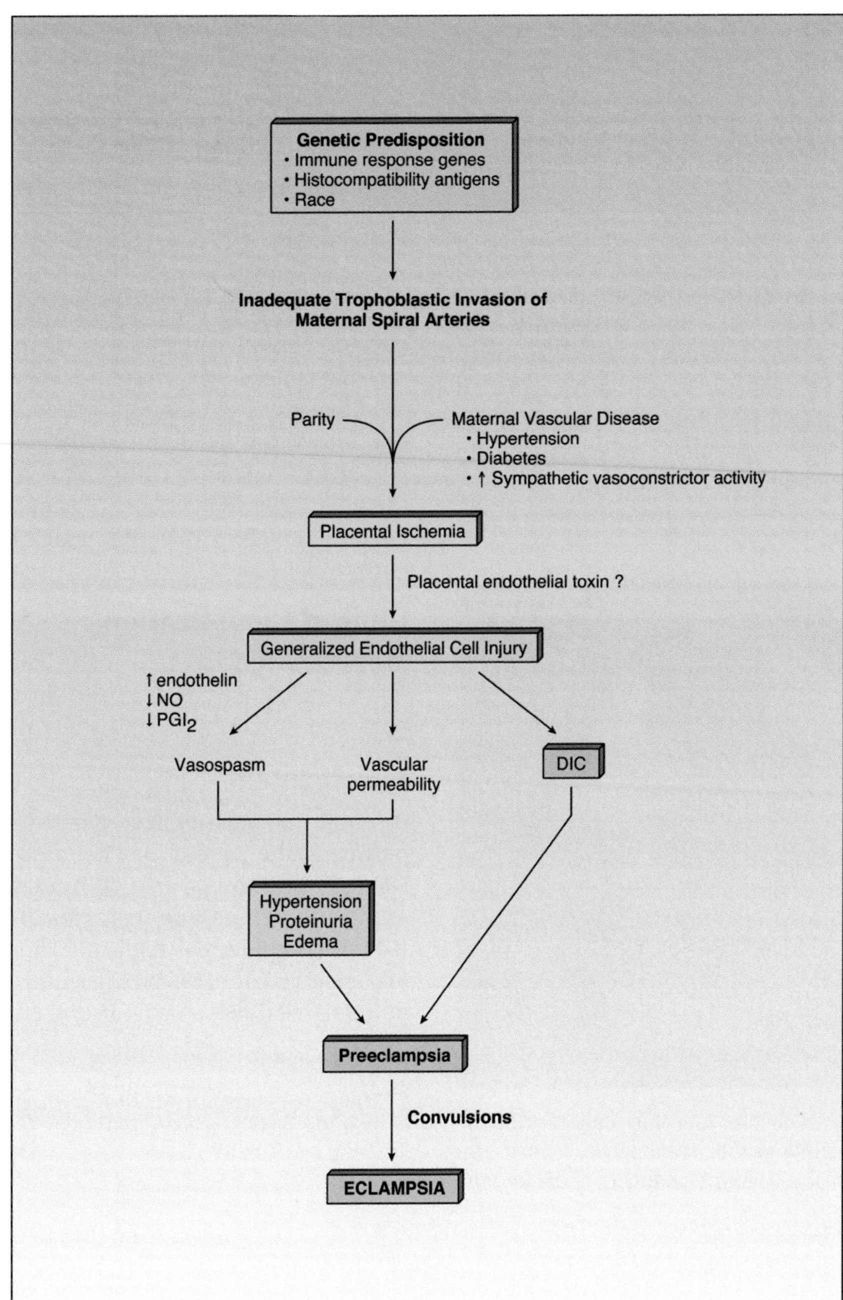

FIGURE 13–2 Pathogenesis of preeclampsia and eclampsia. (From Rubin, with permission.)

13-3

Melasma (Mask of Pregnancy)

Jennifer Hendrickson

Clinical Presentation

Women with melasma typically present during pregnancy with patchy, darkened, macular lesions of the cheeks, forehead, and upper lip. The neck and forearms can also be affected, but lesions are limited to sun-exposed areas.[1]

Pathophysiology

Melasma is an acquired disorder that results in a blotchy hyperpigmentation of the face. It is most frequently seen in pregnant women, earning the name "mask of pregnancy," but can also be seen in women who use oral contraceptives or phenytoin.[1] Although the exact cause of melasma is unknown, a genetic predisposition appears to exist.[1] Ultraviolet (UV) exposure and sex steroids, particularly progesterone, appear to be key mediators.[1] Melanin deposition can occur in either the dermal or the epidermal layer; only the epidermal variant is responsive to topical bleaching agents. The hyperpigmentation tends to increase as the pregnancy progresses, with some regression once delivery occurs. Some or all of the pigmentation may be permanent.

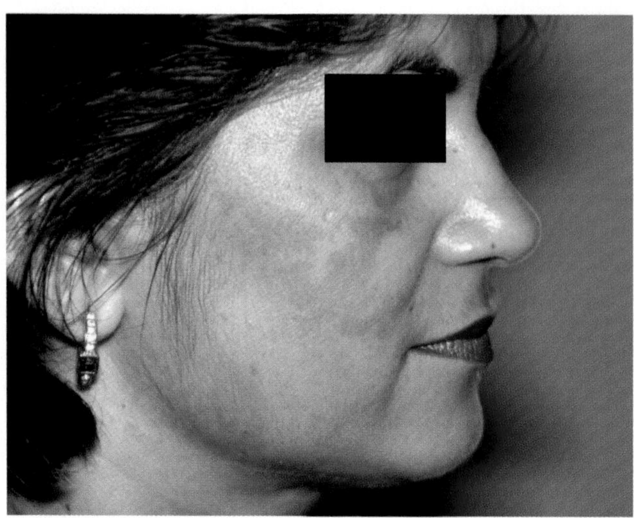

FIGURE 13–3 Melasma of cheeks. Melasma may result from pregnancy, oral contraceptive use, or menopause. It may also arise for no apparent reason. (From Goodheart, with permission.)

Diagnosis

Diagnosis is made on physical examination. Differentiation of dermal from epidermal melasma is important when considering therapy, because dermal melasma does not respond to bleaching agents. A Wood's lamp examination that accentuates the demarcation between normal and hyperpigmented skin suggests epidermal melasma. Differential diagnosis includes erythematic dyschromicum perstans (ashy dermatosis), postinflammatory hyperpigmentation, and vitiligo of the surrounding area.

Clinical Complications

Melasma is strictly a cosmetic alteration. Sensitivity to treatment modalities can result in a worsening of the appearance due to hypersensitivity pigmentation.

Management

Although no treatment is needed in the emergency department, the patient may be informed that avoidance of UV light and liberal use of sunscreen that blocks UV-A and UV-B are first-line therapies. Bleaching regimens are useful for epidermal melasma; however, these are usually reserved for the postpartum period. Laser therapy and chemical peels have also been used.

REFERENCES

1. Halder R, Nandedkar M, Neal K. Pigmentary disorders in ethnic skin. *Dermatol Clin* 2003;21:617–627.

Hyperemesis Gravidarum

Marisa Stumpf and Jacob W. Ufberg

Clinical Presentation

Women with hyperemesis gravidarum may present with intractable vomiting in the first trimester of pregnancy. Although nausea and vomiting are common in early pregnancy (50% to 90%), patients with hyperemesis gravidarum (approximately 0.5%) have persistent, intractable vomiting and may develop weight loss, dehydration, metabolic acidosis and alkalosis, hyponatremia, hypochloremia, and hypokalemia.[1,2] Symptoms usually begin at 5 to 6 weeks of gestation, peak at 9 weeks, and abate by 16 to 18 weeks. However, a small percentage of patients continue to have symptoms until delivery.[1]

Pathophysiology

Hyperemesis gravidarum is a syndrome characterized by intractable vomiting during pregnancy. The cause of hyperemesis gravidarum is unknown and is most likely multifactorial. Several hormones have been implicated (e.g., β-human chorionic gonadotropin [hCG], estradiol, 17-hydroxyprogesterone) because their concentration peaks as the incidence of hyperemesis gravidarum peaks; however, no cause-and-effect relationship has been established.[1] The thyroid hormone concentration may be higher in patients with hyperemesis gravidarum, most likely from an effect of particular subtypes of hCG on the thyroid-stimulating hormone (TSH) receptor. Other possible factors include altered gastrointestinal motility, hepatic function, lipid metabolism, and psychological issues.[1]

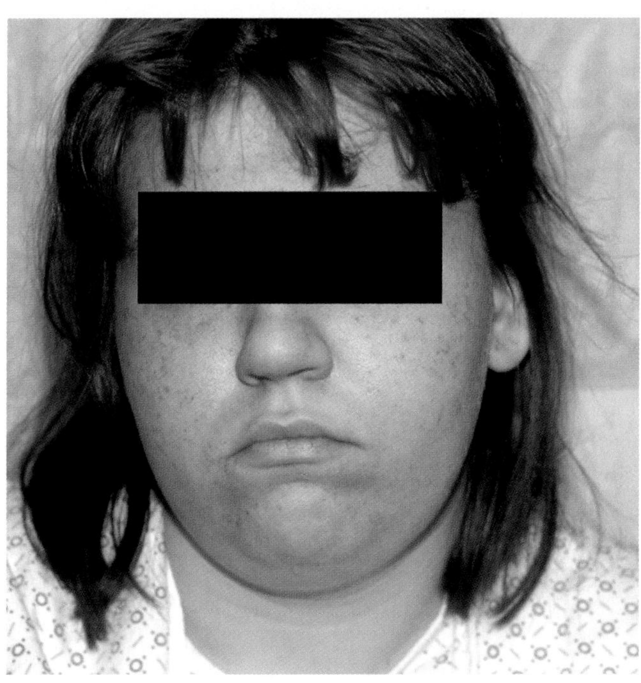

FIGURE 13–4 Facial petechiae secondary to persistent vomiting. (© David Effron, MD, 2004. Used with permission.)

Diagnosis

The diagnosis can be made clinically. Laboratory findings may include ketonemia, ketonuria, elevated hematocrit, and elevated blood urea nitrogen. Hyperemesis gravidarum leads to elevations in liver enzymes in 40% of patients who are hospitalized with hyperemesis.[2] The differential diagnosis includes gastroenteritis, cholecystitis, pancreatitis, hepatitis, peptic ulcer, pyelonephritis, and fatty liver of pregnancy.

Clinical Complications

Clinical complications are related to vomiting (weight loss, syncope, dehydration, pneumothorax, pneumomediastinum, Mallory-Weiss tears).

Management

Management consists of adequate fluid resuscitation, correction of acid–base and electrolyte abnormalities, and thiamine supplementation.[2] Patients with mild symptoms may require only rehydration and antiemetics (oral and suppository) on discharge. Patients with severe symptoms may require intravenous antiemetic and fluid therapy. Patients who are unable to tolerate oral hydration should be admitted to the hospital. The antiemetics, including metoclopramide, promethazine, prochlorperazine, chlorpromazine, and ondansetron, are all effective and there are no data to support one over another.[2] Oral corticosteroids may also be effective in decreasing the frequency of vomiting.[2]

REFERENCES

1. Eliakim R, Abulafia O, Sherer DM. Hyperemesis gravidarum: a current review. *Am J Perinatol* 2000;17:207–218.
2. Goodwin TM. Hyperemesis gravidarum. *Clin Obstet Gynecol* 1998; 41:597–605.

13-5

Pruritic Urticarial Papules and Plaques of Pregnancy

Jennifer Hendrickson

Clinical Presentation

Pruritic urticarial papules and plaques of pregnancy, known as PUPPP, arises most often in the third trimester, with a mean onset at 35 weeks. Eruptions are polymorphous, typically arising from the abdominal striae and spreading to the rest of the trunk and extremities. Patients report rapid onset of intense pruritus that spontaneously resolves shortly after delivery.[1]

Pathophysiology

PUPPP is the most common dermatologic disorder specific to pregnancy. PUPPP affects 1 of every 130 to 300 pregnancies, occurring most frequently in primigravidas and those with multiple gestations.[2] The exact pathophysiology of PUPPP is not clearly defined; some researchers have postulated rapid abdominal distention as a causative factor, whereas the presence of fetal DNA in PUPPP skin lesions has caused others to propose an immune-mediated etiology.[2]

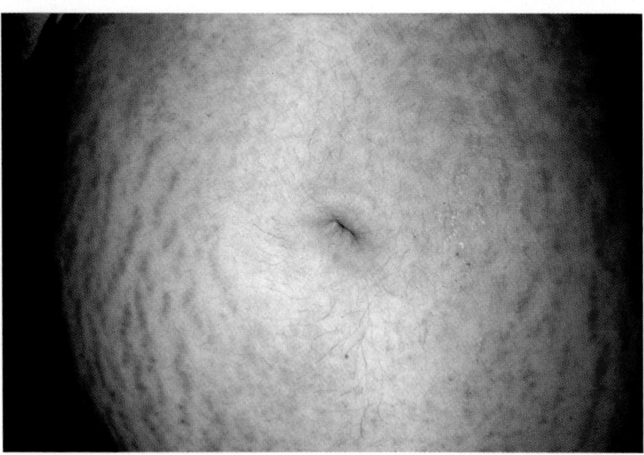

FIGURE 13–5 Rash of pruritic urticarial papules and plaques of pregnancy (PUPPP) in a woman in the third trimester of pregnancy. (© Jeff Callen, MD. Used with permission.)

Diagnosis

PUPPP is mainly a diagnosis of exclusion, because there are no laboratory abnormalities or histopathologic findings specific to this condition. The differential diagnosis includes viral exanthems, drug rashes, herpes gestationis, and intrahepatic cholestasis of pregnancy (ICP).[1] Because of the adverse fetal effects associated with ICP, bile acids should be measured to rule out this diagnosis.

Clinical Complications

With the exception of maternal discomfort from intense pruritus, PUPPP does not appear to cause any adverse effects on the mother or fetus. Spontaneous regression is expected shortly after delivery, and recurrence is rare.[1,2]

Management

Management consists entirely of treating the maternal pruritus. Oral antihistamines and topical steroids are the initial treatment modalities. Some severe cases may require a short course of oral steroids.[1,2]

REFERENCES

1. Sherard GB 3rd, Atkinson SM Jr. Focus on primary care: pruritic dermatological conditions in pregnancy. *Obstet Gynecol Surv* 2001;56:427–432.
2. Kroumpouzos G, Cohen LM. Specific dermatoses of pregnancy: an evidence-based systematic review. *Am J Obstet Gynecol* 2003;188:1083–1092.

Herpes Gestationis

Jennifer Hendrickson

Clinical Presentation

Women with herpes gestationis (HG) typically present with an abrupt onset of urticarial, bullous lesions in the second or early third trimester, although 25% present in the immediate postpartum period.[1] Initially limited to the trunk, these intensely pruritic lesions spread, sparing only the face, palms, soles, and mucous membranes. Most cases resolve spontaneously after delivery; however, postpartum flares and recurrence with menses or with oral contraceptive use have been reported.[2]

Pathophysiology

HG is an autoimmune, dermatologic disorder that occurs in 1 of every 10,000 to 50,000 pregnancies and, rarely, in gestational trophoblastic disease.[1] Some authors have suggested the name *pemphigoid gestationis,* because the disorder is not caused by the herpes virus and bears similarities to bullous pemphigoid.[2] HG is most likely caused by complement fixation that produces dissolution of the dermal–epidermal bond, resulting in bullae formation. Placental tissue appears to be instrumental in the formation of the responsible antibodies.[2]

Diagnosis

The differential diagnosis of HG includes pruritic and urticarial pustules and papules of pregnancy (PUPPP), intrahepatic cholestasis of pregnancy (in which skin lesions arise secondary to scratching), prurigo, and pruritic folliculitis of pregnancy. Drug eruptions and allergic contact dermatitis should also be considered.[1,2] Definitive diagnosis is made by biopsy: a linear band of complement C3 along the basement membrane confirms the diagnosis.[1]

Clinical Complications

Ten percent of neonates of affected mothers are born with HG lesions, secondary to placental transfer of maternal antibodies. Some studies have shown increased risks for premature delivery and small-for-gestational-age infants.[2] Patients with HG may be at risk for development of other autoimmune disorders.[2]

Management

The mainstay of treatment is systemic corticosteroids. Any patient given this type of steroid regimen antenatally should receive "stress doses" of steroids at delivery. Severe cases have been treated with chemotherapeutic agents, plasmapheresis, intravenous immune globulin, cyclosporine, or tetracycline.[1,2] Breast feeding is not only safe but recommended, because it may shorten the duration of the lesions.[2]

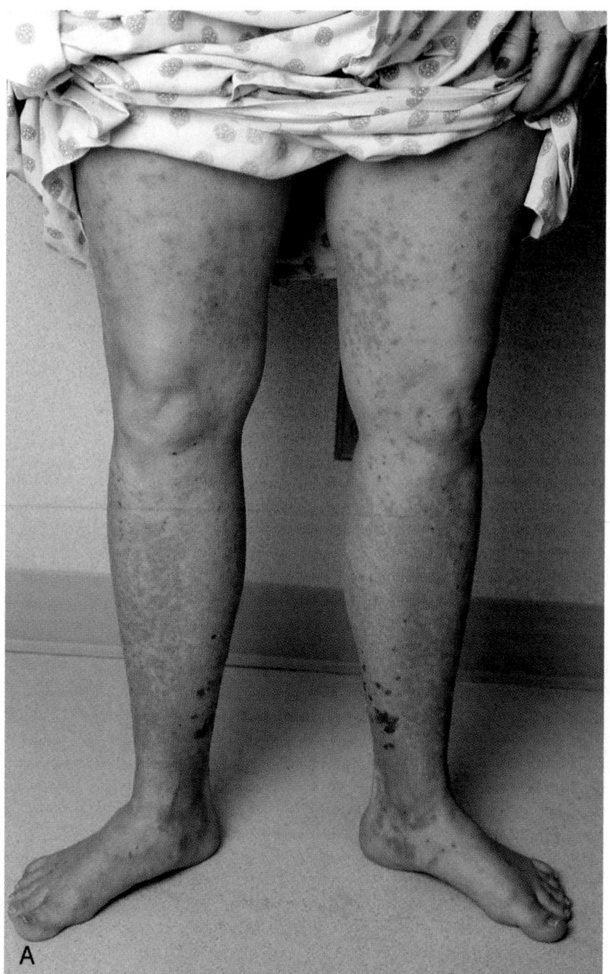

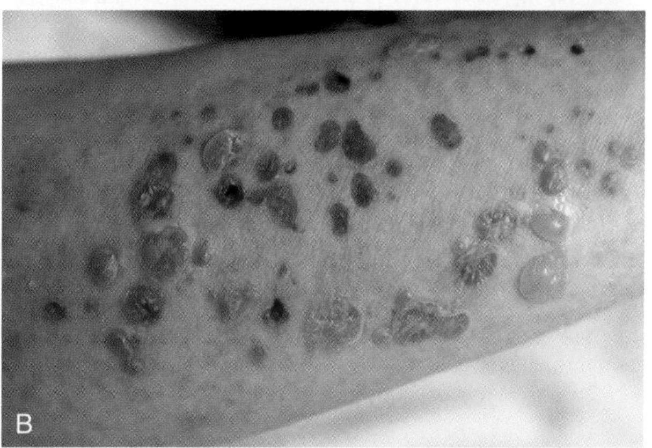

FIGURE 13-6 A and **B:** Herpes gestationis. (Courtesy of Thorsten Lundsgaarde, MD.)

REFERENCES

1. Kroumpouzos G, Cohen LM. Specific dermatoses of pregnancy: an evidence-based systematic review. *Am J Obstet Gynecol* 2003;188: 1083–1092.
2. Sherard GB 3rd, Atkinson SM Jr. Focus on primary care: pruritic dermatological conditions in pregnancy. *Obstet Gynecol Surv* 2001; 56:427–432.

Hydatidiform Mole

Jennifer Hendrickson

Pathophysiology

Hydatidiform mole (HM) is the benign lesion of gestational trophoblastic neoplasms (GTN), a spectrum of disorders that range from HM to invasive malignant disease.[1] HM is further classified as partial or complete HM. Incidence of both types has been reported to be 1/1,000 pregnancies worldwide.[2] Molar pregnancies arise from a genetic event that results in abnormal chromosomes in the conceptus. Complete moles are 46XX or 46XY by karyotype, but both sets of chromosomes are paternal. Partial moles are most commonly triploid.[2]

Diagnosis

Patients typically present in the first trimester of pregnancy with vaginal bleeding. In the case of complete moles, ultrasound reveals no fetal tissue and the classic "snowstorm" appearance in the uterine cavity. Serum β-human chorionic gonadotropin (hCG) often is elevated above expected values (often in excess of 100,000 mIU/mL), and the uterus is larger than expected for gestational age. Classically, patients with molar pregnancy also present with theca-lutein cysts (50%), hyperemesis (26%), preeclampsia before 24 weeks of gestation (27%), and hyperthyroidism (7%); however, with the institution of early and accurate ultrasonography, these presentations are less frequent.[2]

Partial moles have less distinctive findings, and there may be a developing fetus along with the molar tissue. Patients with partial moles most typically present with spontaneous abortion, and the diagnosis is most frequently made on pathologic examination of the conceptus.[2]

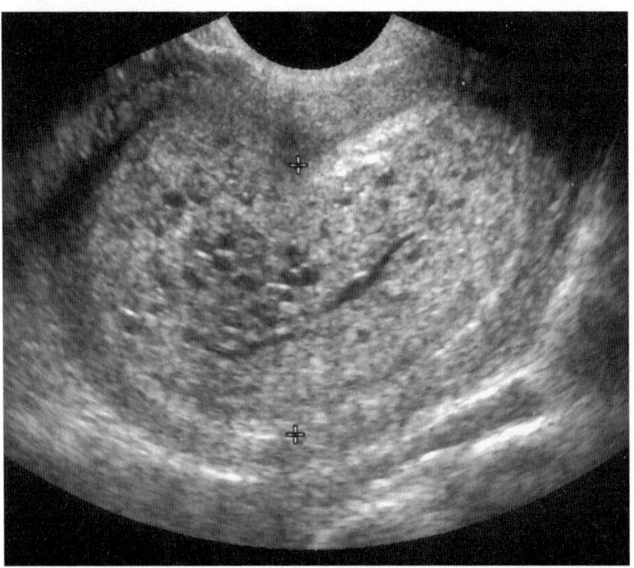

FIGURE 13–7 Ultrasonogram showing uterine mass with hypoechoic areas consistent with hydatidiform mole. (Courtesy of Kristina Vogel, MD.)

Clinical Complications

The main complication of molar pregnancy is the persistence of GTN that can progress to invasive malignancy and metastasis. Because of this, close gynecologic follow-up should be arranged. Trophoblastic embolization and resultant respiratory distress can occur at the time of evacuation.[2]

Management

Once a molar pregnancy is diagnosed, treatment consists of surgical evacuation. This is usually accomplished via suction curettage; however hysterotomy and hysterectomy are considered acceptable options. If the patient is Rh-factor negative, RhoGAM® should be administered. Evacuation is curative in 80% of cases. In those cases considered to carry a high risk for persistent GTN, chemotherapy may be considered.[1] Serum quantitative hCG should be measured at the time of evacuation and weekly thereafter until it is nondetectable for 3 weeks. After this, surveillance of hCG measurements and use of contraception for 6 months is the accepted method of follow-up.[2]

REFERENCES

1. Lawrence LL. Unusual presentations in obstetrics and gynecology. *Emerg Med Clin* 2003;21:649–665.
2. Shapter AP, McLellan R. Gestational trophoblastic disease. *Obstet Gynecol Clin North Am* 2001;28:805–817.

Ectopic Pregnancy

Jennifer Hendrickson

Clinical Presentation

The classic triad of symptoms of ectopic pregnancy (EP) consists of vaginal bleeding, amenorrhea, and abdominal pain, although these symptoms may also be present in intrauterine pregnancies (IUPs). Patients with tubal rupture may develop severe abdominal pain, peritoneal signs, and hypovolemia. Risk factors for EP include prior tubal surgery, previous EP, a history of pelvic inflammatory disease, assisted reproduction, and the presence of an intrauterine device. However, a high level of suspicion must be maintained, because 40% to 50% of EPs occur in patients with no risk factors.[1]

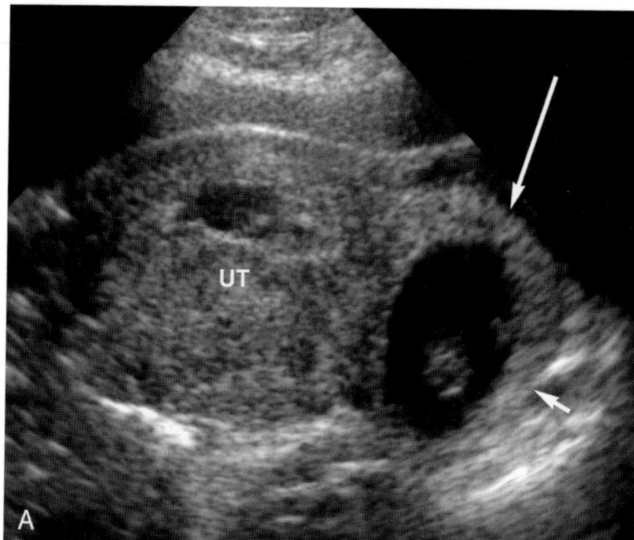

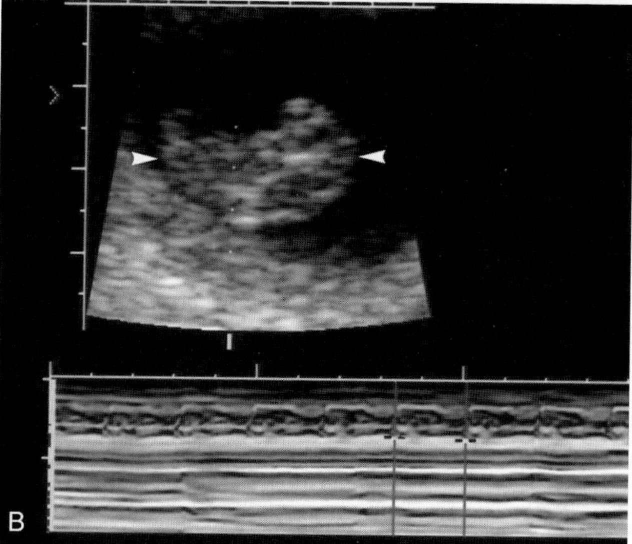

FIGURE 13–8 **A:** Transverse transabdominal ultrasonogram showing cornual gestational sac. **B:** Sagittal M-mode ultrasonogram of gestational sac reveals cardiac activity. (**A** and **B** from Doubilet and Benson, with permission.)

Pathophysiology

EP is defined as any pregnancy implanted outside the uterine cavity. EP occurs in 2% of all pregnancies and account for 9% of all maternal deaths.[2] The implantation of a fertilized ovum can occur at any point along the pathway from the ovary to the endometrium, although 97% of EPs occur in the fallopian tube.[1] Heterotopic pregnancies (coexistence of an IUP and an EP) occur very rarely (1 in 3,000 to 8,000 pregnancies) if no fertility treatments have been performed.[1]

Diagnosis

Transvaginal ultrasonography should detect an IUP if the β-human chorionic gonadotropin (hCG) concentration is greater than 1,500 mIU/mL.[2] An empty uterus with a hCG level beyond this threshold is suspicious for EP. A negative serum hCG essentially rules out EP.[2] In patients with hCG less than 1,500 mIU/mL and no evidence of rupture (e.g., peritoneal signs, hemodynamic instability, peritoneal fluid), obstetric consultation and follow-up in 48 hours for a repeat hCG determination may be appropriate. Inappropriately rising hCG levels (less than 66% in 48 hours) is suspicious for EP. Controversies surrounding the diagnosis are discussed elsewhere.[1]

Clinical Complications

Complications include hypovolemic shock, tubal scarring, and infertility.

Management

Pregnant patients with hemodynamic instability and a history consistent with EP require emergency obstetric consultation, large-bore fluid resuscitation, and, possibly, blood transfusion before diagnostic studies are attempted. Stable patients with evidence of tubal rupture (peritoneal signs or fluid) also require resuscitation and emergency obstetric consultation. Stable patients with no evidence of rupture may be candidates for laparoscopic treatment or medical therapy with methotrexate injection. An obstetrician should be consulted to determine the best course of action. If the diagnosis is uncertain and the patient is stable, follow-up with an obstetrician and a repeat hCG determination in 48 hours may be arranged.

REFERENCES

1. Della-Giustina D, Denny M. Ectopic pregnancy. *Emerg Med Clin North Am* 2003;21:565–584.
2. ACEP Clinical Policies Committee and Clinical Policies Subcommittee on Early Pregnancy. Clinical policy: critical issues in the initial evaluation and management of patients presenting to the emergency department in early pregnancy. *Ann Emerg Med* 2003;41: 123–133.

13-9

Placenta Previa

Jennifer Hendrickson

Clinical Presentation

Patients with placenta previa (PP) classically present with painless vaginal bleeding in the late second or third trimester of pregnancy. The initial episode typically occurs without warning and often is self-limited. This "sentinel" bleed usually is followed by a more significant bleeding episode days to weeks later. If the condition is not addressed and the pregnancy is allowed to proceed to labor, massive maternal hemorrhage and death may result.

Pathophysiology

PP is the abnormal implantation of the placenta, such that the placenta partially or completely covers the internal cervical os. Based on the amount of cervix covered by the placenta, these implantations are further classified as complete, partial, or marginal. The incidence of PP is 1 in 200 births.[1] Implantation of the embryo in the lower uterine segment (LUS) can result in PP. If implantation occurs on the dynamic portion of this highly vascular organ, the placental vascular connections will be disrupted as the LUS thins and the cervix dilates, and bleeding will ensue.[1] Prior cesarean section and multiparity are risk factors for PP. Tobacco and cocaine use have also been implicated.[1]

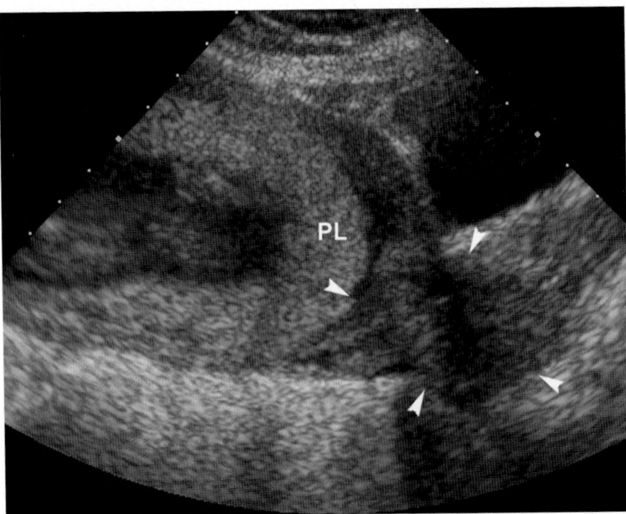

FIGURE 13–9 Complete placenta previa. Sagittal midline view of the lower uterus performed transabdominally demonstrates the placenta (PL) completely covering the cervix *(arrowheads)*. (From Doubilet and Benson, with permission.)

Diagnosis

Any patient who presents with vaginal bleeding after 24 weeks of gestation should be evaluated for PP before a vaginal examination is performed.[1] Diagnosis is made by ultrasonography, which has largely replaced the much-described "double set-up" procedure. Transabdominal ultrasonography has been shown to be 93% accurate in diagnosing PP; in experienced hands, transperineal ultrasound may enhance this accuracy by allowing better visualization of the cervical os.[2]

Clinical Complications

Maternal hemorrhage and fetal morbidity secondary to premature delivery are the most common complications. PP is a risk factor for placenta accreta, a condition in which the placenta is abnormally adherent to the uterus. This condition can increase maternal hemorrhage and necessitate cesarean hysterectomy.

Management

On arrival, the amount of bleeding should be immediately assessed, and fluid resuscitation and blood component therapy should be initiated if indicated. With the exception of some cases of marginal previa, vaginal delivery cannot be accomplished and a cesarean delivery is mandated. Immediate on-site obstetric consultation is essential. Fetal monitoring should be started immediately. Conservative management for preterm pregnancies is possible, with delivery at 36 weeks if conditions allow.[1]

REFERENCES

1. Baron F, Hill WC. Placenta previa, placenta abruptio. *Clin Obstet Gynecol* 1998;41:527–532.
2. Hertzberg BS, Bowie JD, Carroll BA, Kliewer MA, Weber TM. Diagnosis of placenta previa during the third trimester: role of transperineal sonography. *AJR Am J Roentgenol* 1992;159:83–87.

Placental Abruption

Jennifer Hendrickson

Clinical Presentation

Patients with placental abruption (PA) present with painful vaginal bleeding in the third trimester of pregnancy.

Pathophysiology

PA is the partial or total separation of the placenta from the uterus before delivery. The incidence is 6 per 1,000 singleton pregnancies.[1] Bleeding from the small arteries at the interface between the placenta and the uterus results in hematoma formation. Although the exact cause is unknown, vasospasm or vaso-occlusion of these arteries appears to play a key role.[2] Risk factors for PA include hypertension, trauma, maternal use of cocaine or tobacco, prolonged rupture of membranes, thrombophilias, older maternal age, increasing parity, multiple gestations, polyhydramnios, and chorioamnionitis.[2]

Diagnosis

PA must be suspected in any patient presenting with third-trimester bleeding. Diagnosis is confirmed on direct inspection of the placenta after delivery. Ultrasound should be performed to rule out other causes for third-trimester bleeding and to confirm fetal viability in the absence of a fetal monitor; however, the absence of a visible hematoma does not rule out PA.[2] Depending on the severity, bleeding may be minimal and self-limited, or it may progress to massive hemorrhage, maternal disseminated intravascular coagulation (DIC), and fetal death. PA is not ruled out in the absence of vaginal bleeding; retroplacental bleeding within the uterus may manifest as abdominal or low-back pain, with or without fetal compromise. As hemorrhage spreads into the myometrium, the uterus may have a firm, bruised appearance (Couvelaire uterus). Vaginal bleeding and abdominal pain that persists after contractions should raise suspicion of abruption, particularly if fetal heart tones are absent.

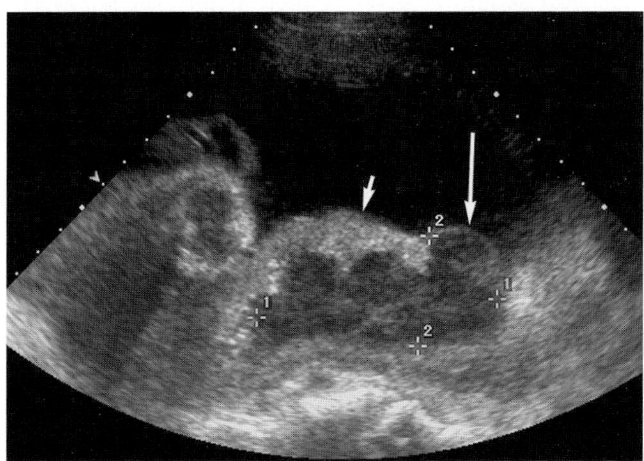

FIGURE 13–10 Placental abruption with retroplacental hematoma. A hypoechoic hematoma *(long arrow and calipers)* is lifting the edge of the placenta *(short arrow)*. (From Doubilet and Benson, with permission.)

Clinical Complications

Complications include maternal hemorrhage, DIC, unplanned hysterectomy, and fetal or maternal death.

Management

Emergency on-site obstetric consultation is mandatory if PA is suspected, because fetal well-being must be assessed as soon as possible. In the event of maternal hemorrhage, fluid resuscitation and preparations for transfusions should be made. Management is tailored to the extent of the abruption; in the event of reassuring fetal status or fetal demise, vaginal delivery can often be accomplished. If fetal compromise is noted or if the status of the mother is unstable, cesarean section should be performed after the initiation of blood component therapy.[2] Coagulation studies should be performed on admission and serially after a PA has been diagnosed.

REFERENCES

1. Ananth CV, Wilcox AJ. Placental abruption and perinatal mortality in the United States. *Am J Epidemiol* 2001;153:332–337.
2. Hladky K, Yankowitz J, Hansen WF. Placental abruption. *Obstet Gynecol Surv* 2002;57:299–305.

13-11

Spontaneous Abortion

Marisa Stumpf and Jacob W. Ufberg

Clinical Presentation

Patients with early pregnancy loss may present to the emergency department with cramping suprapubic pain and vaginal bleeding. Patients with a threatened abortion may complain of continued pain and may have a closed cervical os. Patients with inevitable or incomplete abortions have dilatation of the cervix with pain and bleeding. With incomplete abortions, expelled products of conception may be present in the vaginal vault. Patients with a missed abortion (early fetal demise) may have minimal symptoms or tenderness, a closed cervical os, but no fetal heart motion on ultrasound.[1,2]

Pathophysiology

Spontaneous abortion (loss of pregnancy in the first 20 weeks) may be classified as threatened, inevitable, incomplete, or missed. Early pregnancy loss may be associated with infection, cervical incompetence, genetic anomalies, smoking, or previous miscarriage.

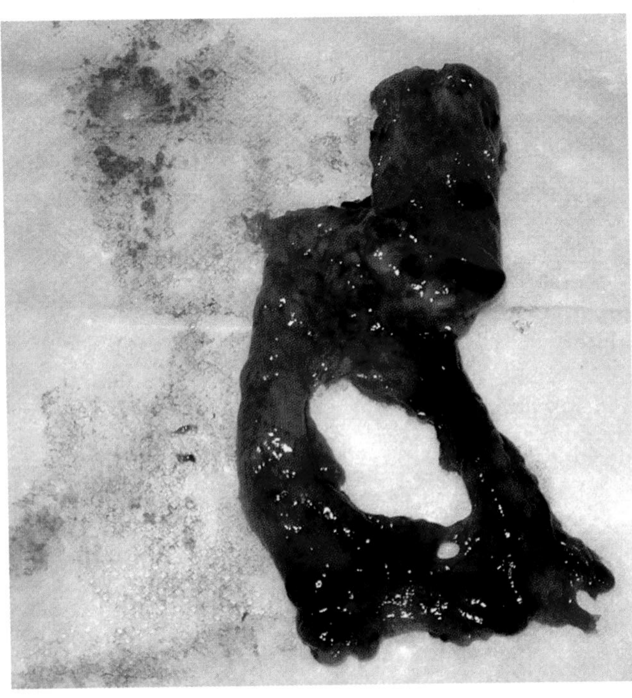

FIGURE 13–11 Products of conception. (Courtesy of Mark Silverberg, MD.)

Diagnosis

The diagnosis is made by history and physical examination and may be confirmed by pelvic ultrasonography. In patients with threatened or missed abortions, the cervical os is closed; these conditions may be differentiated by ultrasonography. In patients with inevitable or incomplete abortions, the cervix is open and there is a mild-to-moderate amount of bleeding.[1,2]

Clinical Complications

Complications from early pregnancy loss include shock (from blood loss) and infection/sepsis.

Management

There is no proven effective therapy for threatened abortion, although bed rest and pelvic rest often are recommended. Patients with inevitable or incomplete abortions require gynecologic consultation and possibly suction curettage.[2] Patients with missed abortions require gynecologic consultation but do not require emergency curettage unless an infection is suspected. A complete blood count with blood and Rh typing should be obtained from all patients with early pregnancy loss. RhoGAM should be given if there is any vaginal bleeding and the patient's blood type is Rh-negative.[1] Kleihauer-Betke cells may be administered after 12 weeks of gestation to determine the dose of RhoGAM.

REFERENCES

1. American College of Emergency Physicians. Clinical policy: critical issues in the initial evaluation and management of patients presenting to the emergency department in early pregnancy. *Ann Emerg Med* 2003;41:123–133.
2. Wieringa-De Waard MW, Hartman EE, Ankum WM, Reitsma JB, Bindels PJ, Bonsel GJ. Expectant management versus surgical evacuation in first trimester miscarriage: health-related quality of life in randomized and non-randomized patients. *Hum Reprod* 2002;17:1638–1642.

Breech Delivery

Marisa Stumpf and Jacob W. Ufberg

Clinical Presentation

Breech presentations occur when the presenting fetal part is not the head. They are more common in preterm deliveries (13%) than in full-term deliveries (3% to 4%).[1] Breech presentations may be classified as frank (hips flexed, knees extended), complete (hips flexed, one or both knees flexed), or incomplete/footling (one or both hips extended).

Pathophysiology

Risk factors for breech presentation include uterine anomalies (bicornuate or septate uterus), placental abnormalities (placenta previa), amniotic fluid abnormalities (polyhydramnios, oligohydramnios), space-occupying lesions (uterine fibroids), altered fetal shape or mobility (anencephaly, hydrocephaly, neurologic impairment, impaired fetal growth), and multiparity.[1,2]

Diagnosis

Breech presentation may be determined by the palpation of the soft buttocks, a foot, or a knee of the fetus through the dilated cervix of a laboring patient. Bedside ultrasonography can quickly confirm any diagnosis made by Leopold's maneuvers and vaginal examination.

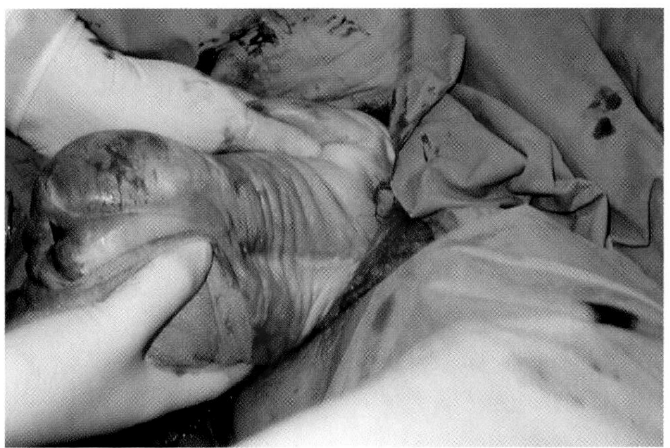

FIGURE 13–12 Breech delivery. (Reprinted with permission from Richard Fischer, MD, and eMedicine.com, Inc., 2003.)

Clinical Complications

Cord prolapse occurs with more frequency in malpresentations and results in fetal hypoxia and the need for emergency cesarean delivery. Complications during delivery such as head entrapment and nuchal arms can lead to brachial plexus injuries and upper-extremity fractures. Head entrapment can also lead to cervical trauma if Dührssen's incisions are performed.[1,2]

Management

Patients presenting to the emergency department (ED) who are in labor should be transported to a labor and delivery suite, or an obstetrician should be consulted on an emergency basis to perform the delivery. Recent studies have confirmed an increased fetal morbidity and mortality rate with vaginal breech delivery[1,2]; therefore, unless delivery is imminent, preparations for cesarean delivery should be made. An anesthesiologist and a pediatrician also should be consulted for a breech delivery. In the event that vaginal delivery is necessary in the ED, care should be taken to ensure that the breeched fetal part, legs, and abdomen are allowed to deliver spontaneously. Once the torso has been delivered, gentle rotation of the trunk can be performed to facilitate delivery of the shoulders. As the axillae come into view, the arms can be swept medially across the torso and delivered. With an assistant placing suprapubic (not fundal) pressure, the head may be delivered by the Mauriceau-Smellie-Veit maneuver. An experienced obstetrician may use forceps to deliver the aftercoming head.[1,2]

REFERENCES

1. Hickok DE, Gordon DC, Milberg JA, Williams MA, Daling JR. The frequency of breech presentation by gestational age at birth: a large population-based study. *Am J Obstet Gynecol* 1992;166:851–852.
2. Hofmeyr GJ, Hannah ME. Planned caesarean section for term breech delivery. *Cochrane Database Syst Rev* 2003;(3):CD000166.

13-13

Nuchal Cord

Marisa Stumpf and Jacob W. Ufberg

Pathophysiology

A nuchal cord occurs when the umbilical cord is wrapped around the neck of the fetus one or more times. The umbilical cord is typically 50 to 60 cm long and consists of three vessels. The umbilical cord may become wrapped around the fetal neck at any time during the pregnancy; this is more common if the cord is long or polyhydramnios is present. Single nuchal cords occur in 25% of pregnancies and usually cause no harm. Multiple nuchal cords are present in about 3.7% of pregnancies.[1]

Diagnosis

After delivery of the anterior shoulder, the neck should be palpated before body is delivered, to feel for a thick cord (separate from the folds in the neck).[1,2]

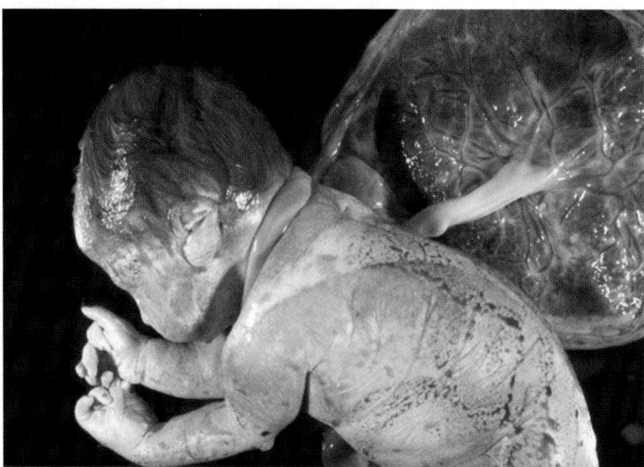

FIGURE 13–13 This tight intrauterine cord led to an umbilical cord accident (death). More commonly, a nuchal cord is detected at birth and must be unlooped around the head or clamped and cut. (Copyright Edward C. Klatt, MD.)

Clinical Complications

Complications of management include rupture of the nuchal cord, possibly leading to exsanguination. Tight or multiple nuchal cords may be associated with fetal distress and the presence of meconium due to an increase in blood-flow resistance and a decrease in oxygen saturation. If the cord is wrapped so tightly that there is inadequate blood flow and/or oxygenation, asphyxia can produce ischemic encephalopathy with neuropathologic changes or even death ("umbilical cord accident").[1,2]

Management

If an umbilical cord is felt around the neck, an attempt should be made to gently slip the cord around the head. If it is too tight to slide over the head, it should be cut between two clamps (metal Kelly clamps) and the fetus quickly delivered. One clamp should be placed 4 to 5 cm from the fetal abdomen, and the second clamp should be placed 2 to 3 cm from the fetal abdomen. The cord can be cut between these clamps and released from the neck. Often if the cord is wrapped many times, it needs to be cut.[1,2]

REFERENCES

1. Ikeda T, Murata Y, Quilligan EJ, et al. Physiologic and histologic changes in near-term fetal lambs exposed to asphyxia by partial umbilical cord occlusion. *Am J Obstet Gynecol* 1998;178:24–32.
2. Collins JH. Nuchal cord type A and type B. *Am J Obstet Gynecol* 1997;177:94.

Postpartum Hemorrhage

Marisa Stumpf and Jacob W. Ufberg

Clinical Presentation

Patients with postpartum hemorrhage (PPH) may present to the emergency department immediately after delivering precipitously at home or while en route to the hospital, with uncontrolled or persistent vaginal bleeding. Patients with late PPH may present up to 6 weeks after delivery with anemia, weakness, hypotension, and syncope related to continued blood loss.

Pathophysiology

The causes of PPH include uterine atony (90%), lacerations, and retained products of conception (POC).[1] Uterine atony usually results from uterine overdistention secondary to hydramnios, multiple gestation, or fetal macrosomia; it is more common in precipitous deliveries.[1] Lacerations of the vaginal wall or cervix can also cause PPH. Retained placental tissue or POC can cause hemorrhage due to inadequate uterine contraction.

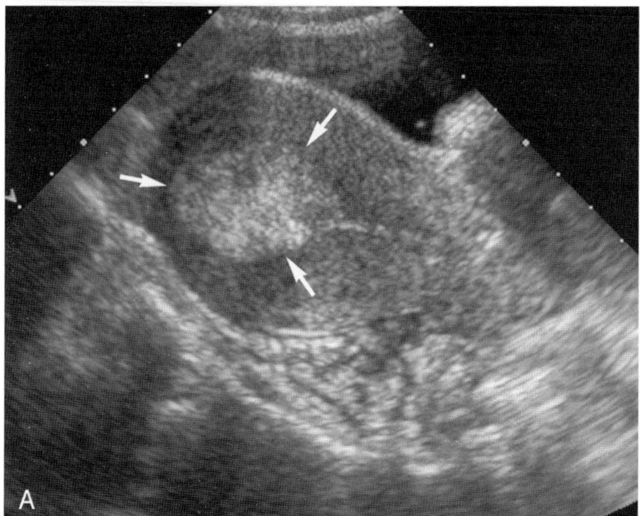

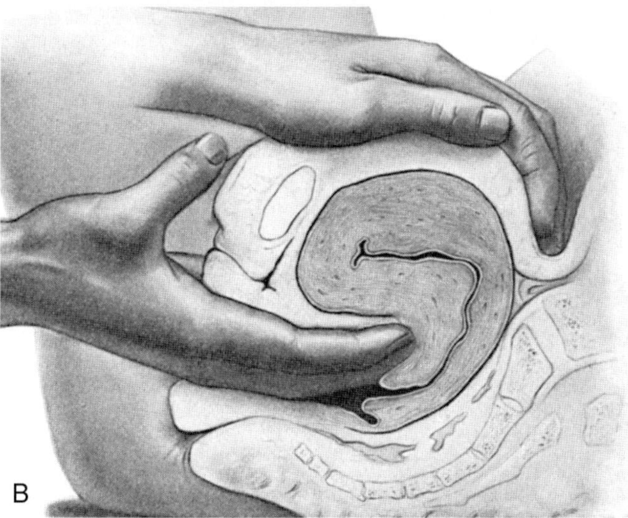

FIGURE 13–14 **A:** Retained products of conception (POC). Ultrasound-guided evacuation of retained POC. Sagittal transvaginal view of the uterus demonstrates a soft-tissue mass *(arrows)* in the uterine cavity, representing retained POC. (From Doubilet and Benson, with permission.) **B:** Bimanual compression of the uterus and massage with the abdominal hand usually controls the hemorrhage effectively. (From Schwartz, with permission.)

Diagnosis

Initial clinical steps should be aimed at determining the cause of the hemorrhage. Vaginal examination may reveal uterine atony or a vaginal/cervical laceration. If appropriate, the placenta should be examined visually to determine whether any segments are missing. Bedside ultrasonography may be used to identify retained POC.[1,2]

Clinical Complications

Hypovolemia can lead to maternal hypotension, shock, acute tubular necrosis, disseminated intravascular coagulation, coagulopathy, cardiac arrest, and death. Sheehan syndrome is a rare complication that is caused by anterior pituitary necrosis; it is characterized by failure of lactation, amenorrhea, hypothyroidism, and adrenal cortical insufficiency.[1,2]

Management

Management of PPH requires rapid establishment of large-bore intravenous access lines, oxygen administration, continuous cardiac monitoring, complete blood count with typing and cross-matching for possible transfusion of blood products, and emergency consultation with an obstetrician. Determining the cause of the hemorrhage is the next step. If uterine atony is suspected (the uterus may feel large and "boggy"), the uterus should be massaged and compressed. A urethral catheter should be placed and oxytocin administered.[1] If the uterus remains atonic and bleeding continues, Methergine or ergonovine may be given, but these drugs are contraindicated in hypertensive states. While the uterotonic medications are given, the physician should compress the uterus by pressing against the anterior uterine wall with a fist in the vagina and pressing on the fundus/posterior uterine wall with a hand on the abdomen. Rectal misoprostol may also be an effective uterotonic.[2] Uterine packs are ineffective and potentially dangerous; however, uterine tamponade (bladder catheter guided into the uterine cavity and inflated) may be effective.[1] Lacerations of the lower genital tract require direct pressure and/or the placement of a suture above the apex of the laceration to control retracted arteries.

REFERENCES

1. Ripley, DL. Uterine Emergencies. Atony, inversion, and rupture. *Obstet Gynecol Clin North Am* 1999;26:419–434.
2. Selo-Ojeme DO. Primary postpartum haemorrhage. *J Obstet Gynaecol* 2002;22:463–469.

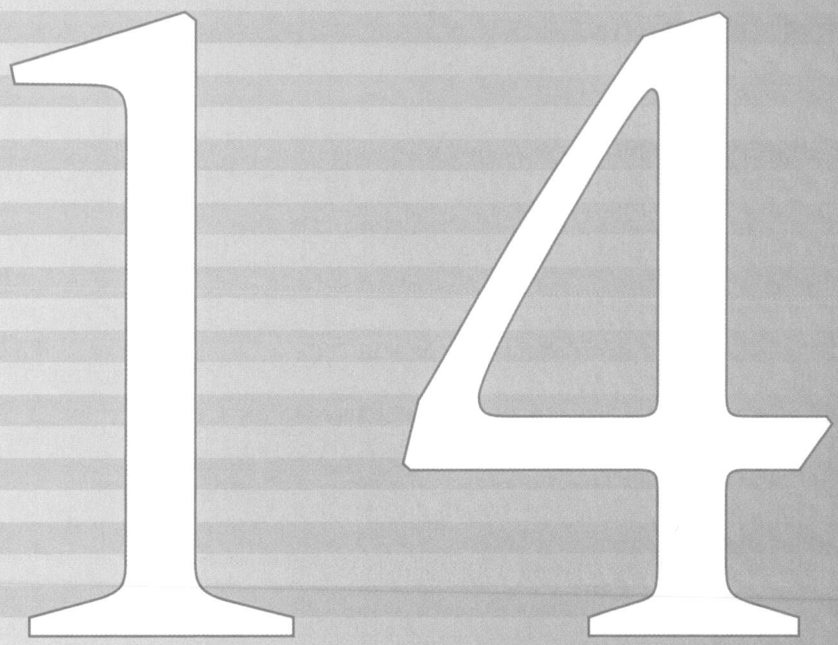

Dermatologic

Rashes

Mark Silverberg

It is imperative to describe correctly any rash found on physical examination of a patient. This facilitates communication among physicians and helps to ensure that the patient will receive appropriate diagnosis and treatment. The following are a number of standard definitions for common rash morphologies[1]:

- *Macule:* A flat, circumscribed change in skin color less than 1 cm in diameter
- *Patch:* A macule that is larger than 1 cm in diameter
- *Papule:* A solid, elevated, superficial lesion smaller than 5 mm in diameter
- *Plaque:* A solid elevated lesion (width greater than height) larger than 5 mm in diameter
- *Nodule:* A solid elevated lesion with depth into the underlying tissue and a diameter between 5 mm and 2 cm
- *Tumor:* A nodule with a diameter greater than 2 cm
- *Vesicle:* An elevated, superficial, fluid-filled blister smaller than 5 mm in diameter
- *Bulla:* An elevated, superficial, fluid-filled lesion larger than 5 mm in diameter
- *Pustule:* A papule or vesicle that contains free pus
- *Wheal:* A rapidly evolving, flat-topped papule or plaque caused by transient cutaneous edema, as seen in an allergic reaction
- *Abscess:* A nodule or tumor containing free pus

REFERENCES

1. Sanfilippo AM, Barrio V, Kulp-Shorten C, Callen JP. Common pediatric and adolescent skin conditions. *J Pediatr Adolesc Gynecol* 2003;16:269–283.

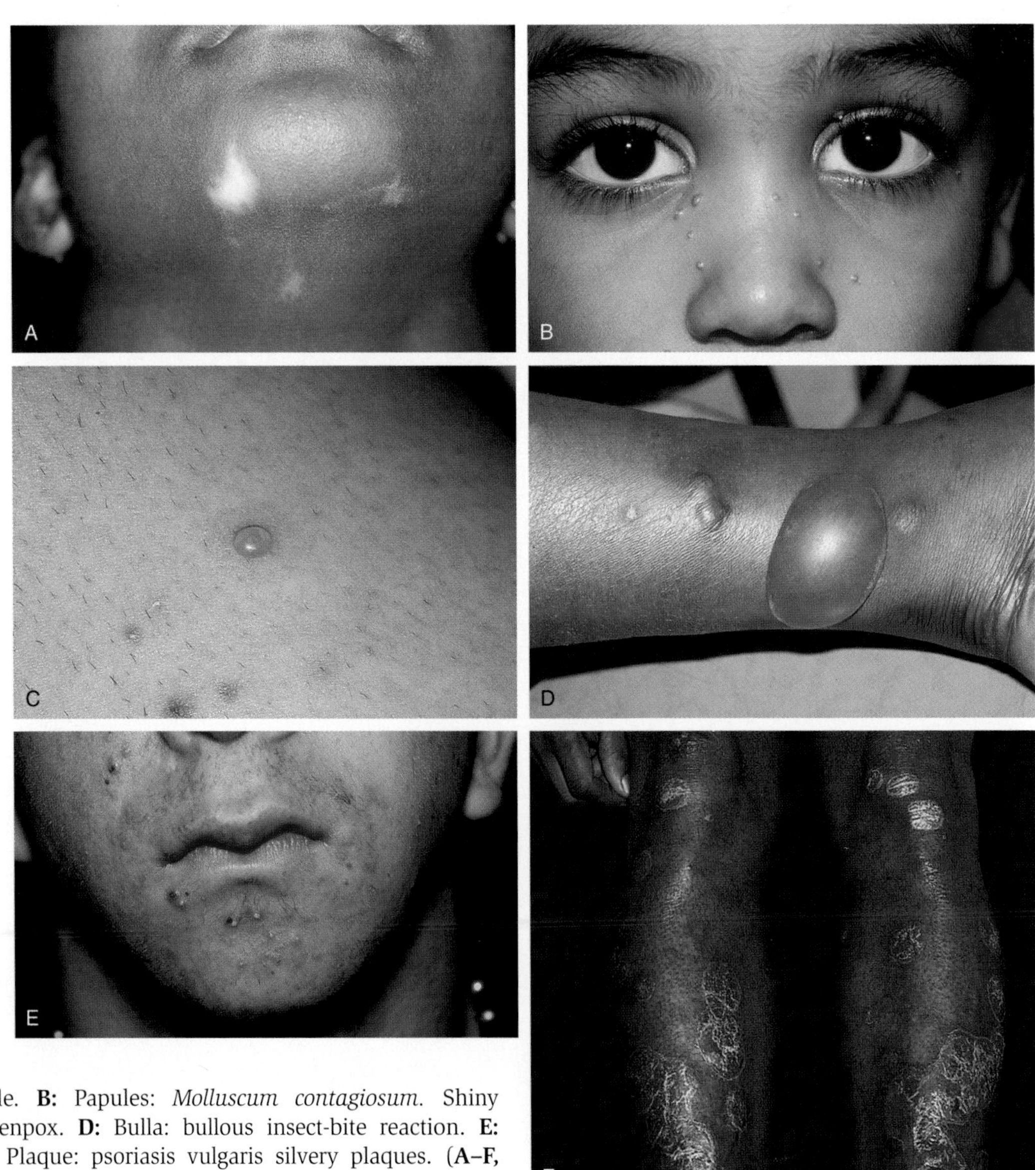

FIGURE 14–1 **A:** Macule. **B:** Papules: *Molluscum contagiosum.* Shiny papules. **C:** Vesicle: chickenpox. **D:** Bulla: bullous insect-bite reaction. **E:** Pustule: acne vulgaris. **F:** Plaque: psoriasis vulgaris silvery plaques. (**A–F,** From Goodheart, with permission.)

Erythema Multiforme

Brenda L. Liu

Clinical Presentation

Patients with erythema multiforme (EM) may present with the classic "target" lesions, which are smaller than 3 cm, with concentric rings of color changes, a well-defined border, and a central grey blister or necrotic area.[1] EM predominantly affects young adults, aged 20 to 40 years.[1,2] Skin lesions are often pruritic and cause burning; oral lesions are painful and can interfere with eating.[1,2]

Pathophysiology

EM results from host immune reactions to antigens.[2] Infectious diseases and pharmacologic agents may precipitate EM.[1,2] Herpes simplex virus (HSV) is the most common cause of EM and has been implicated in 50% of cases.[2] *Mycoplasma* infection is also a potential cause of EM.[1] Histopathology of EM skin lesions reveals dermal edema with epidermal involvement that tends to be limited to the central area of the target lesion.[2]

FIGURE 14–2 Target-like pattern typical of erythema multiforme. (Courtesy of Colleen Campbell, MD.)

Diagnosis

EM is an acute, self-limited process characterized by symmetric, well-demarcated plaques, located predominantly on the extensor surfaces of the extremities.[1] EM is classified into EM minor and EM major, with the latter involving the oral mucosa.[2] The diagnosis is a clinical one, based on physical examination.[1,2] Laboratory studies usually are normal, although in severe EM major, an elevated erythrocyte sedimentation rate (ESR) and a moderate leukocytosis may occur.[2]

Clinical Complications

EM is a self-limited process that usually lasts 1 to 4 weeks.[1,2] Complications involve secondary bacterial infection of the skin.[1,2] Rarely, mortality is seen in patients with severe EM major.[2]

Management

Treatment consists of supportive care. Medications suspected of causing EM should be stopped if possible.[1] Comfort measures include systemic or topical anesthetics for skin lesions and oral anesthetics (e.g., viscous lidocaine rinses) for oral lesions.[2] Patients should be instructed to avoid spicy and acidic foods, and the importance of sufficient fluid intake should be stressed.[2] Topical antibiotics may prevent secondary bacterial infection of the skin. In individuals with recurrent EM and known HSV infection history, acyclovir prophylaxis may be beneficial in preventing recurrences.[1,2]

REFERENCES

1. Ferrera PC, Dupree ML, Verdile VP. Dermatologic problems encountered in the emergency department. *Am J Emerg Med* 1996;14:588–601.
2. Ayangco L, Rogers RS 3rd. Oral manifestations of erythema multiforme. *Dermatol Clin* 2003;21:195–205.

Stevens-Johnson Syndrome

Jennifer Kiss

Clinical Presentation

Patients with Stevens-Johnson syndrome (SJS) present with tenderness and erythema of skin and mucosa, which develops into extensive cutaneous and mucosal exfoliation. This can become life-threatening with multisystem involvement.[1]

Pathophysiology

SJS and toxic epidermal necrolysis (TEN) are part of the same spectrum. Both diseases can be caused by the same drugs, and a disease starting as SJS can lead to full-blown TEN. The histopathologic hallmark of SJS-TEN is epidermal necrosis.[2] The most frequently implicated drugs are sulfa drugs, allopurinol, hydantoins, and carbamazepine.[1] The exact pathogenesis is unknown but is most likely an immune response, such as a cell-mediated cytotoxic reaction against epidermal cells.[3] Onset of SJS in drug-associated cases is usually 7 to 21 days after a new medication is started. SJS has several nondrug associations, including recurrent herpes and *Mycoplasma pneumoniae* infection.[1]

Diagnosis

Diagnosis is mainly clinical but may be confirmed by biopsy. SJS is usually drug-induced. The triad of mucous membrane erosion, target lesions, and epidermal necrosis with skin detachment characterizes SJS. The ultimate extent of full-thickness epidermal detachment is less than 10% in SJS.[1]

Clinical Complications

Delay in recognition and cessation of associated medications are associated with increased mortality.[1] There may be transcutaneous fluid loss with associated electrolyte abnormalities. Other complications include prerenal azotemia, bacterial superinfection, and sepsis.[1]

Management

Suspected inciting agents must be discontinued immediately. Management should include admission to an intensive care unit or burn unit and prompt cessation of potentially associated medications. Intravenous fluids should be managed as for a patient with full-thickness burns, with débridement of devitalized epidermis, burn-type skin care, close monitoring, and prompt treatment of all infections, including sepsis.[1]

REFERENCES

1. Sullivan JR, Shear NH. Drug eruptions and other adverse drug effects in aged skin. *Clin Geriatr Med* 2002;18:21–42.
2. Revuz J. New advances in severe adverse drug reactions. *Dermatol Clin* 2001;19:697–709.
3. Riedl MA, Casillas AM. Adverse drug reactions: types and treatment options. *Am Fam Physician* 2003;68:1781–1790.

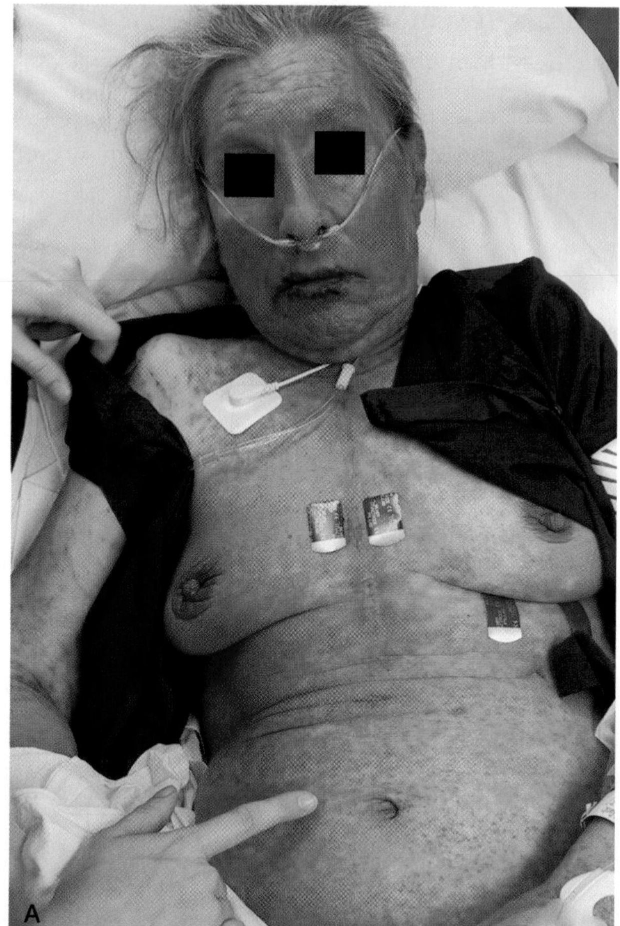

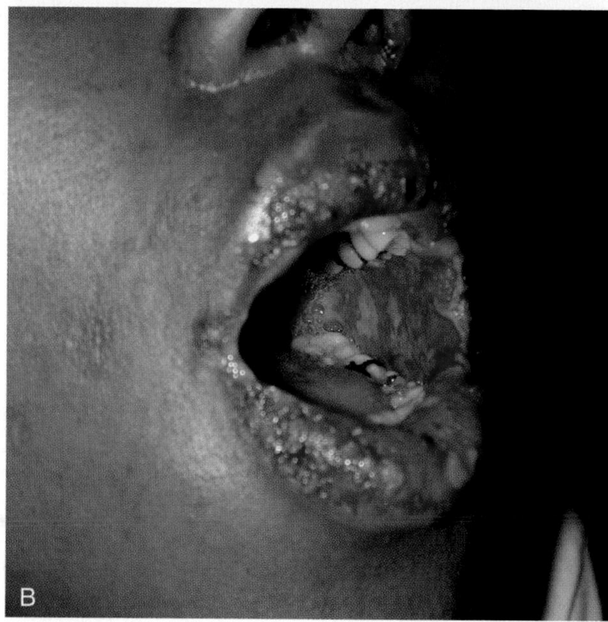

FIGURE 14–3 **A:** Stevens-Johnson syndrome. (Courtesy of Ralph Weiche, MD.) **B:** Mucosal sloughing in a mild form of Stevens-Johnson syndrome. (Courtesy of Robert Hendrickson, MD.)

Toxic Epidermal Necrolysis

Aman Parikh

Clinical Presentation

Patients with toxic epidermal necrolysis (TEN) may report a prodromal phase consisting of fever, upper respiratory tract symptoms, conjunctival burning, and skin tenderness along with fever, headache, muscle aches, joint aches, nausea, vomiting, and diarrhea. Patients present with generalized pain and a rash. Patients may have diffuse involvement with skin sloughing, persistent fevers, and rash. Conjunctival involvement may lead to eye pain and photophobia. The skin manifestations of TEN are acute and progress very rapidly.

Pathophysiology

TEN is believed to be an immunologic reaction that causes disruption of the dermal-epidermal junction. The most common offending agents are antibiotics (penicillin, fluoroquinolones, macrolides, chloramphenicol), cyclooxygenase-1 (COX-1) and COX-2 inhibitors,[1] antiepileptic medications, and allopurinol. Many cases are idiopathic, but causes include lymphoma, leukemia, measles, and viral syndromes. TEN is more common in adults, whereas staphylococcal scalded skin syndrome (SSSS) is more common in children and immunocompromised adults.

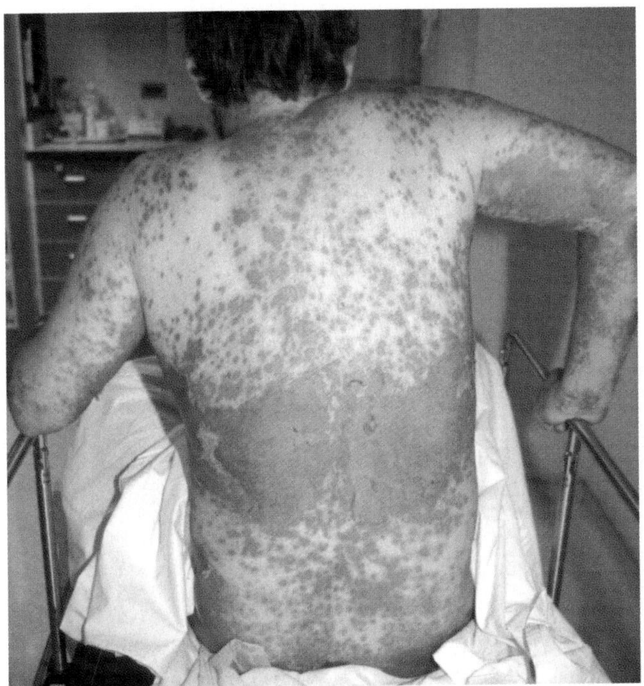

FIGURE 14–4 Extensive exfoliation characteristic of toxic epidermal necrolysis. (© David Effron, MD, 2004. Used with permission.)

Diagnosis

The most important factor leading to diagnosis is strong clinical suspicion. A skin biopsy should be obtained if the diagnosis is being considered. The biopsy shows necrosis of the entire epidermis with minimal inflammatory cells. The epidermis may be completely detached from the dermis, which is characteristic for the disease. The definitive histologic diagnosis requires finding that the TEN blister is "subepidermal with overlying epidermal necrosis."[3] The differential diagnosis should include Stevens-Johnson syndrome (SJS), erythema multiforme (EM), Kawasaki disease, and SSSS.

Clinical Complications

Because of the loss of the skin barrier, bacterial infection and sepsis are common complications. Other complications include electrolyte imbalances, dehydration, hypoxemia, and renal insufficiency. Severe gastrointestinal hemorrhage may result from gastrointestinal mucosal sloughing. Ocular complications may include corneal scar formation, permanent visual impairment, entropions, and pseudomembrane formation.

Management

Discontinuation of the offending medication and meticulous supportive care are essential. Patients with oral involvement are at risk for dehydration and malnutrition, and fluid management is critical. Antibiotics should be started empirically if there are signs of infection. Steroid treatment for TEN is a controversial therapy, and intravenous immunoglobulin G (IVIG) has been proposed as an adjunctive treatment.[2] The mortality rate for drug-induced TEN is approximately 20%, and that of idiopathic TEN is approximately 50%.[3]

REFERENCES

1. Friedman B, Orlet HK, Still JM, Law E. Toxic epidermal necrolysis due to administration of celecoxib (Celebrex). *South Med J* 2002;95:1213–1214.
2. Stella M, Cassano P, Bollero D, Clemente A, Giorio G. Toxic epidermal necrolysis treated with intravenous high-dose immunoglobulins: our experience. *Dermatology* 2001;203:45–49.
3. Ringheanu M, Laude TA. Toxic epidermal necrolysis in children: an update. *Clin Pediatr (Phila)* 2000;39:687–694.

14–5

Erysipelas

Harneet Sethi

Clinical Presentation

Patients with erysipelas present with well-demarcated skin lesions with spreading edges that advance at a rate of 2 to 10 cm per day. Erysipelas is most common on the lower extremities but may also involve the face, upper extremities, and trunk. This disease tends preferentially to afflict the very young and the elderly.

Pathophysiology

Erysipelas is a subset of cellulitis involving the superficial dermis. It is caused by *Staphylococcus pyogenes* or group A streptococci. *Streptococcus agalactiae* (B) and streptococci C and G have also been implicated.[1]

Diagnosis

Erysipelas is diagnosed clinically by the presence of an erythematous rash characterized by an elevated, advancing or spreading margin. Physical findings may include lymphadenopathy and lymphanagitis.[1] The complete blood count (CBC) may reveal an increased white blood cell (WBC) count with leftward shift. An elevated C-reactive protein (CRP) concentration has been associated with erysipelas, but this is a nonspecific finding and may be impractical in the emergency department (ED) setting. It is important to perform a careful search for potential sites of introduction of infection, the most common of which is athlete's foot. Venous stasis ulcers and leg wounds provide additional portals of entry. The area surrounding the lesions is notable for erythema and edema. In the majority of presentations (85%), fever is present.[1]

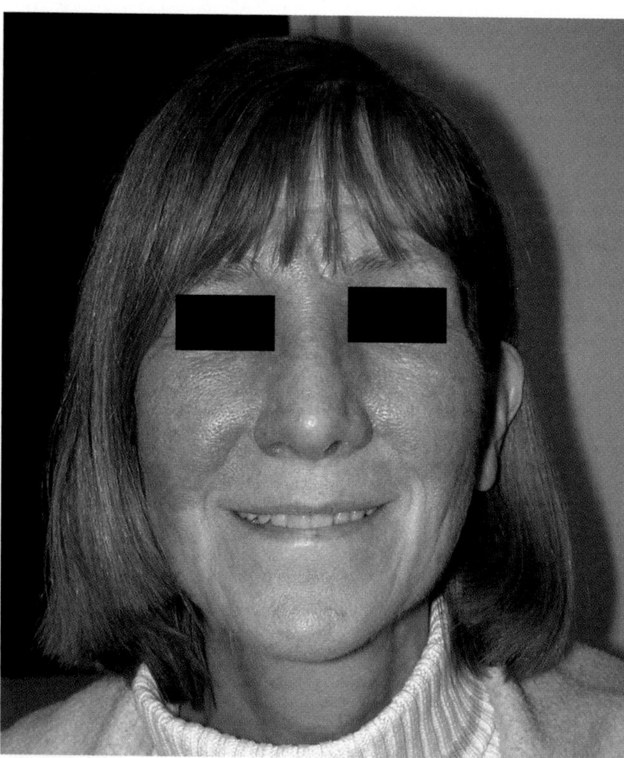

FIGURE 14–5 Erythematous demarcated rash of erysipelas. (Courtesy of Ralph Weiche, MD.)

Clinical Complications

Complications include abscess formation, expanding cellulitis, septicemia, and recurrence. Gangrene, venous thromboemboli, and necrotizing cellulitis also may occur.[1]

Management

Most cases of erysipelas can be treated with penicillin, and oral administration is a first-line treatment, with the intramuscular route reserved for cases of noncompliance.[2] Macrolides and cephalosporins are also effective. The extent of cutaneous involvement, the patient's immune status, and the patient's social situation should be weighed when considering inpatient treatment. Pain and fever control also should be addressed. Follow-up within 48 hours is recommended to ascertain the extent of any possible expansion of swelling and erythema. Failure to respond to antibiotic treatment within 48 hours should raise suspicion of a diagnosis other than erysipelas.[1] Marking the extent of the lesion during the initial visit can provide a baseline from which to measure successful antibiotic treatment or lesion progression.

REFERENCES

1. Bonnetblanc JM, Bedane C. Erysipelas: recognition and management. *Am J Clin Dermatol* 2003;4:157–163.
2. Bishara J, Golan-Cohen A, Robenshtok E, Leibovici L, Pitlik S. Antibiotic use in patients with erysipelas: a retrospective study. *Isr Med Assoc J* 2001;3:722–724.

Shingles

Colleen Campbell

Clinical Presentation

Patients with shingles usually present with a neuropathic pain along the involved dermatome. Patients often describe the pain as tingling or burning, but it can also be itching, lancinating, or sharp. The pain varies from constant to intermittent and can precede the rash by 1 week.[1] In "zoster sine herpete," no rash forms after the prodromal phase.[2] Five percent of patients also have prodromal symptoms of fever, malaise, and headache.[3] The rash is localized to one dermatome and does not cross the midline. It usually involves one area of skin innervated by a single sensory dermatome.[3] In 50% of patients, the rash is found in the thoracic region.[1] The T5 and T6 dermatomes are most commonly affected,[2] followed by the first trigeminal branch. The rash is characterized by clusters of vesicles with underlying erythema.[1] The lesions evolve from macules and papules to vesicles and then pustules, finally forming a crust within 7 to 10 days.

Pathophysiology

Shingles (herpes zoster) is a localized, vesicular, cutaneous eruption caused by reactivation of varicella-zoster virus.

Older patients are more commonly affected than younger, immunocompetent individuals. There is no seasonal prevalence to the disease, and there is no difference in incidence by race or gender.[1]

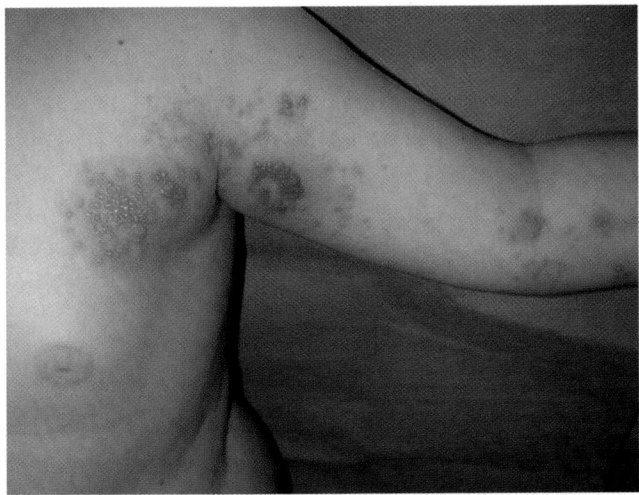

FIGURE 14–6 Shingles in typical C8 dermatomal distribution. (Courtesy of Raymond Moreno, MD.)

Diagnosis

The diagnosis of herpes zoster is largely clinical. The characteristic unilateral vesicular rash is easily identified. There is commonly an accompanying regional lymphadenopathy as well. Hutchinson's sign signals the involvement of the nasociliary branch of the ophthalmic nerve and is characterized by vesicles on the tip of the nose. Ramsey Hunt syndrome signifies involvement of the facial or auditory nerve and is evident with unilateral facial palsy and lesions on the ear or the anterior two thirds of the tongue.[3] A Tzanck smear of early lesions that reveals multinucleated giant cells and intranuclear inclusion bodies confirms the diagnosis.[3]

Clinical Complications

The most common complication of shingles is postherpetic neuralgia, which occurs in 9% to 15% of patients overall,[1] and up to 50% of those older than 65 years of age. Half of the patients with involvement of the ophthalmic branch of the trigeminal nerve (V1) have ophthalmic complications, including cranial nerve palsy (III, IV, VI), mucopurulent conjunctivitis, keratitis, uveitis, and episcleritis.[2] Granulomatous cerebral angitis is a delayed complication of ophthalmic involvement and manifests as transient ischemic attacks (TIAs) or stroke.[3] Up to 0.5% of patients develop meningoencephalitis or myelitis with shingles infection. Rarely, nausea, vomiting, and gastrointestinal distress occurs because of vagus nerve involvement. Motor paralysis can also occur if the infection spreads from the dorsal root ganglia to the anterior horn cells.[3] Widespread dissemination can occur in immunocompromised individuals.

Management

The main therapeutic goal in the treatment of shingles is control of pain. Early treatment with antiviral drugs that inhibit varicella-zoster virus replication has been shown to reduce pain and shorten the time until the rash resolves. The use of oral corticosteroids may increase early healing of the rash, but it has not shown efficacy in reducing the time to resolution of symptoms.

REFERENCES

1. Wallace MS, Oxman MN. Acute herpes zoster and postherpetic neuralgia. *Anesth Clin North Am* 1997;15:371–398.
2. McCarary ML, Severson J, Tyring SK. Varicella zoster virus. *J Am Acad Dermatol* 1999;41:1–14.
3. Stankus SJ, Dlugopolski M, Packer D. Management of herpes zoster (shingles) and post-herpetic neuralgia. *Am Fam Physician* 2000;61:2437–2448.

Urticaria

Colleen Campbell

Clinical Presentation

Patients with urticaria present with dermal papules and plaques that usually are pruritic.[1] The papules may be erythematous, whereas plaques often have white centers with surrounding erythema.[1] These lesions may remain on the skin for longer than 24 hours.[1] Hives may appear round, oval, or serpiginous. Hives may resolve in one area, only to appear in another area shortly thereafter.

Pathophysiology

Urticaria is a raised skin lesion that occurs in response to an immune trigger.[1] This disorder is also known as "hives" or "wheals."

Urticaria reportedly affects up to 20% of the population.[1] It is considered to be acute if symptom duration is less than 6 weeks and chronic if symptoms have been present for longer than 6 weeks.[1] Acute urticarial reactions are more common in children and young adults.[1] Mast cell activation is the primary physiologic mechanism of hives, but urticaria also can be seen in type I, II, or III allergic responses.[1,2] It is believed that the wheal is formed when fluid leaks from blood vessels in response to mast cell degranulation.[1] Urticaria is most commonly idiopathic, but it occurs with a greater frequency in atopic individuals.[2] Other causes are physical, immunologic, or toxic.[1] Physical causes include temperature, pressure, and vibration. Urticaria can be mediated by immunoglobulin E (IgE), such as by aeroallergens. Immunoglobulin G (IgG) and immunoglobulin M (IgM) are mediators in infections. Autoimmune diseases and connective tissue disease induce urticaria through complement-mediated mechanisms.[2] Toxic causes include exposure to nettles, strawberries, and insects.[1] Nonsteroidal antiinflammatory drugs (NSAIDs) can cause histamine release and are also a common cause of urticaria.[1,3]

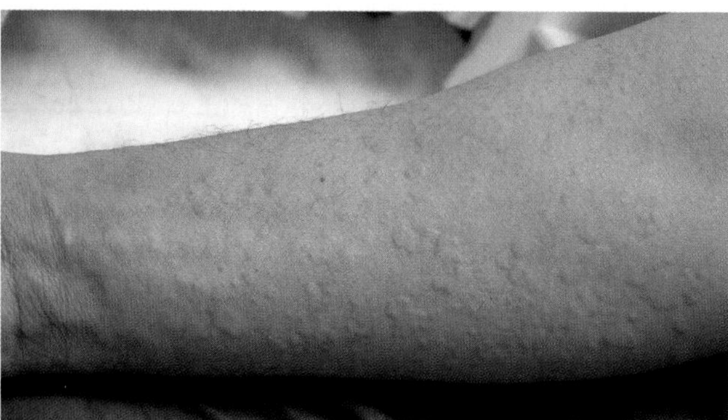

FIGURE 14–7 Urticarial eruption of volar forearm. (Courtesy Mark Silverberg, MD.)

Diagnosis

Diagnosis of urticaria is based on a careful history and physical examination.[2] A history of preexisting atopy and presence of classic wheals confirms the diagnosis. The history must be relied on to determine the inciting cause, although often it is difficult to identify a single significant precipitant.

Clinical Complications

The most dangerous manifestation of urticaria is rapid progression to anaphylaxis, which can lead to death.[2] Superinfection of the skin can occur secondary to scratching of the pruritic areas.

Management

The most important issue in treatment is identification and removal of the cause of the urticaria, if possible.[2] Antihistamines are the mainstay of therapy but are not always effective. It is recommended that antihistamine usage be continued for 96 hours after resolution of symptoms.[2] A nonsedating antihistamine may be used during the day, in combination with diphenhydramine at night.[2] Doxepin lotion may be used in addition to oral medications. Hydroxyzine and doxepin have both been shown to have greater H_1 receptor blockade effects than diphenhydramine, and greater H_2 receptor blockade effects than cimetidine.[2] Oral corticosteroids can be added for a short course (5 days) for severe cases of acute urticaria.[1,2] Alternate-day therapy with low-dose steroids may be useful for those patients whose symptoms recur on steroid withdrawal.[1] Subcutaneous epinephrine injections may be required for sudden severe urticaria. Patients with chronic urticaria should be referred to their primary care physicians for further laboratory work-up and skin testing.[1,3]

REFERENCES

1. Kennedy MS. Evaluation of chronic eczema and urticaria and angioedema. *Immunol Allerg Clin North Am* 1999;19:19–32.
2. Beltrani VS, Thiers BH. Urticaria and angioedema. *Dermatol Clin* 1996;14:171–198.
3. Leung DYM, Boguniewicz M. Advances in allergic skin diseases. *J Allerg Clin Immunol* 2003;111:S805–S812.

Eczema

Yanick Isaac

Clinical Presentation

The eczematous reaction can manifest acutely as erythematous vesicular plaques or as a papulovesicular rash that is oozing, weepy, and intensely pruritic. As lesions progress and become subacute, the vesicles crust over and scale. Chronically, this rash is characterized by lichenification, hyperpigmentation, and scaling. Children older than 2 years of age and adults commonly present with the rash in the antecubital, popliteal, and flexural areas, whereas infants have lesions on the scalp, face, cheeks, and extensor surfaces of the extremities.[1]

Pathophysiology

Eczema is a generic term used to describe a spectrum of inflammatory skin diseases that manifest as a red, itchy rash. These include the subclasses of dermatitis, such as atopic, contact, dyshidrotic, seborrheic, stasis, and phototoxic dermatitis, in addition to lichen simplex chronicus and niacin and riboflavin deficiencies.[1,2]

Both immunologic and nonimmunologic mechanisms have been implicated in the development of eczema.[1] The triggers of this type of response are numerous and include viruses, extremes of temperature, detergents, and cosmetics. These triggers stimulate the production of cytokines, which increase the ratio of type 2 helper (Th2) T cells to Th1 cells. This leads to increased levels of immunoglobulin E (IgE) and eosinophilia, in addition to increased basophil and mast cell degranulation. Despite the cause, biopsy specimens of eczematous lesions reveal epidermal intracellular edema and dermal perivascular intracellular T-cell infiltration.[1]

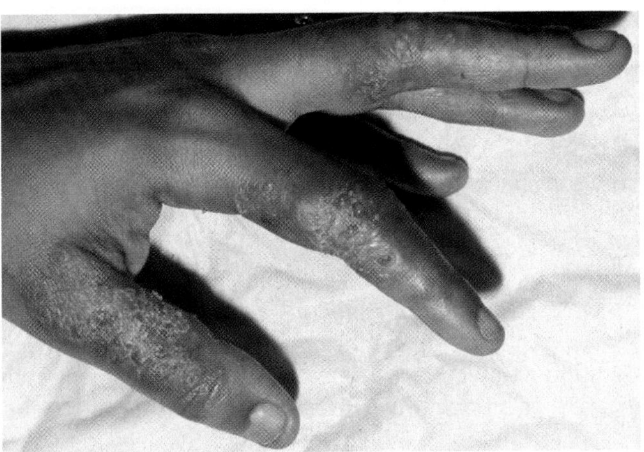

FIGURE 14–8 Eczema of the hand. (© David Effron, MD, 2004. Used with permission.)

Diagnosis

A good history and physical examination are usually adequate to make the diagnosis of eczema. Patients often offer a personal or family history of atopy, allergic rhinitis, or asthma.[1]

Clinical Complications

Complications include bacterial superinfection, typically with *Staphylococcus aureus.* Studies show that use of antibacterial soaps lowers the colonization of eczematous lesions.[2]

Management

Several modalities have been devised for the treatment of eczema. These include skin hydration, short-course topical corticosteroids, antihistamines for symptomatic relief of pruritus, and avoidance of irritants. Maintenance topical corticosteroids are not recommended, because they can potentially cause skin atrophy, hypopigmentation, and immunosuppression.[1] Immunomodulators that block T-cell activation, such as pimecrolimus and tacrolimus, have been shown to be more beneficial than corticosteroids, because they do not appear to induce systemic immunosuppression or cutaneous atrophy.[1,2]

REFERENCES

1. Beltrani V. Clinical features of atopic dermatitis. *Immunol Allergy Clin North Am* 2002;22;25–42.
2. Boguniewicz M. Conventional therapy for atopic dermatitis. *Immunol Allergy Clin North Am* 2002;22;107–124.

Contact Dermatitis

Colleen Campbell

Clinical Presentation

Patients usually present with intense itching in the area of contact. An acutely demarcated area of erythema, edema, papules, and vesicles can be seen in the area of skin contact.[1] In more extreme cases, there may be serous drainage from the involved site. Dry, chapped skin with erythema is seen more often with irritant contact dermatitis.[1] The hands are the most commonly affected site, followed by the face (especially the eyelids).[1] In children, areas commonly affected are the diaper area and the face, especially in the perioral region (i.e., "lip licker dermatitis").[1]

Pathophysiology

Contact dermatitis is a local skin reaction that occurs in response to an immunologic, chemical, mechanical, or physical mediator applied to the skin.[1]

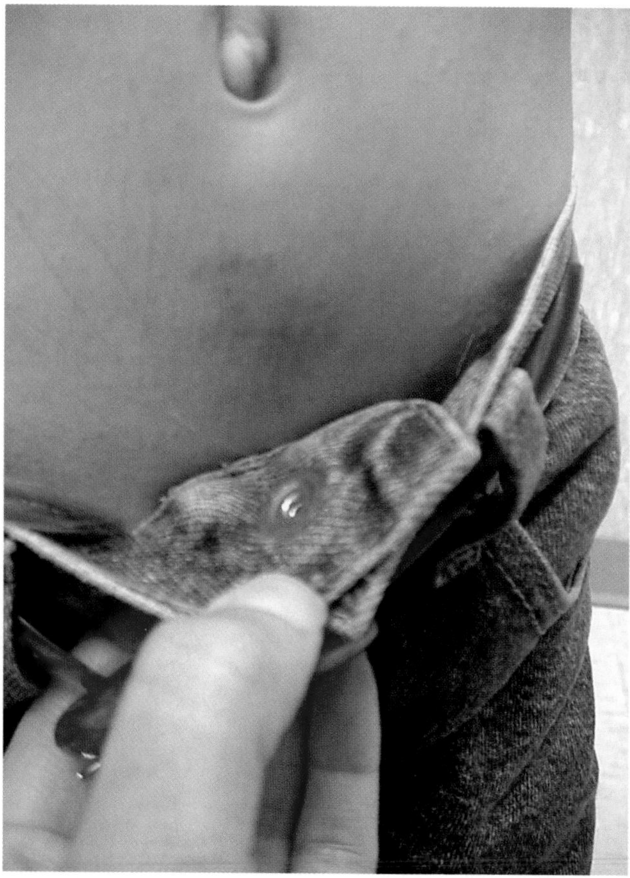

FIGURE 14–9 Contact dermatitis caused by metal snap on jeans. (Courtesy of Christy Salvaggio, MD.)

Contact dermatitis may be allergic- or irritant-mediated.[1] Both types have similar time courses from exposure to reaction, and they are difficult to differentiate.[1] Allergic-mediated contact dermatitis can occur after a single exposure or after years of chronic exposure. This is a type IV allergic reaction.[2] The most common allergic-mediated contact dermatitis in North America is from poison oak or poison ivy exposure.[2] Neomycin, nickel, and components of rubber (especially latex) are common causes of allergic contact dermatitis.[2] Wool is also a common contact irritant.[3] Irritant contact dermatitis is most often the result of repeated contact with low-grade physical, mechanical, or chemical irritants.[1] This may occur as a result of repeated hand washing or from natural irritants such as saliva. Light-skinned individuals are more commonly affected.[2]

Diagnosis

The diagnosis is made largely on the basis of a careful history and physical examination. The exact cause of allergic contact dermatitis often is difficult to determine, because the exposure can antedate the reaction by as much as 2 weeks, as in the case of primary sensitization.[2] Referral back to the patient's primary care doctor for patch testing may be necessary in cases of chronic contact dermatitis.[2]

Clinical Complications

Complications associated with contact dermatitis are not common. However, bacterial superinfection of affected areas is the most common complication.[4]

Management

In most cases, elimination of contact with the irritant suffices. Oral antihistamines may be used for pruritus, in addition to topical corticosteroid creams.[2] In more severe cases with vesicles and serous drainage, Burow's solution (aluminum acetate) with wet-to-dry dressings may further facilitate healing.[2]

REFERENCES

1. Rietschel RL. Comparison of allergic and irritant contact dermatitis. *Immunol Allergy Clin North Am* Aug 1997;17:359–364.
2. Shaw JC. Allergic and non-allergic eczematous dermatitis. *Immunol Allergy Clin North Am* 1996;16:119–134.
3. Beltrani VS. Clinical features of atopic dermatitis. *Immunol Allergy Clin North Am* 2002;22:25.
4. Friedlander SF. Contact dermatitis. *Pediatr Rev* 1998;19:166–171.

Nickel Dermatitis

Colleen Campbell

Clinical Presentation

Patients with nickel dermatitis usually present with an intense itching in the area of contact. An acutely demarcated area of erythema, edema, papules, and vesicles can also be seen in the area of contact.[1] The hands are the most commonly affected area, and nickel dermatitis is an occupational hazard for many workers.[2] Women who wear jewelry composed of nickel may present with erythema of the earlobes or in the neck region. There have been reported cases of inhalation exposure to nickel causing a widespread papuloerythematous rash several hours after exposure.[2]

Pathophysiology

Nickel is the metal that most commonly causes contact dermatitis.[2] Nickel dermatitis can occur after one exposure or after years of exposure. This is a type IV allergic reaction. Women and younger individuals are most commonly affected by nickel dermatitis.[3] Approximately 10% of people who undergo patch testing (using 5% nickel sulfate) are sensitized to nickel.[3] Occupations with risk for nickel sensitization include metal furnace operator and electroplater.[3]

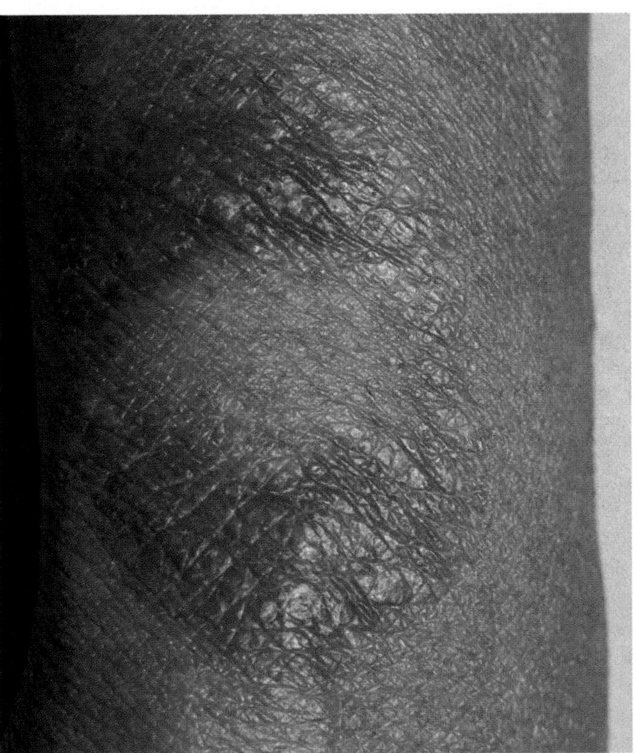

FIGURE 14–10 Nickel dermatitis. (© David Effron, MD, 2004. Used with permission.)

Diagnosis

The diagnosis of nickel dermatitis is suspected by careful history and physical examination. It can be confirmed after referral back to the patient's primary care doctor for patch testing, with results usually available after 3 days.[3]

Clinical Complications

Complications from contact dermatitis are rare. Bacterial superinfection of affected areas is the most common complication.

Management

In most cases, elimination of contact with the nickel suffices. Oral antihistamines may be used for pruritus, in addition to medium- to high-potency topical corticosteroid creams.[1] In more severe cases when vesicles and serous drainage are present, Burow's solution (aluminum acetate) with wet-to-dry dressings may further facilitate healing.[1] Patients with work-related exposures should be referred to an occupational medicine specialist for further follow-up.

REFERENCES

1. Shaw JC. Allergic and non-allergic eczematous dermatitis. *Immunol Allergy Clin North Am* 1996;16:119–134.
2. Candura SM, Locatelli C, Butera R, Gatti A, Fasola D, Manzo L. Widespread nickel dermatitis from inhalation. *Contact Dermatol* 2001;45:174–175.
3. Uter W, Pfahlberg A, Gefeller O, Geier J, Schnuch A. Risk factors for contact allergy to nickel: results of a multifactorial analysis. *Contact Dermatol* 2003;48:33–38.

Psoriasis

Michael Greenberg

Clinical Presentation

Psoriasis afflicts 1% to 2% of the U.S. population. Many patients are aware that they carry the diagnosis of psoriasis. They may present with typically distributed skin lesions that may be itchy, scaly, or painful.[1,2]

Pathophysiology

The precise cause of psoriasis is not known. However, a genetic predisposition is probable, because there is an increased prevalence of this disease among family members. Psoriasis has been associated with specific human leukocyte antigens. Psoriasis clearly involves excessive proliferation of keratinocytes, as well as a substantial decrease in the time required for epidermal cells located within psoriatic plaques to divide. Altered immune mechanisms are probably involved, because activated T cells, and upregulation of immune-mediated adhesion molecules on keratinocytes have been observed. In addition, psoriasis may improve with treatments that modify cutaneous T-cell infiltration.[1,2]

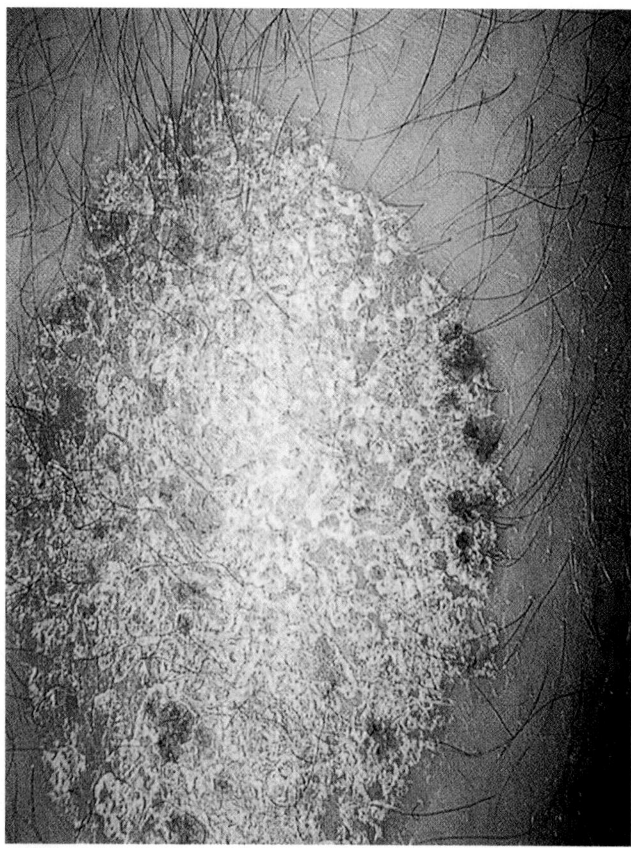

FIGURE 14–11 Typical plaque-like lesion of psoriasis; note oval shape, defined borders, and "silvery" scales. (From Dockery and Crawford, with permission.)

Diagnosis

Psoriasis is a chronic skin disease with distinctive cutaneous lesions. Usually, the diagnosis is easily made on clinical examination by finding erythematous and well-demarcated cutaneous plaques, commonly located on the extensor surfaces of the elbows and knees, on the scalp, and in the lumbosacral region.[1,2] The most common form of psoriasis is the chronic plaque form known as psoriasis vulgaris, which accounts for approximately 90% of cases. Characteristic nail findings include pits and areas of yellowish discoloration known as "oil spots." Thickened and yellow nail plates occur in up to 50% of patients.[1,2]

Clinical Complications

Complications include local skin infections, and psoriatic arthritis, which occurs in up to 20% of cases. Psoriatic arthritis appears to be more common in patients who have nail and scalp psoriasis. Mechanical, chemical, or ultraviolet (UV) injury to the skin may result in the Koebner phenomenon (local skin damage followed by development of the disease state in that previously normal area of skin).[1,2] Various infections, including streptococcal and acute viral infections, may trigger the development of psoriatic lesions.[1,2]

Management

Although no treatment is curative, various therapies may be effective. The emergency physician is rarely called upon to initiate or alter therapy. Current treatment regimens may include emollients, keratolytics, corticosteroids, tar, anthralin, vitamin D analogues, retinoids, phototherapy, acitretin, methotrexate, cyclosporine, and the Goeckerman treatment, or a combination of these.[3]

REFERENCES

1. Espinoza LR, van Solingen R, Cuellar ML, Angulo J. Insights into the pathogenesis of psoriasis and psoriatic arthritis. *Am J Med Sci* 1998;316:271–276.
2. Peters BP, Weissman FG, Gill MA. Pathophysiology and treatment of psoriasis. *Am J Health Syst Pharm* 2000;57:645–659.
3. Witman PM. Topical therapies for localized psoriasis. *Mayo Clin Proc* 2001;76:943–949.

Atopic Dermatitis

Harneet Sethi

Clinical Presentation

Patients with atopic dermatitis (AD) present with a rash, which is pruritic, on fields of skin that may be inflamed, swollen, and dry. AD is often found in conjunction with other atopic entities.[1-3]

Pathophysiology

The precise causes and mechanisms involved in AD are not fully understood. The role of provoking allergens has been suggested, but in some studies refuted. AD appears to be an immune disturbance that involves increased immunoglobulin E (IgE) levels in conjunction with T-cell dysregulation.[1] Histamine release is not involved in AD.

Diagnosis

Criteria for the diagnosis of AD include the presence of a pruritic skin rash within the past 12 months (obligatory), plus three or more of the following: history of flexural dermatitis, onset before the age of 2 years, personal history of asthma or hay fever, history of dry skin, and visible flexural dermatitis.[2] More detailed criteria have been delineated in the past, but they are too burdensome to be used in the emergency department (ED). Laboratory testing is of limited value in the ED setting; however, an elevated serum IgE value may be helpful in making the diagnosis.[3]

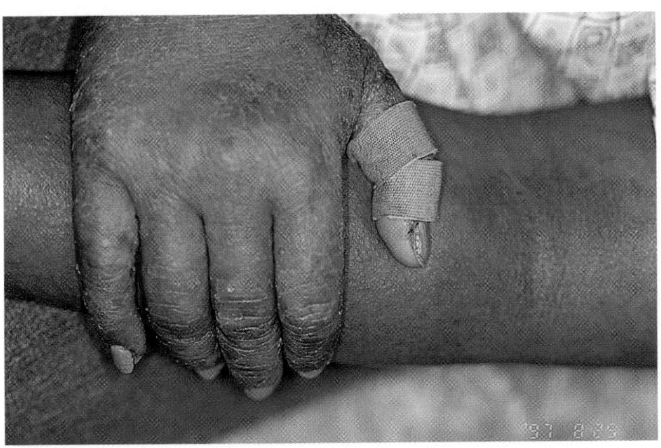

FIGURE 14–12 Typical findings of atopic dermatitis include eczematous eruptions and lichenification or thickening of the skin, particularly in the antecubital and popliteal fossae. (From Fleisher, Baskin, and Ludwig, with permission.)

Clinical Complications

Complications include bacterial and viral superinfections.

Management

Dermatologic referral is appropriate in all cases. Sweat and skin heat are often provoking factors, and avoidance is recommended. Bathing in lukewarm water and use of mild soaps are recommended; emollients may be applied to moist skin to maximize moisture retention.[1] Midpotency steroids may be applied twice daily for AD exacerbations. Antibiotics should be reserved for use with evidence of infection.

REFERENCES

1. Borirakchanyavat K, Kurban AK. Atopic dermatitis. *Clin Dermatol* 2000;18:649–655.
2. Thestrup-Pedersen K. Clinical aspects of atopic dermatitis. *Clin Exp Dermatol* 2000;25:535–543.
3. Williams HC, Burney PG, Pembroke AC, et al. The UK Working Party's diagnostic criteria for atopic dermatitis: derivation of a minimum set of discriminators for atopic dermatitis. *Br J Dermatol* 1994;131:383–396.

Hidradenitis Suppurativa

Michael Greenberg

Clinical Presentation

Many patients present knowing that they carry the diagnosis of hidradenitis suppurativa (HS), and that history is forthcoming. These patients present with pain, swelling, itching, bleeding, and purulent drainage from multiple sinus tracts in the axillae and/or anogenital areas. Other patients first present at the onset of puberty with tender subcutaneous nodules and deep abscesses that are characteristically round in shape. HS-related abscesses tend to manifest initially with symmetric lesions in the axillary or anogenital regions.[1–3]

Pathophysiology

Women are more commonly affected than men (3:1). The disease incidence peaks in the second and third decades of life and declines by the fifth decade. The precise cause of HS is not certain; however, genetic predisposition and various endocrine factors appear to be important. Obesity is an exacerbating factor. There appears to be an association between HS development and smoking. Coagulase-negative staphylococci and *Staphylococcus aureus* organisms are frequently isolated from patients with HS.[1]

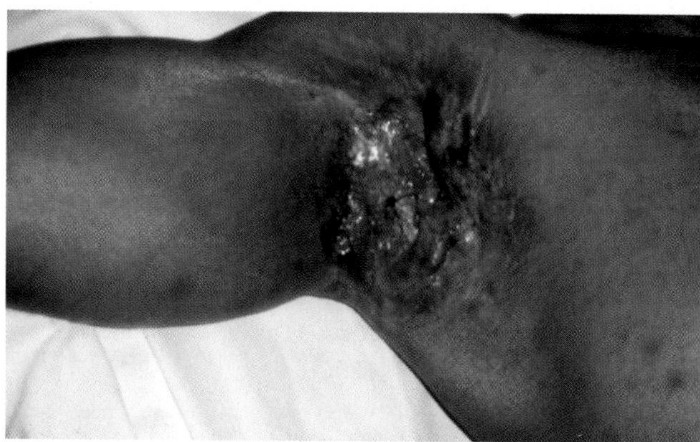

FIGURE 14–13 Hidradenitis suppurativa. (Courtesy of Richard Hamilton, MD.)

Diagnosis

The diagnosis is made based on clinical findings of multiple recurrent anogenital and axillary abscesses, purulent draining sinus tracts, and fistulas.

Clinical Complications

Complications include fibrosis and scarring with contracture formation and decreased mobility of extremities. Fistulas may develop in the anorectal and urethral areas. Other complications include frequent recurrences, anemia, squamous cell carcinoma, arthropathies, amyloidosis, renal failure, and death.

Management

Medical management involves encouraging weight loss, smoking cessation, and meticulous local care of abscesses and fistulas. Topical and enteral clindamycin is helpful in many cases. Antiandrogen therapy and finasteride may be helpful. Retinoids and immunosuppressive doses of corticosteroids may also be useful. Recent reports of radiotherapy for HS are impressive but unconfirmed. Surgical treatment is probably the best option for severe cases; it may range from simple drainage to radical excision procedures.[1,2]

REFERENCES

1. Slade DE, Powell BW, Mortimer PS. Hidradenitis suppurativa: pathogenesis and management. *Br J Plast Surg* 2003;56:451–461.
2. Tanaka A, Hatoko M, Tada H, Kuwahara M, Mashiba K, Yurugi S. Experience with surgical treatment of hidradenitis suppurativa. *Ann Plast Surg* 2001;47:636–642.
3. Silverberg MA, Rahman MZ. Axillary breast tissue mistaken for suppurative hidradenitis: an avoidable error. *J Emerg Med* 2003;25: 51–55.

Cutaneous Abscess

Matthew Pius

Clinical Presentation

Patients with cutaneous abscess may present with localized swelling that may or may not be painful or tender. Fever generally is not reported unless bacteremia has occurred.

Pathophysiology

Abscesses typically arise after a break in the skin, which provides bacteria a portal of entry through the protective, cornified layers of the epidermis.[1] Intertriginous areas, where the skin may become macerated, and shaved areas, where there may be microabrasions, are particularly prone to abscess formation.[1,2] Skin flora (e.g., *Staphylococcus aureus*) are commonly responsible for skin abscess formation, although most collections contain a mixture of aerobic and anaerobic bacteria.[1] Lesions in the inguinal and perineal area may contain a predominance of anaerobes (especially *Bacteroides* species) and other normal flora of the anorectal region.[2]

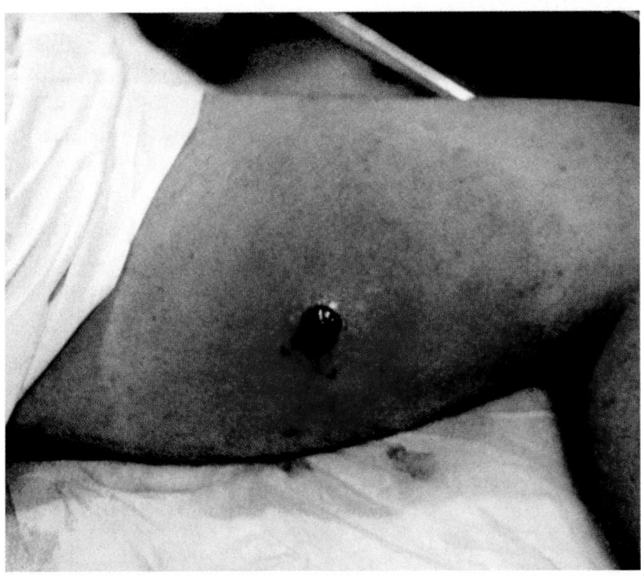

FIGURE 14–14 Cutaneous abscess resulting from transdermal injection of street drugs. (Courtesy of B. Zane Horowitz, MD.)

Diagnosis

On physical examination, a fluctuant mass may be present. These are often exquisitely tender to palpation. There may be erythema and warmth of the surrounding skin if cellulitis has also developed. Spontaneous drainage of pus may be seen. Lymphangitis and lymphadenopathy may also be present.[1]

Clinical Complications

Abscesses may spread to the surrounding skin, resulting in localized cellulitis. They may also track through the skin, forming fistulas that may or may not persist. The collection can penetrate the skin into deeper structures, resulting in abscess formation within the muscle or osteomyelitis. Untreated abscesses can also result in bacteremia, sepsis, and death.

Management

The definitive treatment for an abscess is surgical incision and drainage. If the abscess cavity is sizable, it should be packed with sterile packing material to prevent resealing of the incision site and reaccumulation of pus. Because the abscess cavity itself has very little vascular supply, systemic antibiotics are not well delivered to the site of infection. However, those patients whose clinical picture suggests bacteremia or other systemic infection, those with immunocompromise, and those with overlying cellulitis may benefit from systemic antibiotics.[1,2] Impending abscess formation (i.e., advanced cellulitis that has not yet organized into a collection of pus) should be treated with 10- to 15-minute soaks in warm water every 2 hours, to accelerate organization of the pus collection and to stimulate possible spontaneous drainage.[1,2]

REFERENCES

1. Caruthers LD, Griggs R, Snell GF. Office management of epithelial cysts and cutaneous abscesses. *Prim Care* 1986;13:477–491.
2. Meislin HW, McGehee MD, Rosen P. Management and microbiology of cutaneous abscesses. *JACEP* 1978;7:186–191.

Scabies

Aman Parikh and Colleen Campbell

Clinical Presentation

Patients with scabies complain of an intensely pruritic rash. The pruritus may be more severe at night and may affect any part of the body, but the most commonly affected areas are the interdigital web spaces, axillae, genital area, buttocks, and breasts.[1]

Pathophysiology

Sarcoptes scabiei var. *hominis* is a mite, approximately 0.5 mm in length, that causes human scabies. The female mite burrows under the skin and produces eggs and scybala. A type IV delayed hypersensitivity reaction occurs after approximately 1 month in unsensitized patients or within hours in sensitized patients. This leads to the severe pruritus that is characteristic of scabies infection.

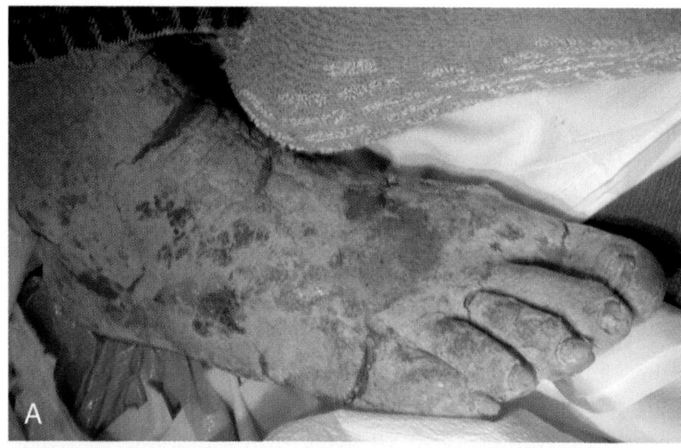

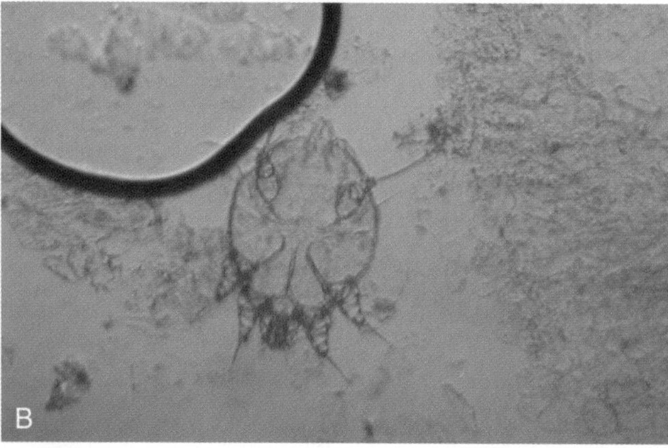

FIGURE 14–15 **A:** Severe scabies of the foot. **B:** Skin scraping shows scabies mite. (**A** and **B**, Courtesy of Robert Hendrickson, MD.)

Diagnosis

If scabies is suspected, the diagnosis can be confirmed by opening of a burrow or other skin lesion with a number 15 scalpel blade. The contents are placed on a slide, and a drop of oil is applied. Diagnosis is confirmed with identification of mites, eggs, or scybala (feces) on microscopic examination.

Clinical Complications

Complications are usually limited to secondary infection, and are usually a problem only in immunocompromised patients. A generalized form of scabies (Norwegian or "crusted" scabies) is associated with severe secondary infections in immunocompromised patients.[2] This form of scabies caused hyperkeratosis and an erythematous rash of the face, trunk, and extremities. Crusted scabies is highly contagious and is a special risk for health care workers. Pruritus may last for months after successful treatment of the infection.

Management

Treatment of scabies involves topical application of lindane, permethrin, or a sulfur agent. Lindane 1% lotion is not recommended for children younger than 2 years of age, because of the potential neurotoxicity and risk of aplastic anemia. Patients who are allergic to chrysanthemums, as well as pregnant and lactating women, should not be given lindane. Permethrin (5%) can be used for infants as young as 2 months of age and should be applied for 8 to 14 hours. This is considered the treatment of choice, with a cure rate in excess of 90%.[1] Sulfur ointment 6% (applied for three consecutive nights) is an alternative treatment.[2] Patients need to be advised to wash and dry all clothing and sheets to prevent reinfection. Sulfur ointment has not yet been approved by the U.S. Food and Drug Administration (FDA) for treatment of scabies. Close household contacts and sexual contacts should be treated to avoid reinfection.[3]

REFERENCES

1. Morgan-Glenn PD. Scabies. *Pediatr Rev* 2001;22:322–323.
2. Brook I. Secondary bacterial infections complicating skin lesions. *J Med Microbiol* 2002;51:808–812.
3. Buffet M, Dupin N. Current treatments for scabies. *Fundam Clin Pharmacol* 2003;17:217–225.

Head Lice

Edgar Collazo

Clinical Presentation

Patients with head lice present with scalp pruritus, although some patients are asymptomatic. Head lice infestation is usually discovered by another person, who sees the nits or lice. The eggs or nits are tiny, white ovals less than 1 mm in length that adhere to the hair shaft. The louse is 2 to 3 mm in length, has six legs, and may be seen on the scalp.

Pathophysiology

Pediculosis capitis is the infestation of a human scalp by the tiny head louse, *Pediculus humanus capitis.* It is common in children 3 to 12 years of age. A female louse can lay more than 100 eggs during the span of 3 to 4 weeks. The eggs are attached to the hair shaft close to the scalp by a glue-like substance.[1-3] Head lice do not jump from person to person, nor can they fly, so transmission comes from close, prolonged head-to-head contact such as co-sleeping, sharing hats, and sharing combs or brushes.[1-3]

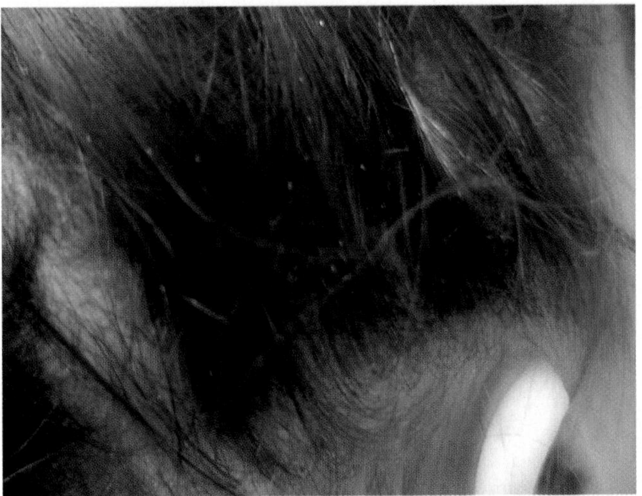

FIGURE 14–16 **A:** Extensive infestation with head lice. Note shiny, white nits on the hair shafts. (Courtesy of Christy Salvaggio, MD.)

Diagnosis

A positive diagnosis can be made on seeing a live, active head louse. Visualization of nits on the scalp of a child is not sufficient to diagnose active lice infestation, because the eggs tend to remain attached long after the louse has hatched.

Clinical Complications

There are no clinical complications; however, most children are sent home from school on discovery of the infestation.

Management

Over-the-counter topical pyrethroids are available. These usually destroy the lice but not the eggs; therefore, a second treatment is recommended after 7 to 10 days. Persistent scalp itching without visualization of live lice does not warrant reapplication. Prescription lice treatment is available in the form of malathion 0.5% lotion or lindane 1%. Lindane is absorbed through the skin and can cause seizures or death if applied improperly, applied too often, or given to the very young. Bed linens, towels, and clothes must be washed in hot water. Items that cannot be washed should be dry cleaned. Brushes and combs must be soaked in hot, soapy water for at least 1 hour. Floors and furniture must be vacuumed, including the car seats of younger children. Stuffed animals should be washed if the child sleeps with them.[1-3]

REFERENCES

1. Dolianitis C, Sinclair R. Optimal treatment of head lice: is a no-nit policy justified? *Clin Dermatol* 2002;20:94–96.
2. Meinking TL, Burkhart CG, Burkhart CN. Head lice. *N Engl J Med* 2002;347:1381–1382.
3. Hill N. Treatment of head lice. *Lancet* 2000;356:2007.

Pubic Lice

Colleen Campbell

Clinical Presentation

The most common clinical symptom of pubic lice infestation is pruritus, which occurs in 85% of cases.[1] Patients often have very few lice during infection, so pubic hair must be inspected carefully for the presence of 1- to 2-mm, brown-colored lice.[2] Other findings suggestive of infestation are maculae caeruleae, bluish-gray macules that appear at feeding sites; rust-colored fecal material may be evident as well.[2]

Pathophysiology

Phthirus pubis are approximately 1 mm in size and have three sets of legs. They can live away from human hosts for up to 24 hours.[1] Pubic lice are easily transmitted via physical contact.[2] The most common mode of transmission is through sexual contact. Rarely, they can also be found in facial hair, thigh hair, and eyelashes.[3] Men are infected more commonly than women, possibly because women typically have less pubic hair.[3] Eggs are attached to the base of hair follicles and mature over the next 3 weeks to become adults. Adults can lay up to 100 eggs during their lifespan of 1 month.[2]

Diagnosis

The diagnosis of pubic lice is based on clinical evidence of disease. To confirm the diagnosis, hair follicles may be examined under low-power microscopy.[2]

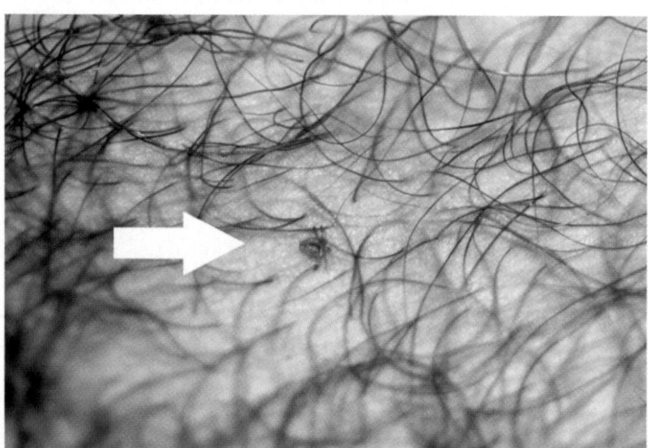

FIGURE 14–17 Pubic lice are well camouflaged among the hair shafts. (From Goodheart, with permission.)

Clinical Complications

The most common complication of infestation is spread to other individuals. Bacterial superinfection can occur as a result of excoriation.

Management

Treatment of pubic lice is with topical lindane, permethrin, or pyrethrins. Lindane 1% is applied to the affected area for 4 minutes.[4] Complications from lindane use for this limited amount of time are very rare. However, this treatment is contraindicated in women who are pregnant or lactating and in children younger than 2 years of age because of the risk of seizures and aplastic anemia.[2] Treatment with permethrin (1% crème) or pyrethrins should be for 10 minutes. Treatment may need to be repeated in 1 week if symptoms persist.[4]

All clothing and bedding should be washed to prevent reinfestation. Nits can be removed with a fine-toothed comb. Because one third of patients infested with pubic lice have a concomitant sexually transmitted disease, all patients should be screened and treated appropriately.[2] Urethritis and vulvovaginitis were the most commonly associated sexually transmitted diseases in one study.[3] All sexual partners (contacts within the previous month) should be treated as well.[4]

REFERENCES

1. Ko WT, Adal KA, Tomecki KJ. Infectious diseases. *Med Clin North Am* 1998;82:1001–1031.
2. Brown TJ, Yen-Moore A, Tyring SK. An overview of sexually transmitted diseases: part II. *J Am Acad Dermatol* 1999;41:661–677.
3. Varela JA, Otero L, Espinosa E, Sanchez C, Junquera ML, Vazquez F. *Phthirus pubis* in a sexually transmitted disease unit: a study of 14 years. *Sex Transm Dis* 2003;30:292–296.
4. Workowski KA, Levine WC. CDC STD treatment guidelines 2002. *MMWR Morb Mortal Wkly Rep* 2002;51(RR-6):1–78.

Pityriasis Rosea

Anthony S. Mazzeo

Clinical Presentation

Patients with pityriasis rosea (PR) usually present in the second or third decade of life complaining of a diffuse and itchy rash, which may be associated with a viral prodrome that includes fever, headache, fatigue, malaise, and arthralgias.

Pathophysiology

Various factors support a viral origin, including a predilection for fall and spring months, increased incidence among immunocompromised persons, lifelong immunity after the rash, and case clusters.[1] Human herpes virus-6 (HHV-6) or HHV-7 may be the inciting factor, although a definitive association remains controversial.[2] A PR-like rash may appear in conjunction with use of medications such as captopril, metronidazole, clonidine, and barbiturates.[3]

Diagnosis

Diagnosis is based on clinical examination; 50% of patients have or recall having a "herald patch," which is a lone, erythematous area, 2 to 10 cm in diameter, with raised, edematous borders. This lesion is usually on the trunk, but it may be located elsewhere. Between 7 and 10 days after the appearance of the herald patch, a diffuse eruption of smaller, pink, oval-shaped, papulosquamous patches appears along the skin tension lines. This distribution of the lesions leads to the so-called "Christmas tree" pattern on the back. They have a fine scale that may be located around the edges. The lesions can coalesce and recur.

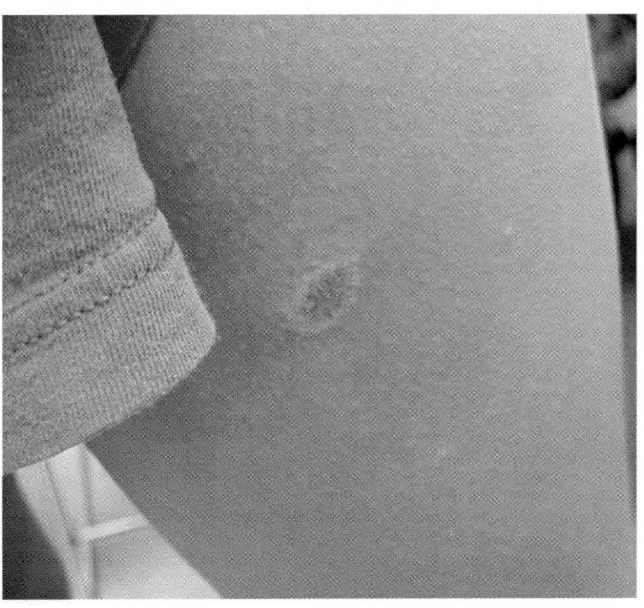

FIGURE 14–18 "Herald patch" seen in pityriasis rosea. (Courtesy of Christy Salvaggio, MD.)

Clinical Complications

PR can last for months, with a waxing and waning course. The course is generally benign and healing complete, although patients should be informed that postinflammatory pigmentation changes may persist.[3] If lesions persist for longer periods or are associated with other symptoms, the patient should be referred for dermatologic evaluation for psoriasis guttata and other conditions that mimic PR.

Management

Education and reassurance are the most important aspects of treatment for this benign, self-limited entity. Ultraviolet (UV) light has been reported anecdotally to shorten the duration, but it has no documented long-term benefit and in some cases may worsen changes in pigmentation. For those patients who experience pruritus, standard oral antihistamines may ease symptoms. Topical steroids may also provide symptomatic relief. Despite the recent evidence of HHV association and studies showing that erythromycin may hasten resolution, at this time antimicrobial therapy is not indicated.[2]

REFERENCES

1. Chuh AA, Lee A, Molinari N. Case clustering in pityriasis rosea: a multicenter epidemiologic study in primary care settings in Hong Kong. *Arch Dermatol* 2003;139:489–493.
2. Watanabe T, Kawamura T, Jacob SE, et al. Pityriasis rosea is associated with systemic active infection with both human herpesvirus-7 and human herpesvirus-6. *J Invest Dermatol* 2002;119:793–797.
3. Allen RA, Janniger CK, Schwartz RA. Pityriasis rosea. *Cutis* 1995;56:198–202.

14-19

Bullous Impetigo

Dziwe Ntaba

Clinical Presentation

Bullous impetigo (BI) is a common cutaneous infection that is seen primarily in infants and children. Presenting signs are typically flaccid blisters and bullae measuring between 0.5 and 3 cm in diameter.[1] Their distribution can be either local or diffuse, and they typically occur on the face. The trunk, perineum, and extremities can also be affected.[1,2]

Pathophysiology

BI is caused almost exclusively by coagulase-positive *Staphylococcus aureus,* although involvement of streptococcal species has been reported. The staphylococcal epidermolytic toxin is thought to be responsible for the tenderness and bullae formation that are characteristic of the disease.[1] Infection usually occurs in the absence of any apparent prior injury to the skin. If untreated, the bullae rupture in 1 to 2 days, leaving a honey-colored crust and superficial erosions.

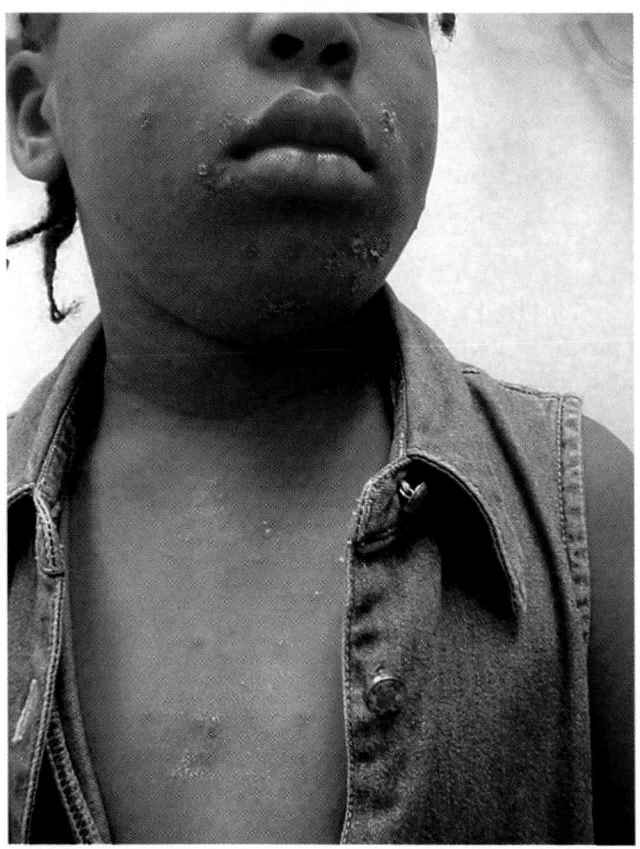

FIGURE 14–19 Bullous impetigo. (Courtesy of Christy Salvaggio, MD.)

Diagnosis

The diagnosis can usually be made on clinical grounds, but atypical presentations may resemble thermal or chemical burns.[1] Definitive diagnosis may be established by biopsy; however, this is reserved for unusual cases.

Clinical Complications

Complications (usually seen in infants) include local extension of infection that leads to osteomyelitis or septic arthritis. If the infection involves phage-group II, type-71 *Staphylococcus,* then larger bullae (up to 8 cm) may form as the toxin produces intradermal cleavage.[2] More severe but unusual presentations of this spectrum include staphylococcal scalded skin syndrome (SSSS), which involves generalized epidermolysis with desquamation.[3]

Management

Azithromycin and cephalosporins are the currently recommended drugs of choice. Dicloxacillin and first-generation cephalosporins are acceptable alternatives. Some fluoroquinolones have been shown to be effective, but they currently are approved only for adults. Erythromycin is no longer recommended because of microbial resistance.[2]

REFERENCES

1. Scales JW, Fleischer AB Jr, Krowchuk DP. Bullous impetigo. *Arch Pediatr Adolesc Med* 1997;151:1168–1169.
2. Stulberg DL, Penrod MA, Blatny RA. Common bacterial skin infections. *Am Fam Physician* 2002;66:119–124.
3. Edlich RF, Horowitz JH, Nichter LS, Silloway KA. Morgan, RF. Clinical syndromes caused by staphylococcal epidermolytic toxin. *Compr Ther* 1985;11:45–48.

Pemphigus Vulgaris

Reid Brackin

Clinical Presentation

Patients with pemphigus vulgaris (PV) may present with blisters or erosions of the skin, lesions in the mouth, secondary complications of the disease, or poor control of symptoms.

Pathophysiology

PV is a rare autoimmune disease involving mucocutaneous blister formation. Immunoglobulin G (IgG) antibody is targeted against desmoglein-3, an adhesion protein found in desmosomes, disturbing these main adhesion structures of the epidermis. The result is acantholysis (separation between keratinocytes), suprabasilar blister formation, and mild superficial dermal inflammatory infiltrate. The exact mechanism remains controversial.[1,2]

PV is the most common form of pemphigus. Other major types include pemphigus foliaceus and paraneoplastic pemphigus. Frequency is increased in people of Mediterranean or Jewish descent. The mean age at onset is between 50 and 60 years. Men and women are equally affected.[1,3]

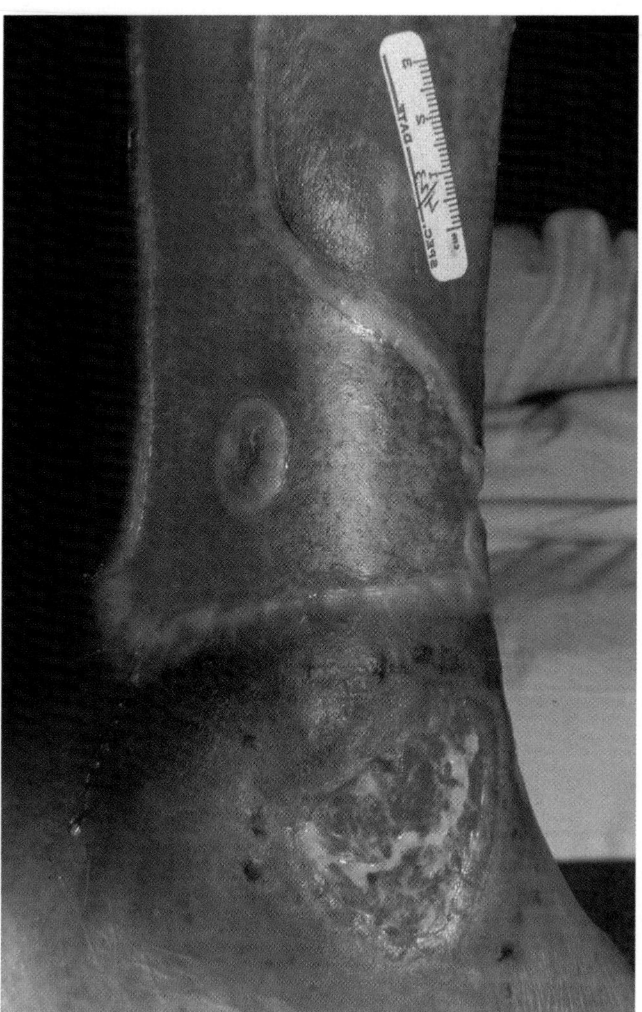

FIGURE 14–20 Intraepidermal blistering and dermal disruption characteristic of pemphigus vulgaris. (© David Effron, MD, 2004. Used with permission.)

Diagnosis

Blisters (bullae) are the primary lesions of PV. Cutaneous lesions commonly start on the head and trunk. The bullae are usually clear and tense at onset and become turbid and flaccid within 2 to 3 days. Ensuing rupture results in painful, denuded erosions and crusted ulcerations that may be pruritic. Pressure applied by a finger to skin at the edge of active lesions results in blister extension or new blister formation; this reaction is known as Nikolsky's sign and is characteristic of PV.[3] Oral lesions are the first sign of disease in more than half of patients. These lesions typically are painful erosions or chronic ulcerations, frequently on the lips, gums, and buccal mucosa, with possible extension to the pharynx and larynx. Intact bullae in the mouth are rare. Misdiagnosis as herpes simplex virus (HSV) infection is a potential pitfall.[1] PV is confirmed by intraepidermal vesicles and acantholysis on histologic examination and by direct or indirect immunofluorescence studies.[1-3]

Clinical Complications

Untreated PV is fatal in most patients due to spread of disease, sepsis, malnutrition, dehydration, debilitation, and thromboembolism.[3]

Management

Treatment involves pain control, wound care, administration of intravenous fluids, and appropriate antibiotics. The mainstay of long-term therapy is systemic corticosteroids, which have reduced the mortality rate from 95% to less than 10%.[1,2] Mild disease may be treated with a trial of topical corticosteroids or lower doses of prednisone. Dermatology consultation is essential.[1,3]

REFERENCES

1. Fellner MJ, Sapadin AN. Current therapy of pemphigus vulgaris. *Mt Sinai J Med* 2001;68:268–278.
2. Martel P, Joly P. Pemphigus: autoimmune diseases of keratinocyte's adhesion molecules. *Clin Dermatol* 2001;19:662–674.
3. Cotell S, Robinson ND, Chan LS. Autoimmune blistering skin diseases. *Am J Emerg Med* 2000;18:288–299.

Pyogenic Granuloma

Dziwe Ntaba

Clinical Presentation

Pyogenic granuloma (PG) occurs most commonly in children and young adults, with a distinctive variant in pregnant women.[1] Patients present with a rapidly growing nodule in the skin or mucous membranes. These are often friable and may lead to bleeding as part of the chief complaint.

Pathophysiology

The term *pyogenic granuloma* is a misnomer, because the lesion is neither purulent nor granulomatous. PG is actually a benign acquired vascular lesion.[2] It has been known to occur in response to injury or hormonal factors, although not exclusively so.[1] Debate exists as to whether the underlying lesion is a hemangioma or a hyperplastic proliferation of granulation tissue.[3]

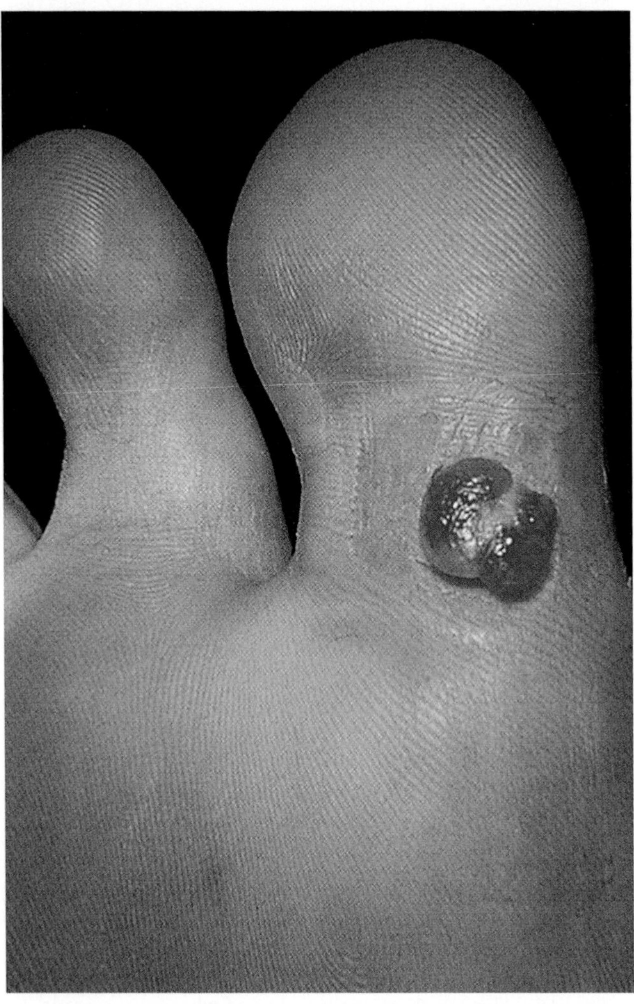

FIGURE 14–21 Pyogenic granuloma, a dome-shaped lesion with a moist and fragile surface that may bleed with minimal trauma. (From Dockery and Crawford, with permission.)

Diagnosis

PG lesions typically are small (less than 1 cm in diameter), rapidly evolving, solitary, yellow to bright red nodules. The surface may be lobular or ulcerated, with a moist or scaly texture. Lesions often become pedunculated with the development of a scaly stalk or "collarette." The most common distribution involves the head and neck region (62.5%), followed by the trunk (19.7%), and extremity (upper greater than lower; 17.9%).[1,2] Within this pattern, mucous membranes and fingers are common sites of localization. When found in pregnancy, PG lesions typically occur on the gingiva and are referred to as "pregnancy tumors."[1] The differential diagnosis of PG includes malignant conditions such as amelanotic melanoma (particularly if found along the nail bed), angiosarcoma, basal cell carcinoma (BCC), and squamous cell carcinoma (SCC). Biopsy for histopathologic characteristics confirms the diagnosis.

Clinical Complications

The most common complication is copious bleeding from the lesion that is refractory to pressure. Recurrence is also seen if any abnormal tissue remains after initial treatment. Rarely, multiple satellite lesions occur after excision of a solitary primary lesion.[1]

Management

Chemical cauterization with silver nitrate is an effective means of hemostasis in the emergency department (ED); excision, curettage, and laser therapy are available means for removal of the lesion. If appropriate, referral to a dermatologist, otolaryngologist, or capable primary physician is an acceptable disposition.[2]

REFERENCES

1. Mooney MA, Janniger CK. Pyogenic granuloma. *Cutis* 1995;55:133–136.
2. Luba MC, Bangs SA, Mohler AM, Stuhlberg DL. Common benign skin tumors. *Am Fam Physician* 2003;67:729–738.
3. Mills SE, Cooper PH, Fechner RE. Lobular Capillary Hemangioma: the underlying lesion of pyogenic granuloma. *Am J Surg Pathol* 1980;4:471–479.

Diabetic Dermopathy

Sigrid Wolfram

Clinical Presentation

Diabetic dermopathy (DD) is the most common dermatosis associated with diabetes. It develops in as many as 70% of diabetics, predominantly men older than 50 years of age.[1,2] The typical clinical presentation involves multiple, small (0.5 to 1 cm), asymmetric, annular or irregularly shaped, reddish-brown papules or plaques on the extensor surface of the lower legs, which slowly progress into atrophic, hyperpigmented, finely scaled macules.[1] These "spots" gradually resolve to leave a brown, atrophic scar. Lesions may also be found on the forearms, thighs, and lateral malleoli. New lesions may appear while older ones persist or resolve.[1]

Pathophysiology

The cause of DD is unclear. Microangiopathic changes and trauma are thought to predispose to DD-type lesions.[1,2] No correlation has been found between DD development and the extent of diabetes, duration of diabetes, or degree of glycemic control. In some patients, shin spots appear before abnormal glucose metabolism becomes evident.

Diagnosis

DD is a clinical diagnosis. Histologic examination reveals a thin epidermis with thickened vessels in the dermis and increased periodic acid–Schiff–positive material.[1] Lymphohistiocytic infiltrates with a few hemosiderin deposits may also be seen.[1] Differential diagnosis includes stasis dermatitis, necrobiosis lipoidica, pigmented purpuric eruption, and posttraumatic scarring.

Clinical Complications

No associated dermatologic or systemic complications have been described secondary to DD other than cosmetic disruption.

Management

The lesions of DD often resolve spontaneously, even as new ones arise. No treatment is effective or is recommended for these generally asymptomatic, cutaneous blemishes.[1,2] If the patient is concerned with their appearance, cosmetics may be used to hide the lesions. All medical therapy should be directed toward the patient's underlying diabetes mellitus.

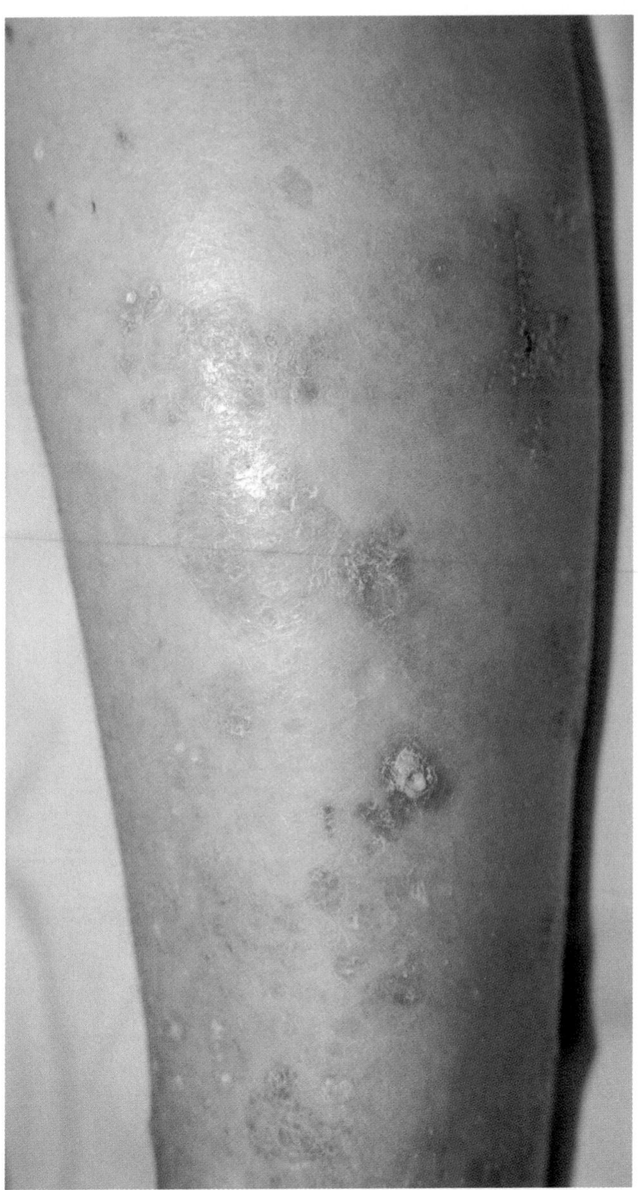

FIGURE 14–22 Patchy lesions of the lower leg associated with diabetes mellitus. (© David Effron, MD, 2004. Used with permission.)

REFERENCES

1. Ferringer T, Miller F 3rd. Cutaneous manifestations of diabetes mellitus. *Dermatol Clin* 2002;20:483–492.
2. Stulberg DL, Clark N, Tovey D. Common hyperpigmentation disorders in adults: part II. Melanoma, seborrheic keratoses, acanthosis nigricans, melasma, diabetic dermopathy, tinea versicolor, and postinflammatory hyperpigmentation. *Am Fam Physician* 2003;68: 1963–1968.

Necrobiosis Lipoidica

Anita Lynn Haynes

Clinical Presentation

Necrobiosis lipoidica (NL) usually is seen in patients with diabetes mellitus, who present with chronic granulomatous skin changes located bilaterally on the pretibial areas, face, hands, scalp, and forearms.[1] NL lesions begin as painless, reddish-brown papules that transform into a yellowish, atrophic plaque with a peripherally elevated purple ring and a central area that appears to be depressed.[1]

Pathophysiology

The presumptive mechanisms of NL include chronic inflammatory, microangiopathic, and structural disorders.[1] The abnormal accumulation of macrophages with subsequent granuloma formation may be a contributing cause of NL. Increased levels of prostaglandins, platelet aggregation, and small vessel disease are thought to be associated as well.[1] Microangiopathy, the thickening of dermal vessel walls, and occasional vessel occlusion are commonly seen in NL. Chronic venous insufficiency in obese, sedentary adults and in elderly individuals with diabetes mellitus may be precipitating factors.[1] Previous trauma in patients already predisposed to NL (i.e., obese diabetics) may lead to lesion formation.

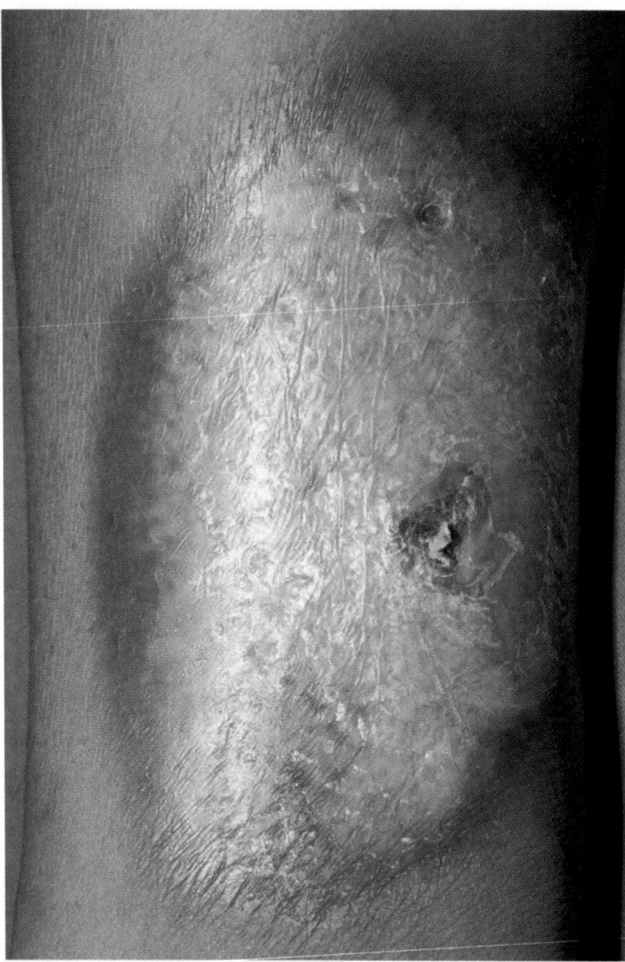

FIGURE 14-23 Oval violaceous plaque of necrobiosis lipoidica on anterior lower leg. (© David Effron, MD, 2004. Used with permission.)

Diagnosis

The diagnosis is clinical and is confirmed by biopsy to determine the depth of involvement of NL and the specific histologic categorization (i.e., granulomatous or necrobiotic or both). Vascular Doppler studies may demonstrate the level of venous stasis, suggesting local valvular dysfunction.[2]

Clinical Complications

Complications of NL include delayed wound healing, prolonged immobilization, subsequent accelerated weight gain, and superinfection.[2]

Management

Although NL is a chronic condition, it has been reported to resolve spontaneously in 10% to 20% of cases.[2] Endocrine consultation is appropriate for patients who have diabetes mellitus and cutaneous markers of the disease. Topical and/or intralesional corticosteroids, systemic corticosteroids, nicotinamide, cyclosporine, pentoxifylline, acetylsalicylic acid, oral ticlopidine, topical tretinoin, hyperbaric oxygen, porcine dressings, skin grafts, and pressure garments may help patients with NL.[1] Chronic NL usually does not require emergency therapy, and often patients may be discharged from the emergency department (ED) with timely follow-up by their primary care physicians.

REFERENCES

1. Nguyen K, Washenik K, Shupack J. Necrobiosis lipoidica diabeticorum treated with chloroquine. *J Am Acad Dermatol* 2002;46(2 Suppl Case Reports):S34–S36.
2. Yigit S, Estrada E. Recurrent necrobiosis lipoidica diabeticorum associated with venous Insufficiency associated in adolescent with poorly controlled type 2 diabetes mellitus. *J Pediatr* 2002;141: 280–282.

Lichen Planus

Kevin Y. Lin

Clinical Presentation

Patients with lichen planus (LP) may present with pruritic papules and plaques located over the flexor surfaces of the extremities.[1-3]

Pathophysiology

LP is an inflammatory cutaneous and mucous membrane disease of unknown cause. Current theories have focused on genetic issues and immune dysfunction as potentially causative. Exposure to some medications, including gold, antimalarial agents, penicillamine, thiazide diuretics, β-adrenergic blockers, nonsteroidal antiinflammatory drugs (NSAIDs), quinidine, and angiotensin-converting enzyme inhibitors, may produce a lichenoid eruption.[1]

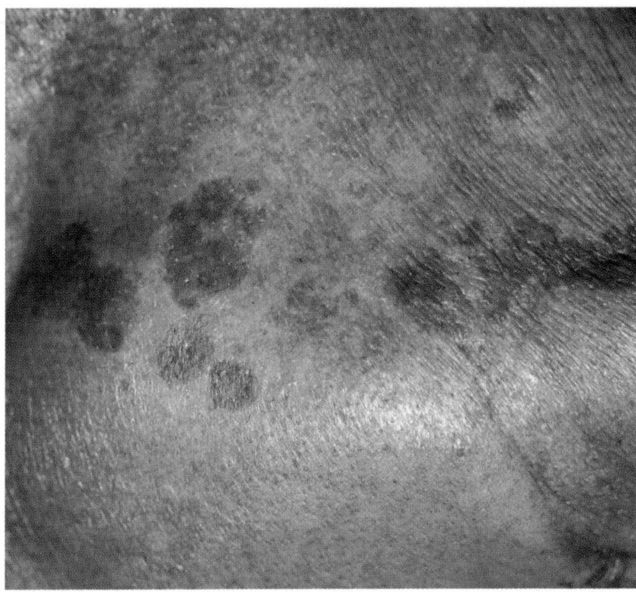

FIGURE 14–24 Typical lacy, reticular pattern of criss-crossed white lines (Wickham's striae) in lichen planus. (© David Effron, MD, 2004. Used with permission.)

Diagnosis

The diagnosis of LP is based on clinical inspection and biopsy of the lesion. LP lesions tend to be "violaceous polygonal flat-topped papules and plaques," sometimes characterized as "the six Ps": pruritic, polygonal, planar, purple papules and plaques.[1] LP lesions begin on the flexor surface of the extremities, most commonly the wrists, and may last from months to years. LP may also involve the genital mucosa, mucus membranes, hair, and nails.

Clinical Complications

Complications include involvement of oral mucosa, painful oral erosions, candidal infections, and squamous cell carcinoma (SCC).

Management

Clinical suspicion of LP warrants prompt dermatologic consultation. For localized cutaneous LP, topical corticosteroid creams such as clobetasol, halobetasol, betamethasone dipropionate, or diflorasone can be used. Less potent corticosteroids, such as hydrocortisone 2.5%, should be used on the face and genitalia. For generalized cutaneous LP, systemic corticosteroids should be considered.[3]

REFERENCES

1. Katta R. Lichen planus. *Am Fam Physician* 2000;61:3319–3324, 3327–3328.
2. Boyd AS, Neldner, KH. Lichen planus. *J Am Acad Dermatol* 1991;25:593–619.
3. Eisen D. The clinical manifestations and treatment of oral lichen planus. *Dermatol Clin* 2003;21:79–89.

Phytophotodermatitis

Anthony Morocco

Clinical Presentation

Patients initially develop an erythematous, vesicular rash in sun-exposed areas such as the face, upper chest, and dorsum of forearms and hands. The rash may appear as streaks, in the pattern of contact with the plant. Symptoms peak 36 to 72 hours after exposure. In severe cases, blistering and systemic symptoms may be present, including nausea and vomiting. The initial rash is followed by the development of raised, uniformly hyperpigmented lesions that can last for several months or longer.[1,2]

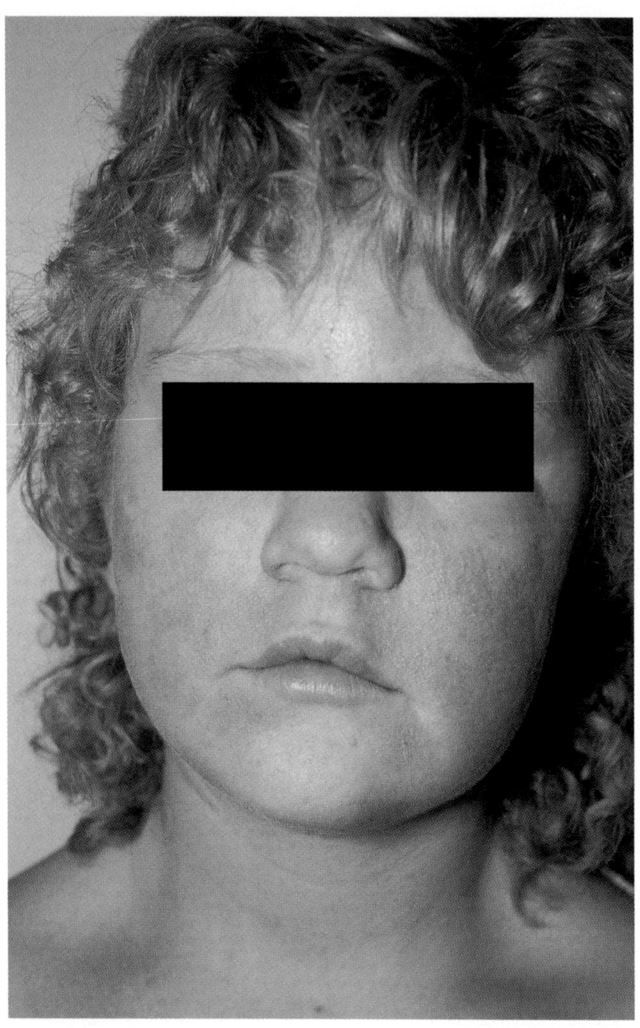

FIGURE 14–25 Exposure to plants containing light-sensitizing chemicals may result in intense skin reactions. (© David Effron, MD, 2004. Used with permission.)

Pathophysiology

Phytophotodermatitis is a nonallergic skin reaction that occurs after exposure to certain plants in combination with sunlight. The condition is commonly seen in workers such as gardeners, farmers, chefs, and grocers. Many common plants contain psoralens, the class of compounds responsible for the reaction. These include lemon, lime, celery, wild carrot, parsley, parsnip, fennel, dill, fig, buttercup, and mustard.[1] Psoralens are used therapeutically in combination with ultraviolet light (PUVA) for treatment of psoriasis, vitiligo, and mycosis fungoides (cutaneous T-cell lymphoma). Berloque dermatitis occurs on the upper body after use of perfume made from psoralen-containing oil of bergamot lime.[2]

When exposed to sunlight, psoralens cause DNA cross-linking and inhibition of cell division and growth. This injury stimulates keratin and melanin synthesis as well as thickening of the stratum corneum.[1]

Diagnosis

Diagnosis is based on the history, appearance, and location of the skin lesions. A careful exposure history should be obtained. Patients may not remember seemingly trivial exposures to psoralens, such as making mixed drinks with limes. Misdiagnosis of child abuse has occurred when children developed hyperpigmented lesions in the shape of handprints. In these cases, parents with lemon or lime juice on their hands touched the children, who were subsequently exposed to sun and developed the condition.[1]

Management

Acute treatment consists of topical corticosteroids and cool compresses. Hyperpigmentation generally resolves over time, but treatment with tretinoin or a skin-bleaching agent may improve the appearance.[1]

REFERENCES

1. Weber IC, Davis CP, Greeson DM. Phytophotodermatitis: the other "lime" disease. *J Emerg Med* 1999;17:235–237.
2. Gould JW, Mercurio MG, Elmets CA. Cutaneous photosensitivity diseases induced by exogenous agents. *J Am Acad Dermatol* 1995; 33:551–576.

Pilonidal Cyst

Jason Sundseth

Clinical Presentation

Pilonidal cysts typically affect young adults (before age 40 years), with a 4:1 male predominance.[1,2] Patients may present with a painful, fluctuant mass, approximately 5 cm cephalad from the anus in the midline, that may be associated with fluid drainage.[1]

Pathophysiology

Pilonidal cysts are granulomatous reactions to small nests of hair in the midline sacrococcygeal area that progress into abscesses and tracts of infection.[1]

Pilonidal disease is most likely an acquired disease, although a congenital origin has been argued.[1] The disease develops from penetration of the skin by hair. An inflammatory, granulomatous reaction of pilosebaceous glands and hair follicles results in a granulomatous cyst. Epithelialized sinuses form from entrapped hairs that accumulate in the original tract and start a foreign body reaction. Bacteria may enter the sterile follicle and produce inflammation and edema, as well as occluding the follicle. The contents may expand until the follicle ruptures and the infection extends into the subcutaneous tissue, leading to abscess formation. Ninety percent of the tracts extend cephalad from the inciting follicle; they may track to the midline or laterally.[1,2]

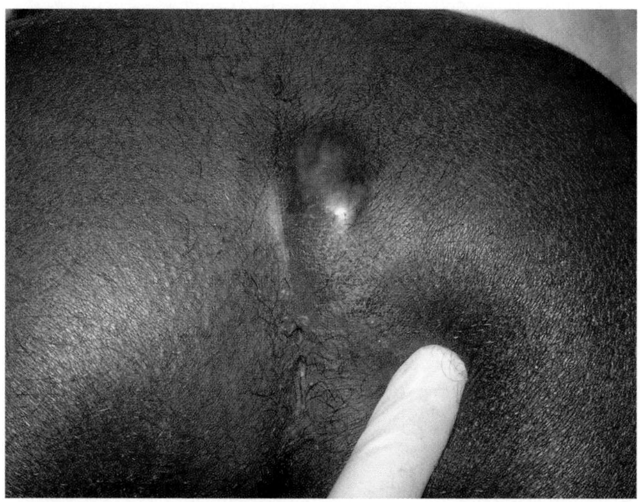

FIGURE 14–26 Pilonidal cyst in a typical location at the base of the spine. (Courtesy of Mark Silverberg, MD.)

Diagnosis

The diagnosis of pilonidal disease is made by finding a painful, fluctuant area in the presacral region. Chronic or recurrent disease is appreciated when there is recurrence after incision and drainage for a pilonidal abscess has been performed.[1]

Clinical Complications

The most common complication is recurrence of pilonidal abscesses (1% to 19% of cases).[2]

Management

Pilonidal abscesses may be treated with incision and drainage in the emergency department (ED). The wound should be packed, and the patient should receive follow-up with a surgeon for definitive treatment. Until recently, definitive therapy for pilonidal abscesses was an open excision that required weeks to months to heal. Simple incision and curettage, with minimal tissue loss, is now a more common surgical option.[1] Additional definitive options include injection with phenol, marsupialization, excision and primary closure, and excision with plastic closure (e.g., Z-plasty, skin graft).[2] Patients may be instructed to shave the hairs within 3 to 4 cm of the cyst every 1 to 3 weeks to prevent recurrence.[2]

REFERENCES

1. da Silva JH. Pilonidal cyst: cause and treatment. *Dis Colon Rectum* 2000;43:1146–1156.
2. Hull TL, Wu J. Pilonidal disease. *Surg Clin North Am* 2002;82: 1169–1185.

Tinea Cruris

Lorenzo Paladino

Clinical Presentation

Tinea cruris is a common fungal infection that is seen almost exclusively in men. It often occurs concurrently with tinea infections of the feet.[1] Pruritus is common, and pain may be present if the involved area is macerated or secondarily infected.[1] The infection starts with scaling and erythema from the inguinal fold and advances to involve the anterior aspect of the thighs.[1] The rash may also spread to the anal cleft. Tinea cruris is well-defined and rarely involves the scrotum; both of these features distinguish it from candidiasis.[1]

Pathophysiology

Tinea cruris is a fungal infection involving the groin, sometimes referred to as "jock itch."[1]

Common dermatophytes associated with groin infections are *Trichophyton rubrum, Epidermophyton floccosum,* and *Trichophyton mentagrophytes.*[1]

Diagnosis

The organism can be seen in potassium hydroxide (KOH) preparations from scrapings of the advancing, scaling border.[1] A fungal culture can also help confirm the diagnosis. Tinea cruris does not fluoresce under the light from a Wood's lamp.

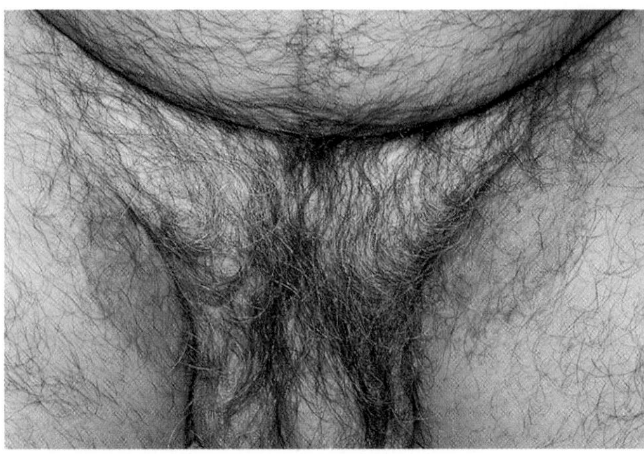

FIGURE 14–27 Tinea cruris. Note the scalloped border. (From Goodheart, with permission.)

Clinical Complications

Clinical complications are rare, but superinfection of the area by cellulitis-causing bacteria may occur. This is more commonly seen in immunocompromised individuals.[1]

Management

Dermatophyte infections can be curtailed in two ways: altering their environment to make it unfavorable for propagation, and using topical antifungal agents. In order to reduce the humidity of the local environment, loose-fitting cotton or moisture-"wicking" clothing should be recommended. Topical antifungals include the azole class of medications, such as clotrimazole, ketoconazole, or miconazole. These have a broad spectrum of activity, with some gram-positive coverage as well. The allylamines are the other main class of antifungals and include terbinafine and naftifine. These agents require daily application and remain active in the skin for 1 week after application. Newer agents such as ciclopirox, butenafine, and haloprogin have been tried with mixed results. Mycostatin (nystatin) has not been found to be effective in the treatment of tinea cruris. These topical treatments should extend 2 cm beyond the affected borders of the lesion. Topical steroids may be used as an adjunct in cases of severe inflammation. For immunosuppressed patients, those with extensive disease, and those for whom topical treatment has failed, fluconazole, itraconazole, or terbinafine may be given orally. Concomitant treatment of tinea pedis in affected individuals is necessary to prevent recurrence.[1]

REFERENCES

1. Gupta AK, Chaudhry M, Elewski B. Tinea corporis, tinea cruris, tinea nigra, and piedra. *Dermatol Clin* 2003;21:395–400.

Tinea Capitis

Colleen Campbell

Clinical Presentation

Tinea capitis is common in infants and small children, and it is the most common dermatophyte infection in this age group.[1] Patients usually present with pruritic scalp lesions that appear as papules, pustules, or plaques. Nodules also may be present on the scalp. Scaling, erythema, exudates, and alopecia occur secondary to the inflammatory response. Patients often have associated cervical and occipital lymphadenopathy. Patients may present with a kerion, which is a soft, erythematous, and inflammatory scalp nodule associated with hair loss.[2]

Pathophysiology

Tinea capitis may be transmitted from fomites, person-to-person, or from animals to people.[1] It is commonly found in preschool-aged children and is reportedly more common in African American and Hispanic children.[2] *Trichophyton* species, most commonly *Trichophyton tonsurans* and *T. mentagrophytes,* cause 80% of cases.[2] Infection with these species is asymptomatic in up to 30% of patients.[2] *Microsporum* species are zoophilic and are also commonly found.[1] Keratin is used as the nutrient source of dermatophytes; therefore, invasion of live tissue is rare.

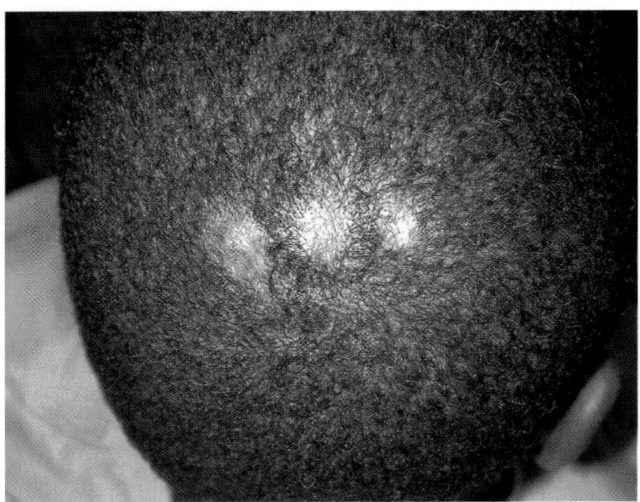

FIGURE 14–28 Tinea capitis occurs most frequently in children between the ages of 3 and 7 years. (Courtesy of Raymond Moreno, MD.)

Diagnosis

Physical examination revealing at least three of four criteria (scalp scaling, pruritus, occipital adenopathy, and alopecia) are accurate in 92% of culture-confirmed cases.[1] Diagnosis is confirmed by extracting a hair sample and performing a potassium hydroxide (KOH) preparation, and by checking the sample for hyphae. Culture results can also be obtained from the hair sample, using Sabouraud's dextrose agar with cycloheximide.[3] Wood's lamp examination shows blue-green fluorescence if the genus is *Microsporum.*[1]

Clinical Complications

Because dermatophyte infections tend to be superficial, the main complication is hair loss. Spread to other individuals is also prevalent and occurs more frequently in those with depressed cell-mediated immunity.[1]

Management

To prevent spread to other family members, all grooming utensils should be washed thoroughly. It is recommended that family members use a selenium sulfide shampoo three times a week as well.[2] Oral antifungals are then prescribed to the patient for cure of disease.[1] Griseofulvin is the only FDA-approved treatment for tinea capitis in children. Terbinafine is also effective. Other available treatments include ketoconazole, itraconazole, and fluconazole.

REFERENCES

1. Hainer BL. Dermatophyte infections. *Am Fam Physician* 2003;67: 101–108.
2. Vander Straten MR, Hossain MA, Ghannoum MA. Cutaneus infections: dermatophytosis, onychomycosis, and tinea versicolor. *Infect Dis Clin North Am* 2003;17:87–112.
3. Weinstein A, Berman B. Topical treatment of common superficial tinea infections. *Am Fam Physician* 2002;65:2095–2102.

Tinea Barbae

Colleen Campbell

Clinical Presentation

Tinea barbae manifests as nodular, boggy lesions that often are associated with exudates. Lesions may appear as erythematous pustules or scaly patches. The infection involves the hair shafts and is exacerbated by ingrown hairs. Hair removal in affected areas is characteristically painless.[2] Patients may complain of associated itching or burning in the region.

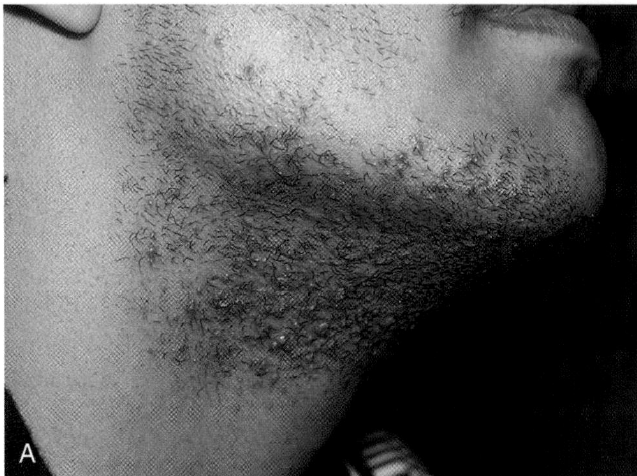

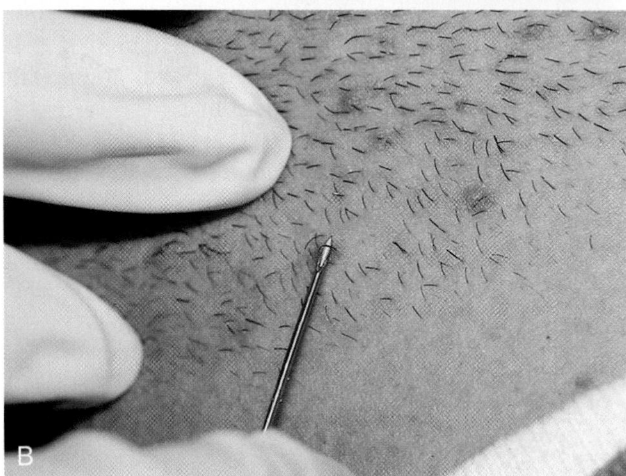

FIGURE 14–29 **A:** Tight, curly hairs that have been sharpened by shaving penetrate the skin. Inflammatory papules and pustules that resemble acne are evident. **B:** A curled hair that had penetrated the skin is lifted with a fine needle. (**A** and **B**, From Goodheart, with permission.)

Pathophysiology

Tinea barbae is a dermatophyte infection of the beard area.[1]

Tinea barbae is caused by *Trichophyton verrucosum*. This organism, like other dermatophytes, colonizes the keratinized stratum corneum. It forms on the outside of hair shafts and subsequently destroys the cuticle.[3] Because the infection is more common in men who work with animals, it is thought to have zoophilic spread.[2]

Diagnosis

Diagnosis of tinea barbae usually is based on the clinical presentation alone. Microscopic examination of a potassium hydroxide (KOH) preparation of a hair sample often reveals fungal hyphal elements. Diagnosis of tinea barbae is confirmed with culture from affected hair.

Clinical Complications

Superinfection of the affected area with bacteria is the most common complication of tinea barbae.

Management

Patients should be advised to shave regularly and to wash the face frequently with antibacterial soap.[3] Treatment of tinea barbae infection involves the use of orally administered antifungal drugs.[1,2] The agent most commonly used is griseofulvin, which should be continued for 2 to 4 weeks after resolution of infection. For resistant cases, itraconazole, terbinafine, or fluconazole may be used.

REFERENCES

1. Weinstein A, Berman B. Topical treatment of common superficial tinea infections. *Am Fam Physician* 2002;65:2095–2102.
2. Hainer BL. Dermatophyte infections. *Am Fam Physician* 2003;67: 101–108.
3. Vander Straten MR, Hossain MA, Ghannoum MA. Cutaneus infections: dermatophytosis, onychomycosis, and tinea versicolor. *Infect Dis Clin North Am* 2003;17:87–112.

Tinea Versicolor

Colleen Campbell

Clinical Presentation

Patients present with involvement of sebaceous glands of the upper trunk, neck, and arms. Children may present with facial lesions. Lesions appear erythematous; they may consist of hypopigmented or hyperpigmented macules, or they may appear patchy. Scaling and pruritus are variably present. Affected areas do not tend to tan as much as unaffected areas do.[2] The rash does not typically clear spontaneously, so patients may present with long-standing symptoms.

Pathophysiology

Tinea versicolor, or pityriasis versicolor, is a superficial mycotic infection. It is not a true tinea infection, because the organism causing infection is not a dermatophyte but a yeast.[1]

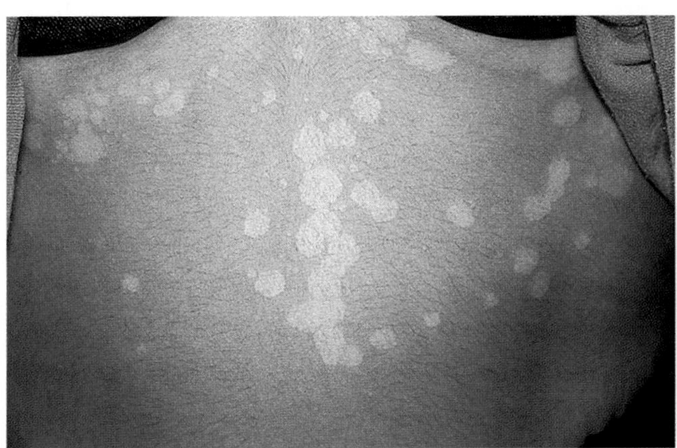

FIGURE 14–30 Hypopigmented lesions consistent with tinea versicolor. (From Goodheart, with permission.)

Tinea versicolor is caused by *Malassezia furfur*, a lipophilic yeast. High temperature and humidity contribute to the development of infection, as do occlusive clothing and greasy skin.[2]

Diagnosis

Diagnosis is often made in the emergency department (ED) on the basis of appearance of the rash alone. This can be confirmed by Wood's light examination or microscopic examination of a potassium hydroxide (KOH) preparation.[3] A Wood's lamp reveals the pale yellow fluorescence of *M. furfur*.[3] Short, angular hyphae and budding yeast can be seen on microscopic evaluation.[2]

Clinical Complications

The most common complication of tinea versicolor is reinfection. Reinfection rates are reported to be as high as 80% after 2 years.[2]

Management

Treatment of tinea versicolor involves topical or oral antifungal therapy. Topical agents include selenium sulfide lotion or shampoo, left on for 15 minutes, applied daily for 2 weeks and then once a month thereafter. Other topical treatments include terbinafine or treatment with econazole or ketoconazole. Recurrence may be less frequent if oral therapy is used.[2]

REFERENCES

1. Weinstein A, Berman B. Topical treatment of common superficial tinea infections. *Am Fam Physician* 2002;65:2095–2102.
2. Vander Straten MR, Hossain MA, Ghannoum MA. Cutaneus infections: dermatophytosis, onychomycosis, and tinea versicolor. *Infect Dis Clin North Am* 2003;17:87–112.
3. Hainer BL. Dermatophyte infections. *Am Fam Physician* 2003;67:101–108.

14-31

Tinea Pedis

Colleen Campbell

Clinical Presentation

There are three recognized forms of tinea pedis: interdigital, moccasin, and vesiculobullous.[1] Interdigital tinea pedis is the most common, often occurring between the fourth and fifth toes. The skin appears either macerated and moist or dry and scaly. In the moccasin variety, there is a nonpruritic, scaly white, or silvery rash that may be seen on the plantar aspect of the foot. This scale often has a thickened, erythematous base. Vesiculobullous tinea is most commonly seen on the heel or sole, and pustules are often present.

Pathophysiology

Tinea pedis is a dermatophyte infection involving the skin of the toes and feet.

Tinea pedis is the most common dermatophyte infection of humans, occurring in 70% of adults.[1] The most commonly identified agent is *Trichophyton rubrum*. This organism was reported to be responsible for 76% of all superficial fungal diseases in one study.[2] Other dermatophytes causing this infection include *T. mentagrophytes* and *Epidermophyton floccosum*. These fungal organisms are common in humid, warm environments such as athletic or other occlusive shoes and locker rooms.[1] Most infections are spread from person to person, but they can also be spread through contact with fomites.[1]

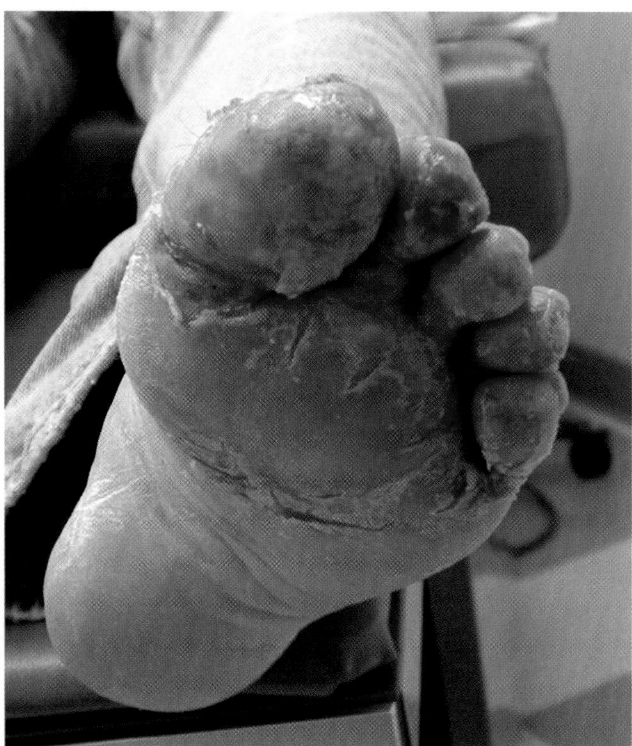

FIGURE 14–31 Tinea pedis with secondary infection. (Courtesy of Robert Hendrickson, MD.)

Diagnosis

The diagnosis of tinea pedis usually is made on the basis of clinical presentation alone but can be confirmed with a potassium hydroxide (KOH) preparation taken from the leading edge of the lesion or from the roof of pustules or vesicles, if present.[3] Fungal hyphae are visible on microscopic examination of the slide.

Clinical Complications

Bacterial superinfection is the most common complication of tinea pedis. Recurrent tinea infection is also commonly seen, especially in the presence of onychomycosis.[1]

Management

Patients should be advised to wear moisture-wicking socks and to keep their feet open to the air as much as possible. The mainstay of treatment is the use of topical antifungal drugs. The primary types of antifungal agents used to treat infection are the azoles and the allylamines. Azoles include clotrimazole, econazole, and miconazole. The allylamine group includes terbinafine and naftifine. Ciclopirox is a broad-spectrum agent that is effective against dermatophytes and yeasts and has some antibacterial activity as well.[2] Polyenes, including nystatin, are less effective in the treatment of tinea pedis.[2] All agents should be used one to two times daily for 7 days after the resolution of symptoms, or for a total of 4 weeks. A steroid antifungal agent may be used if patients have a significant inflammatory component to their infection. Concomitant onychomycosis should be treated with an oral agent.[3]

REFERENCES

1. Vander Straten MR, Hossain MA, Ghannoum MA. Cutaneus infections: dermatophytosis, onychomycosis, and tinea versicolor. *Infect Dis Clin North Am* 2003;17:87–112.
2. Weinstein A, Berman B. Topical treatment of common superficial tinea infections. *Am Fam Physician* 2002;65:2095–2102.
3. Hainer BL. Dermatophyte infections. *Am Fam Physician* 2003;67:101–108.

Intertriginous Candidiasis

Allon Amitai

Clinical Presentation

Intertriginous candidiasis may be an incidental finding, or the patient may complain of pain, pruritus, and maceration of the affected region. Such areas are generally "beefy" red and patchy, with satellite lesions.[1] They are often found in the axillae, the groin, and the inframammary or pannus folds. The corners of the mouth (angular cheilitis or perlèche) and finger and toe web spaces are also periodically infected.[1] Diaper dermatitis can be seen in infants and in the incontinent elderly.[1]

Pathophysiology

Candida species are normal commensal flora, but pathogenicity may be facilitated by the warm, moist microenvironments of skin folds. Intertriginous regions experience chronic friction rubbing, which can break down the epidermis and permit candidal tissue invasion. Decreased host resistance in patients who are elderly, diabetic, or immunocompromised increases the likelihood of infection. Other predisposing factors include obesity, humid living environment, poor hygiene, antibiotic use, pregnancy, skin trauma, topical steroid use, and inflammatory skin disorders such as psoriasis. Pustules may be found intact as satellites. Chronic maceration can lead to fissuring.[1]

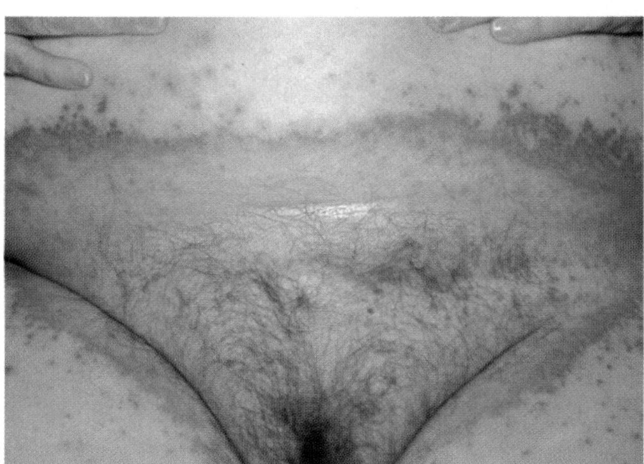

FIGURE 14–32 Candidiasis. Note the "beefy" erythematous plaques and satellite lesions. (© David Effron, MD, 2004. Used with permission.)

Diagnosis

The clinical diagnosis of a fungal infection may be confirmed by a potassium hydroxide (KOH) mount of skin scrapings, which demonstrates budding spores and pseudohyphae or true hyphae. Candidal skin disease may be indistinguishable from dermatophyte infection.[1]

Clinical Complications

Complications include persistent or recurrent candidal infection and bacterial superinfection, which may be related to increasing resistance to azole antimicrobial agents. In severely immunocompromised patients, candidemia and systemic candidosis may develop.[1]

Management

Coexisting systemic diseases such as impaired cell-mediated immunity, malnutrition, endocrinopathy, and neoplasia should be sought.[1] The patient should be advised to keep the skin dry with antifungal powder and the regular use of a hair dryer, lamp, or towel. Tight-fitting clothing should be avoided. Local treatment may include topical application of one of the azole creams or ciclopirox olamine. Oral Diflucan (fluconazole) may be used in severe cases or if topical medications cannot be used easily in specific patients.[1]

REFERENCE

1. Martin ES, Elewski BE. Cutaneous fungal infections in the elderly. *Clin Geriatr Med* 2002;18:59–75.

14-33

Tinea Corporis

Alex Paxson

Clinical Presentation

Patients with tinea corporis (TC) present with annular, erythematous patches with scaly borders on the arms, chest, back, or legs.[1-3] Most annular lesions have central clearing ("ringworm"), whereas others have concentric rings of scales within the external border. Severity varies with the offending species, with zoophilic species (transmitted by animals) causing a more intense inflammatory, suppurative, pustular eruption. Dermatophyte infection is common among high school and college wrestlers (tinea corporis gladiatorum).[2]

Pathophysiology

TC, also known as "ringworm," is caused by dermatophytes from the *Trichophyton, Microsporum,* and *Epidermophyton* genera. *T. rubrum* and *T. mentagrophytes* are most commonly isolated by culture.[1-3] The infection is normally confined to the stratum corneum of the epidermis, where the organisms are attracted to keratin and colonize keratinocytes.

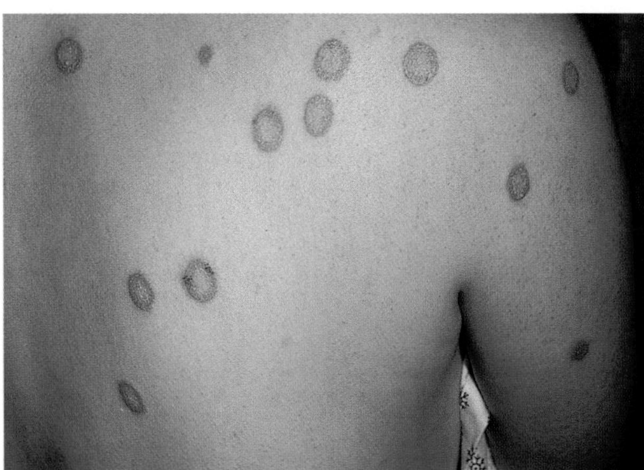

FIGURE 14–33 Tinea corporis with typical annular lesions ("ringworm"). Note the inflammatory reaction, which is more often seen when the source of the tinea is zoophilic. (From Ostler, with permission.)

Diagnosis

TC may be misdiagnosed as eczema or psoriasis. Definitive diagnosis requires visualization of microscopic hyphae on a potassium hydroxide (KOH) preparation.

Clinical Complications

Complications may include reoccurrence, superinfection, and cellulitis.

Management

Topical antifungal agents such as miconazole, clotrimazole, and ketoconazole require 4 to 6 weeks of treatment, whereas the newer agent, terbinafine, requires 3 to 4 weeks. All topical antifungals should be applied twice daily after washing of the affected area, and treatment should continue until all lesions are gone. Occasionally, systemic antifungals such as ketoconazole or fluconazole are needed for resistant infections or in more severe cases. Because of side effects (hepatic/bone marrow suppression), oral treatment should be reserved for resistant cases, as opposed to cases in which patients discontinue treatment early. Topical steroids should not be applied, because they may worsen the lesion and make the diagnosis more difficult.[1-3]

REFERENCES

1. Papa CA, Maroon MS, Clark CC. Picture of the month. Trichophyton verrucosum tinea corporis. *Arch Pediatr Adolesc Med* 1999;153: 201–202.
2. Perri BR, Lynch SA. Common injuries in the skilled wrestler. *Curr Opinion Orthop* 2003;14:109–113.
3. Ginsburg CM. Superficial fungal and mycobacterial infections of the skin. *Pediatr Infect Dis* 1985;4[3 Suppl]:S19–S23.

Viral Warts

Colleen Campbell

Clinical Presentation

The common wart initially appears as a smooth, well-circumcised papule that evolves over time to a dome-shaped papule with an irregular surface.[1,2] They may appear grayish or brownish in color and hyperkeratotic in form. They may be firm, nodular, or polypoid.[2] Most commonly, they are found in the periungual region of the hands, although they can be found anywhere.[1] Filiform warts are a variant of the common wart; they appear with finger-like projections and are often found near the eyes.[1] Flat warts appear as flattened papules in areas that are frequently shaved and on the face and dorsum of the hands.

Pathophysiology

Warts, or verrucae, are benign epithelial tumors caused by the DNA virus known as human papillomavirus (HPV).[1]

Viral warts are divided into common warts (verrucae vulgaris), flat warts (verrucae planus), and plantar warts (verrucae plantaris). Common warts represent 70% of the HPV cases seen in clinical practice.[1] Warts can be transmitted from person to person, by autoinoculation, or through contact in a warm, moist environment.[1] Infection is increased in those patients with decreased T-cell immunity.[3] HPV types 1, 2, and 4 cause both common and plantar warts, whereas types 3 and 10 are more commonly found in flat warts. Flat warts are the least common type of common wart, occurring in 4% of patients with warts.[1]

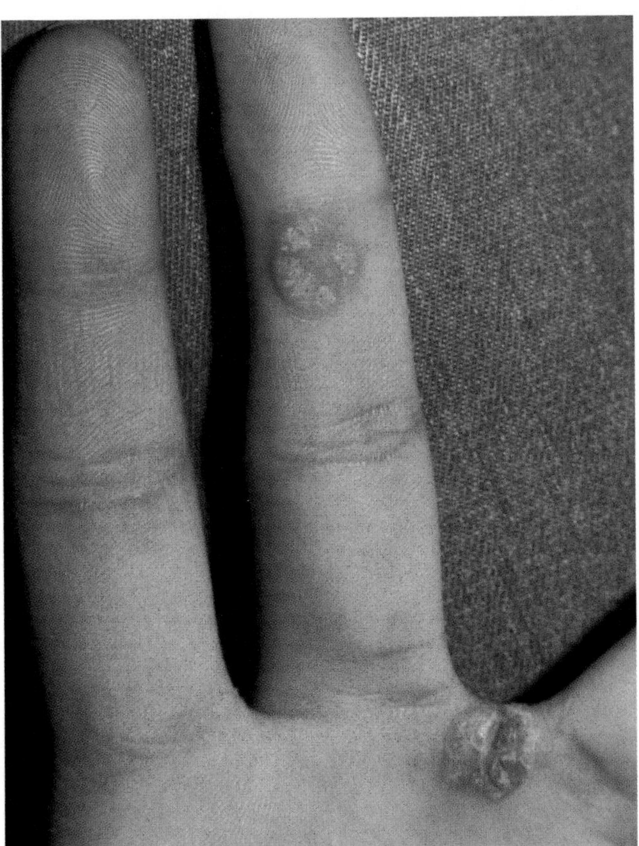

FIGURE 14–34 Wart with typical mosaic surface. (© David Effron, MD, 2004. Used with permission.)

Diagnosis

The diagnosis of warts is made on clinical grounds. Diagnosis may be improved by débridement of the affected skin area, because warts are often mistaken for corns or calluses. After débridement of skin, the wart has an appearance of having "seeds."[1] These seeds represent capillary hemorrhages in the area of the wart. Warts do not retain the usual handprint or footprint lines, another feature that is helpful in differentiating them from calluses or corns.[1]

Clinical Complications

The most important complications of warts are resistant infection, autoinoculation, and pain at the site of infection.

Management

Treatment of warts is through chemical, surgical, or chemotherapeutic measures. The most common treatment involves the use of salicylic acid, which is available over the counter. This treatment comes in the form of a liquid, a gel, or a transdermal patch. Soaking the affected area in warm water and débriding it before application of salicylic acid is recommended for optimal effect.[1] Treatment may take weeks to months, but salicylic acid has a 70% to 80% cure rate.[1] Other chemical agents include formaldehyde, glutaraldehyde, and cantharidin.[1] Surgical measures include electrosurgery, cryotherapy, and blunt dissection.[1] Cryogens used include liquid nitrogen, nitrous oxide, and carbon dioxide. Cryotherapy requires a temperature of at least −50°C.[3] A repeat treatment after thawing has been shown to be more effective than a single cryotherapy treatment.[2] Bleomycin, interferon, podophyllin, and 5-fluorouracil injections into the wart are also used in treatment of resistant warts.[1,2] Cimetidine, which has been shown to boost cell-mediated immunity, may be used in children who have multiple warts.[2]

REFERENCES

1. Plasencia JM. Cutaneous warts: diagnosis and treatment. *Prim Care* 2000;27:423–434.
2. Stulberg DL, Hutchinson AG. Molluscum contagiosum and warts. *Am Fam Physician* 2003;67:1233–1240.
3. Tyring SK. Human papillomavirus infections: epidemiology, pathogenesis, and host immune response. *J Am Acad Dermatol* 2000;43: S18–S26.

Herpetic Whitlow

Colleen Campbell

Clinical Presentation

Herpetic whitlow usually occurs on the digits of the dominant hand.[2] It first appears as a large vesicle with surrounding erythema; however, multiple small vesicles may also be seen.[2] Multiple lesions on several fingers were reported in 19% of pediatric cases.[1] The vesicles are initially filled with clear fluid but may become cloudy as white blood cells (WBCs) infiltrate the region.[1] There often is a history of a burning sensation for 2 or 3 days before the appearance of the vesicle. Patients may also complain of systemic symptoms, including fever and malaise.[1] The digital pulp space is the most commonly affected site.[1] Herpetic whitlow usually resolves spontaneously within approximately 3 weeks.[1]

Pathophysiology

Herpetic whitlow is an infection of the digits caused by herpes simplex virus (HSV)-1 or -2.[1]

HSV is the viral organism responsible for herpetic whitlow. In adults, HSV-2 is more commonly identified, whereas in children HSV-1 is the most common isolate.[2] Typically, infection is caused by autoinoculation, with the incubation period ranging 2 and 20 days.[1] Autoinoculation usually occurs from gingivostomatitis or herpes labialis in children.[1] Health care workers may contract herpetic whitlow from exposure to oral secretions of their patients if universal precautions are not strictly followed.[2]

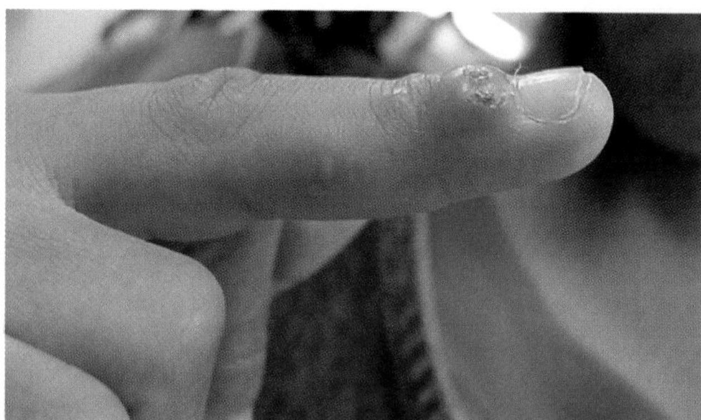

FIGURE 14-35 Herpetic whitlow. (Courtesy of Christy Salvaggio, MD.)

Diagnosis

Herpetic whitlow can be diagnosed initially based on the clinical appearance and confirmed with PCR or viral culture.[2] The Tzanck smear is no longer recommended because of its low sensitivity.[1] Care should be taken not to unroof the vesicles, because this may cause spread of the disease.[1] Instead, a small needle should be used to aspirate vesicle contents for diagnostic testing.

Clinical Complications

Bacterial superinfection is the most common complication of herpetic whitlow; it occurred in more than 25% of reported cases in one series.[1] Other complications of herpetic whitlow include lymphadenitis, hypoesthesia, keratitis, and, rarely, systemic viremia.[2] Recurrence rates of whitlow are quite high. In one review, it was found to reemerge in more than 20% of patients.[1]

Management

Topical application of idoxuridine has been used in treatment, but it is unclear whether this agent reduces the duration of infection.[2] Systemic acyclovir may shorten the disease course and decrease multifocal lesions in pediatric patients.[1,3] Acyclovir is recommended in immunocompromised patients to reduce the risk of systemic spread.[1,3]

REFERENCES

1. Szinnai G, Schaad UB, Heininger U. Multiple herpetic whitlow lesions in a 4 year-old girl: case report and review of the literature. *Eur J Pediatr* 2001;160:528–533.
2. Avitzur Y, Amir J. Herpetic whitlow infection in a general pediatrician: an occupational hazard. *Infection* 2002;30:234–236.
3. Trizna Z, Tyring SK. Antiviral treatment of diseases in pediatric dermatology. *Dermatol Clin* 1998;16:539–552.

Plantar Warts

Colleen Campbell

Clinical Presentation

Patients present with a hyperkeratotic, thick, flattened wart, usually located on the weight-bearing aspects of the foot. The heel and metatarsal heads are most commonly affected.[1] Warts are often found at sites of callus. Thrombosed capillaries may be visible within the lesion as multiple small "seeds." There may be a plaquelike area of coalesced warts, or the lesion may have a mosaic appearance, referred to as myrmecia.

Pathophysiology

Plantar warts, or verrucae plantaris, are caused by human papillomavirus (HPV) and are located on the plantar surface of the foot.

Adolescents and young adults are most commonly affected with plantar warts. The virus is a DNA virus and is limited to the epidermis. HPV types 1, 2, 4, and 63 most commonly cause plantar warts.[2] Plantar warts are spread easily in warm, moist environments, such as a locker room floor. Microtrauma and autoinoculation are the major factors in propagation of the disease.[1] The incubation period is 1 to 8 months.[1]

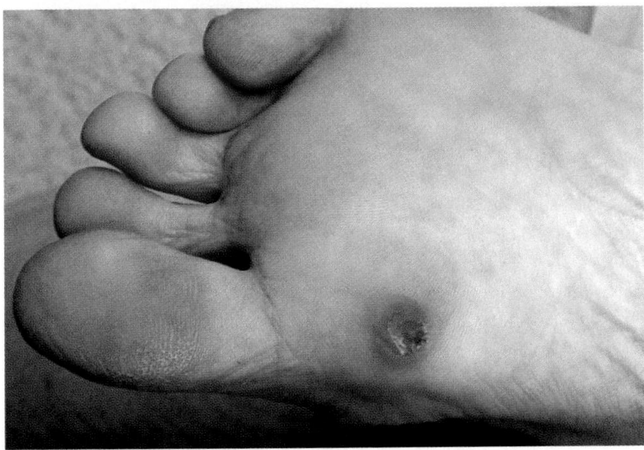

FIGURE 14–36 Plantar wart in typical location. (Courtesy of Michael Greenberg, MD.)

Diagnosis

The diagnosis of plantar warts may be difficult on the basis of physical examination, because they are often mistaken for a callus. If the area is débrided to the core, the characteristic "seeds" will be visible. Another finding on pathologic examination is "rete pegs," or epidermal ridges that go in the direction of the core of the wart.[1] Another useful way to discriminate a wart from a callus is that warts do not retain the normal fingerprint or footprint lines, whereas calluses do.[3]

Clinical Complications

Painful ambulation is the most common complication associated with plantar warts. The area may become superinfected after treatment or débridement of the wart.[2]

Management

Treatment of plantar warts can be through chemical, surgical, or chemotherapeutic measures. Chemicals used to treat warts topically include salicylic acid, formaldehyde, glutaraldehyde, and cantharidin.[2] Daily treatment with salicylic acid, a keratolytic agent, has a cure rate of 70% to 80%.[2]

REFERENCES

1. Esterowitz D, Greer KE, Cooper PH, Edlich RF. Plantar warts in the athlete. *Am J Emerg Med* 1995;13:441–443.
2. Plasencia JM. Cutaneous warts: diagnosis and treatment. *Prim Care* 2000;27:423–434.
3. Stulberg DL, Hutchinson AG. Molluscum contagiosum and warts. *Am Fam Physician* 2003;67:1233–1240.

Malignant Melanoma

Mark Mossey

Clinical Presentation

Patients with malignant melanoma present with hyperpigmented, irregular, macular cutaneous lesions; they often occur on the back in men, on the legs in women, and on the nail bed or nail fold in African-Americans and Asians. Less commonly, melanoma may occur on mucosal surfaces.[1,2]

Pathophysiology

In America, the lifetime risk of malignant melanoma is approximately 1 in 87.[1,2] Risk factors include a family history of melanoma, fair skin, light hair and blue eyes, as well as atypical nevi, which are larger than typical moles, have irregular borders, are variegated in color, and appear after age 35 years.

Diagnosis

Specific features suggesting melanoma can be summarized by the mnemonic "ABCD": **a**symmetry, **b**order irregularity, **c**olor irregularity (brown, tan, black, red, white, or blue), and **d**iameter greater than 6 mm. The differential diagnosis includes freckles, which are more commonly present from birth and unchanging in terms of size and appearance. Biopsy provides the definitive diagnosis.

Clinical Complications

Malignant melanoma commonly metastasizes to the central nervous system and can cause emergency complications. Between 6% and 10% of patients develop brain metastases, and 23% develop leptomeningeal metastases causing carcinomatous meningitis.[1]

Management

Referral to a dermatology specialist is essential for all patients with suspicious lesions. The prognosis is good for thin lesions without metastasis but extremely poor if distant metastases are present, in which case the median survival time is 6 months.[2] Primary prevention measures include limiting sun exposure by using protective clothing and wearing sunscreen. All patients should perform monthly self-examinations, and patients with atypical nevi should have screening examinations performed by a dermatologist every 6 to 12 months.

REFERENCES

1. Wen PY, Schiff D. Neurologic complications of solid tumors. *Neurol Clin* 2003;21:107–140.
2. Koh HK. Cutaneous melanoma. *N Engl J Med* 1991;325:171–182.

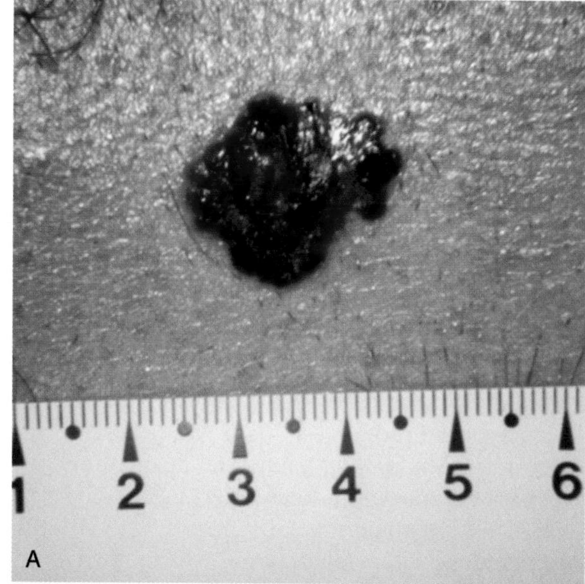

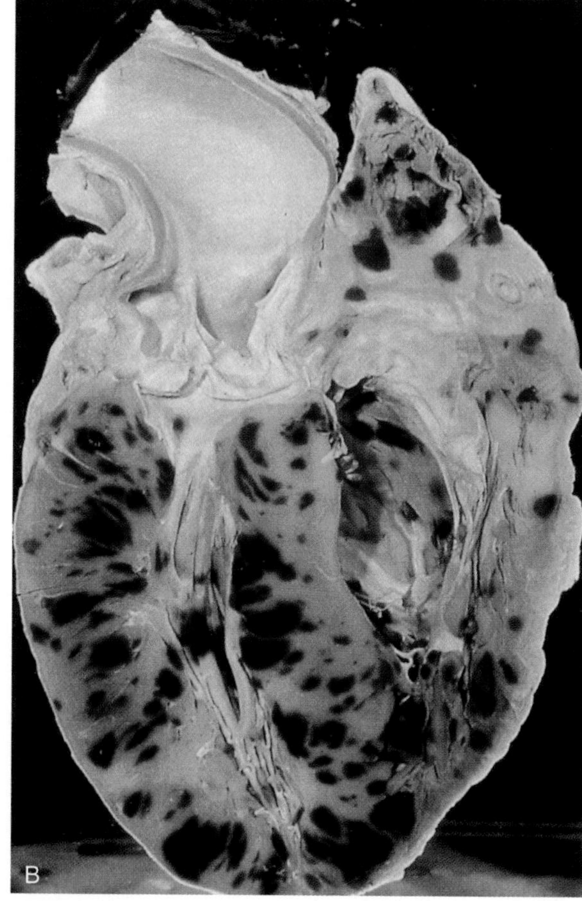

FIGURE 14–37 **A:** Superficial spreading melanoma. Note the "ABCD" features: asymmetry, notched border, varied colors, and diameter greater than 6 mm. (From Goodheart, with permission.) **B:** Untreated melanoma can metastasize to the heart, as seen here. (From Skarin AT. *Atlas of diagnostic oncology.* New York: Gower, 1991, with permission.)

Squamous Cell Carcinoma

Reid Brackin

Clinical Presentation

Patients with squamous cell carcinoma (SCC) present to the emergency department (ED) with complaints of skin lesions or ulceration. SCC may also be discovered incidentally on skin examination.

Pathophysiology

SCC develops from actinic keratoses in areas of chronic sun exposure. Atypical keratinocytes from these potential precursor lesions may invade the dermis. SCC *in situ* (intraepidermal SCC) demonstrates full-thickness atypia histologically. Further progression results in frankly invasive SCC.[1] Alternatively, SCC may develop in areas of scarring, repetitive trauma, or burns. Chemical carcinogens (including arsenic and tobacco) and medical conditions (e.g., human papillomavirus [HPV] infection, internal malignancy) are additional risk factors.[2]

SCC is the second most common cutaneous malignancy, after basal cell carcinoma (BCC). The annual incidence of SCC in the United States is estimated at 100,000 to 150,000 cases. SCC occurs more commonly in men (4:1) and with advancing age (most patients are older than 50 years of age, and there is an especially increased risk after age 75 years). Caucasians have a 10% lifetime risk. The disease is uncommon in African American, Hispanic, and Asian populations.[2]

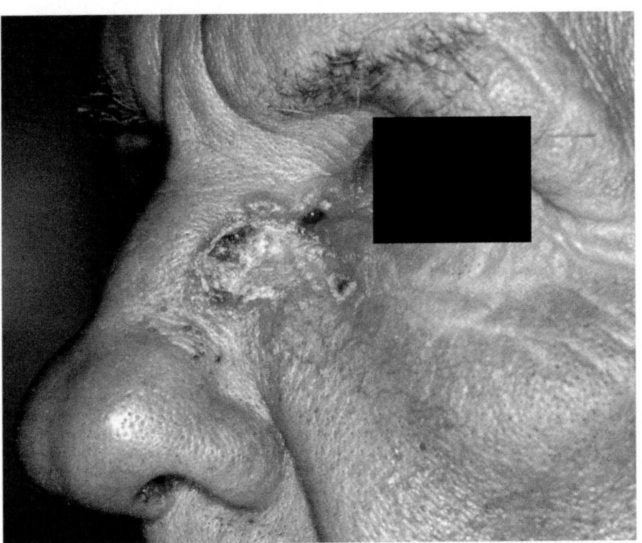

FIGURE 14–38 Squamous cell carcinoma in typical location. (© David Effron, MD, 2004. Used with permission.)

Diagnosis

Clinical suspicion is the mainstay of ED diagnosis. Actinic keratoses are small, erythematous, keratotic papules or scaly patches often discovered by palpation. SCC *in situ* is recognized as an erythematous, slightly keratotic, and mildly elevated papule or plaque with a velvet-like texture and a distinct, irregular border. It may be mistaken for eczema. SCC is a keratotic papule or nodule. It grows slowly and may show crusting or central ulceration as it enlarges. The most common locations for SCC are the head, the neck, and the back of the hands. A cutaneous "horn" reflective of hyperkeratosis may be present.[1] If the diagnosis is uncertain, evaluation in follow-up care may include a diagnostic excisional, punch, or shave biopsy.[3]

Clinical Complications

Complications of SCC include metastasis and recurrence. Common sites of metastasis are lymph nodes, lungs, and liver.

Management

Patients with high-risk lesions (as described here) should be referred to a dermatologist. Surgical excision is the first-line treatment for suspected skin malignancies. Any and all tissue excised in the ED must be sent for pathologic evaluation, no matter how benign the lesion may appear. Curettage and electrodesiccation, as well as other treatment options, may be considered on an individual basis.[3]

REFERENCES

1. Shelton RM. Skin cancer: a review and atlas for the medical provider. *Mt Sinai J Med* 2001;68:243–252.
2. Diepgen TL, Mahler V. The epidemiology of skin cancer. *Br J Dermatol* 2002;146[Suppl61]:1–6.
3. Reynolds PL, Strayer SM. Treatment of skin malignancies. *J Fam Pract* 2003;52:456–464.

Basal Cell Carcinoma

Jennifer Harris

Clinical Presentation

Patients with basal cell carcinoma (BCC) present with a lesion that typically has been present for some time, and they may report a history of persistent bleeding at the site. Typical locations are sun-exposed areas of the skin, such as the head (most commonly the nose), neck, and upper trunk.[1]

Pathophysiology

BCC is the most common cutaneous malignancy, accounting for more than 70% of nonmelanoma skin cancers.[1,2] BCC has been linked to ultraviolet (UV) radiation exposure, especially UV-B, and 99% of cases occur in Caucasians, particularly those with fair skin that burns easily with sun exposure.[1] UV radiation has been shown to cause mutations in the DNA of epidermal cells. Failure to repair these mutations is the first step in the carcinogenic pathway that, after a latency period of several years to decades, eventually leads to skin cancer. Certain genetic syndromes are also predisposing factors for BCC, including albinism, xeroderma pigmentosum, basal cell nevus syndrome, and epidermodysplasia verruciformis.[2]

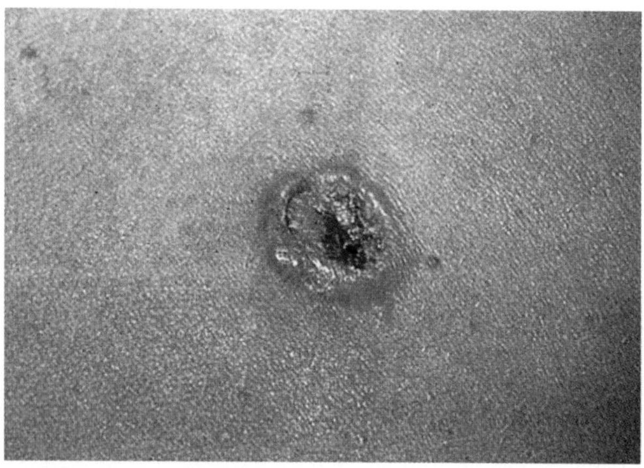

FIGURE 14–39 Basal cell carcinoma. (From *Basal cell carcinoma: the most common skin cancer.* New York: The Skin Cancer Foundation. Copyright © 1986, Revised 1999.)

Diagnosis

Suspicious lesions should be identified by physical examination, and definitive diagnosis should be made by biopsy and histologic confirmation.

Clinical Complications

Morbidity from BCC is most commonly secondary to local invasion of the lesion and destruction of adjacent tissues. Because BCC commonly occurs on the face (30% on the nose), cosmetic disfigurement is a frequent complication. Metastatic disease is rare, with an incidence of less than 0.1%. Metastasis is two times more common in men than in women and preferentially affects the regional lymph nodes, lungs, liver, bone, and other skin sites. Death from BCC is rare.[2]

Management

BCC can be treated with either destructive or excisional therapy. The former includes electrodesiccation and curettage, and cryotherapy with liquid nitrogen. Conventional surgical excision offers the benefit of identification of clear tumor margins.[1] Patients with suspected malignancy should be referred to a dermatologist for further evaluation and therapy.

REFERENCES

1. Humphreys TR. Skin cancer: recognition and management. *Clin Cornerstone* 2001;4:23–32.
2. Padgett JK, Hendrix JD Jr. Cutaneous malignancies and their management. *Otolaryngol Clin North Am* 2001;34:523–553.

Mycosis Fungoides

Michael Greenberg

Clinical Presentation

Patients with mycosis fungoides (MF) present with pruritic, irregularly shaped, scaly patches and plaques that may appear erythematous. Over time, these lesions may become rather thick-appearing cutaneous tumors with a "mushroom-like" ("fungoides") appearance. MF progresses at a variable rate. Consequently, patients may present initially with cutaneous patches, plaques, and tumors in various locations, as well as extracutaneous involvement.[1-3]

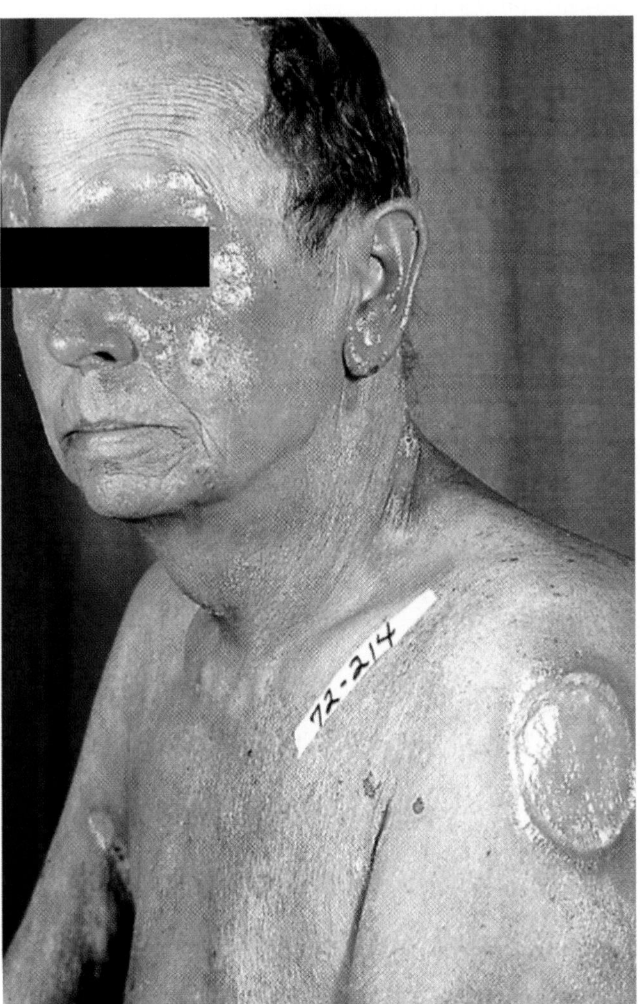

FIGURE 14–40 Mycosis fungoides. Note plaques and ulcerative nodules. (From Handin, with permission.)

Pathophysiology

MF is a primary cutaneous lymphoma; it is a malignant lymphoproliferative T-cell disorder usually found in middle-aged adults and rarely in children and adolescents.[2] Involvement of the lymph nodes or viscera occurs with advanced disease; the lungs, spleen, and liver are the most common noncutaneous sites. Atypical T cells with hyperconvoluted cerebriform nuclei (Sézary's cells) are characteristic for the disease. The incidence of MF in the United States appears to have increased over the last decade, with approximately 1,000 new cases annually.[3] Various viruses, environmental toxicants, and ionizing radiation have been implicated in the pathogenesis; however, the precise cause has yet to be elucidated.

Diagnosis

The gold standard for diagnosis of MF is light microscopy of histologic specimens. However, a high index of clinical suspicion is necessary to trigger biopsy and tissue examination.[1-3]

Clinical Complications

Complications include disseminated disease and death.[1-3]

Management

Psoralen ultraviolet A therapy, UV-B, topical nitrogen mustard, and topical steroids are used to treat MF.[2] Late-stage disease requires systemic chemotherapy in conjunction with radiation; a multidisciplinary team is needed, including dermatologists, oncologists, and radiation oncologists.

REFERENCES

1. de Coninck EC, Kim YH, Varghese A, Hoppe RJ. Clinical characteristics and outcome of patients with extracutaneous mycosis fungoides. *J Clin Oncol* 2001;19:779–784.
2. Hoang MT, Friedlander SF. Rare cutaneous malignancies of childhood. *Curr Opin Pediatr* 1999;11:464–470.
3. Cook DL. Early mycosis fungoides: can the diagnosis be made reliably? *Adv Anat Pathol* 2001;8:240–244.

Kerion

Jennifer Kiss

Clinical Presentation

Patients with kerion present with large areas of boggy, tender, raised skin on the scalp that often are covered with multiple pustules.[1] Cervical and occipital lymphadenopathy may be present. Kerion is preceded by a more typical tinea capitis infection characterized by alopecia, pruritus, and scaling.[2]

Pathophysiology

Kerion is caused by an intense cell-mediated immune response to tinea capitis infection.[2] Ninety percent of tinea capitis infections are caused by *Trichophyton tonsurans,* and it is almost endemic among African American children.[1] A less common cause of kerion is *Microsporum* species.

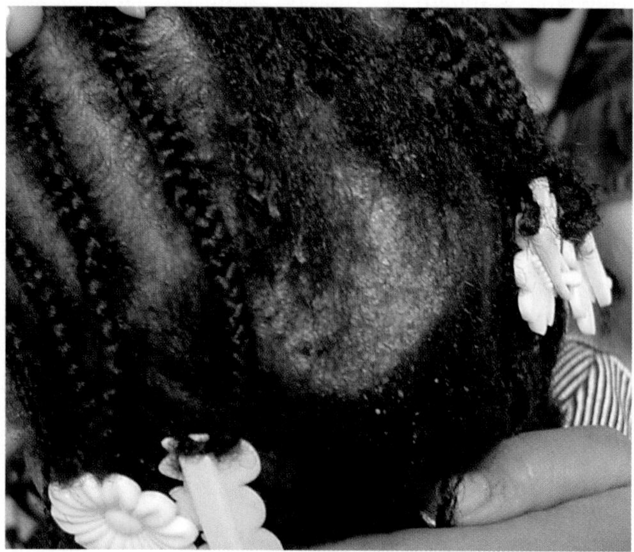

FIGURE 14–41 Centrally located kerion. (Courtesy of Christy Salvaggio, MD.)

Diagnosis

Diagnosis is clinical but may be confirmed by potassium hydroxide (KOH) examination of infected skin or scalp hair to look for branching hyphae and spores.[1] Infected skin fluoresces under a Wood's lamp if it is caused by *Microsporum,* but the more common *Trichophyton* infection does not fluoresce.[2] If KOH microscopy and Wood's lamp examination are negative, a fungal culture may be considered if tinea capitis is highly suspected.[2]

Clinical Complications

Clinical complications of kerion include permanent scarring and hair loss.[1]

Management

Although kerion appears very similar to abscesses, incision and drainage is not recommended.[1] Topical treatment is not effective for tinea capitis. Systemic antifungal therapy is required to penetrate hair follicles.[2] Griseofulvin is the only agent that the U.S. Food and Drug Administration (FDA) has labeled for treatment of tinea capitis, and it remains the gold standard. However, griseofulvin is less than ideal because the treatment requires 6 to 12 weeks, relapse rates are high, and the liquid children's form is bitter-tasting. Itraconazole, fluconazole, and terbinafine all may be as effective as 6 weeks of griseofulvin therapy.[2] Adjunctive therapy with selenium shampoo may decrease spore shedding and lower the risk of spreading infection to others.[1]

REFERENCES

1. Bhumbra NA, McCullough SG. Skin and subcutaneous infections. *Prim Care* 2003;30:1–24.
2. Hainer BL. Dermatophyte infections. *Am Fam Physician* 2003;67:101–108.

Erythema Nodosum

Lorenzo Paladino

Clinical Presentation

Patients (usually young adult women) who have erythema nodosum (EN) present with well-localized, red, tender subcutaneous nodules, 1 to 5 cm in diameter.[1]

Pathophysiology

EN is a hypersensitivity reaction causing a localized inflammatory infiltrate that involves the septae of subcutaneous fat.[1] There are few, if any, systemic manifestations.[1] On histologic examination, Miescher's radial granulomas are noted; these consist of small, well-defined nodular aggregations of small histiocytes around a central stellate or banana-shaped cleft.[1] EN may be associated with a variety of medical disorders, although up to 50% of cases are idiopathic.[1] In children, the most common causes are infectious, with streptococcal illnesses being most common.[1] In adults, drugs, sarcoidosis, and inflammatory bowel disease are the leading causative factors.[1,2] Coccidioidomycosis, or San Joaquin Valley fever, is an important cause of EN in the western and southwestern United States.[2] Other, less common causes of EN include fungal infection, malignancies, pregnancy, lymphogranuloma venereum, syphilis, and chancroid.[1,3]

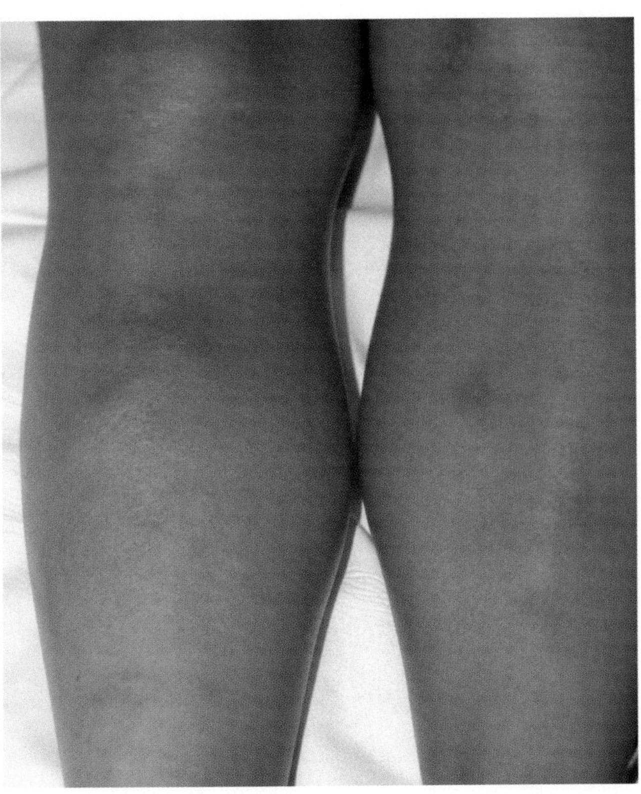

FIGURE 14–42 Erythema nodosum with healing "contusiform" lesions. (© David Effron, MD, 2004. Used with permission.)

Diagnosis

The diagnosis is made clinically in most cases. However, for individuals in whom the diagnosis is uncertain, excisional biopsy may be helpful.[1] A careful history usually reveals prodromal symptoms of fever, malaise, and arthralgia preceding the eruption by 1 to 3 weeks.[2] One or more lesions develop simultaneously and may last several weeks. They are usually found on the extensor aspects of the extremities, and they occur bilaterally in most cases.[1] The lesions usually do not suppurate or form ulcers, but they often involute, leaving yellow-purple bruises.[1]

Management

The eruption is usually self-limited if the underlying cause can be eliminated. Therefore, clinical and laboratory evaluations should be directed at determining the causative etiology. If the cause cannot be identified or treated, symptomatic therapy with aspirin, nonsteroidal antiinflammatory drugs (NSAIDs), oral potassium iodide, or a short course of systemic steroids may provide symptomatic relief.[1]

REFERENCES

1. Requena L, Yus ES. Panniculitis. Part 1: mostly septal panniculitis. *J Am Acad Dermatol* 2001;45:163–183.
2. Soderstrom RM, Krull EA. Erythema nodosum: a review. *Cutis* 1978;21:806–810.
3. Fox MD, Schwartz RA. Erythema nodosum. *Am Fam Physician* 1992;46:818–822.

Acanthosis Nigricans

Benjamin Roemer

Clinical Presentation

Patients with acanthosis nigricans (AN) usually present with a benign dermatosis. Occasionally, patients present with complications of an underlying endocrine disorder or malignancy.

Pathophysiology

AN is a nonspecific dermatologic reaction caused by excess insulin and insulin-like growth factor, which "hyperstimulate" keratinocytes and dermal fibroblasts. The resulting dermatosis is composed of hyperkeratosis, papillary hypertrophy, and increased numbers of melanocytes. AN is associated with obesity, Cushing's syndrome, acromegaly, diabetes, genetic variants, pineal tumors, endocrine disorders, use of drugs such as nicotinic acid, estrogens, and corticosteroids, and adenocarcinoma.[1] The incidence of AN is unknown, but more than 50% of patients who weigh more than 200% of their ideal body weight manifest this dermatosis.[2] AN is common among African-Americans and Hispanics, and the incidence is equal in males and females. Some cases are genetically inherited.

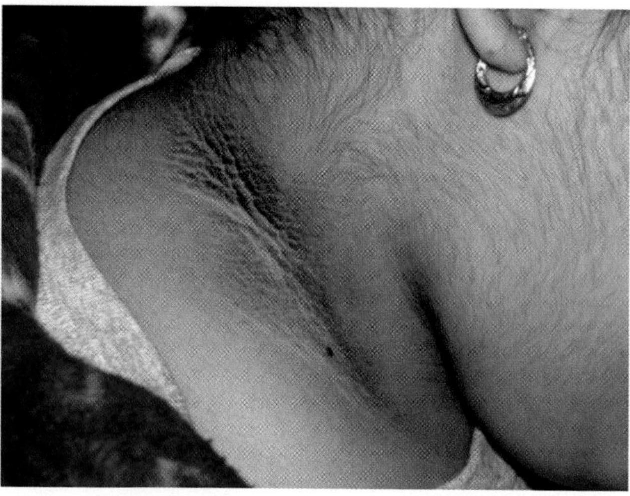

FIGURE 14–43 Linear, alternating dark and light pigmentation becomes more apparent when the skin is stretched. (From Goodheart, with permission.)

Diagnosis

AN manifests as a symmetric, brown, velvety thickening of the skin. The hyperkeratosis and hyperpigmentation of the skin may thicken and develop a leathery, warty, or papillomatous surface. It most often occurs in skin folds, including the axilla, antecubital fossa, neck, and groin.[1] Adult-onset AN requires a workup for malignancy and for diabetes mellitus.

Clinical Complications

Complications are rare and are limited to consequences of the underlying malignancy or endocrine disorder.

Management

The majority of cases are idiopathic and are associated with obesity. Patients should be instructed regarding dietary changes and weight loss. Treatment of an underlying endocrine disorder or malignancy is sometimes necessary. Topical retinoids may reduce the dermatosis.[3] Patients with nonobese or adult-onset AN must be evaluated for underlying malignancy.[4]

REFERENCES

1. Kihiczak NI, Leevy CB, Krysicki MM, et al. Cutaneous signs of selected systemic diseases. *J Med* 1999;30:3–12.
2. Hud JA Jr, Cohen JB, Wagner JM, Cruz PD Jr. Prevalence and significance of acanthosis nigricans in an adult obese population. *Arch Dermatol* 1992;128:941–944.
3. Darmstadt GL, Yokel BK, Horn TD. Treatment of acanthosis nigricans with tretinoin. *Arch Dermatol* 1991;127:1139–1140.
4. Braverman IM. Skin manifestation of internal malignancy. *Clin Geriatr Med* 2002;18:1–19.

Dermatographia

Colleen Campbell and Arthur Chang

Clinical Presentation

Patients present with a wheal-and-flare skin lesion in response to manipulation of the skin.[1] The classic lesion is a raised erythematous plaque surrounded by erythema visible in the area of applied skin pressure.[1] Patients usually complain of accompanying pruritus or burning.[2] Lesions can last from minutes up to 24 hours.[2]

Pathophysiology

Dermatographia is a physically induced urticarial reaction in response to stroking of the skin.[1]

Dermatographia is more common in young adults and may be found in 4% to 5% of the population.[3] It is believed that intraepithelial mast cells release their contents in response to physical stimulation.[1] This represents a type I allergic reaction, in which histamines, arachidonic acids, and leukotrienes are the mediators of response.[3] Although no specific immunoglobulin E (IgE) antibody has been identified, dermatographia has been passively transferred by infusion of the serum of an afflicted patient into another individual.[3] Some believe that substance P also plays a role in dermatographia.[3]

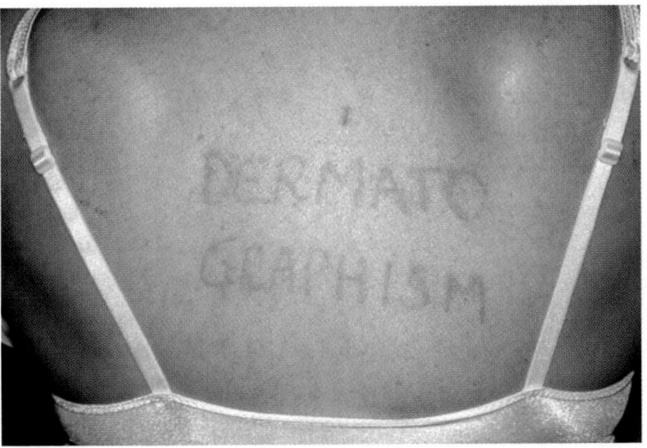

FIGURE 14–44 These lesions occurred 3 minutes after the skin was stroked with the wooden tip of a cotton swab. (From Goodheart, with permission.)

Dermatographia has reportedly been associated with other medical conditions, such as urticaria pigmentosa, diabetes, viral illness, and late pregnancy, and with certain drugs such as penicillin, codeine, and sulfonamides.[3]

Diagnosis

The diagnosis is based on history and physical examination. The best physical location in which dermatographia may be induced is on the back.[3] The skin turns red when firm pressure is applied and then develops the "triple response of Lewis"—a red line that expands until a wheal forms.[3]

Clinical Complications

Dermatographia is a benign disease process, and complications are rare. However, superinfection of the involved area may occur due to scratching and excoriation associated with pruritus, and patients may also experience headaches, flushing, lightheadedness, or hypotension.[4]

Management

Ultraviolet (UV) light may prevent occurrences, but oral antihistamines are the treatment of choice.[3] Doxepin, tricyclic antidepressants, or hydroxyzine may be used; all have H_1 and H_2 receptor blocking properties.[1] Corticosteroids do not inhibit cutaneous mast-cell degranulation and therefore do not have a role in the treatment of dermatographism or other physical urticarias.[3] Follow-up is essential, because dermatographia has been associated with other disorders, such as Behçet's disease and chronic rheumatic fibrositis.[1,2]

REFERENCES

1. Kennedy MS. Evaluation of chronic eczema and urticaria and angioedema. *Immun Allerg Clin North Am* 1999;19:19–32.
2. Leung DYM, Boguniewicz M. Advances in allergic skin diseases. *J Allerg Clin Immun* 2003;111[Suppl 3]:S805–S812.
3. Beltrani VS, Thiers BH. Urticaria and angioedema. *Dermatol Clin* 1996;14:171–198.
4. Mahmood T. Physical urticarias. *Am Fam Physician* 1994;49: 1411–1414.

Actinic Keratosis

In-Hei Hahn

Clinical Presentation

People with actinic keratosis (AK) may complain of scaly, rough patches of skin on the sun-exposed parts of the body, such as the head, face, neck, arms, and hands.[2] Occasionally, these lesions are palpable before they can be visualized. If similar lesions develop on the lips, they are termed actinic cheilitis.[2] Pigmentation ranges from flesh-colored to reddish-brown, and the lesions can range from 1 mm to more than 1 inch in size. They may appear flat to slightly depressed, with a distinct border.

Pathophysiology

AK, also known as solar keratosis, is a dermatologic condition that manifests with localized patches of thickened, scaly skin and is caused by damage from exposure to solar radiation.[1]

Some risk factors for development of AK include age older than 40 years, fair skin color, working outdoors, and history of sunburn.[2] UV-B radiation is responsible for most cases of AK formation. UV-B causes thymidine-dimer formation in the DNA, which leads to mutations in the keratinocytes. This results in a loss of orderly differentiation between the basal cell layer and the stratum corneum.[1] Most researchers believe that AK is an intraepidermal focus of malignancy and represents the earliest clinical stage in the continuum of squamous cell carcinoma (SCC). The only histologic difference between AK and SCC is the level of invasiveness.[1,2] According to one study, there is at least a 10% frequency of progression of these lesions to SCC.[2]

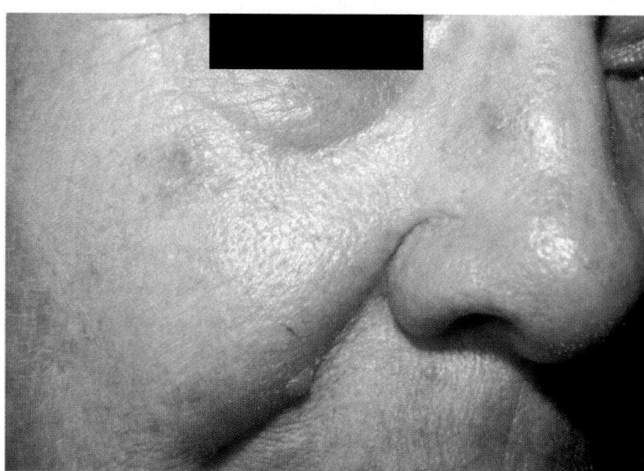

FIGURE 14–45 Actinic keratosis is a sun-induced squamous cell carcinoma limited to the epidermis. (© David Effron, MD, 2004. Used with permission.)

Diagnosis

The diagnosis of AK usually is made clinically. A biopsy may be performed to confirm the diagnosis and to exclude the possibility of deeper involvement, especially if the lesion is bleeding, pruritic, large, erythematous, ulcerated, or otherwise unusual in presentation.[1,2]

Clinical Complications

Complications include progression to SCC, trauma to and bleeding of lesions, and infection.[1]

Management

AK lesions should be removed, either surgically with a laser or by cryotherapy with liquid nitrogen.[2] Other topical therapies approved by the U.S. Food and Drug Administration (FDA) include 5-fluoruracil, diclofenac 3% gel, and imiquimod.

REFERENCES

1. Cockerell CJ. Pathobiology and pathophysiology of actinic (solar) keratosis. *Br J Dermatol* 2003;149[Suppl 66]:34–36.
2. Webster GF. Common skin disorders in the elderly. *Clin Cornerstone* 2001;4:39–44.

Radiodermatitis

Eric Adar

Clinical Presentation

Patients usually present after diagnostic or interventional fluoroscopy procedures.[1] Several hours after exposure, erythema of the skin can be seen at the site of beam entry. The reaction usually peaks within 24 hours and subsides by 48 hours.[1] Presenting complaints include pain, burning, and itching of the affected area.

Pathophysiology

Radiodermatitis refers to a range of inflammatory skin reactions that occur after exposure to ionizing radiation.[1]

Ionizing radiation can damage DNA either directly or as a result of free radical formation. The amount of damage depends on the dose of radiation absorbed. A typical angiographic study exposes a patient to 2.5 Gy, whereas percutaneous transluminal coronary angiography (PTCA) with coronary stenting may deliver up to 6.5 Gy. With these procedures, the right axillary region is the most common site affected due to preferential fluoroscopy beam paths.[1] Exposure to a large dose of radiation from other sources may manifest initially as skin injury, but significant damage to other organ systems may subsequently develop.[1] A second hyperemic phase associated with cell proliferation peaks approximately at day 14.[1] Sebaceous glands are particularly sensitive to radiation, and their destruction may cause dry, scaly skin. The skin may develop hyperpigmentation or hypopigmentation, depending on the radiation dose. After 1 or 2 weeks, the process of healing begins from the wound edges and progresses centrally.[1]

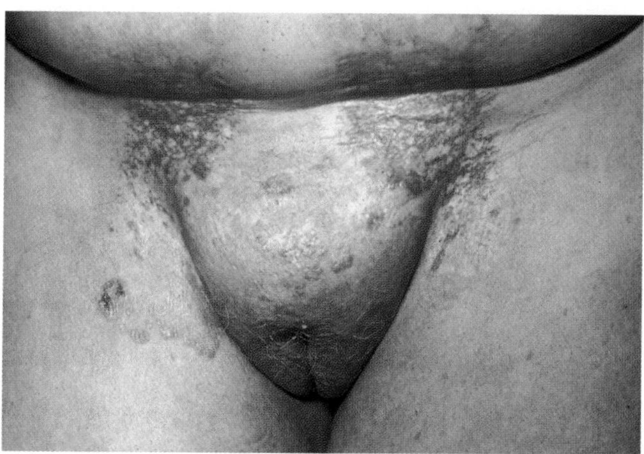

FIGURE 14–46 Radiodermatitis. (© David Effron, MD, 2004. Used with permission.)

Diagnosis

The diagnosis is made clinically and is based on the presence of characteristic skin changes after exposure to ionizing radiation.[1]

Clinical Complications

One month after irradiation and desquamation, the skin may appear scaly and flaky, a condition known as dry desquamation. With doses exceeding 18 Gy, blistering and skin weeping is typical and is known as moist desquamation.[1] Thin epithelial regrowth may occur because of initial capillary damage. A long, protracted healing course is typical, with frequent ulcerations and skin infections being common. Full healing can take months to years.[1]

Management

Treatment of radiodermatitis consists of prevention of superinfection after the superficial skin layer is disrupted. This is accomplished with the use of superficial antibiotic creams and regular application of sterile dressings.[1] Nonhealing ulcers may require wound excision and skin grafting.[1] Healed skin is at risk for neoplastic changes, so regular dermatologic examinations are recommended.[1] Depending on symptomatology and time of injury, further testing may be necessary.

REFERENCES

1. Koenig TR, Wolff D, Mettler FA, Wagner LK. Skin injuries from fluoroscopically guided procedures. Part 1: characteristics of radiation injury. *AJR Am J Roentgenol* 2001;177:3–11.

Vitiligo

Lorenzo Paladino

Clinical Presentation

Patients with vitiligo present with a symmetric pattern of well-circumscribed, depigmented macules.[1,2] The loss of pigmentation may be subtle on fair skin, but it can be disfiguring in darker-skinned individuals.[2]

Pathophysiology

Vitiligo occurs in up to 1% of the population and affects both sexes equally.[1,2] In most cases, onset is before age 20 years.[1,2] The cause remains elusive, but genetic factors, autoimmunity, autocytotoxic agents, neurologic factors, toxic metabolites, and lack of melanocyte growth factors have all been proposed.[1,2] Evidence points to theories involving autoantibodies to melanocytes as most probable.[2] Family history is positive in as many as 33% of cases, suggesting that, whatever the mechanism, it is inherited in a multifactorial fashion.[2] Vitiligo has been associated with hypothyroidism, Graves' disease, Addison's disease, alopecia areata, pernicious anemia, insulin-dependent diabetes mellitus, uveitis, inflammatory bowel disease, and melanoma.[2]

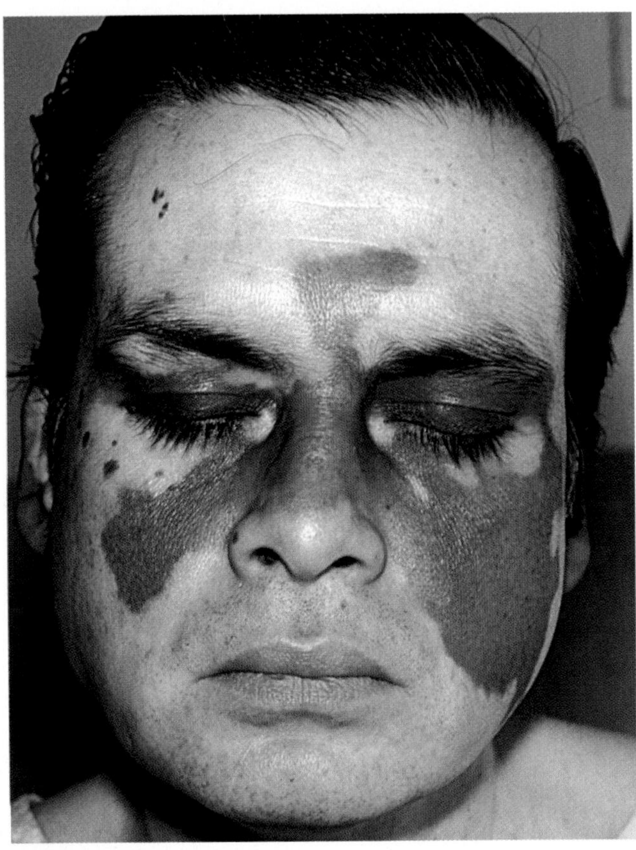

FIGURE 14–47 Extensive depigmentation associated with vitiligo. (From Goodheart, with permission.)

Diagnosis

The diagnosis is made clinically and can be assisted by inspection with a Wood's lamp, which accentuates the hypopigmented regions.[2] In uncertain cases, a biopsy may be helpful to differentiate vitiligo from other hypopigmentary disorders.[2] The disease usually begins in localized macules but progresses slowly over years.[2] The most common sites of involvement are the face, scalp, dorsum of the hands, distal phalanges, body folds, and genitalia.[2] Body orifices (eyes, nostrils, mouth, nipples, umbilicus, and anus) are frequently affected, as are areas that are subjected to repeated trauma, such as bony prominences.[2] Vitiligo of the scalp usually manifests as leukotrichia, a localized patch of white or gray hair.[2]

Clinical Complications

Vitiligo, particularly in darker-skinned individuals, can be a cosmetically disfiguring condition with substantial psychological impact.[1,2] The lack of melanin pigment makes the affected skin more sensitive to sunburn and its complications.[1] Patients with vitiligo are prone to the development of halo nevi.[2]

Management

Patients with vitiligo should be referred to a dermatologist. Topical psoralens, ultraviolet (UV)-A and -B light, and topical steroids have all been used with varying success.[1,2] In extensive cases, depigmentation therapy and surgical treatments may achieve some improvement.[1,2] Sunscreens, camouflage products, and good physician direction may help patients better cope with the psychological ramifications of the disease process.[1,2]

REFERENCES

1. Njoo MD, Westerhof W. Vitiligo: pathogenesis and treatment. *Am J Clin Dermatol* 2001;2:167–181.
2. Kovacs SO. Vitiligo. *J Am Acad Dermatol* 1998;38:647–666.

Decubitus Ulcers

Mark Mossey

Clinical Presentation

In the emergency department (ED), decubitus ulcers are usually incidental findings in chair-bound or bed-bound patients presenting for another complaint.

Pathophysiology

Pressure ulcers develop when subcutaneous tissues are compressed against bony prominences such as the ischium, trochanter, sacrum, and heel. Hyperemia leads to ischemia and necrosis. Risk factors include age, inactivity, and smoking.[1]

Diagnosis

The National Pressure Ulcer Advisory Panel classifies pressure sores into four stages. In stage I, pressure sores appear as intact skin with blanching erythema. Stage II pressure sores appear as blistering skin, representing partial-thickness loss of skin to the level of dermis. In stage III ulcers, fatty subcutaneous tissue is visible, and this represents full-thickness skin loss. In stage IV ulcers, muscle or bone is visible.

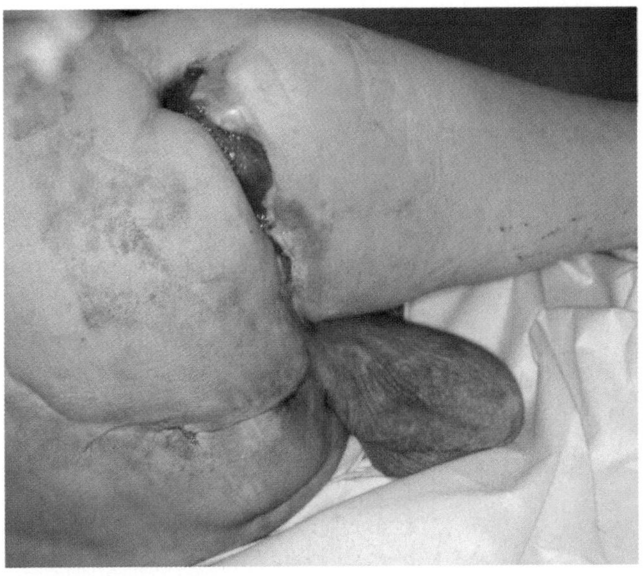

FIGURE 14–48 Decubitus ulcer of proximal leg. (© David Effron, MD, 2004. Used with permission.)

Clinical Complications

Infection is common, especially in incontinent patients at risk for fecal contamination of wounds. Cellulitis, osteomyelitis, or sepsis may develop.

Management

Stage I pressure sores can be managed with an ointment-based skin barrier to prevent fecal contamination. Stage II pressure sores should be covered with an occlusive dressing that functions essentially as a blister, providing a sterile, moist environment in which granulation and epithelialization can occur. These dressings typically are left in place for several days at a time. Stage III ulcers can be débrided with a scalpel, with a topical enzyme preparation, or with serial wet-to-dry dressings. A patient with stage IV ulcers should be referred for care to a plastic surgeon.

Any wound that appears to be locally infected should be treated with a topical antibiotic, such as silver sulfadiazine. All decubitus ulcers should be managed with padding and frequent repositioning. Additionally, several studies have shown that dietary intake of protein correlates directly with primary prevention of decubitus ulcers and with wound healing.[2] Local heat applications have a positive effect on wound healing.[3]

REFERENCES

1. Guralnik JM, Harris TB, White LR, Cornoni-Huntley JC. Occurrence and predictors of pressure sores in the National Health and Nutrition Examination survey follow-up. *J Am Geriatr Soc* 1988;36: 807–812.
2. Bourdel-Marchasson I, Barateau M, Rondeau V, et al. A multicenter trial of the effects of oral nutritional supplementation in critically ill older inpatients. *Nutrition* 2000;16:1–5.
3. Kloth LC, Berman JE, Dumit-Minkel S, Sutton CH, Papanek PE, Wurzel J. Effects of a normothermic dressing on pressure ulcer healing. *Adv Skin Wound Care* 2000;13:69–74.

Alopecia

Michelle C. Peters and Benjamin Roemer

Clinical Presentation

Patients with alopecia present with hair loss over varying periods. A variety of medical problems and traumatic events may be associated with alopecia.

Pathophysiology

Tinea capitis may lead to a scarring type of alopecia, known as kerion tinea capitis. Tinea capitis is a dermatophyte infection of the scalp that is common in African-American children. Alopecia areata is a nonscarring, potentially reversible form of alopecia with an unknown cause. Telogen effluvium is hair loss caused by a major stressful event (e.g., crash diet, major surgery, pregnancy and delivery). Infants who spend a significant amount of time supine can experience occipital hair loss. Tight braids may promote traction alopecia. The recent trend of placing headbands on infants has given rise to a new form of hair loss called circumferential alopecia.[1] Cicatricial alopecia is permanent hair loss caused by repetitive trauma or by autoimmune, neoplastic, or hereditary disorders. Patients should be referred to a physician who specializes in hair loss disorders. Trichotillomania is a psychiatric disorder involving voluntary hair removal by pulling. Hair loss follows bizarre patterns with incomplete clearing. Psychiatric referral is essential.[2]

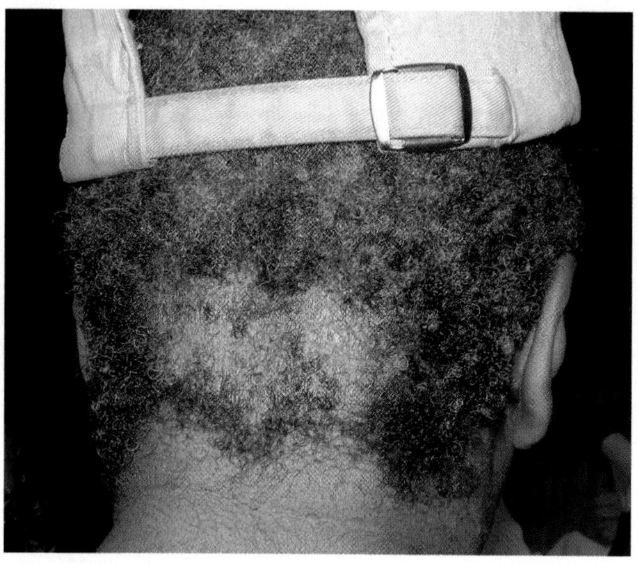

FIGURE 14–49 Alopecia from chronic wear of baseball hat. (Courtesy of Mark Silverberg, MD.)

Diagnosis

The diagnosis is clinically based, and it is important to elicit detailed historical information, including recent chemotherapy, childbirth, major surgery, new "fad" diets, past medical and family history, past and present medications, and psychological stressors.

Clinical Complications

If a thorough history, physical examination, and laboratory evaluation are not carried out, a serious illness such as hyperthyroidism/hypothyroidism, anemia, syphilis, or fungal infection may be missed.

Management

Patients with tinea capitis may be treated with griseofulvin and Nizoral (ketoconazole) shampoo. Localized alopecia areata usually resolves within 2 to 6 months; however, extensive disease may not resolve completely. In many cases, no satisfactory treatment is available. Patients with alopecia due to stressful circumstances need firm reassurance, and all patients should be referred to a dermatologist.[3]

REFERENCES

1. Marino RV. Headband alopecia. *Pediatrics* 1995;96:1174.
2. Messinger ML, Cheng TL. Trichotillomania. *Pediatr Rev* 1999;20:249–250.
3. Price VH. Treatment of hair loss. *N Engl J Med* 1999;341:964–973.

Neurofibromatosis

Raffi Kapitanyan

Clinical Presentation

Patients with neurofibromatosis type 1 (NF1) present as newborns with multiple flat, hyperpigmented "café-au-lait spots" that increase in size throughout infancy.[1] Axillary or groin freckling is also commonly seen. Patients present with three distinct types of neurofibromas: benign lesions of the dermis, nodular lesions arising in peripheral nerves, and plexiform neurofibromas.[1] Patients may have ocular complaints secondary to optic nerve gliomas or Lisch nodules, which are hamartomas of the iris.[1] Less frequent presentations include hypertension secondary to pheochromocytoma, intestinal tumors, and learning disabilities.[1]

Patients with neurofibromatosis type 2 (NF2) present with hearing loss (with or without tinnitus) secondary to bilateral vestibular schwannomas.[2] Dizziness and imbalance also occur, in addition to skin tumors, the most frequent being a raised, plaque-like hyperpigmented lesion with excess hair.[2] Ocular complaints are often secondary to cataracts. Intracranial meningiomas and spinal tumors may also be seen.[2]

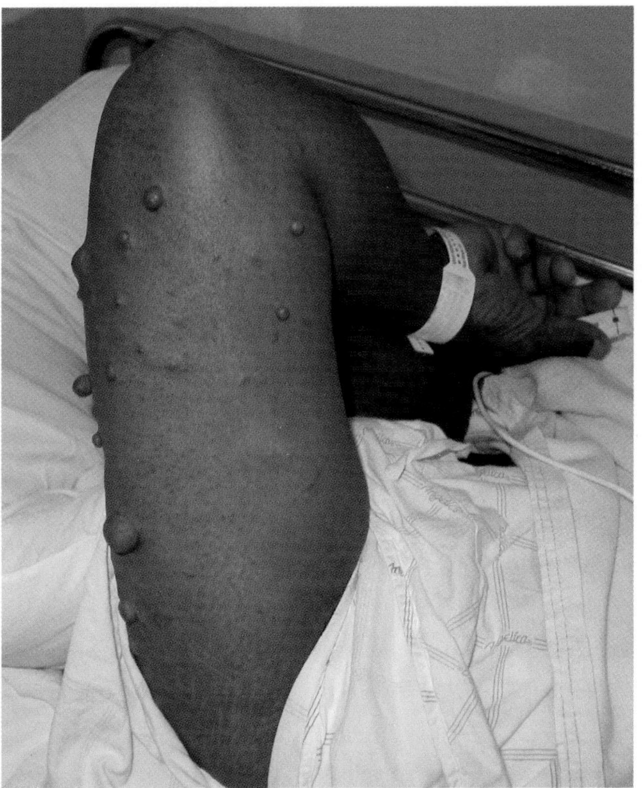

FIGURE 14–50 Multiple neurofibromas. (Courtesy of Colleen Campbell, MD.)

Pathophysiology

The neurofibromatoses are inherited autosomal dominant disorders and consist of two distinct forms: NF1, von Recklinghausen's disease, and NF2.[1]

The *NF1* gene encodes a tumor suppressor protein known as neurofibromin.[1] Inactivation of this gene leads to development of the distinct tumors seen in NF1 disease.[1] Mutation of the *NF2* gene leads to the classic vestibular schwannomas and other tumors of NF2.[2]

Diagnosis

Diagnostic criteria for NF1 require the presence of two or more of the following: six or more café-au-lait spots, two or more neurofibromas of any type, one or more plexiform neurofibroma, and axillary/groin freckling.[1] Diagnostic criteria for NF2 include bilateral vestibular schwannomas or a family history of NF2, plus either unilateral vestibular schwannomas or any two of the following: meningioma, glioma, neurofibroma, and posterior subcapsular opacities.[2]

Clinical Complications

Complications in NF1 are secondary to invasion of nerve sheaths or surrounding tissue by neurofibromas, which results in disfigurement and motor disability.[1] About 10% of these tumors become malignant. The mean age at death is 54 years.[1] The most common complication of NF2 is deafness, followed by poor balance, visual problems, and weakness secondary to spinal tumors.[2] Death may occur prematurely between age 20 and 30 years.[2]

Management

For both NF1 and NF2, supportive measures and genetic counseling are required. Recent advances in NF1 biology have led to the possibility of treatment with RAS inhibitors.[1] Surgery plus radiation, together with cochlear implants for deafness, has had limited success in patients with NF2.[2]

REFERENCES

1. Reynolds RM, Browning GG, Nawroz I, Campbell IW. Von Recklinghausen's neurofibromatosis: neurofibromatosis type 1. *Lancet* 2003;361:1552–1554.
2. Evans DG, Sainio M, Baser ME. Neurofibromatosis type 2. *J Med Genet* 2000;37:897–904.

Lipoma

Benjamin Roemer

Clinical Presentation

Patients with lipoma present with one or more painless masses located between the skin and deep fascia. Occasionally, patients present with complaints related to mass effect, but most are asymptomatic. The overlying skin is uninvolved.

Pathophysiology

Lipomas are the most common benign soft tissue tumors in adults, occurring in about 1% of the population. Lipomas first appear between 40 and 60 years of age. Malignant progression of lipomas is uncommon. Lipomas are collections of mature adiposities arranged in lobules. Many lipomas are surrounded by a fibrous capsule. Infiltrating lipomas are nonencapsulated and can infiltrate into muscle. Variations may be noted on biopsy specimens. Angiolipomas arise after puberty, develop vascularization, and may be painful. Pleomorphic lipomas occur in men 50 to 70 years of age and contain normal adiposities and bizarre, multinucleated giant cells.[1] Spindle lipomas contain both normal lipid cells and slender spindle cells.[2] Adenolipomas contain eccrine sweat glands and are often located proximally on the limbs.[3]

Malignancy is rare. Liposarcoma manifests similarly to a lipoma but is more common on the shoulder, lower extremities, and retroperitoneum.[3] Liposarcoma should be considered in nonhomogenous or fast-growing lesions.

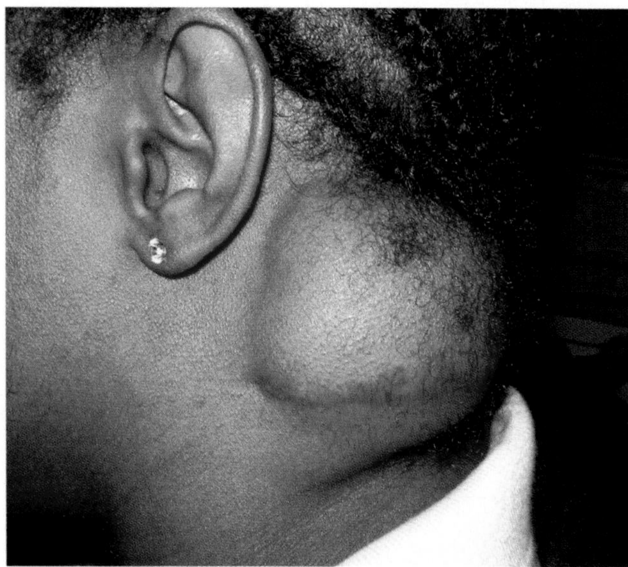

FIGURE 14–51 Neck lipoma. (Courtesy of Moshe Weizberg, MD.)

Diagnosis

Lipomas are diagnosed by their clinical appearance. Lipomas are round, nonmobile, nonpainful masses that are soft and doughy to palpation.[3] The overlying skin is normal. Contraction of muscle may alter the shape of the lesion. Lipomas appear radiographically as homogenous, radiolucent masses with sharp margins.

Clinical Complications

Complications are rare and usually are limited to patient discomfort and anxiety. Complications may occur due to mass effect, because lipomas can develop anywhere in the body.

Management

No intervention is necessary for most lipomas, although they can be excised or injected with steroids. Patients with lipomas that are growing rapidly, are painful, are larger than 5 cm, are tethered to fascia, or are located on the lower extremities should be referred to specialists for evaluation of possible liposarcoma.[4]

REFERENCES

1. Digregorio F, Barr RJ, Fretzin DF. Pleomorphic lipoma: case reports and review of the literature. *J Dermatol Surg Oncol* 1992;18:197–202.
2. Fanburg-Smith JC, Devaney KO, Miettinen M, Weiss SW. Multiple spindle cell lipomas: a report of 7 familial and 11 nonfamilial cases. *Am J Surg Pathol* 1998;22:40–48.
3. Salam GA. Lipoma excision. *Am Fam Physician* 2002;65:901–904.
4. Rydholm A, Berg NO. Size, site and clinical incidence of lipoma: factors in the differential diagnosis of lipoma and sarcoma. *Acta Orthop Scand* 1983;54:929–934.

Hemangioma

Raffi Kapitanyan

Clinical Presentation

Approximately 55% of hemangiomas are present at birth, with the remainder developing during the first weeks of life.[1] Lesions usually originate as pale macules with radiating, thread-like telangiectases.[1] As they grow, they become bright red, slightly elevated, noncompressible plaques that range in size from a few millimeters to several centimeters.[1]

Pathophysiology

Hemangiomas are vascular tumors with a growth phase marked by endothelial proliferation, hypercellularity, and an involutional phase.[2] Although their origin is not clearly understood, both vasculogenesis (precursors of endothelial cells giving rise to blood vessels) and angiogenesis (the development of new vessels from existing vasculature) seem to occur.[1] Although most tumors are solitary, as many as 20% of infants have multiple lesions.[1] With time, the lesions involute through a process characterized by a change in color, from bright red to purple or grey, and eventually on to complete resolution in many cases.[1] Rarely, fully-grown tumors may be present at birth and resolve rapidly, leaving atrophic skin changes in their place.[1]

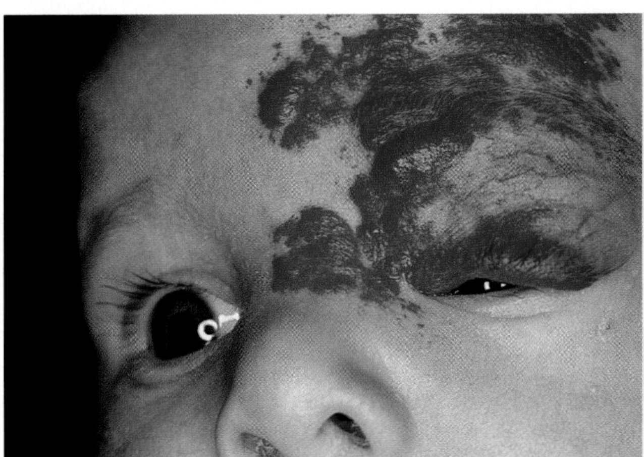

FIGURE 14–52 Capillary hemangioma. The surface is raised and irregular, with a bright red color characteristic of superficial hemangiomas. (Reprinted from Tasman, with permission.)

Diagnosis

The diagnosis of hemangioma is made clinically, based on their classic appearance. However, ultrasonography with Doppler studies may demonstrate a high-flow pattern that can differentiate a hemangioma from solid tumors and malformations of the veins, lymph vessels, and capillaries.[1]

Clinical Complications

The most frequent complication associated with these lesions is ulceration.[1] They can be very painful and bleed when traumatized, leaving residual scarring. Superinfection of these ulcers may lead to cellulitis, osteomyelitis, or septicemia. Hemangiomas of the periorbital region may lead to astigmatism from compression on the globe.[1] Children with multiple cutaneous tumors may develop visceral components, with those of the liver associated with 40% morbidity secondary to high-output cardiac failure.[1]

Management

Treatment depends on many factors, including location, depth of lesion, age of patient, presence or likelihood of complications, and parental preference.[1] Support for parents is important; before-and-after pictures of involution can be reassuring. For larger lesions, daily injections of steroids have been used, resulting in dramatic shrinkage in one third of subjects.[1] Patients with hemangioma identified in the emergency department (ED) should be referred to a pediatrician or dermatologist for follow-up and continuing care.

REFERENCES

1. Drolet BA, Esterly NB, Frieden IJ. Hemangiomas in children. *N Engl J Med* 1999;341:173–181.
2. Mulliken JB, Glowacki J. Hemangiomas and vascular malformations in infants and children: a classification based on endothelial characteristics. *Plast Reconstr Surg* 1982;69:412–422.

Angular Cheilitis (Perlèche)

In-Hei Hahn

Clinical Presentation

Angular cheilitis, or perlèche, may develop at any age. Patients present with macerated deep fissures or cracks at the corners of the mouth and complain of dryness with a painful, burning sensation. This disorder often is accompanied by either oral candidiasis or denture stomatitis.[1]

Pathophysiology

Perlèche is caused by continuous irritation, such as from lip licking, biting the corners of the mouth, thumb sucking, and even aggressive dental manipulation (including the use of dental floss).[1] This combination of repeated insults leads to fissuring and ulceration of the oral commissures. *Candida* species can be cultured from most lesions, but it is unknown whether this is a causative organism or simply a superinfection. Less common causes of angular cheilitis include vitamin deficiency, iron deficiency, herpes simplex virus (HSV), and contact dermatitis (e.g., from exposure to nickel in braces).[2] Underlying medical conditions may predispose patients to angular cheilitis; these include the xerostomia of Sjögren's syndrome and the oral candidiasis commonly seen in patients with diabetes, human immunodeficiency virus (HIV) infection, or malignancy. Congenital anomalies and aging can also lead to perlèche when excessive skin folds or an abnormal jaw line lead to the accumulation of saliva at the corners of the mouth.[1,2]

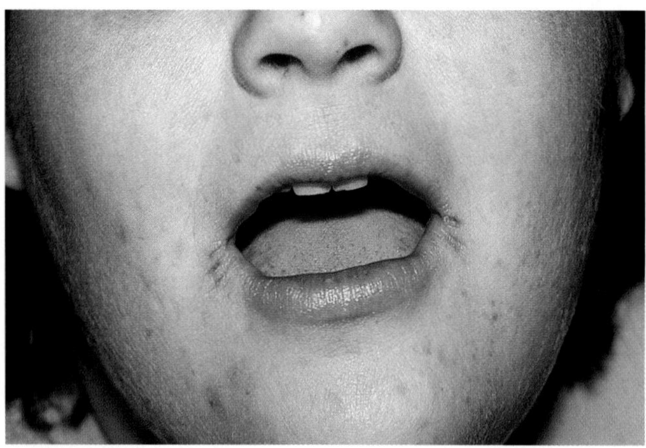

FIGURE 14–53 Typical of angular cheilitis, this patient has scaling, fissuring, and crusting at the corners of her mouth. She has atopic dermatitis elsewhere on her skin. (From Goodheart, with permission.)

Diagnosis

Angular cheilitis is diagnosed clinically; however, identification of a superinfection requires visualization of the organism on Gram staining or isolation of it from a scraping of the site.[1]

Clinical Complications

The most common complication is superinfection, especially by staphylococcal and candidal species.[1]

Management

Treatment depends on the cause of the disease. For candidal infections, use of topical nystatin or clotrimazole, in addition to intraoral or systemic antifungals, is effective.[1] Bacterial infections respond to topical or systemic antibiotics. Topical antifungal or antibacterial agents should be followed by a steroid cream with a nongreasy base (e.g., triamcinolone acetonide) until the area is dry and free of inflammation.[1] A thick, protective lip balm may help to keep the lips moist and prevent aggravation of the healing ulcers. Associated thrush should be treated appropriately. It is imperative to keep the oral commissures dry to expedite healing.[1]

REFERENCES

1. Martin ES, Elewski BE. Cutaneous fungal infections in the elderly. *Clin Geriatr Med* 2002;18:59–75.
2. Yesudian PD, Memon A. Nickel-induced angular cheilitis due to orthodontic braces. *Contact Dermatitis* 2003;48:287–288.

Rhinophyma

Colleen Campbell

Clinical Presentation

Rhinophyma appears as thickened, erythematous or purple-hued nasal skin.[1] The skin may have fissures, pits, and scarring, with a distortion of the usual curves of the nose.[2] Telangiectases may be present as well.[1] The tip of the nose appears enlarged and bulbous, with pilosebaceous pores containing foul-smelling sebum.[2] Papules and pustules are commonly seen, whereas multiple firm, smooth nodules may be more prominent in severe disease.[2] Tumors may also grow from the affected area in severe cases.[1]

Pathophysiology

Rhinophyma is a severe manifestation of rosacea that affects the nose.[1]

Rhinophyma is considered the fourth stage of rosacea. The first two stages are characterized by increased vascularity, which leads to skin hypertrophy and erythema. The third stage is acne rosacea, which is marked by papule and pustule formation. Hypertrophy of the dermal and sebaceous glands results in clogged pores and buildup of sebum. Although women are more commonly affected with rosacea than men, men develop rhinophyma at least five times more frequently.[1] People of Irish or English descent have a greater risk than those of other ethnicities.[1] Sun exposure and alcohol consumption have been linked to the disease.[3]

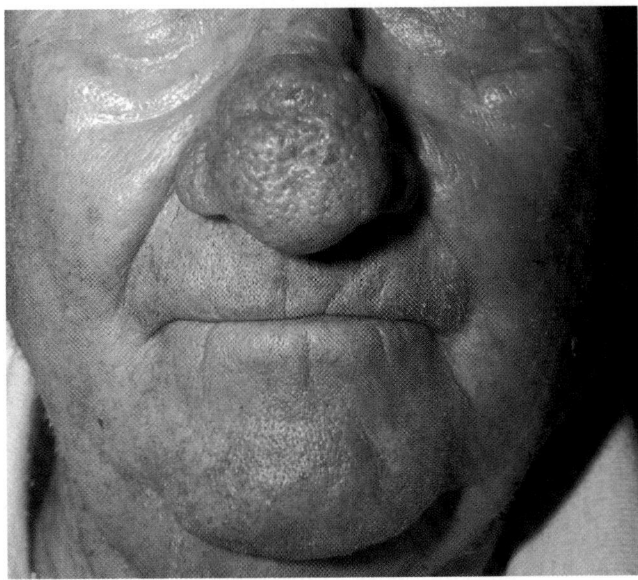

FIGURE 14–54 Typical nasal cosmetic deformity of rhinophyma. (© David Effron, MD, 2004. Used with permission.)

Diagnosis

Rhinophyma is largely a clinical diagnosis based on the characteristic erythematous, nodular, and enlarged appearance of the nose.[1] However, referral for surgical evaluation is warranted, because some studies have shown a 3% incidence of occult basal cell carcinoma (BCC) of the nose in affected patients.[1]

Clinical Complications

Nasal obstruction may result from the morphologic changes in the nose, although bony structures usually are unaffected.[1] Skin cancers and tumors appear more frequently on the nose in patients with rhinophyma. Ocular complications of rosacea are common and require referral to an ophthalmology specialist to evaluate for corneal involvement.[1]

Management

The treatment for rosacea centers on topical and oral antibiotics and retinoids.[1] Antibiotics used include metronidazole and, secondly, tetracyclines. Topical clindamycin is a reasonable alternative in pregnant women.[3] Accutane (isotretinoin) has the advantage of decreased skin irritation and erythema in comparison with Retin-A (tretinoin); however, it must be used with extreme caution in women of child-bearing age, because its use has been associated with a substantial incidence of teratogenicity.[1] Patients are advised to avoid Accutane for 1 year before surgery, because it impairs reepithelialization.[1] Because of the extreme appearance of rhinophyma, dermabrasion and dermaplaning remain the main treatments. Other surgical options include carbon dioxide and argon laser therapy, cryotherapy, and excision with heated knives and an ultrasonic scalpel.[1]

REFERENCES

1. Rohrich RJ, Griffin JR, Adams WP Jr. Rhinophyma: review and update. *Plast Reconstr Surg* 2002;110:860–869.
2. Aloi F, Tomasini C, Soro E, Pippione M. The clinicopathologic spectrum of rhinophyma. *J Am Acad Dermatol* 2000;42:468–472.
3. Blount BW, Pelletier AL. Rosacea, a common, yet commonly overlooked, condition. *Am Fam Physician* 2002;66:435–440.

Complications of Body Piercing

Colleen Campbell

Clinical Presentation

Patients may present after a piercing procedure for a variety of reasons, including excessive postprocedure bleeding, acute infection, evaluation for the transmission of blood-borne pathogens, and evaluation of the spread of other infectious diseases as a result of the piercing procedure. Patients with acute local infections may present with redness, purulent drainage, or increasing pain at the site of the piercing. Infection often occurs in the early postprocedural period. However, some piercings take up to 8 months to heal and can become infected at any time during that period.[1]

As genital and other body-site piercings become more common in the United States, it is important for practitioners to be aware of the various types of piercings and the potential complications that may arise. By way of example, there are three popular types of penile piercings. The most common is known as the "Prince Albert."[2] This is a piercing that enters through the urethra and then turns out of the penis on the undersurface of the shaft. This piercing may result in a spray of urine during micturition. The second type is the Apabravya, in which the urethra is speared top to bottom. This is described as "two screws tightening around the head."[2] The third common type is the Ampallang, in which the glans is pierced from side to side and the urethra remains intact.[2] Other, less common types include pubic or scrotal piercing, a Dydoe or coronal ridge piercing, and frenulum piercing.

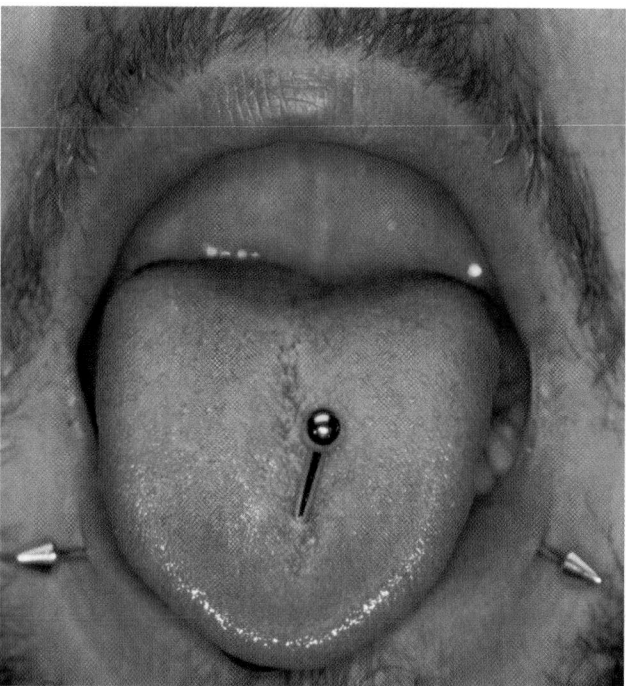

FIGURE 14–55 Extensive oral piercing. (© David Effron, MD, 2004. Used with permission.)

Pathophysiology

The pathophysiology of piercing-related problems depends on the specific problem and the anatomic location of the piercing.

Diagnosis

Diagnosis of complications of body piercing is based on careful history taking and clinical observation. Infection may be evidenced by the classic findings of redness at the site of the piercing, purulent drainage, and induration. Urinalysis is essential to evaluate infection involving the urinary tract. A complete blood count (CBC) with differential and C-reactive protein (CRP) measurement, and an erythrocyte sedimentation rate (ESR) determination may be useful in evaluating systemic involvement of infection.

Clinical Complications

Local infections secondary to piercing are reported to occur in up to 30% of cases and are, to some degree, site-dependent.[3] The most common complication from piercing is wound infection, which may progress to cellulitis or, rarely, to necrotizing fasciitis or even endocarditis or sepsis. These infections are largely caused by common skin flora, such as *Staphylococcus aureus* and *Streptococcus* species.[3] Staphylococcal endocarditis has been reported after nasal piercing.[3] It is suspected that certain types of infection, such as *Condyloma acuminatum*, hepatitis B, and human immunodeficiency virus, have been spread through piercings done without sterile instrumentation.[3] Urinary tract infection may occur in association with piercings involving the urethra. Urethral stricture with obstruction and paraphimosis are potential complications of penile piercings.[2] Granulation tissue can form in reaction to the foreign object, or there may be allergic reactions to the various metals and alloys used in body jewelry.[3] Priapism has been reported in response to penile piercing.[2] Sexual partners of those with piercings may present with complications such as chipped teeth, choking, foreign bodies getting stuck between the partner's teeth, and mucosal injury to receptive partners.[3] Additional complications may arise when patients are unable to remove pieces of body jewelry on their own. Such removal at times requires the attention of a surgeon and conscious sedation or general anesthesia, depending on the complexity of the removal.[3]

Complications of Body Piercing

Colleen Campbell

Management

Treatment of severe infection requires antistreptococcal and staphylococcal antibiotics, such as intravenous cefazolin. Milder infections may be treated with parenteral cephalosporins, such as cephalexin. Quinolones are the drugs of choice for infections involving the urinary tract. The body jewelry in an infected piercing should be removed with a metal or ring cutter if it cannot be removed in a simple fashion. An urgent urology consultation is necessary in the case of an extensive genital infection, or if a stricture or obstruction of the urinary tract is present.[1–4]

REFERENCES

1. Anderson WR, Summerton DJ, Sharma DM, Holmes SA. The urologist's guide to genital piercing. *BJU Int* 2003;91:245–251.
2. Hansen RB, Olsen LH, Langkilde NC. Piercing of the glans penis. *Scand J Urol Nephrol* 1998;32:219–220.
3. Stirn A. Body piercing: medical consequences and psychological motivations. *Lancet* 2003;361:1205–1215.
4. Marcoux D. Appearance cosmetics, and body art in adolescents. *Dermatol Clin* 2000;18:667–673.

ID Reaction

Michael Greenberg

Clinical Presentation

Patients present after the acute onset of an intensely pruritic erythematous, maculopapular, or vesicular rash within about 14 days after a primary episode of dermatitis or cutaneous infection.[1–3] The ID eruption is often symmetric and may involve the upper and lower extremities, trunk, face, and neck. Some patients may also have fever, leukocytosis, generalized adenopathy, and enlargement of the spleen. The prevalence of ID reaction is equal in men and women.

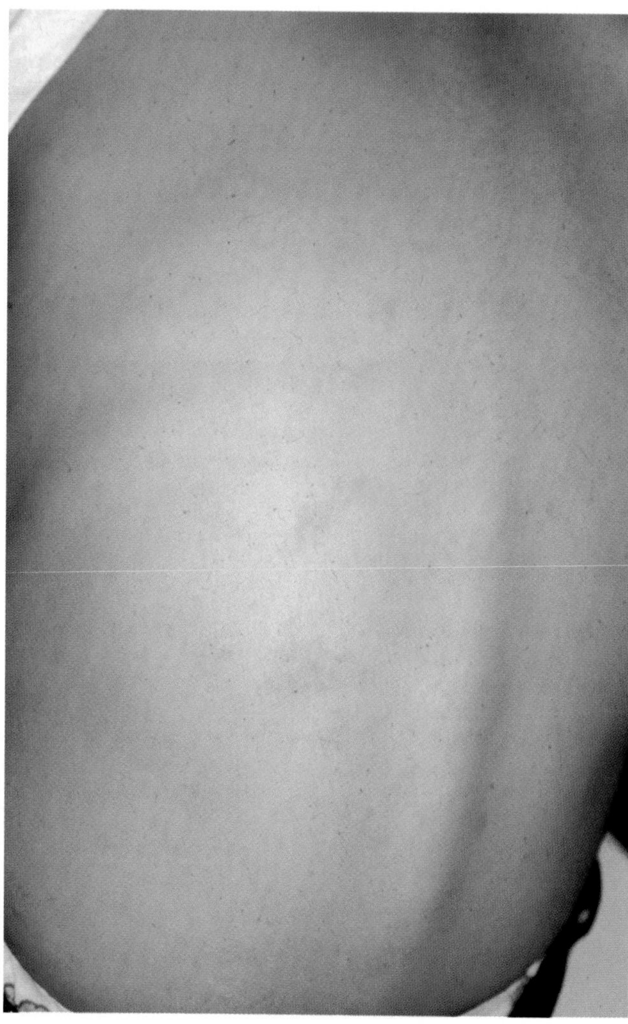

FIGURE 14–56 Itchy, dyshidrotic vesicular eruption of ID reaction. (Copyright James R. Roberts, MD.)

Pathophysiology

The ID reaction is a generalized acute reaction to various skin conditions of an inflammatory or infectious nature.[1–3]

ID reactions are probably immunologic in origin, and the pathology of a given ID reaction depends on the cause of the primary insult. Specifically, the ID process may be identified by the primary inciting process as dermatophytid, pediculid, or bacterid. In any case, the ID reaction is essentially a secondary allergic skin eruption in sensitized persons that results from the hematologic spread of fungi, bacteria, parasites, or products therefrom.[3]

Diagnosis

The clinical findings associated with ID reactions are variable and depend on the primary inciting cause. However, ID lesions always occur at anatomic locations removed from the primary infection or dermatitis site and tend to be symmetric.[1–3]

Clinical Complications

The most common complication is reoccurrence, especially if the primary lesion is incompletely treated. Other complications include secondary infection and secondary allergic contact dermatitis.[1–3]

Management

The inciting infection or dermatitis must be eradicated in order to effectively treat the ID reaction. Systemic and topical steroids and systemic antihistamines can be very helpful in the treatment of this condition. Patients with severe underlying infections as the trigger for an ID reaction may require hospital admission.

REFERENCES

1. Gonzalez-Amaro R, Baranda L, Abud-Mendoza C, Delgado SP, Moncada B. Autoeczematization is associated with abnormal immune recognition of autologous skin antigens. *J Am Acad Dermatol* 1993;28:56–60.
2. Brenner S, Wolf R, Landau M. Scabid: an unusual ID reaction to scabies. *Int J Dermatol* 1993;32:128–129.
3. Derebery J, Berliner KI. Foot and ear disease: the dermatophytid reaction in otology. *Laryngoscope* 1996;106:181–186.

Sporotrichosis

Anthony S. Mazzeo

Clinical Presentation

Patients present with nonhealing, relatively painless skin lesions in an area that was pricked by a thorn during the preceding 1 to 4 weeks. However, many patients do not recall the inciting trauma.[1]

Pathophysiology

Sporotrichosis is a chronic fungal infection of the cutaneous/subcutaneous tissues caused by *Sporothrix schenckii,* an organism that lives on decaying plant matter but has also been isolated from the nails of animals.[1-3] *S. schenckii* is a thermally dimorphic fungi that exists as a mold at room temperature and as a yeast in host tissues.[2] Patients suffer a traumatic inoculation of the mold, which sparks a local granulomatous response, resulting in nodule development locally and along the regional lymphatic system.[3] *S. schenckii* is pathogenic even in immunocompetent hosts.

Diagnosis

Diagnosis relies on recognition of the cutaneous manifestation. The fixed cutaneous form begins as a papule at the site of inoculation that slowly enlarges and becomes nodular.[1,2] This nodule may ulcerate and produce a nonpurulent drainage. Because of lymphangitic spread, there may be additional lesions and lymphadenopathy proximal to the initial lesion; this is termed the lymphocutaneous form. Fungal culture is the gold standard for diagnosis, because the lesions may resemble other infections, such as nocardial, staphylococcal, and mycobacterial infections, syphilis, and basal cell carcinoma (BCC).[3] Culture of actual tissue specimens is required, because wound drainage culture has proven to be insufficient.

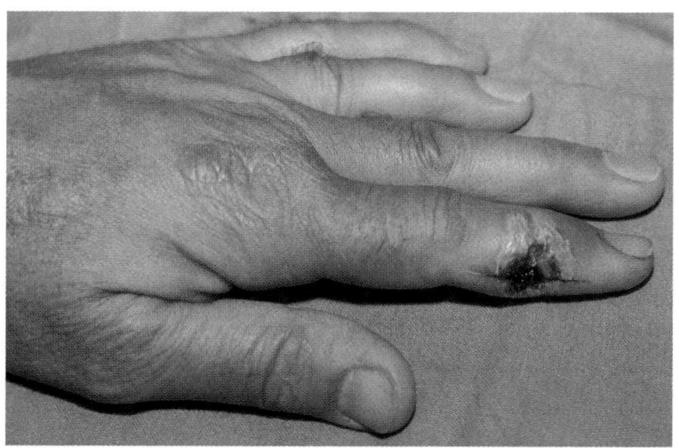

FIGURE 14–57 Typical lesions caused by *Sporothrix schenckii.* (© David Effron, MD, 2004. Used with permission.)

Clinical Complications

Complications include chronicity, superinfection, and systemically disseminated disease. Immunocompromised individuals are at risk for life-threatening systemic, arthritic, and meningitic forms of the disease. Pulmonary sporotrichosis has been reported secondary to inhalation of the organism.

Management

Local heat has been shown to improve healing.[3] Almost all patients require pharmacologic treatment to clear the infection, because spontaneous improvement is rare even in normal hosts. In developed countries, itraconazole is the preferred treatment for nondisseminated disease in situations in which cost does not preclude its use.[1] Potassium iodide (SSKI), terbinafine, and fluconazole are also treatment options, although somewhat less effective. For disseminated or meningitic sporotrichosis, hospital admission and intravenous amphotericin B are required. Bone or joint disease may require débridement in addition to antifungal therapy.

REFERENCES

1. Morris-Jones R. Sporotrichosis. *Clin Exp Dermatol* 2002;27:427–431.
2. De Araujo T, Marques AC, Kerdel F. Sporotrichosis. *Int J Dermatol* 2001;40:737–742.
3. Queiroz-Telles F, McGinnis MR, Salkin I, Graybill JR. Subcutaneous mycoses. *Infect Dis Clin North Am* 2003;17:59–85.

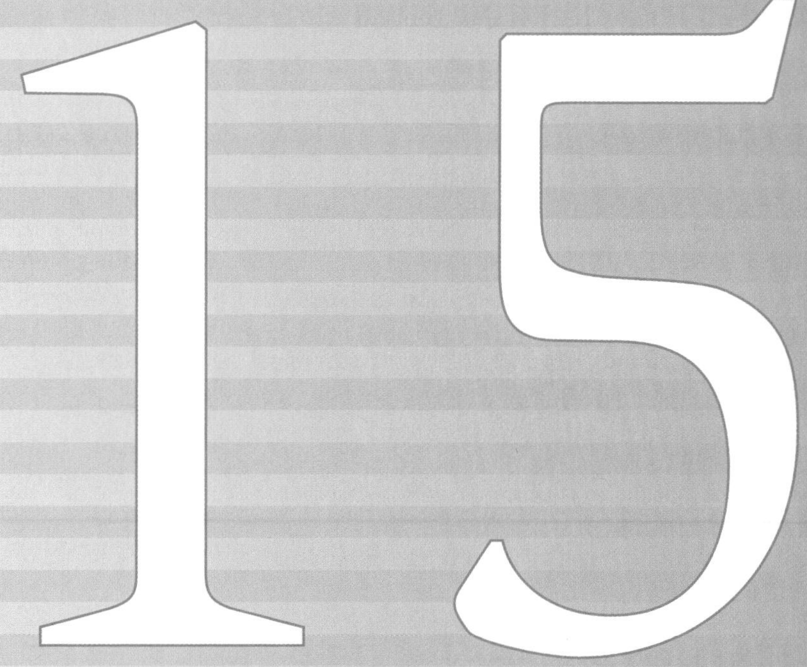

Orthopedic

Salter-Harris Classification

Robert Hendrickson

Clinical Presentation

Patients with fractures described by the Salter-Harris (SH) classification system present with pain, tenderness, and possibly swelling. Injuries may occur after minimal trauma, because the growth plate is II to V times weaker than the surrounding bone.[1] SH II–V fractures should be readily recognizable on radiographs. An SH 1 fracture may not be detectable on radiographs, and conservative therapy for a presumed fracture may be needed.[1,2]

Pathophysiology

Fractures may occur via direct trauma or rotational pressure. The SH classification of fractures is a system of grouping childhood fractures that involve the epiphyseal growth plate (physis). SH I is a fracture through the growth plate only. These fractures may or may not be recognizable on radiographs. In SH II, the fracture is through the metaphysis as well as the physis. SH III fractures are intraarticular fractures through the physis as well as the epiphysis. SH IV fractures traverse both the epiphysis and the metaphysis. SH V is a crush injury to the growth plate and is noted as a compression of the physis.[1,2]

Diagnosis

Diagnosis is suspected by recognition of clinical symptoms and confirmed by radiography. Comparison views of the contralateral extremity are sometimes helpful in detecting fractures.

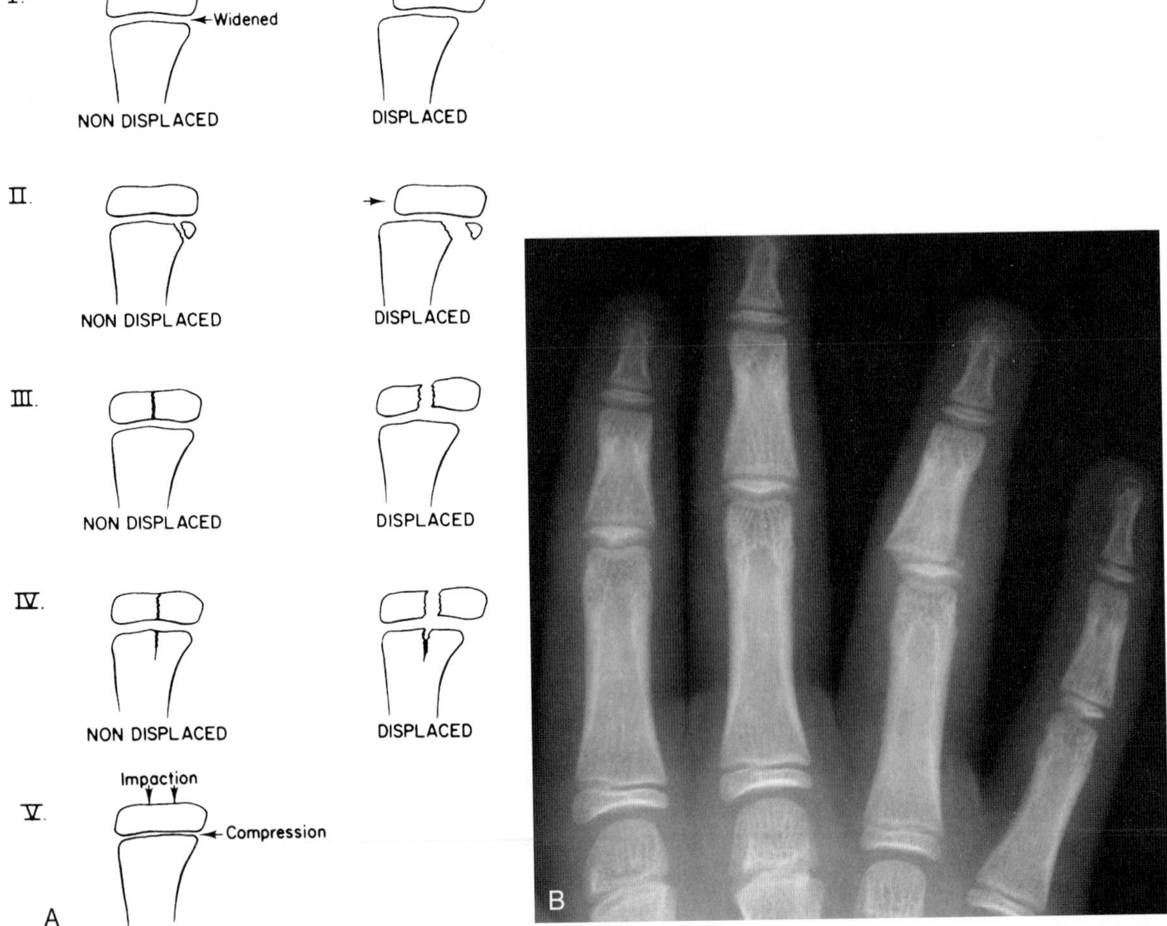

FIGURE 15–1 **A:** Salter-Harris (SH) classification of fractures. (From Swischuk, with permission.) **B:** SH I fracture of the middle phalanx. (Courtesy of Mark Silverberg, MD.)

Salter-Harris Classification

Robert Hendrickson

Clinical Complications

Complications include premature growth plate closure, bony growth arrest, angular deformity, nonunion, and chronic pain.[2] Prognosis is indirectly related to classification number. For example, SH V has a worse prognosis than SH IV, which has a worse prognosis than SH III, and so on.

Management

If a patient has pain and tenderness of a growth-plate area, the involved part should be immobilized with a splint, and follow-up with an orthopedist or primary doctor should be sought, because SH I fractures are extremely difficult to detect on radiography and usually are diagnosed clinically. Patients with SH II–V fractures also require splinting and an orthopedic consultation.

REFERENCES

1. Brown JH, DeLuca SA. Growth plate injuries: Salter-Harris classification. *Am Fam Physician* 1992;46:1180–1184.
2. Rogers LF, Poznanski AK. Imaging of epiphyseal injuries. *Radiology* 1994;191:297–308.

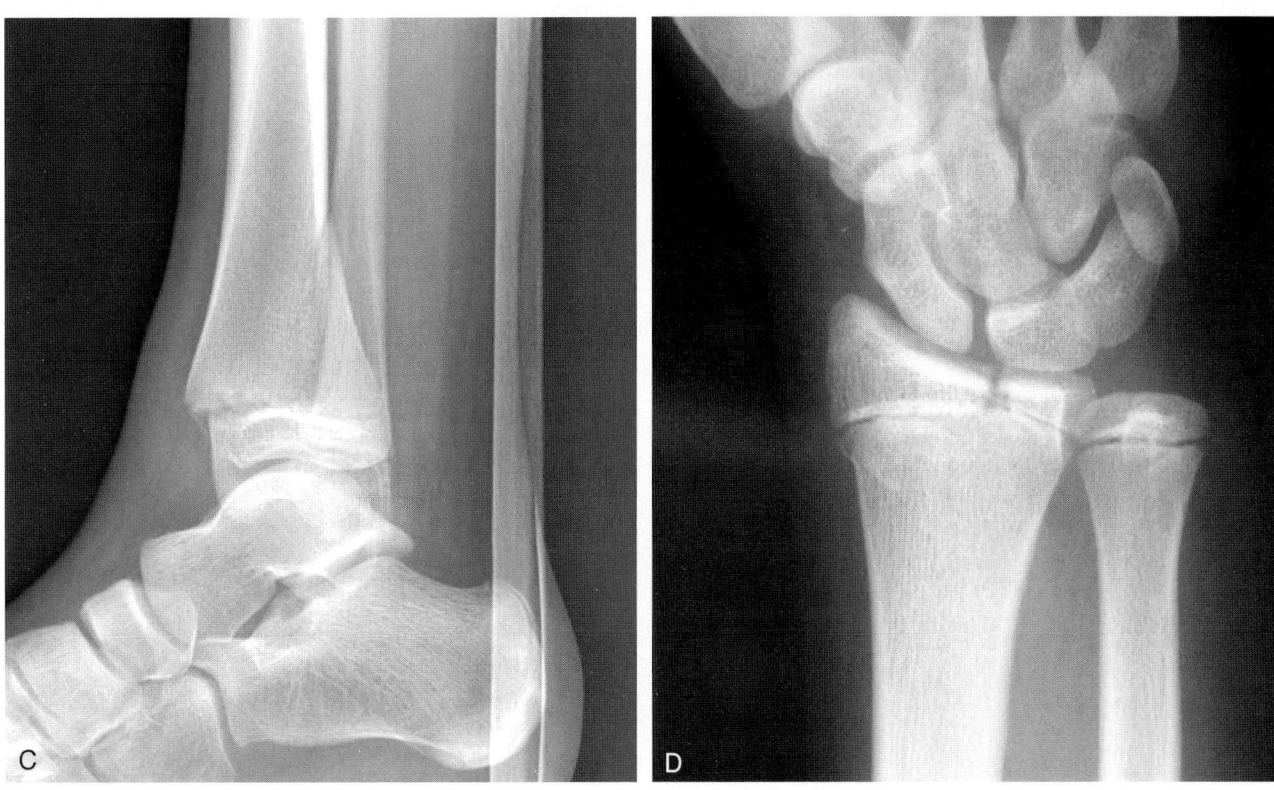

FIGURE 15–1, cont'd. C: Lateral view of SH II fracture of the tibia. (Courtesy of Kevin Reinhard, MD.) **D:** SH III fracture. (Courtesy of Mark Silverberg, MD.)

15-2

Open Fractures

Colleen Campbell

Clinical Presentation

Patients with open fractures (OFs) present with pain in the involved extremity, along with an overlying laceration or puncture wound.

Pathophysiology

An OF is a fracture in which there is an overlying disruption of the normal skin barrier, with a resultant exposure or tract from the skin to the fracture or its hematoma. One classification of open fractures is as follows. Grade I is a clean puncture wound of less than 1 centimeter. Grade II is a laceration of less than 5 cm that does not involve extensive soft tissue injury or loss. Grade III injuries have extensive soft tissue damage by crush injury or involve extensive loss of tissue. Grade IIIA injuries have adequate soft tissue coverage of bone; IIIB injuries have associated periosteal stripping and bone exposure; and Grade IIIC injuries involve extensive arterial injury.[1]

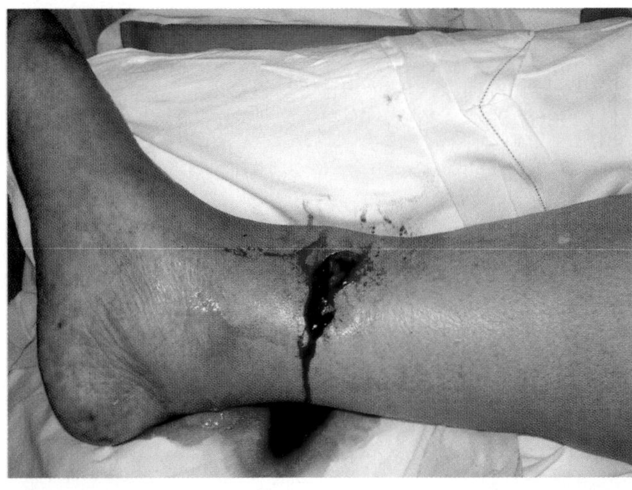

FIGURE 15-2 Open fracture with bone protruding through skin. (Courtesy of Mark Silverberg, MD.)

Diagnosis

The diagnosis of an OF is made on the basis of a careful history and physical examination, along with radiographic evaluation of the involved underlying bone. A careful examination and documentation of the neurovascular status of the affected limb is essential.[1]

Clinical Complications

OFs are complicated by infection, osteomyelitis, nonunion, and delayed union. The underlying bone and soft tissue may be devascularized to the extent that amputation is necessary. Because of the large forces that cause OFs, there is often associated myonecrosis and rhabdomyolysis.[1]

Management

Initial treatment of OFs involves immobilization and emergency orthopedic referral. Antibiotics effective against skin organisms should be given intravenously in the emergency department (ED). First-generation cephalosporins are the drugs of choice. Tetanus prophylaxis should be provided if indicated. Débridement of the wound, followed by copious high-pressure irrigation, should be done in a timely manner in the ED if surgery will be delayed for longer than 1 hour.[1] Sterile dressings should then be applied. Treatment of OFs involves high-pressure irrigation and débridement in the operating room, as well as fracture fixation. Intramedullary nails are used with increasing frequency in the treatment of open tibia and femur fractures. External fracture fixation may be necessary if there is a large amount of soft tissue injury or if hemorrhage must be controlled quickly, as in the case of pelvic fractures.[1]

REFERENCES

1. Musgrave DS, Mendelson SA. Pediatric Orthopedic Trauma: Principles in management. *Crit Care Med* 2002;30[11 Suppl]:S431–S443.

Paronychia

Jennifer Harris

Clinical Presentation

Patients with paronychia present with acute or chronic pain and tenderness of the perionychium, the fingers, or the toes. Acutely, patients report symptoms arising spontaneously or after trauma or manipulation of the nail bed. Chronic symptoms usually are present for longer than 6 weeks and may be episodic, typically occurring after exposure to water or a moist environment.[1]

Pathophysiology

Paronychia is a localized, superficial infection or abscess of the epidermis bordering the nails that develops when a disruption occurs between the seal of the proximal nail fold and the nail plate. Acute paronychia is caused by trauma, nail biting, finger sucking, aggressive manicuring, or a hangnail. The most common offending organism is *Staphylococcus aureus,* followed by *Streptococcus* and *Pseudomonas* species, but gram-negative organisms, herpes simplex virus, and yeast also have been reported.[1] In chronic infections, separation of the cuticle from the nail plate occurs secondary to overexposure to water, solvents, or chemicals. The infecting organism is typically *Candida albicans.*[2] In addition, metastatic cancer, subungual melanoma, and squamous cell carcinoma can manifest as chronic paronychia.[1]

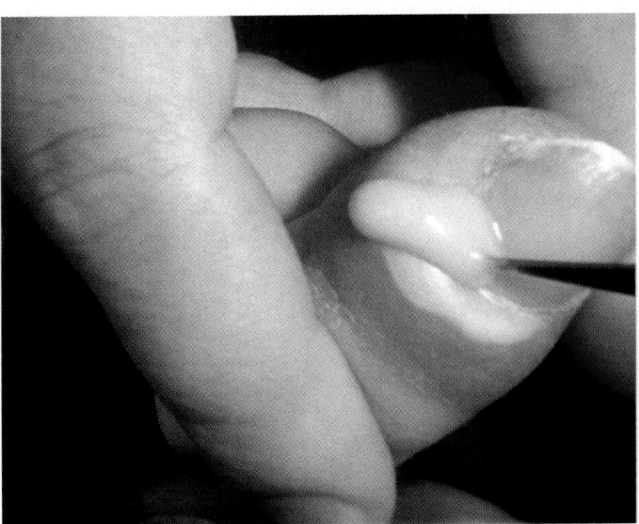

FIGURE 15-3 Excision and drainage of paronychia. (Courtesy of Michael Greenberg, MD.)

Diagnosis

Diagnosis of acute or chronic paronychia is made by physical examination and history. Because chronic paronychia typically is caused by *C. albicans* (95% of cases), a wet mount with potassium hydroxide from a scraping or sample of the purulent drainage may reveal hyphae.[1]

Clinical Complications

Neglected paronychia, although painful, has few long-term complications. If chronic paronychia does not resolve with appropriate therapy, unusual and potentially serious causes such as malignancy must be explored.[1]

Management

Acute paronychia in which abscess formation has not occurred may resolve with conservative treatment (e.g., warm-water soaks). Antibiotics, if used, should cover *S. aureus* as well as anaerobes; amoxicillin-clavulanate potassium (Augmentin) or clindamycin (Cleocin) is the drug of choice. Once abscesses have formed, incision of the nail fold to promote drainage is required to clear the infection.[1] The treatment of chronic paronychia should include avoidance of exposure to the offending agent (water, solvents) and application of topical antifungal drugs and steroids. If secondary bacterial infection is suspected, antibiotic ointment or oral agents should be added to the regimen.[2] Long-standing paronychia may require more invasive treatment (e.g., removal of the entire nail for adequate drainage) but usually responds once addressed.

REFERENCES

1. Rockwell PG. Acute and chronic paronychia. *Am Fam Physician* 2001;63:1113–1116.
2. Rich P. Nail disorders: diagnosis and treatment of infectious, inflammatory, and neoplastic nail conditions. *Med Clin North Am* 1998;82:1171–1183.

Felon

Colleen Campbell

Clinical Presentation

Patients with felons present complaining of throbbing pain and swelling in the fingertip. Pain usually develops over a few days. On examination, there is a reddened, warm fingertip with fluctuance evident.

Pathophysiology

A felon is an abscess of the pulp space of the distal phalanx. Most felon infections are caused by introduction of *Staphylococcus aureus* into the pulp space through microtears in the skin. Infections with streptococci and gram-negative organisms also occur in the pulp space. Septations in the pulp usually isolate the infection to the pulp space.[1] Splinters or other foreign bodies may precipitate infection, but usually felons arise without any identifiable source of trauma.

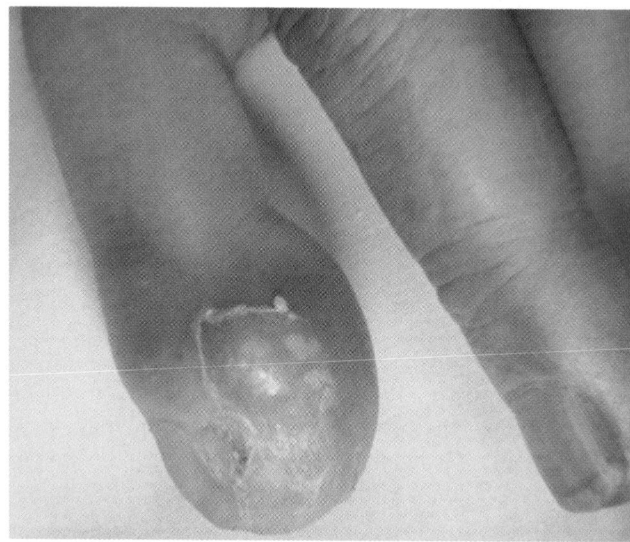

FIGURE 15–4 Digital felon. (Courtesy of Michael Greenberg, MD.)

Diagnosis

Diagnosis of felon is made on the basis of history and classic physical findings. Cultures may be useful if there is evidence of underlying osteomyelitis. Plain radiographs are reserved for those cases in which a foreign body or osteomyelitis is suspected.[1]

Clinical Complications

Osteomyelitis of the distal phalanx may occur if the infection in the pulp space is left untreated. Skin, soft tissue, and nerve necrosis may also occur if the infection is not promptly treated.[1]

Management

Treatment of felon involves incision and drainage of the infected pulp space. A digital block is used for anesthesia. A high lateral incision is made, starting just distal to the distal fold of the nail and continuing parallel to the nail plate. Curved hemostats are then used to gently break up loculations. This incision preserves the neurovascular bundle. An alternative approach is through a longitudinal incision in the volar aspect of the fingertip (the fatpad), ending distal to the distal interphalangeal (DIP) joint to avoid inadvertent injury to the flexor sheath or flexor digitorum profundus insertion. The drawback of this incision is the potential for a painful fingertip scar. The wound should be thoroughly irrigated and then packed if necessary. The patient should be prescribed oral antistaphylococcal antibiotics for 1 week and seen again in 2 days for follow-up.[1]

REFERENCES

1. Harrison BP, Hilliard MW. Emergency department evaluation and treatment of hand injuries. *Emerg Med Clin North Am* 1999;17:793–822.

Digit Amputation

Mark Silverberg

Clinical Presentation

Patients with digit amputation (DA) present after industrial or agricultural accidents, high-speed trauma events, or assaults with sharp weapons.

Pathophysiology

A complete DA denotes a finger or toe that is completely severed from the body, whereas an incomplete DA implies that the digit is still partially attached by a pedicle but the arterial circulation has been disrupted.[1] Amputation is better tolerated in children than in adults.[1] Guillotine-type, clean amputations are best suited for reimplantation, but most DAs result from crush or avulsion mechanisms.[1] The viability of an amputated digit may be maintained for up to 6 hours of warm ischemia and more than 12 hours of cold ischemia.[1]

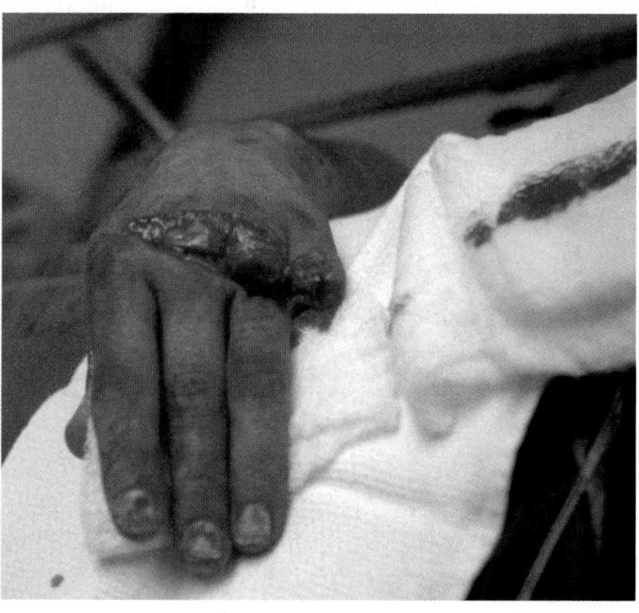

FIGURE 15–5 Partial and complete digital amputations from a power-saw accident. (Courtesy of B. Zane Horowitz, MD.)

Diagnosis

DAs can be classified according to the anatomic location of the amputation. Zone I DAs occur distal to the bony structures of the digit. Injuries classified as zone II are located distal to the lunula of the nail bed and are complicated by bone exposure. Zone III injuries involve the nail matrix and usually result in loss of the entire nail.[2]

Clinical Complications

Complications include reimplantation failure, permanent loss of function, infection, osteomyelitis, reflex sympathetic dystrophy, and permanent sensory changes that include paresthesias, hyperesthesia, or a sensation of coldness.[2]

Management

The patient should be assessed for other injuries, and the digit should be wrapped in gauze moistened with saline and placed inside a plastic bag. That bag should then be placed on ice. The digit must not be allowed to freeze.[1] The patient should be transferred to a reimplantation center if the hospital does not have that service.[1,2] Attempts at digital reattachment should take place at a specialized reimplantation center.[1] The order of reimplantation is bone first, followed by tendons, arteries, veins, and then nerves.[2] The entire site should be wrapped in a compression dressing, and skin grafts may or may not be used. Tetanus prophylaxis should be checked and updated if necessary, and parenteral antibiotics should be administered.[1]

REFERENCES

1. Michalko KB, Bentz ML. Digital replantation in children. *Crit Care Med* 2002;30[11 Suppl]:S444–S447.
2. Jackson EA. The V-Y plasty in the treatment of fingertip amputations. *Am Fam Physician* 2001;64:455–458.

15-6

Nail Avulsion

James Nelson and Colleen Campbell

Clinical Presentation

Patients with nail avulsion present with pain and bleeding at the nail bed after trauma. A laceration of the nail bed often accompanies avulsion injuries. In partial avulsions, an underlying nail-bed injury should be suspected if there is a subungual hematoma occupying more than 25% of the nail-bed area.[1]

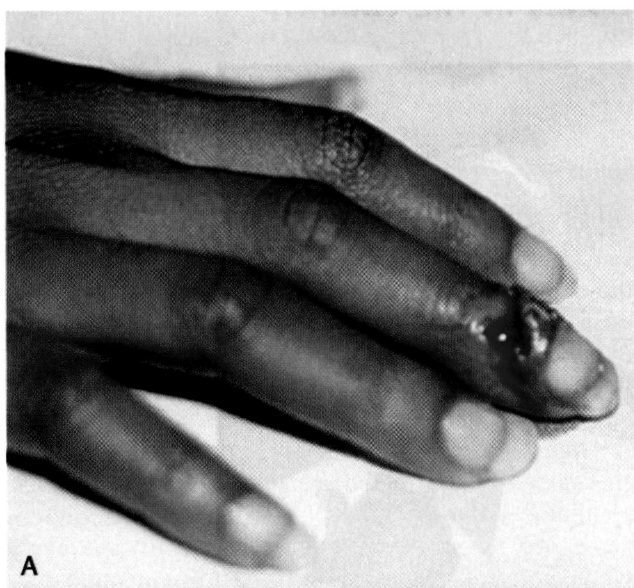

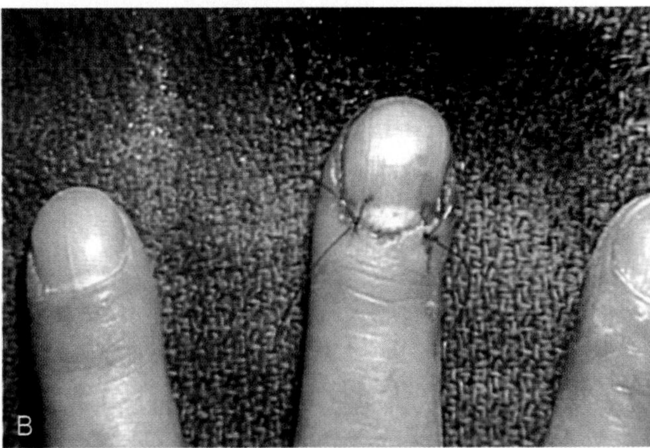

FIGURE 15–6 **A:** Fingernail avulsion. The root of the nail lies on top of the eponychium and must be implanted back to its original position under the eponychium (cuticle). **B:** Repair of fingernail avulsion. Without trimming or débriding, the base of the avulsed nail is carefully replaced in the nail fold (between the eponychium and the nail bed). This step is critical to avoid synechia formation and a resulting split nail. (**A** and **B,** From Roberts, with permission.)

Pathophysiology

Simple separation of the nail from its nail bed does not disrupt the underlying germinative centers. The germinative matrix forms the new nail proximally to distally, at a rate of 1 mm/day, so that it often takes 6 months for complete nail formation after injury.

Diagnosis

Nail avulsion is a clinical diagnosis. Radiographs should be obtained if a tuft fracture is suspected.[1]

Clinical Complications

Failure to adequately repair the nail bed can cause irregularities in the new nail. There may be permanent loss of the nail if the injury is severe.[1]

Management

The most effective treatments have not been completely elucidated. Nail-bed lacerations should be thoroughly cleansed and irrigated, especially if there is an underlying tuft fracture. If laceration of the nail bed is suspected, the nail should be removed for further inspection and repair. Repair of the nail bed can be done with the use of 6-0 or 7-0 absorbable suture.[1] Some recommend using the nail, if it is intact, as a splint for 2 to 3 weeks. Alternatively, the nail bed may be covered with a nonadhesive dressing shaped like a nail. Antibiotics directed at skin organisms are used prophylactically if an open tuft fracture is present.[1]

REFERENCES

1. Harrison BP, Hilliard MW. Emergency department evaluation and treatment of hand injuries. *Emerg Med Clin North Am* 1999;17:793–822.

Nail Bed Injury

Tyler Vadeboncoeur

Clinical Presentation

Patients with nail bed lacerations present after high-force crush injuries or lacerations. A grossly deformed nail, with or without a nail-bed laceration, is evident.[1]

Pathophysiology

Crush injuries range from subungual hematomas to amputation. An additional mechanism of injury is catching and ripping off the nail plate, with resultant laceration or avulsion of the nail bed. Approximately 50% of injuries involve fracture to the distal phalanx.[1]

Diagnosis

Simple injuries are diagnosed by history, examination, and radiography to assess the presence of fracture or foreign body. Complex injuries may require digital block followed by cleansing and a close evaluation with loupe magnification.[1-3]

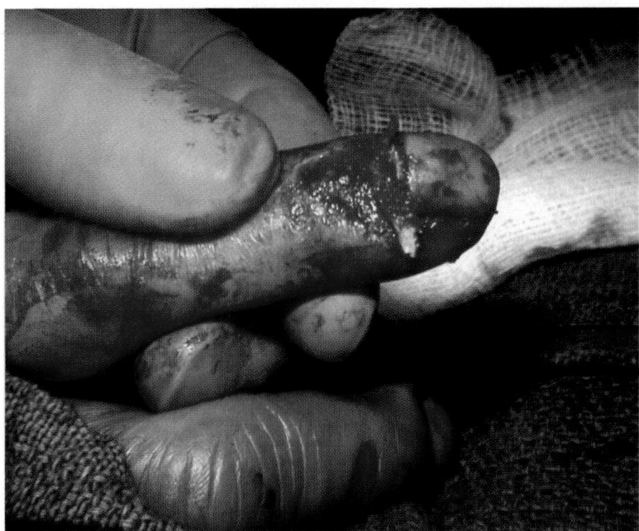

FIGURE 15–7 Avulsed nail bed with underlying injury caused by a crush mechanism. (Copyright James R. Roberts, MD.)

Clinical Complications

Nail-plate deformity affecting permanent nail growth is a common complication.[2]

Management

Subungual hematomas with partially adherent nail plates that are still aligned in the nail fold may be treated with trephination, regardless of the size of the hematoma.[3] Nail-bed lacerations may be repaired after a digital block and exsanguination of the finger. If the nail plate is still attached and is still within the nail fold, it generally does not need to be removed. If the nail is displaced, it should be removed and the nail bed further examined. Repair of lacerations is performed with 6-0 or 7-0 absorbable suture under loupe magnification. The nail may then be sutured in place or taped as a temporary splint to protect the underlying nail bed and maintain the fold for new nail growth. If the nail is not available, a single thickness of nonadherent gauze may be used in its place.[1] Complex injuries in which the nail bed cannot be accurately repaired, or in which nail-bed fragments are lost, should be referred to a hand surgeon. Tuft fractures do not alter the management of nail-bed injuries, but more proximally displaced fractures might require reduction.[1] Tetanus prophylaxis should be administered as needed.[1-3]

REFERENCES

1. Brown RE. Acute nail bed injuries. *Hand Clin* 2002;18:561–575.
2. Hart RG, Kleinhart HE. Fingertip and nail bed injuries. *Emerg Med Clin North Am* 1993;11:755–765.
3. Roser SE, Gellman H. Comparison of nail bed repair versus nail trephination for subungual hematomas in children. *J Hand Surg Am* 1999;24:1166–1170.

Subungual Hematoma

Colleen Campbell

Clinical Presentation

Patients with subungual hematomas present with throbbing pain at the fingertip and purple-red discoloration underlying the nail after trauma to the hand.

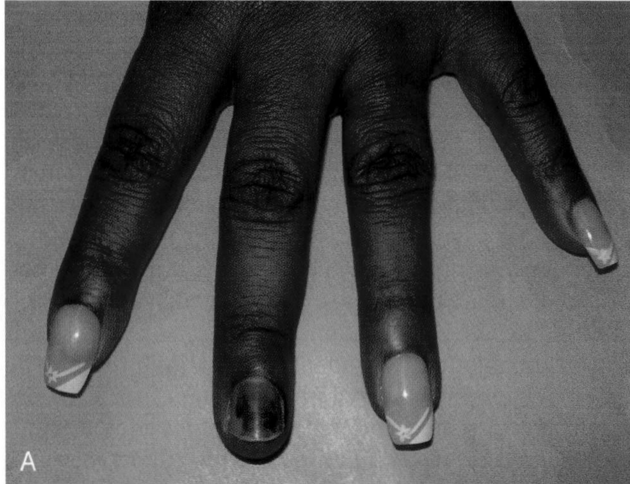

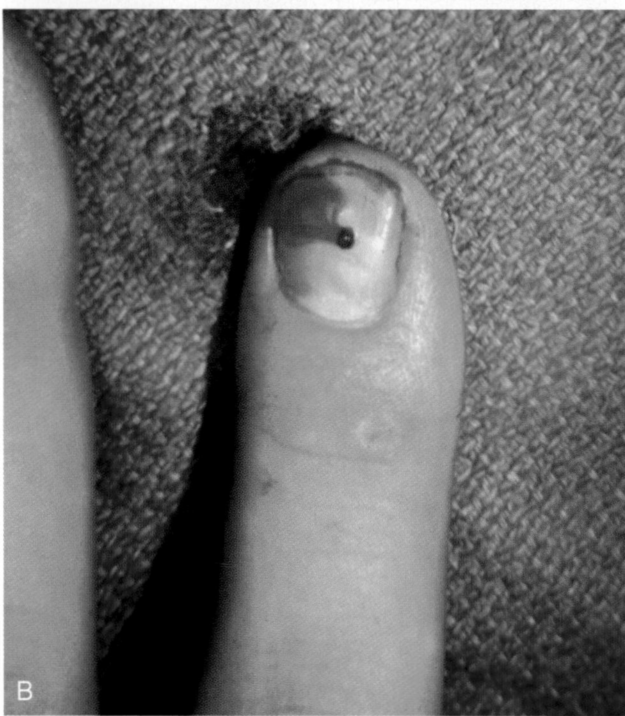

FIGURE 15–8 **A:** Nail polish removed to diagnose subungual hematoma. (Courtesy of Teresa Liu, MD.) **B:** Trephination of nail to decompress and treat subungual hematoma. (Copyright James R. Roberts, MD.)

Pathophysiology

Most subungual hematomas result from crush injuries. If the hematoma involves greater than half of the nail bed, a nail-bed laceration is likely.[1] Concomitant tuft fractures are common and are considered to be open.[2]

Diagnosis

Diagnosis of subungual hematoma is made on the basis of history, physical examination, and the finding of blood visible under the nail. Radiographs of the finger (anteroposterior, lateral, and oblique) are necessary to evaluate possible underlying fractures of the distal phalanx.[1]

Clinical Complications

Loss of the overlying nail is common after a large subungual hematoma. Subungual abscess or infection may also result from retained blood.

Management

Subungual hematomas involving more than 25% of the nail, as well as those associated with substantial pain, require trephination. This may be accomplished with the use of an electrocautery tip, a heated paperclip, or a sterile large-bore needle.[1] The needle is carefully twisted through the overlying nail until blood is released from under the nail through the hole. If the hematoma involves more than half of the nail bed, it may be necessary to remove the nail to repair the nail bed. Digital anesthesia is administered, followed by nail bed removal. The nail may be replaced and secured with a suture, or the nail bed may be covered with petrolatum-impregnated gauze.[1] A padded aluminum splint is then applied for added protection of the fingertip.

REFERENCES

1. Wang QC, Johnson BA. Fingertip injuries. *Am Fam Physician* 2001;63:1961–1966.
2. Harrison BP, Hilliard MW. Emergency department evaluation and treatment of hand injuries. *Emerg Med Clin North Am* 1999;17:793–822.

Clenched-Fist Injury ("Fight Bite")

Michael Greenberg

Clinical Presentation

Some patients with clenched-fist injuries present immediately after the injury with swelling and pain around a laceration over the dorsum of the third through fifth metacarpal joints. Other patients present 1 to 3 days after the initial injury with swelling, redness, severe pain, and decreased range of motion.[1]

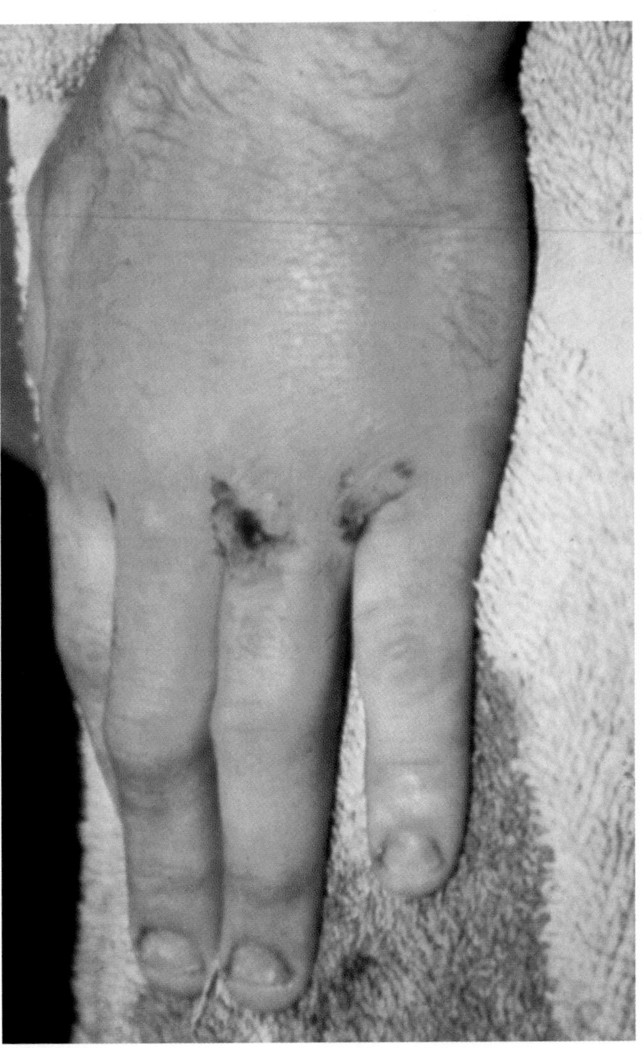

FIGURE 15–9 "Fight bite." Laceration over the fourth metacarpal, with associated swelling and early cellulitis. (Copyright James R. Roberts, MD.)

Pathophysiology

Clenched-fist injuries result when a person strikes another individual in the mouth region with the fist. If the soft tissue injury includes a break in the integrity of the skin on the dorsum of the hand, infection can complicate the original injury.[1] Fist-to-mouth contact may be the most common cause of human bite wounds. These "fight bite" wounds have the highest incidence of complications of any closed-fist injury, as well as any type of bite wound.[1]

Diagnosis

A high index of suspicion for "fight bite" is essential in any injury involving lacerations, abrasions, or bruising over the metacarpophalangeal (MCP) joints.[1] The wound must be thoroughly explored to rule out joint capsule violation and a retained foreign body, such as a tooth fragment or piece of jewelry. Exploration must be done throughout the range of motion, because the injury may be noted only when the hand is flexed, as in a fist. The wound should be copiously irrigated. If the joint space was violated, it should be thoroughly irrigated as well. The wound should be left open. No primary closure should be attempted, because such an approach increases the possibility of infection.[1]

Management

After careful examination, these wounds should be infiltrated with local anesthetic, soaked and vigorously scrubbed, and then carefully explored. Patients should receive a parenteral broad-spectrum antibiotic in the emergency department, as well as continued outpatient oral antimicrobial agents.[1] Early follow-up (24 to 48 hours) with a physician skilled in the management of these injuries is encouraged. If the patient appears noncompliant, consideration should be made for initial inpatient care. Early range of motion exercise is initiated, and the wound is allowed to heal-in secondarily or closed as a delayed primary closure.[1]

REFERENCES

1. Perron AD, Miller MD, Brady WJ. Orthopedic pitfalls in the ED: fight bite. *Am J Emerg Med* 2002;20:114–117.

15-10

Flexor Tendon Laceration

Michael Greenberg

Clinical Presentation

Patients with flexor tendon lacerations (FTLs) present after lacerations or punctures of the volar surface of one or more digits. Patients may complain of pain and inability to flex all or part of the digits distal to the injury. Other patients may be unaware of their inability to flex the digits until function is fully tested by the physician.

Pathophysiology

FTLs may be partial or complete, depending on the nature of the injury and the depth of the wound. Injury to the tissue around the tendon can result in decreased nutrition to the tendon due to inadequate blood flow, decreased synovial fluid, or other factors.[1] Many factors can influence effective healing and result in weak repairs, postrepair adhesions, or postrepair scarring. All of these issues make flexor tendon repair "one of the most challenging problems in orthopedic surgery."[1] The flexor tendons are weakest at approximately 21 days after repair.

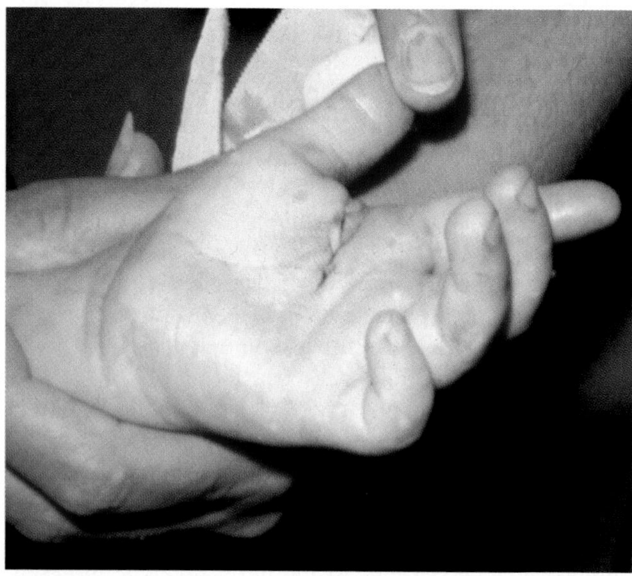

FIGURE 15–10 Flexor tendon laceration of the second digit. (Courtesy of Michael Greenberg, MD.)

Diagnosis

Accurate diagnosis hinges on a complete history and careful physical examination. The emergency physician is usually the first physician to see the patient who has sustained an FTL and must take caution never to miss the diagnosis. Any laceration involving the volar surface of the digits or hand must be considered suspect for flexor tendon injury. The examination must include placing the injured digits through both passive and active range of motion. In many cases, accessory muscles provide functionality, creating the appearance that no tendon injury has occurred. However, the diagnosis will not be missed if the physician uses careful sterile, bloodless, extension of the wound with a scalpel to allow full visualization. The examination must also include a careful assessment of the neurovascular aspects of the injured areas.

Clinical Complications

Complications include missing the diagnosis of FTL, infection, posttreatment digital stiffness, functional disability, and peritendinous adhesions.

Management

Surgical repair usually is required. Therefore, the primary role for the emergency physician is accurate diagnosis, wound cleansing, and prompt referral. Antibiotics should be given in consultation with the consulting surgeon. Tetanus immunization should be updated as needed.

REFERENCES

1. Beredjiklian PK. Biologic aspects of flexor tendon laceration and repair. *J Bone Joint Surg Am* 2003;85:539–550.

Extensor Tendon Laceration

Michael Greenberg

Clinical Presentation

Patients with extensor tendon lacerations (ETLs) present with inability to normally extend one or more digits or the hand at the wrist.

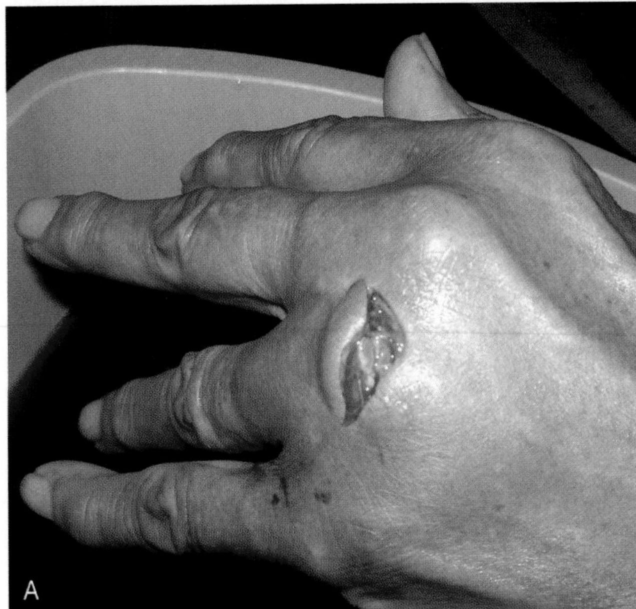

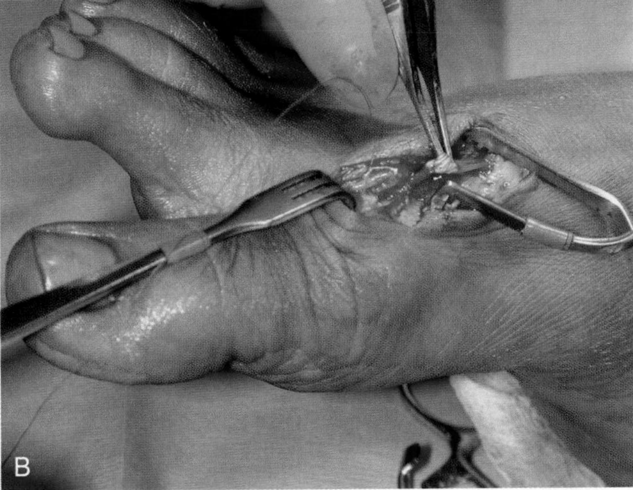

FIGURE 15–11 **A:** Extensor tendon laceration with distal end showing. (Courtesy of Mark Silverberg, MD.) **B:** Laceration of the extensor hallucis longus tendon laceration. (Courtesy of Anthony Morocco, MD.)

Pathophysiology

ETLs may result from punctures or lacerations to the dorsal surfaces of the hand, wrist, or digits.

Diagnosis

The diagnosis may be made or suspected by having the patient extend the affected digits or the hand at the wrist, both passively and against gentle resistance. With an open wound, it may be necessary to widely extend the wound, using a sterile scalpel and sterile technique, to allow maximal visualization of the tendon and its sheath. Direct inspection should then be performed under both passive and resistive full range of motion. The temporary use of a blood-pressure cuff may facilitate inspection in this manner by creating a relatively bloodless field.

Clinical Complications

Complications include missing the diagnosis of ETL, infection, chronic pain, and disability.

Management

In some cases, partial laceration of one or more extensor tendons located proximal to the metacarpophalangeal (MCP) joint does not require surgical repair. These injuries are often treated expectantly, with immobilization and early rehabilitation. Many lacerations that extend through less than 30% of the tendon width may be treated in this fashion, but partial lacerations of the extensor tendons at, or distal to, the MCP joint uniformly require suture repair. The strength of a tendon repair, once healing has occurred, depends on the number and size of sutures crossing the laceration site. The most efficient repair technique involves the use of running horizontal mattress sutures. Simple ETL repair may be accomplished in the emergency department but should be performed by a physician with training and experience in the surgical treatment of this injury.

REFERENCES

1. Russell RC, Jones M, Grobbelaar A. Extensor tendon repair: mobilise or splint? *Chir Main* 2003;22:19–23.
2. Calabro JJ, Hoidal CR, Susini LM. Extensor tendon repair in the emergency department. *J Emerg Med* 1986;4:217–225.

Trigger Finger

Michael Greenberg

Clinical Presentation

The age distribution for trigger finger is bimodal: before 6 years of age, and after 40 years of age.[1] Patients present with difficulty in flexing or extending the digit, and pain may be present. A snapping sensation is reported when the finger is extended.

Pathophysiology

Trigger finger is characterized by snapping or locking of the thumb or fingers. This condition is also known as flexor tendon entrapment of the digits.[1] Most cases of trigger finger are related to thickening of the digit's first annular pulley, but other causes include trauma, inflammatory response, diabetes, or heredity.[2] The condition generally occurs in the palm at the metacarpophalangeal (MCP) joint. Triggering results from a disproportion between the diameter of the flexor tendons and the diameter of the fibro-osseous canal. Trigger finger may occur rarely at the level of the other annular pulleys, the carpal tunnel, or the dorsal compartments.[1]

Diagnosis

Palpation during motion may reveal a snapping sensation. A nodule may also be felt on the palmar side of the MCP joint. Radiographic evaluation is not helpful in diagnosing this condition.[1]

Clinical Complications

Trigger finger is usually a minor condition for most patients, who report it to be only an annoyance. However, depending on the patient's occupation, trigger finger can be disabling (e.g., musicians, technicians). Trigger finger can be chronic and progressive, with the digit eventually becoming locked in flexion.[1]

Management

Corticosteroid injection may be used to treat trigger finger, especially in patients with rheumatoid arthritis. It may be used in conjunction with a 3-week course of splinting that extends the MCP joint while allowing the interphalangeal joints to remain mobile. Surgical treatment for severe trigger finger may become necessary.[1,3]

REFERENCES

1. Moore J. Flexor tendon entrapment of the digits (trigger finger and trigger thumb). *J Occup Environ Med* 2000;42:526–545.
2. Gaffield J, Mackay D. A-3 pulley trigger finger. *Ann Plastic Surg* 2001;46:352–353.
3. Bain G, Wallwork N. Percutaneous A1 pulley release: a clinical study. *J Bone Joint Surg Br* 1998;80:131.

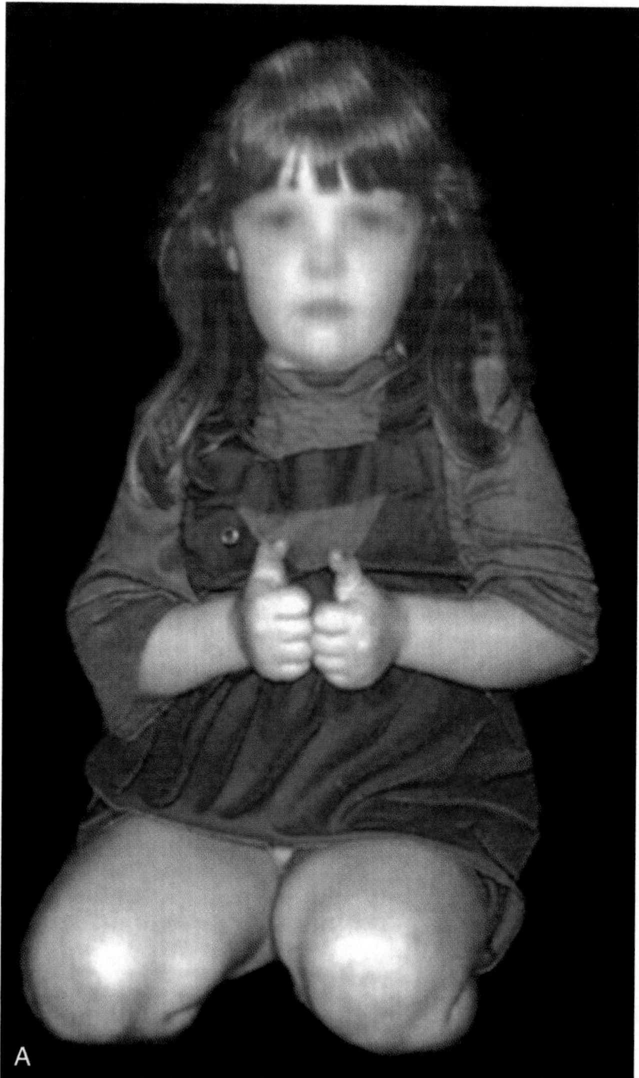

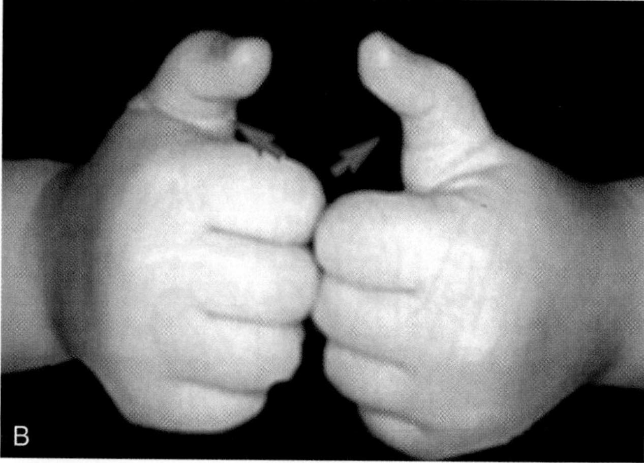

FIGURE 15–12 **A** and **B:** Trigger thumbs. Bilateral trigger thumbs locked in flexion. Operative release of the pulleys allowed free movement of the tendons and extension of the thumbs. (**A** and **B,** From Staheli, with permission.)

Finger Dislocations

Colleen Campbell

Clinical Presentation

Patients with finger dislocations present with pain in the affected finger.

Pathophysiology

Dislocations often occur as a result of injuries sustained during ball sports. Dislocations occur most frequently at the proximal interphalangeal (PIP) joint, followed by the metacarpophalangeal (MCP) joint and, rarely, the distal interphalangeal (DIP) joint.[1] Most dislocations are dorsal, but they can be lateral or volar. Dorsal dislocations are caused by longitudinal compression during a hyperextension injury.[1] Full dislocation occurs as a result of bilateral splitting of the collateral ligaments in combination with avulsion of the volar plate.[1] There are three different types of dislocations. Type I is a hyperextension injury that results in a partial slip of the collateral ligament, with avulsion of the volar plate of the middle phalanx. Type II is a full dislocation and volar-plate avulsion, and type III is a fracture-dislocation.

Diagnosis

Dislocation usually is suspected on the basis of physical examination findings. Radiographs of the finger, including anteroposterior, lateral, and oblique views, are necessary to confirm dislocation and to evaluate for associated fracture. Tenderness and obvious deformity of the affected joint are present on examination. The joint may appear hyperextended.

Clinical Complications

Joint stiffness is common after dislocations, which is why early movement of the joint through its range of motion is advocated. Chronic instability may follow if the injury is not properly treated.

Management

Reduction usually can be achieved with gentle traction distal to the dislocation. For MCP dislocations, distally directed pressure should be applied to the base of the proximal phalanx, with simultaneous gentle distraction of the proximal phalanx.[2] A digital block using lidocaine may be useful before reduction. Type I and II dislocations require dynamic splinting (buddy tape) for 3 weeks, with range-of-motion exercises afterward. Treatment of type III injuries depends on the stability of the joint in flexion. If the joint is stable, treatment with dynamic splinting for 6 weeks is often successful. Joints are more prone to instability if the fracture involves more than 40% of the articular surface.[1] In these cases, extension block splinting, joint arthroplasty, or rigid fixation with Kirschner wiring may be necessary.[1]

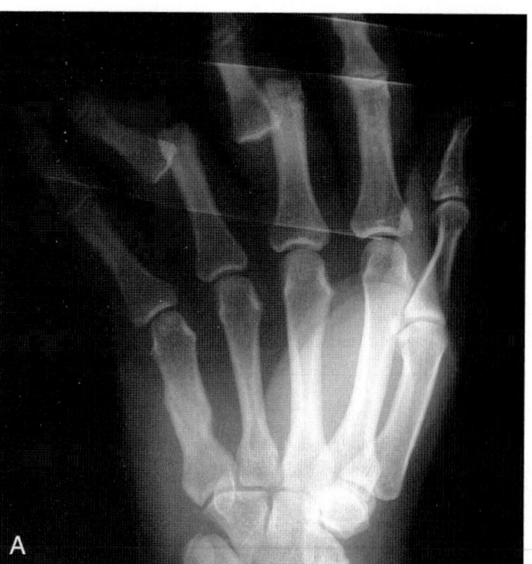

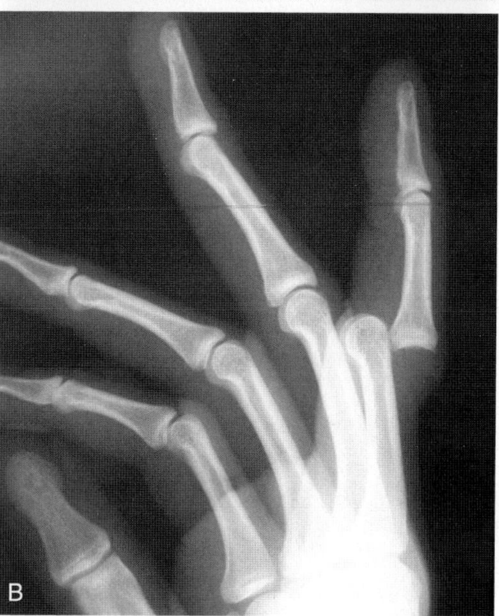

FIGURE 15–13 Digital dislocations. **A:** Proximal interphalangeal joint dislocation of the third and fourth digits. (Courtesy of Robert Hendrickson, MD.) **B:** Dorsal dislocation of the middle phalanx. (Courtesy of Colleen Roberts Campbell, MD.)

REFERENCES

1. Palmer RE. Joint injuries of the hand in athletes. *Clin Sports Med* 1998;17:513–531.
2. Young CC, Raasch WG. Dislocations: diagnosis and treatment. *Clin Fam Pract* 2000;2:613–635.

15-14

Lunate Dislocation

Catherine Pelletier

Clinical Presentation

Patients with lunate dislocations present with swelling of the dorsum of the wrist and pain associated with range of motion. Symptoms consistent with neuropathy in the distribution of the median nerve may also be present.

Pathophysiology

Lunate dislocations usually are associated with a mechanism of injury that produces forceful dorsiflexion of the wrist, such as those associated with falls onto an outstretched hand or motor vehicle crashes.[1]

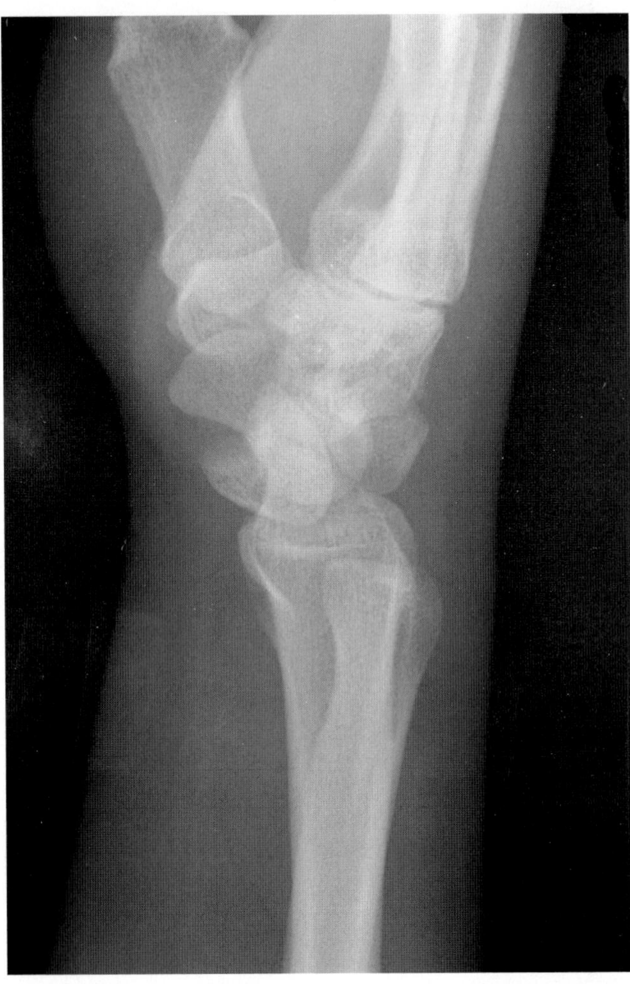

FIGURE 15–14 The "spilled teacup" (lunate dislocation) can be seen on this lateral wrist radiograph. (Courtesy of Mark Silverberg, MD.)

Diagnosis

The diagnosis of lunate dislocation is based on clinical examination in conjunction with posteroanterior (PA) and lateral wrist radiographs. On the PA view of the wrist, the volar dislocation of the lunate appears as a wedged-shaped "piece of pie," as opposed to its usual quadrangle appearance. As the lunate tips toward the palmar aspect of the wrist, the lateral wrist radiographic appearance is that of a "spilled teacup." The capitate slips behind the lunate and may even move proximally, toward the radius. Care must be taken when reviewing wrist radiographs, because up to 20% of all carpal pathologic conditions are erroneously interpreted as being normal.[1,2]

Clinical Complications

Complications include chronic pain and disability, scapholunate collapse secondary to avascular necrosis, and damage to the median nerve.

Management

Orthopedic consultation from the emergency department is the critical step in management of lunate dislocations, because patients require admission with urgent open reduction and internal fixation for definitive care of this injury.[1,3,4] Careful splinting is required while awaiting the arrival of the orthopedist.

REFERENCES

1. Yaghoubian R, Goebel F, Musgrave DS, Sotereanos DG. Diagnosis and management of acute fracture-dislocation of the carpus. *Orthop Clin North Am* 2001;32:295–305.
2. Perron AD, Brady WJ, Keats TE, Hersh RE. Orthopedic pitfalls in the ED: lunate and perilunate injuries. *Am J Emerg Med* 2001;19: 157–162.
3. Cooney WP, Bussey R, Dobyns JH, Linscheid RL. Difficult wrist fractures: perilunate fracture-dislocations of the wrist. *Clin Orthop* 1987;(214):136–147.
4. Ferenz CC. Acute perilunate dislocations. *Orthop Rev* 1986;15: 213–217.

Perilunate Dislocations

Catherine Pelletier

Clinical Presentation

Patients with perilunate dislocations present to the emergency department with wrist pain, swelling over the dorsum of the wrist, and limited range of motion secondary to pain. Physical deformity of the wrist may also be present.

Pathophysiology

Perilunate dislocations are a specific type of carpal instability representing 1.5% of all carpal fractures.[1] Perilunate dislocations are associated most commonly with a fall onto an outstretched hand, although it can be caused by any mechanism of injury that produces forceful dorsiflexion of the wrist. A high level of clinical suspicion must be maintained in the setting of these types of injuries, because up to 20% of radiographs of carpal pathologic conditions are initially misinterpreted as normal.[1]

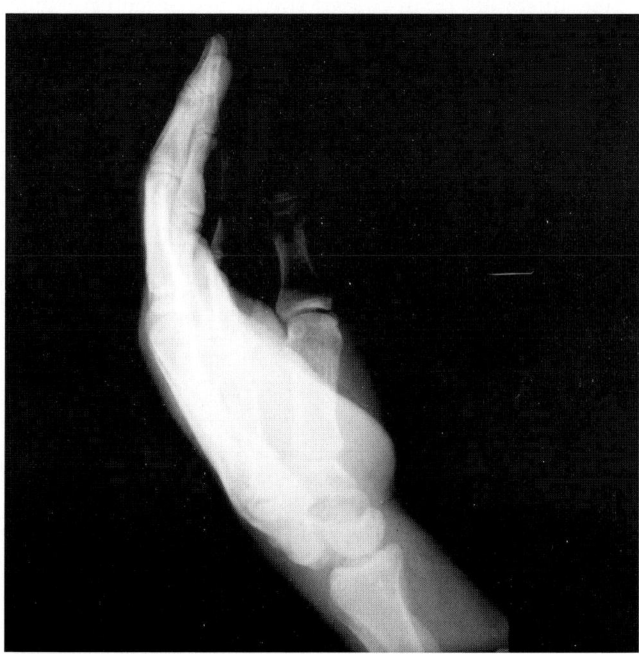

FIGURE 15–15 Perilunate dislocation is best diagnosed on the lateral radiographic view. (Courtesy Robert Hendrickson, MD.)

Diagnosis

Diagnosis is made via posteroanterior (PA) and lateral wrist radiographs. On a lateral wrist radiograph, the capitate no longer forms the fourth "C" in a linear row formed by the distal radius, the proximal aspect of the lunate, the distal aspect of the lunate, and the proximal aspect of the capitate. This obscures the separation between the proximal and distal rows of the carpal bones on the PA view. This injury is often associated with fracture or subluxation of the scaphoid. The median nerve is also commonly injured because of its proximity to the carpal bones.[1,2]

Clinical Complications

Complications include median-nerve injury, posttraumatic arthritis, avascular necrosis of the lunate and/or scaphoid, and chronic pain.

Management

Early radiographic recognition of these injuries is necessary. Closed reduction and long-arm splint application was once the standard of care and may still be attempted, although better outcomes result after open reduction and internal fixation, especially in high-risk, noncompliant populations.[2–5]

REFERENCES

1. Perron AD, Brady WJ, Keats TE, Hersh RE. Orthopedic pitfalls in the ED: lunate and perilunate injuries. *Am J Emerg Med* 2001;19:157–162.
2. Herzberg G, Comtet JJ, Linscheid RL, Amadio PC, Cooney WP, Stalder J. Perilunate dislocations and fracture-dislocations: a multicenter study. *J Hand Surg Am* 1993;18:768–779.
3. Cooney WP, Bussey R, Dobyns JH, Linscheid RL. Difficult wrist fractures: perilunate fracture-dislocations of the wrist. *Clin Orthop* 1987;(214):136–147.
4. Ferenz CC. Acute perilunate dislocations. *Orthop Rev* 1986;15:213–217.
5. Yaghoubian R, Goebel F, Musgrave DS, Sotereanos DG. Diagnosis and management of acute fracture-dislocation of the carpus. *Orthop Clin North Am* 2001;32:295–305.

Phalanx Fractures (Hand)

Colleen Campbell

Clinical Presentation

Patients with phalanx fractures present after trauma to the hand with pain and swelling of the fingers or thumb. Deformity may be present as well. Rotational deformity is usually evident on examination of flexed fingers in the palm. All fingers should be aligned and pointed toward the scaphoid tubercle.[1]

Pathophysiology

Phalanx fractures occur as a result of crush or shearing forces. The distal phalanx is injured most often.[2] Fractures are usually transverse, longitudinal, or comminuted.[3] Transverse fracture patterns are the most common, because most injuries are the result of a direct blow.[1] Proximal phalanx fractures often have a degree of volar angulation because of the action of the interosseous muscles. Sports-related injuries are the most common cause of phalanx fractures in teenagers and young adults.[1]

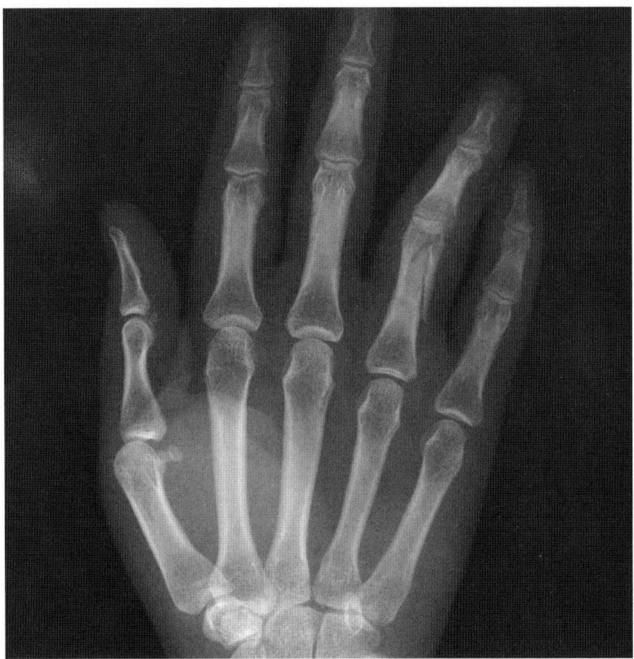

FIGURE 15–16 Minimally displaced fracture of the fourth proximal phalanx. (Courtesy of Mark Silverberg, MD.)

Diagnosis

Bony point tenderness is evident on examination. Diagnosis is confirmed by plain radiography, including anteroposterior, lateral, and oblique views of the finger. If multiple fingers are injured, a splayed view of the hand may be necessary. Brewerton views can be used to further visualize the base of the proximal phalanx.[1]

Clinical Complications

Malunion is the most common complication of phalanx fractures. Other complications include post-traumatic arthritis, decreased range of motion, and deformity of the finger.[2]

Management

Fractures of the distal phalanx may be treated with a hairpin splint that extends to the middle phalanx. K-wires or plates may be necessary to fix severely angulated, unstable, or displaced fragments.[1] Fractures with associated nail bed injuries are considered to be open. Treatment with antistaphylococcal antibiotics is controversial.[3] Stable, nondisplaced proximal and middle phalanx fractures are treated with "buddy" taping.[2] Other fractures may be treated after reduction with a radial gutter splint (index and long fingers) or an ulnar gutter splint (small and ring fingers) in a position of function. The wrist is placed in 30 degrees of extension, the metacarpophalangeal (MCP) joints in 90 degrees of flexion, and the interphalangeal (IP) joints in extension.[1] Orthopedic referral is indicated for all unstable, angulated, and intraarticular fractures.[3]

REFERENCES

1. Capo JT, Hastings H II. Metacarpal and phalangeal fractures in athletes. *Clin Sports Med* 1998;17:491–511.
2. Harrison BP, Hilliard MW. Emergency department evaluation and treatment of hand injuries. *Emerg Med Clin North Am* 1999;17:793–822.
3. Wang QC, Johnson BA. Fingertip injuries. *Am Fam Physician* 2001;63:1961–1966.

Metacarpal Fractures

Robert Hendrickson

Clinical Presentation

Patients with metacarpal (MC) fractures present as a result of blunt trauma sustained to the hand, with swelling, pain, and tenderness in the area of injury.

Pathophysiology

MC fractures can occur at various locations in the MC bones, including the base, shaft, neck, and head of the bone. Force may be transferred to the MC bones by a direct blow to the hand, either perpendicularly, longitudinally, or rotationally.

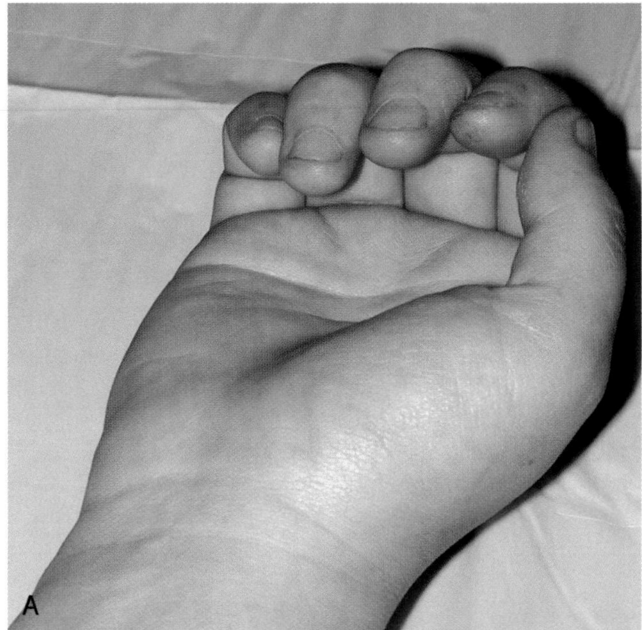

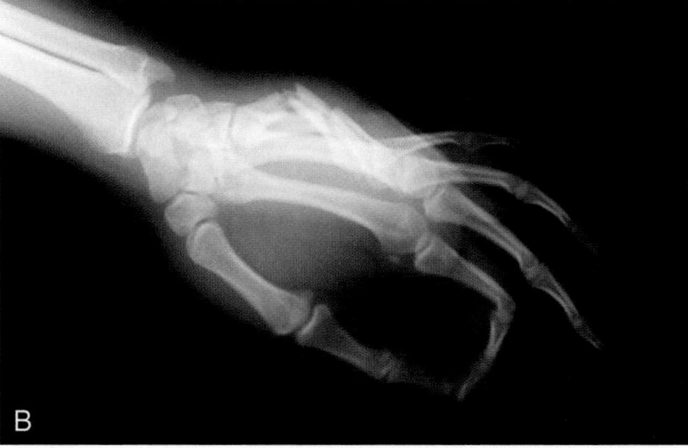

FIGURE 15-17 **A:** Moderately severe swelling associated with metacarpal fracture. (Courtesy of Robert Hendrickson, MD.) **B:** Multiple metacarpal fractures. (Courtesy of Christy Salvaggio, MD.)

Diagnosis

The diagnosis may be suspected by recognizing swelling, pain, and tenderness on examination and should be confirmed with radiography. The integrity of the neurovascular aspects of the affected areas should be evaluated and the hand should be examined for rotational deformities. Fractures usually are visible on radiography. A Bennett's fracture is an intraarticular fracture/dislocation of the thumb metacarpal. Rolando's fractures are Y-shaped, comminuted Bennett's fractures.

Clinical Complications

Complications include chronic pain, arthritis, open fracture, and significant occupational and functional disability.

Management

Open fractures of the MC bones require immediate sterile irrigation and débridement, often best done in the operating theater.[1] Treatment decisions regarding reduction, splinting, and consultation depend primarily on the location of the fracture.

Fractures of the head of the MC typically occur after a direct blow or crush injury. These fractures should be splinted with a gutter splint, and the patient should be referred to a hand surgeon, because the outcome for these injuries tends to be poor, regardless of treatment. Fractures of the metacarpal neck should be treated with closed reduction if there is angulation greater than 15, 15, 35, or 45 degrees in the second, third, fourth, or fifth metacarpophalangeal (MCP), respectively. The injury should be splinted in a gutter splint from the elbow up to, but not including, the proximal interphalangeal joint, and the patient should be referred to a hand surgeon. Fractures of the MC shaft require closed reduction if there is any angulation of the second or third MC, or if the angulation of the fourth or fifth MC is greater than 10 or 20 degrees. The gutter splint should extend up to, but should not include, the MCP joint, and the patient should be referred to a hand surgeon. Patients with fractures of the second through fifth MC bases require a volar splint and referral to a hand surgeon. Fractures of the first MC may require reduction if they are either intraarticular or extraarticular with greater than 20% to 30% angulation. After reduction, a thumb spica splint may be applied, and the patient is referred to a hand surgeon for open reduction and internal fixation.[1]

REFERENCES

1. Harrison BP, Hilliard MW. Emergency department evaluation and treatment of hand injuries. *Emerg Med Clin North Am* 1999;17: 793–822.

Scaphoid Fracture

Mark Silverberg

Clinical Presentation

Patients with scaphoid fractures present with moderate to severe wrist pain, usually after a fall on an outstretched hand. Swelling and ecchymosis may also be present, and wrist motion is commonly limited.

Pathophysiology

The scaphoid is the most commonly fractured carpal bone, accounting for 70% to 80% of all carpal fractures.[1] The most common mechanism of injury is a fall onto an outstretched hand.

Diagnosis

Physical examination reveals exquisite tenderness in the anatomic snuff box and pain when the thumb is axially loaded. In addition, pain with resisted supination or pronation is typical.[1] Normal wrist radiographs are usual. However, a scaphoid view showing the scaphoid on its long axis should also be obtained. In 85% of scaphoid fractures, the navicular fat stripe (a radiolucent line parallel to the radial surface of the scaphoid bone on the anteroposterior projection) is laterally displaced or completely obliterated.[1] Negative radiographic findings do not necessarily rule out a scaphoid fracture. If the patient appears to have a fracture clinically and the radiographs are negative, the patient should be placed in a short-arm thumb spica cast, and the radiographs should be repeated in 10 to 14 days. A bone scan or magnetic resonance imaging scan performed 72 hours after the injury may reveal scaphoid fractures that do not appear on plain films.[1]

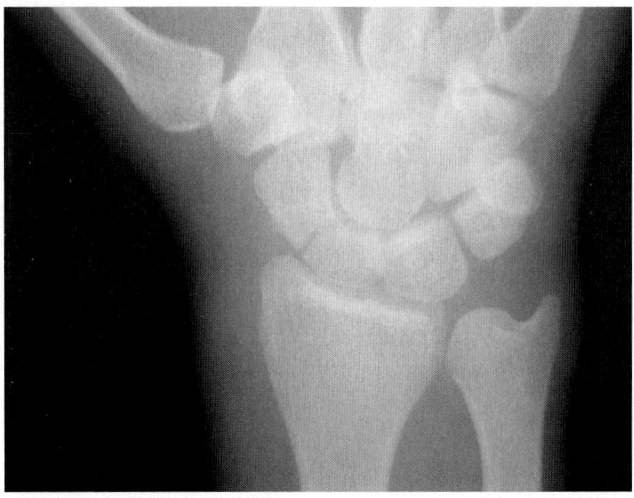

FIGURE 15–18 Nondisplaced, transverse fracture of the scaphoid. (Courtesy of Colleen Campbell, MD.)

Clinical Complications

Because of the distal-to-proximal blood supply of the scaphoid bone, fractures through the wrist and proximal region are prone to ischemia. This increases the risk for prolonged healing and nonunion, as well as avascular necrosis resulting in chronic wrist pain.[1]

Management

Nondisplaced fractures of the distal third or scaphoid tubercle usually heal well and may be splinted, with the patient sent for follow-up with an orthopedic surgeon. These fractures usually are placed in a short-arm thumb spica cast for 10 to 12 weeks. Some orthopedists obtain follow-up radiographs every 2 to 3 weeks until radiographic healing is demonstrated.[1] Rapid orthopedic consultation should be obtained for proximal fractures, comminuted fractures, and fractures displaced more than 2 mm, because of the high risk of complications. These patients usually require a long-arm thumb spica and should be monitored closely by an orthopedist.[1]

REFERENCES

1. Paras RD. Upper extremity fractures. *Clin Fam Pract* 2000;2: 637–659.

Scapholunate Dislocation

Tyler Vadeboncoeur

Clinical Presentation

Patients with scapholunate dislocations present with wrist pain and swelling as a result of a dorsiflexion injury to the wrist. A clicking sensation may be present with wrist movement.[1,2]

Pathophysiology

Scapholunate dislocations are the most common ligamentous injury of the wrist; they occur when the scapholunate interosseous ligament and the long radiolunate ligaments tear. This causes the scaphoid to be displaced to a more vertical position relative to the lunate.[1,2]

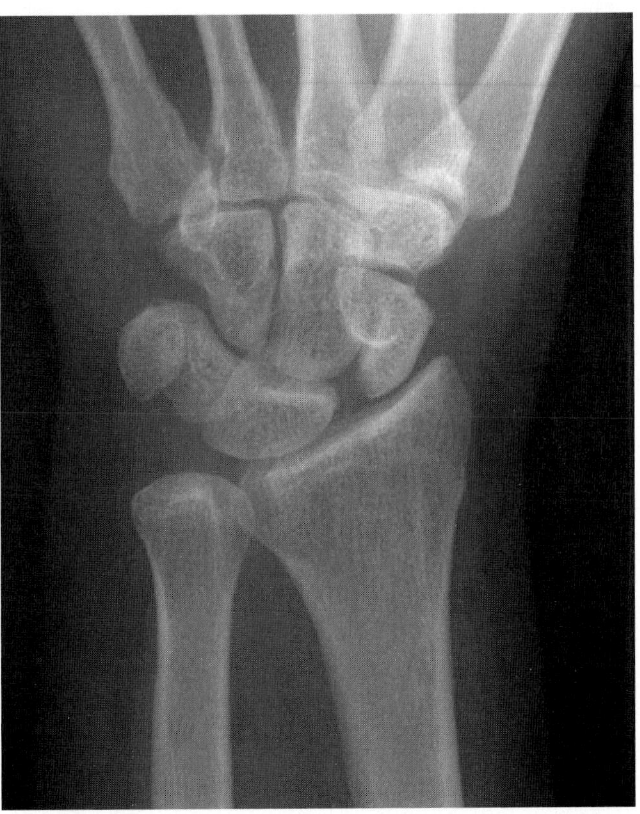

FIGURE 15–19 Scapholunate dislocation. (Courtesy of Mark Silverberg, MD.)

Diagnosis

The diagnosis is made radiographically. The "signet ring" sign results with volar rotation of the scaphoid. The radiographic criteria for dissociation include a scapholunate angle greater than 60 degrees; a scapholunate space wider than 2 mm (the Terry Thomas sign); and the scaphoid ring sign, either singly or in any combination. In the case of suspected dissociation with normal-appearing routine radiographs, additional stress views should be taken with a clenched fist in ulnar deviation, which accentuates the widening of the scapholunate joint.[2] Acute scapholunate dislocations may be asymptomatic or mildly symptomatic.

Clinical Complications

Complications include chronic instability, degenerative arthritis, poor wrist function, and chronic pain.[1,2] Approximately 50% of scapholunate dislocations are associated with distal radius fractures.[2]

Management

Acute scapholunate dislocations require hand surgery consultation in the emergency department. The injury should be splinted in a radial gutter splint or posterior mold. Subacute or chronic injuries may be casted or splinted, and they also require hand surgery referral.[1] These injuries may require radiographically guided reduction and pinning and usually require open reduction with internal fixation for ligamentous repair.[1]

REFERENCES

1. Lee JS, Gaala A, Shaw R, Harris JH Jr. Signs of acute carpal instability associated with distal radius fracture. *Emerg Radiol* 1995;2: 77–83.
2. Mayfield JK, Johnson RP, Kilcoyne RK. Carpal dislocations: pathomechanics and progressive perilunar instability. *J Hand Surg Am* 1980;5:226–241.

Swan Neck Deformity

Colleen Campbell

Clinical Presentation

Patients with swan neck deformity (SND) present with only the flexion deformity of the distal interphalangeal (DIP) joint after injury. On examination, the acutely injured patient has pain at the DIP joint with swelling, tenderness, and inability to actively extend the DIP of the affected digit. Over time, patients develop hyperextension at the proximal interphalangeal (PIP) joint. SND usually is not painful.

Pathophysiology

SND occurs as a progression of mallet finger, when there is a flexion deformity of the DIP combined with a hyperextension of the PIP. Mallet finger occurs when there is forced flexion of the extended DIP.[1] Mallet finger, the most common finger injury in athletes, is caused by blunt trauma. SND occurs when a mallet finger goes untreated; the flexion deformity of the DIP causes chronic strain and eventually failure of the lateral bands. The PIP is hyperextended when the lateral bands are displaced dorsally and proximally.[1]

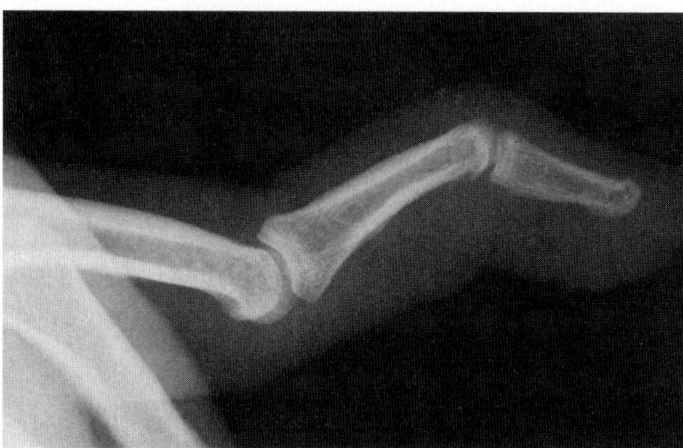

FIGURE 15–20 Untreated terminal tendon injury with persistent distal interphalangeal (DIP) joint flexion may combine with compensatory hyperextension of the proximal interphalangeal (PIP) joint, leading to a "swan neck" pattern of extensor mechanism imbalance. (From Bucholz, with permission.)

Diagnosis

Diagnosis of SND is made on the basis of physical examination. Anteroposterior, lateral, and oblique radiographs of the finger are necessary to reveal an associated fracture.

Clinical Complications

Complications of SND include post-traumatic arthritis and chronic deformity or chronic subluxation and associated chronic disability.

Management

Treatment of mallet fingers initially involves splinting the DIP in extension for 6 to 8 weeks.[1] For SND, prompt orthopedic referral is warranted, given the chronic nature of the condition.

REFERENCES

1. Wang QC, Johnson BA. Fingertip injuries. *Am Fam Physician* 2001;63:1961–1966.
2. Palmer RE. Joint injuries of the hand in athletes. *Clin Sports Med* 1998;17:513–531.

Mallet Finger

Michael Greenberg

Clinical Presentation

Mallet finger injuries usually are not excessively painful, and therefore presentation may be delayed. Patients may have ecchymosis over the dorsum of the distal interphalangeal (DIP) joint. There may not be any tenderness, swelling, or discoloration. However, all patients demonstrate an extensor lag at the DIP joint.[1]

Pathophysiology

Mallet finger, also known as "baseball finger" or "drop finger," is a flexion deformity that is caused by the detachment of the extensor tendon from the base of the distal phalanx.[2] Mallet injuries are classified into four types. Type I is closed, with or without associated avulsion fracture. Type II involves a laceration proximal to the DIP joint with loss of tendon continuity. Type III mallet fingers are deep abrasion injuries with the loss of skin, subcutaneous cover, and tendon substance. Type IV mallet fingers can involve either pediatric transepiphyseal plate fractures or fractures of the articular surface.[3] The mechanism of injury usually involves direct trauma that forces an extended finger into flexion. The direct blow could also occur to the dorsum of the finger.[1]

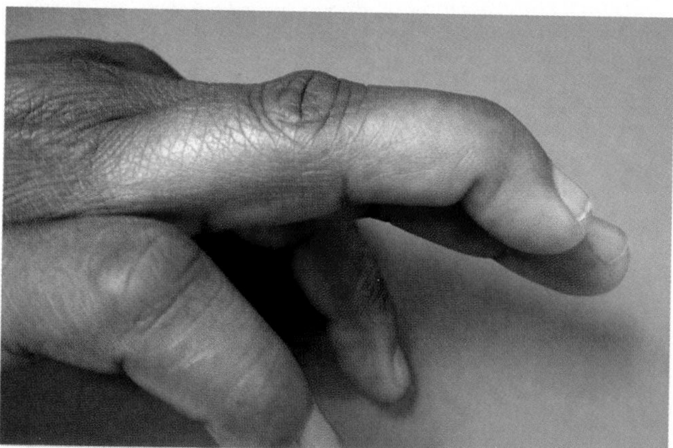

FIGURE 15–21 Mallet finger, or "baseball finger." (Courtesy of Mark Silverberg, MD.)

The extensor tendon is ruptured, and there is often an associated bony avulsion.[1,3]

Diagnosis

On clinical evaluation, patients exhibit an extensor lag at the DIP joint. This lag may not develop for several days after injury, so patients may present to the emergency department late in the course of events. The magnitude of the lag can vary according to the severity of the mallet injury. Diagnosis is confirmed by plain radiography.[1]

Clinical Complications

Patients may believe that mallet injuries are simple problems that have minor complications. If the injury is left untreated, however, a "swan neck" deformity may develop in the digit due to hyperextensive compensation at the proximal interphalangeal (PIP) joint. Untreated mallet injuries can become chronically painful.[2]

Management

Surgical treatment reportedly has a higher morbidity than conservative, nonsurgical treatment.[2] Splinting alone may be satisfactory in most cases. Type I injuries can be treated with continuous DIP joint splinting for up to 8 weeks. Type II injuries may be corrected with suturing, followed by splinting. Type III mallet fingers require immediate soft-tissue coverage and grafting reconstruction. Type IV injuries that involve transepiphyseal plate fractures may be treated with closed reduction.[3] Patients must understand that if they remove the splinting before clinical follow-up, they cannot let the DIP joint fall into flexion.[1]

REFERENCES

1. Perron A, Brady W, Keats T, Hersh R. Orthopedic pitfalls in the emergency department: closed tendon injuries of the hand. *Am J Emerg Med* 2001;19:76–80.
2. Okafor B, Mbubaegbu C, Munshi I, Williams D. Mallet deformity of the finger: five-year follow-up of conservative treatment. *J Bone Joint Surg Br* 1997;79:544–547.
3. Rockwell W, Butler P, Byrne B. Extensor tendon: anatomy, injury, and reconstruction. *Plastic Reconstruct Surg* 2000;106:1592–1603.

Gamekeeper's Thumb

Grant Wei

Clinical Presentation

Patients with so-called gamekeeper's thumb present with either acute or chronic injury, with pain and swelling over the metacarpophalangeal (MCP) joint and pain and weakness of pinch-grasp.[1,2]

Pathophysiology

Gamekeeper's thumb, also known as "skier's thumb," is an injury of the ulnar collateral ligament of the thumb. Originally described as a chronic injury in Scottish gamekeepers, it is now commonly seen as an acute-phase injury after sudden forced extension and abduction of the thumb against an object (e.g., ski pole) or as a football injury; this results in a partial or complete disruption of the ulnar collateral ligament of the thumb.[1-3] Chronic injuries occur from repetitive thumb and hand movements, which result in gradually increasing laxity of the ulnar collateral ligament over time.[1,2]

Diagnosis

The diagnosis is suspected based on the clinical history and physical examination. Radiographs should be obtained to rule out underlying avulsion or condylar fractures.[1,2] Once fracture has been ruled out, the thumb should be flexed at 30 degrees and stressed radially (abduction) to test for laxity and the lack of a defined end point. A complete tear should be considered if radial stress results in greater than 35 degrees of angulation, compared with the uninvolved side, with no defined end point.[1-3]

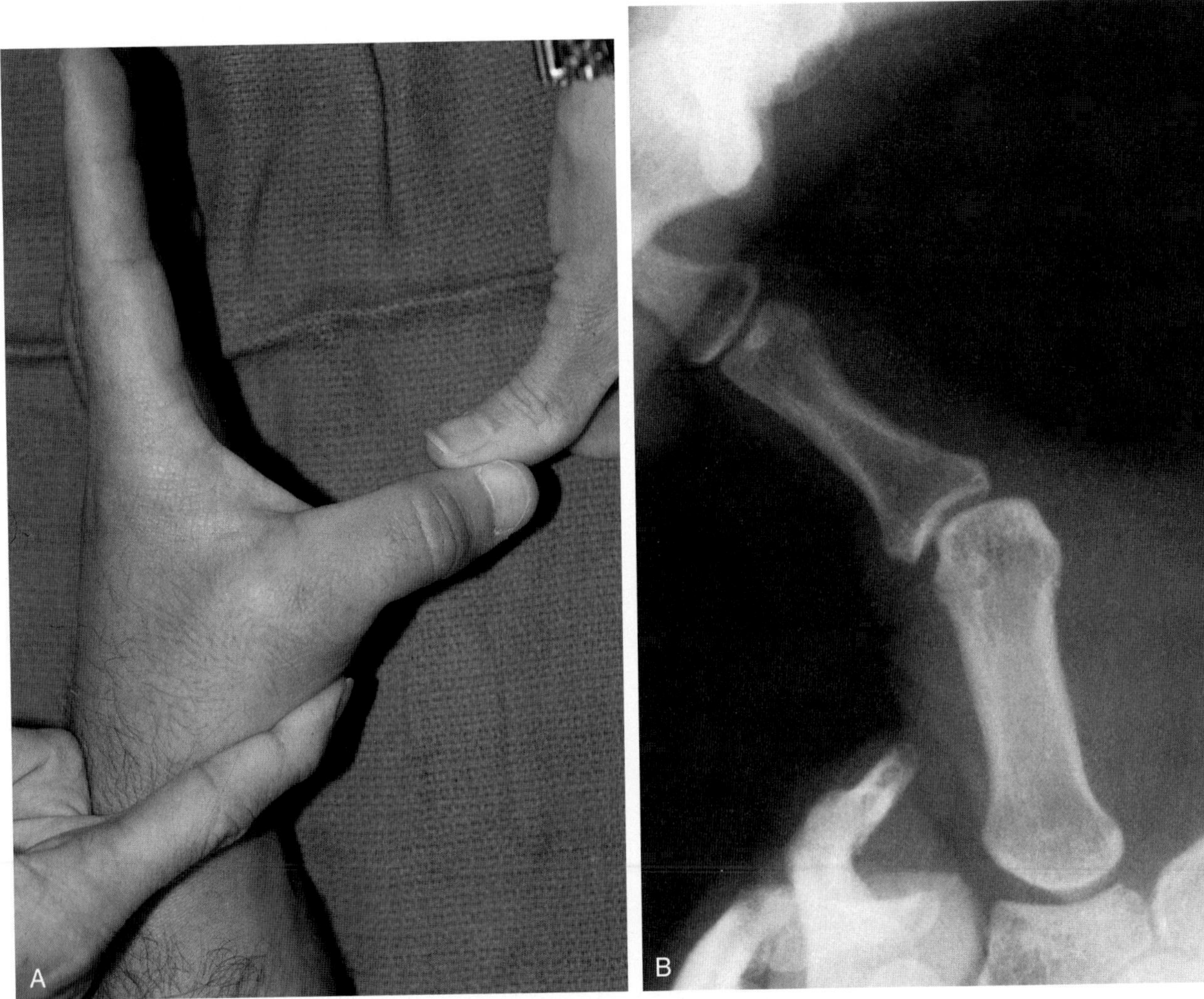

FIGURE 15–22 **A:** A clinical stress examination is best performed under local anesthesia and with the thumb in 30 degrees of flexion, to avoid a false-negative test due to an intact volar plate when the test is performed with the thumb in full extension. Comparison with the opposite side (15 degrees) is more valid than the absolute amount of angulation. **B:** Uncertainty in the clinical deviation test can be clarified by stress radiography, following the same rules as for the stress examination. (**A** and **B,** From Bucholz, with permission.)

Gamekeeper's Thumb

Grant Wei

Clinical Complications

With acute partial tears, healing is often complete. However, the so-called Stener lesion, which results from entrapment of a completely torn ulnar collateral ligament outside the adductor aponeurosis, may result in chronic pain and decreased range and strength of motion.[1,2]

Management

For partial tears, a thumb spica splint should be applied for 2 to 6 weeks, after which flexion exercise is prescribed.[1-3] Complete tears also should be placed in a thumb spica, although an early orthopedic referral is needed for possible surgical exploration and repair.[1-3] The presence of an avulsion fracture larger than 5 mm, or a fracture involving the articular surface, also warrants early orthopedic follow-up for potential surgical treatment.[1]

REFERENCES

1. Richard JR. Gamekeeper's thumb: ulnar collateral ligament injury. *Am Fam Physician* 1996;53:1775–1781.
2. Harrison BP, Hilliard MW. Emergency department evaluation and treatment of hand injuries. *Emerg Med Clin North Am* 1999;17: 793–822.
3. Lee SJ, Montgomery K. Athletic hand injuries. *Orthop Clin North Am* 2002;33:547–554.

Bennett's and Rolando's Fractures

Colleen Campbell

Clinical Presentation

Patients present with pain at the base of the thumb after a direct axial compression injury, usually as a result of sports. Swelling and dorsal deformity of the metacarpal may be evident. Bony point tenderness at the base of the first metacarpal (MC) is present.

Pathophysiology

A Bennett's fracture is an oblique, intraarticular fracture involving the volar edge of the first metacarpal base. A Rolando's fracture is similar, except that the intraarticular component is "Y"- or "T"-shaped.[1,2]

In Bennett's fracture, the abductor pollicis longus (APL) and the abductor pollicis brevis (APB) pull the shaft of the MC dorsal and radial, while the volar fracture fragment remains aligned.[1] This is caused by an axial force to a partially flexed thumb.[2]

Diagnosis

Diagnosis of Bennett's or Rolando's fractures usually is based on plain films of the finger, including anteroposterior and lateral views. The shaft of the MC appears dorsally dislocated, with the volar lip held in place. A posteroanterior stress view with the thumbs pressed

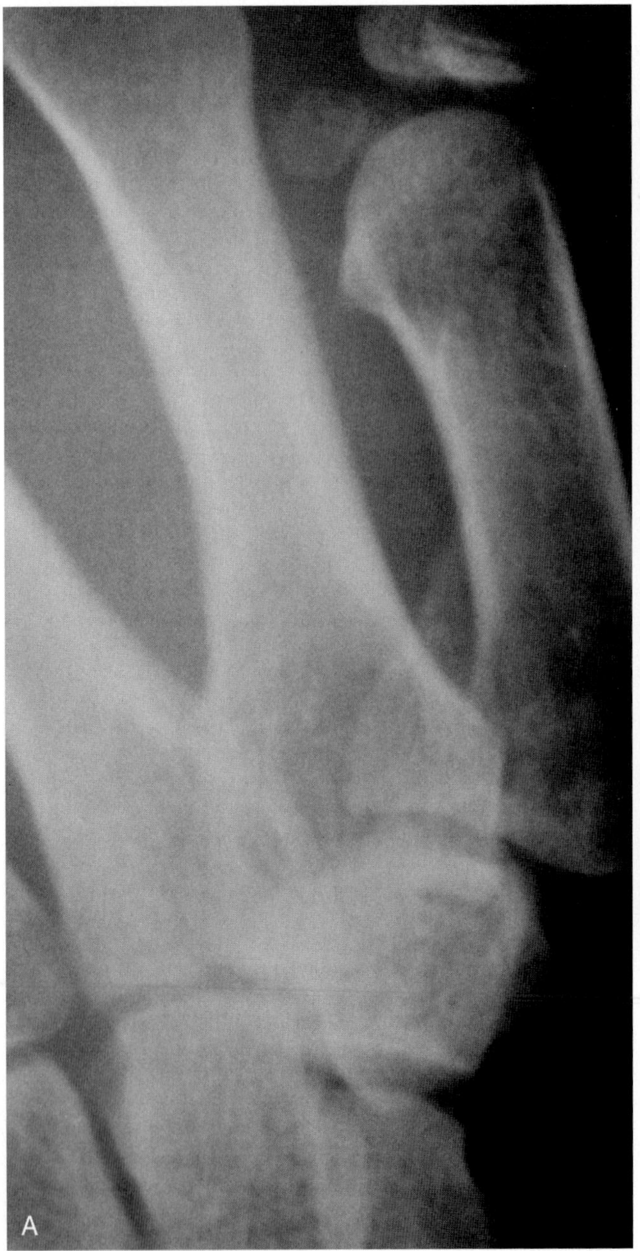

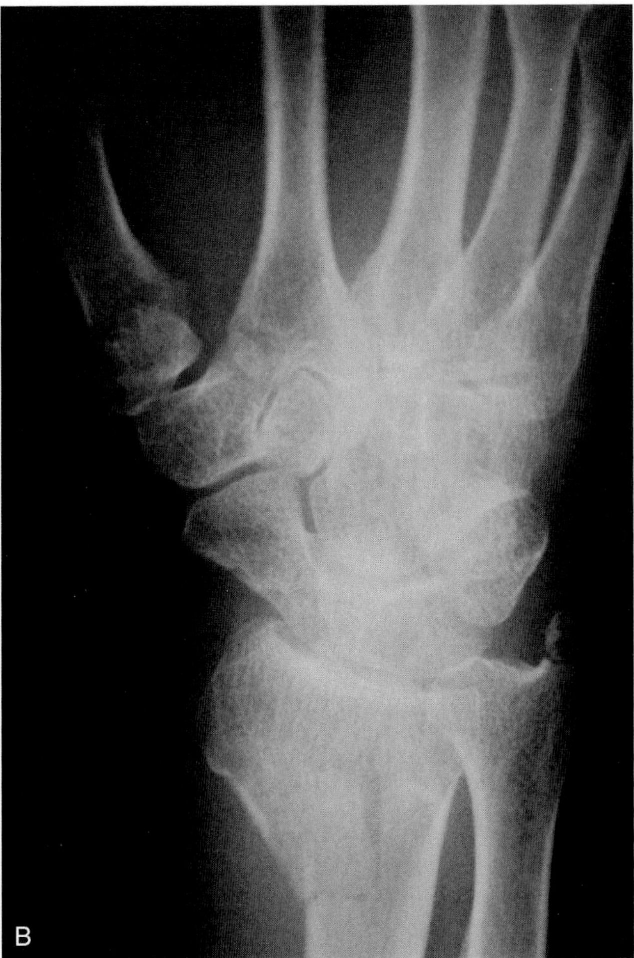

FIGURE 15–23 **A:** Bennett's fracture-dislocation of the base of the thumb metacarpal is seen here with a large articular fragment. **B:** Rolando's fracture at the base of the thumb metacarpal presents an unstable configuration that frequently does not lend itself well to rigid internal fixation and may be too distal to achieve satisfactory fixation with Kirschner wires. (**A** and **B,** From Bucholz, with permission.)

Bennett's and Rolando's Fractures

Colleen Campbell

against each other at their radial borders reveals partial dislocations.[2] Computed tomography may be necessary to fully visualize the articular surface.[1]

Clinical Complications

Complications include malunion, nonunion, chronic dislocation, arthritis, and chronic pain.

Management

Bennett's fracture usually is treated by closed reduction, with Kirschner wiring used to fix the joint in abduction and extension.[2] A cortical screw is used if the volar fragment is large (greater than 20% of the joint space).[2] This is followed by immobilization in a thumb spica cast for 6 weeks.[1] Treatment of Rolando's fracture usually requires open reduction with multiple Kirschner wires through the trapezium and MC. Skeletal traction or external fixation occasionally is necessary for severely comminuted fractures.[1] If the capsule is torn, it is reconstructed with the radial portion of the flexor carpi radialis tendon.[2]

REFERENCES

1. Palmer RE. Joint injuries of the hand in athletes. *Clin Sports Med* 1998;17:513–531.
2. Langford SA, Whitaker JH, Toby EB. Thumb injuries in the athlete. *Clin Sports Med* 1998;17:553–566.

Triquetral Fracture

Tyler Vadeboncoeur

Clinical Presentation

Triquetral fractures are the third most common carpal bone fracture, after scaphoid and lunate fractures.[1,2] Patients present with wrist pain after a direct blow to the wrist or a fall on an outstretched hand.

Pathophysiology

Dorsal cortical triquetral fractures occur by one of two mechanisms. A fall on the wrist in dorsiflexion and ulnar deviation can lead to impingement of the hamate or ulnar styloid on the dorsal triquetrum, or palmar flexion injury can cause the dorsal radiotriquetral and scaphotriquetral ligaments to produce a ligamentous avulsion of the dorsal cortex.[3] Fractures of the triquetral body occur less frequently and are caused by a direct blow to the hand.[2,3]

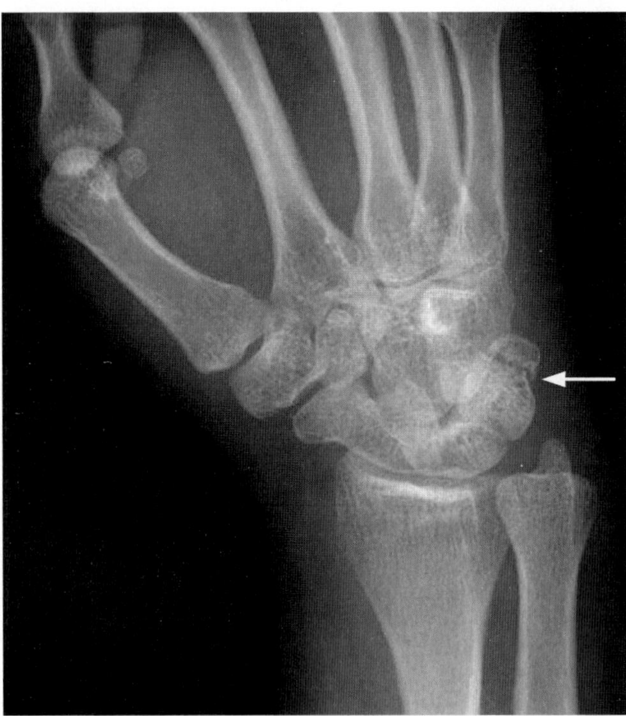

FIGURE 15-24 Triquetral fracture. (Courtesy of Elzbieta Pilat, MD.)

Diagnosis

The diagnosis of a triquetral fracture depends on a high index of suspicion. A complete wrist series should be obtained. Dorsal chip fractures of the triquetrum often are seen on standard lateral radiographs of the wrist, but they are best seen on a pronated lateral view that projects the dorsal triquetrum away from adjacent carpal bones.[3] Triquetral body fractures are best visualized on anteroposterior and oblique radiographs. There is localized tenderness over the dorsum of the wrist, just distal to the ulnar styloid.[3]

Clinical Complications

The deep branch of the ulnar nerve lies in close proximity to the triquetrum and may be compromised in triquetral fractures, with resultant motor impairment. Nonunions of triquetral body fractures occur, but avascular necrosis has not been reported.[1-3]

Management

Dorsal chip and triquetral body fractures require immobilization of the wrist with a short-arm splint or cast for 4 to 6 weeks.[2] Orthopedic follow-up is recommended. Displaced fractures may require internal fixation.[3]

REFERENCES

1. Bryan RS, Dobyns JH. Fractures of the carpal bones other than lunate and navicular. *Clin Orthop* 1980;149:107–111.
2. Hocker K, Menschik A. Chip fractures of the triquetrum: mechanism, classification, and results. *J Hand Surg Br* 1994;19: 584–588.
3. Cohen MS. Fractures of the carpal bones. *Hand Clin* 1997;13: 587–599.

Carpal Tunnel Syndrome

Colleen Campbell

Clinical Presentation

Patients with carpal tunnel syndrome (CTS) present with wrist pain and a feeling that the hand is "falling asleep." Symptoms may be worse at night and on awakening. Pain may radiate from the wrist to the proximal arm and forearm.[1]

Pathophysiology

CTS is an entrapment neuropathy of the medial nerve that causes pain, numbness, and weakness in the wrist and hand. The median nerve becomes entrapped by the overlying flexor retinaculum in the wrist. Repetitive motion, diabetes, connective tissue disorders, trauma, and pregnancy are associated with CTS. The digital sensory branch of the median nerve supplies sensation to the first three digits on the palmar aspect, and the thenar eminence is supplied by the palmar cutaneous sensory branch.[2] The motor branch of the median nerve supplies the first and second lumbricals and gives off a recurrent thenar motor branch, which supplies the thenar muscles. The median nerve sensory branch supplies the lateral half of the ring finger as well.

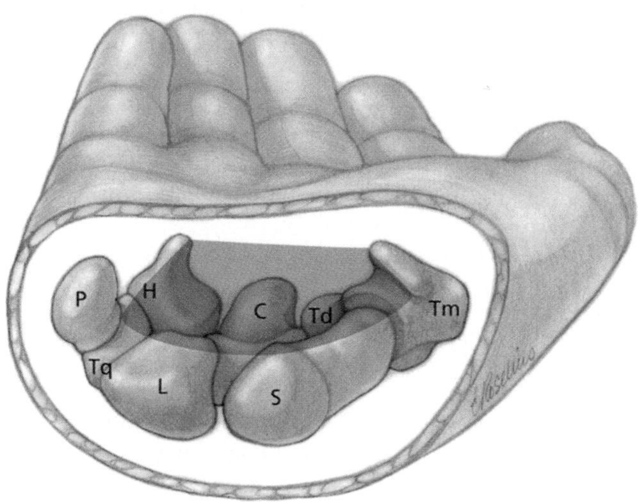

FIGURE 15–25 The carpal tunnel is a fibro-osseous canal. Associated bones that contribute to its boundaries include the hook process of the hamate (H), capitate (C), trapezoid (Td), pisiform (P), triquetrum (Tq), lunate (L), scaphoid (S), and trapezium (Tm). The roof is formed by the flexor retinaculum. (From Berger, *Atlas,* with permission.)

Diagnosis

Diagnosis of CTS is based on history and physical examination findings. Classic findings in CTS include Tinel's sign—increased pain and paresthesias when the flexor retinaculum is percussed over the median nerve at the wrist—and Phalen's sign—exacerbation of symptoms when the patient actively flexes the wrists against each other for 30 to 240 seconds. Phalen's sign is more sensitive and specific for CTS, but neither is highly sensitive nor specific.[1,2] The diagnosis may be confirmed with evidence of prolonged sensory and motor latencies of the median nerve on electromyography (EMG). Up to 20% of patients have a "normal" EMG result unless internal comparison myography is performed on the ulnar or radial nerve.[2] Extremes of wrist flexion or extension may exacerbate the pain. The thenar eminence may be visibly atrophied, with weakness noted in thumb abduction and opposition.[2]

Clinical Complications

Complications include chronic weakness of the thenar muscles and associated disability.

Management

Treatment involves limiting repetitive activities. Wrist splints that hold the wrists in neutral position and a short course of nonsteroidal antiinflammatory drugs (NSAIDs) may be helpful. Depo-Medrol injections adjacent to the carpal tunnel may be used only once or twice to alleviate symptoms. Surgical decompression of the carpal tunnel is successful in 90% of refractory cases.[2]

REFERENCES

1. Campbell WW. Diagnosis and management of common compression and entrapment neuropathies. *Neurol Clin* 1997;15:549–567.
2. Preston DC. Distal median neuropathies. *Neurol Clin* 1999;17: 407–424.

DeQuervain's Tenosynovitis

Colleen Campbell

Clinical Presentation

Patients with DeQuervain's tenosynovitis present with pain in the base of the thumb that is exacerbated by repetitive motion. There is pain on palpation of the first dorsal compartment of the hand. In some cases, crepitus or triggering may be evident with thumb movement. If symptoms are chronic, the tendons may be noticeably thickened, and there may be a ganglion cyst.[1]

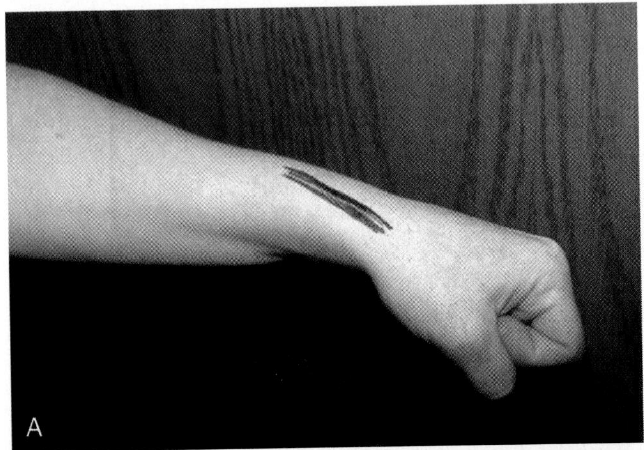

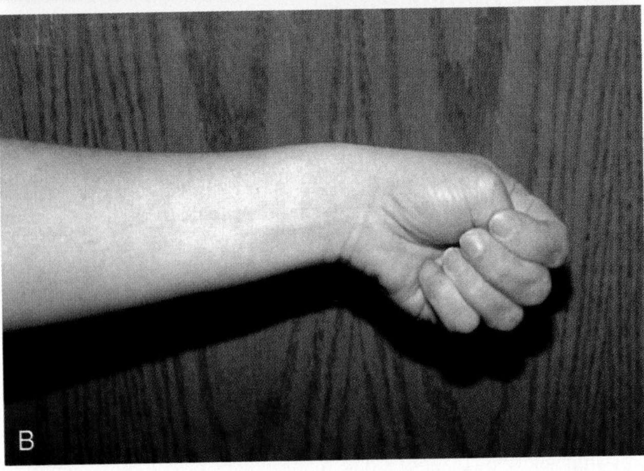

FIGURE 15–26 **A:** DeQuervain's tenosynovitis produces pain in the radial aspect of the wrist due to inflammation of the abductor pollicis longus and extensor pollicis brevis tendons. Pain may radiate up the forearm or into the thumb, but it is maximal at the radial styloid *(area marked)*. **B:** Finkelstein's test involves grasping the thumb in the palm and applying ulnar deviation of the wrist. If the pain is reproduced, this test is sensitive for, but not specific for, deQuervain's disease. (**A** and **B,** From Roberts, with permission.)

Pathophysiology

DeQuervain's disease is a stenosing tenosynovitis that involves the abductor pollicis longus (APL) and the extensor pollicis brevis (EPB) of the thumb. DeQuervain's is the most common tendonitis of the wrist in athletes.[1] Repetitive activities that involve forceful grasping with ulnar deviation cause this type of tendonitis. Initially, the condition was described in middle-aged washer women.[2] People involved in activities such as golf, fly fishing, and racquet sports (squash, racquetball) may be susceptible.[2] It is unclear which is inflamed first, the tendon and synovium or the overlying sheath.[1]

Diagnosis

The diagnosis is made on the basis of the history and physical examination. There are two tests that help identify this disease process. In Finkelstein's test, which is considered pathognomonic, maximal pain is elicited when the thumb is held flexed in the fist while the wrist is pulled into ulnar deviation by the examiner.[1] In the alternative test, the wrist is held in radial deviation while the examiner actively resists thumb extension.

Clinical Complications

Complications from DeQuervain's tenosynovitis include weakened grip strength and disability from pain.

Management

Initial treatment of DeQuervain's tenosynovitis involves application of ice, rest, and use of nonsteroidal antiinflammatory drugs (NSAIDs). A thumb spica splint is indicated for persistent symptoms. One or two injections of corticosteroids (0.5 mL of dexamethasone and 0.5 mL of lidocaine 2%) in the first dorsal compartment, administered 6 weeks apart, usually provide relief of symptoms. Rehabilitation measures include stretching and strengthening of the APL and EPB tendons. Surgical release of the sheath is reserved for those rare cases in which conservative measures fail.[1]

REFERENCES

1. Rettig AC. Wrist and hand overuse syndromes. *Clin Sports Med* 2001;20:591–611.
2. Fulcher SM, Kiefhaber TR, Stern PJ. Upper-extremity tendinitis and overuse syndromes in the athlete. *Clin Sports Med* 1998;17:433–448.

Colles' and Smith's Fractures

Mark Silverberg

Clinical Presentation

Most patients with Colles' or Smith's fracture patterns present after low-energy mechanisms such as a fall onto an outstretched hand. Patients complain of pain in the distal forearm and may or may not have an obvious deformity. If a Colles' fracture is grossly displaced, some refer to it as a "dinner fork" deformity, because its bent appearance resembles the shape of a fork.[1]

Pathophysiology

Colles' fracture is an extraarticular fracture of the distal forearm with dorsal displacement of the distal fragment, whereas Smith's fracture is an intraarticular or extraarticular fracture of the same region with palmar displacement of the distal wrist.[1,2] The mechanism of injury is similar in both types; both are usually caused by a fall onto an outstretched hand. Many patients presenting with these injuries are elderly women with some degree of osteoporosis. Osteoporosis is thought to contribute substantially to the fragility of the distal radius, making the elderly female population more likely to sustain these sorts of fractures.[1]

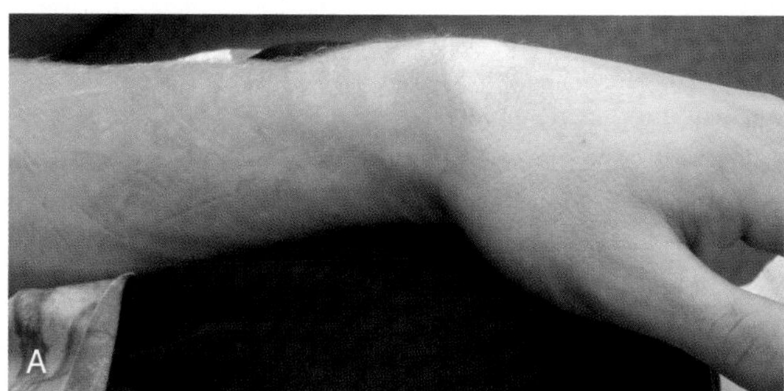

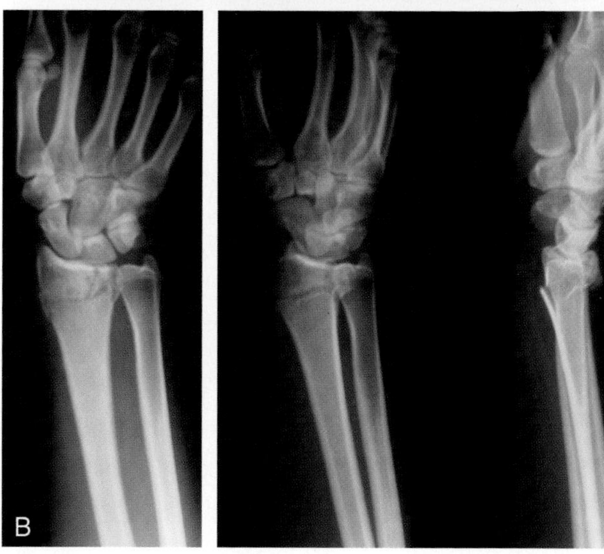

FIGURE 15–27 **A:** Minimal "dinner fork" deformity of Colles' fracture. **B:** Colles' fracture. (Courtesy of Seth Mehr, MD.)

Diagnosis

The diagnosis should be suspected clinically if the wrist is displaced or very tender. However, anteroposterior, lateral, and oblique radiographs of the region should be obtained to confirm clinical suspicions.[1,2] Physical examination elicits tenderness in the region.

Clinical Complications

Soft tissue injuries of the cartilages, ligaments, and joint capsule may not be seen on radiographs but can make realignment difficult.[2] Injuries to tendons or nerves (most commonly the median nerve) may be present and may necessitate open reduction with internal fixation and simultaneous carpal tunnel release.[1] Vascular compromise rarely occurs, but nonunion, malunion, and post-traumatic arthritis are common complications.[1,2]

Management

In the event of an open fracture, immediate surgical treatment is necessary.[2] If doubt exists regarding the complexity of the fracture and the treating physician is unsure whether surgical treatment is necessary, a computed tomographic scan may be helpful.[1] Treatment modalities include closed reduction with plaster immobilization and open reduction with internal fixation.[1,2] After closed reduction, radiographs should be repeated to ensure acceptable fragment alignment.[1,2] Neurologic status should be checked carefully before and after reduction, because median nerve injuries are common with these fractures.[1,2]

REFERENCES

1. Hanel DP, Jones MD, Trumble TE. Wrist fractures. *Orthop Clin North Am* 2002;33:35–57.
2. Hanker GJ. Radius fractures in the athlete. *Clin Sports Med* 2001;20: 189–201.

15-28

Monteggia Fracture-Dislocation

Anthony S. Mazzeo

Clinical Presentation

Patients with Monteggia fracture-dislocations (MFDs) present with forearm pain after a fall or direct trauma.

Pathophysiology

The MFD injury involves a proximal ulnar fracture associated with dislocation of the radial head. Because of the close proximity of the radius and ulna, forces that cause fracture of one bone may result in dislocation of the proximate neighboring bone.[1,2] In MFD, the annular ligament and the interosseus membrane are often injured as well. In cases of falls, the mechanism is most often a fall onto an outstretched hand with the hand pronated or the elbow flexed. Trauma to the proximal forearm, such as from a "nightstick injury" (in which the recipient attempts to block a downward-moving blow from a hard, stick-like object), may also result in MFD.[1,2]

Diagnosis

Radiographic imaging reveals the proximal ulnar fracture and should then prompt an assessment of the radial head. A true lateral radiograph of the elbow may demonstrate the radial head dislocation. A line drawn through the center of the radial head should pass through the center of the humeral capitellum.[1] Comparison views may be necessary in some cases. In addition to diagnosing MFD, the physician must perform a complete neurovascular examination to rule out associated limb-threatening injury and to document nerve function.[1,2]

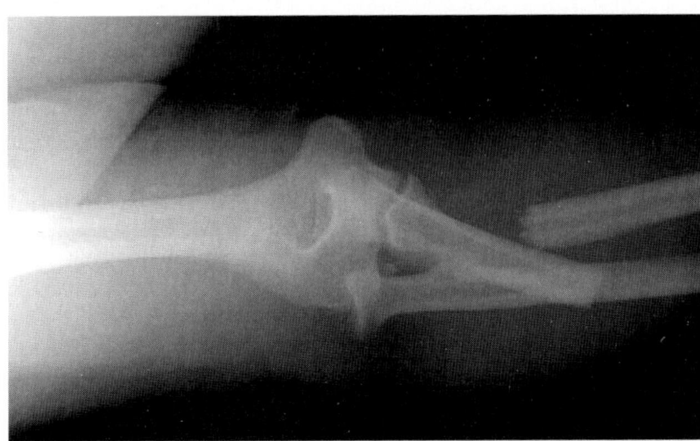

FIGURE 15–28 Monteggia fracture-dislocation. (Courtesy of Jerrica Chen, MD.)

Clinical Complications

The posterior interosseus nerve courses around the proximal radius and may be damaged in MFD injuries.[1,2] This may result in weakness of finger/thumb extension.[1] This impairment usually resolves over the course of several months. Compartmental syndrome is always a potential complication.

Management

The initial reduction and treatment regimen must be determined in conjunction with an orthopedic surgeon, because of the potential for long-term pain and disability if this injury is not appropriately managed.[1] Most MFDs in adults require open reduction and operative repair. Most pediatric cases heal well with a closed approach after appropriate reduction.[2] Adequate analgesia is essential, and antibiotics should be administered if there is an open fracture.[1,2]

REFERENCES

1. Perron AD, Hersh RE, Brady WJ, Keats TE. Orthopaedic pitfalls in the ED: Galeazzi and Monteggia fracture-dislocation. *Am J Emerg Med* 2001;19:225–228.
2. Wilkins KE. Changes in the management of Monteggia fractures. *J Pediatr Orthop* 2002;22:548–554.

Galeazzi Fracture-Dislocation

Anthony S. Mazzeo

Clinical Presentation

Patients with Galeazzi fracture-dislocations (GFDs) present with arm pain and swelling and, at times, deformity at the distal radioulnar joint (DRUJ) after falling onto an outstretched, "hyperpronated" hand or after direct trauma to the dorsal aspect of the wrist.[1,2]

Pathophysiology

GFDs involve fractures of the radius at the junction of the middle and distal thirds, with concomitant dislocation.[1] In most cases, the dislocation is dorsal. Because of the anatomic proximity of the radius and ulna, forces that are capable of fracturing one bone may result in dislocation of the proximate neighboring bone.

Diagnosis

Physical examination reveals pain and swelling at the radial fracture site. Visible deformity or swelling over the DRUJ may also be present.[1,2] Radiographs reveal the fracture near the junction of the distal and middle thirds of the radius. The presence of this fracture should prompt the clinician to look closely for DRUJ dislocation. Radiographic evidence of DRUJ dislocation, however, may be subtle.[1,2] DRUJ dislocation should be suspected if radiographs reveal either shortening of the radius compared with the ulna, or a space greater than 2 mm between the two bones on anteroposterior view.[1] Comparison views are often helpful. Computed tomographic imaging may help in assessing for DRUJ dislocation.

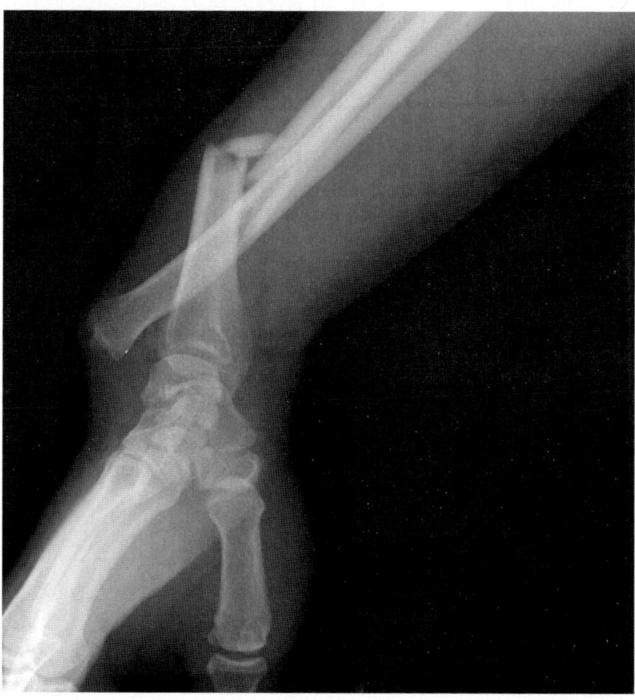

FIGURE 15–29 Galleazzi fracture-dislocation. (Courtesy of Mark Silverberg, MD.)

Clinical Complications

A complete vascular and neurosensory examination must be done in all cases. The anterior interosseus branch of the median nerve, which innervates the flexor pollicis longus and flexor pollicis brevis, is susceptible to injury and should be assessed carefully.[1,2] Physical examination reveals a weak pinch between the index finger and the thumb if this nerve is injured. Without prompt surgical intervention, GFD has a high rate of complications, including malunion, nonunion, nerve injuries, limitations in pronation and supination, chronic pain, and weakness.[1] Compartment syndrome is a rare complication that must be watched for.[1,2]

Management

GFD management in the emergency department should be done in consultation with an orthopedic surgeon. In adults, open surgical reduction and internal fixation is the usual treatment, because closed reduction is ineffective.[2] In children, however, closed reduction carries a higher degree of success. Adequate analgesia is essential, and antibiotics should be administered for open fractures.[2]

REFERENCES

1. Perron AD, Hersh RE, Brady WJ, Keats TE. Orthopaedic pitfalls in the ED: Galeazzi and Monteggia fracture-dislocation. *Am J Emerg Med* 2001;19:225–228.
2. Macule Beneyto F, Arandes Renu JM, Ferreres Claramunt A, Ramon Soler R. Treatment of Galeazzi fracture-dislocations. *J Trauma* 1994;36:352–355.

Nightstick Fracture

Mark Silverberg

Clinical Presentation

Patients with nightstick fractures present with forearm pain after receiving a direct blow to the radial aspect of the forearm.

Pathophysiology

A nightstick fracture is an isolated, nondisplaced fracture of the ulna.[1,2] The fracture gets its name from injuries that result when the forearm is placed in a defensive posture to fend off downward-moving assaultive blows inflicted with a blunt object such as a baseball bat, club, or nightstick. The ulna is struck on the external surface and usually fractures inward under the force of the trauma. The injuries may be closed or open, depending on the degree of force brought to bear against the forearm.

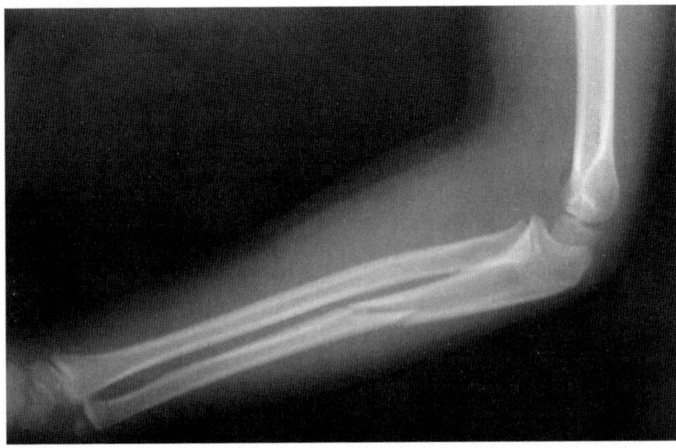

FIGURE 15–30 Nightstick fracture, showing an isolated ulna fracture. (Courtesy of Christy Salvaggio, MD.)

Diagnosis

The diagnosis of a nightstick fracture should be suspected based on the clinical presentation but needs to be confirmed with anteroposterior and lateral radiographs of the forearm.[1,2] The elbow and wrist should also be filmed to rule out other injuries. On physical examination, the elbow and wrist may or may not exhibit gross deformity, but they are almost always tender and bruised in the region. The distal radial-ulna joint (DRUJ) is not usually unstable.[1]

Clinical Complications

Complications include posttreatment loss of motion at the wrist and elbow and loss of forearm rotation, as well as fracture malunion and nonunion.[1,2]

Management

All ulna fractures should be treated in consultation with an orthopedic surgeon to arrange definitive care. The preferred treatment modality for nightstick fractures occurring in the distal third of the ulna is a plaster splint for 7 to 10 days or until the swelling is relieved, and then a short-arm cast until bone healing is stabilized.[2] Fractures involving the middle and proximal thirds of the ulna are more likely to progress to malunion or other complications and often require both surgical correction and longer periods of immobilization in a long-arm cast.[2]

REFERENCES

1. Villarin LA Jr, Belk KE, Freid R. Emergency department evaluation and treatment of elbow and forearm injuries. *Emerg Med Clin North Am* 1999;17:843–858.
2. Dymond IW. The treatment of isolated fracture of the distal ulna. *J Bone Joint Surg Br* 1984;66:408–410.

Greenstick Fracture

Mark Silverberg

Clinical Presentation

Patients with greenstick fractures present with complaints of pain and swelling at the site of injury. Younger children may be brought in after a parent notices that they are unwilling to move an extremity.

Pathophysiology

A greenstick fracture is an incomplete transverse fracture pattern seen in children.[1] Greenstick fractures occur when an injuring force applied to a bone exceeds the limits of elasticity of that bone. This results in the bone's bending to the point of bony disruption and fracture on the side opposite to the applied force. However, a greenstick fracture is, in actuality, an incomplete fracture, in which the compressed cortex and periosteum remain intact.[1] Greenstick fractures of the radius and ulna are common fractures in children and often result from a fall onto an outstretched hand.[1]

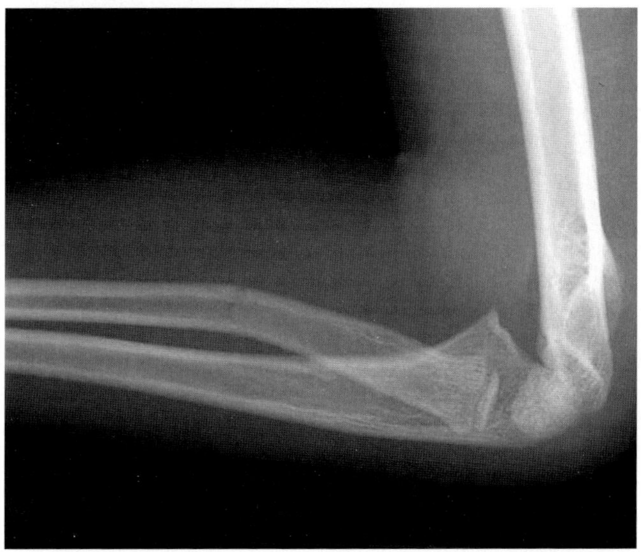

FIGURE 15–31 Greenstick fracture of the radius. (Courtesy of Mark Silverberg, MD.)

Diagnosis

Greenstick fractures may be suspected clinically, especially if a gross deformity of the limb is visible. However, anteroposterior, lateral, and occasionally oblique radiographs should be obtained to confirm and classify the injury.[1] On physical examination, gross deformity may be apparent but point tenderness over the fracture site is more common.[1] Examination should include careful evaluation of the joints above and below the fracture to identify other injuries.

Clinical Complications

Because of skeletal immaturity, fractures in children may affect the potential growth of the injured bone. Limb asymmetry or angular deformity may result if the fracture affects the bony growth area.[1] Additionally, all the complications potentially associated with adult fractures may be seen in children with greenstick fractures. Complications include nonunion, malunion and arthritis.[1]

Management

Minimally displaced and nondisplaced greenstick fractures are treated in the same manner as torus fractures, employing immobilization with a short-limb cast for up to 4 weeks.[1] Because the pediatric periosteum is more biologically active than that in adults, remodeling and callus formation tend to be more pronounced in children. For this reason, perfect anatomic alignment of fracture fragments is less important than in adult fractures.[1] However, orthopedic referral should be obtained if the fracture is more than mildly angulated or if rotational deformity exists.[1]

REFERENCES

1. Della-Giustina K, Della-Giustina DA. Emergency department evaluation and treatment of orthopedic injuries. *Emerg Med Clin North Am* 1999;17:895–922.

15–32

Torus Fracture

Christy Salvaggio

Clinical Presentation

A torus fracture manifests similarly to other pediatric fractures, with swelling and point tenderness. Obvious deformities are unusual.

Pathophysiology

A torus fracture is a fracture of the metaphyseal bone that involves buckling or compression of the bone rather than an actual break in both cortices of the bone. The distinctive quality of pediatric bones renders torus fractures a uniquely pediatric entity.[1,2] The bone structure of pediatric bones is different from that of mature adult bones. Comminuted fractures are rare in children. The bone's ability to remodel is significant, and nonunion is also rare. In contrast to the thin periosteum surrounding adult bone, immature bone is covered by a thick periosteum. Additionally, immature bone is more porous and more flexible than adult bone. Consequently, immature bones can bend without breaking, and incomplete fractures can result in greenstick fractures as well as torus or "buckle" fractures.[1,2]

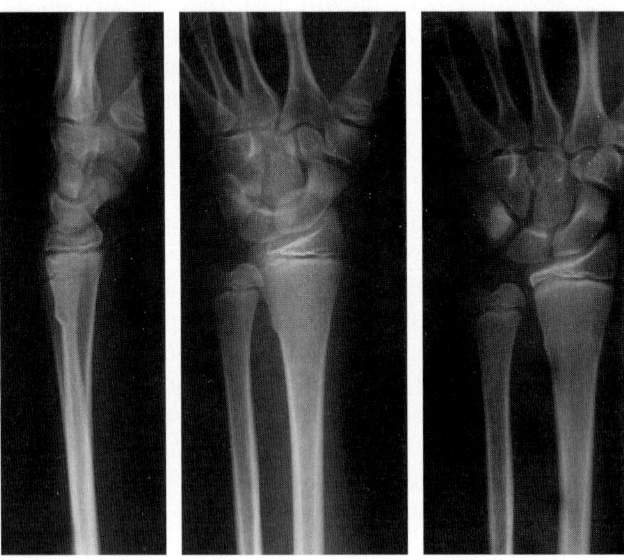

FIGURE 15–32 Torus fracture of the radius. (Courtesy of Seth Mehr, MD.)

Diagnosis

Radiographs reveal a wrinkling or compression of the distal bone. Subtle torus fractures can easily be overlooked and must be actively sought when evaluating pediatric radiographs for possible fractures.

Clinical Complications

With appropriate orthopedic follow-up and casting, torus fractures routinely heal well without complications.

Management

The specific management of a torus fracture varies, depending on the anatomic site of the fracture. An appropriately padded splint should be applied in the emergency department, and orthopedic follow-up for evaluation and casting should be arranged. The need for casting of some buckle fractures (e.g., distal radius fractures) is controversial. Because these fractures do not displace, simple splinting rather than casting may be all that is required to facilitate healing.[1,2]

REFERENCES

1. Davidson JS, Brown DJ, Barnes SN, Bruce CE. Simple treatment for torus fractures of the distal radius. *J Bone Joint Surg Br* 2001;83:1173–1175.
2. Solan MC, Rees R, Daly K. Current management of torus fractures of the distal radius. *Injury* 2002;33:503–505.

Radial Head Fracture

Michael Greenberg

Clinical Presentation

Patients with radial head fractures (RHFs) present with pain about the elbow after a fall onto an outstretched upper extremity or, in some rare cases, after direct trauma to the elbow.[1-3]

Pathophysiology

RHFs account for as many as one third of all fractures involving the elbow. Because the radial head is a stabilizing element for the elbow and forearm, RHFs can seriously interfere with upper-extremity function. RHFs are classified as Mason type 1 (nondisplaced), Mason type 2 (minimally displaced/partial articular), and Mason type 3 (complete articular).[1,2]

Diagnosis

The diagnosis is suspected based on the mechanism of injury and physical examination, which may reveal decreased range of motion as well as point tenderness directly over the radial head. Plain radiographs are usually confirmatory; however, in some cases, presumptive findings consistent with fracture (anterior fat pad sign) are all that can be discerned.

Clinical Complications

Complications include postinjury/posttreatment decreased range of motion (extension) and chronic pain.

Management

Acute treatment includes ice, elevation, and analgesia. Patients with minimally displaced or nondisplaced fractures can usually be successfully treated nonoperatively with short-term sling immobilization for 7 to 10 days.[2] Open reduction with internal fixation has been recommended for "partial articular fractures with a single fragment and for complete articular fractures with three or fewer fragments."[1] Comminuted fractures and fracture-dislocations usually require excision of the radial head.[1,3]

REFERENCES

1. Ring D, Quintero J, Jupiter JB. Open reduction and internal fixation of fractures of the radial head. *J Bone Joint Surg Am* 2002;84:1811–1815.
2. Liow RY, Cregan A, Nanda R, Montgomery RJ. Early mobilization for minimally displaced radial head fractures is desirable: a prospective randomized study of two protocols. *Injury* 2002;33:1801–806.
3. Lee DH. Treatment options for complex elbow fracture dislocations. *Injury* 2001;32[Suppl 4]:SD41-SD69.

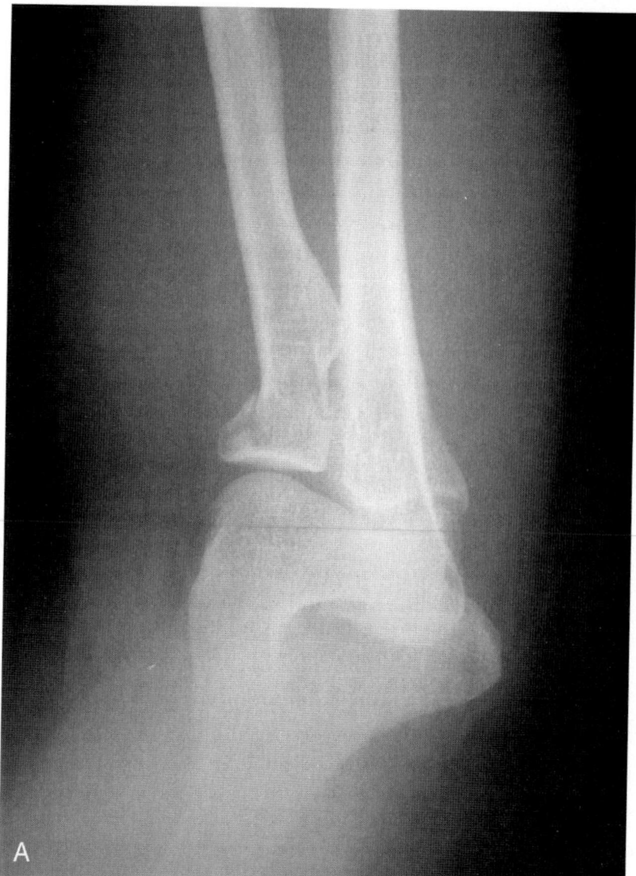

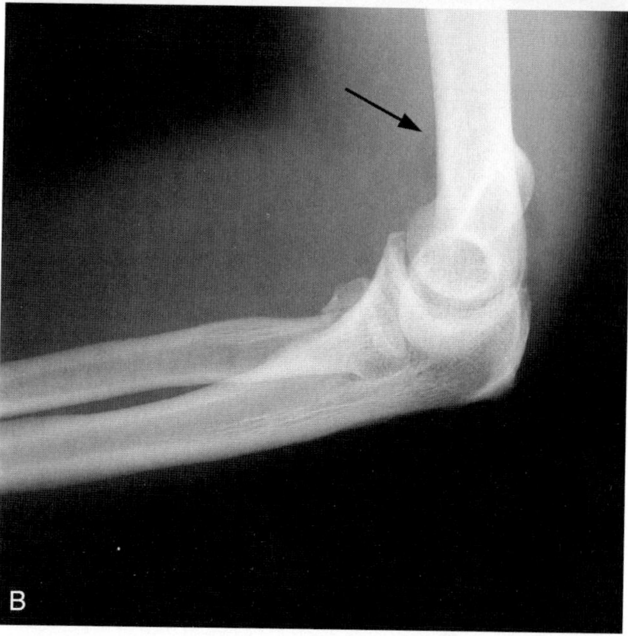

FIGURE 15–33 **A:** Minimally displaced radial head fracture. (Courtesy of Mark Silverberg, MD.) **B:** Radial head fracture. Note anterior fat pad sign. (Courtesy of John Fojtik, MD.)

Ossification Centers of the Elbow

Colleen Campbell

Pathophysiology

Ossification of the elbow is initiated from the diaphyses of the bones and progresses distally.[1] The capitellum is the first to appear, at about 1 year of age in both sexes. In general, the remaining ossification centers appear 2 years later in boys than in girls.[2] The radial head and medial epicondyle appear at 5 years of age in girls and at 6 to 7.5 years in boys, with the radial head appearing first.[2] Next, the olecranon appears at 8.7 years in girls and 10.5 years in boys. The trochlea ossifies at 9 years in girls and 10.7 years in boys. Older studies evaluating white American children showed that the olecranon fused after the trochlea; the newer studies were done on children of Chinese descent.[3] The lateral epicondyle is last to ossify, at 10 years of age in girls and 12 years in boys.[2] A mnemonic to remember the order of appearance of the six ossification centers is "**C**ome **r**ake **m**y **o**ak **t**ree **l**eaves." The capitellum, lateral epicondyle, and trochlea fuse before growth is completed (age 11 to 12 years). They then fuse with the distal humeral metaphysis at 12 to 14 years in girls and 13 to 16 years in boys. The medial epicondyle is the last to fuse, at 14 years in girls and 17 years in boys.[1]

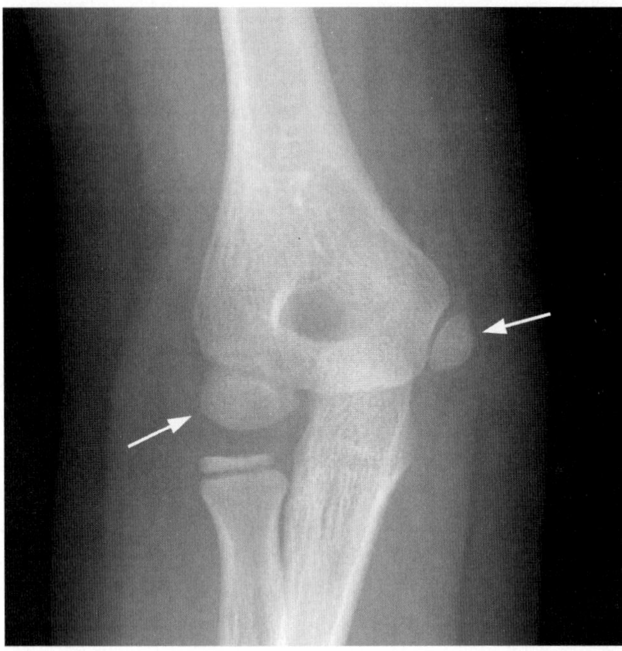

FIGURE 15–34 Ossification centers about the elbow. (Courtesy of Jay Itzkowitz, MD.)

Diagnosis

Standard radiographs of the elbow include anteroposterior and lateral views. The Jones view is used if the patient is unable to fully extend the elbow. This is an axial view that is helpful in evaluation of the distal humerus. The trochlea often has an irregular, fragmented appearance and is easily mistaken for a fracture. Routine use of comparison films has not been shown to make the diagnosis of elbow fractures more accurate.[3]

REFERENCES

1. Spinseller PD, Stanitski CL. Osgood Schlatter lesion. In: Beaty JH, Kasser JR, eds. *Rockwood and Wilkins' fractures in children.* Philadelphia: Lippincott Williams & Wilkins, 2001:563–575.
2. Cheng JC, Wing-Man K, Shen WY, Xia G, et al. A new look at the sequential development of elbow-ossification centers in children. *J Pediatr Orthop* 1998;18:161–167.
3. Chacon D, Kissoon N, Brown T, Galpin R. Use of comparison radiographs in the diagnosis of traumatic injuries of the elbow. *Ann Emerg Med* 1992;21:895–899.

Supracondylar Fractures

Michael Greenberg

Clinical Presentation

Patients with supracondylar fractures (SFs) present with pain, swelling, and limitation of motion at the elbow after a fall, direct trauma, or multiple high-speed trauma events. SFs are more common in children.[1-3]

Pathophysiology

SFs account for 3% to 7% of all fractures in children and for the majority (up to 80%) of all elbow fractures in children. The most common of SFs involve an extension mechanism wherein the condylar complex shifts posteromedially or posterolaterally after a fall onto an outstretched arm.[1-3] Only about 2% of SFs involve a so-called flexion mechanism, in which the condylar bony components shift anterolaterally.[1,2] Up to 15% of SFs involve initial vascular compromise from swelling, bleeding, or impingement of displaced fracture fragments.[1-3]

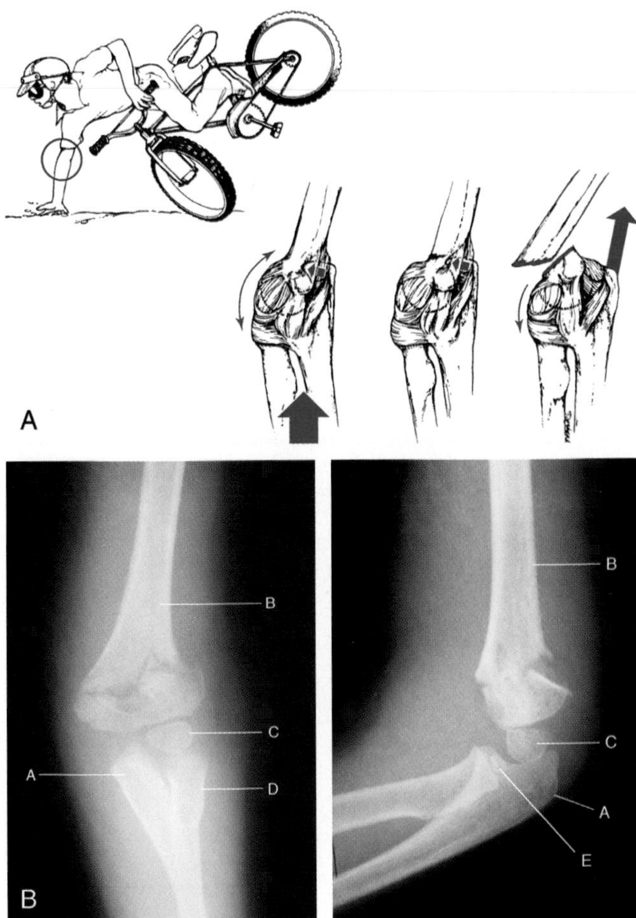

FIGURE 15-35 **A:** Most young children attempt to break falls with the upper extremity extended. Because of the laxity of the ligaments, the elbow becomes locked into hyperextension. (From Beaty, with permission.) **B:** Type II extension supracondylar humerus fracture (left elbow). A, anteroposterior view. B, lateral view. A, ulna; B, humerus; C, capitellar epiphysis; D, radius; E, radial head. (From Koval, with permission.)

Diagnosis

The diagnosis is based on the history of the injury and the clinical findings. Radiographic imaging is required for definitive diagnosis and to determine the positions of fracture fragments. Vascular compromise associated with these fractures represents an orthopedic emergency.[1-3]

Clinical Complications

SFs are serious fractures and may be complicated by injury to the brachial artery, median nerve, or radial nerve; nerve entrapment; neurovascular injury due to sharp fracture fragments; Volkmann's contracture due to vascular compromise; compartmental syndrome; and permanent disability. Nerve injury occurs in up to 20% of all SFs.[1-3]

Management

Ice, immobilization in a comfortable splint, and careful elevation are essential components of the management of SFs in the emergency department (ED). In addition, a careful and complete documentation of the neurovascular status of the injured extremity is essential. This assessment should be repeated frequently while the patient remains in the ED and before and after the patient is taken to the x-ray suite. All patients with SFs need to be hospitalized for observation. Most will require operative fixation, and these fractures should all receive the on-site attention of an orthopedic consultant.[1-3]

REFERENCES

1. Gosens T, Bongers KJ. Neurovascular complications and functional outcome in displaced supracondylar fractures of the humerus in children. *Injury* 2003;34:267–273.
2. Garbuz DS, Leitch K, Wright JG. The treatment of supracondylar fractures in children with an absent radial pulse. *J Pediatr Orthop* 1996;16:594–596.
3. McLauchlan GJ, Walker CR, Cowan B, Robb JE, Prescott RJ. Extension of the elbow and supracondylar fractures in children. *J Bone Joint Surg Br* 1999;81:402–405.

Elbow Dislocations

Colleen Campbell

Clinical Presentation

Patients with elbow dislocations often present with a history of a fall onto an outstretched hand.[1,2] Patients may complain of numbness or paresthesias in the median or ulnar nerve distribution.[1]

Pathophysiology

Elbow dislocations are the second most common type of dislocation and are classified as simple (with no bony fractures) or complex.[2] Simple dislocations are further divided into posterior, anterior, lateral, and divergent types.[2] Divergent dislocations occur when the radius and the ulna are separated. Complex dislocations are classified as anterior or posterior.[2] Most elbow dislocations are posterior. The anterior capsule and collateral ligaments are torn as the ulna is forced out of the trochlea.[1]

Diagnosis

Neurovascular status must be assessed before reduction is attempted. Radiographic evaluation of the elbow, with anteroposterior and lateral projections, is necessary to diagnose elbow dislocations.[2]

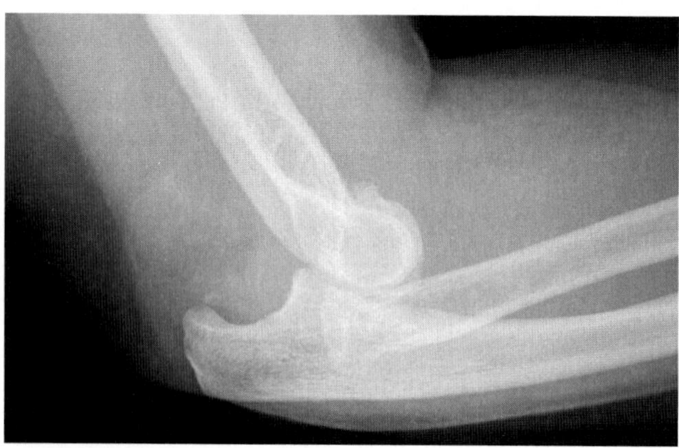

FIGURE 15–36 Posterior dislocation of the olecranon. This dislocation usually is evident clinically. (Courtesy of Robert Hendrickson, MD.)

Clinical Complications

Injury to the brachial artery and compartment syndrome may accompany elbow dislocations. The median or ulnar nerve may become entrapped during the injury. Radial head fractures, coronoid process fractures, and fractures of the distal humerus are associated with elbow dislocations.[1] Half of all patients complain of reduced range of motion or arthritis symptoms after elbow dislocation.[2] Heterotopic ossification after injury is common.[2] Recurrent dislocation may occur after complex dislocations.[2]

Management

Posterior dislocations may be reduced in the emergency department with the use of conscious sedation. The elbow is held in about 30 degrees of flexion with traction on the forearm. Countertraction is applied to the arm while the olecranon is pushed distally.[2] The reduced elbow is tested for range of motion, then splinted in 90 degrees of flexion. It is preferable to reduce anterior and divergent dislocations in the operating room. Open reduction with internal fixation may be necessary for complex dislocations and unstable injuries.[2]

REFERENCES

1. Mezera K, Hotchkiss RN. Fractures and dislocations of the elbow. In: Bucholz RW, Heckman JD, eds. *Rockwood and Green's fractures in adults.* Philadelphia: Lippincott Williams & Wilkins, 2002: 920–933.
2. Hilldebrand KA, Patterson SD, King GJ. Acute elbow dislocations: simple and complex. *Orthop Clin North Am* 1999;30:63–79.

Nursemaid's Elbow

Carla Valentine

Clinical Presentation

Children 1 to 6 years of age are most commonly affected by nursemaid's elbow.[1] The child typically refuses to use the arm and keeps the affected extremity adducted, with the elbow flexed and the arm pronated. The neurovascular examination is normal, and there should be no deformity, swelling, or ecchymosis.

Pathophysiology

Nursemaid's elbow occurs when there is a sudden pull on the extremity with longitudinal traction while the elbow is fully extended and the arm pronated.[2] The annular ligament slips over the radial head and becomes lodged within the radiocapitellar joint.[3]

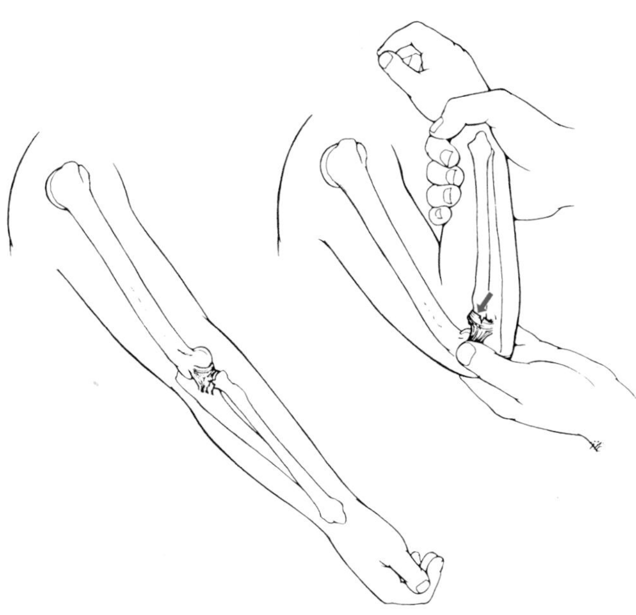

FIGURE 15–37 Reduction technique for nursemaid's elbow. *Left:* The forearm is first supinated. *Right:* The elbow is then hyperflexed. The surgeon's thumb is placed laterally over the radial head to feel the characteristic snapping as the ligament is reduced. (From Beaty, with permission.)

Diagnosis

With the proper clinical history and physical examination, radiographs are not necessary. However, in the presence of swelling, ecchymosis, deformity, bony tenderness (except over the radial head), unsuccessful reduction, an uncharacteristic history, or concern for abuse, radiographs should be obtained to evaluate for alternative diagnoses.[3]

Clinical Complications

Complications are rare; however, approximately 27% of cases recur.[3]

Management

Reduction usually is achieved by the supination technique. The clinician's thumb is placed on the radial head; the other hand is used to supinate the forearm and flex the elbow while applying gentle pressure over the radial head. There usually is a palpable click with appropriate reduction. The clinician should then leave the room; the child typically begins to use the arm within 30 minutes after appropriate reduction. Immobilization is not required after the first episode. After a recurrence, the arm should be immobilized with a sling or posterior long-arm splint, and prompt orthopedic follow-up should be arranged.[1–3]

REFERENCES

1. McDonald J, Whitelaw C, Goldsmith LJ. Radial head subluxation: comparing two methods of reduction. *Acad Emerg Med* 1999;6: 715–718.
2. Macias CG, Bothner J, Wiebe R. A Comparison of supination/ flexion to hyperpronation in the reduction of radial head subluxations. *Pediatrics* 1998;102:e10.
3. Schunk JE. Radial head subluxation: epidemiology and treatment of 87 episodes. *Ann Emerg Med* 1990;19:1019–1023.

Olecranon Bursitis

Colleen Campbell

Clinical Presentation

Patients with olecranon bursitis may report a history of trauma to the elbow or repetitive motion; they present with swelling and soft tissue prominence at the olecranon area. Fluctuance may be evident. Patients usually exhibit full range of motion of the elbow.[1] Infected bursitis manifests with warmth and erythema overlying the olecranon.

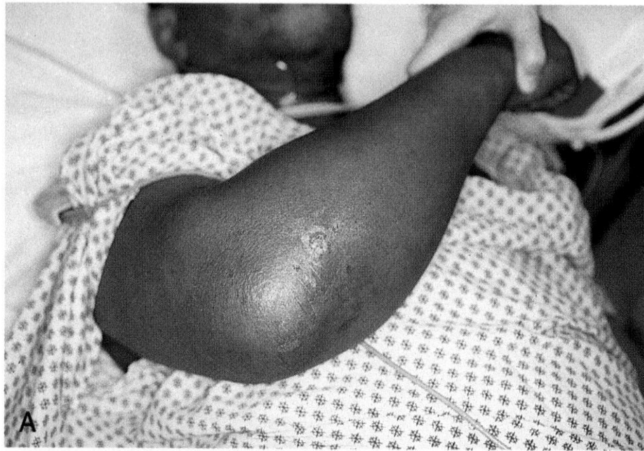

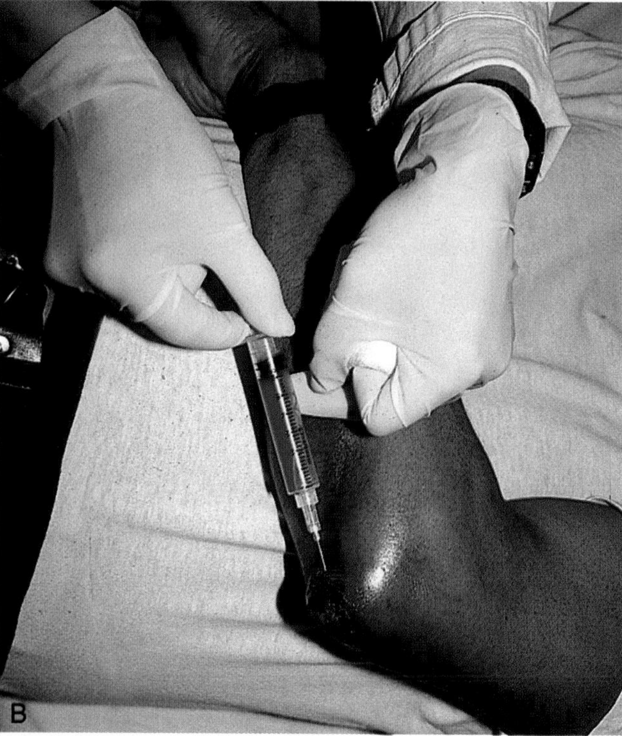

FIGURE 15–38 **A:** Swollen, warm, tender olecranon bursitis. **B:** Needle aspiration of the olecranon bursa. (**A** and **B,** From Roberts JR. Olecranon bursitis: the technique of bursal aspiration. *Emergency Medicine News* 2002;24:20–21, with permission.)

Pathophysiology

Olecranon bursitis may result from infectious processes, gout, or an overuse syndrome.[2]

Diagnosis

The diagnosis is made on the basis of history and physical examination. Radiographs usually are normal.[1] The cause of olecranon bursitis may be ascertained by synovial fluid analysis.[2] Gram staining, culture, white blood cell (WBC) count, and crystal analysis should be performed. If the WBC count is greater than 10,000/mm^3, an infectious cause is likely.[2] Traumatic bursitis typically has a WBC count of less than 1,000/mm^3.[1,2]

Management

Treatment involves drainage of accumulated bursal fluid. A penicillinase-resistant antibiotic should be administered. Inflammatory bursitis is treated with supportive care, including nonsteroidal antiinflammatory drugs (NSAIDS), ice, and compressive dressings.[1,2]

REFERENCES

1. Chumbley EM, O'Connor FG, Nirschl RP. Evaluation of overuse elbow injuries. *Am Fam Physician* 2000;61:691–700.
2. Villarin LA Jr, Belk KE, Freid R. Emergency department evaluation and treatment of elbow and forearm injuries. *Emerg Med Clin North Am* 1999;17:843–858.

Olecranon Fractures

Colleen Campbell

Clinical Presentation

Patients with olecranon fractures present with pain and swelling of the elbow with or without an effusion.

Pathophysiology

Olecranon fractures result from direct trauma to the elbow or from a fall onto an outstretched hand with the elbow held in flexion.[1,2] Avulsion fractures can also occur from an excessive pull of the triceps muscle on its insertion.[3] Stress fractures occasionally are seen in baseball players and gymnasts.[3]

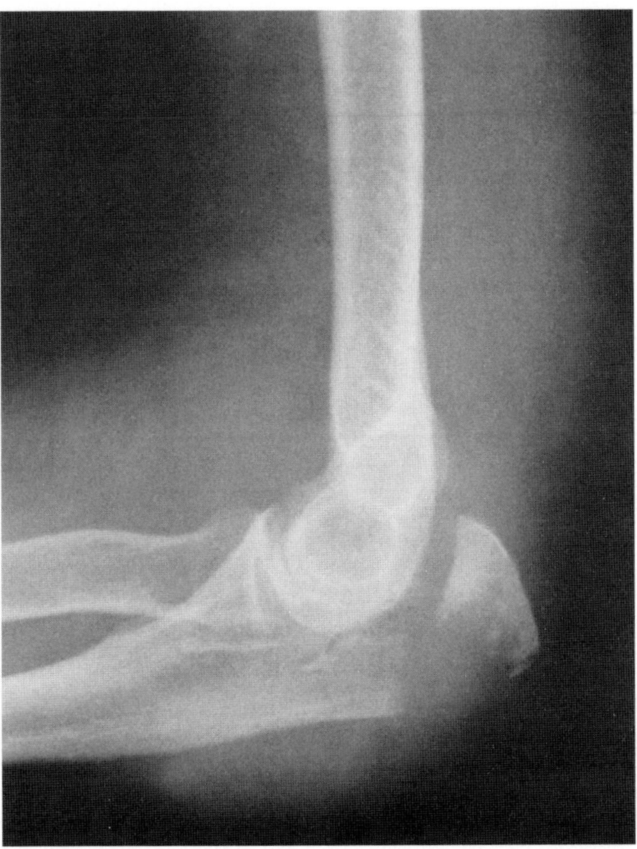

FIGURE 15–39 Fracture of the olecranon. Note the comminution and disruption of the articular surface; a true lateral view is necessary to visualize this damage adequately. The pull of the triceps tendon is the displacing force on the proximal fragment. (From Bucholz, with permission.)

Diagnosis

The diagnosis is made based on anteroposterior and lateral films of the elbow. The lateral view is most useful in assessing displacement and comminution.[2] Fracture fragments may be palpable at the olecranon.[1] A careful neurovascular examination should be performed to evaluate the ulnar nerve, including motor function of the interosseous muscles and sensation over the palmar aspect of the fifth finger.[2]

Clinical Complications

Open fractures can become infected. Associated injuries include fracture and dislocation of the radial head, elbow dislocation, and instability.[1] The ulnar nerve may be injured.[2] Patients may lose up to 15 degrees of flexion after an olecranon fracture. Nonunion and post-traumatic arthritis are other complications.[1–3]

Management

Olecranon fractures require orthopedic consultation from the emergency department. Nondisplaced fractures may be treated nonoperatively and splinted in a position of 30 degrees of flexion.[2] Displaced fractures require open reduction with internal fixation or pinning with tension bands.[1]

REFERENCES

1. Kuntz DG Jr, Baratz ME. Fractures of the elbow. *Orthop Clin North Am* 1999;30:37–61.
2. Villarin LA Jr, Belk KE, Freid R. Emergency department evaluation and treatment of elbow and forearm injuries. *Emerg Med Clin North Am* 1999;17:843–858.
3. Rettig AC. Traumatic elbow injuries in the athlete. *Orthop Clin North Am* 2002;33:509–522.

Humeral Head Fractures

Colleen Campbell

Clinical Presentation

Patients with humeral head fractures (HHFs) present with swelling and ecchymoses overlying the shoulder area. If there is a delayed presentation, the swelling may extend to the fingers. Range of motion may be limited secondary to pain. With concomitant injury to the axillary nerve, patients have numbness or tingling overlying the lateral deltoid muscle.[1,2]

Pathophysiology

Most HHFs occur in osteoporotic elderly women after falls.[1] Fractures in younger patients result from high-energy trauma. The Neer classification system divides these fractures into four groups: one-part, two-part, three-part, and four-part fractures. A 1-cm displacement or 45 degrees of angulation defines displacement. A one-part fracture is a nondisplaced two-part fracture. Eighty-five percent of HHFs are nondisplaced or minimally displaced.[2]

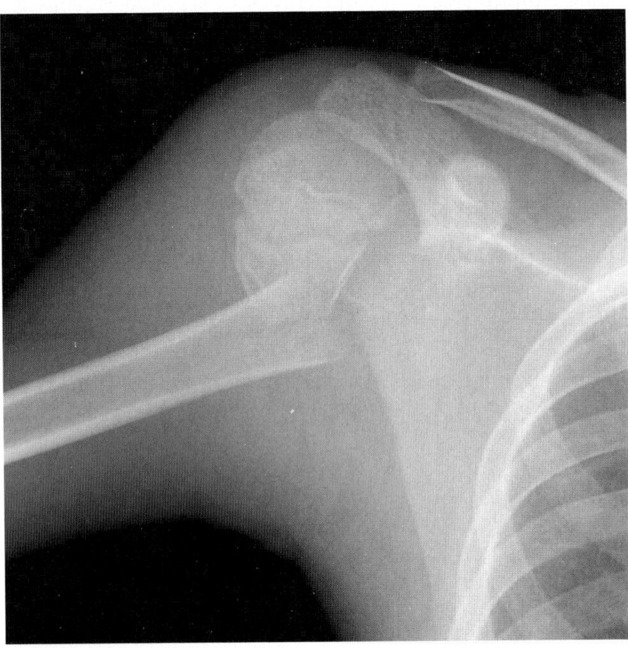

FIGURE 15–40 Fracture of the proximal humerus. (Courtesy of Mark Silverberg, MD.)

Diagnosis

Diagnosis is based on radiographic evaluation with anteroposterior, axillary lateral, and scapular "Y" views. The Velpeau axillary view, obtained with the patient leaning backward while the arm is held in the sling, is an alternative axillary view that affords more comfort for the patient.[2]

Clinical Complications

The axillary nerve may be injured as a result of a proximal humerus fracture. This may manifest as a sensory deficit overlying the lateral deltoid. Arterial injury may occur to the axillary artery or its branches in displaced fractures. Avascular necrosis of the humeral head occurs more often in four-part fractures, as does post-traumatic arthritis. Inferior shoulder dislocation may result from muscular atrophy secondary to fracture. Other complications include malunion and nonunion.

Management

Treatment of nondisplaced lesser tuberosity fractures is generally nonoperative, with sling immobilization and gradually increased range-of-motion exercises. Most other HHFs require percutaneous pinning or open reduction with internal fixation. Extensive rehabilitation is required for all proximal humerus fractures.[1,2]

REFERENCES

1. McKoy BE, Benson CV, Hartsock, LA. Fractures about the shoulder: conservative management. *Orthop Clin North Am* 2000;31:205–216.
2. Williams GR Jr, Wong KL. Two-part and three-part fractures: open reduction and internal fixation versus closed reduction and percutaneous pinning. *Orthop Clin North Am* 2000;31:1–21.

Anterior Shoulder Dislocation

Carla Valentine

Clinical Presentation

Patients with anterior shoulder dislocations (ASDs) present with flattening of the normal shoulder contour, and the arm held in abduction and external rotation, after a fall or other trauma.[1-3]

Pathophysiology

There are four types of ASD: subcoracoid (most common), subglenoid, subclavicular, and intrathoracic (rare). Dislocation occurs when the shoulder is abducted, hyperextended, and externally rotated. ASDs may result from direct force to the shoulder.[1-3]

Diagnosis

The diagnosis is made by history and physical examination, although standard shoulder radiographs, including anteroposterior, lateral, and scapular "Y" views, are required before reduction to evaluate for associated fractures. A defect over the lateral aspect of the shoulder may be palpable, and the humeral head may be visibly displaced.

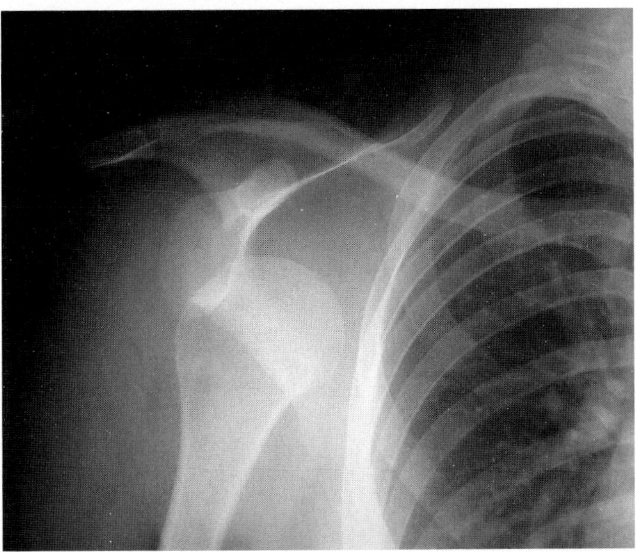

FIGURE 15–41 Anterior dislocation of the shoulder. (Courtesy of Shoma Desai, MD.)

Clinical Complications

The most common complication is recurrent dislocation.[1] Associated fractures may include avulsion of the greater tuberosity, acromioclavicular fractures, glenoid lip fractures, Hill-Sachs lesions, and Bankart lesions. Rotator cuff injuries may also occur and may be associated with axillary nerve injury or neurapraxias.[2]

Management

There are many techniques for reducing ASDs. The traction-countertraction method is performed with firm, steady traction on the affected abducted arm while a sheet is wrapped around the patient's chest for countertraction. After reduction, a repeat neurovascular examination and repeat shoulder films are necessary. The shoulder should be immobilized with a sling or sling and swathe for 2 to 6 weeks. Immobilization times should be controlled to minimize the risk of adhesive capsulitis.[2]

REFERENCES

1. Hayes K, Callanan M, Walton J, Paxinos A, Murrell GA. Shoulder instability: management and rehabilitation. *J Orthop Sports Phys Ther* 2002;32:497–509.
2. Wen DY. Current concepts in the treatment of anterior shoulder dislocations. *Am J Emerg Med* 1999;17:401–407.
3. Liu SH, Henry MH. Anterior shoulder instability: current review. *Clin Orthop* 1996;(323):327–337.

Posterior Shoulder Dislocation

Carla Valentine

Clinical Presentation

Posterior shoulder dislocations (PSDs) are uncommon, occurring in fewer than 5% of patients with glenohumeral dislocations.[1] The affected arm is held in adduction and internal rotation.

Pathophysiology

There are three varieties of PSD: subacromial (most common), subglenoid, and subspinous. Falls onto a flexed, adducted, and internally rotated arm is one mechanism of injury. PSDs may also result from indirect forceful internal rotation and adduction after a seizure or electrocution, because the internal rotator muscles are much stronger than the external rotators.[2] PSDs may result from blunt trauma to the anterior shoulder.

Diagnosis

Prominence of the coracoid process, posterior shoulder fullness, and anterior flatness may be noted on examination. The patient may report severe pain and resists abduction, external rotation, and supination. Chronic dislocations may be misdiagnosed as adhesive capsulitis.[2] Standard shoulder radiographs, including anteroposterior, axillary, and scapular "Y" views, are required before reduction to evaluate for associated fractures. The scapular "Y" view is useful for differentiating anterior from posterior dislocations.[2]

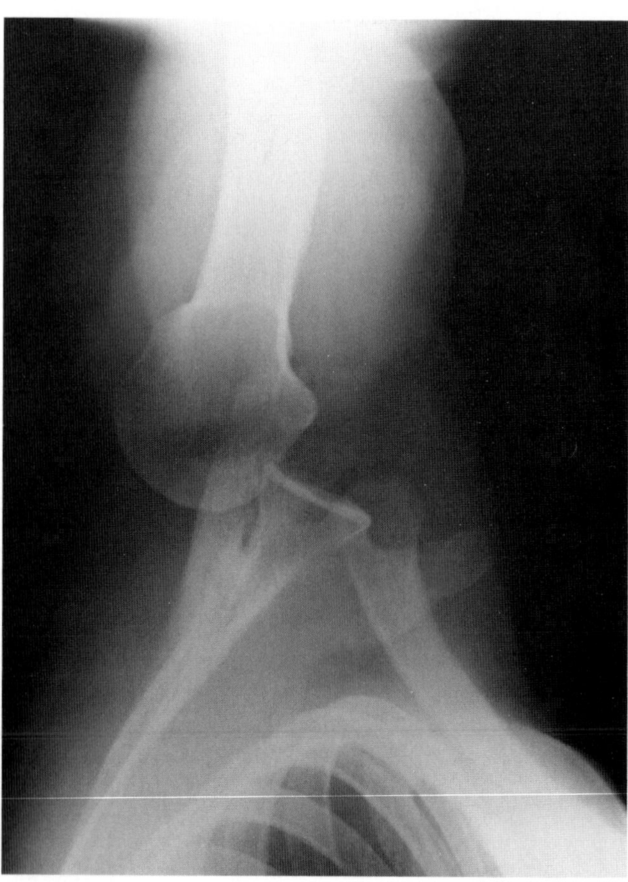

FIGURE 15–42 The axillary view of a posterior shoulder dislocation. (Courtesy of Mark Silverberg, MD.)

Clinical Complications

Common complications include missed diagnosis of PSD and PSD recurrence.[3] Associated fractures may include reversed Hill-Sachs deformity (anteromedial fracture of the humeral head), greater and lesser tuberosity fractures, proximal humerus fractures, and posterior glenoid rim fractures.[3] Neurovascular complications are uncommon.[3]

Management

An orthopedist should be consulted for all patients with PSD. Reduction may be achieved with conscious sedation in the emergency department. With the patient supine, axial traction is applied with gentle external rotation. Posterior pressure may be applied to the humeral head to achieve reduction. A postreduction neurovascular examination and repeat radiographs should be performed. If reduction is not successful, operative reduction is required. The shoulder should be immobilized for 1 to 4 weeks, with orthopedic follow-up.[1-3]

REFERENCES

1. Gosens T, Poels PJ, Rondhuis JJ. Posterior dislocation fractures of the shoulder in seizure disorders: two case reports and a review of literature. *Seizure* 2000;9:446–448.
2. Perrenoud A, Imhoff AB. Locked posterior dislocation of the shoulder. *Bull Hosp Jt Dis* 1996;54:165–168.
3. Beeson MS. Complications of shoulder dislocation. *Am J Emerg Med* 1999;17:288–295.

Hill-Sachs Deformity

Colleen Campbell

Clinical Presentation

Patients with the Hill-Sachs deformity usually present with shoulder pain after an anterior dislocation of the shoulder. Physical examination is consistent with anterior dislocation; there is often a palpable defect in the lateral aspect of the shoulder, and the humeral head is palpable in the axilla.

Pathophysiology

Hill-Sachs deformity is a defect of the humeral head caused by impaction against the glenoid rim during a shoulder dislocation.[1] Almost 70% of patients who have had a shoulder dislocation have a Hill-Sachs deformity. It is a compression fracture of the posterolateral aspect of the humeral head that occurs in association with shoulder dislocation. The classic lesion is caused by an anterior shoulder dislocation.[1]

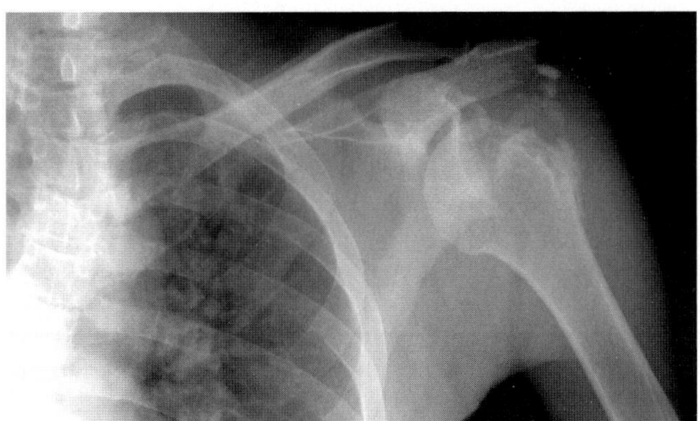

FIGURE 15–43 Hill-Sachs deformity. Note proximal humeral head fragment. (Courtesy of Mark Silverberg, MD.)

Diagnosis

Diagnosis of a Hill-Sachs deformity is made on the basis of plain radiographs of the shoulder, including anteroposterior, lateral, and scapular "Y" views. A flattening in the contour of the posterolateral aspect of the humerus is evident. If the lesion is not apparent, an anteroposterior film performed with the shoulder in internal rotation will make the lesion more obvious.

Clinical Complications

Intraarticular foreign bodies may result from the Hill-Sachs deformity.[1]

Management

No specific treatment of the Hill-Sachs deformity is necessary, unless there is an articular bone chip. Arthroscopic removal is indicated if a bone chip is present.[1]

REFERENCES

1. Beeson MS. Complications of shoulder dislocation. *Am J Emerg Med* 1999;17:288–295.

Luxatio Erecta

Colleen Campbell

Clinical Presentation

Patients with luxatio erecta present with severe shoulder pain, and with the affected arm held above the head in a hyperabducted position, after indirect forces applied to abduct the shoulder, or after a direct axial load applied to the abducted shoulder.[1]

Pathophysiology

Inferior dislocation accounts for only 1% of all shoulder dislocations.[2] This injury results from extreme hyperabduction. It may occur as a result of falls, motor vehicle accidents, or sports injuries.[1]

Diagnosis

Diagnosis is made on the basis of physical examination and radiographic evaluation. The humeral head is often palpable along the upper lateral aspect of the chest wall. Careful examination is necessary to evaluate for any neurovascular injuries. Plain radiographs of the shoulder (anteroposterior, lateral, and scapular "Y" views) confirm the diagnosis. The entire humeral head and neck is viewed inferior to the glenoid fossa.[1]

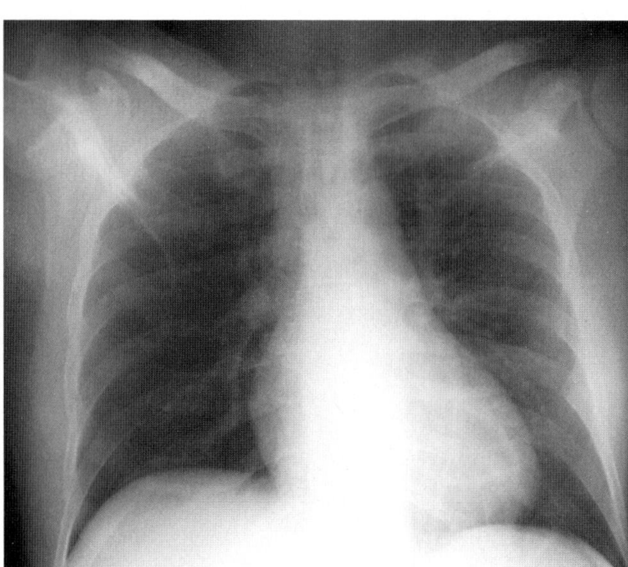

FIGURE 15–44 Right-sided luxatio erecta. (Courtesy of Mark Silverberg, MD.)

Clinical Complications

The rotator cuff is injured in as many as 80% of cases. Vascular injuries occur commonly and may include indirect injury of the axillary artery and subclavian vein thrombosis.[2] The nerve most commonly injured is the axillary nerve; the brachial plexus and the suprascapular, musculocutaneous, radial, and ulnar nerves also may be injured.[2] Fractures of the inferior glenoid rim, the greater tuberosity, and the acromion may result.[1] Adhesive capsulitis may also result from this injury.

Management

Reduction requires conscious sedation and a traction-countertraction method. An assistant exerts inferiorly directed pressure using a sheet draped around the superior shoulder. The physician brings the arm superiorly and applies gentle abduction to dislodge the humeral head from the rim of the glenoid. After reduction, the arm is immobilized by sling. Patients require orthopedic referral for follow-up.[1]

REFERENCES

1. Grate I Jr. Luxatio erecta: a rarely seen, but often missed shoulder dislocation. *Am J Emerg Med* 2000;18:317–321.
2. Beeson MS. Complications of shoulder dislocation. *Am J Emerg Med* 1999;17:288–295.

Acromioclavicular Joint Separation

Colleen Campbell

Clinical Presentation

Patients with acromioclavicular (AC) joint separation present with pain over the AC joint after a direct force with the humerus adducted, sometimes associated with a fall onto an outstretched hand.

Pathophysiology

The AC joint relies on ligamentous strength to maintain its anatomic location. Superiorly, this is provided by the AC ligament and reinforced by the deltoid and trapezoid muscles. This ligament is first to tear in dislocation.[1] The coracoclavicular and coracoacromial ligaments lend extracapsular support. The Rockwood classification of AC injuries has six categories, based on the amount of joint-space widening and the direction of clavicular displacement.[1] Type I is an AC ligament sprain with a normal radiograph; type II is a torn AC ligament and a sprained coracoclavicular ligament, with slight widening of the AC space on the radiograph. Types III through VI have torn AC and coracoclavicular ligaments with clavicular displacement in different directions and are often associated with disruption of the trapezius and deltoid muscles.[1]

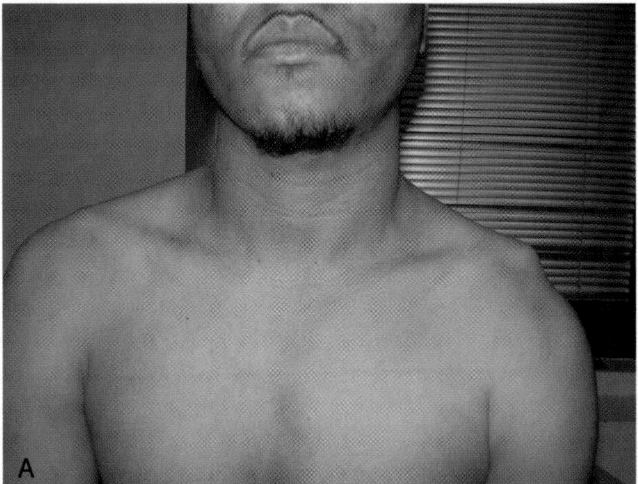

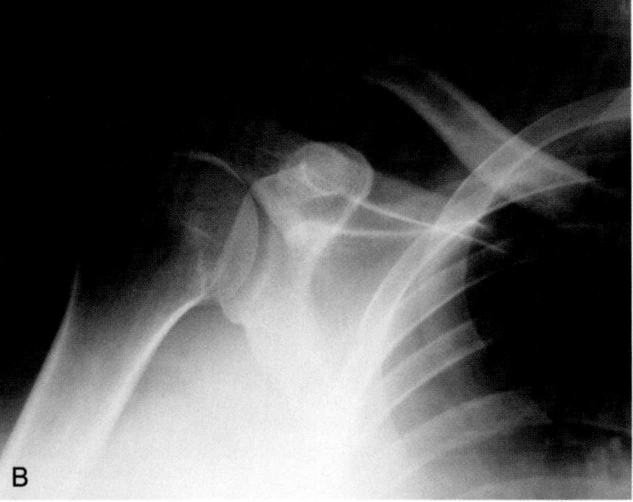

FIGURE 15–45 **A:** Obvious left-sided acromioclavicular (AC) separation. (Courtesy of Mark Silverberg, MD.) **B:** AC separation. (Courtesy of Seth Mehr, MD.)

Diagnosis

Diagnosis is based on the history and physical examination in conjunction with radiographs specifically directed at the AC joint. These include anteroposterior views of both AC joints, axillary views, and 10- to 15-degree cephalad views. Weighted stress views may not be as useful as previously thought.[1]

Clinical Complications

Patients frequently complain of pain and clicking in the AC joint after AC separation.[1] Weakness of shoulder abduction may result from more severe injury types. Skin breakdown and infection may result if the clavicle is significantly displaced.[1] Osteoarthritis is a common long-term complication. Coracoclavicular ossification and osteolysis of the distal clavicle are uncommon complications. There are rare reports of associated brachial plexus neuropraxia after AC separations.

Management

Treatment of AC separations involves a simple sling for type I through III injuries, with operative repair reserved for types IV and VI. Ice, rest, and pain control are essential.[1]

REFERENCES

1. Clarke HD, McCann PD. Acromioclavicular joint injuries. *Orthop Clin North Am* 2000;31:177–187.

Scapular Winging

Christian Sloane

Clinical Presentation

Strenuous upper-extremity activity or a history of lifting heavy weights is present in most patients with scapular winging. A history of backpacking or shoveling may also be given. On examination, an abnormal deflection of the scapula posteriorly or laterally (or both) is observed with reaching of the shoulder. It is most evident when the patient pushes against a wall or does a push-up. Elevation of the arm is limited to 110 degrees.[1]

Pathophysiology

There are several causes of scapular winging. Perhaps most common is injury to the long thoracic nerve, which leads to a palsy of the serratus anterior muscle. Any injury caused by trauma or direct compression of the nerve as it comes from the nerve roots of the brachial plexus and courses through the muscles can lead to the palsy; most commonly, it is a stretching phenomenon, as can occur during vigorous sporting activity.[1] Less commonly, injuries to the fifth cervical root or a brachial plexus injury (causing rhomboid palsy) or injury to the spinal accessory nerve (leading to trapezius muscle weakness) can cause scapular winging. Weakness of the trapezius may take several weeks to become evident, because it takes time for the trapezius to stretch out. Any painful condition of the glenohumeral joint can lead to scapular winging, because the patient splints to prevent pain. Voluntary winging has also been described and has psychogenic causes.[1]

Diagnosis

Diagnosis is entirely clinical. Electromyographic testing on an outpatient basis can determine the exact cause.

Clinical Complications

The complications of scapular winging occur as a result of the altered biomechanics of the shoulder. The muscles supporting the scapula are weakened, and the compensatory muscular activity required to improve shoulder stability may lead to pain and spasm, or to tendonitis around the shoulder joint.[1]

Management

Conservative management is the cornerstone of initial treatment, including ice, nonsteroidal antiinflammatory drugs (NSAIDs), and the recommendation to cease the suspected offending activity. Simple neuropraxias or stretching injuries usually resolve within 12 to 18 months. Patients should follow-up with an orthopedic specialist, because surgical stabilization may be required for persistent deficits. The orthopedic literature describes several techniques for surgical stabilization, including tendon transfers and scapulothoracic arthrodeses.[1]

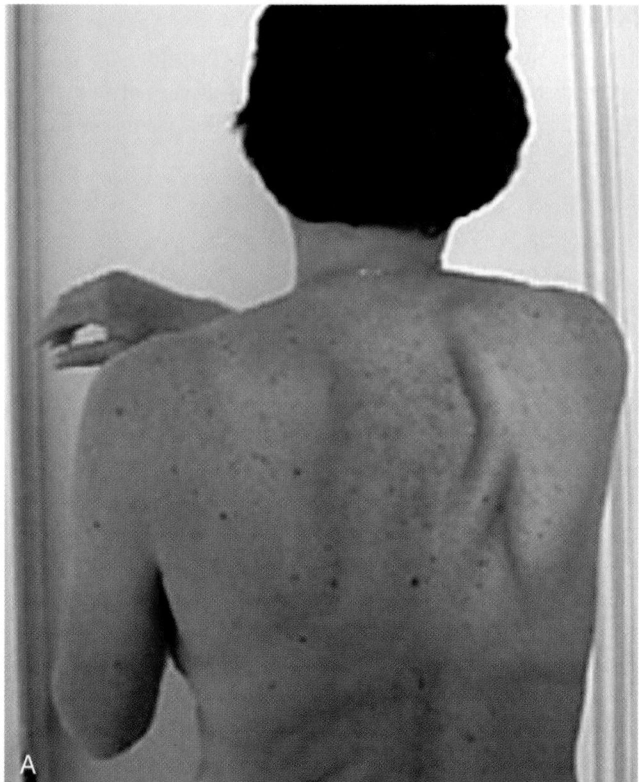

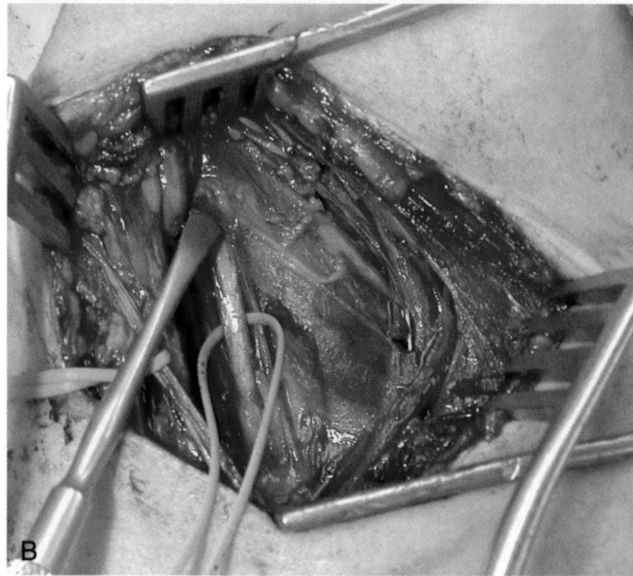

FIGURE 15-46 **A:** Image of woman's back showing winging of right scapula. **B:** The long thoracic nerve is shown exiting the middle scalene muscle before surgical decompression. (Courtesy of Rahul Nath, MD.)

REFERENCES

1. Owens S, Itamura JM. Differential diagnosis of shoulder injuries in sports. *Orthop Clin North Am* 2001;32:393–398.

Scapulothoracic Dissociation

Robert Hendrickson

Clinical Presentation

Patients with scapulothoracic dissociation present to the emergency department after events involving high-force trauma. This injury is characterized by soft-tissue swelling of the shoulder and lateral displacement of the scapula.[1,2]

Pathophysiology

Scapulothoracic dissociation, also known as "closed traumatic forequarter amputation," is a distinctly uncommon injury involving dissociation of the shoulder girdle from the thorax secondary to the application of overwhelming shearing forces to the shoulder.[1,2] The injury occurs when strong rotational forces are applied to the shoulder girdle, essentially "shearing" the shoulder from the thorax.[1]

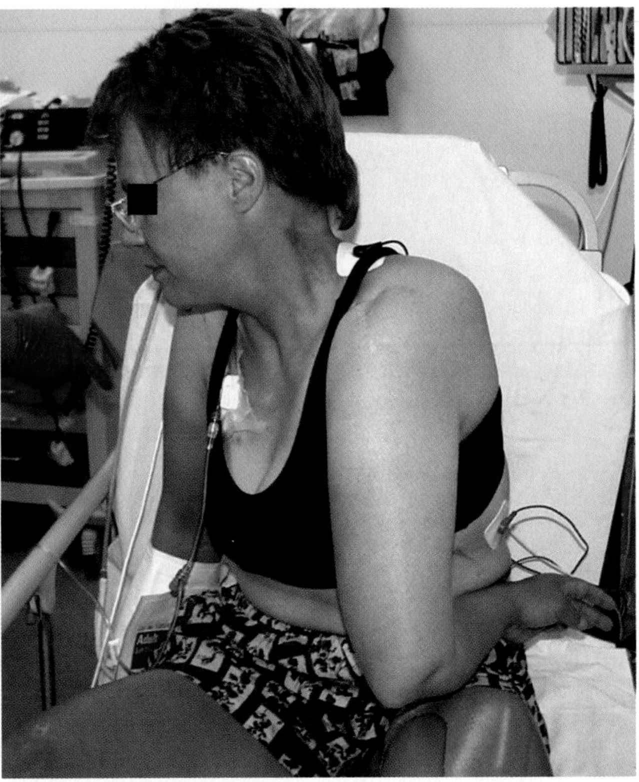

FIGURE 15–47 Scapulothoracic dislocation. The patient is demonstrating her chronic complications of a previous scapulothoracic dissociation. (Courtesy of Nicole Delorio, MD.)

Diagnosis

The diagnosis may be clinically suspected after massive shoulder trauma, but it must be confirmed with typical findings on radiography and, possibly, computed tomography. Patients may have concomitant neurologic injury, as well as vascular insufficiency of the affected upper extremity. The pattern of injury is generally noted on radiologic evaluation. Typical findings include lateral displacement of the scapula, acromioclavicular separation, and a displaced clavicle fracture.[2]

Clinical Complications

Acute clinical complications include neurologic injury, which may be permanent, and, more rarely, vascular injury and amputation. Chronic complications include permanent neurologic and orthopedic injuries.

Management

Patients with scapulothoracic dissociation often have sustained severe multisystem trauma and may require aggressive resuscitation and trauma care. Careful evaluation for concomitant injuries, including blunt chest injury, is essential. In addition, patients should be assessed for brachial plexus and subclavian artery injuries.[2] Emergency on-site evaluation by trauma surgery and orthopedic surgery specialists is critical, because patients with scapulothoracic dissociation require surgical repair of the shoulder girdle.

REFERENCES

1. Witz M, Korzets Z, Lehmann J. Traumatic scapulothoracic dissociation. *J Cardiovasc Surg (Torino)* 2000;41:927–929.
2. Tuzuner S, Yanat AN, Urguden M, Ozkaynak C. Scapulothoracic dissociation: a case report. *Isr J Med Sci* 1996;32:70–74.

Distal Clavicle Fractures

Michael Greenberg

Clinical Presentation

Most patients present with focal pain over the top of the shoulder, with discrete swelling. On physical evaluation, the fracture may resemble an acromioclavicular joint dislocation or separation. There may also be trapezius muscle spasm and tenderness.[1]

Pathophysiology

Clavicle fractures can occur at several points along the bone, including the middle third, distal third, and medial third regions.[2] Type I fractures occur laterally to the coracoclavicular (CC) ligament and are only minimally displaced; type II fractures occur when the proximal fragment detaches from the CC ligament, making it unstable; and type III fractures extend into the acromioclavicular joint.[1]

The common mechanism of injury usually involves a direct, high-energy blow to the clavicle or a fall onto the top portion of the shoulder.[1] Fractures that cannot be attributed to traumatic injury may indicate the presence of a pathologic fracture.

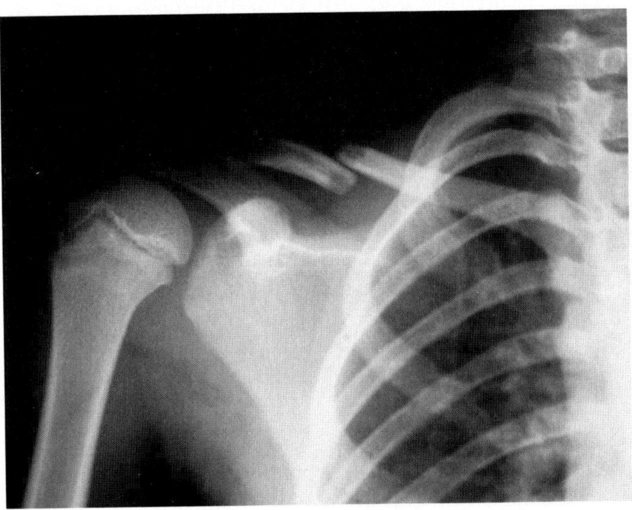

FIGURE 15-48 Clavicular fracture (middle third). (Courtesy of Matthew Spencer, MD.)

Diagnosis

The clavicle is fully palpable through its entire length, thus facilitating diagnosis based on local pain and swelling. The diagnosis is confirmed radiographically. The skin may appear taut in severely displaced fractures.[1]

Clinical Complications

Complications are uncommon in most simple fractures. However, malunion or nonunion of the bone, clavicular osteomyelitis, osteoarthritic change, and ankylosis are associated with surgical treatment of distal clavicle fractures.[2]

Management

Management of distal clavicle fractures mirrors management strategies for other clavicular fractures. Type I fractures are stable and may require only nonsurgical treatment. A sling is placed to support the weight of the arm, and rotation is encouraged, as well as passive range-of-motion exercises, as pain allows.[1] Type II fractures may involve detachment of the CC ligament, which necessitates surgical intervention. If osteoarthritis develops, late resection of the clavicle end may also be required.[2] Open reduction with internal fixation is the preferred surgical procedure for type II fractures, using an intramedullary pin and fixation with a Kirschner wire.[2]

REFERENCES

1. Anderson K. Evaluation and treatment of distal clavicle fractures. *Clin Sports Med* 2003;22:319–326.
2. Kao FC, Chao EK, Chen CH, Yu SW, Chen CY, Yen CY. Treatment of distal clavicle fracture using Kirschner wires and tension-band wires. *J Trauma* 2001;51:522–525.

Sternoclavicular Dislocation

Colleen Campbell

Clinical Presentation

Patients with sternoclavicular dislocations present with pain that is increased with lateral compression of both shoulders or when the patient is placed in a supine position. The shoulder may appear shortened and may be held in an anterior position. The medial end of the clavicle is prominent and palpable in anterior dislocations.[1] The lateral edge of the sternum is prominent in posterior dislocations. Posterior dislocations may be accompanied by dyspnea, hoarseness, dysphagia, or frank respiratory distress if a pneumothorax is present.[1]

Pathophysiology

The most common mechanism of acute dislocation is an indirect force applied to the lateral aspect of the shoulder from an anterior or posterior angle. Substantial forces applied to the medial aspect of the clavicle can cause posterior dislocation. Anterior dislocations are more common than posterior dislocations.[1]

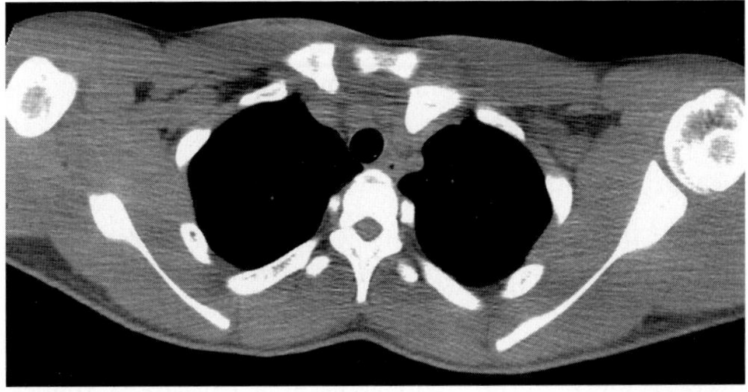

FIGURE 15–49 Computed tomogram showing left-sided sternoclavicular dislocation. (Courtesy of Mark Silverberg, MD.)

Diagnosis

The diagnosis is made on the basis of examination with radiographic confirmation. A plain chest radiograph is useful, along with special projections. A Heinig view is obtained with the beam directed at the joint and parallel to the opposite clavicle, whereas a Hobbs view is performed with the patient leaning forward over the cassette. A serendipity view is performed with the beam directed at the sternoclavicular joint with a 40-degree cephalic tilt. Computed tomography of the sternoclavicular joints is the most useful study to evaluate these injuries.[1]

Clinical Complications

Posterior dislocations can result in potentially life-threatening injuries to underlying structures. Thoracic outlet obstruction or venous congestion and brachial plexus injury may result.[1]

Management

Closed reduction can be accomplished with conscious sedation and a direct pressure to the proximal clavicle in anterior dislocations. Mild anterior dislocations are treated nonoperatively with a figure-of-eight clavicle strap, pain control, ice, and rest. Operative repair is reserved for those cases that fail closed reduction.[1]

REFERENCES

1. Yeh GL, Williams GR Jr. Conservative management of sternoclavicular injuries. *Orthop Clin North Am* 2000;31:189–203.

Calcaneal Fractures

Robert Hendrickson

Clinical Presentation

Patients with calcaneal fractures present with pain, swelling, and tenderness of the heel, usually after a fall or jump.

Pathophysiology

The calcaneus is the most frequently fractured bone of the foot; the injury typically occurs after landing on the feet after a fall from height.[1] An axial loading force is transferred to the calcaneus, causing a compression fracture of the midcalcaneus, a posterior tuberosity fracture, or an anterior process fracture.[1]

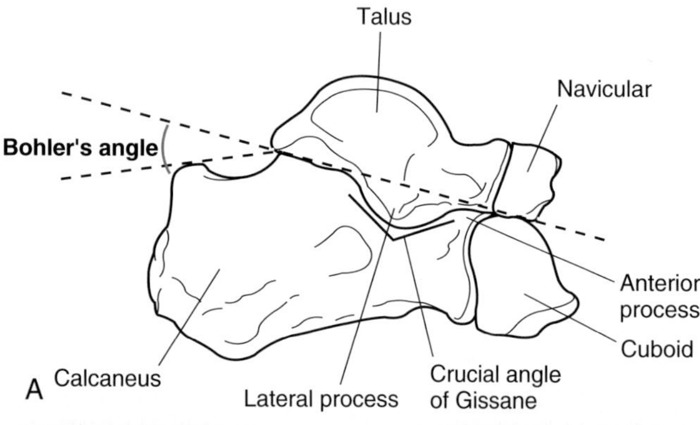

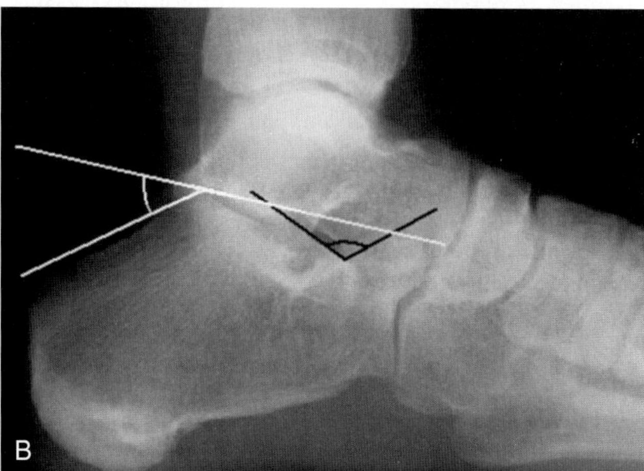

FIGURE 15–50 Calcaneal fracture. **A:** Schematic lateral anatomy of the calcaneus with surrounding structures. Note the angle of Bohler and the crucial angle of Gissane. **B:** Standing lateral radiograph of the same structures, with the angles of Bohler and Gissane depicted. (**A** and **B**, From Bucholz, with permission.)

Diagnosis

The diagnosis is made by recognition of the clinical signs, and confirmation is obtained by radiography. Bohler's angle should be measured, because occasionally it is the only sign of fracture. Draw a line along the superior aspect of the posterior tuberosity through the superior aspect of the subtalar calcaneus. Another line, from the superior surface of the anterior process through the superior aspect of the subtalar calcaneus, should form an angle between 20 and 40 degrees. If Bohler's angle is less than 20 or greater than 40 degrees, a fracture should be suspected. If the clinical suspicion is high and radiographs are normal, a computed tomographic (CT) scan of the foot should be performed. The hips and back should be carefully examined for injury, because up to 20% of patients with calcaneal fractures have vertebral compression fractures as well.[1]

Clinical Complications

Complications include nonunion, chronic pain, gait abnormalities, and chronic disability.

Management

If there is high suspicion for a fracture and radiographs are normal, a CT scan should be performed. The management of calcaneus fractures is controversial. Patients with gross displacement of the heel, horizontally depressed talus, intraarticular fractures with more than 2 mm of displacement, or skin tenting should be considered for early surgery.[1] Most other fractures require delayed surgical intervention, usually in 1 week after the swelling has subsided. Patients may be placed in a bulky dressing and a surgical boot, with crutches, and scheduled for follow-up with an orthopedist for delayed surgery.[1] Elevation, ice, and avoidance of weight bearing may be helpful in decreasing pain and swelling.

REFERENCES

1. Barei DP, Bellabarba C, Sangeorzan BJ, Benirschke SK. Fractures of the calcaneus. *Orthop Clin North Am* 2002;33:263–285.

Ganglion Cyst

Mark Silverberg

Clinical Presentation

Some patients with ganglion cysts present when the cyst first appears. Others present complaining that a preexisting ganglion cyst is cosmetically undesirable or has grown in size and become painful.

Pathophysiology

A ganglion cyst represents a herniation of synovial membranes through the joint capsule.[1] These lesions usually develop spontaneously in adults 20 to 50 years of age.[2] The dorsal wrist ganglion arises from the scapholunate joint, whereas the volar wrist ganglion usually originates from the distal aspect of the radius.[2]

Diagnosis

The diagnosis is made clinically by recognizing the usual appearance and physical characteristics of the ganglion cyst. If the diagnosis is in question, it may be confirmed by aspiration of the classic thick, clear to straw-colored fluid from the structure. On physical examination, most ganglion cysts are found on the dorsal or volar aspects of the wrist, are noted to be soft and ballotable, and may or may not be tender.[1,2]

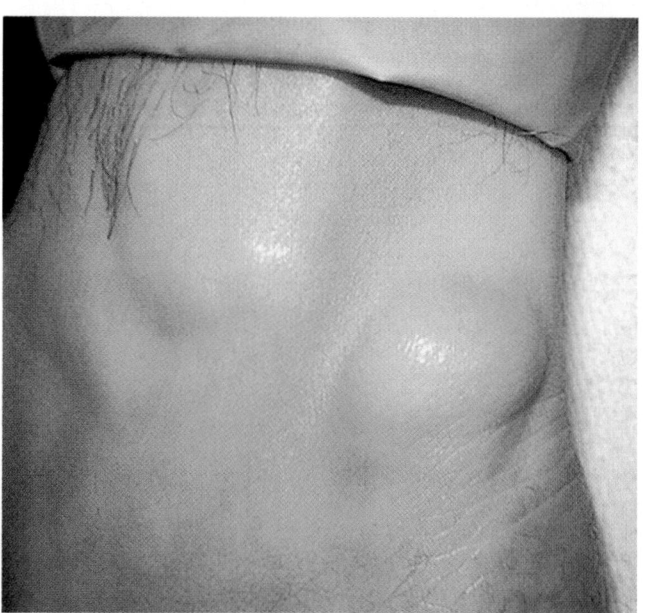

FIGURE 15–51 Ganglionic cyst. Multiple ganglionic cysts may be seen in the same area of the foot or ankle. (From Dockery and Crawford, with permission.)

Clinical Complications

Most ganglion cysts do not develop any complications other than occasionally becoming painful or rarely impinging on a nearby nerve or tendon. However, complications can arise after the cyst is injected. Cyst infection is possible but can be avoided by use of proper sterile technique. A local reaction of swelling, tenderness, and warmth may occur within a few hours after lidocaine/steroid injection and can last up to 2 days.[2] Alterations in taste have also been reported after injection. Hyperglycemia is possible in any diabetic patient who is injected with corticosteroids.[3]

Management

Most ganglion cysts resolve spontaneously and do not require treatment. If pain or paresthesias develop, aspiration with or without injection of a corticosteroid is usually effective, although cysts have been known to recur in about one third of cases.[2] A 20- or 30-mL syringe with an 18-gauge needle should be used to provide adequate suction for aspiration, given the high viscosity of cyst contents.[2]

REFERENCE

1. Siegel MJ. Magnetic resonance imaging of musculoskeletal soft tissue masses. *Radiol Clin North Am* 2001;39:701–720.
2. Tallia AF, Cardone DA. Diagnostic and therapeutic injection of the wrist and hand region. *Am Fam Physician* 2003;67:745–750.
3. Cardone DA, Tallia AF. Joint and soft tissue injection. *Am Fam Physician* 2002;66:283–288.

Primary and Metastatic Pathologic Fractures

Colleen Campbell

Clinical Presentation

Patients with pathologic fractures often complain of gradual onset and increasing intensity of bone pain in affected bones. Pain may awaken patients at night. If the affected bone is non-weight bearing, patients may be asymptomatic until a fracture occurs. Neurologic impairment may worsen gradually in patients with spinal metastasis.[1] Pathologic fractures tend to occur with minimal or no trauma.

Pathophysiology

Pathologic fractures may occur as a result of osteoporosis, osteomalacia, Paget's disease, osteogenesis imperfecta, benign bone lesions, or malignancy. Osteoporosis is the most common cause of pathologic fractures overall. Primary bone malignancy usually is found in the metaphysis and occurs in patients younger than 50 years of age. Osteosarcoma and Ewing's sarcoma are the most common types. Metastatic lesions of the bone are more common than primary bone lesions. Prostate, breast, lung, kidney, and thyroid cancer commonly metastasize to bone. The spine, ribs, pelvis, and proximal femur are the most common sites of metastasis.[1]

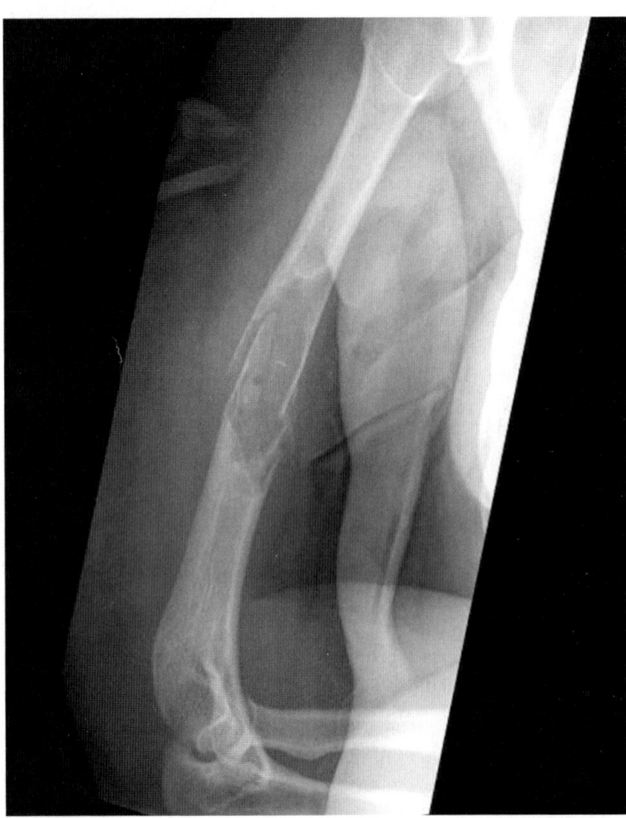

FIGURE 15–52 Unicameral bone cyst of the humerus with pathologic fracture. (Courtesy of Kevin Reinhard, MD.)

Diagnosis

The diagnosis is made on the basis of history and physical examination, as well as radiographic evaluation. Radiographs may show periosteal reaction, abnormal radiodensity, or soft-tissue shadows. Radiographic signs of malignancy include eccentric bone deposits, broad transitional borders, "sunburst" or "onion-skin" patterns, or "Codman's triangle." Further laboratory workup undertaken to determine the type of bone lesion may include alkaline phosphatase, prostate-specific antigen, and calcium determinations; serum immunoelectrophoresis; a complete blood count; and blood urea nitrogen (BUN)/creatinine measurement with liver function testing.

Clinical Complications

Delayed healing is common in pathologic fractures and often leads to fixation device failure. Pulmonary embolism, deep venous thrombosis, and blood loss are other complications of pathologic fracture.[1]

Management

Definitive treatment is determined by the orthopedist. All pathologic fractures require urgent orthopedic consultation.

REFERENCES

1. Hage WD, Aboulofia AJ, Aboulofia DM. Incidence and location and diagnostic evaluation of metastatic bone disease. *Orthop Clin North Am* 2000;31:515–528.

Scoliosis

Michael Greenberg

Clinical Presentation

Early identification of spinal deformity in patients with neuromuscular disease is important. Large numbers of adults are treated for scoliosis, and it has been estimated that up to 500,000 adults have spinal curves greater than 30 degrees.[1] Scoliosis can also be characteristic of underlying syringomyelia, which is a cyst filled with cerebrospinal fluid located within the spinal cord. Patients often report pain, peripheral neurologic deficits, pes cavus, and wasting of the intrinsic hand muscles. Scoliosis secondary to syringomyelia may also manifest with abnormal abdominal reflexes.[2]

Pathophysiology

Spinal scoliosis involves lateral curvature of the spine measuring greater than 10 degrees. Vertebral rotation is also associated with scoliosis, and adolescent idiopathic scoliosis is one of the most common childhood congenital orthopedic deformities.[3] Many factors contribute to scoliosis, such as asymmetric paraplegia or neuropathic spinal arthropathy. The deformity may also develop in compensation for pelvic asymmetry. Other underlying pathologies may include congenital spinal anomalies, genetic disorders involving connective tissue, developmental conditions, trauma, infection, neoplasia, radiation, prior surgery, and postural disorders.[4]

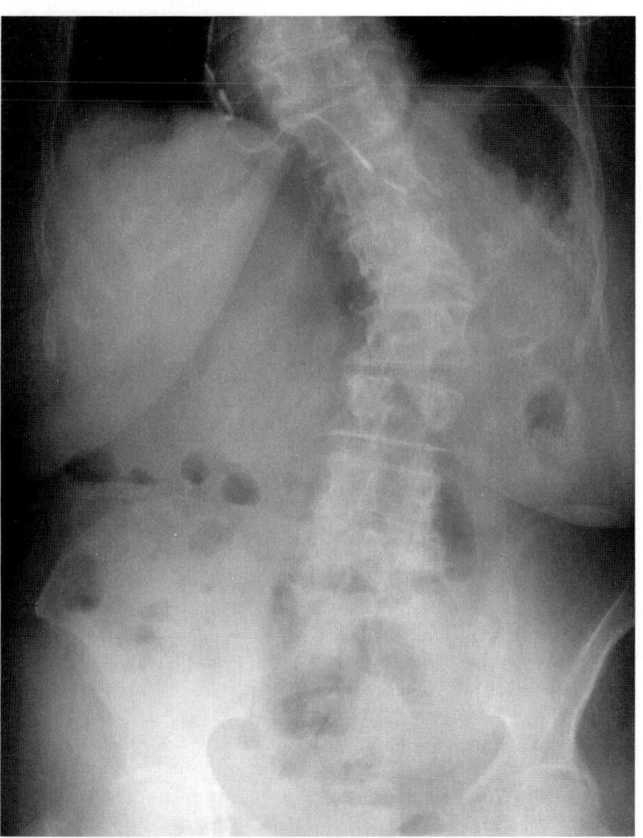

FIGURE 15–53 Scoliosis. (Courtesy of Mark Silverberg, MD.)

Diagnosis

Patient evaluation with a comprehensive history is useful because of the multiple, convergent systems involved in scoliosis. The history should include information about the perinatal period, developmental markers, family history, age at which scoliosis was first detected, and medical history including cardiac and renal abnormalities. Physical findings such as rib prominence, shoulder asymmetry, trunk imbalance, and pelvic obliquity are important findings. A functional assessment should also be made, and radiographic evaluation is important in making a definitive diagnosis.[4]

Clinical Complications

Patients with scoliosis usually have progressive curvature of the spine, which can be associated with other neuromuscular disorders, muscular dystrophy, or cerebral palsy. Such associations make it difficult to predict the progressive rate of degeneration. Morbidities that can accompany scoliosis progression include pulmonary and cardiac compromise.

Management

Both nonoperative and operative interventions are available for patients with scoliosis. Nonoperative management is useful for neuromuscular-scoliosis patients who need to improve sitting balance and functional independence. Spinal orthoses can provide external support to the trunk and delay surgical intervention. Functional strengthening is another useful way to improve patients' activity tolerance.[4]

REFERENCES

1. Shapiro G, Taira G, Boachie-Adjei O. Results of surgical treatment of adult idiopathic scoliosis with low back pain and spinal stenosis: a study of long-term clinical radiographic outcomes. *Spine* 2002;28: 358–363.
2. Kontio K, Davidson D, Letts M. Management of scoliosis and syringomyelia in children. *J Pediatr Orthop* 2002;22:771–779.
3. Goldberg C, Fogarty EE, Moore DP, Dowling FE. Scoliosis and developmental theory: adolescent idiopathic scoliosis. *Spine* 1997;22: 2228–2237.
4. Berven S, Bradford D. Neuromuscular scoliosis: deformity and principles for evaluation and management. *Semin Neurol* 2002;22: 167–178.

Vertebral Fractures

Robert Hendrickson

Clinical Presentation

Young, nonosteoporotic individuals with vertebral fractures may present after a major traumatic event complaining of back pain. The "jumper's syndrome" includes fractures of the calcaneus and vertebrae after a fall from a height.

Pathophysiology

Osteoporotic vertebral fractures may or may not cause significant pain, and they may not involve trauma. Up to 70% of osteoporotic vertebral fractures are not acutely diagnosed.[1] Typical locations for these fractures are at the thoracolumbar junction (T12–L2) and in the midthoracic region (T6–8).[1] Vertebral fractures may occur after a traumatic event or as a result of osteoporotic bone disease with or without trauma.

Diagnosis

Diagnosis is made on the basis of anteroposterior and lateral vertebral radiographs or computed tomographic (CT) scans. Patients with a high clinical suspicion of fracture and normal radiographs should be further evaluated with a CT scan.

Clinical Complications

Complications include chronic pain, spinal cord compression with permanent neurologic deficits, decreased height, inability to bend, kyphosis, and instability.[1]

Management

Patients with fractures that compress the spinal canal and those with neurologic findings require prompt consultation with a neurosurgeon. Patients who have experienced significant traumatic events and exhibit alterations of mental status, distracting injuries, neurologic signs, or pain or tenderness in the back should have radiographs of the thoracolumbar spine. CT is more sensitive than radiography in detecting fractures and should be performed if clinical suspicion is high or in lieu of radiography.[2] Patients with traumatic fractures should be carefully examined for associated injuries.

Patients with vertebral fractures that do not affect the spinal canal should be treated with acetaminophen and opioids. Early movement with stretching and light exercise should be encouraged.[1] Intranasal calcitonin is effective in decreasing pain for patients with osteoporotic vertebral fractures.[1]

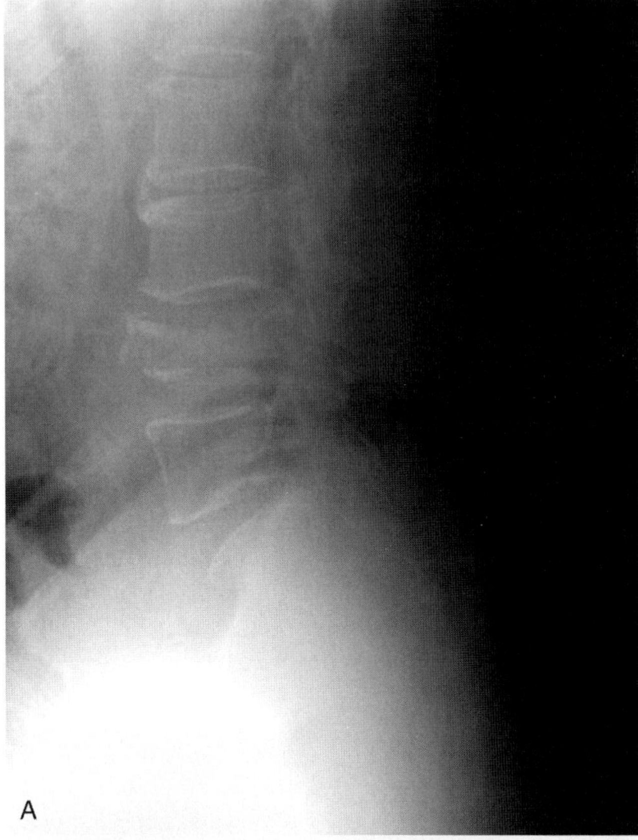

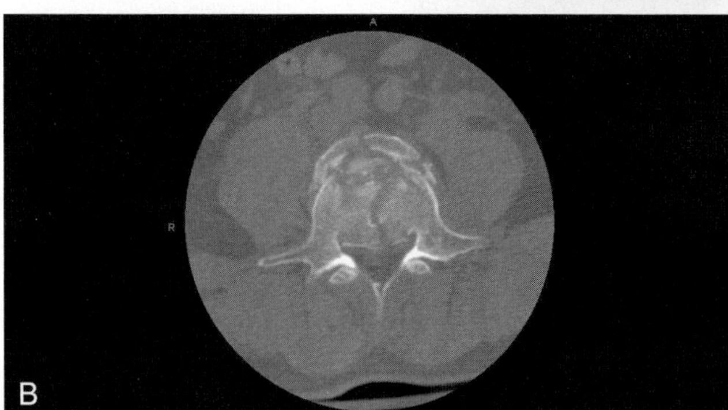

FIGURE 15–54 **A:** Lateral view of L4 vertebral compression fracture. **B:** Computed tomogram of L4 vertebral compression fracture. (Courtesy of Kevin Reinhard, MD.)

REFERENCES

1. Papaioannou A, Watts NB, Kendler DL, Yuen CK, Adachi JD, Ferko N. Diagnosis and management of vertebral fractures in elderly adults. *Am J Med* 2002;113:220–228.
2. Rhee PM, Bridgeman A, Acosta JA, et al. Lumbar fractures in adult blunt trauma: axial and single-slice helical abdominal and pelvic computed tomographic scans versus portable plain films. *J Trauma* 2002;53:663–667.

Spondylolisthesis

Colleen Campbell

Clinical Presentation

Athletic children and adolescents with spondylolisthesis present with a chief complaint of low back pain. Hyperextension of the low back may worsen symptoms.

Pathophysiology

Spondylolisthesis is the anterior dislocation of a superior vertebral body on an inferior vertebral body. Spondylolisthesis may result from a congenital defect of the pars interarticularis or from trauma.[1] It may result from a combination of flexion and torsion forces.[2] Several types of spondylolisthesis have been recognized. Congenital disease is associated with a superior articular facet defect, whereas isthmic spondylolisthesis involves a pars interarticularis defect. Other types include degenerative, traumatic, pathologic, and postsurgical spondylolisthesis.[2] Four classifications, based on the amount of dislocation, have been recognized: grade I is less than 25% dislocation, grade II is less than 50%, grade III is less than 75%, and grade IV is more than 75% dislocation.[1] The lumbosacral spine (L5–S1) is the most commonly affected area, followed by the lumbar (L4–5) region. Slippage usually occurs during childhood or adolescence and rarely progresses in adulthood.[2]

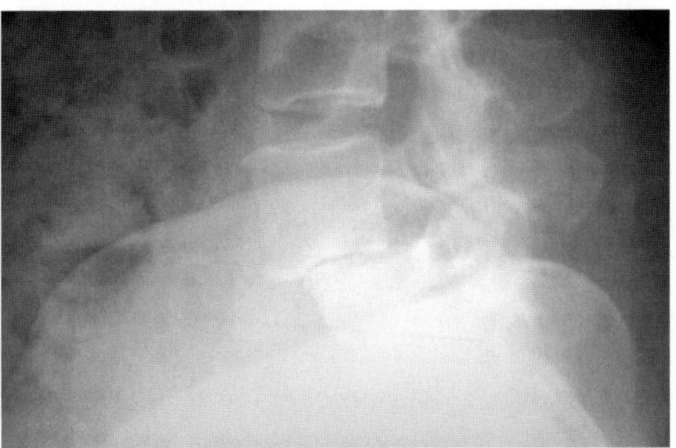

FIGURE 15–55 Spondylolisthesis. (Courtesy of Colleen Campbell, MD.)

Diagnosis

The diagnosis is based on radiographic evidence. Standard anteroposterior and lateral views of the spine are revealing. The classic teaching is to "look for the collar of the Scottie dog," signifying a pars defect on oblique films.[2] Computed tomography may be helpful in severe disease for operative planning. Magnetic resonance imaging should be used if neurologic deficits are present.[1] Patients may have symptoms of sciatica and a positive straight-leg test on examination. A step-off may be palpable if it is significant. The stride may be shortened in patients with advanced disease.[1] In patients with sciatic symptoms, the Achilles reflex may be diminished.

Clinical Complications

Spondylolisthesis predisposes patients to sciatica. Neurologic compromise, especially cauda equina syndrome, may result as the slip progresses.[2] Permanent restriction of sports and other activities rests on the stability of the disease and the treating physician's judgment.

Management

Treatment of grade I and II lesions usually involves antilordotic bracing, activity restriction, and rehabilitation. Operative repair is indicated for patients who are without improvement after 6 months of conservative management, those with a neurologic deficit, and those with grade III or higher defects. L5–S1 posterolateral fusion is indicated in these cases. L4–5 bilateral fusion and a pantaloon spica cast may also be needed in severe cases.[1,2]

REFERENCES

1. Herman MJ, Pizzutillo PD, Cavalier R. Spondylolysis and spondylolisthesis in the child and adolescent athlete. *Orthop Clin North Am* 2003;34:461–467.
2. Wimberly RL, Lauerman WC. Spondylolisthesis in the athlete. *Clin Sports Med* 2002;21:133–145.

Jumper's Syndrome

Paul Ishimine

Clinical Presentation

Patients who fall or jump from heights may present with a triad of injuries, including bilateral calcaneal fracture, thoracolumbar fractures, and bilateral wrist fractures; this is known as jumper's syndrome.[1–4]

Pathophysiology

The extent and severity of a fall victim's injuries depends on a number of variables. An important factor that contributes to a person's injury is the height of the fall; adults have a 50% mortality rate with falls of 4 stories (48 feet), whereas children have a 50% mortality rate with falls of 5 to 6 stories.[1] Other important factors are the characteristics of the surface on which the patient lands and the position of the patient's body when it strikes the surface. The patient's age and overall health status are important as well. Two thirds of patients with a fractured foot or ankle have associated lumbar vertebral fractures.[2]

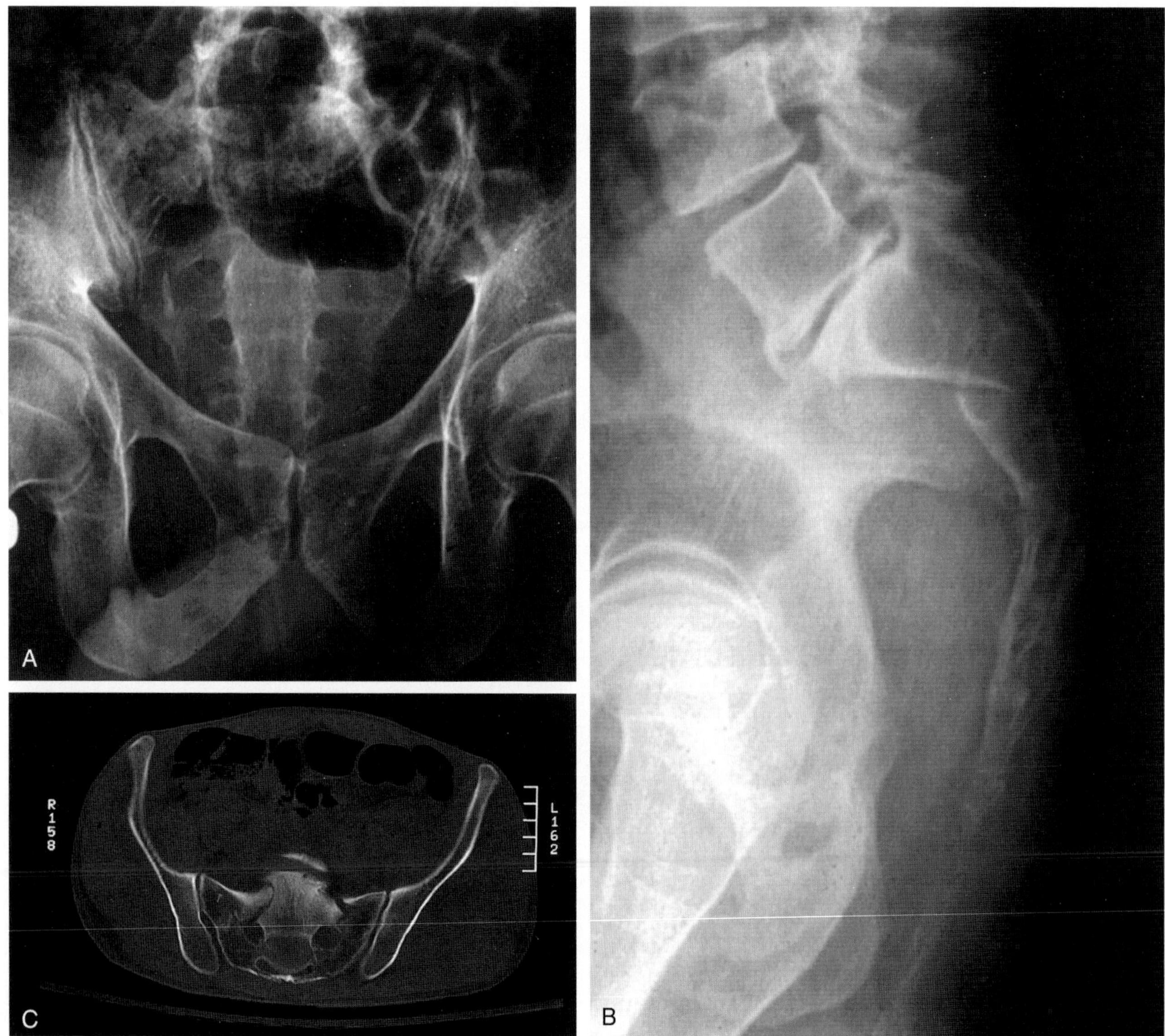

FIGURE 15–56 Jumper's syndrome. Anteroposterior **(A)** and lateral **(B)** radiographs demonstrate transverse component of the fracture. Computed tomographic scan **(C)** demonstrates bilateral, vertically oriented sacral fractures. (**A, B** and **C,** From Bucholz, with permission.)

Jumper's Syndrome

Paul Ishimine

Diagnosis

Obtaining a detailed history is essential. Falls may be precipitated by a medical emergency, or they may be the result of a suicide attempt or nonaccidental trauma. Because these patients frequently have multiple injuries, careful attention to advanced trauma life support (ATLS) protocols and evaluation standards is essential. The presence of lower extremity fractures and spinal fractures is highly correlated. Given this association, the presence of a calcaneus or other lower-extremity fracture should prompt consideration for obtaining imaging of the entire spine; likewise, the presence of a vertebral fracture necessitates consideration for imaging of the lower extremities.

Clinical Complications

Complications include open fractures, infection, fracture nonunion, chronic pain/disability, and other complications related to concomitant intrathoracic, intraabdominal, and other potentially serious injuries.

Management

Treatment depends on the nature of the patient's injuries. As with all multiply traumatized patients, the primary survey needs to be performed rapidly, with attention to immobilizing and protecting the spine. Once the airway, breathing, and circulation are stabilized, diagnosis and treatment is then directed at specific injuries.

REFERENCES

1. Buckman RF Jr, Buckman PD. Vertical deceleration trauma: principles of management. *Surg Clin North Am* 1992;71:331–344.
2. Velmahos GC, Demetriades D, Theodorou D, et al. Patterns of injury in victims of urban free-falls. *World J Surg* 1997;21:816–821.
3. Richter D, Hahn MP, Ostermann PA, Ekkernkamp A, Muhr G. Vertical deceleration injuries: a comparative study of the injury patterns of 101 patients after accidental and intentional high falls. *Injury* 1996;27:655–659.
4. Scalea T, Goldstein A, Phillips T, et al. An analysis of 161 falls from a height: the "jumper syndrome." *J Trauma* 1986;26:706–712.

Coccyx Fractures

Paul Ishimine

Clinical Presentation

Patients with coccyx fractures present for evaluation of pain after direct trauma to the coccyx, often after a fall in the sitting position. Fractures may also occur during the birth process. The pain typically is worsened with prolonged sitting or with straining at bowel movements.

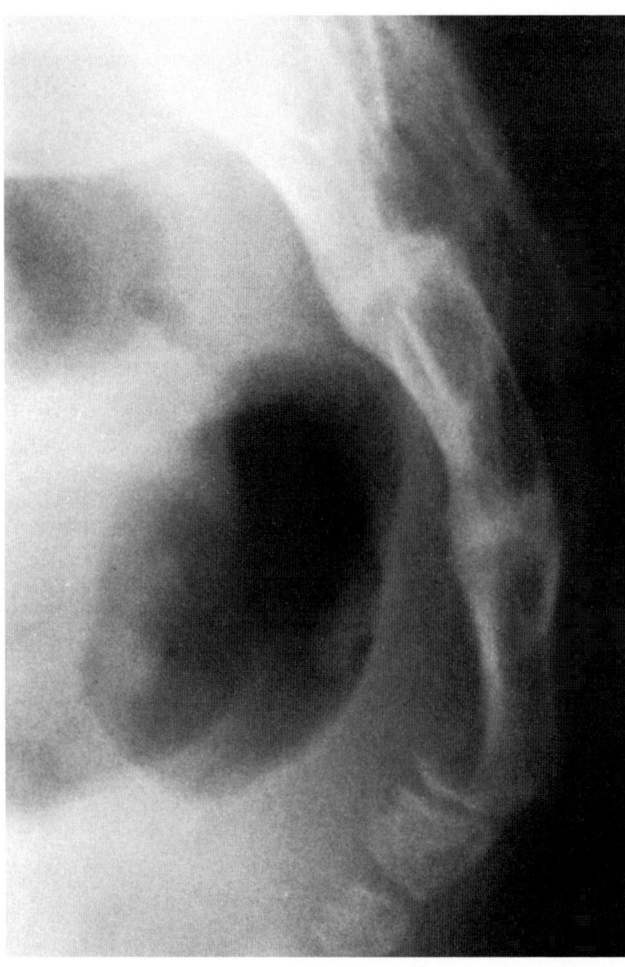

FIGURE 15–57 Lateral radiograph with the hips maximally flexed reveals displaced coccygeal fracture in a 14-year-old boy. (From Beaty, with permission.)

Pathophysiology

The coccyx is relatively well protected by the glutei maximi. However, because the coccyx serves as the attachment point for these and other pelvic muscles, healing can be prolonged due to the muscular tension exerted on the fracture fragments. Fractures are more likely in women, because the female pelvis is broader and the coccyx is more exposed.

Diagnosis

This diagnosis usually is made clinically. Because the treatment usually is nonoperative, it is unclear whether radiographic evidence changes management. Although these fractures are sometimes detected on plain radiographs with anteroposterior and lateral views, computed tomography may be required to detect subtle injuries not seen on radiography. Physical examination reveals ecchymosis and local tenderness to palpation in the gluteal crease. Tenderness, and occasionally coccygeal instability, can be elicited on rectal examination.

Clinical Complications

Recent coccygeal trauma may lead to coccydynia, a chronic pain syndrome associated with pain in or around the coccyx.[1,2] One case report described hemorrhage and edema from a coccyx fracture that caused a cauda equina syndrome.[2]

Management

Coccyx fractures generally are managed conservatively. Treatment includes stool softeners, analgesics, and the use of rubber donut cushions when sitting. Healing is often prolonged. Patients with refractory pain are sometimes referred for steroid injections or coccygectomy.[1,2]

REFERENCES

1. Maigne JY, Doursounian L, Chatellier G. Causes and mechanisms of common coccydynia: role of body mass index and coccygeal trauma. *Spine* 2000;25:3072–3079.
2. Davis DP, Bruffey JD, Rosen P. Coccygeal fracture and Paget's disease presenting as acute cauda equina syndrome. *J Emerg Med* 1999;17:251–254.

Hip Dislocation

Mark Silverberg

Clinical Presentation

The posterior hip dislocation is the most common clinical variant; patients usually present with the affected extremity held in flexion and obviously shortened, internally rotated, and adducted. Other hip dislocations may appear in a similar position.[1]

Pathophysiology

First-time hip dislocations (not involving a prosthesis) generally reflect traumatic incidents exerting enormous forces against the body. Most hip dislocations result from high-energy vehicular trauma, except in the case of young children or adults with prostheses, in whom reduced forces are capable of dislocating the hip. Anterior, posterior, and central dislocations have been reported. Posterior dislocations commonly occur when the flexed knee and hip strike the dashboard in a vehicular accident—hence, the term, "dashboard dislocation."[1] This force essentially pushes the femoral head through or over the posterior acetabular rim. Central dislocations result from a force applied to the lateral aspect of the hip that drives the femoral head centrally through the acetabulum.[1]

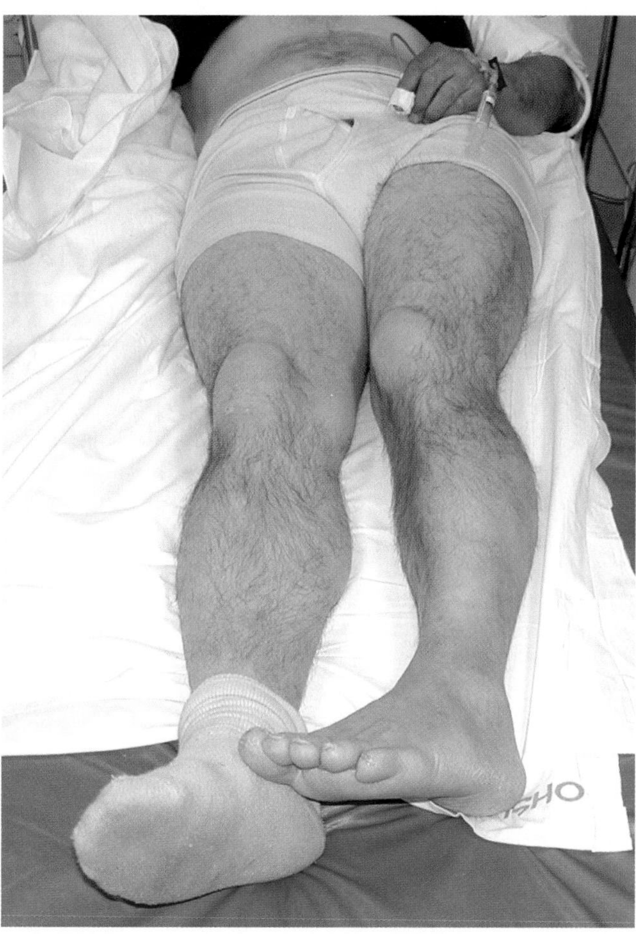

FIGURE 15-58 Posterior dislocation of the left hip. Note shortening and internal rotation. (Courtesy of Robert Hendrickson, MD.)

Diagnosis

This diagnosis usually can be made clinically, based on the history and physical examination. However, plain radiographs of the hip in two views should be obtained before attempts at reduction are made, to identify associated fractures of the acetabulum or femur.[1]

Clinical Complications

Complications include avascular necrosis of the femoral head and post-traumatic arthritis, as well as fractures of the acetabulum and femur. Sciatic nerve injury has been reported approximately 10% of cases involving posterior dislocations.[1] Central dislocations are especially prone to excessive blood loss.[1]

Management

As soon as the patient has been stabilized following the advanced trauma life support (ATLS) protocols, an attempt at close reduction, facilitated by conscious sedation, should be made. The only exception to this rule is in the setting of an associated femoral neck or shaft fracture, in which case open reduction with internal fixation is the treatment of choice. Inability to reduce the dislocation easily is usually due to interposed soft tissue, cartilage, or bone and is also an indication for open reduction. Once the hip has been reduced clinically, radiography or computed tomography should confirm its correct position and help to identify occult fractures and interposed bone chips and soft tissues.[1]

REFERENCES

1. Rudman N, McIlmail D. Emergency department evaluation and treatment of hip and thigh injuries. *Emerg Med Clin North Am* 2000;18:29–66.

Hip and Femur Fractures

Colleen Campbell

Clinical Presentation

Patients with hip or femur fractures complain of inability to bear weight and have pain in the hip or knee region after a fall or other trauma.

Pathophysiology

Most patients with hip fractures are elderly individuals who present after a simple fall. Impaired vision and reflexes, loss of bone density, and weak muscle tone all contribute to the frequency of hip fracture in the elderly population.[1] Hip fractures in younger patients occur as a result of high-energy trauma, such as a motor vehicle accident or a fall from height.[2] These fractures often are associated with femoral shaft fractures and frequently are missed on initial evaluation. Fractures of the hip are divided into femoral head, neck, trochanteric, intertrochanteric, and subtrochanteric fractures.[1] Ninety percent of hip fractures are femoral neck fractures or intertrochanteric fractures.[1] Subtrochanteric fractures are defined as those that occur below the lesser trochanter to within 5 cm distal to the lesser trochanter. Pathologic fractures are commonly seen in this area.

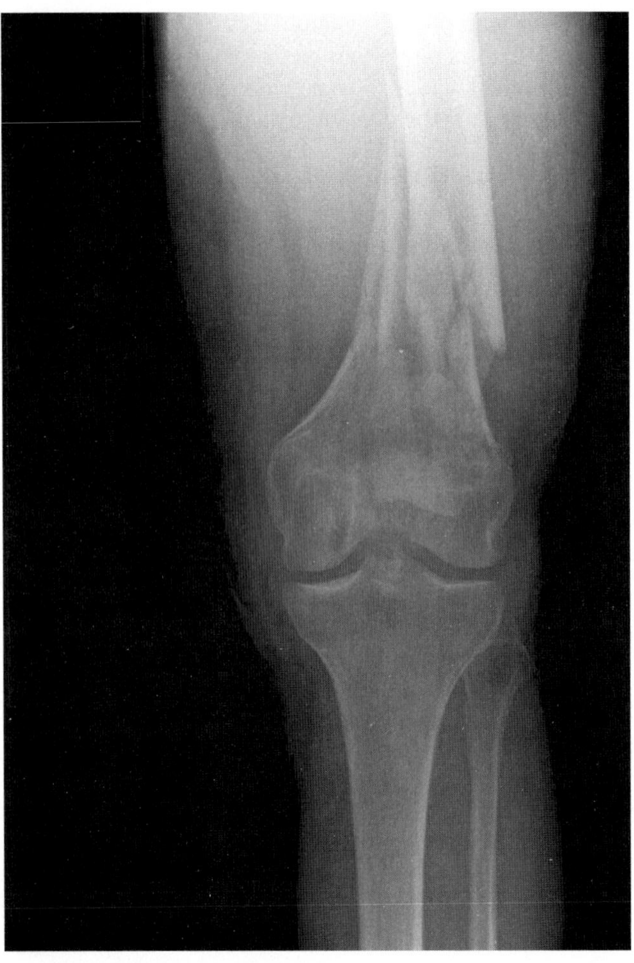

FIGURE 15-59 Comminuted fracture of the distal femur. (Courtesy of Robert Hendrickson, MD.)

Most femur fractures result from high-energy trauma, such as motor vehicle accidents, industrial accidents, gunshot wounds, and falls from height. Femur fractures may result in loss of 1 to 1.5 L of blood in the thigh, but this was not shown (in a retrospective review) to cause hypotensive shock in trauma patients. Stress fractures occur in the femur but are often misdiagnosed initially.[1] Fractures are classified into proximal, middle, and distal thirds, and they are described as transverse, oblique, spiral, or comminuted.[3] Comminuted fractures are further subdivided into four grades by the Winquist classification.[3]

Diagnosis

The diagnosis of hip fracture is based on radiographic findings on anteroposterior and lateral views of the hip. If the plain radiograph is unrevealing and there is a high index of suspicion, magnetic resonance imaging (MRI) or a bone scan may be warranted. Patients may present with the affected leg shortened and externally rotated, especially in intertrochanteric fractures. On examination, swelling, ecchymoses, and focal tenderness may be evident. There is severely limited range of motion secondary to pain.

Diagnosis of femur fracture is made on the basis of radiologic evaluation of the femur, including anteroposterior and lateral views. Both the knee and the pelvis should be imaged as well. Bone scan, MRI, or computed tomography may be necessary to diagnose stress fractures, because plain radiographs usually are negative for 10 to 14 days after the injury.[3] Swelling and deformity are present on examination. Shortening of the affected leg is common. It is imperative to examine the femoral pulses, the dorsalis pedis pulses, and the posterior tibial pulses, and to assess the neurologic status of the leg.

Hip and Femur Fractures

Colleen Campbell

Clinical Complications

Hip fractures in the elderly have an associated 1-year mortality rate of 14% to 36%.[1] Deep venous thrombosis and pulmonary embolus are common complications and are associated with significant morbidity and mortality. Avascular necrosis of the femoral head occurs in 25% of femoral neck fractures.[1] Post-traumatic arthritis is also a common complication. Significant bleeding may result from hip fractures, especially intertrochanteric fractures. Femur fractures can cause significant bleeding and can result in compartmental syndrome.[1] The sciatic nerve or peroneal nerve is rarely injured. Deep venous thrombosis and pulmonary embolus are common complications and have significant associated morbidity and mortality. Fat embolism may occur as well. The superficial femoral artery is rarely injured. Refracture and nonunion are uncommon.[3]

Management

Patients with hip fractures generally require orthopedic consultation for admission and operative repair. Operative repair may employ a variety of hardware, including cannulated screws, compression hip screws, and hemiarthroplasty.[2] Some isolated trochanteric fractures may be managed initially with rest and crutches.[2] Pain control can be achieved through use of intravenous medications or a femoral nerve block. A femoral nerve block may be achieved by injecting 20 mL of 0.5% bupivacaine 2 cm below the inguinal ligament and lateral to the femoral artery.[1]

Traction splints should be applied by emergency medical services (EMS) personnel for suspected femur fractures, to reduce the risk of neurovascular injury. Pneumatic antishock garments are sometimes applied by EMS to limit bleeding. Loss of pulse necessitates immediate reduction. Closed intramedullary nailing and retrograde nailing are the most common techniques used to repair fractures of the femoral shaft. External fixators are used for severely comminuted open fractures.[3] Fractures secondary to gunshot wounds are treated as closed fractures and do not require the same degree of irrigation and débridement that open fractures do.[1,3]

REFERENCES

1. Rudman N, McIlmail D. Emergency department evaluation and treatment of hip and thigh injuries. *Emerg Med Clin North Am* 2000;18:29–66.
2. Schmidt AH, Swiontkowski MF. Femoral neck fractures. *Orthop Clin North Am* 2002;33:97–111.
3. Ostrum RF, Verghese GB, Santner TJ. The lack of association between femoral shaft fractures and hypotensive shock. *J Orthop Trauma* 1993;7:338–342.

Slipped Capital Femoral Epiphysis

Carla Valentine

Clinical Presentation

Slipped capital femoral epiphysis (SCFE) occurs most commonly in young people 10 to 15 years of age, with boys affected more often than girls.[1] African-Americans are affected more commonly than Caucasians.[1] The most common scenario is an obese, teenage African-American male with antalgic gait presenting with knee, hip, or groin pain after an activity. The affected extremity is adducted and externally rotated with limited abduction and internal rotation. In some cases, the disorder is bilateral.

Pathophysiology

The cause of SCFE is unclear. During the periadolescent period, the growth plate shifts from a horizontal to an oblique position and overweight conditions may add strain. Associated endocrine abnormalities (e.g., hypothyroidism) may delay puberty and bone maturity. Genetic predisposition may also play a role.

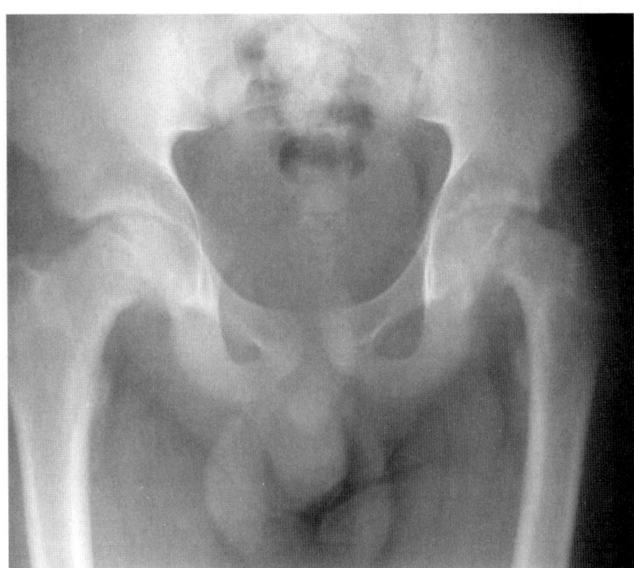

FIGURE 15-60 Slipped capital femoral epiphysis. (Courtesy of Christy Salvaggio, MD.)

Diagnosis

A hip radiographic series, including anteroposterior view (to evaluate for medial slip), lateral view, and frog-leg lateral view (to evaluate for posterior slip), should be obtained. Inferoposterior slippage of the femoral head with loss of Shenton's line may be visible.

Clinical Complications

Diagnosis may be difficult because of referral of pain to distant sites. The most common complication of SCFE is avascular necrosis of the femoral head, which is reported in approximately 15% of patients.[2] Chondrolysis secondary to pinning treatment may occur, with associated osteoarthritis.[3] Coxa vara is another complication with resultant leg-length discrepancy.

Management

Orthopedic consultation should be obtained. The child should remain non-weight bearing to prevent further slippage and should be admitted for open reduction with internal fixation, with hip immobilization.[2]

REFERENCES

1. Richards BS. Slipped capital femoral epiphysis. *Pediatr Rev* 1996; 17:69–70.
2. Perron AD, Miller MD, Brady WJ. Orthopedic pitfalls in the ED: slipped capital femoral epiphysis. *Am J Emerg Med* 2002;20: 484–487.
3. Loder RT. Slipped capital femoral epiphysis in children. *Curr Opin Pediatr* 1995;7:95–97.

Avascular Necrosis

James Nelson and Colleen Campbell

Clinical Presentation

The most common sites for avascular necrosis (AVM) are the femoral head, talus, and scaphoid, but the presentation of AVM varies according to location of infarction. Physical examination reveals limitation of range of motion and pain over the involved bone.

Pathophysiology

AVN, or osteonecrosis, is characterized by ischemic bone death. It is sometimes called aseptic necrosis.[1,2] Important risk factors include vascular disruption, corticosteroids, vascular pathology, alcoholism, renal failure, and hemoglobinopathy. In 20% of cases, no cause is identifiable.[2] Regardless of the contributing factors, AVN is characterized by ischemic bone death. Vascular injury leads to focal ischemia of the bone. This may occur secondary to mechanical insult, as in fractures and dislocations, or secondary to corticosteroid use.[2] Other causes include thrombosis, microangiopathy (i.e., sickle cell disease), embolism, and vasculitis.

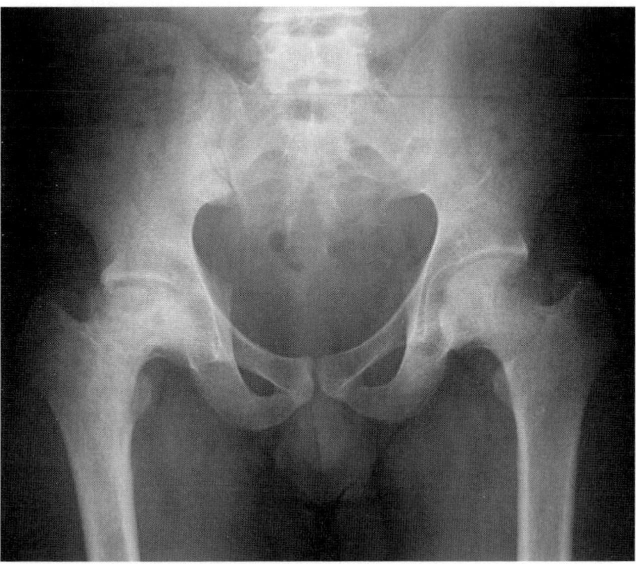

FIGURE 15–61 Bilateral avascular necrosis of the femoral heads. (Courtesy of Mark Silverberg, MD.)

Diagnosis

Anteroposterior pelvis and lateral frog-leg radiographs may reveal sclerosis as one of the earliest radiographic signs of AVN. Subchondral collapse is identifiable by the crescent sign, which is a radiolucency under the cartilage rim.

Clinical Complications

The opposite hip is affected in 50% of patients, and it should be included in radiographic studies.[1] The disease tends to progress despite medical interventions.

Management

Treatment varies according to severity. Conservative therapy with nonsteroidal antiinflammatory drugs (NSAIDs) and partial weight bearing with crutches does not prevent the progression of the disease. With collapse of the femoral head, arthroplasty is indicated.[1,2]

REFERENCES

1. Arlet J. Nontraumatic avascular necrosis of the femoral head: past, present, and future. *Clin Orthop* 1992;(277):12–21.
2. Lee CC, Syed H, Crupi RS. Avascular necrosis of common bones seen in the ED. *Am J Emerg Med* 2003;21:336–338.

Osteochondritis Dissecans

Colleen Campbell

Clinical Presentation

Most patients with osteochondritis dissecans (OD) present with knee pain that has been insidious in onset and intermittent in nature.[1] Patients give a history of being involved in sports with repetitive motions. Joint stiffness and sensations of "catching" or "giving away" are common presenting complaints.[2]

Pathophysiology

OD is an inflammatory disorder of the bone and cartilage that affects adolescents. OD occurs when a focal area of subchondral bone undergoes necrosis, resulting in breakdown of the underlying cartilage.[1,3] This may occur before or after physeal closure.[2] Onset of symptoms occurs between the ages of 11 and 18 years, with 13 being the most common age at presentation. Between 20% and 30% of cases are bilateral.[2] The femoral condyle is affected in 75% of cases.[1] Less commonly, the talar dome or capitellum of the humerus is affected. This condition can affect the humeral capitellum in baseball pitchers and gymnasts. If the humerus is affected, the condition is known as "little leaguers' elbow" and is thought to arise from a repetitive valgus stress on the elbow.[1]

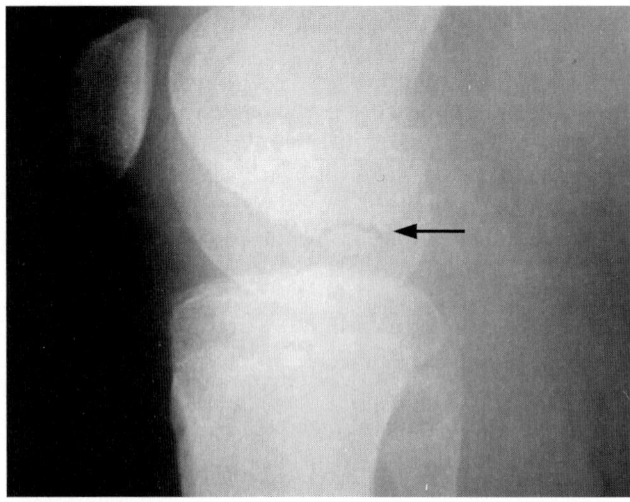

FIGURE 15-62 Osteochondritis dissecans of the distal femur. (Courtesy of Mark Silverberg, MD.)

Diagnosis

Diagnosis is made by radiographic evaluation of the involved joint. A tunnel view is required in addition to anteroposterior and lateral radiographs of the knee.[2] Radiographs show bony lucencies within the joint and cystic changes within the involved area of bone.[3] Magnetic resonance imaging (MRI) is used to evaluate the stability of the lesion.[3] Swelling and joint-line tenderness are evident on physical examination, with limited extension being the most important finding. Crepitus and hemarthrosis may also be present. Patients with elbow involvement have a similar limitation of extension, pain to palpation of the elbow, and possible joint effusion.[1]

Clinical Complications

Complications include osteoarthritis and chronic limitation of motion.

Management

Most cases are treated conservatively, with rest and restriction from athletic activity. If MRI findings classify the lesion as unstable, operative repair may be necessary. This can usually be accomplished via arthroscopy.[2]

REFERENCES

1. Hogan KA, Gross RH. Overuse injuries in pediatric athletes. *Orthop Clin North Am* 2003;34:405–415.
2. Hickson AL, Gibbs LM. Osteochondritis dissecans: a diagnosis not to miss. *Am Fam Physician* 2000;61:151–156.
3. Wall E, Von Stein D. Juvenile osteochondritis dissecans. *Orthop Clin North Am* 2003;34:341–353.

Tenosynovitis

Michael Greenberg and Tyler Vadeboncoeur

Clinical Presentation

Patients with tenosynovitis present with pain, swelling, and decreased range of motion at or near the course, origin, or insertion of a tendon. One of the most common forms of tenosynovitis is DeQuervain's stenosing tenosynovitis, which is tenosynovitis involving the first dorsal compartment.[1,2]

Pathophysiology

Tenosynovitis is an inflammatory condition involving tissues of the tendon sheath. In most instances, it is caused by repetitive friction due to mechanical overuse. Several forms of tenosynovitis have been recognized, including acute inflammatory conditions such as gout or arthritis, infectious tenosynovitis (e.g., disseminated gonorrhea), and stenosing tenosynovitis (e.g., DeQuervain's).[1,2]

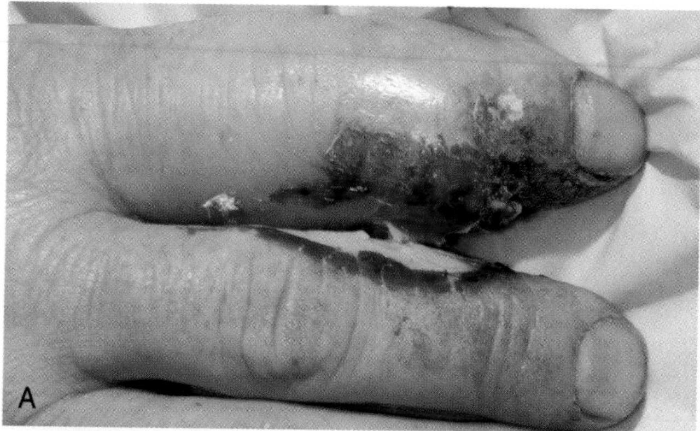

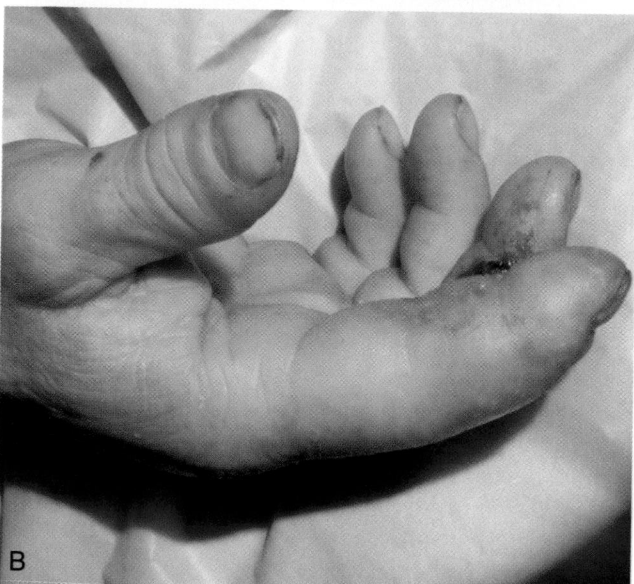

FIGURE 15–63 **A:** Tenosynovitis. **B:** Note fusiform swelling, redness, and digit held in slight flexion. (**A** and **B,** Courtesy of Robert Hendrickson, MD.)

Diagnosis

The diagnosis is based on history and physical examination; there are no specific laboratory or imaging studies. On examination, the patient has tenderness along the course of the tendon, which may be swollen and slightly warm. Crepitations may be appreciated if the tendon is gently palpated while being put through a range of motion. Exquisite pain on passive extension of the tendon may also be present. DeQuervain's tenosynovitis is characterized by a positive Finklestein test (pain on active flexion with the thumb volarly flexed within the fist).[1,2] In many cases involving the digits, Kanavel's four cardinal signs of tenosynovitis may be present and may help differentiate tenosynovitis from other soft-tissue infections. These signs are tenderness along the course of the flexor tendon, fusiform swelling of the digit, pain on passive extension, and a flexed resting position of the finger. All four signs may not be present in every case.

Clinical Complications

Complications include chronicity and disability. If the cause is infectious, complications include abscess formation, spread to contiguous structures, destruction of tendons, osteomyelitis, and systemic spread.[1,2]

Management

For infectious causes, hospitalization with open débridement and irrigation in the operating theater is frequently necessary. Tenosynovitis of inflammatory origin may be treated with elevation, frequent moist-heat applications, nonsteroidal antiinflammatory drugs (NSAIDs), and resting of the injured part with rigid splinting.[1,2]

REFERENCES

1. Moore JS. De Quervain's tenosynovitis: stenosing tenosynovitis of the first dorsal compartment. *J Occup Environ Med* 1997;39: 990–1002.
2. Almekinders LC, Temple JD. Etiology, diagnosis, and treatment of tendonitis: an analysis of the literature. *Med Sci Sports Exerc* 1998; 30:1183–1190.

Knee Dislocations

Mark Silverberg

Clinical Presentation

Knee dislocations (KDs) are uncommon injuries that may be associated with substantial traumatic mechanisms.

Pathophysiology

A KD is a complete disruption of the joint such that the articular surfaces of the tibia and femur are no longer touching. Subluxation is similar, but the articular surfaces remain partially opposed.[1] The most commonly reported cause is motor vehicle collision, although industrial accidents, farm-related injuries, and sports injuries are also common causes for KD. Forces directed against the flexed knee may displace the tibia posteriorly (dorsally), leaving the knee posteriorly dislocated.[1] Anterior KDs result from an axial load applied against a hyperextended knee, such as may occur in a fall in a vertical position or even under the stress of severe obesity.[1] Substantial valgus and varus stresses may lead to lateral and medial dislocations when both collateral ligaments are disrupted.[1]

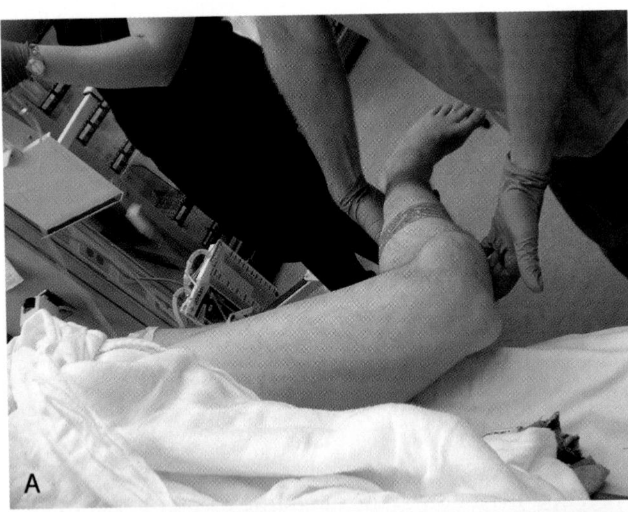

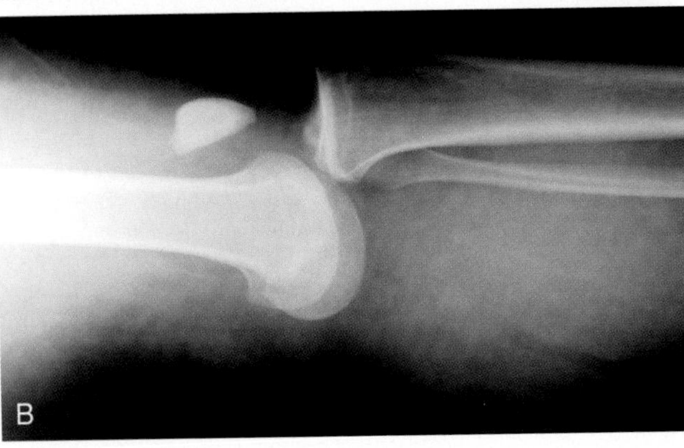

FIGURE 15–64 **A:** Posterior knee dislocation. (Courtesy of Robert Hendrickson, MD.) **B:** Anterior knee dislocation. (Courtesy of John Fojtik, MD.)

Diagnosis

KDs are usually diagnosed clinically. However, if spontaneous reduction has occurred before arrival at the emergency department, diagnosis can be problematic. Physical examination may reveal instability of the knee's ligamentous structures, with the tibia dislodged anteriorly (most common), posteriorly, medially, or laterally. Because vascular injuries are common with KDs, distal pulses may be diminished or absent.[1] Consequently, all bicruciate ligament tears should be considered to be KDs until proven otherwise.[1]

Clinical Complications

KDs usually result in disruption of two or more of the major knee ligaments.[1] The popliteal artery can be stretched, torn, or transected, which can cause limb-threatening vascular compromise. Tibial and peroneal nerve injuries have been reported, along with tibial plateau and supracondylar femur fractures.

Management

Rapid orthopedic consultation is imperative for these injuries, and a vascular surgeon may also be required if popliteal-artery injury is suspected. Once reduced, the knee should be splinted in a neutral position. If a vascular injury is suspected, angiography is recommended. However, in the presence of obvious vascular deficits, time should not be wasted getting angiography; rather, the patient should be taken directly to the operating room for limb-saving vascular repair. Patients who have consistently good pedal pulses and no signs or symptoms of ischemia may be closely monitored and do not require arteriography, although pulses must be checked hourly.[1] The patient should be given analgesics but should not be overmedicated, because overmedication might interfere with the ability to accurately report limb-threatening ischemic pain.[1]

REFERENCES

1. Brautigan B, Johnson DL. The epidemiology of knee dislocations. *Clin Sports Med* 2000;19:387–397.

Patellar Dislocations

Mark Silverberg

Clinical Presentation

Many patients with a patellar dislocation (PD) have spontaneous reduction before arrival at the emergency department. However, if the patella remains dislocated, it can easily be seen and palpated outside its correct anatomic location, usually lateral to its normal position while the knee is stuck in a flexed position.[1,2] Patella alta is often seen after reduction, and the medial retinaculum may be tender along the patellofemoral ligament or at the patella-quadriceps junction. Hemarthrosis may also be present.[2] Generalized ligamentous laxity should be evaluated to assure that additional knee ligaments have not been disrupted, and neurovascular status should be checked.[2]

Pathophysiology

PDs result from noncontact mechanisms with the knee flexed and the limb rotated.[1] Specific anatomic conformations may predispose to PD. The "patella at risk" may display patella alta, flattening of the femoral sulcus angle, trochlear dysplasia, quadriceps muscular weakness or imbalance, and excessive passive lateral patellar mobility.[1,2]

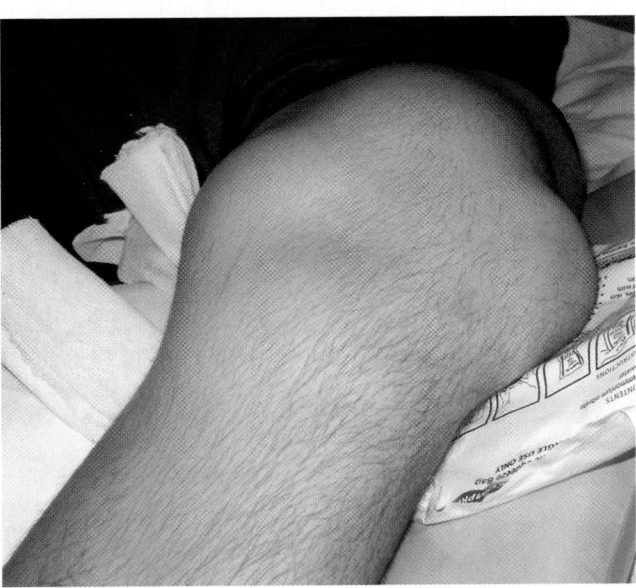

FIGURE 15–65 Lateral patella dislocation (prereduction). (Courtesy of Madelyn Garcia, MD.)

Diagnosis

The diagnosis usually can be made clinically. However, radiographic confirmation should include anteroposterior, lateral, and axial radiographs of the knee. A computed tomographic (CT) scan may be used to analyze the patellofemoral joint with the knee in less than 30 degrees of flexion. Additional knee injuries may occur in conjunction with PD, so other modalities, such as ultrasonography, arthrography, cine CT, CT arthrography, static and ultrafast magnetic resonance imaging (MRI), radionuclide imaging, and single-photon emission computed tomography (SPECT) scanning, may assist clinicians in diagnosing and characterizing the injury.[1]

Clinical Complications

Complications include recurrence (17% to 44% of cases), failure to return to previous levels of sports activity (55% of cases), osteochondral fractures, ligament tears, and cartilage injuries.[2]

Management

Reduction of PDs usually occurs spontaneously with knee extension. However, slight medial traction on the patella may be applied if flexion alone fails.[2] Nonoperative management of first-time PDs in a knee immobilizer is the preferred method of treatment. If that fails or redislocation occurs, various surgical techniques are available to resolve patellar laxity.

REFERENCES

1. Arendt EA, Fithian DC, Cohen E. Current concepts of lateral patella dislocation. *Clin Sports Med* 2002;21:499–519.
2. Iobst CA, Stanitski CL. Acute knee injuries. *Clin Sports Med* 2000; 19:621–635.

Tibial Plateau Fractures

Colleen Campbell

Clinical Presentation

Patients with tibial plateau fractures (TPFs) present with knee pain, effusion, and inability to bear weight.

Pathophysiology

A TPF is a fracture of the proximal tibia that involves the articular surface. The mechanism of injury involves axial compression combined with a lateral force at the knee (varus or valgus).[1] The distal femur compresses on the tibial plateau to create the fracture. In most cases (55% to 75%), the lateral tibial plateau is involved.[1] This injury most often occurs in victims of motor vehicle accidents and in older patients, but it is also seen after sports injuries, including skiing, soccer, and football.[1]

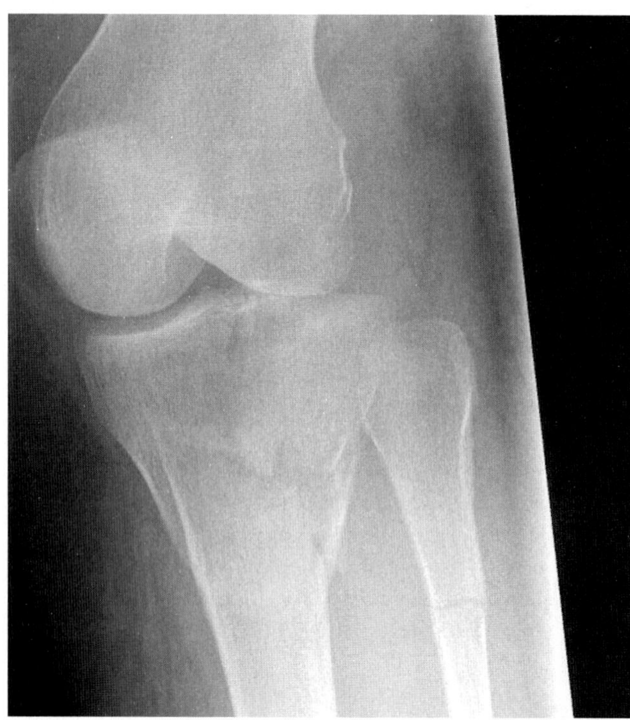

FIGURE 15–66 Anteroposterior view of comminuted tibial plateau fracture and proximal fibula fracture. (Courtesy of Eric Rueckmann, MD.)

Diagnosis

Joint-line tenderness is elicited on examination. On physical examination, patients have limited range of motion (less than 90 degrees of flexion) and pain with range of motion. Ecchymoses may also be present on examination. Care must be taken to examine soft tissues and skin for evidence of open fracture. The diagnosis is made using standard anteroposterior and lateral plain radiographs. Additional views to show the condyles include 40-degree internal and external oblique views.[1] Computed tomography with a spiral scanner (2-mm cuts) may be especially helpful. Magnetic resonance imaging is more useful in the evaluation of associated soft-tissue injury.[2]

Clinical Complications

In 25% to 50% of cases, high-energy TPFs are associated with soft-tissue injuries, most commonly meniscal and anterior cruciate injuries.[1,2] The medial collateral ligament also is commonly injured. It is important to recognize the potential for peroneal nerve injury associated with TPF. Deep venous thrombosis is a common complication of TPF, and prophylaxis is recommended routinely.[1] Compartment syndrome is another common complication of TPF, and post-traumatic arthritis of the knee also occurs.

Management

Nondisplaced TPFs may be treated nonoperatively in a long-leg cast with no weight bearing for 6 weeks. Operative treatment is indicated for arterial injury, compartment syndrome, or significant depression (3 mm or more).[1]

REFERENCES

1. Bharam S, Vrahas MS, Fu FH. Knee fractures in the athlete. *Orthop Clin North Am* 2002;33:565–574.
2. Pretorius ES, Fishman EK. Spiral computed tomography and three-dimensional CT of musculoskeletal pathology: emergency room applications. *Radiol Clin North Am* 1999;37:953–974.

Hemarthrosis

Mary Anne Fuchs

Clinical Presentation

Patients with hemarthrosis present with joint pain, swelling, and diminished range of motion, either spontaneously or after a traumatic injury.[1]

Pathophysiology

The rapid development of joint swelling after trauma suggests a major ligamentous injury or an intraarticular fracture.[2] In the absence of trauma, an acute hemarthrosis is most likely related to a bleeding diathesis.[1,2] In rare cases, joint neoplasm or pigmented villonodular synovitis may cause bleeding.[2] The knee is the most commonly affected joint, followed by the elbow and the ankle, but any large joint may be involved.

Diagnosis

Hemorrhagic synovial fluid in these cases is diffusely bloody, generally has high viscosity, has a white blood cell count of less than 5,000/mm[1,2], and has less than 25% polymorphonuclear neutrophils. The glucose level should be almost equal to the serum concentration, and the lactate level should be less than 6. There should be no apparent crystals, no organisms on Gram staining, and negative cultures.[1] The presence of a bleeding diathesis may be confirmed with a prothrombin time and partial thromboplastin time.[1] In traumatic hemarthrosis, mechanism of injury and physical examination often serve to diagnose the injury. Aspiration of a hemarthrosis may be necessary for pain relief and to allow adequate examination of the joint for ligamentous injuries. The presence of fat globules in the joint aspirate is diagnostic of a cortical fracture.[2] Radiographs are indicated, and magnetic resonance imaging may be useful.[1,2]

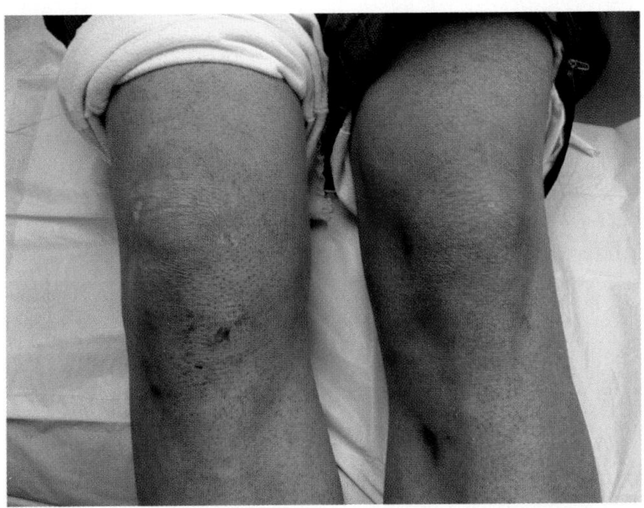

FIGURE 15–67 Clinically obvious effusion of the right knee. (Courtesy of Robert Hendrickson, MD.)

Clinical Complications

Blood is a synovial-fluid irritant, and elevated pressure in the joint can damage cartilage.[1,2] Large hemarthroses may lead to persistent pain and chronic joint dysfunction if not aspirated.[1]

Management

With traumatic hemarthroses, in the absence of joint instability requiring early surgical intervention, immobilization and rest are adequate initial therapy.[2] Aspiration of the fluid may be done to aid diagnosis and to alleviate pain.[1,2] Treatment of hemarthroses associated with bleeding diatheses involves replacement of the deficient clotting factor, aspiration of the hemarthrosis, analgesia, and immobilization. Aspiration should be performed immediately after factor replacement to avoid excessive bleeding and coagulation of the hemarthrosis. Patients should be referred for follow-up. Ice and analgesics are important adjuncts to treatment, but salicylates and nonsteroidal antiinflammatory drugs (NSAIDs) can aggravate bleeding by inhibiting platelet function.[2]

REFERENCES

1. Baker CL. Acute hemarthrosis of the knee. *J Med Assoc Ga* 1992;81:301–305.
2. Preslar AJ 3rd, Heckman JD. Emergency department evaluation of the swollen joint. *Emerg Med Clin North Am* 1984;2:425–440.

Patellar Fractures

Colleen Campbell

Clinical Presentation

Patients with patellar fracture present with pain and swelling directly over the patella. Crepitus and a palpable defect, as well as hemarthrosis, are often evident on examination. Athletes may present with pain over the patella after activities involving rapid jumping or powerful quadriceps flexion, such as in basketball or volleyball. Patients with avulsion injuries may demonstrate weakness on straight-leg extension.[1]

Pathophysiology

Patellar fractures may be stellate, transverse, vertical, or avulsive. Athletes often present with transverse fractures, whereas older people who have fallen directly on the patella are more likely to have stellate fractures.[1] Many patellar fractures occur as a result of motor vehicle accidents, when the flexed knee is compressed against the dashboard.[2] Vertical fractures occur in association with patellar dislocation.[1] Open fractures may result from the superficial location of the patella.

Diagnosis

The diagnosis is made based on the history, physical examination, and radiographic evaluation. Radiographs include anteroposterior and lateral views. A 45-degree tangential view, or "sunrise" view, can further elucidate nondisplaced fractures.[2] Removal of a hemarthrosis using sterile technique and arthrocentesis, followed by injection of lidocaine, may facilitate examination and range-of-motion testing.[2] If an open fracture cannot be confirmed based on examination alone, arthrocentesis and injection of sterile saline may be necessary to determine whether the joint is involved.

Clinical Complications

Retinacular tears occur in association with patellar fractures. Loss of reduction can occur after fixation, or hardware can cause soft-tissue irritation, necessitating eventual removal. Osteoarthritis and loss of range of motion also occur.[2]

Management

Nondisplaced fractures are treated initially with a knee immobilizer and crutches, followed by full extension casts for 4 to 6 weeks. Open reduction and internal fixation is required if more than 2 mm of displacement is present.[1]

REFERENCES

1. Bharam S, Vrahas MS, Fu FH. Knee fractures in the athlete. *Orthop Clin North Am* 2002;33:565–574.
2. Roberts DM, Stallard TC. Emergency department evaluation and treatment of knee and leg injuries. *Emerg Med Clin North Am* 2000; 18:67–84.

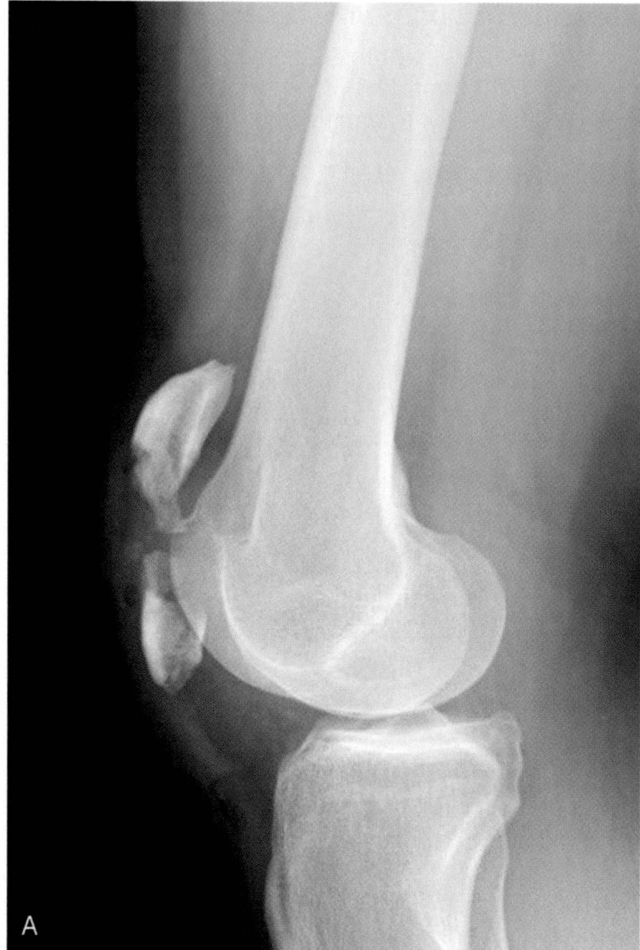

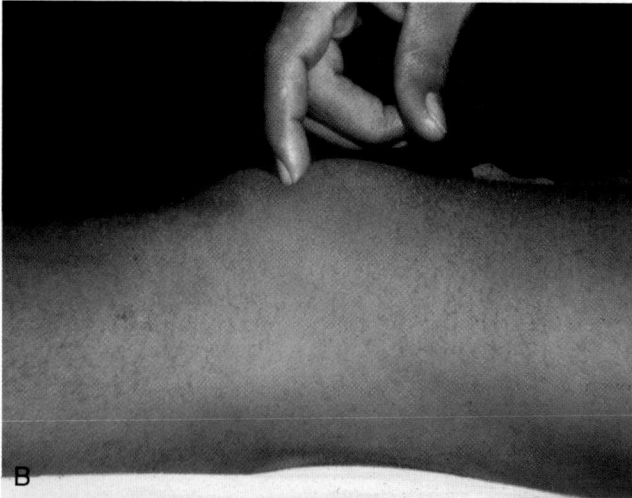

FIGURE 15–68 **A:** Patellar fracture, lateral. (Courtesy of Tim Lum, MD.) **B:** Clinically obvious patellar fracture. (Courtesy of David K. Wagner, MD.)

Patellar Tendon Rupture

Colleen Campbell

Clinical Presentation

Patients with patellar tendon ruptures present with pain in the knee area and inability to walk. Men younger than 40 years of age are most often affected.[1]

Pathophysiology

Patellar tendon ruptures may result from chronic inflammation and weakness, sometimes in association with steroid injections or systemic steroid use. Rupture can occur on forceful contraction of the quadriceps while the leg is held in a relatively fixed position. Bilateral rupture occurs infrequently and is more common in diabetics.[1]

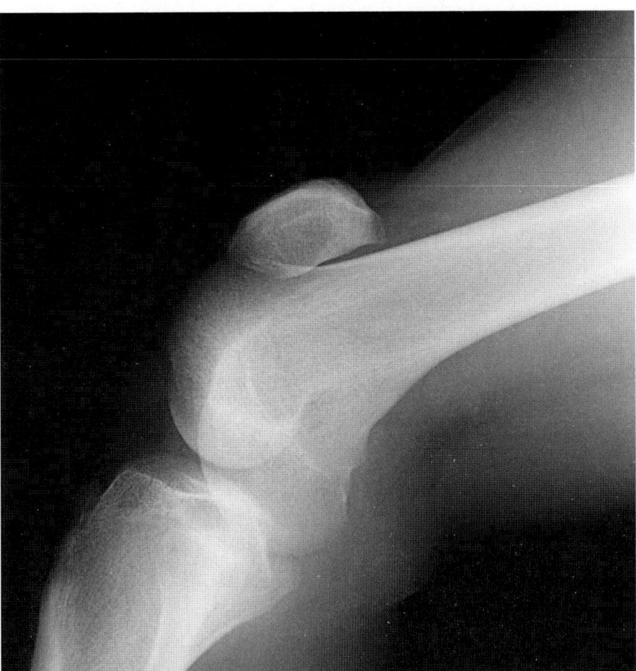

FIGURE 15–69 Note high-riding patella, consistent with patellar tendon rupture. (Courtesy of Mark Silverberg, MD.)

Diagnosis

Diagnosis is made on the basis of physical examination and is confirmed by magnetic resonance imaging. Patients may report a history of sports-related injury after jumping. Other consistent histories include that of chronic pain at the patellar tendon or steroid injections in the area. Swelling is evident around the patellar tendon, and a palpable defect may be present, usually at the inferior aspect of the tendon. On physical examination, the patella appears "high-riding." Plain radiographs should be performed to exclude accompanying patellar avulsion fractures. Weakness or inability to perform unassisted straight-leg raising is evident on examination.

Clinical Complications

Patellar avulsion fractures may be associated with patellar tendon tears. Associated retinacular tears are almost always present.[1] Limited flexion of the knee, patella baja, or chronic pain and weakness may complicate patellar rupture, and patellar tracking may be altered after this injury.[1]

Management

Patellar tendon ruptures require orthopedic consultation. Treatment of patellar tendon rupture is surgical unless the tear is incomplete. Incomplete lesions are treated with a cylindrical cast in extension for 6 weeks.[1]

REFERENCES

1. Marder RA, Timmerman LA. Primary repair of patellar tendon rupture without augmentation. *Am J Sports Med* 1999;27:304–307.

Tibial Tubercle Avulsion (Watson-Jones Fracture)

Colleen Campbell

Clinical Presentation

Patients with tibial tubercle avulsions present with swelling and tenderness at the tibial tubercle after violent quadriceps contraction.

Pathophysiology

Tibial tubercle avulsions are classified by the Watson-Jones system. Most of these fractures occur during sports or other play with forceful quadriceps contraction.[1] Boys present with this injury usually between the ages of 14 and 17 years, corresponding to the epiphyseal stage of fusion of the proximal tibia.[1] The Watson-Jones classification system divides these fractures into three types. Type I is a distal physis avulsion through the secondary ossification center. Type II involves an anterior extension of the fracture through to the proximal tibial epiphysis at the junction of the primary and secondary ossification centers. Type III extends through the primary ossification center proximally and is intraarticular; it is a Salter-Harris type III variant.[2]

Diagnosis

Standard radiographs of the knee are required. Diagnosis is made from a lateral knee film with the tibia in slight internal rotation.[2] Soft-tissue films delineate the margins of the patellar ligament.[2] The tubercle fragment may be palpable and freely moving, with a corresponding palpable defect in the tubercle. The knee is held flexed at 20 to 40 degrees. Joint effusion is often present.[1]

Clinical Complications

Complications include compartment syndrome, malunion, nonunion, and deep venous thrombosis.[1] Patients may have associated meniscal tears or anterior cruciate tears. Genu recurvatum can result if the anterior growth plate fuses prematurely. Loss of knee flexion is a long-term complication.

Management

Urgent orthopedic referral is necessary. For minimally displaced fractures, the leg is immobilized with the knee in extension and the hips partially flexed.[2] Patients remain non–weight bearing for 4 to 6 weeks. Open reduction with internal fixation is necessary for type II and III fractures.[1]

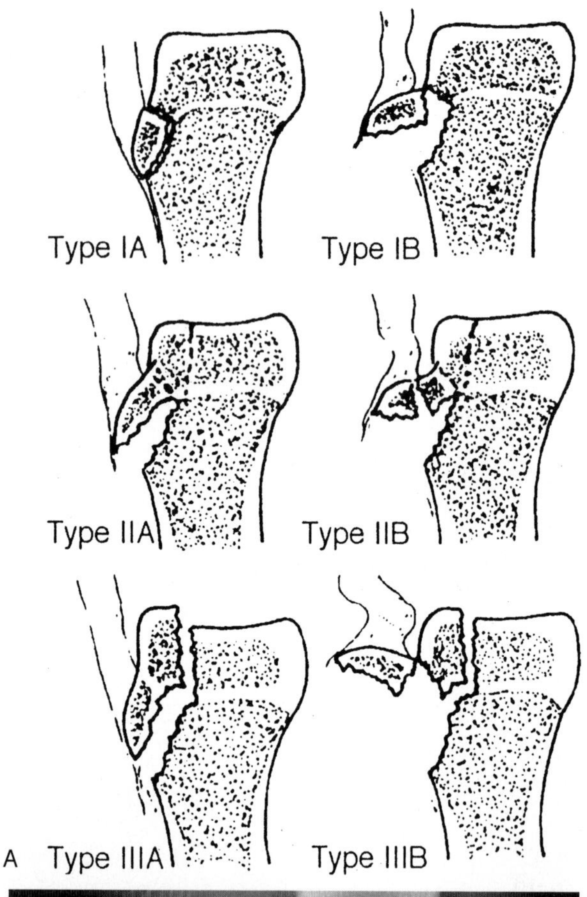

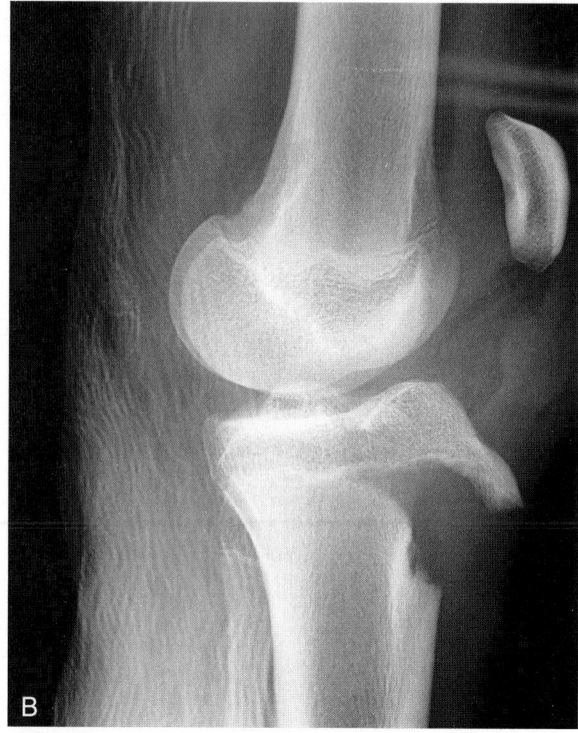

FIGURE 15–70 **A:** Ogden classification of tibial tuberosity fractures in children. (From Ogden, with permission.) **B:** Type IIA (Ogden) tibial tuberosity fracture. (Courtesy of Mark Silverberg, MD.)

REFERENCES

1. McKoy BE, Stanitski CL. Acute tibial tubercle avulsion fractures. *Orthop Clin North Am* 2003;34:397–403.
2. Spinseller PD, Stanitski CL. Tibial tubercle fractures. In: Beaty JH, Kasser JR, eds. *Rockwood and Wilkins' fractures in children.* Philadelphia: Lippincott Williams & Wilkins, 2001:1019–1026.

Plantaris Tendon Rupture

Colleen Campbell

Clinical Presentation

Patients with plantaris tendon ruptures may present after sudden twisting associated with an audible "snap" perceived in the calf. This is accompanied by an acute onset of pain or burning in the calf and variable amounts of swelling.[1]

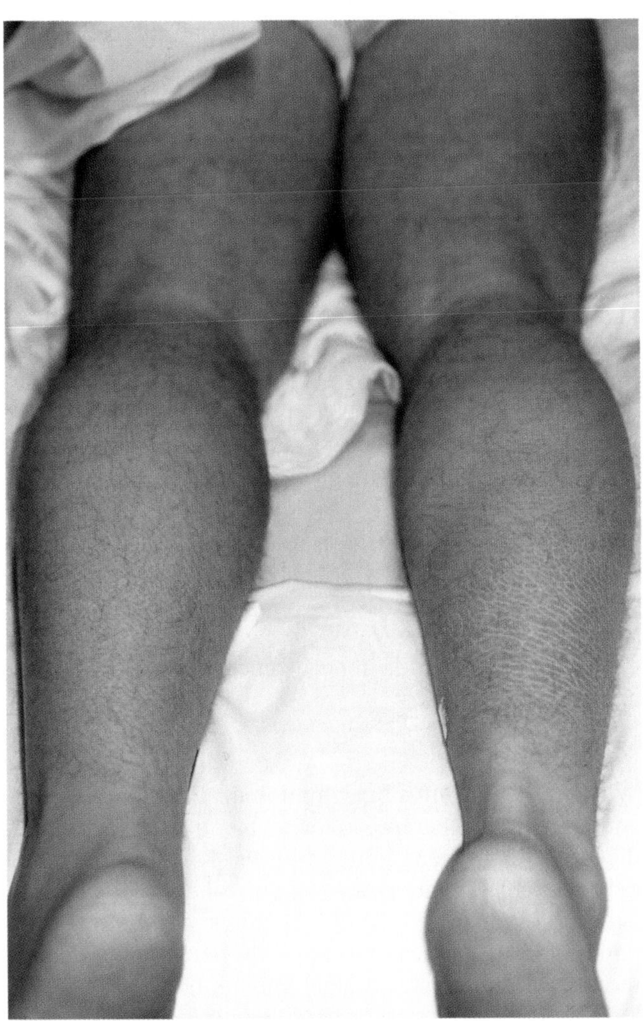

FIGURE 15–71 Note swelling of the calf, consistent with plantaris tendon rupture. (Copyright James R. Roberts, MD.)

Pathophysiology

Patients with this disorder are often described as "weekend warriors." Patients are often in their fourth decade of life. This injury occurs frequently in tennis and is sometimes referred to as "tennis leg." This injury may be confused with a tear of the medial head of the gastrocnemius.[1]

Diagnosis

Diagnosis is made on the basis of history and physical examination and can be confirmed by magnetic resonance imaging or ultrasonography. A partial rupture of the Achilles tendon and a tear of the medial gastrocnemius are the main diagnoses that must be differentiated from this entity. Patients have maximal pain between the heads of the gastrocnemius. The Thompson test, or hyperdorsiflexion test, should be performed to rule out Achilles tendon rupture. The hyperdorsiflexion test is done against resistance while the patient is prone, with weakness indicating a tear of the Achilles tendon.[1]

Clinical Complications

Compartment syndrome may complicate plantaris tendon rupture and subsequent calf swelling. Because the plantaris is a vestigial muscle, no long-term weakness is evident after this injury.[1]

Management

Treatment of plantaris tendon rupture requires rest, ice, elevation, and non–weight bearing as needed.[1]

REFERENCES

1. Feied C, Smith M, Handler J, Gillam M. Plantaris Tendon Rupture. Available at: http://www.ncemi.org/cse/cse0928.htm. Accessed June 23, 2004.

Knee Effusion

Mary Anne Fuchs

Clinical Presentation

Patients with knee effusions present with painful or painless swelling of the knee.

Pathophysiology

Traumatic causes of knee effusion include ligamentous, osseous, and meniscal injuries and overuse syndromes. Atraumatic causes include arthritis, infection, crystal deposition, gout, bleeding diatheses, pseudogout, and tumor.[1,2]

Diagnosis

If substantial joint fluid is present, the knee is held in 15 to 25 degrees of flexion.[1] "Milking" of the fluid distally from the suprapatellar pouch and palpation of the area adjacent to the patellar tendon for fluid accumulation facilitate detection of small effusions, and causes the patella to be ballotable.[1] Radiographs are indicated if the patient is unable to bear weight or if an effusion or ecchymosis is present.

Arthrocentesis is the essential tool in diagnosis of atraumatic effusions. Fluid obtained should be sent for cell count, determination of glucose and protein levels, Gram staining, bacterial culture, and special tests (e.g., crystals) as indicated. Joint fluid characteristics can be classified as follows: noninflammatory (200 to 2,000 white blood cells [WBCs]/mm^3), inflammatory (2,000 to 100,000 WBCs/mm^3), septic (more than 50,000 WBCs/mm^3, mostly polymorphonuclear neutrophils), or hemorrhagic (bloody, with a variable WBC count). Presence of organisms on Gram staining and positive cultures indicate an infection. In crystal-induced arthritis, the synovial-fluid WBC count typically ranges from 2,000 to 10,000 WBCs/mm^3 but may be higher in severe cases.[2] The presence of urate crystals is diagnostic of gout. Calcium pyrophosphate crystals, seen in pseudogout, appear as weakly birefringent rectangles or rhomboids. The presence of crystals does not rule out a coexisting infection.[1]

An effusion that develops within 4 to 6 hours after an acute injury is most likely a hemarthrosis and is indicative of a major osseous, ligamentous, or meniscal injury.[1] A cut, deceleration, or hyperextension mechanism of injury, commonly with a "pop," and a sensation of knee instability are typical of anterior cruciate ligament (ACL) injuries. Collateral ligament injuries occur with medial or lateral force to the knee. Postexertional swelling, clicking, and locking and pain with rotational movements are indicative of a meniscal injury.[1]

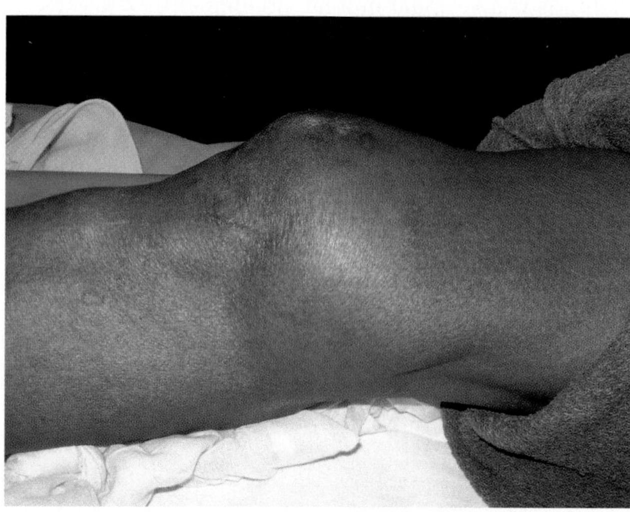

FIGURE 15–72 Knee effusion filling normal median concavity. (Courtesy of Mark Silverberg, MD.)

Clinical Complications

Complications include reoccurrence, joint destruction, and chronic pain.

Management

With traumatic effusions, immobilization and rest are adequate initial therapy, followed by outpatient orthopedic referral. Open joint injuries require operative débridement, irrigation, and parenteral antibiotic administration. Infectious arthritis requires admission, with parenteral antibiotics started in the emergency department, and immediate surgical intervention.

REFERENCES

1. Johnson MW. Acute knee effusions: a systemic approach to diagnosis. *Am Fam Physician* 2000;61:2391–2400.

Osgood-Schlatter Lesion

Colleen Campbell

Clinical Presentation

Symptoms of the Osgood-Schlatter lesion (OS) begin intermittently and are exacerbated by activities involving the quadriceps, such as jumping and running. Half of all patients are able to identify a specific injury, and 25% of patients have bilateral lesions. On examination, tenderness and swelling are localized to the insertion of the patellar ligament.[1] If symptoms have been ongoing, the tibial tubercle may appear prominent. Pain is elicited on forced resistance to quadriceps flexion.[1]

Pathophysiology

OS is a subacute avulsion of an osteochondral fragment of the tibial tubercle. Avulsion of the tibial tubercle occurs as a result of repetitive forceful contraction of the quadriceps. Fibers of the patellar ligament avulse a part of the surface cartilage and secondary ossification center of the tibial tubercle. Subsequent new bone growth occurs between the fragment and the tibial tubercle. The appearance of the lesion corresponds to the apophyseal development in the tibial tubercle, which occurs between the ages of 8 and 12 years in girls and 9 and 14 years in boys.[1]

Diagnosis

Diagnosis is clinical, but radiographs may be helpful. Fragments of the secondary ossification center may be visibly displaced anteriorly and superiorly on a lateral radiograph.[1] Ultrasonography is useful in identifying soft-tissue changes around the knee, including swelling around the tendon and ossification center fragmentation.[2] Magnetic resonance imaging demonstrates a thickened patellar tendon.[2]

Clinical Complications

Complete avulsion of the tibial tubercle may accompany OS. Restricted activity may be necessary for up to 2 years after diagnosis. OS-related knee pain may extend into adulthood.[1,2]

Management

Treatment involves rest and supportive care.[1] Tight hamstrings and quadriceps may contribute to symptoms, so patients should undertake a stretching and strengthening program.[1] If symptoms are severe, a knee immobilizer is required for up to 6 weeks.[1] Some authors recommend steroid injections into the area to reduce scarring.[1] Shaving of the tibial tubercle, after growth is completed, may be necessary for persistent symptoms.[2]

REFERENCES

1. Spinseller PD, Stanitski CL. Osgood Schlatter lesion. In: Beaty JH, Kasser JR, eds. *Rockwood and Wilkins' fractures in children.* Philadelphia: Lippincott Williams & Wilkins, 2001:1026–1028.
2. Hogan KA, Gross RH. Overuse injuries in pediatric athletes. *Orthop Clin North Am* 2003;34:405–407.

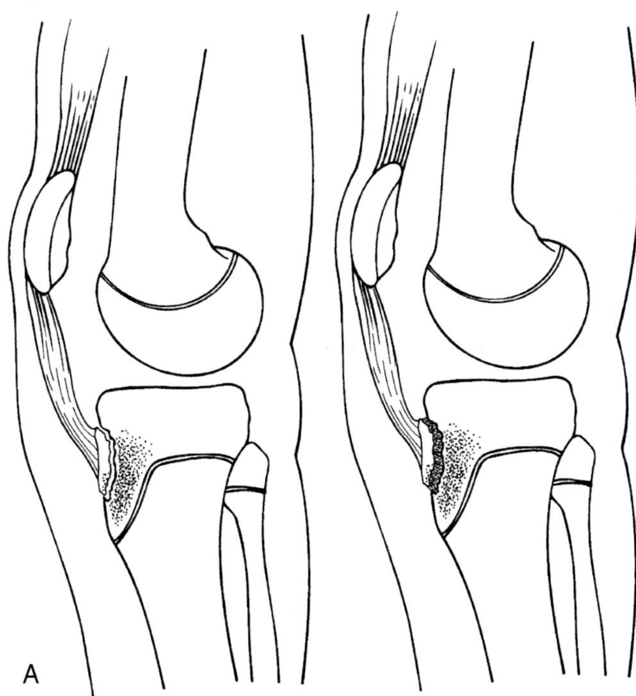

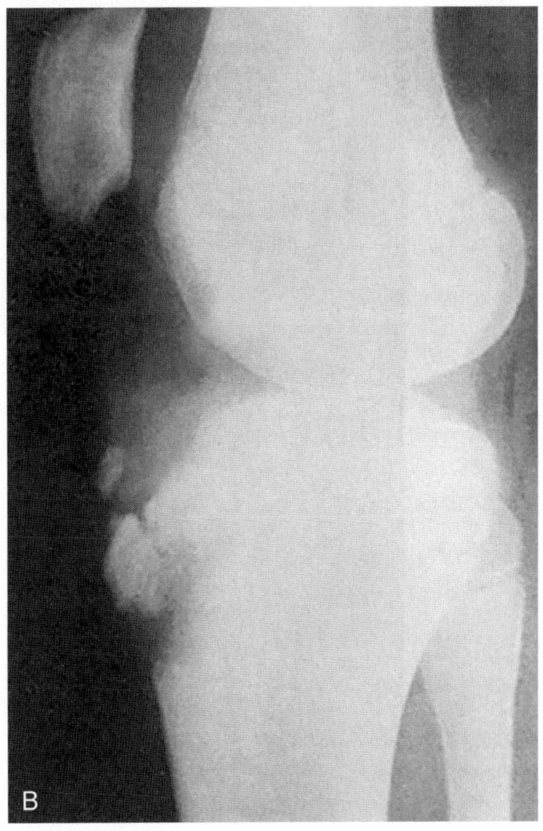

FIGURE 15–73 A: Development of Osgood-Schlatter lesion. Left: Avulsion of osteochondral fragment that includes surface cartilage and a portion of the secondary ossification center of the tibial tubercle. Right: New bone fills in the gap between the avulsed osteochondral fragment and the tibial tubercle. **B:** Extreme example of Osgood-Schlatter lesion. Lateral radiograph shows enlargement of the tibial tubercle, nonunited ossicles, and patella alta. (**A** and **B**, From Beaty, with permission.)

15-74

Maisonneuve Fracture

Colleen Campbell

Clinical Presentation

Patients with Maisonneuve fractures present with ankle swelling, pain, ecchymosis, and inability to bear weight. They may describe a twisting force applied to the planted foot.[1] On examination, there is proximal fibular pain, as well as pain radiating to the ankle when the proximal tibia and fibula are compressed together. There is usually bony point tenderness overlying the medial malleolus. Particular attention to examination of the skin and neurovascular structures is necessary to avoid missing open fractures or damage to peripheral nerves, especially the perineal nerve as it crosses over the head of the fibula.[1]

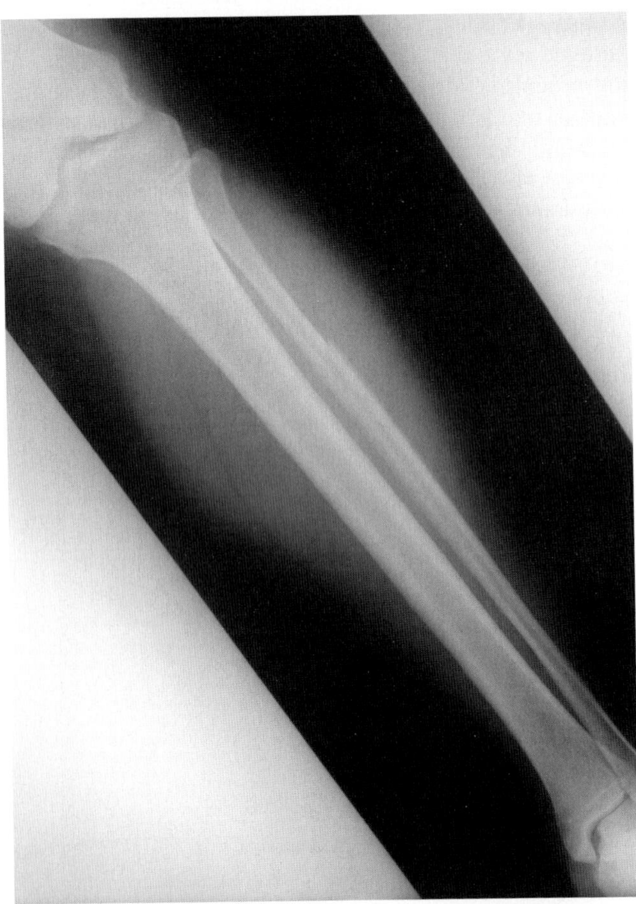

FIGURE 15–74 Maisonneuve fracture. (Courtesy of Robert Hendrickson, MD.)

Pathophysiology

The Maisonneuve fracture is a fracture of the medial malleolus or deltoid ligament disruption combined with an oblique fracture of the proximal fibula and an interosseous ligament disruption.[2] Five percent of ankle fractures are Maisonneuve fractures. The force causing this fracture type is usually pronation combined with external rotation.[3] These injuries often result from participation in sports or from motor vehicle trauma.

Diagnosis

Standard anteroposterior, lateral, and mortise radiographic views of the ankle, combined with full-length tibia/fibula films, are necessary to make the diagnosis. All patients with bimalleolar pain should have full-length tibia/fibula films made. On plain radiographs, the medial joint space of the ankle often appears widened.[1]

Clinical Complications

Complications include compartment syndrome, nonunion, malunion, infection (either postoperatively or as a result of an open fracture), degenerative joint disease, reflex sympathetic dystrophy, and vascular injury.[3] The severity of degenerative joint disease is largely determined by the anatomic alignment of the mortise.[3]

Management

If there is no joint space widening and the mortise is intact, the fracture may be treated with casting and immobilization for 6 to 12 weeks.[1] The medial malleolus requires open reduction with internal fixation in most cases.

REFERENCES

1. Roberts DM, Stallard TC. Emergency department evaluation and treatment of knee and leg injuries. *Emerg Med Clin North Am* 2000; 18:67–84.
2. Wedmore IS, Charette S. Emergency department evaluation and treatment of ankle and foot injuries. *Emerg Med Clin North Am* 2000;18:85–113.
3. Donnato KC. Ankle fractures and syndesmosis injuries. *Orthop Clin North Am* 2001;32:79–90.

Acetabular Fracture

Colleen Campbell

Clinical Presentation

Patients with acetabular fractures often are the victims of high-energy trauma and consequently may have multiple injuries. Older patients often present after a fall and are unable to bear weight on the affected side.[1,2]

Pathophysiology

Acetabular fractures result from a direct compressive force applied at the flexed knee while the hip is flexed.[2] The Judet-LeTournel system is used to classify acetabular fractures into five groups: posterior column, posterior wall, anterior wall, anterior column, and transverse. More complex fractures are classified as T-shaped, posterior wall and column, transverse posterior wall, anterior-posterior hemitransverse, or posterior and anterior column. The most common type of fracture involves the posterior wall.[1] The posterior column, viewed by the ilioischial line, is fractured when the femoral head is internally rotated; the anterior column, viewed by the iliopectineal line, is fractured when it is externally rotated.

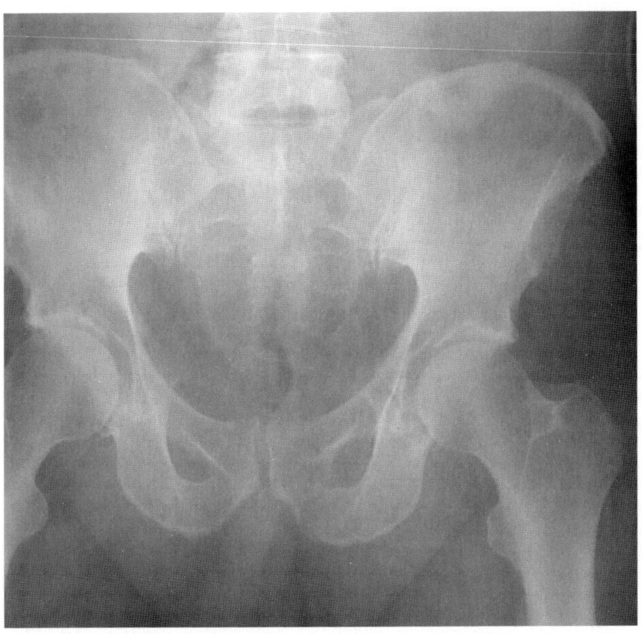

FIGURE 15–75 Acetabular fracture. (Courtesy of Samara Soghoian, MD.)

Diagnosis

Diagnosis is suspected clinically and confirmed with anteroposterior views of the pelvis, along with 45-degree oblique views, or Judet views.

Clinical Complications

Posterior hip dislocations are associated with this injury.[2] Complications include excessive bleeding, with the superior gluteal artery at risk for injury.[1] Deep venous thrombosis is very common with this injury. However, anticoagulation is often contraindicated because of the bleeding associated with these injuries. The sciatic, lateral femoral cutaneous, peroneal, or pudendal nerves may be injured during fracture fixation.[1] Late complications include heterotopic ossification, pseudoarthrosis, and arthritis.[1]

Management

Emergency department treatment requires hemodynamic stabilization and fracture immobilization. Acetabular fractures require specialized management by an orthopedic surgeon.[1] Treatment usually requires open reduction with internal fixation. Total hip arthroplasty may be necessary in older patients with complex fractures.

REFERENCES

1. Perry DC, DeLong W. Acetabular fractures. *Orthop Clin North Am* 1997;28:405–417.
2. Coppola PT, Coppola M. Emergency department evaluation and treatment of pelvic fractures. *Emerg Med Clin North Am* 2000;18: 1–27.

Fractures of the Ankle: Bimalleolar and Trimalleolar

Tyler Vadeboncoeur

Clinical Presentation

Patients with fractures of the ankle present with pain and swelling of the ankle and inability to bear weight after a high-force mechanism of injury. Ankle deformity, ecchymosis, edema, and instability of the ankle may be evident. Vascular and nerve injuries may coexist.[1-3]

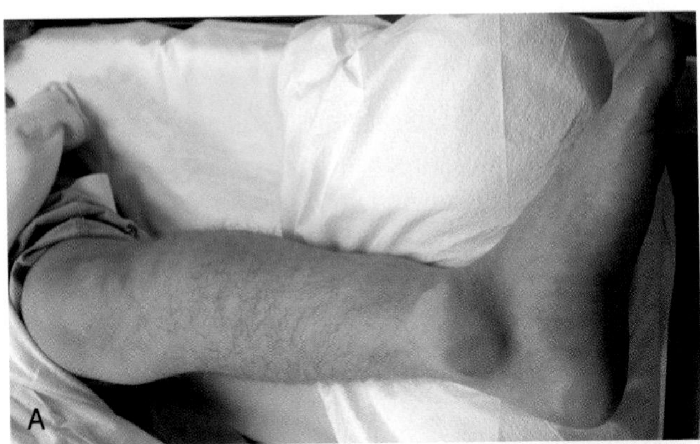

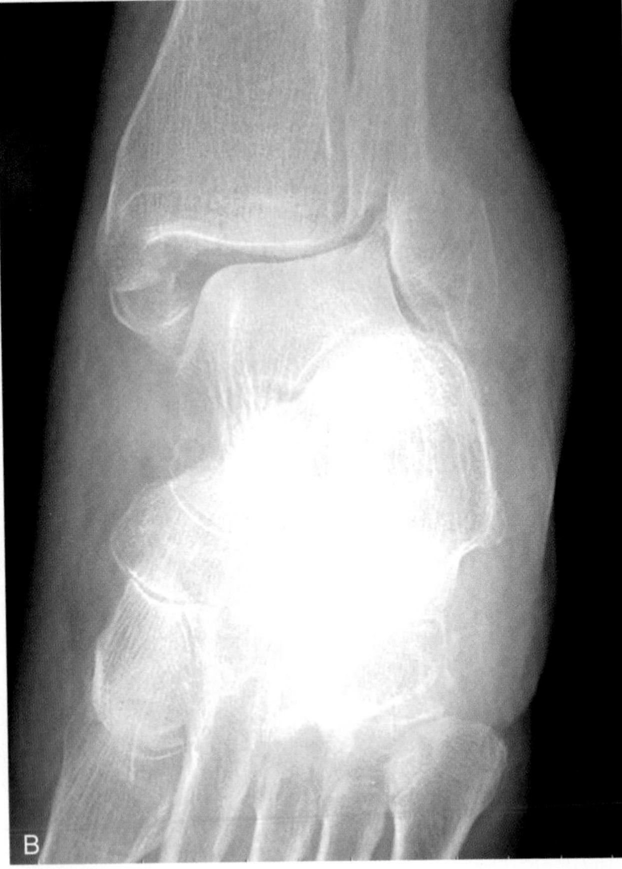

FIGURE 15-76 **A:** Trimalleolar fracture. (Courtesy of Alex Lapidus, MD.) **B:** Anteroposterior view of bimalleolar ankle fracture. (Courtesy of Greg Hunt, MD.)

Pathophysiology

It is helpful to conceptualize the ankle as a stable, ring-like structure around the talus. The ring is composed of the tibia, tibiofibular ligament, fibula, lateral ligaments of the ankle, the calcaneus, and the deltoid ligament. An isolated fracture or ligamentous disruption to one element of the ring is a stable fracture, but if two or more elements are disrupted, as in bimalleolar and trimalleolar fractures, the fracture is considered unstable.[1]

Diagnosis

Anteroposterior, lateral, and oblique ankle radiographic films should be obtained. Computed tomographic scanning is useful in evaluating complex bony injuries. A thorough foot and leg examination should always be performed to rule out neurovascular, bony, and associated injuries.[1-3]

Clinical Complications

Osteochondral disruption of the talar dome is not evident on plain radiographs and can result in arthritis and chronic pain.[1] Wound complications may occur with delayed fracture reduction and excessive handling of the traumatized soft tissues. The infection rate in operative management of closed ankle fractures is 2%.[3] Malunion may result from nonanatomic reduction of the fibula.[1]

Management

Both bimalleolar and trimalleolar fractures require emergency orthopedic consultation. Fractures with associated neurovascular compromise should be reduced immediately, before obtaining radiographs, and without waiting for orthopedic specialists.[3] Open fractures should be covered with saline-soaked sterile dressings and should be reduced and splinted to prevent further soft-tissue injury. Tetanus prophylaxis should be updated if needed, and a first-generation cephalosporin should be administered, together with an aminoglycoside in grossly contaminated wounds.[2]

REFERENCES

1. Donatto KC. Ankle fractures and syndesmosis injuries. *Orthop Clin North Am* 2001;32,1:79–90.
2. Sanders R, Swiontkowski M, Nunley J, Spiegel P. The management of fractures with soft tissue disruptions. *J Bone Joint Surg Am* 1993;75:778–789.
3. Stiehl JB. Open fractures of the ankle joint. *Instr Course Lect* 1990; 39:113–117.

Compartment Syndrome

Carla Valentine

Clinical Presentation

Compartment syndrome may manifest clinically with one or more of the so-called "5 Ps": pain, paresthesias, paralysis, pallor, and pulselessness. Pain is the earliest sign. Typically, the patient has pain out of proportion to the physical examination findings, as well as pain with active or passive stretch. Pulselessness is a late finding. Seventy-five percent of compartment syndrome cases occur as a complication of fractures, most commonly fractures of the tibia.[1]

Pathophysiology

The lower leg and forearm are the most common sites for compartment syndrome. This typically occurs when the intracompartmental pressure rises above capillary pressure. Edema followed by ischemia and necrosis ensues if treatment is not rendered in a timely fashion. Causes of compartment syndrome include fractures, crush injuries, improper casting, circumferential burns, intracompartmental hemorrhage (e.g., hemophilia, Coumadin, arterial injury), and prolonged compression (as in alcohol or drug overdoses). Myoneural components may survive up to 4 hours of ischemia, with 6 hours being the upper limit of viability.[2] After 8 hours, permanent ischemic damage occurs.[1,2]

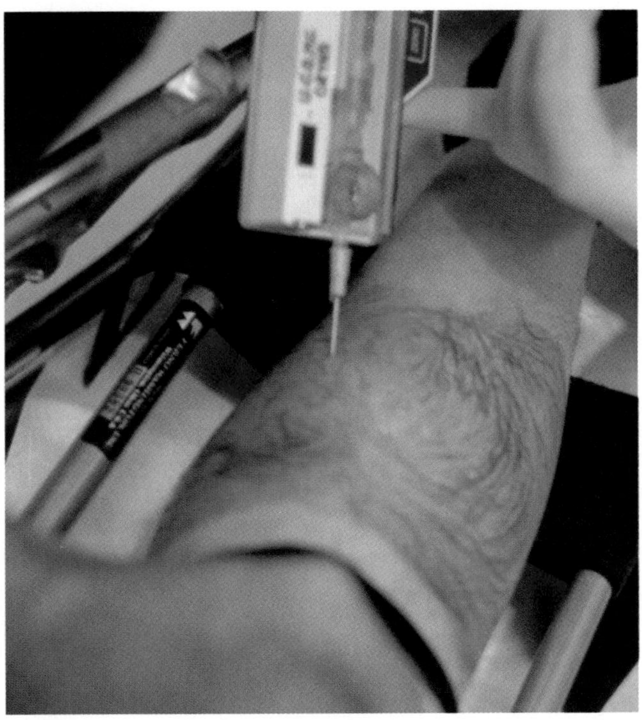

FIGURE 15–77 Striker kit being used to measure compartment pressure. (Courtesy of B. Zane Horowitz, MD.)

Diagnosis

Diagnosis is based on clinical suspicion and quantification of the intracompartmental pressure by the use of various devices. A measurement of 30 mm Hg or greater is significant (normal compartment pressure is less than 10 mm Hg) and is an indication for fasciotomy, although the exact pressure at which fasciotomy should be performed is controversial.[2]

Clinical Complications

Neurovascular necrosis may occur with resultant loss of the limb. Reperfusion injuries include acidosis, hyperkalemia, myoglobinuria, renal failure, acute respiratory distress syndrome, and diffuse intravascular coagulation.[3] Volkmann's ischemic contracture is another complication of compartment syndrome.[3]

Management

Compartment syndrome is a true emergency, and emergency decompressive fasciotomy is the definitive treatment. The extremity should not be elevated above the level of the heart, because this decreases arterial perfusion and is detrimental.[1] Ice should not be used, because it causes local vasoconstriction and may decrease perfusion.[1]

REFERENCES

1. Perron AD, Brady WJ, Keats TE. Orthopedic pitfalls in the ED: compartment syndrome. *Am J Emerg Med* 2001;19:413–416.
2. Whitesides TE, Heckman MM. Acute compartment syndrome: update on diagnosis and treatment. *J Am Acad Orthop Surg* 1996;4:209–218.
3. Velmahos GC, Toutouzas KG. Vascular trauma and compartment syndromes. *Surg Clin North Am* 2002;82:125–141.

Achilles Tendon Rupture

Michael Greenberg

Clinical Presentation

Achilles tendon rupture is a common tendinous lesion that occurs more commonly in men.[1] The incidence of total Achilles tendon rupture is increasing, and reruptures occur in approximately 2% to 8% of patients.[2] Patients often present with a history of sudden pain in the affected leg and report that they thought they were struck with an object or kicked in the posterior aspect of the distal part of the leg. Sometimes an audible snap is reported. Examination may show diffuse edema and bruising, and possibly a palpable gap along the length of the tendon.[3]

Pathophysiology

The Achilles tendon is the strongest, thickest tendon in the human body. The cause of Achilles tendon rupture remains unknown, and it is likely that the healthy fibrillar structure of the tendon is lost after rupture.

Spontaneous rupture of the Achilles tendon has been associated with inflammatory and autoimmune conditions, infectious diseases, and neurologic conditions. The normal Achilles tendon is composed predominantly of type I collagen; however, a ruptured Achilles tendon also contains type III collagen. It has been shown that fibroblasts from ruptured Achilles tendons produce both type I and type III collagen. Because the type III collagen cannot withstand tensile forces as well as type I collagen does, its presence may predispose the tendon to spontaneous rupture. Genetically determined abnormalities in collagen production may contribute to spontaneous Achilles tendon rupture.[3]

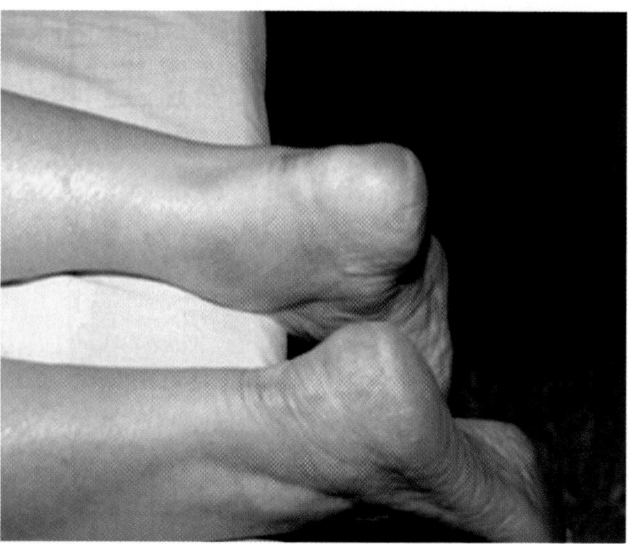

FIGURE 15–78 Achilles tendon rupture. Note discontinuity of the right Achilles tendon. (From Roberts, with permission.)

Diagnosis

The diagnosis usually is obvious. Several clinical tests are available to aid in diagnosing Achilles tendon rupture, including the calf-squeeze test, knee-flexion test, needle test, and sphygmomanometer test.[3]

Clinical Complications

Achilles tendon rupture may be associated with fluoroquinolone administration.[4] Deep infections are reported to occur postsurgically in 1% to 2% of patients, and other minor complications occur in 15% to 20% of patients. Nonoperative treatment results in more frequent reruptures than does surgical treatment.

Management

Various procedures may be employed in the treatment of ruptured Achilles tendon. The three main categories are open operative, percutaneous operative, and nonoperative procedures. The choice of treatment is largely dependent on the preference of surgeon and patient. Surgery is often elected by younger, active patients.[5] Patients can bear weight on the affected leg as tolerated, but elevation is suggested to prevent postoperative swelling.

REFERENCES

1. Bhandari M, Guyatt GH, Siddiqui F, et al. Treatment of acute Achilles tendon reruptures: a systemic overview and meta-analysis. *Clin Orthop* 2002;(400):190–200.
2. Pajala A, Kangas J, Ohtonen P, Leppilahti J. Rerupture and deep infection following treatment of total Achilles tendon rerupture. *J Bone Joint Surg Am* 2002;84:2016–2021.
3. Maffulli N. Rupture of the Achilles tendon. *J Bone Joint Surg Am* 1999;81:1019–1036.
4. Haddow L, Chandra Sekhar M, Hajela V, Gopal Rao G. Spontaneous Achilles tendon rupture in patients treated with levofloxacin. *J Antimicrob Chemother* 2003;51:747–748.
5. Bleakney RR, Tallon C, Wong JK, Lim KP, Maffulli N. Long-term ultrasonographic features of the Achilles tendon after rupture. *Clin J Sport Med* 2002;12:273–278.

Fibula Fractures

Colleen Campbell

Clinical Presentation

Patients with fractures of the fibula usually present with localized pain and tenderness in the lateral aspect of the leg.

Pathophysiology

Isolated fibula fractures usually occur as a result of a direct blow to the lateral aspect of the leg. Oblique or avulsion fractures of the fibula occur as a result of indirect forces.[1] Stress fractures also occur rarely in the fibula.[2] Maisonneuve fractures are an ankle injury associated with a proximal fibular fracture caused by external rotation forces. Proximal fibula fractures are also associated with ligamentous knee injuries (usually the lateral collateral ligament), as well as tibial plateau fractures.[1]

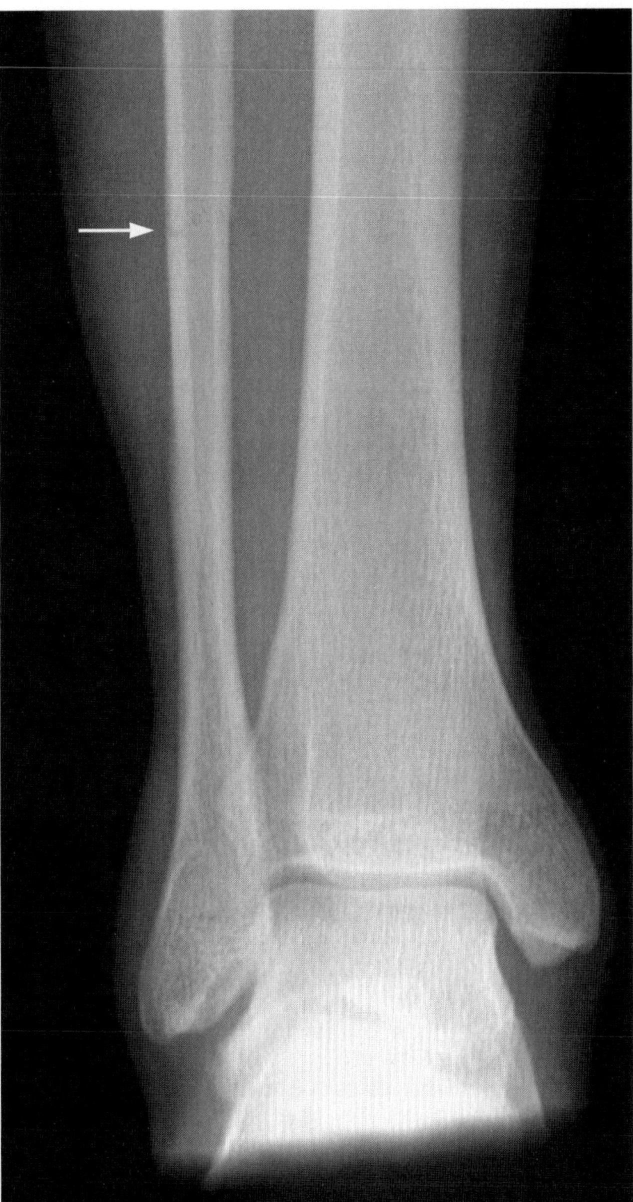

FIGURE 15–79 Nondisplaced midshaft fibular fracture. (Courtesy of Robert Hendrickson, MD.)

Diagnosis

Diagnosis is made on the basis of history and physical examination, in conjunction with radiographs of the lower leg. Anteroposterior and lateral views of the tibia and fibula, as well as the ankle and knee, confirm the diagnosis. Deformity is usually obvious if a tibial fracture is present. Swelling may be evident. The physical examination should include a full evaluation of the ligamentous structures of the knee and ankle.

Clinical Complications

Complications are rare, because the fibula is largely a non–weight-bearing bone. Proximal fibular fractures can cause superficial peroneal nerve damage. Nonunion can cause chronic pain at the fracture site.[3] Refracture and delayed healing have been reported in athletes sustaining isolated nondisplaced fractures of the fibular shaft.[2]

Management

Treatment of isolated fibula fractures involves pain control, ice, rest, and elevation.[1] Patients may be placed in Ace® bandage wraps or short-leg walking casts for midfibular or distal fractures, or given a knee brace for proximal fibular fractures. Crutches are used in conjunction with weight bearing as tolerated. Orthopedic consultation is warranted for severe displacement or comminution.[1]

REFERENCES

1. Steele PM, Bush-Joseph C, Bach B. Management of acute fractures of the knee, ankle, and foot. *Clin Fam Pract* 2000;2:661–705.
2. Slauterbeck JR, Shapiro MS, Liu S, Finerman GA. Traumatic fibular shaft fractures in athletes. *Am J Sports Med* 1995;23:751–754.
3. Roberts DM, Stallard TC. Emergency department evaluation and treatment of knee and leg injuries. *Emerg Med Clin North Am* 2000; 18:67–84.

Ankle Dislocations

Michael Greenberg

Clinical Presentation

Patients with ankle dislocations (ADs) present with pain, swelling, and obvious deformity after injury to the lower leg or ankle. AD is most commonly caused by motorcycle and other motor vehicle injuries; it has also been associated with sports injuries.[1]

Pathophysiology

AD that is not accompanied by malleolar or other associated fractures is uncommon, the ankle mortise architecture creates a somewhat tight recess. This, in conjunction with the fact that healthy ankle ligaments have tensile strength that exceeds bone strength, makes isolated dislocations at the ankle very unusual. AD is usually associated with high-speed trauma that creates a situation of forced plantar flexion in conjunction with forced eversion or inversion.[1] Previous ankle sprains may predispose to AD. In addition, malleolar hypoplasia, laxity of ligaments, and peroneal muscle weakness may also predispose to AD.[1]

Diagnosis

The diagnosis is made clinically and confirmed by plain radiography. On presentation, a careful neurovascular examination of the injured leg and foot must be performed and documented. This should be repeated frequently.

Clinical Complications

Complications include vascular injuries to the anterior tibialis artery, the dorsal pedis artery, or both, and neurologic injury to the tibial nerve, the superficial peroneal nerve, or the sural nerve.[1] Severe injury has resulted in the need for amputation in some cases.[1]

Management

Successful reduction of AD usually requires general anesthesia in the operating theater. The technique involves the application of longitudinal traction followed by pronation or supination of the foot, based on the position of the injury.[1]

REFERENCES

1. Rivera F, Bertone C, De Martino M, Pietrobono D, Ghisellini F. Pure dislocation of the ankle: three case reports and literature review. *Clin Orthop* 2001;(382):179–184.

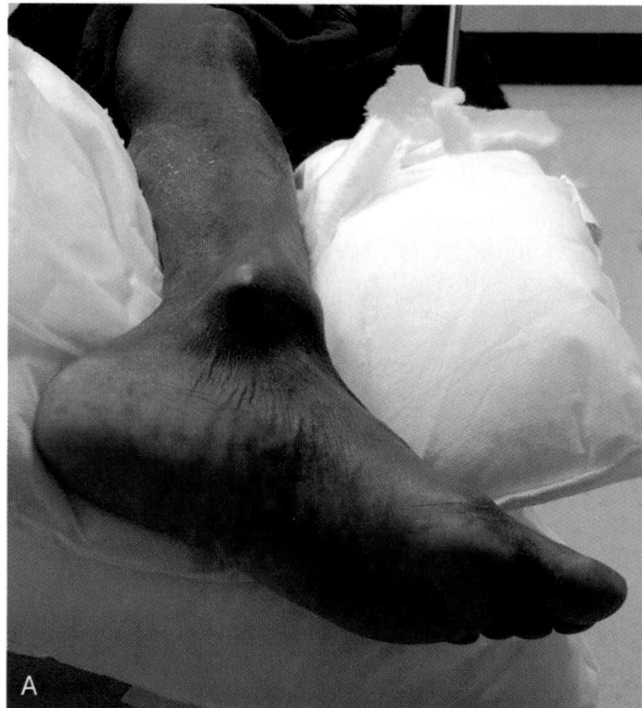

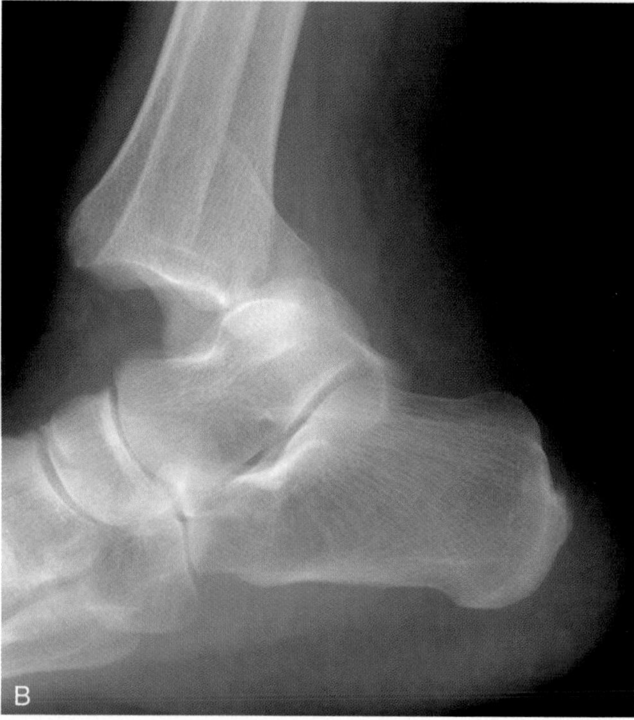

FIGURE 15–80 **A:** Ankle dislocation with "tenting" of the skin. **B:** Ankle dislocation. (**A** and **B,** Courtesy of Mark Silverberg, MD.)

Subtalar Dislocations

Michael Greenberg

Clinical Presentation

Patients with subtalar dislocations present with ankle pain and deformity after inversion or eversion injury to the ankle in conjunction with falls, motor-vehicle crashes, or other causes of high-impact trauma.

Pathophysiology

Subtalar or peritalar dislocations are characterized by the position the foot assumes in relation to the talus, after the traumatic injury—medial, lateral, anterior, or posterior. Seventy-six percent of cases involve medial displacement of the foot due to inversion forces. Eversion forces result in lateral subtalar dislocations.[1-3]

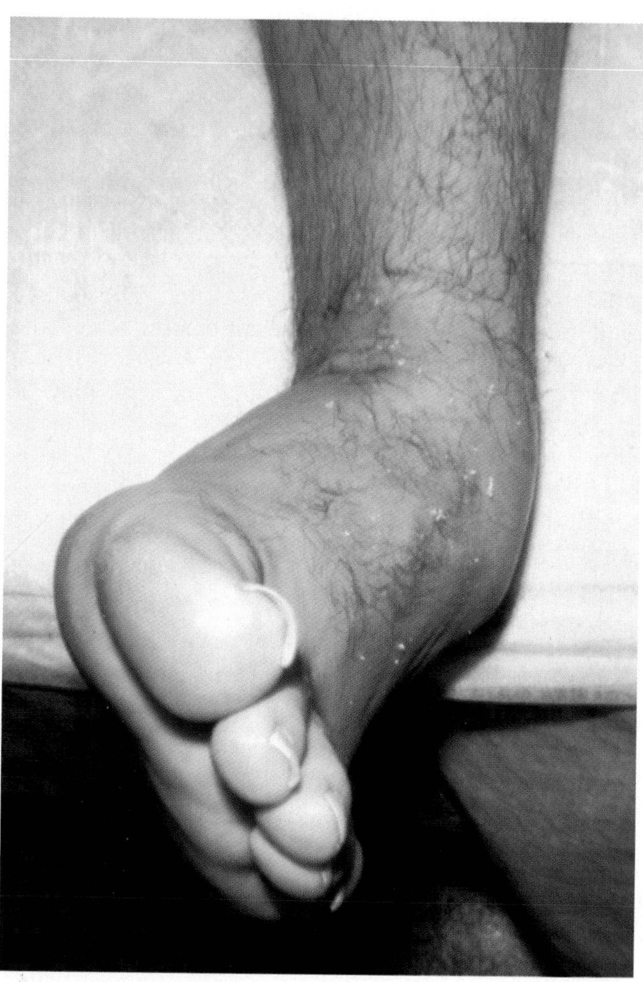

FIGURE 15–81 Obvious subtalar dislocation. (Courtesy of Michael Greenberg, MD.)

Diagnosis

The diagnosis usually is obvious on clinical examination, which reveals a grossly deformed ankle with an obviously displaced distal foot in relation to the ankle. At times the overlying skin is tented or excessively taut and pale. Either of these circumstances may predispose to skin necrosis. Plain radiographs are essential to determine the presence of associated injuries.[1]

Clinical Complications

Complications include vascular compromise, conversion of a closed injury to an open injury, necrosis of overlying skin, neurologic injury, avascular necrosis of the talus, chronic arthritis, chronic joint instability, and reflex sympathetic dystrophy.[1-3]

Management

If pulses are absent, reduction of this injury requires emergency action. If pulses are present, on-site emergency orthopedic consultation should be summoned, and plain radiographs should be obtained after the administration of appropriate pain medication. The same treatment paradigms apply to open dislocations. In addition, these injuries should be covered with moist sterile dressings, and consideration should be given to supplying parenteral antibiotic coverage. Emergency reduction is accomplished by flexing the knee to relax the gastrocnemius and then firmly applying traction to the foot with countertraction to the lower leg. The foot is then manipulated into the normal anatomic position and immobilized with a plaster splint. Ice, elevation, and analgesia should be supplied. Hospitalization and prompt orthopedic consultation are recommended.[1]

REFERENCES

1. Love JN, Hayden DK, Dhindsa HS. Subtalar dislocation: evaluation and management in the emergency department. *J Emerg Med* 1995; 13:787–793.
2. Bibbo C, Anderson RB, Davis WH. Injury characteristics and the clinical outcome of subtalar dislocations: a clinical and radiographic analysis of 25 cases. *Foot Ankle Int* 2003;24:158–163.

Pseudofractures of the Os Trigonum

Mary Anne Fuchs

Clinical Presentation

The presentation of os trigonum injury is similar to that of fractures of the lateral tubercle of the posterior process of the talus. The pseudofracture usually results from hyperplantar flexion or inversion of the ankle.[1] Patients present with posterior lateral ankle pain, tenderness, and swelling.[2]

Pathophysiology

Hyperplantar flexion causes impingement of the lateral facet or os trigonum against the posterior tibia and calcaneus.[1] Inversion can cause an avulsion injury.[1] The os trigonum, a common accessory ossicle seen in 8% of the population,[2] is located posterior to the lateral tubercle of the posterior process of the talus and is often confused with a fracture of the lateral tubercle. Injury to the fibrous attachment between the os trigonum and the posterior process of the talus can be a source of pathology.[2] These injuries may be misdiagnosed as ankle sprains.

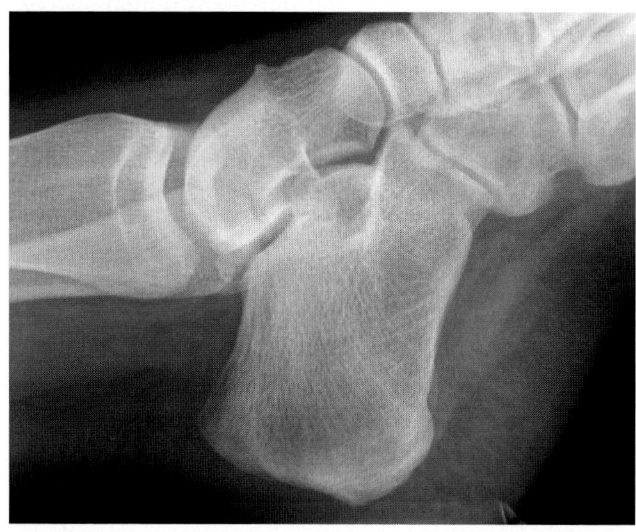

FIGURE 15–82 Os trigonum in a patient who twisted his ankle. (Courtesy of Robert Hendrickson, MD.)

Diagnosis

Physical examination and correlation with radiographic findings help to differentiate a fracture of the lateral tubercle, a fracture of a fused os trigonum, a tear in the fibrous attachment of the os trigonum to the lateral tubercle, and a normal os trigonum.[1] Pain may be elicited with ankle plantar flexion or, occasionally, with dorsiflexion of the great toe.[1] A lateral radiograph of the foot best visualizes the lateral tubercle and, if present, the os trigonum.[2] A rough, irregular cortical surface suggests the presence of an acute fracture, whereas the os trigonum usually has a smooth, rounded cortical surface. In chronic cases, these differences may be less distinct. If the diagnosis is uncertain, magnetic resonance imaging or computed tomography may be helpful.[2]

Clinical Complications

Delay in treatment may result in long-term disability and results in the need for surgery.

Management

Initial treatment consists of ice, elevation, and immobilization in a splint or cast in 15 degrees of equinus, with referral for follow-up.[2] These injuries often can be managed nonsurgically, with non–weight-bearing status and a short-leg cast worn for approximately 4 weeks.[1] If conservative measures fail, then surgical excision may be needed.

REFERENCES

1. Blake RL, Lallas PJ, Ferguson H. The os trigonum syndrome: a literature review. *J Am Podiatr Med Assoc* 1992;82:154–161.
2. Judd DB, Kim DH. Foot fractures frequently misdiagnosed as ankle sprains. *Am Fam Physician* 2002;66:785–794.

Plantar Fasciitis

Colleen Campbell

Clinical Presentation

The pain of plantar fasciitis (PF) is historically insidious in nature, is worse after rest, and may radiate to the medial ankle or lateral aspect of the foot.[1] The pain is most severe with the first few steps of the day, or when the toes are dorsiflexed. It is often relieved by walking on the lateral aspect of the foot.[1]

Pathophysiology

The plantar fascia originates at the medial tubercle of the calcaneus and extends to the longitudinal foot arch. PF is the most common cause of heel pain.[2] This inflammation may actually represent collagen degeneration involving the plantar fascia.[3] PF may be associated with a "tight" Achilles tendon, or with pes planus or cavus.[3] This is a common ailment of long-distance runners.[2] A valgus hindfoot and pronation are more common in patients who have PF.[1] Elderly people with weak gastrocnemius or soleus muscles are also at risk for PF.

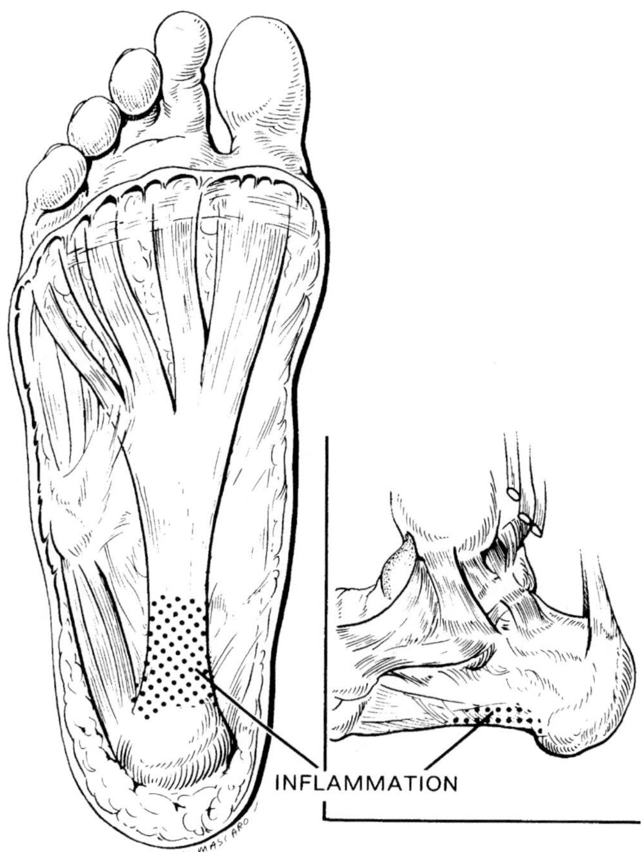

FIGURE 15-83 Plantar fasciitis. Plantar surface of foot with skin removed, showing inflammation as an area of pain and tenderness just above the tuberosity of calcaneus. (MediClip image copyright 2003 Lippincott Williams & Wilkins. All rights reserved.)

Diagnosis

Diagnosis of PF is made on the basis of history and physical examination. Radiographs are obtained to rule out stress fractures and bone spurs of the calcaneus.[1] On examination, pain is elicited by palpation at the anteromedial aspect of the heel on the plantar surface.

Clinical Complications

The most common complication is restriction of activities secondary to pain.[2] The first branch of the lateral plantar nerve may become entrapped, resulting in chronic heel pain.[1]

Management

Treatment involves stretching of the Achilles tendon. Ankle splints (90 degrees, or slight dorsiflexion) that are worn at night may be used to passively stretch the Achilles while the patient is resting, in conjunction with nonsteroidal antiinflammatory drugs (NSAIDs), rest, and heel support.[3] Motion-control running shoes, heel cups, medial foot wedges, arch taping, and elevation of the first metatarsal with the use of orthotics all provide symptomatic relief.[3] Infrequent (once or twice per year) use of steroid injections has been successful in high-level athletes during training periods but is not recommended for routine use.[1] Operative treatment is reserved for the rare case in which conservative measures fail.

REFERENCES

1. Clanton TO, Porter DA. Primary care of foot and ankle injuries in the athlete. *Clin Sports Med* 1997;16:435–466.
2. Barret SL, O'Malley R. Plantar fasciitis and other causes of heel pain. *Am Fam Physician* 1999;59:2200–2206.
3. Young CC, Rutherford DS, Niedfeldt MW. Treatment of plantar fasciitis. *Am Fam Physician* 2001;63:467–474, 477–478.

Jones and Pseudo-Jones Fractures

Robert Hendrickson

Clinical Presentation

Patients with Jones or pseudo-Jones fractures may present with pain, tenderness, ecchymosis, swelling, and the inability to bear weight. Patients with tuberosity fractures may occasionally complain only of ankle pain, because this injury occurs during foot inversion with plantar flexion. It is essential to specifically examine the fifth metatarsal of all patients with ankle complaints.

Pathophysiology

Fractures of the base (proximal 1.5 cm) of the fifth metatarsal have been described as Jones fractures (proximal fifth metatarsal fracture) and pseudo-Jones fractures (fifth metatarsal tuberosity fracture).[1] The use of eponyms in this case is confusing and should be avoided in practice. Tuberosity fractures may be caused by avulsion of the attachment of the peroneus brevis muscle and the lateral band of the plantar fascia on inversion of the hindfoot.[1] Metatarsal base fractures may be caused by direct trauma to the foot, repetitive trauma, or inversion.[1,2]

Diagnosis

The diagnosis can be suspected by recognition of the typical clinical signs and examination of the fifth metatarsal area in patients with ankle "sprains." Confirmation is made from radiographs of the foot (ankle radiographs may not visualize fractures of the fifth metatarsal).[1]

Clinical Complications

Complications include nonunion and chronic pain.

Management

Patients with nondisplaced, nonarticular tuberosity fractures may be treated conservatively with the use of hard-soled shoes, bulky dressings, or a cast with weight bearing as tolerated. These injuries are typically pain free within 3 weeks and healed within 8 weeks.[1,2] Displaced fractures and fractures involving more than 30% of the cubometatarsal articular surface may require surgical fixation.[2] Fractures of the proximal 1.5 cm of the fifth metatarsal may be treated with 6 to 8 weeks of strict non–weight bearing or with surgical fixation. Orthopedic referral and surgical fixation may be considered for patients who are athletes, young, active, or prefer surgery to non–weight bearing.[2]

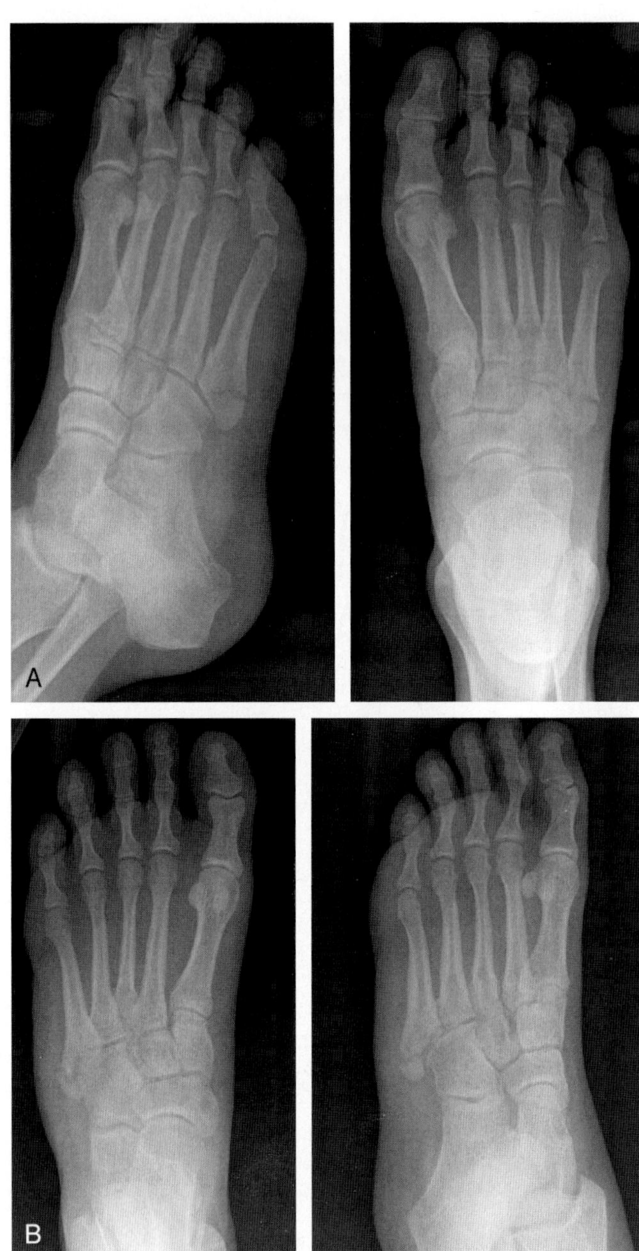

FIGURE 15–84 **A:** Jones fracture. **B:** Pseudo-Jones fracture (fifth metatarsal tuberosity fracture). (**A** and **B**, Courtesy of Robert Hendrickson, MD.)

REFERENCES

1. Nunley JA. Fractures of the base of the fifth metatarsal: the Jones fracture. *Orthop Clin North Am* 2001;32:171–180.
2. Strayer SM, Reece SG, Petrizzi MJ. Fractures of the proximal fifth metatarsal. *Am Fam Physician* 1999;59:2516–2522.

Lisfranc's Fracture

Katherine Douglass

Clinical Presentation

Patients with Lisfranc's fracture present with midfoot tenderness, swelling, or pain with ambulation after direct trauma to the dorsal foot or after high-speed, complex injury to the lower extremity.[1-3]

Pathophysiology

Disruption of the tarsometatarsal joint may occur secondary to direct or indirect forces. Direct traumatic forces may cause dorsal or plantar displacement, comminuted fracture, vascular compromise, or compartment syndrome. Indirect injuries are more common, involving the transmission of a rotational force to the forefoot with a fixed hindfoot, or axial load to a plantar flexed foot. The ligamentous and bony anatomy of the tarsometatarsal joint predisposes the dislocation of the second through fifth metatarsals from the first.[1-3]

Diagnosis

There is a high index of suspicion for disruption of the tarsometatarsal joint in patients with post-traumatic pain in the midfoot area. Standard radiographs include anteroposterior, lateral, and oblique views, in addition to comparison films of the opposite foot. If these standard films are nondiagnostic, further studies may include weight-bearing films, stress radiographs, or computed tomograms. Clinicians must carefully evaluate the second metatarsal for evidence of fracture, avulsion, or displacement. Any midfoot bone fracture should raise suspicion of joint disruption. The normal anteroposterior and oblique views should display alignment from the medial border of the second metatarsal along the edge of the middle cuneiform, and from the medial border of the fourth metatarsal along the cuboid. Any loss of alignment is abnormal. The lateral film may show dorsal displacement of the metatarsal shaft to the midfoot bones, again indicative of significant injury.[1-3]

Clinical Complications

Missed or delayed diagnosis of Lisfranc's fracture can lead to joint arthrosis, long-term disability, and poor functional outcome. Compartmental syndrome may cause significant morbidity if it is not recognized and treated in a timely fashion.[1-3]

Management

The most important component of effective treatment is early diagnosis and referral. Orthopedic consultation is essential for proper treatment of Lisfranc's fracture, and operative management is indicated in most cases. A stable midfoot sprain (confirmed by stress radiographs) may be treated with immobilization for 6 to 8 weeks. Open reduction with internal fixation or closed reduction is indicated in any case of instability.[1-3]

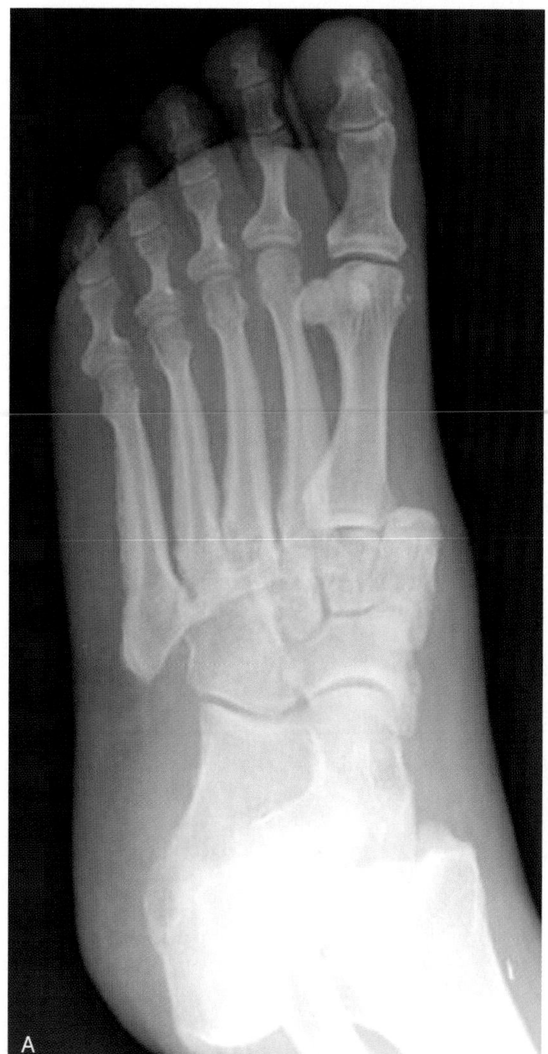

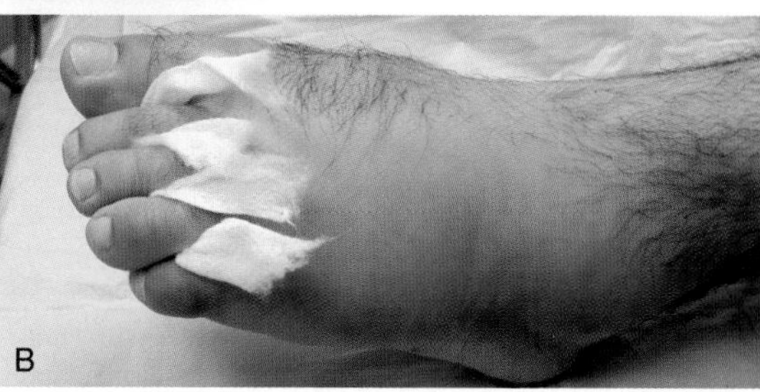

FIGURE 15-85 **A:** Oblique view showing midfoot fracture-dislocation (Lisfranc's fracture). (Courtesy of George Lin, MD.) **B:** Midfoot swelling associated with Lisfranc's fracture. (Courtesy of Robert Hendrickson, MD.)

REFERENCES

1. Perron AD, Brady WJ, Keats TE. Orthopedic pitfalls in the ED: Lisfranc fracture-dislocation. *Am J Emerg Med* 2001;19:71–75.
2. Burroughs KE, Reimer CD, Fields KB. Lisfranc injury of the foot: a commonly missed diagnosis. *Am Fam Physician* 1998;58:118–124.
3. Chiodo CP, Myerson MS. Developments and advances in the diagnosis and treatment of injuries to the tarsometatarsal joint. *Orthop Clin North Am* 2001;32:11–20.

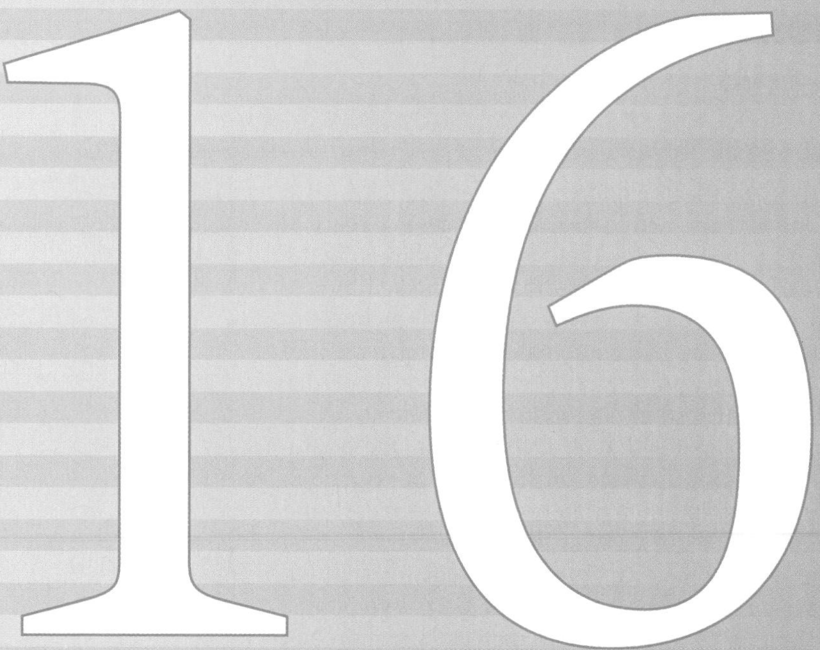

Pediatrics

Croup

Christy Salvaggio

Clinical Presentation

Croup typically affects children between the ages of 6 months and 6 years, with a peak incidence at 2 years of age. Croup occurs year-round but is most common in the fall and early winter. Male children are affected almost 1.5 times more often than female children.[1] The onset of the illness is marked by prodromal symptoms typical of a viral upper respiratory tract infection (URTI), such as a runny nose, congestion, and mild cough. Fever is common. On approximately day 3 of the illness, the classic symptoms of croup develop, including a barky cough that may sound like a barking seal, hoarseness, and varying degrees of stridor with possible respiratory distress. The severity may vary greatly. The majority of patients have only a barky cough and URTI symptoms. Most of these patients never seek medical attention and are treated with supportive care at home. Patients with more severe disease have stridor when crying or agitated, and those most severely affected have stridor at rest, with marked increased work of breathing, hypoxia, or both. Classically, croup symptoms are exacerbated at night, and the second night of croup symptoms is often worse than the first night. Children typically improve if they are exposed to cool or humidified air while crying; other distress exacerbates the symptoms.

Pathophysiology

Croup, or acute laryngotracheobronchitis, is a viral infection most commonly caused by parainfluenza virus. It manifests with URTI symptoms and varying degrees of a barky cough, hoarseness, and stridor. Parainfluenza type 1 is the main cause of croup; however, other viruses are occasionally identified, including respiratory syncytial virus, parainfluenza types 2 and 3, influenza A and B, and adenovirus. Bacterial causes (e.g., *Mycoplasma pneumoniae*) are rare.[1] Croup causes respiratory distress secondary to subglottic edema. Older children infected with parainfluenza or other croup-causing viruses are likely to present with laryngitis. Younger children manifest symptoms of croup because of the smaller diameter of their upper airway. Croup is rare before 6 months of age, probably because of the presence of maternal antibodies.

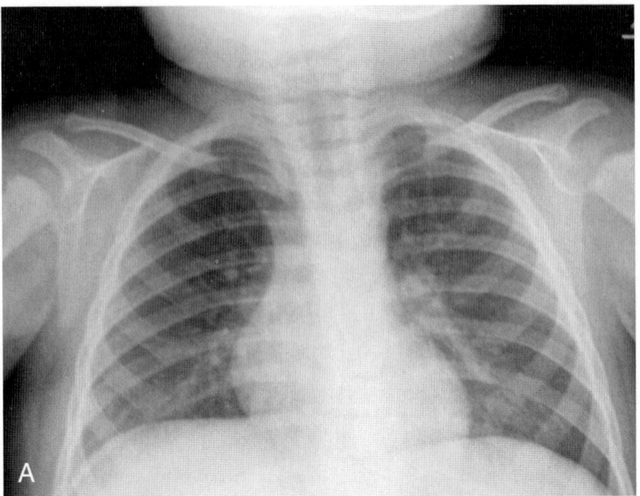

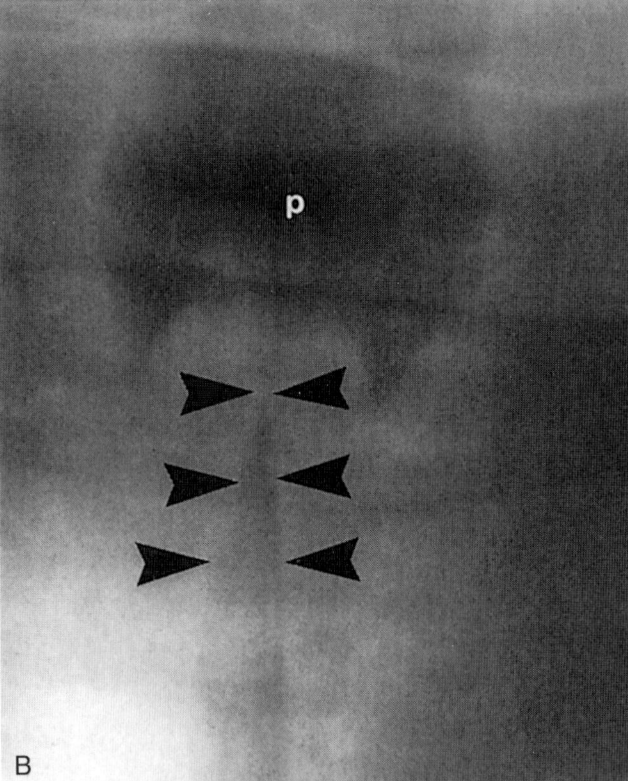

FIGURE 16–1 **A:** "Steeple sign." (Courtesy of Robert Hendrickson, MD.) **B:** Croup. The airway is smoothly narrowed or tapered *(arrowheads)*. As a result, the hypopharynx is dilated (p). (From Ovassapian, with permission.)

Croup

Christy Salvaggio

Diagnosis

Croup is a clinical diagnosis. Patients classically present with URTI symptoms, a barky cough, and stridor that are not difficult to diagnose. For patients with unusual presentations, those with severe symptoms not responding to treatment, or croup in a child older than 6 years of age, additional work-up may be required to rule out other upper airway obstruction. A complete medical history, including any history of intubations, recent choking episodes, or the presence of hemangiomas, should be elicited. The differential diagnosis for croup includes foreign body obstruction, airway hemangiomas, epiglottitis, tracheitis, and anterior mediastinal masses. A soft-tissue lateral neck radiograph to evaluate for possible upper airway obstruction may be helpful; however, in children with classic croup symptoms, a posteroanterior neck radiograph looking for the classic "steeple sign" is not necessary or recommended.

Acute spasmodic croup should also be considered as a possible diagnosis. It affects children 3 months to 3 years of age. Its presentation is almost identical to that of viral croup, with the acute onset of hoarseness, a barky cough, and inspiratory stridor; however, patients with spasmodic croup lack the prodrome of infectious URTI symptoms that includes fever.

Clinical Complications

Croup is usually a self-limited illness that resolves within 1 week. More than 90% of children with croup never develop symptoms more severe than mild stridor and dyspnea. In more severe cases, patients may have severe respiratory distress secondary to marked subglottic edema and inflammation; however, respiratory failure secondary to croup is rare. Viral laryngotracheobronchitis may predispose patients to secondary bacterial infections, including bacterial tracheitis.

Management

Mild cases of croup, involving a well-appearing child with URTI symptoms and a barky cough without stridor, may be treated with supportive care (e.g., cool or humidified air). Placing the child in the bathroom with a hot running shower may provide the humidified air. Alternatively, in cool weather, the child may be taken outside or placed near an open window to be exposed to cool air. Stridor that is present only with crying or other distress should be treated with a one-time dose of oral dexamethasone. Some studies have shown equal efficacy with lower Decadron doses (0.15 to 0.3 mg/kg). Oral Decadron is as efficacious as intramuscular Decadron; the latter should be reserved for patients who are unable to take oral medications.[2] Nebulized budesonide, 2 to 4 mg, may be used instead of or in addition to Decadron.

Children who have stridor at rest are more concerning and need urgent care. Few data support the use of cool humidified air in the emergency department setting; however, it may be tried as long as it does not cause more distress in the child. Subcutaneous (s.c.) racemic epinephrine, 0.05 mL/kg to a maximum of 0.5 mL, should be administered immediately. Alternatively, 0.5 mL of 1:1000 of L-epinephrine may be administered, with equal efficacy.[1] Oral or intramuscular Decadron should also be given. Racemic epinephrine may provide an acute improvement in symptoms, but the improvement is transient and patients' symptoms may return or "rebound," sometimes with increased intensity. All patients who require s.c. racemic epinephrine should be monitored for at least 3 hours.[1] Well-appearing patients who have adequate follow-up and no stridor at rest may be discharged after 3 hours of observation. Any patient who has persistent stridor at rest or who requires a second dose of s.c. racemic epinephrine should be admitted for observation and s.c. racemic epinephrine on an as-needed basis. The s.c. racemic epinephrine may be administered as often as every 30 minutes for severe symptoms, but multiple doses should be administered with caution. Patients require careful monitoring for side effects.

REFERENCES

1. Wright RB, Pomerantz WJ, Luria JW. New approaches to respiratory infections in children: bronchiolitis and croup. *Emerg Med Clin North Am* 2002;20:93–114.
2. Rittichier KK, Ledwith CA. Outpatient treatment of moderate croup with dexamethasone: intramuscular versus oral dosing. *Pediatrics* 2000;106:1344–1348.

Bronchiolitis

Maria McColgan

Clinical Presentation

Bronchiolitis begins as an upper respiratory tract infection with rhinorrhea and mild cough, which may progress to respiratory compromise. Young infants may present with apnea. Patients may also present with feeding intolerance and signs of dehydration. Clinical signs include fever of 38.5 to 39° C (101 to 102° F), tachypnea, inspiratory and expiratory wheezing, crackles, retractions, hypoxemia, nasal flaring, and grunting. In severe cases, respiratory failure may ensue.

Pathophysiology

Bronchiolitis is an acute, inflammatory, obstructive disease of the bronchioles, often caused by a viral infection, in children younger than 2 years of age. Respiratory syncytial virus (RSV) is the leading cause of bronchiolitis (up to 80% of cases). Other causes include influenza, adenovirus, parainfluenza, and mycoplasma. Winter is the peak season for bronchiolitis. The peak incidence is between 3 and 6 months of age.[1–3]

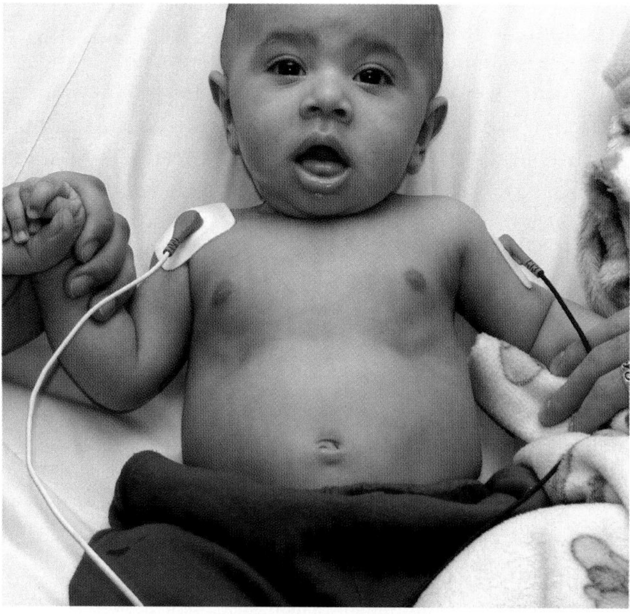

FIGURE 16–2 Note respiratory distress with substernal retractions in this child with bronchiolitis. (© David Effron, MD, 2004. Used with permission.)

Diagnosis

The diagnosis is based on clinical findings. A chest radiograph should be obtained if clinically indicated, to rule out bacterial pneumonia. Typical radiographic findings include hyperinflation, hyperlucency, and flattened diaphragm. Patchy, interstitial infiltrates, representing areas of atelectasis, may be seen in 30% of patients. The white blood cell count usually is normal. Viral cultures usually are not helpful.[1–3]

Clinical Complications

Respiratory failure from hypoxemia or hypercarbia may occur. Mortality is highest in infants younger than 2 months of age, premature infants, and infants with bronchopulmonary dysplasia or congenital heart disease. Bronchiolitis may be complicated by secondary bacterial pneumonia or bacterial infection, especially in hospitalized infants.

Management

Treatment is supportive, including hydration, supplemental oxygen, and mechanical ventilation if necessary. Nebulized albuterol, racemic epinephrine, or both are commonly used. However, studies have shown only brief improvement in clinical score, and no effect on the duration of illness or hospitalization, with the use of these agents.[1–3] Corticosteroids are generally considered not effective in bronchiolitis. Antibiotics should be used only if secondary bacterial infection is suspected. Criteria for hospital admission typically include respiratory rate greater than 60 breaths per minute, apnea, color changes, hypoxia, and inability to take adequate oral solutions. Hospitalization should be strongly considered for high-risk infants, including infants younger than 2 months of age, those with cardiac or pulmonary disease, and those who were born prematurely.[1–3]

REFERENCES

1. Flores G, Horowitz RI. Efficacy of beta2-agonists in bronchiolitis: a reappraisal and meta-analysis. *Pediatrics* 1997;100:233–239.
2. Dobson JV, Stephens-Groff SM, McMahon SR, et al. The use of albuterol in hospitalized infants with bronchiolitis. *Pediatrics* 1998; 101:361–368.
3. Garrison MM, Christakis DA, Harvey E, et al. Systemic corticosteroids in infant bronchiolitis: a meta-analysis. *Pediatrics* 2000;105: e44.

Diphtheria

Mark Silverberg

Clinical Presentation

Diphtheria classically manifests in children 1 to 9 years of age, but it may be seen in nonimmunized adults.[1] The disease has an insidious onset, beginning with a sore throat and low-grade fever accompanied by nausea, vomiting, and diarrhea. The pharynx is initially red, but grayish-white lesions develop and coalesce into a single membrane covering the tonsils, soft palate, and uvula within 24 hours.[1] This membrane is not easily removed and bleeds when forcefully removed.

Pathophysiology

Corynebacterium diphtheriae is a club-shaped, gram-positive rod with an incubation period of 2 to 5 days. Toxigenic strains produce diphtheria toxin that inactivates the translocase of ribosomes, preventing translation of messenger RNA into cellular peptides.[1]

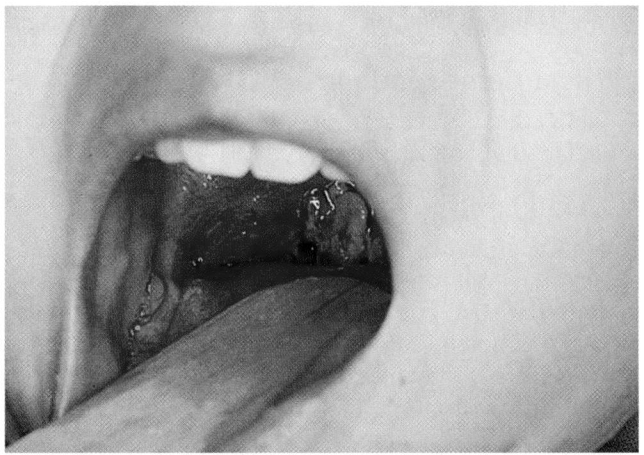

FIGURE 16–3 Pharyngeal pseudomembrane in diphtheria. (Copyright CW Leung, Princess Margaret Hospital, Lai Chi Kok, Kowloon, Hong Kong.)

Diagnosis

The diagnosis of diphtheria is clinical, based on the presence of the classic gray/white pseudomembrane covering a mucosal surface. In every suspected case, samples should be cultured on Loeffler's medium and analyzed for virulence by a gel diffusion test for toxigenicity.[1] Diphtheria may develop on any mucosa surface, giving rise to nasal, laryngeal, and cutaneous diphtheria. Cervical lymphadenopathy usually is present. In cases of moderate disease, symptoms begin to resolve in 5 to 6 days even without the use of antitoxin, although it does increase the rate of symptom resolution.[1] In severe disease ("bullneck diphtheria"), the symptoms are very severe and the entire neck becomes swollen, giving rise to its characteristic shape with airway compromise a danger.

Clinical Complications

Dehydration is often present due to dysphagia. Airway obstruction may develop and may progress to death in severe cases. Myocarditis is commonly encountered, and degenerative changes occur in the central nervous system in almost all fatal cases.[1] Serum sickness may occur after treatment with the horse antitoxin.[1]

Management

Airway management is paramount in all suspected cases of pharyngeal diphtheria. Intravenous hydration should be initiated to prevent dehydration. Patients with suspected diphtheria should be placed in isolation and should receive diphtheria antitoxin.[1] Penicillin and erythromycin are the drugs of choice; either is active against *C. diphtheriae* as well as streptococcal species, which are found in a large proportion of diphtheria cases.

REFERENCES

1. Hodes HL. Diphtheria. *Pediatr Clin North Am* 1979;26:445–459.

Pertussis

Rakesh D. Mistry

Clinical Presentation

Pertussis has three phases—catarrhal, paroxysmal, and convalescent. The catarrhal stage lasts approximately 1 to 2 weeks; symptoms resemble those of a simple upper respiratory tract illness. The paroxysmal stage is characterized by harsh, prolonged coughing spells, or paroxysms. It is during this stage that patients develop the classic "inspiratory whoop." This inspiratory sound is usually limited to older toddlers and children. Infants and young children with pertussis cannot generate sufficient inspiratory strength to create this "whoop." The paroxysmal stage typically lasts 1 to 2 weeks, after which symptoms wane. The convalescent stage of pertussis infection may last several weeks. Fever is absent in most cases of pertussis.[1]

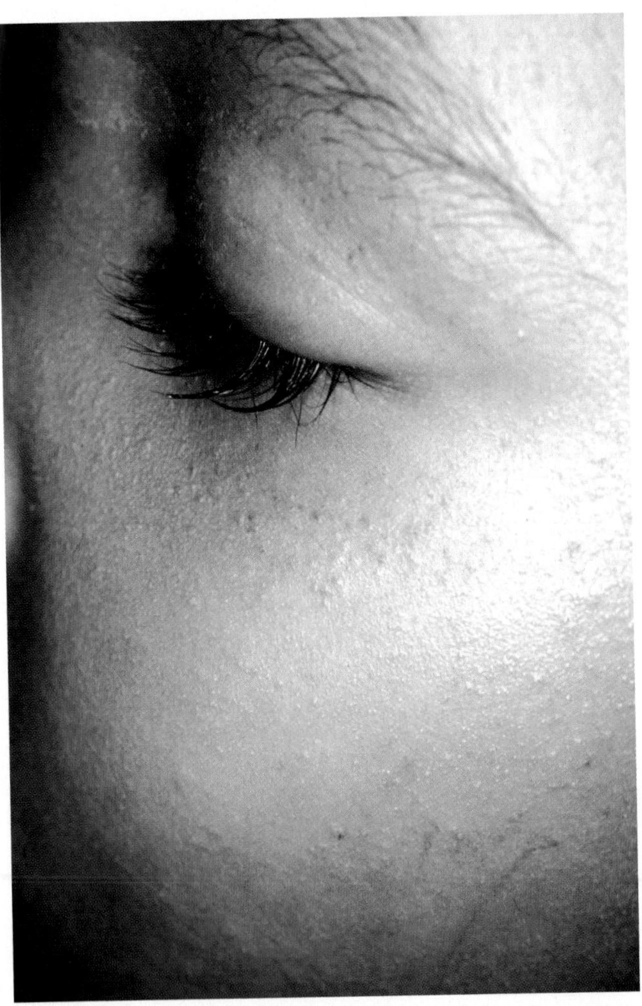

FIGURE 16–4 Facial petechiae are common in patients with pertussis as a result of continued, forceful coughing. (© David Effron, MD, 2004. Used with permission.)

Pathophysiology

The organism responsible for pertussis is the gram-negative rod, *Bordetella pertussis. B. pertussis* has selective tropism for ciliated epithelial cells of the human respiratory tract, and local inflammation is the rule; invasive infection is not characteristic. Transmission is by aerosolized droplets, with transmission rates approaching 80% in close contacts.[1]

Diagnosis

Diagnosis is usually made during the paroxysmal stage. A complete blood count showing an absolute lymphocytosis supports the diagnosis, and the degree of lymphocytosis correlates with disease severity. The gold standard for diagnosis is isolation of *B. pertussis* in culture. This is accomplished by collecting mucus from the posterior nasopharynx with a Dacron or calcium alginate swab (cotton inhibits growth of *B. pertussis*). Direct fluorescent antibody (DFA) testing is the preferred modality for identification of *B. pertussis* in many institutions.

Clinical Complications

Complications include pneumonia, seizures, encephalopathy, apnea, and death.[1,2]

Management

Treatment of active pertussis infection in all stages consists of oral erythromycin. Erythromycin decreases infectivity of the host, but it diminishes disease severity only if it is instituted during the catarrhal stage. Patients younger than 12 months of age are at greatest risk for complications from pertussis infection, and inpatient management is prudent.[1,2]

REFERENCES

1. Waggoner-Fountain L, Hayden GF. Pertussis in primary care practice: recent advances in diagnosis, treatment, and prevention. *Pediatr Clin North Am* 1996;23:793–804.
2. Vitek CR, Pascual FB, Baughman AL, Murphy TV. Increase in deaths from pertussis among young infants in the United States in the 1990s. *Pediatr Infect Dis J* 2003;22:628–634.

Measles

Mark Silverberg

Clinical Presentation

Patients with measles may present with a prodrome of fever, cough, coryza, malaise, and conjunctivitis. Before 1968, an inactivated vaccine was used to prevent measles, and patients immunized before this date may present with "atypical measles," which includes a magnified prodrome and a rash that spreads centripetally.[1] An incubation period of 6 to 19 days exists between the time the viral infection occurs and the beginning of the classic clinical prodrome.[1]

Pathophysiology

Measles is caused by a highly contagious single-stranded RNA paramyxovirus and is spread via respiratory droplets. The virus multiplies in the respiratory mucosa and is then carried to the bloodstream in lymphoid cells.[1] In 2001, 30 million cases of measles were reported worldwide; however, the disease is relatively uncommon in the United States since the introduction of a two-dose immunization program in 1963.[1]

Diagnosis

The diagnosis usually is made clinically. However, a number of serologic tests exist to confirm clinical suspicions.[1] Koplik's spots are pathognomonic for measles. Koplik's spots (white spots that look like "grains of sand on a red background") appear on the buccal mucosa approximately 2 days before the rash appears.[1] The classic measles rash is maculopapular in nature; it starts on the face and progresses down the body. It then becomes brownish and fades in the same order as it appeared.

Clinical Complications

Complications of measles may occur in healthy persons but are more common in the very young, the malnourished, and those with suppressed immunity (e.g., patients with human immunodeficiency virus infection [HIV], those undergoing radiotherapy or chemotherapy).[1] Complications include pneumonia, diarrhea, otitis media, premature labor, croup, hepatitis, encephalitis, seizures, and death.[1,2] Other complications include idiopathic thrombocytopenia and subacute sclerosing panencephalitis, which usually is fatal and occurs 7 to 10 years after the initial measles infection.[1]

Management

The management of measles is supportive. Antipyretics should be given to prevent febrile seizures, and the patient should be encouraged to increase oral intake to prevent dehydration. Many patients become sensitive to light and benefit from muted lighting. Some authors believe that vitamin A helps decrease the complication rate associated with measles, but this is believed to be helpful only in individuals who are vitamin A deficient.[1] Measles is a notifiable disease.[1]

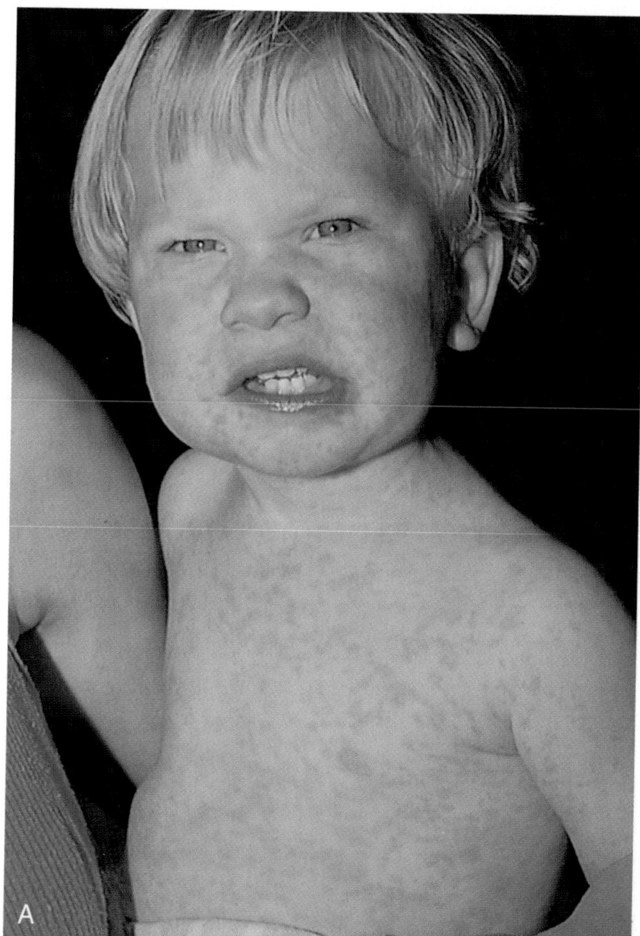

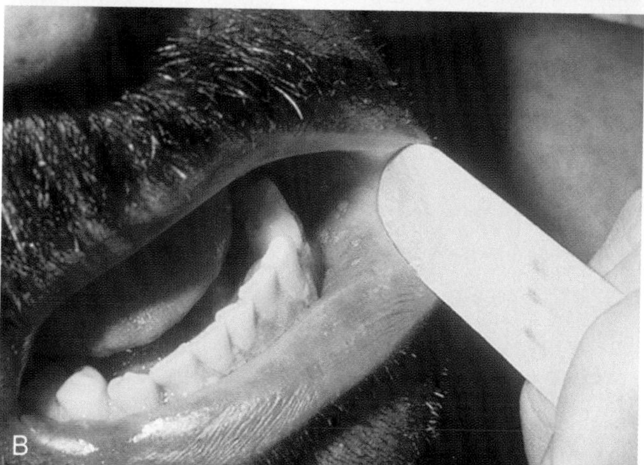

FIGURE 16–5 **A:** Skin rash of measles. Note periorbital edema and photophobia. (From Ostler, with permission.) **B:** Koplik's spots in an adult patient. (From Goodheart, with permission.)

REFERENCES

1. Stalkup JR. A review of measles virus. *Dermatol Clin* 2002;20:209–215.
2. Rall GF. Measles virus 1998–2002: progress and controversy. *Annu Rev Microbiol* 2003;57:343–37.

Mumps

Michael Greenberg

Clinical Presentation

Patients with mumps may present with prodromal symptoms including malaise, fever, chills, headache, and sore throat. This prodrome is followed by uncomfortable swelling of one or both parotid glands. Mumps orchitis, a common complication of the disease, manifests with unilateral pain and swelling of the scrotum. Approximately 30% of cases are subclinical and asymptomatic.[1-3]

Pathophysiology

Mumps is caused by the mumps paramyxovirus, which may invade tissues including the parotid glands, testicles, pancreas, and eyes.[1,2] The period for incubation is 2 to 3 weeks, and the patient is contagious for approximately 10 days, from a few days before swelling is noted until the swelling resolves. Death from mumps is not a common event, but it is more common in young adults.[1,2]

Mumps orchitis, which is common in preadolescent boys, is usually unilateral in nature. It rarely causes sterility unless the condition is bilateral. Mumps orchitis should be considered in the differential diagnosis for any patient who presents with scrotal swelling. Mumps is also one of the most frequent causes of unilateral hearing loss.[1-3]

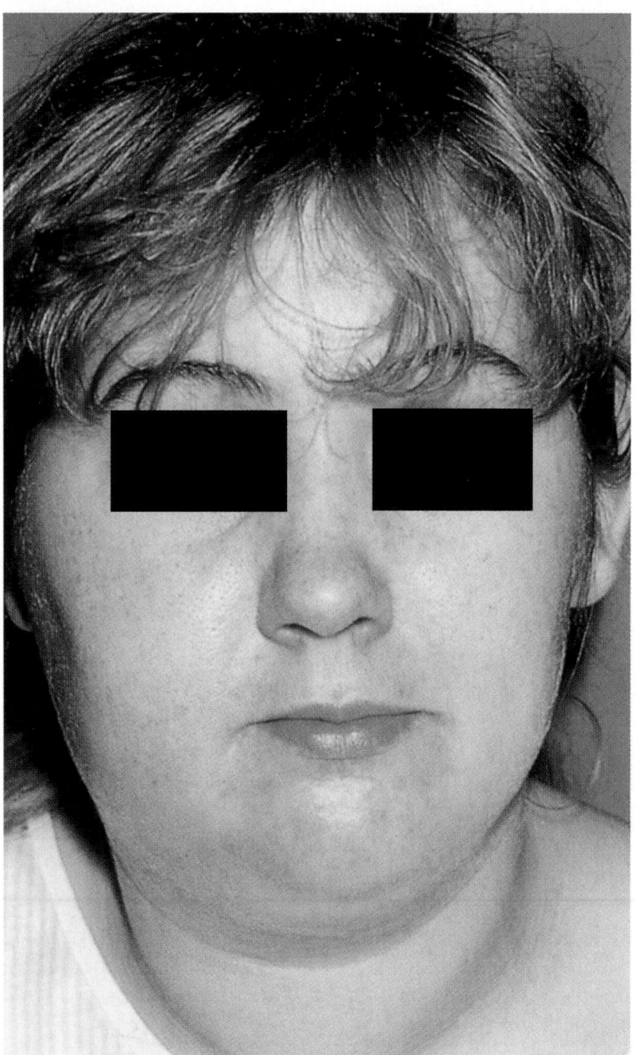

FIGURE 16–6 Parotitis (mumps). This teenager has bilateral parotid swellings as a result of mumps. (From Benjamin, with permission.)

Diagnosis

The diagnosis is based on clinical examination. Patients usually manifest fevers up to 103° F in conjunction with nonindurated swelling in the area of the parotid glands. The area overlying the parotids usually is not red or warm, unless a secondary bacterial parotitis has developed. In many cases of mumps parotidis, Stensen's duct is erythematous and swollen. In some cases, facial edema spreads to include the anterior chest, resulting in obvious presternal edema. The diagnosis of mumps may be confirmed by serologic testing. Viral cultures may be obtained in some cases.[1-3]

Clinical Complications

Complications include orchitis, pancreatitis, unilateral hearing loss, cerebellar ataxia, cranial neuritis, meningitis, cerebritis, cerebellitis, polyradicular neuritis, encephalitis, transverse myelitis, spontaneous abortion, nephritis, and myocarditis. Among patients who develop the rare complication of meningoencephalitis, the mortality rate is approximately 2%.[1-3]

Management

Treatment is primarily supportive and directed at preventing dehydration and relieving discomfort. Scrotal pain may be addressed with scrotal support, cold compresses, and antiinflammatory medications. If dehydration has occurred, or if serious complications such as central nervous system infection are suspected, the patient should be promptly hospitalized.

REFERENCES

1. McQuone SJ. Acute viral and bacterial infections of the salivary glands. *Otolaryngol Clin North Am* 1999;32:793–811.
2. Nussinovitch M, Volovitz B, Varsano I. Complications of mumps requiring hospitalization in children. *Eur J Pediatr* 1995;154:732–734.
3. Kabakus N, Aydinoglu H, Yekeler H, Arslan IN. Fatal mumps nephritis and myocarditis. *J Trop Pediatr* 1999;45:358–360.

Rubella

Christy Salvaggio

Clinical Presentation

Children with rubella first present with a pruritic, maculopapular, erythematous rash that starts on the face and spreads to the extremities.[1] The rash typically lasts 3 days, with the face clearing first. Adults may present with prodromal symptoms (fever, malaise, cough, sore throat, lymphadenopathy) several days before the rash appears. Lymphadenopathy lasts about 1 week and is most prominent in the posterior auricular, suboccipital, and posterior cervical chains. Arthralgias and arthritis, infrequently seen in children, are more common in adolescents and adults, especially women.

Pathophysiology

Humans are the only host for the RNA togavirus that causes rubella. Transmission is primarily by nasopharyngeal, airborne, or droplet spread. Patients are infectious 5 to 7 days before and up to 2 weeks after onset of symptoms. Congenitally infected infants may remain infectious for months after birth. Rubella is typically a mild infection in children and is often subclinical in adults. The incubation period ranges from 1 to 21 days.

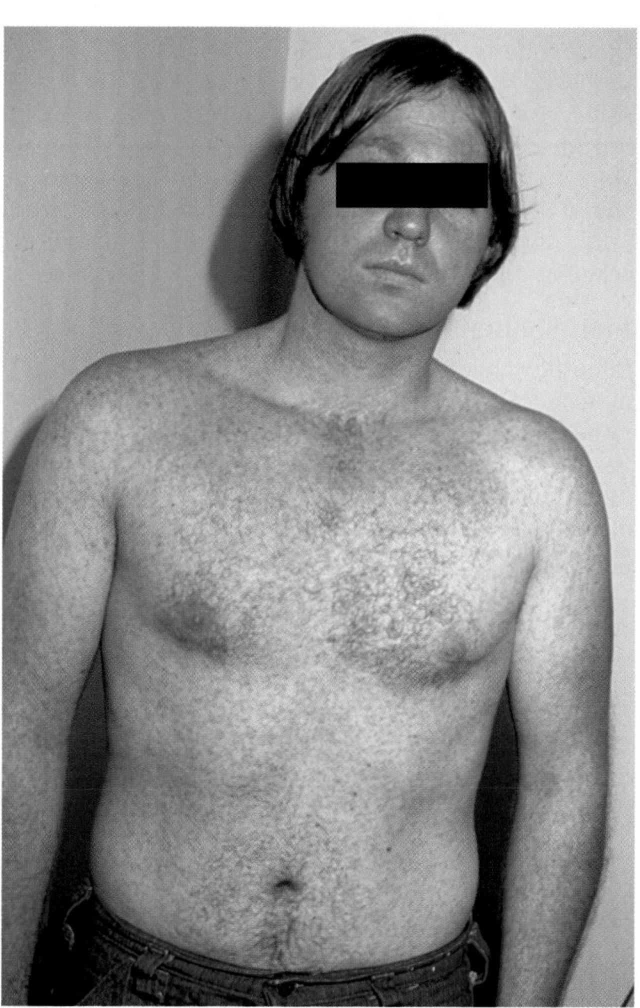

FIGURE 16–7 Rubella. This patient has a viral exanthem. This rash is not distinctive enough to allow a definitive diagnosis based on the clinical presentation alone. (From Goodheart, with permission.)

Diagnosis

Serum immunoglobulin M (IgM) and acute and convalescent serum IgG levels usually confirm the diagnosis. Rubella virus may be cultured from nasopharyngeal or pharyngeal swabs, urine, blood, and cerebrospinal fluid. Notification to laboratory personnel of possible rubella infection may increase culture sensitivity.

Clinical Complications

Most infections are self-limited, and clinical complications are rare; however, congenital infections are associated with significant morbidity and mortality. Maternal infection in the first trimester results in fetal infection in most cases and congenital defects in 100% of infected infants. In contrast, there is almost no risk of fetal infection or congenital defects after the second trimester.[1]

Congenital infection may result in spontaneous abortion, intrauterine growth retardation, or stillbirth. Congenital rubella syndrome (CRS) may include mental or physical retardation, hearing loss, cardiac anomalies, ocular anomalies, hepatomegaly and jaundice, purpura, and thrombocytopenia.

Management

Preventative care consists of a two-dose vaccine regimen (part of the measles-mumps-rubella MMR vaccine). The rubella vaccine is a live-attenuated vaccine and is contraindicated in pregnancy. Management of rubella infection generally consists of supportive care, because rubella is usually mild and self-limited. Nonsteroidal antiinflammatory drugs (NSAIDS) are effective for patients with arthralgias.

Postexposure prophylaxis for women exposed early in pregnancy who do not desire pregnancy termination consists of intramuscular immune globulin (20 mL). Consultation with an obstetric or infectious disease specialist (or both) is recommended. Administration of immune globulin within 72 hours after exposure is most effective in preventing infection. There is no effective treatment for infection during pregnancy or for infants with CRS. Contact isolation must be provided for any infant with suspected CRS.

REFERENCES

1. Vander Straten MR, Tyring SK. Rubella. *Dermatol Clin* 2002;20: 225–231.

Varicella (Chickenpox)

Kimberly J. Center

Clinical Presentation

Varicella (chickenpox) manifests as a characteristic generalized, purpuric, vesicular exanthem occurring about 14 days after infection (incubation period, 10 to 21 days). Lesions appear on the head and trunk and spread centrifugally to cover the body and mucous membranes; the average number of lesions is 300. Lesions begin as red macules that evolve to form clear vesicles on an erythematous base ("dew drop on a rose petal"); over the next 24 to 48 hours, the fluid becomes cloudy and crusting begins. New crops of lesions appear for 1 to 7 days. Typically, lesions in various stages of evolution are evident. Crusts are eventually sloughed, leaving minimal scars, although changes in pigmentation may persist for several weeks. Varicella in vaccinated patients may be less severe, with fewer, nonvesiculopustular lesions and milder systemic symptoms.[1] Constitutional symptoms, including fever (100 to 102° F), malaise, anorexia, and mild abdominal pain, occur 24 to 72 hours after the rash appears.

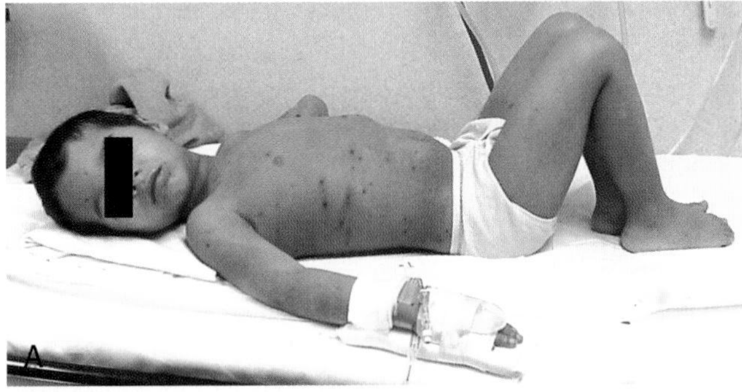

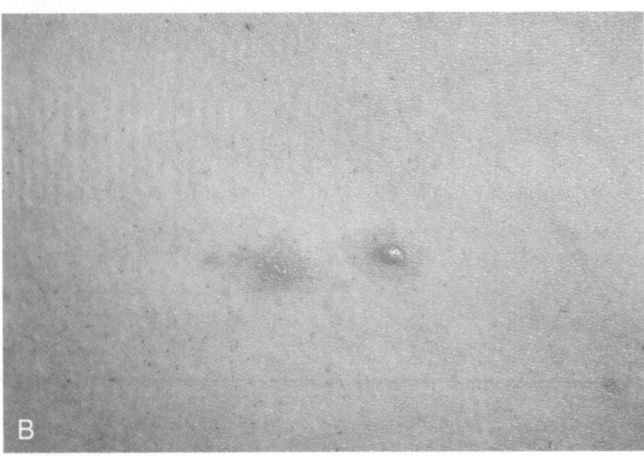

FIGURE 16–8 **A:** Varicella. Note truncal distribution. (Courtesy of Kimberly J. Center, MD.) **B:** Varicella. "Dewdrops on rose petals." (From Goodheart, with permission.)

Pathophysiology

Varicella-zoster virus (VZV) is the causative agent of chickenpox (primary infection) and zoster (reactivation of latent infection). VZV is highly contagious. Transmission occurs via direct contact with skin lesions or by airborne spread. Respiratory secretions are infectious before the rash appears. The virus remains in the dorsal root ganglia as an inevitable consequence of primary infection, and reactivation results in zoster. After infection, immunity is generally lifelong, and symptomatic reinfection is uncommon in healthy people.

Diagnosis

Diagnostic testing is not required in healthy children. If testing is desired, the direct fluorescent antibody test, polymerase chain reaction testing of a lesion scraping, or viral culture is available.

Clinical Complications

Complications include bacterial superinfection, encephalitis, seizures, cerebellar disease, varicella hepatitis, Reye's syndrome, thrombocytopenia, and varicella pneumonia (in adolescents and adults).[2] Pregnant women may have severe disease, and infection may result in congenital varicella syndrome (cutaneous defects, limb atrophy, microcephaly, mental retardation, seizures, and chorioretinitis).

Management

In healthy children, antiviral therapy is not routinely recommended.[2] Antiviral treatment (e.g., acyclovir) is warranted in patients who are older than 12 years of age, have chronic skin or pulmonary conditions, are receiving long-term salicylate therapy, or are taking corticosteroids. Acyclovir should be started within the first 24 to 72 hours of illness.[1] A live-attenuated varicella vaccine is recommended for healthy people older than 12 months of age.[2]

REFERENCES

1. Feder HM Jr, LaRussa P, Steinberg S, Gershon AA. Clinical varicella following varicella vaccination: don't be fooled. *Pediatrics* 1997;99:897–899.
2. American Academy of Pediatrics Committee on Infectious Diseases: The use of oral acyclovir in otherwise healthy children with varicella. *Pediatrics* 1993;91:674–676.

Pediatric Foreign Body Aspiration

Mark Waltzman

Clinical Presentation

If foreign body aspiration (FBA) in a child is witnessed, the clinical presentation is easily identified as a brief period of choking, gagging, or wheezing, followed by hoarseness, aphonia, or dysphonia. However, up to 50% of patients with FBA do not have a contributing history.[1] These patients may present with a variety of respiratory complaints, including cough, dyspnea, and chest pain. FBA should be considered in all pediatric patients who have unilateral lung findings, particularly unilateral wheezing.

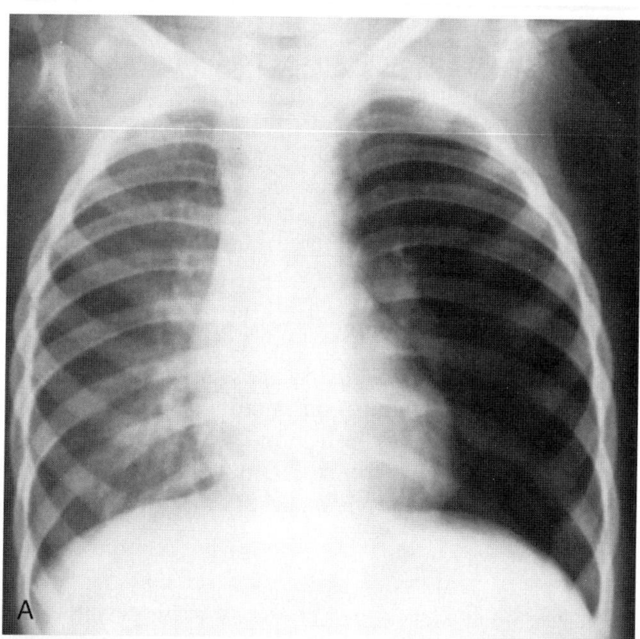

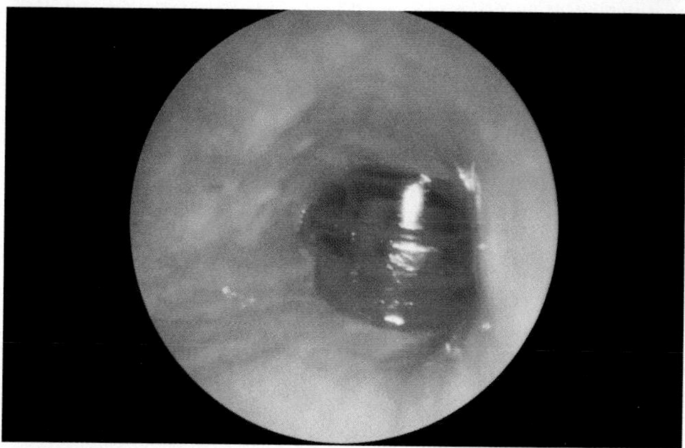

FIGURE 16–9 A: Hyperinflation of the left lung and mediastinal shift to the right. (From Swischuk, with permission.) **B:** Inhaled plastic foreign body lodged in airway as seen on endoscopy. (From Benjamin, with permission.)

Pathophysiology

Foreign bodies in the trachea or in a bronchus may lead to air trapping, inflammation, and consolidation. Of special note are complications associated with aspiration of nuts such as peanuts or cashews. The salt and oil may cause an inflammatory response and subsequent pneumonitis.[1] In addition, peanuts and similar organic materials may swell, fragment, and crumble, making them difficult to remove.

Diagnosis

Patients may be asymptomatic, initially developing delayed symptoms related to the area of obstruction. Tracheal foreign bodies may produce a "brassy" cough with or without abnormal voice, bidirectional stridor, or complete airway obstruction.[2] Bronchial foreign bodies may produce cough, asymmetric wheezing, diminished breath sounds, and hyperresonance to percussion. Because many FBAs are radiolucent, radiographs are useful primarily in detecting indirect signs of a foreign body, such as air trapping, mediastinal shift, atelectasis, or pneumonia.[3] Forced expiratory or lateral decubitus chest radiographs may be used in the evaluation of air trapping (the obstructed lung remains inflated during expiration). Absence of physical or radiographic findings does not preclude the possibility of an FBA, and, if clinical suspicion is high, bronchoscopy should be considered.

Clinical Complications

Complications include pneumonia, respiratory distress, and respiratory arrest.[4]

Management

Once the diagnosis of an FBA has been confirmed, or if the history is compelling for a foreign body, referral to an ear, nose, and throat specialist is recommended, and removal by bronchoscopy in the operating theater, as opposed to the emergency department, should be considered.[1–4]

REFERENCES

1. Cataneo AJ, Reibscheid SM, Ruiz RL Jr, Ferrari GF. Foreign body in the tracheobronchial tree. *Clin Pediatr (Phila)* 1997;36:701–706.
2. Verghese ST, Hannallah RS. Pediatric otolaryngologic emergencies. *Anesthesiol Clin North Am* 2001;19:237–256.
3. Rovin JP, Rodgers BM. Pediatric foreign body aspiration. *Pediatr Rev* 2000;21:86–90.
4. Swanson KL, Prakash UB, Midthun DE, et al. Flexible bronchoscopic management of airway foreign bodies in children. *Chest* 2002;121:1695–1700.

Pediatric Pneumonia

Carolyn Trend

Clinical Presentation

Pediatric patients with pneumonia present with a history that is typical of pneumonia. The child is usually acutely ill, with fever, cough, tachypnea, and leukocytosis, although some children present with only mild respiratory symptoms.

Diagnosis

The radiographic appearance of "round pneumonia" and the thymus are relatively unique to pediatrics. "Round pneumonia" is a pulmonary infection that appears as a round, water-density shadow on chest radiograph.[1,2] The thymus may produce opacities in the upper lung field that may be evident in very young children. Chest radiography of a "round pneumonia" shows an infiltrate with irregular margins and air bronchograms. The infiltrate, commonly found in the posterior portions of the lungs, usually appears round on frontal projection but may look triangular on lateral views. Some patients have additional parenchymal densities in the ipsilateral or contralateral lung fields. Many patients have hilar enlargement as well.[1,2] A child with signs and symptoms consistent with respiratory infection who has radiographic findings consistent with round pneumonia does not require additional diagnostic studies.

The thymus may produce a shadow in bilateral upper lung fields (the so-called "sail sign") that should not be mistaken for an infiltrate. The thymus is typically symmetric on the anteroposterior or posteroanterior film and is not present in the upper lung fields of the lateral image.

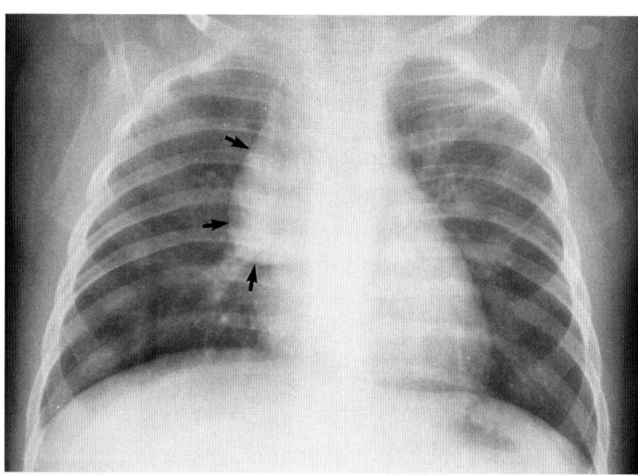

FIGURE 16–10 This well-defined, right mediastinal mass is actually the thymus shadow *(arrows)*. (From Harris and Harris, with permission.)

Clinical Complications

Complications of pneumonia include empyema, lung abscess, pneumatocele, respiratory failure, sepsis, and metastatic infection.

Management

Patients with pneumonia should be treated with antibiotics to cover *Streptococcus pneumoniae*, the most common organism causing round pneumonia.[2] Other organisms that may cause infection presenting as round pneumonia include group A streptococci, *Klebsiella pneumoniae*, and staphylococcal species.

REFERENCES

1. Rose RW, Ward BH. Spherical pneumonias in children simulating pulmonary and mediastinal masses. *Radiology* 1973;106:179–182.
2. Camargos PA, Ferreira CS. On round pneumonia in children. *Pediatr Pulmonol* 1995;20:194–195.

Cystic Fibrosis

Robert Hendrickson

Clinical Presentation

Patients with cystic fibrosis (CF) may present to the emergency department (ED) with infectious, pulmonary, or gastrointestinal manifestations of CF. Patients with CF may have chronic productive cough, obstructive airway disease, sinusitis, and nasal polyps, as well as pulmonary colonization with *Staphylococcus aureus, Haemophilus influenzae, Pseudomonas aeruginosa,* and *Burkholderia cepacia.*[1] Exacerbations of their pulmonary disease may be obstructive or infectious (e.g., pneumonia, bronchitis). Patients with CF may have chronic pancreatitis, with acute exacerbations presenting as abdominal pain and increased steatorrhea.

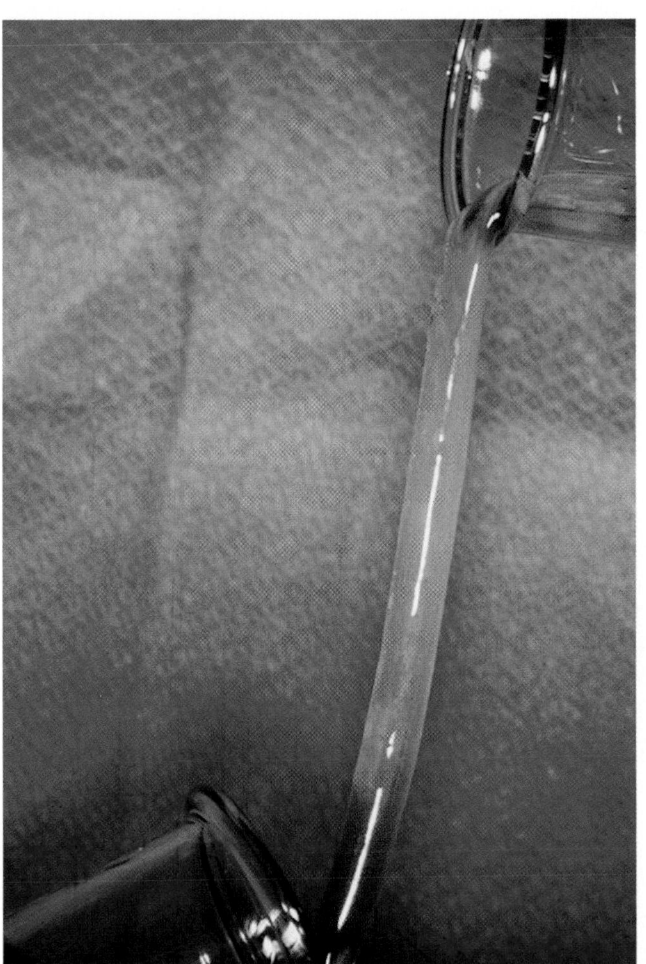

FIGURE 16–11 Duodenal mucus from a patient with cystic fibrosis obtained by means of intraduodenal intubation. Extremely viscid mucus retains its elastic properties even when poured from flask to flask. (From Yamada, with permission.)

Pathophysiology

CF is an autosomal recessive disorder of chloride channels that is associated with disorders of the pulmonary, gastrointestinal, and urogenital systems.[1] A variety of mutations of the cystic fibrosis transmembrane conductance regulator (CFTR) gene on chromosome 7 may lead to an altered chloride channel and CF. Alteration in the chloride channel leads to decreased absorption of water and sodium in epithelial cells (e.g., in the pulmonary tree) and decreased mucociliary clearance.[2] This leads to chronic thickening of bronchial secretions and edema, as well as inhibited pulmonary immunity (obstructive and infectious pulmonary disease) and obstruction of seminal vesicles (oligospermia) and the pancreatic duct (pancreatitis).

Diagnosis

Most CF patients seen in the ED already carry the diagnosis of CF. The diagnosis may be made at birth through perinatal screening or in early childhood by recognition of the typical chronic symptoms. The diagnosis may be confirmed by quantitative pilocarpine iontophoresis, or the "sweat test."[2]

Clinical Complications

Complications include acute and chronic obstructive airway disease, suppurative pulmonary infections, hepatitis, biliary cirrhosis, sinusitis, pancreatitis, oligospermia, protein-calorie malnutrition, intestinal obstruction, and ileus.[1,2]

Management

Patients with infectious or obstructive pulmonary exacerbations may require airway control, ventilation, fluid resuscitation, and antibiotics. Obstructive airway symptoms may be treated with inhaled β-adrenergic agonists and anticholinergic agents. Patients with suspected infections should be treated with parenteral antistaphylococcal and antipseudomonal antibiotics.[2] Several weeks of antibiotic therapy is required; the specific antibiotic should be based on the patient's prophylactic regimen and personal and local resistance and should be coordinated with the primary physician. Gastritis or gastroesophageal reflux disease may be treated with proton-pump inhibitors. Mild, chronic pancreatitis may require oral pancreatic enzymes. Severe pancreatitis may require bowel rest, pain control, and intravenous hydration.

REFERENCES

1. Rosenstein BJ, Zeitlin PL. Cystic fibrosis. *Lancet* 1998;351:277–282.
2. Ratjen F, Doring G. Cystic fibrosis. *Lancet* 2003;361:681–689.

16–12

Kawasaki Disease

Christy Salvaggio

Clinical Presentation

Patients with Kawasaki disease are typically children aged 1 to 2 years who are irritable and have the following symptoms: fever lasting 5 days or longer (high and unresponsive to antipyretics), cervical lymphadenopathy greater than 1.5 cm, nonsuppurative conjunctivitis, mucous membrane lesions (dry, cracked lips; strawberry tongue), hand and/or foot swelling (diffuse erythema/ swelling), and an erythematous rash (truncal maculopapular).[1,2]

Pathophysiology

Kawasaki disease, or "mucocutaneous lymph node syndrome," is a medium- and large-vessel vasculitis of uncertain origin that has a propensity for coronary arteries.[1,2] The cause of Kawasaki disease is most likely multifactorial, including genetic factors (Asian children are at highest risk) as well as seasonal, infectious, and environmental influences.

Diagnosis

The criteria for Kawasaki disease are fever (5 days or longer) with at least four of the following symptoms: lymphadenopathy, conjunctivitis, mucous membrane involvement, hand/feet erythema or swelling, and an erythematous rash. Children are typically quite irritable and uncomfortable. Children with fever who have fewer than four of the diagnostic criteria may represent "atypical" Kawasaki presentations. Resting tachycardia out of proportion to the fever is common, and most children show some degree of myocarditis and effusion on initial echocardiography. Some children have overt congestive heart failure. Although cardiovascular symptoms predominate, Kawasaki disease may involve multisystem (gastrointestinal, renal, rheumatologic, neurologic) pathology. Symptoms may include vomiting, diarrhea, hepatitis, cholestasis, hydrops of the gallbladder, sterile pyuria, arthritis, arthralgias, and aseptic meningitis. Acute phase reactants, including erythrocyte sedimenta-

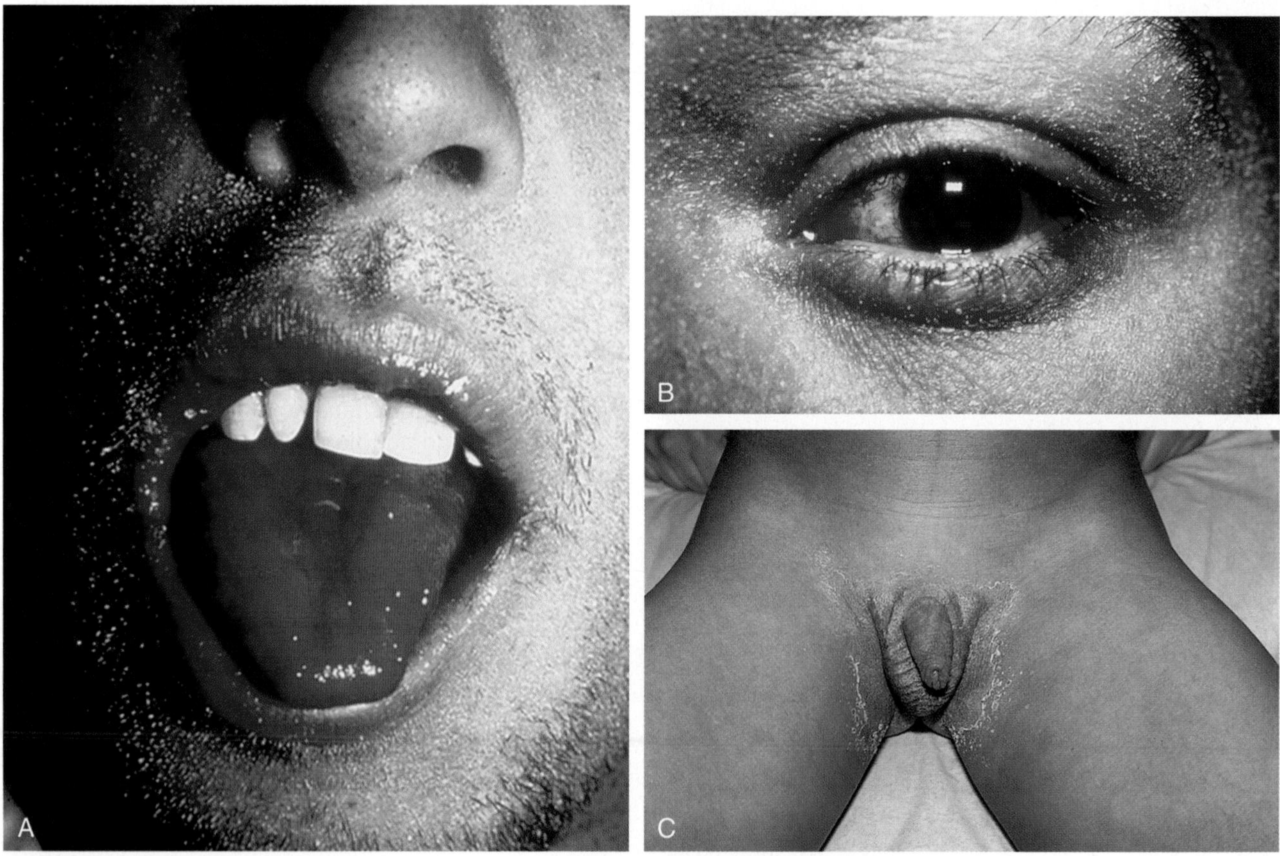

FIGURE 16–12 **A:** "Strawberry tongue." **B:** Conjunctivitis of Kawasaki disease. **C:** Erythema and desquamation may occur in the genital area and on the hands and feet. (**A–C**, From Goodheart, with permission.)

Kawasaki Disease

Christy Salvaggio

tion rate (ESR) and C-reactive protein level (CRP), are elevated, and patients may have a leukocytosis and a cerebrospinal fluid pleocytosis.

Clinical Complications

Complications include aneurysm formation (from vasculitis), especially of the coronary arteries, with thrombosis. Patients ultimately need long-term cardiology follow-up with serial echocardiograms.[1,2]

Management

A pediatric and/or cardiology consultation should be obtained for any patient with a constellation of symptoms concerning Kawasaki disease, even if not all of the criteria for diagnosis are met.[1] Patients with Kawasaki disease may be treated with intravenous immune globulin (IVIG) and acetylsalicylic acid (ASA) therapy. Single-dose IVIG given within 10 days after symptom onset decreases the incidence of coronary artery pathology from 17% to 4%.[1] The response to IVIG may vary, but most children are markedly improved and afebrile within 24 hours. The white blood cell count and CRP decrease significantly, but the ESR remains elevated for several weeks after IVIG. Patients may be treated with high-dose aspirin therapy until they are at least 14 days into the illness and have been afebrile for 48 hours, followed by low-dose aspirin until the ESR normalizes and a repeat echocardiogram is normal.[1]

REFERENCES

1. Newburger JW, Takahashi M, Burns JC, et al. The treatment of Kawasaki syndrome with intravenous gamma globulin. *N Engl J Med* 1986;315:341–347.
2. Rowley AH. Incomplete (atypical) Kawasaki disease. *Pediatr Infect Dis J* 2002;21:563–565.

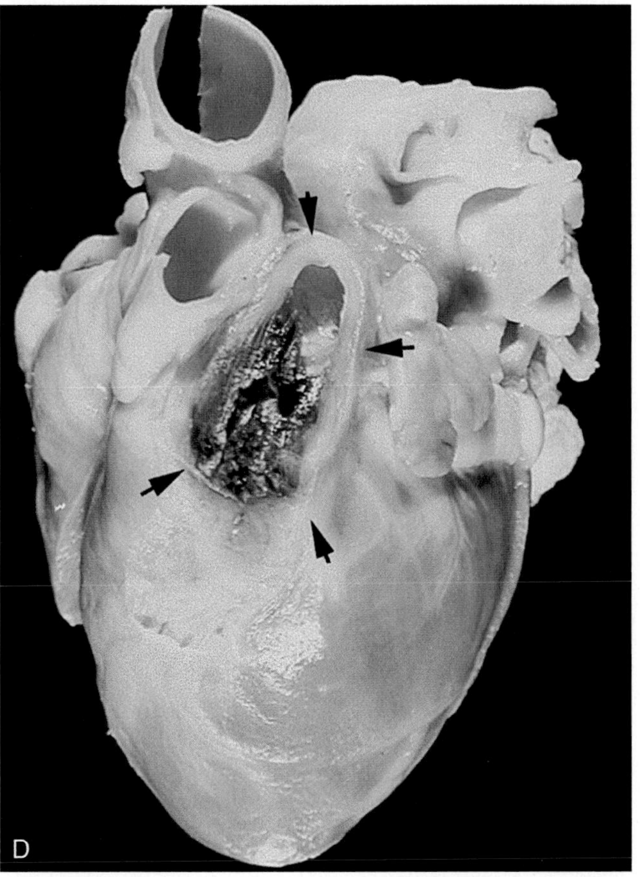

FIGURE 16–12, cont'd D: Coronary artery aneurysm with thrombosis. (From Reece, with permission.)

Hand-Foot-and-Mouth Disease

Christy Salvaggio

Clinical Presentation

The large majority of coxsackie infections are asymptomatic. Symptomatic patients with hand-foot-and-mouth disease present with fever, malaise, oral ulcers, and papular cutaneous lesions. The oral lesions are erythematous macules that may evolve into vesicles or ruptured ulcers on the buccal and glossal mucosa and hard palate. Children may complain of a sore throat, refuse to eat, or be drooling secondary to painful oral ulcers.[1,2] Cutaneous lesions consist of 3- to 5-mm, tender, gray papules or vesicles with surrounding erythema. The lesions are most concentrated on the distal extremities and the buttocks. Palm and sole involvement is common. The timing of the appearance of cutaneous lesions is variable, and they may precede the appearance of oral ulcers. Oral and cutaneous lesions usually resolve within 1 week.[1,2]

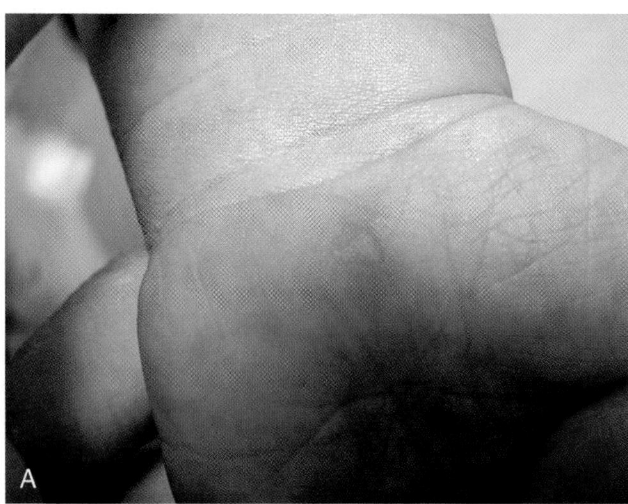

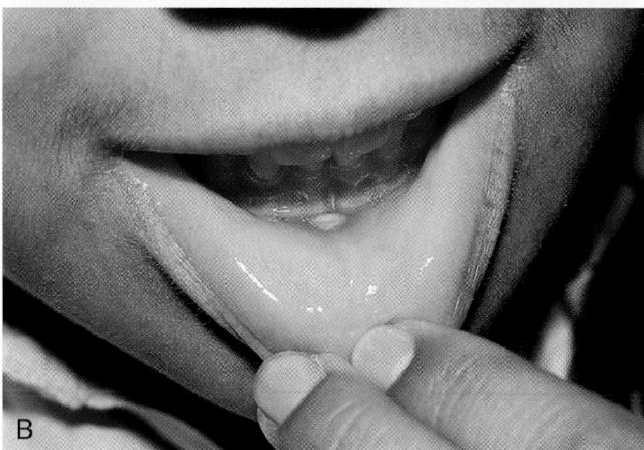

FIGURE 16–13 **A:** Typical 3- to 7-mm, oval, gray vesicle of the palm. (Courtesy of Christy Salvaggio, MD.) **B:** Oral lesion of hand-foot-and-mouth disease. Note the oval shape and rim of erythema. (From Goodheart, with permission.)

Pathophysiology

Hand-foot-and-mouth disease is an enterovirus infection, most commonly caused by coxsackie A16, that manifests as oral mucosal ulcerations and cutaneous papular lesions, especially on the hands and feet.[1,3] This is primarily a disease of childhood, usually affecting children younger than 10 years of age. Children younger than 5 years of age are at highest risk. High-risk adults include caretakers and household contacts of infected children. Most enteroviruses are shed in the stool, and hand-foot-and-mouth disease is predominantly spread by the fecal-oral route. Infection rates are high, approaching 100% for close contacts. Hand-foot-and-mouth disease occurs year-round, but infection rates are highest during the summer and fall.[1–4]

Diagnosis

Hand-foot-and-mouth disease is essentially a clinical diagnosis. If oral ulcers and classic cutaneous lesions are present, the disease is easy to diagnosis; however, cutaneous lesions may precede any mucosal involvement, making the diagnosis more challenging. Viral cultures or determination of circulating antibodies is rarely needed for diagnosis.[1,2] The differential diagnosis for oral ulcers and gingival inflammation includes herpangina, which is also caused by coxsackie viruses, and gingivostomatitis, which is caused by herpes simplex viruses. Neither herpangina nor gingivostomatitis has the cutaneous manifestations classic for hand-foot-and-mouth disease. The oral ulcers of herpangina are more concentrated in the posterior oropharynx. Gingivostomatitis often has significant gingival inflammation, erythema, and tenderness that may precede the appearance of ulcers. Coalescence of ulcers and bleeding mucosa may also be seen. An accurate clinical diagnosis is important, because there is no effective antiviral therapy for hand-foot-and-mouth disease, but acyclovir is effective for herpes gingivostomatitis.[1,2]

Clinical Complications

Dehydration is the most common complication and may usually be avoided with persistent efforts to encourage oral hydration and adequate pain management. Rarely, hand-foot-and-mouth disease progresses to more serious disease, such as pneumonia, myocarditis, acute flaccid paralysis, encephalitis, or meningitis.[1–4]

Management

Although this is usually a self-limited disease, caregivers must be aware that fever may persist for several days and more lesions may appear before symptoms start to resolve. Oral lesions may be painful, and oral hydration may be difficult. For patients who are moderately to severely symptomatic, topical anesthetics, such as diphenhydramine with or without topical lidocaine, are the mainstay of treatment. A popular combination, called "magic mouthwash," includes equal parts of 1% viscous lidocaine, diphenhydramine, and aluminum/magnesium hydroxide (e.g., Maalox). Older patients can gargle and spit the solution. For young children, caregivers can paint the solution on the lesions. Because of the potential for lidocaine toxicity, patients should not be prescribed more than 2 mL/kg of the mixed solution (no more than 0.6 mL/kg of 1% lidocaine). Greater quantities may produce seizures or confusion if taken all at once by the child.[2,4] Dehydrated children who are refusing liquids should receive intravenous hydration and topical oral anesthetics. Children who continue to refuse liquids may need hospitalization for continued intravenous hydration.[4]

REFERENCES

1. Stalkup J. Enterovirus infections: a review of clinical presentation, diagnosis, and treatment. *Dermatol Clin* 2002;20:217.
2. Amir J. Clinical aspects and antiviral therapy in primary herpetic gingivostomatitis. *Paediatr Drugs* 2001;3:593–597.
3. Glick M. Viral and fungal infections of the oral cavity in immunocompetent patients. *Infect Dis Clin North Am* 1999;13:817–831.
4. Amir J, Harel L, Smetana Z, et al. Treatment of herpes simplex gingivostomatitis with aciclovir in children: a randomised double blind placebo controlled study. BMJ 1997;314:1800–1803.

Erythema Infectiosum

Mark Silverberg

Clinical Presentation

Erythema infectiosum (EI) typically afflicts children 5 to 15 years of age, with seasonal peaks in late winter and early spring. It begins with a mild prodrome of low-grade fever and symptoms of an upper respiratory tract infection, soon followed by a symmetric facial rash, giving the "slapped cheek" appearance.[1] The rash then spreads to the trunk and extremities in a reticulated pattern. In adults and adolescents, the rash is less common. They are more likely to present after parvovirus B19 infection with arthralgias that are self-limited and resolve within a few weeks.[1]

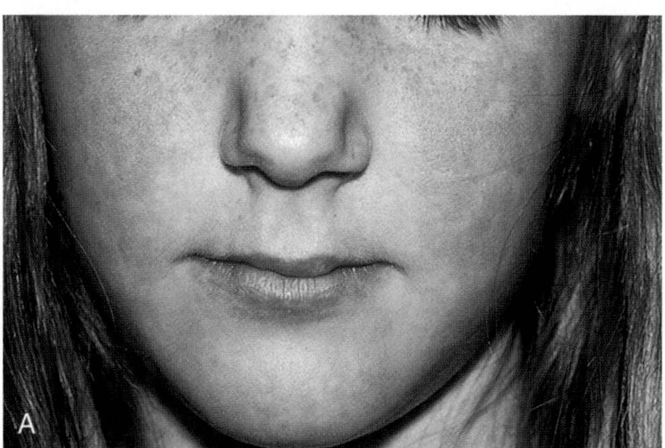

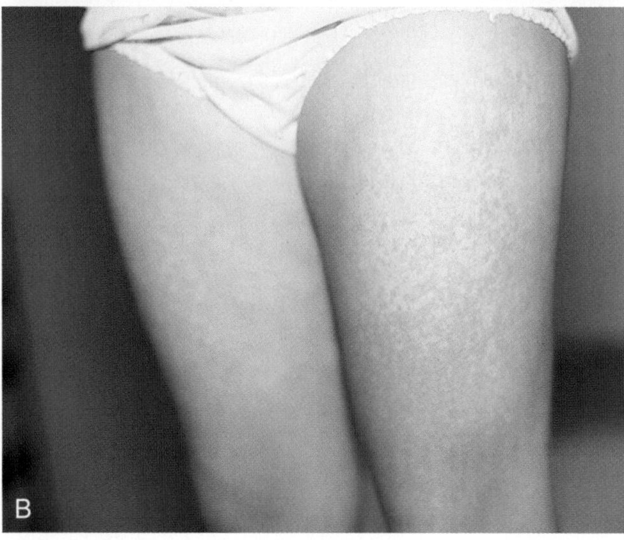

FIGURE 16–14 **A:** Malar rash of fifth disease ("slapped cheek"). **B:** Typical reticular pattern on the legs of this patient with fifth disease. (**A** and **B**, From Goodheart, with permission.)

Pathophysiology

EI, also known as "fifth disease," is an acute infectious illness of childhood caused by parvovirus B19, a nonenveloped, single-stranded DNA virus,[2] that results in a characteristic prodrome and rash.[1] It is transmitted through respiratory secretion droplets, but infection through blood products has been documented.[1,2] Parvovirus B19 has a tendency to attack erythroid precursor cells, especially in individuals who already have chronic hemolytic anemias.[1] The distinctive rash of fifth disease is associated with the clearance of viremia and the production of a specific antibody to the virus particles; it is thought to be caused by immune complex deposition.[1] In immunocompromised individuals, chronic infection with parvovirus B19 may persist.[1,2]

Diagnosis

The diagnosis has traditionally been based on the clinical appearance of the typical rash, although reliable serologic tests have recently been developed. A test for anti-B19 immunoglobulin M has been marketed, and a serologic assay for B19 viral antigens is also available.[1,2]

Clinical Complications

Complications may include transient aplastic crisis in hemolytic anemia, arthropathy, myocarditis, encephalitis, idiopathic thrombocytopenic purpura, hemophagocytic syndrome, dermatologic syndromes, rheumatologic diseases, renal disease, and hepatitis.[1] Maternal infection during pregnancy usually leads to fetal infection, which has been shown to cause nonimmune hydrops fetalis and fetal death.[1] Chronic infection in immunocompromised individuals has brought about chronic anemia.[1]

Management

The treatment of EI is usually symptomatic. In patients with chronic hemolytic anemias such as sickle cell disease, aplastic crisis may require blood transfusions. Intravenous immune globulin (IVIG) has been successful in treating chronic infection associated with inadequate humoral responses. IVIG has also been used to treat chronic anemia due to B19 infection in immunocompromised individuals.[1]

REFERENCES

1. Koch WC. Fifth (human parvovirus) and sixth (herpesvirus 6) diseases. *Curr Opin Infect Dis* 2001;14:343–356.
2. Katta R. Parvovirus B19: a review. *Dermatol Clin* 2002;20:333–342.

Henoch-Schönlein Purpura

Adriana Klucar Stoudt

Clinical Presentation

Henoch-Schönlein purpura (HSP) is a self-limited disease that lasts approximately 1 to 2 weeks and has a tendency to recur. The median age at onset is 4 years (range, 6 months to 86 years).[1–3] The common triad of symptoms consists of purpura, colicky abdominal pain, and arthritis. Hallmark skin findings include symmetric, palpable, nonblanching purpura or petechiae (or both), most commonly on the buttocks and lower extremities. Edema (feet, hands, scalp, and periorbital), gastrointestinal symptoms (colicky abdominal pain, nausea, vomiting, and gastrointestinal bleeding), and muscular complaints (transient lower-extremity arthralgias and arthritis) are common. HSP vasculitis may affect any organ system. Renal involvement may be noted at the time of diagnosis, or it may develop months later. Transient hematuria with or without proteinuria is the most common renal manifestation. Rarely, patients develop hypertension, nephrotic syndrome, rapidly progressive glomerulonephritis, renal insufficiency, or renal failure. Acute scrotal swelling due to inflammation and hemorrhage may occur (2% to 35% of cases). Central nervous system manifestations, including headache, subtle encephalopathy, and seizures, are rare.[1] Constitutional symptoms such as malaise and low-grade fever are present in half of patients with HSP. Fever is usually an early sign and is often caused by a precipitating respiratory infection.[2]

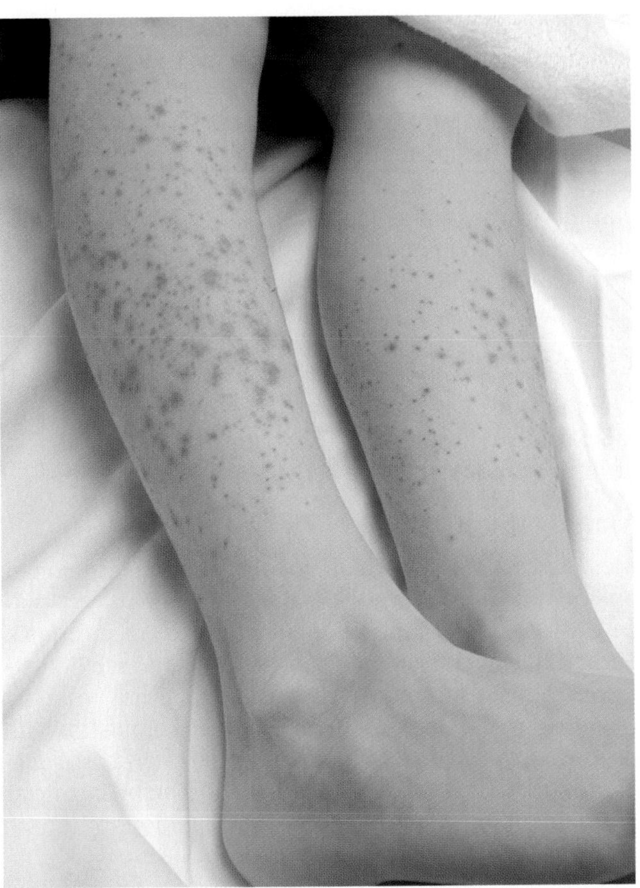

FIGURE 16–15 Lower-extremity purpura in a child with Henoch-Schönlein purpura. (Courtesy of Robert Hendrickson, MD.)

Pathophysiology

HSP is an immunoglobulin A–mediated vasculitis.

Diagnosis

The diagnosis is made based on recognition of the typical clinical symptoms. In children, palpable purpura with a normal platelet count is adequate to make the diagnosis.[1] Routine laboratory findings are typically normal.

Clinical Complications

Approximately 2% of patients develop ileoileal or ileocolic intussusception because of an intestinal wall hematoma lead point.[1] Abdominal ultrasonography is the study of choice, because enema studies may miss ileoileal intussusception. Renal complications are rare but may include persistent hypertension and end-stage kidney disease.[3]

Management

Treatment of HSP is largely supportive. Nonsteroidal antiinflammatory drugs (NSAIDs) may be used to treat joint involvement unless renal insufficiency is present. A short course of corticosteroids may be used, particularly in children with severe abdominal pain, but the efficacy of this treatment is unproven.[1] Patients with severe abdominal pain or renal failure should be hospitalized for observation. Mild renal insufficiency may be monitored closely with outpatient urinalysis and serum creatinine values. If the patient does not present with nephritis, serial outpatient urinalysis and serum creatinine levels should be monitored to observe for the development of late-onset renal involvement.[1]

REFERENCES

1. Szer IS. Henoch-Schonlein purpura: when and how to treat. *J Rheumatol* 1996;23:1661–1665.
2. Saulsbury FT. Henoch-Schonlein purpura in children. *Medicine (Baltimore)* 1999;78:395–409.
3. Robson WL, Leung AK. Henoch-Schonlein purpura. *Adv Pediatr* 1994;41:163–194.

Juvenile Rheumatoid Arthritis

Leo Ho

Clinical Presentation

Common initial symptoms of juvenile rheumatoid arthritis (JRA) include morning joint stiffness, which usually lasts at least 1 hour, stiffness after periods of inactivity (gel phenomenon), and easy fatigability. Single or multiple joints may be affected. Patients typically present to the emergency department with objective signs of arthritis (joint swelling or limited range of motion accompanied by pain). Oligoarthritis involves fewer than five joints and usually involves the lower extremities (knees, ankles). The mean age at onset is 2 years. Forty percent of patients develop anterior uveitis.[1] Polyarthritis involves five or more joints (both large and small joints). Two subtypes exist. Rheumatoid factor (RF)–negative polyarthritis (85%) has a median age at onset at 3 years. RF-positive polyarthritis has a later onset, usually in adolescence.[1] Firm, nontender, subcutaneous nodules may develop on extensor skin areas, most commonly the elbow. Systemic-onset disease (10% to 20% of cases) may manifest with arthritis with high-spiking fevers (greater than 39° C), often occurring twice daily for a minimum of 2 weeks. A salmon-pink evanescent rash (2- to 5-mm macules on the trunk and proximal extremities) may be precipitated by scratching or pressure (Koebner's phenomenon).[1]

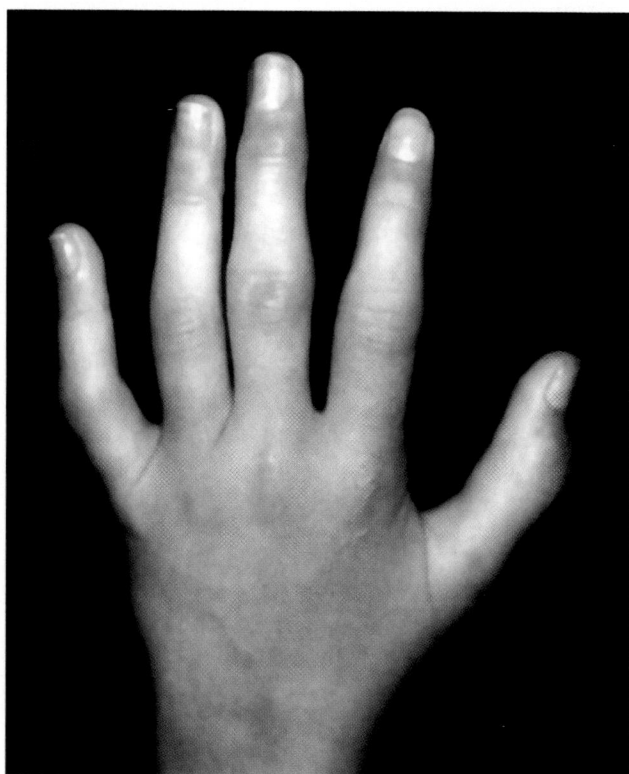

FIGURE 16–16 Hand involvement in systematic juvenile rheumatic arthritis. Note the swelling of multiple joints. (From Staheli, with permission.)

Pathophysiology

JRA is characterized by synovitis of the peripheral joints and has a strong female predominance. The three principle types of JRA are oligoarthritis (persistent or extended type), polyarticular arthritis, and systemic-onset disease (Still's disease).[1] Less common types include enthesitis arthritis, psoriatic arthritis, and unclassified arthritis.[1] The cause of JRA is unknown. However, immunogenetic susceptibility and external triggers may be involved. Possible triggers include viruses (e.g., parvovirus B19, rubella, Epstein-Barr), specific self-antigens (type II collagen), and external trauma.

Diagnosis

Diagnostic criteria include age at onset less than 16 years, oligoarticular or polyarticular arthritis, duration 6 weeks or longer, and exclusion of other forms of juvenile arthritis. Laboratory abnormalities include elevated erythrocyte sedimentation rate and C-reactive protein level, leukocytosis, thrombocytosis, and anemia of chronic disease. Radiographic findings include soft-tissue swelling and periarticular osteopenia adjacent to the involved joint. Late findings include narrowing of the joint space, erosions, subluxations, and ankylosis.

Clinical Complications

Complications include pericarditis, myocarditis, atlantoaxial subluxation, pleural effusions, cricoarytenoid arthritis, and macrophage activation syndrome.

Management

Most cases of oligoarticular JRA respond to nonsteroidal antiinflammatory drugs (NSAIDs), but children with polyarticular disease may require additional medications. Second-line agents include sulfasalazine and methotrexate. Azathioprine and cyclophosphamide are reserved for resistant cases. Intraarticular corticosteroids may be used in some patients, and intravenous corticosteroids are used for systemic illness.[1] Physical therapy is crucial for maintaining strength and range of motion.

REFERENCES

1. Woo P, Wedderburn LR. Juvenile chronic arthritis. *Lancet* 1998; 351:969–973.

Scarlet Fever

Rakesh D. Mistry

Clinical Presentation

Scarlet fever (SF) manifests abruptly with high fever, severe sore throat, vomiting, chills, and malaise in children. A fine, papular, erythematous rash is initially seen in the flexural areas on the second day of illness. Within 24 hours, the exanthem rapidly becomes generalized and begins to take on a maculopapular, "sandpaper-like" quality, often referred to as scarlatiniform.

Pathophysiology

Infection with group A β-hemolytic streptococcus (GABHS) usually occurs via direct contact or transmission of large nasal droplets. This is followed by an incubation period of 1 to 7 days, during which time the index case often manifests signs of infection. The GABHS organism typically causes direct infection of the affected site—pharynx, skin, or wound. Infecting strains then elicit streptococcal pyrogenic exotoxins A and C, which circulate systemically and produce the characteristic rash and strawberry tongue of scarlet fever.[1]

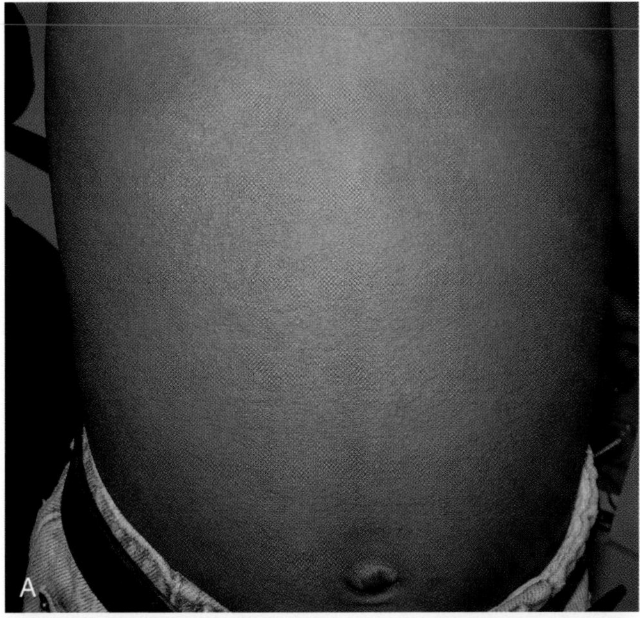

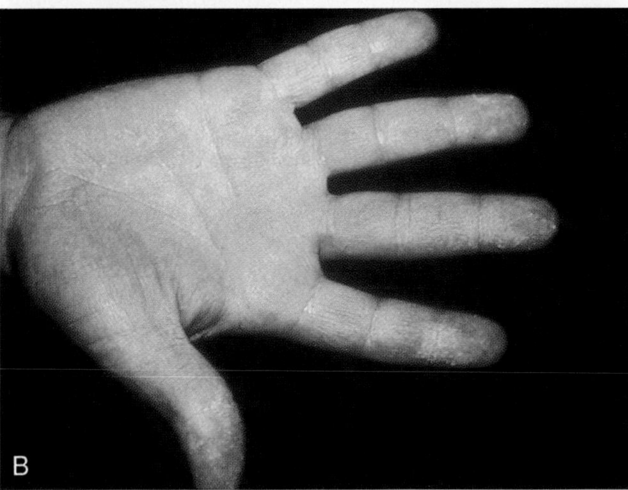

FIGURE 16–17 **A:** The "sandpaper" rash of scarlet fever. (Courtesy of Mark Silverberg, MD.) **B:** Scarlet fever. Note skin peeling from the fingertips. (From Goodheart, with permission.)

Diagnosis

Clinical diagnosis of scarlet fever is based on findings of classic GABHS pharyngitis, accompanied by signs associated with toxin-producing strains, such as "strawberry tongue" and the characteristic exanthem.[2] Throat culture is the gold standard of diagnosis. The oropharynx reveals diffuse erythema with palatal petechiae, significant tonsillar enlargement, and purulent exudates of the tonsils or posterior pharynx or both. The rash usually is accentuated in the flexural creases of the neck, elbows, and groin. This is best demonstrated in the antecubital areas, where lines of papules, known as Pastia's lines, may be seen. The rest of the skin becomes diffusely erythematous; however, the perioral area may be spared, and patients are frequently described as having "circumoral pallor."[1–3]

Clinical Complications

Complications include otitis media, sinusitis, retropharyngeal or parapharyngeal abscess, cervical adenitis, and sepsis. Poststreptococcal glomerulonephritis may develop despite treatment. A unique complication of scarlet fever is progression to the life-threatening toxic shock syndrome.

Management

Children with scarlet fever require supportive therapy, including hydration, pain control, and antipyresis. Antibiotic therapy may shorten the duration of illness and reduce symptoms; more importantly, it prevents suppurative complications and rheumatic fever. GABHS is susceptible to standard penicillin, which remains the first-line therapy, although studies have documented similar efficacy of easier-dosed penicillins and cephalosporins.[2] For penicillin-allergic patients, a course of clindamycin or a macrolide antibiotic is efficacious.[1–3]

REFERENCES

1. Corneli HM. Rapid strep tests in the emergency department: an evidence-based approach. *Pediatr Emerg Care* 2001;17:272–288.
2. Pichichero ME. Group A streptococcal tonsillopharyngitis: cost-effective diagnosis and treatment. *Ann Emerg Med* 1995;25:390–403.
3. Kline JA, Runge JW. Streptococcal pharyngitis: a review of pathophysiology, diagnosis, and management. *J Emerg Med* 1994;12:665–680.

Rickets

Michael Greenberg

Clinical Presentation

Patients usually first present between 6 and 24 months of age with orthopedic problems, inability to walk, and/or failure to thrive and grow. Modern cases of rickets involve children with darker skin who live in northern areas and therefore may have inadequate sunlight exposure.[1–3]

Pathophysiology

Rickets involves inadequate mineralization of bone due to imbalances of phosphorus and calcium metabolism, related to inadequate intake of vitamin D or inadequate exposure to sunlight or both. The poor bone mineralization results in long-bone weakness and inadequate development of bony growth plates.[1–3] Human milk does not supply vitamin D sufficient to prevent rickets without the concomitant exposure to adequate sunlight.

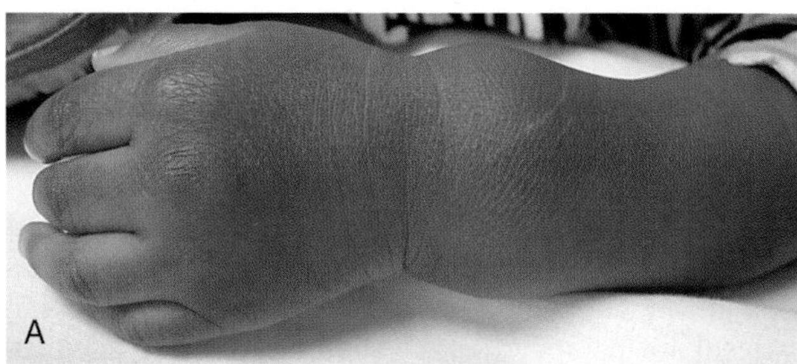

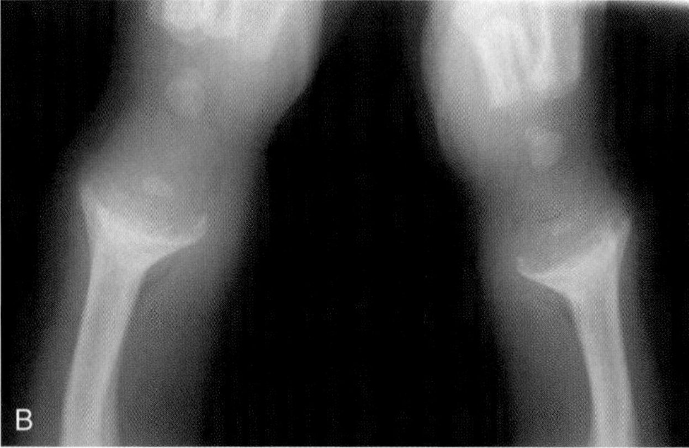

FIGURE 16–18 **A:** Characteristic widening of the wrist in a child with rickets. **B:** Widening of the epiphyseal plates and metaphyseal cupping is also characteristic of rickets. (**A** and **B**, Courtesy of Christy Salvaggio, MD.)

Diagnosis

Rickets is a clinical diagnosis and should be suspected in pediatric patients with frontal bossing of the skull, wide metaphyses, thick wrists and knees, and clinically prominent and easily palpable costochondral junctions ("rachitic rosary"). Laboratory studies reveal elevated alkaline phosphatase, secondary hyperparathyroidism, and low vitamin D and calcium levels. Nutritional rickets involves a deficiency of vitamin D, resulting from poor diet and inadequate gastrointestinal absorption in conjunction with inadequate exposure to sunlight. Vitamin D is a fat-soluble chemical that may be provided in the diet or synthesized in the skin with sunlight exposure, after which it is hydroxylated in the kidneys and liver. It is important for calcium absorption and metabolic usage.

Children who may have rickets require the taking of a careful history, including a dietary, medication, vitamin use, and social history. The physical examination must include evaluation of growth and development. Laboratory studies should include serum calcium, phosphorus, parathyroid hormone, 25-hydroxy (OH) vitamin D levels, and a complete blood count. Chest radiography may be diagnostic.

Management

A complete work-up of patients with rickets in the emergency department may not be appropriate. However, it is incumbent on emergency physicians to recognize the potential for this disease and to take steps to ensure that the child will receive a prompt and complete work-up. If the disease is suspected, patients should receive vitamin D therapy in the emergency department, and parents should be instructed to provide increased sunlight exposure for the child. Admission may be warranted, based on the patient's clinical findings or social situation.[1–3]

REFERENCES

1. Chesney RW. Rickets: the third wave. *Clin Pediatr* 2002;41:137–139.
2. Bishop N. Rickets today: children still need milk and sunshine. *N Engl J Med* 1999;341:602–604.
3. Pattaragarn A, Alon US. Antacid-induced rickets in infancy. *Clin Pediatr* 2001;40:389–393.

Hemolytic-Uremic Syndrome

Douglas Thompson

Clinical Presentation

Two forms of hemolytic-uremic syndrome (HUS) are recognized. Typical (diarrhea-positive) HUS is heralded by the onset of diarrhea that is most commonly bloody. Symptoms of anemia and thrombocytopenia, including pallor, weakness, and petechiae, present 5 to 7 days after the onset of diarrhea. Within a few days, oliguria with associated uremia occurs. Worsening renal failure ensues over the next few days, followed by a period of resolution in most patients. Hypertension is common. In atypical (diarrhea-negative) HUS, the preceding diarrheal illness is absent.[1]

Pathophysiology

HUS is defined by the clinical triad of microangiopathic hemolytic anemia, thrombocytopenia, and renal failure.[2] *Escherichia coli* O157:H7 is the usual etiologic agent, but other *E. coli* species and *Shigella dysenteriae* are also possible.[1] Potential sources include animal feces at petting zoos, undercooked beef (particularly ground beef), and unpasteurized milk and cheeses. Infection results in attachment of the bacteria to the intestinal mucosa and secretion of shiga toxin 1, which causes damage to the intestinal epithelial cells and bloody diarrhea. Systemic absorption of this toxin damages the renal epithelial and tubular cells, resulting in platelet deposition, thrombus formation, and thrombocytopenia. Anemia results when red blood cells pass through these distorted blood vessels, become sheared, and are subsequently removed from circulation by the spleen. The combination of the epithelial cell pathology and tubular cell damage leads to renal failure. In the diarrhea-negative form, there is a genetic and frequently familial basis for this disease.

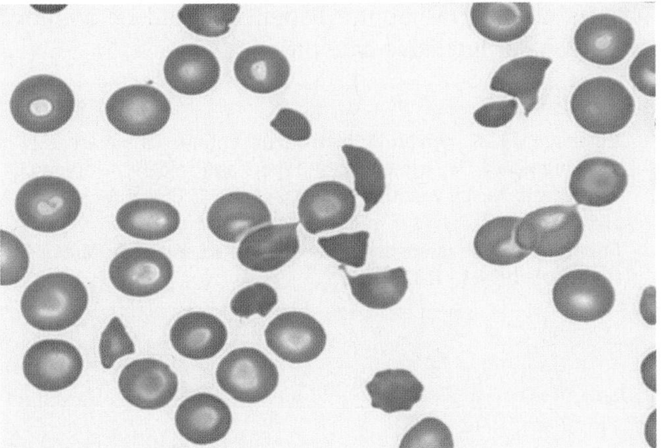

FIGURE 16–19 Microangiopathic hemolytic anemia and thrombocytopenia. (From Anderson, with permission.)

Diagnosis

The diagnosis is made when the characteristic clinical triad coincides with anemia (median hemoglobin concentration, 8 g/dL), an elevated reticulocyte count, schistocytes on blood smear, and a negative Coombs' test. Hematuria, proteinuria, uremia, and electrolyte imbalances are evidence of renal dysfunction. Shiga toxin may be identified in the stool.[1]

Clinical Complications

Between 9% and 30% of children infected with *E. coli* O157:H7 develop HUS. The use of antimotility agents and antimicrobials may increase the risk.[1] In addition to the classic clinical triad, encephalopathy, seizures, pancreatic insufficiency, myocarditis, cardiomyopathy, and hepatic involvement have been associated with HUS. Mortality is low; 5% of patients with acute renal failure require life-long dialysis, 10% to 15% of patients develop end-stage renal disease on long-term follow-up.[1] Atypical disease predicts a worse prognosis.

Management

Management requires careful monitoring and supportive care in the inpatient setting. Transfusions of red blood cells and platelets are sometimes required. Fluid and electrolyte imbalances need to be corrected. Dialysis is needed in some patients. Hypertension is controlled with antihypertensives. Plasmapheresis may be beneficial in atypical disease.[1,2]

REFERENCES

1. Siegler RL. The hemolytic uremic syndrome. *Pediatr Clin North Am* 1995;42:1505–1529.
2. Corrigan JJ Jr, Boineau FG. Hemolytic-uremic syndrome. *Pediatr Rev* 2001;22:365–369.

16–20

Necrotizing Enterocolitis

Robert Hendrickson

Clinical Presentation

Although most of the patients with necrotizing enterocolitis (NEC) are premature infants, approximately 10% of cases develop in full-term infants.[1] Patients present with relatively acute onset of feeding intolerance and bilious vomiting, followed by abdominal distention and hypotension.

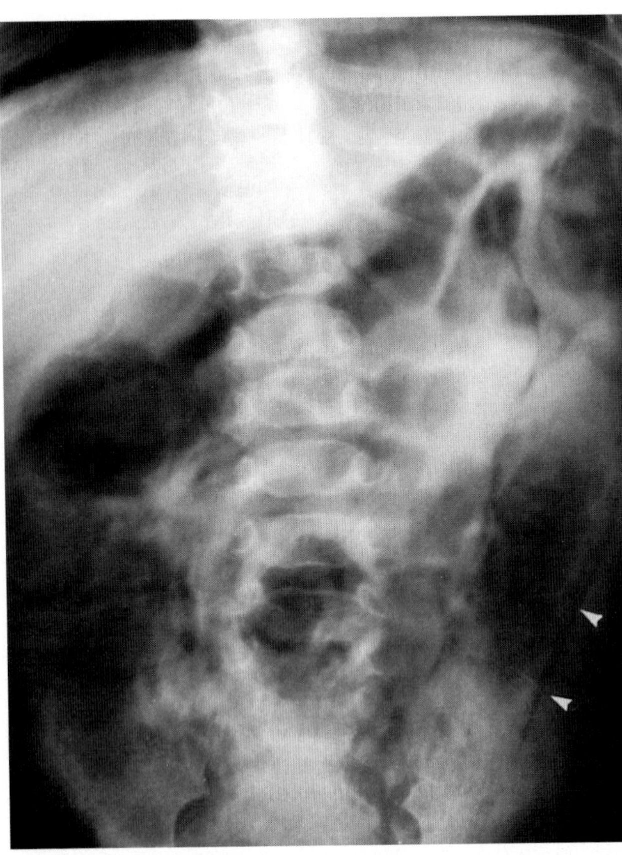

FIGURE 16–20 Note intramural air in the descending colon and thickened bowel loops in the splenic flexure (pneumatosis intestinalis). (From Swischuk, with permission.)

Pathophysiology

NEC is an inflammatory disease of the intestines that occurs in neonates. Focal mucosal inflammation leads to transmural inflammation, necrosis of the bowel, and perforation. The major risk factor for NEC is prematurity.

Diagnosis

The diagnosis may be made by recognition of the typical history and confirmed by radiography. Affected children may develop hematemesis, melena, acidosis, and disseminated intravascular coagulation (DIC).[1] Radiographs of the abdomen may reveal dilated loops of bowel, air–fluid levels, and pneumatosis intestinalis (air within the wall of the intestines).[2] Pneumatosis may also be found in the gastric wall and portal system.[1,2] Free air may be evident after bowel perforation.[1]

Clinical Complications

NEC has a mortality rate of 10% to 50%.[1] Complications include bowel necrosis, shock, DIC, bowel resection, and death. Survivors are at increased risk for strictures, fistulas, and short-gut syndrome.[1]

Management

Children should receive intravenous fluid boluses, antibiotics, orogastric tube decompression, bowel rest, as well as nothing by mouth. Patients should be admitted to a neonatal intensive care unit.

REFERENCES

1. Hostetler MA, Schulman M. Necrotizing enterocolitis presenting in the Emergency Department: case report and review of differential considerations for vomiting in the neonate. *J Emerg Med* 2001;21:165–170.
2. Buonomo C. The radiology of necrotizing enterocolitis. *Radiol Clin North Am* 1999;37:1187–1198.

Erythema Toxicum Neonatorum

Christy Salvaggio

Clinical Presentation

Erythema toxicum neonatorum (ETN) manifests within the first 72 hours of life in full-term infants and is uncommon in premature infants. The rash is diffuse, with typical 1- to 2-mm white/yellow pustular lesions that may be surrounded by blanching erythema.[1,2]

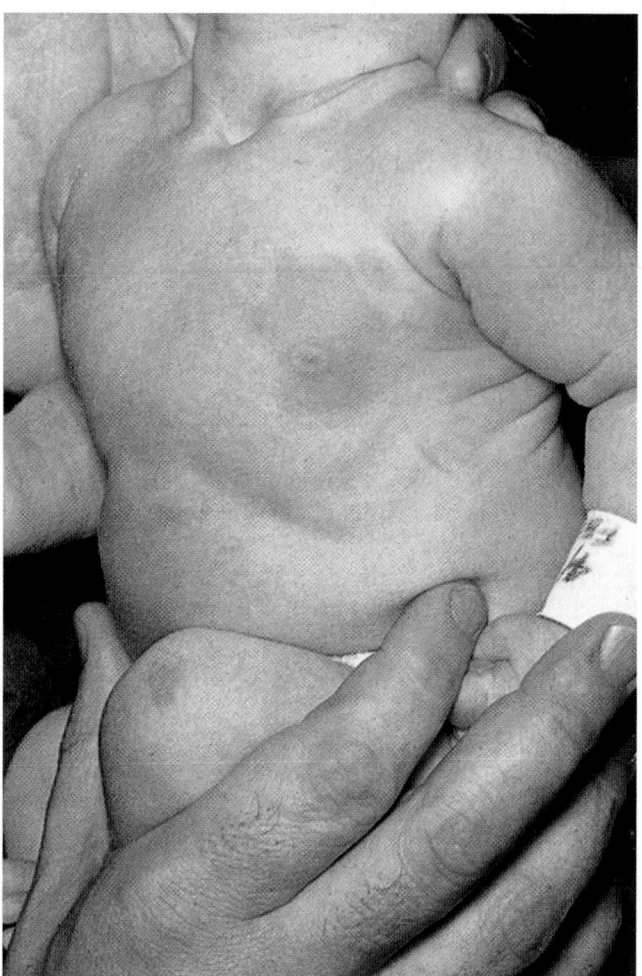

FIGURE 16–21 Papules on an erythematous base consistent with erythema toxicum. (From O'Doherty N. *Atlas of the newborn.* Philadelphia: JB Lippincott, 1979:32, with permission.)

Pathophysiology

ETN is a benign, self-limited pustular rash that occurs in healthy neonates. It is one of the most common neonatal rashes and manifests shortly after birth. The cutaneous lesions contain an accumulation of eosinophils.[3] ETN may represent the neonate's immunologic response to the microorganisms present on skin flora. However, the specific cause of ETN is not known.[3]

Diagnosis

ETN is common in healthy neonates, and the diagnosis is made by recognizing the classic lesions that manifest within the first 48 to 72 hours of life. Other diagnoses, including sepsis, herpes, and impetigo, must be considered with late presentations. The lesions are most common on the trunk but may be diffusely distributed on the head, trunk, and extremities. The palms and soles are typically spared. ETN has no associated systemic symptoms, and infants with erythema toxicum are otherwise healthy. A definitive diagnosis may be made by noting the predominance of eosinophils and the lack of neutrophils or organisms on a smear of the pustular contents.

Management

The rash of ETN resolves spontaneously, usually within the first week, and is not associated with permanent scarring.[1,2]

REFERENCES

1. Nanda S, Reddy B, Ramji S, Pandi D. Analytical study of pustular eruptions in neonates. *Pediatr Dermatol* 2002;19:210–215.
2. Van Praag MC, Van Rooij RW, Folkers E, et al. Diagnosis and treatment of pustular disorders in the neonate. *Pediatr Dermatol* 1997; 14:131–143.
3. Marchini G, Ulfgren A, Lore K, et al. Erythema toxicum neonatorum: an immunohistochemical analysis. *Pediatr Dermatol* 2001;18: 177–187.

16-22

Cradle Cap

Sharon McGregor

Clinical Presentation

Cradle cap manifests between the second and tenth week of life as an erythematous, scaly dermatitis of the scalp. The scales may be flaky and thin, or there may be well-demarcated patches covered with greasy, thick, yellow to brown scale. The rash may spread to the forehead, eyebrows, ears, face, and neck. The diaper area and flexural folds may also be involved with scaly, greasy, well-demarcated, salmon-colored to erythematous lesions.

Pathophysiology

Seborrheic dermatitis (SD) of the infant scalp, known as cradle cap, is an erythematous, scaly rash that begins in the first 3 months of life and resolves spontaneously by 12 months of age.[1-3] The cause of SD is not clear, but it appears to be an inflammatory reaction to dysfunctional sebaceous glands in a predisposed individual, and it occurs in areas of the body with a high density of sebaceous glands.[1-3]

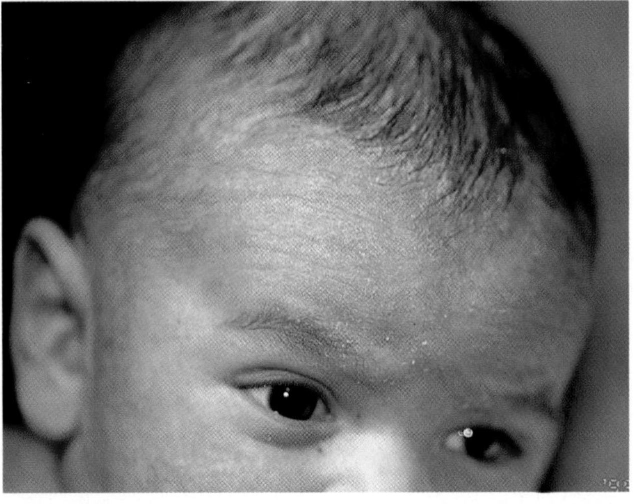

FIGURE 16–22 Scaly oily rash of the scalp (cradle cap). (From Fleisher, with permission.)

Diagnosis

The diagnosis is based on the typical appearance and distribution of the rash and the age of the patient. The primary disorder from which SD must be distinguished is atopic dermatitis (eczema). SD tends to have an earlier onset, is not pruritic, and does not involve a family history of atopy. Also, the skin is not generally dry, and there is no thickening or lichenification. Involvement of intertriginous areas as well as the diaper area indicates seborrhea.[1-3]

Clinical Complications

SD is generally an uncomplicated and self-limited rash, but if it affects the diaper area or intertriginous areas, secondary bacterial or yeast infection may occur. Secondary yeast infection in the postauricular area is also common.[1-3]

Management

Treatment involves shampooing with an antiseborrheic shampoo (containing sulfur, salicylic acid, or both) or an antidandruff shampoo (containing selenium sulfide or zinc pyrithione) two or three times a week. A preparation of 1% or 2% hydrocortisone may be used on the skin lesions three times a day, then decreased as the rash improves. An anti-yeast cream, such as nystatin, may be added if rash located behind the ears, in the diaper area, or in intertrigonal areas does not respond to hydrocortisone alone. Studies linking SD to *Malassezia* species have shown clearing of the scalp with the use of ketoconazole shampoo (Nizoral 2% shampoo), and some authors recommend the use of topical antifungals routinely.[1-3]

REFERENCES

1. Faergemann J. Management of seborrheic dermatitis and pityriasis versicolor. *Am J Clin Dermatol* 2000;1:75–80.
2. Kristal L, Klein PA. Atopic dermatitis in infants and children: an update. *Pediatr Clin North Am* 2000;47:877–895.
3. Ruiz-Maldonado R, Lopez-Martinez R, Perez Chavarria EL, et al. Pityrosporum ovale in infantile seborrheic dermatitis. *Pediatr Dermatol* 1989;6:16–20.

Candidal Diaper Dermatitis

Christy Salvaggio

Clinical Presentation

Candidal diaper dermatitis presents with erythematous papules and vesiculopustular lesions in the diaper region. Coalescence of these lesions may lead to markedly erythematous plaques with irregular, sharply demarcated borders. With severe infections, skin excoriation with bleeding may occur. Although infections occur as early as the first week of life, the peak incidence is in the second to fourth month of life.

Candidal diaper dermatitis may be differentiated from contact dermatitis by the predisposition of candida to cause lesions in intertriginous areas and in the perianal region. The presence of "satellite lesions," papules or pustules outside the immediate diaper rash region, are also classic findings of candidal infections.[1]

Pathophysiology

Candidal diaper dermatitis is a variant of cutaneous candidiasis caused by the yeast species, *Candida albicans. C. albicans* thrives in the moist environment of an infant's wet diaper.[1] Candidal diaper dermatitis is most commonly caused by *C. albicans* that is harbored in the gastrointestinal tract. Infants with oropharyngeal candidal infections ("thrush") are predisposed to candidal diaper dermatitis, because swallowed yeast is excreted in the stool. One third to one half of the infants with thrush develop candidal diaper dermatitis. Although not all infants with candidal diaper dermatitis have thrush, a thorough examination of the oropharynx needs to be performed to rule out concomitant infection.[1]

Diagnosis

Candidal diaper infections are easily recognized by their classic, markedly erythematous, macular-papular lesions that are concentrated on intertriginous skin. Satellite lesions are often present on the inner thighs or lower abdomen and may help make the diagnosis. Although rarely needed, a potassium hydroxide slide may be prepared, ideally from a satellite lesion; the presence of branching hyphae or pseudohyphae is diagnostic.[1]

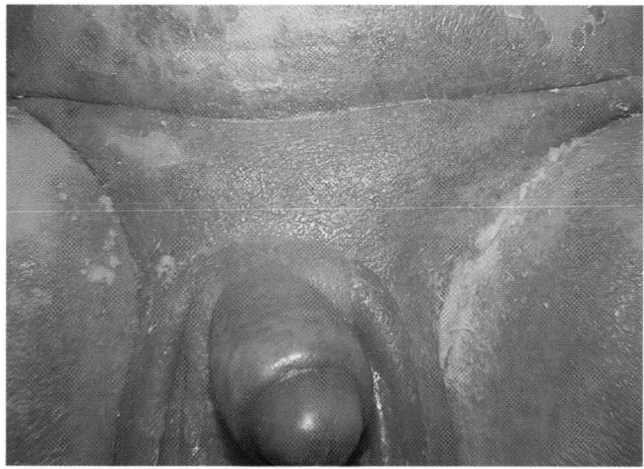

FIGURE 16–23 Candidal diaper dermatitis. Note involvement of the inguinal folds, which usually are spared in contact dermatitis. (From Ostler, with permission.)

Clinical Complications

Clinical complications are rare. With appropriate antifungal treatment, most infections significantly improve or clear within 1 to 2 weeks. Infrequently, secondary bacterial infections may arise. Transient skin hypopigmentation may occur after candidal diaper dermatitis. Hypopigmentation is most common in infants with darker pigmentation, such as African-American or Latino infants, and may take several months to resolve. If left untreated, candidal diaper dermatitis may spread outside the diaper region and evolve into a diffuse erythematous, macular-papular rash across the trunk and extremities. Hypersensitivity reactions, or ID reactions, to the candidal infection may also cause a similar diffuse rash.[1]

Management

Candidal infections flourish in a moist environment. Efforts to decrease skin moisture, such as meticulous attention to frequent diaper changing, help clear the infection. Keeping the infant out of diapers for several hours a day and exposing the skin directly to air is especially helpful. Diapers with impermeable linings should be avoided, because they trap moisture against the infant's skin.[1] Candidal infections should be treated with topical antifungal agents such as nystatin, miconazole, ketoconazole, or clotrimazole ointment. Antifungal ointments should be applied after each diaper change and at least four times daily until the infection has resolved. The addition of low-potency topical steroid creams should be considered only for severe infections that involve significant skin inflammation. Topical steroids should be continued for no longer than 1 week. Commercially available combination antifungal and topical steroid creams should be avoided, because they often contain high-potency steroid preparations.[1] Because *C. albicans* is harbored in the stool, concomitant use of oral antifungal agents such as nystatin suspension may improve both clinical and mycologic cure rates; however, definitive studies to support this practice are lacking.[1]

REFERENCES

1. Hoppe JE. Treatment of oropharyngeal candidiasis and candidal diaper dermatitis in neonates and infants: review and reappraisal. *Pediatr Infect Dis J* 1997;16:885–894.

Diaper Dermatitis

Robert Hendrickson

Clinical Presentation

Diaper dermatitis (contact dermatitis) manifests with erythematous macular and papular lesions that typically spare the creases. Diaper dermatitis may occur at any age, but it is most common between 9 and 12 months of age. Most diaper dermatitis is mild and transient, usually resolving within 1 day. However, if severe, it may cause skin excoriation and bleeding. Diaper dermatitis usually is secondary to friction with the diaper and contact with urine and feces. It may also occur after changing brands of diapers, wipes, or diaper cream. Occasionally, infants present with a ring of contact dermatitis, around the legs and waist only, that is secondary to irritation from the elastic edging of a new diaper brand.[1]

Pathophysiology

Diaper dermatitis, one of the most common skin rashes of infancy, results from skin irritation and inflammation after contact with wet or irritating diapers.[1,2]

Diagnosis

Diaper dermatitis is not a difficult clinical diagnosis. However, the differential diagnosis for diaper dermatitis is extensive, and other possible causes should be considered. Candidal diaper dermatitis is also a common rash of infancy. Unlike diaper dermatitis, candidal diaper dermatitis is concentrated in the inguinal creases or gluteal cleft, and its hallmark symptom is the presence of "satellite" lesions. Scaly lesions are suggestive of seborrheic dermatitis, whereas pustules and yellow crusting are suggestive of bacterial infections. Group A streptococcus causes a unique pattern of well-demarcated erythema, commonly in the perianal region. The differential diagnosis for diaper dermatitis also includes vitamin deficiencies, such as biotin or zinc deficiencies, and a brief diet history should be elicited. Histiocytosis X (Letterer-Siwe disease) should be considered in cases of severe, recurrent diaper dermatitis.[1,2]

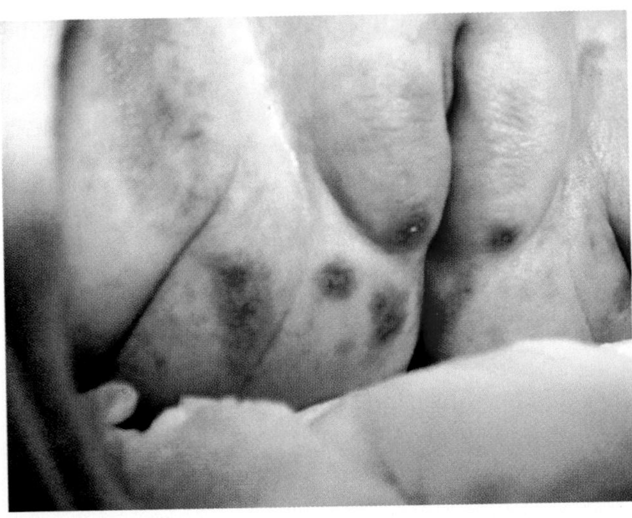

FIGURE 16–24 Contact dermatitis. Note sparing of the skin folds. (Courtesy of Christy Salvaggio, MD.)

Clinical Complications

Diaper dermatitis is rarely serious, although, in cases of severe infection, skin breakdown may lead to secondary bacterial infections or candidal yeast infections.[2]

Management

Although contact with urine and feces is the usual cause of diaper dermatitis, a history of new diapers, wipes, or creams should be sought as a possible cause. To resolve diaper dermatitis, the skin should be kept as dry as possible and contact with urine and feces as brief as possible. Super-absorbent disposable diapers keep the skin drier and are preferred to cloth diapers. The skin should be bathed with mild soap and water. Barrier diaper creams, such as petroleum-based products or zinc oxide preparations, should be applied with each diaper change. Complete removal of all of the barrier cream with each diaper change is not necessary and may cause more skin irritation. Commercial diaper wipes, especially those containing alcohol, may exacerbate the dermatitis. With the use of barrier diaper creams and meticulous attention to changing diapers promptly, most diaper dermatitis resolves or markedly improves within 1 week.[2]

REFERENCES

1. Kazaks EL. Diaper dermatitis. *Pediatr Clin North Am* 2000;47: 909–919.
2. Boiko S. Treatment of diaper dermatitis. *Dermatol Clin* 1999;17: 235–240.

Neonatal Gonococcal Conjunctivitis

Christy Salvaggio

Clinical Presentation

Gonococcal conjunctivitis (GC) typically manifests with copious purulent yellow-green eye discharge within the first 2 to 7 days of life. However, as a result of partial treatment by routine prophylactic eye antibiotics or postnatal infection, GC may have a delayed presentation. The hallmark of GC is the severity of the conjunctival erythema, swelling, and purulent discharge.[1,2]

Pathophysiology

Neonatal GC is an infection of the bulbar and palpebral conjunctiva caused by *Neisseria gonorrhoeae*, a gram-negative intracellular diplococcus.[1–4] Perinatal infections are most commonly transmitted from an infected mother during delivery. High-risk infants include those born to mothers with prior sexually transmitted diseases or limited prenatal care and infants who did not receive routine ophthalmic antibiotic prophylaxis at delivery.[1–4]

Diagnosis

Although neonatal GC is rare, physicians should maintain a high index of suspicion, because the clinical course may be quite aggressive. GC infection should be considered in any case of neonatal conjunctivitis and strongly considered in any hyperpurulent neonatal conjunctivitis. A Gram stain and culture should be obtained in all cases of neonatal conjunctivitis. In GC, the Gram stain reveals numerous white blood cells and gram-negative intracellular diplococci. GC specimens should immediately be cultured on chocolate agar and incubated in 5% to 10% carbon dioxide.[3,4]

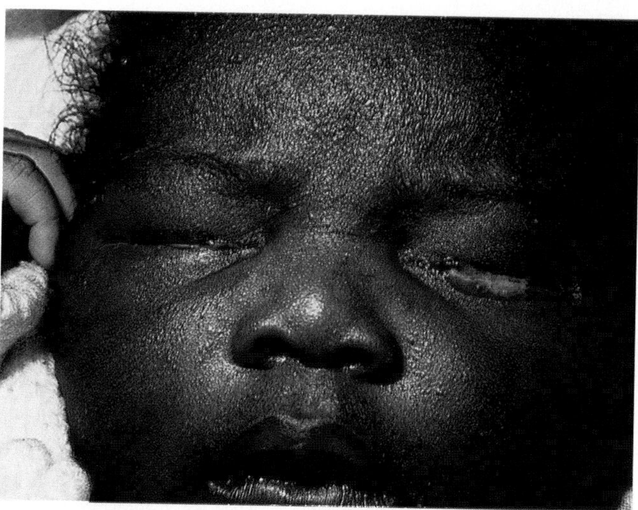

FIGURE 16–25 Gonococcal ophthalmia neonatorum. (From Ostler, with permission.)

Clinical Complications

GC is a medical emergency. GC may spread to the cornea, with subsequent corneal ulceration, perforation, and possible blindness.[1–4]

Management

Treatment, including systemic antibiotics and hourly saline eye irrigation, must be initiated immediately. Single-dose intravenous or intramuscular ceftriaxone is usually adequate treatment for uncomplicated cases. For infants with hyperbilirubinemia, single-dose intravenous or intramuscular cefotaxime, 100 mg/kg, is recommended instead of ceftriaxone. Topical antibiotic treatment is inadequate and is not recommended. All neonates with GC should be hospitalized, and sepsis evaluations should be considered for these infants, because they are at increased risk for systemic gonococcal infections. Infants should be screened for other sexually transmitted infections, including chlamydia, syphilis, and human immunodeficiency virus. Testing and treatment of the mother and her partners must also be initiated.[3,4]

REFERENCES

1. Darville T. Gonorrhea. *Pediatr Rev* 1999;20:125–128.
2. American Academy of Pediatrics. *AAP 2000 Red book: report of the Committee on Infectious Diseases,* 25th ed. Elk Grove Village, IL: AAP, 2000:254–256.
3. Diamant JI. Therapy for bacterial conjunctivitis. *Ophthalmol Clin North Am* 1999;12:15–20.
4. Workowski KA. Sexually transmitted diseases: treatment guidelines 2002. *MMWR Morb Mortal Wkly Rep* 2002;51:1.

Neonatal and Infantile Acne

Sharon McGregor

Clinical Presentation

In neonatal acne (NA), lesions of cephalic pustulosis generally appear in the first 1 to 2 weeks of life. They manifest as small, erythematous follicular papules or pustules without comedones, usually concentrated on the cheeks. They may also appear on the forehead, chin, neck, scalp, upper torso, and upper arms. They usually disappear in days to weeks, with or without treatment.[1]

Infantile acne may manifest by 1 month of age but usually occurs after 3 to 4 months, with comedones, inflammatory papules, pustules, and even cysts. There is often a strong family history of acne.[1]

Pathophysiology

NA may be caused by stimulation of the neonatal sebaceous glands by maternal hormones or by an inflammatory reaction to the yeast, *Malassezia furfur* or *Malassezia sympodialis,* that colonizes the neonatal skin.[1,2]

Infantile acne is a variant of true acne vulgaris, with increased sensitivity of the sebaceous glands to endogenous hormones, followed by changes in the pilosebaceous unit, leading to open and closed comedones, papules, pustules, and nodules.

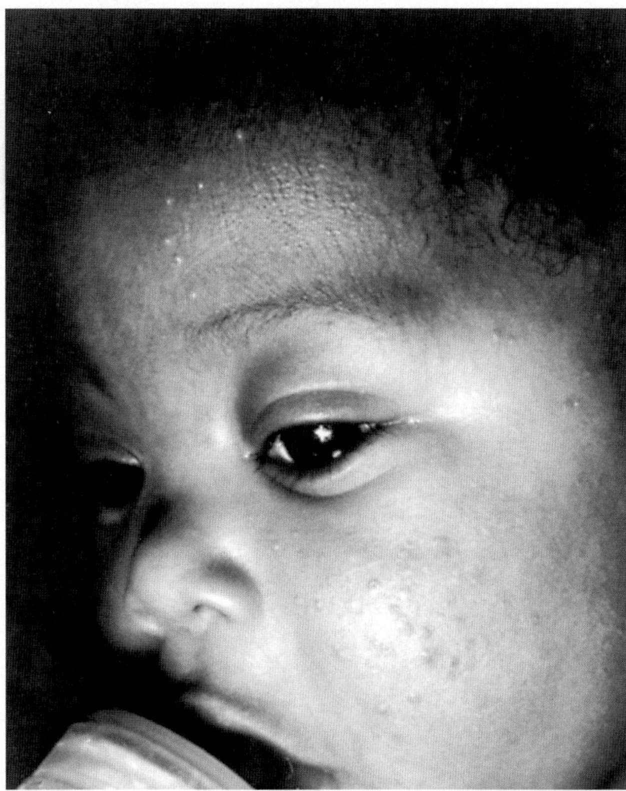

FIGURE 16–26 Neonatal acne. (From Avery GB, Fletcher MA, MacDonald MG. *Neonatology: pathophysiology and management of the newborn,* 5th ed. Philadelphia: Lippincott Williams & Wilkins, 1999:1326, with permission.)

Diagnosis

The diagnosis of NA is made clinically by the typical appearance and distribution of the lesions and the age at onset. Neonatal acne can be differentiated on clinical grounds from milia (white/yellow papules without inflammation), miliaria (vesicles with surrounding erythema), and seborrheic dermatitis (erythematous, greasy, scaly rash that may also affect the diaper area).[1,2] The diagnosis of infantile acne is made clinically by the age at onset and the appearance, which resembles that of typical adolescent acne vulgaris.

Clinical Complications

Infantile acne may lead to scarring and may predict severe acne during adolescence.

Management

NA is usually mild and self-limited and resolves without intervention. Reassurance, daily washing with mild soap and water, and the avoidance of oils on the affected skin are recommended. Clotrimazole has been used experimentally, but it is not currently recommended.[1,2]

Infantile acne may be very mild and resolve on its own in several weeks. Severe or persistent cases should be referred to a pediatric dermatologist for treatment with topical agents (tretinoin, benzoyl peroxide, or benzoyl peroxide/antibiotic). Patients with severe infantile acne should be referred to an endocrinologist.

REFERENCES

1. Lucky AW. A review of infantile and pediatric acne. *Dermatology* 1998;196:95–97.
2. Bernier V, Weill FX, Hirigoyen V, et al. Skin colonization by *Malassezia* species in neonates: a prospective study and relationship with neonatal cephalic pustulosis. *Arch Dermatol* 2002;138: 215–218.

Transient Neonatal Pustular Melanosis

Edgar Collazo

Clinical Presentation

Children with transient neonatal pustular melanosis (TNPM) may be born with diffuse pustules up to 2 mm in diameter on the skin that rupture within the first 2 days of life, leaving a hyperpigmented spot. More often, the infant is born with melanotic spots on the face, neck, and trunk, representing pustules that most likely ruptured in utero. Over a period of weeks to months, these hyperpigmented macules fade. TNPM is more common in infants with deeper skin pigmentation; African-American infants are more likely to present with this benign rash than Hispanic children, who are more likely to present than Caucasian infants. Premature infants are rarely affected, regardless of race.

Pathophysiology

TNPM is a benign, self-limited rash observed at birth that is characterized by multiple discrete pustules. When these pustules rupture, they leave hyperpigmented macules with rings of fine scale, which tend to self-resolve with time.[1] If unroofed, these lesions reveal a collection of neutrophils within each pustule.

Diagnosis

The diagnosis is made clinically by recognition of the classic rash in an otherwise well newborn. The diagnosis may be supported microscopically by identification of neutrophils within each pustule, although this is rarely necessary. Gram staining and culture, although rarely necessary, are negative for bacteria. The differential diagnosis includes other benign neonatal rashes, such as erythema toxicum neonatorum, milia neonatorum, and miliaria rubra, as well as infectious rashes such as staphylococcal folliculitis and herpes simplex. Negative findings on Gram stain, Tzanck smear, and culture rule out the latter two. Erythema toxicum appears after birth as areas of erythema with a central papule or pustule that does not leave any residual pigmented changes. Milia tends to be limited to the nose and cheeks of the neonate and presents with whitish-yellow pinpoint papules that also disappear with time. Miliaria rubra, also known as "prickly heat," is similar to milia, but it may appear anywhere on the body where sweating has occurred. The skin around the pinpoint papule of miliaria is erythematous, thus giving the rash its last name.[1]

Clinical Complications

This is a benign rash with no systemic effects and no complications. Although resolution of the melanosis may take weeks to months, ultimately there is no residual scar.[1]

Management

Parents should be reassured that TNPM will resolve spontaneously without any specific treatment.

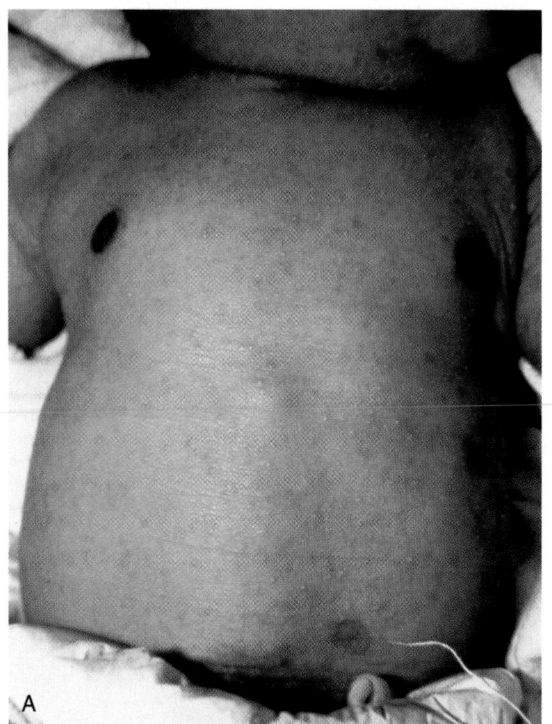

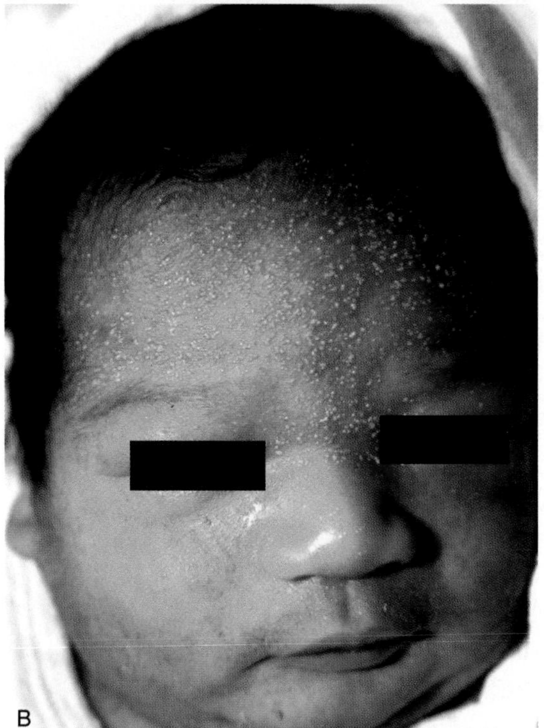

FIGURE 16–27 **A** and **B:** Transient neonatal pustular melanosis. Note the vesicular pustules that tend to rupture, readily forming pigmented macules. (Courtesy of Tor Shwayder, MD.)

REFERENCES

1. Van Praag MCG, Van Rooij RWG, Folkers E, et al. Diagnosis and treatment of pustular disorders in the neonate. *Pediatr Dermatol* 1997;14:131–143.

Neonatal Mastitis

Christy Salvaggio

Clinical Presentation

Neonatal mastitis occurs during the first 2 to 5 weeks of life. Girls are affected twice as often as boys, and most cases are unilateral.[1] The neonatal breast tissue is swollen, erythematous, and often warm. It may be possible to express purulent discharge from the nipples. The infection is usually localized, and the infant is typically otherwise well-appearing.

Pathophysiology

Secondary to maternal hormones, neonatal breast tissue is often palpable and at times engorged. A clear or slightly cloudy discharge is sometimes seen. This occurs in both male and female neonates. The breast tissue significantly decreases over the first 2 weeks and completely resolves over the first month or two, as maternal estrogen levels fall. Engorged breast tissue may become infected, with the potential for abscess formation. Local trauma (e.g., from a caretaker's trying to express "milk") may be an inciting incident. The usual pathogens are skin flora, especially *Staphylococcus aureus*. Occasionally, gram-negative enteric bacteria are the cause.[1]

Diagnosis

The key to diagnosis is to differentiate normal hypertrophied glandular breast tissue from a true mastitis. In contrast to neonatal mastitis, normal engorged breast tissue is nontender, cool, and not erythematous. Normal nipple discharge is clear or milky, not purulent. Gram staining of normal nipple discharge does not reveal the polymorphonuclear cells or bacteria seen with neonatal mastitis.[1]

Clinical Complications

Neonatal mastitis is most often a focal infection that resolves without sequelae if treated with appropriate antibiotics. Only 25% of infants are ill-appearing or febrile at presentation. Abscess formation may occur and may require surgical drainage. Because neonates have less mature immune systems, focal infections are more likely to disseminate and cause systemic disease. The risk of bacteremia and subsequent hematogenous spread (e.g., to the kidneys or meninges) must always be considered.[1]

Management

Patient management hinges on the extent of the infection and the appearance of the infant. Localized infections in well-appearing, healthy, afebrile, full-term in-

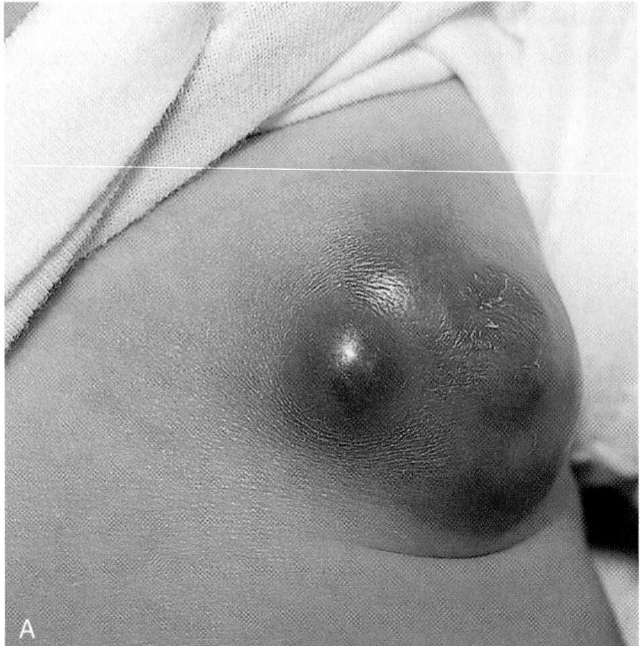

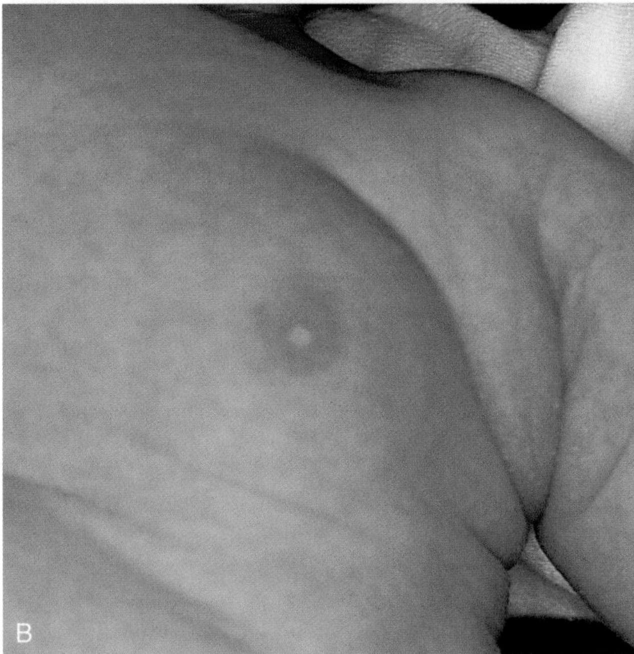

FIGURE 16–28 Mastitis. **A:** This infant has mastitis. The breast is swollen and erythematous, with some areas suggesting abscess formation. **B:** In contrast, this newborn has physiologic gynecomastia and lactation ("witch's milk"). Note that the breast shows no erythema. (**A** and **B**, From Fleisher, with permission.)

fants may be treated with intravenous antibiotics effective against staphylococcal and streptococcal species (e.g., nafcillin). If the infant has reliable caretakers and 24-hour follow-up can be assured, outpatient treatment with adequate antibiotics may be considered. Careful discharge instructions should include the need for the patient to return immediately if symptoms worsen, including fever, change in activity or feeding, or worsening infection. A screening complete blood count and differential may be considered.[1] Any discharge should be cultured. If there is fluctuance, pediatric surgical consultation should be considered; needle aspiration may be as effective as incision and drainage. A full sepsis evaluation, including blood, urine, and cerebrospinal fluid studies, is required for ill-appearing or febrile neonates.[1]

REFERENCES

1. Walsh M, McIntosh K. Neonatal mastitis. *Clin Pediatr* 1989;25: 395–399.

Cold Panniculitis ("Popsicle Panniculitis")

Christy Salvaggio

Clinical Presentation

Cold panniculitis occurs in response to poor peripheral circulation after cold exposure. Patients present with subcutaneous, well-circumcised, slightly mobile nodules that represent fat necrosis. A single nodule or several nodules may be present. The overlying skin is often erythematous with irregular borders. Although the nodule may be mildly tender at onset, patients are usually asymptomatic and otherwise healthy and well-appearing.[1-4] The classic presentation of cold panniculitis occurs in young children who present with a cheek nodule with overlying ill-defined erythema after sucking on a popsicle or ice cube ("popsicle panniculitis"). Cold panniculitis has also been reported in infants treated with ice application after vaccinations or to break supraventricular tachycardia.[1-4]

Although cold panniculitis is most common in infants and young children, it is not limited to childhood. There have been case reports of young women developing cold panniculitis in their thighs after equestrian riding in cold temperatures ("equestrian panniculitis"). It is hypothesized that, in addition to cold temperatures, tight-fitting riding pants decrease perfusion to the thighs and place these patients at increased risk for cold panniculitis.[1-4]

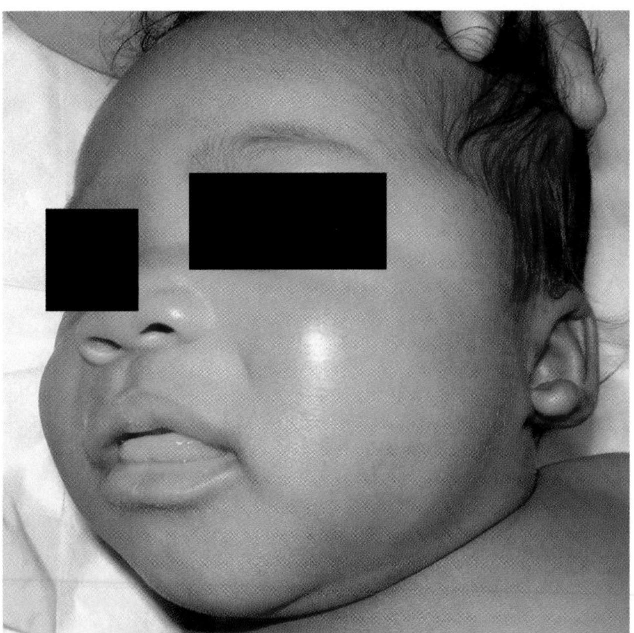

FIGURE 16–29 Buccal erythema from cold panniculitis. (Courtesy of Mark Silverberg, MD.)

Pathophysiology

Cold panniculitis is a cold-induced fat necrosis. It occurs most commonly in infants and children and manifests as benign subcutaneous nodules.[1-4] Infants are especially at risk for cold-induced panniculitis, perhaps because of differences in their fat composition. Compared to older children and adults, infants have an increased percentage of saturated fat; saturated fat has a higher melting point and is more likely to solidify at cool temperatures.

Diagnosis

Cold panniculitis is typically a clinical diagnosis. If a healthy, well-appearing patient presents with classic subcutaneous nodules, a history of cold exposure should be sought. Biopsy specimens are rarely needed but are diagnostic. Biopsies reveal a predominantly lobar panniculitis, often with an inflammatory infiltration of lymphocytes and histiocytes. Fat necrosis and calcium deposits may be seen.[1-4]

In addition to cold panniculitis, two related variants of panniculitis occur in infants: subcutaneous fat necrosis and sclerema neonatorum. Although hypothermia is implicated as a potential cause, both subcutaneous fat necrosis and sclerema neonatorum occur without direct cold exposure.[1-4] Infants with subcutaneous fat necrosis often have a history of a difficult perinatal course, but as in cold panniculitis, they are classically well-appearing and healthy at the time of diagnosis. Subcutaneous nodules manifest within the first 2 to 6 weeks of life and are most common over bony prominences of the cheeks, buttocks, back, or extremities.[1-4] In contrast, sclerema neonatorum may be seen in seriously ill or premature infants and manifests with areas of firm, mottled skin, usually starting on the buttocks or lower extremities. In these ill infants, poor peripheral circulation and hypothermia are the likely causes, and sclerema neonatorum is often considered a premorbid condition.[1-4]

The clinical presentations of cold panniculitis, subcutaneous fat necrosis, and sclerema neonatorum differ. If the diagnosis is uncertain, biopsy specimens may differentiate between these three variants of panniculitis.

Clinical Complications

Complications are very uncommon, and cold panniculitis usually resolves without sequelae. Uncommonly, overlying skin breakdown may lead to scarring. Subcutaneous fat necrosis usually self-resolves without sequelae; however, this condition has been associated with hypercalcemia, probably secondary to resorption of calcified plaques. Infants with hypercalcemia after subcutaneous fat necrosis may have significant morbidity and mortality. These infants should be monitored closely for signs of hypercalcemia, such as poor feeding, lethargy, vomiting, or irritability. Screening of these high-risk infants with serial calcium levels for several months should be considered.[1–4]

Management

The affected area should be kept warm, but no additional therapy is needed. The plaque or nodule gradually softens and resolves over weeks to months. Aggressive rewarming, including use of heating pads or warm soaks, is neither necessary nor recommended. Vasodilatory drugs are not effective prophylaxis or treatment for cold panniculitis.[1–4]

REFERENCES

1. Ter Poorten JC, Hebert AA, Ilkiw R. Cold panniculitis in a neonate. *J Am Acad Dermatol* 1995;33:383–385.
2. Ter Poorten M. Panniculitis. *Dermatol Clin* 2002;20:421.
3. Requena L. Panniculitis: part II. Mostly lobular panniculitis. *J Am Acad Dermatol* 2001;45:325–361.
4. Day S, Klein BL. Popsicle panniculitis. *Pediatr Emerg Care* 1992;8:91–93.

Mongolian Spots

Christy Salvaggio

Clinical Presentation

Mongolian spots are present at birth. They are most common on the back, buttocks, or shoulders, and are rarely seen on the face.[1,2] Their incidence varies greatly among different populations of children: 90% in African-American infants, 80% in Asian infants, 70% in Latin-American infants, and less than 10% in Caucasian infants.[1,2]

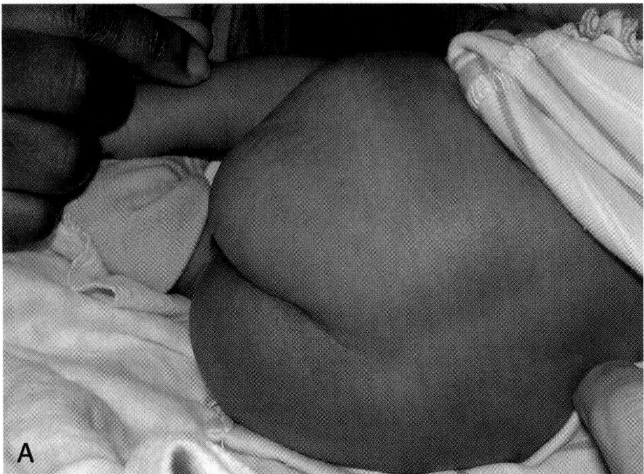

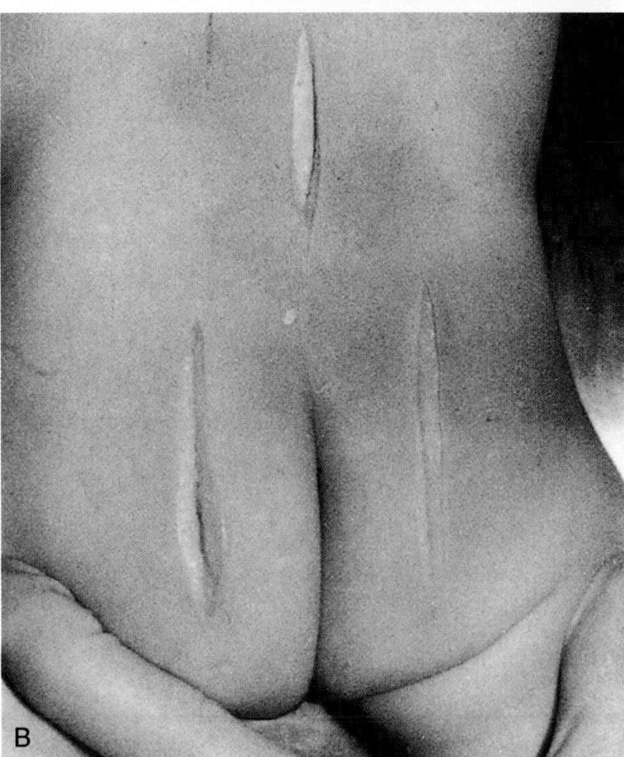

FIGURE 16–30 **A:** Mongolian spots. (Courtesy of Mark Silverberg, MD.) **B:** Incisions have been made through multiple Mongolian spots, or birth marks, found on the buttocks and sacral area of a victim of child abuse to demonstrate the lack of hemorrhage in the underlying soft tissue. (From Jones, with permission.)

Pathophysiology

Mongolian spots are benign, hyperpigmented, macular skin lesions commonly seen in infancy. Their primary clinical significance is that they may be confused with bruises that are suggestive of child abuse.[3] Mongolian spots represent areas of dermal melanocytosis, and their cause is unknown.

Diagnosis

Mongolian spots may easily be recognized by their characteristic blue-green or blue-black coloration, their common lumbosacral distribution, and their presence at birth. Unlike bruises, Mongolian spots do not change in appearance over several days.

Clinical Complications

Because Mongolian spots are benign, there are no complications associated with these lesions.

Management

Mongolian spots are benign discolorations that require no treatment. They most commonly fade within the first 4 to 5 years of life, but they persist into adulthood in approximately 5% of patients. Mongolian spots are not associated with an increased malignant potential, and their persistence later in life has no clinical significance. Their primary relevance is that they must not be confused with bruises that are suggestive of child abuse.

REFERENCES

1. Cordova A. The Mongolian spot: a study of ethnic differences and a literature review. *Clin Pediatr* 1981;20:714–719.
2. Osburn K, Schosser RH, Everett MA. Congenital pigmented and vascular lesions in newborn infants. *J Am Acad Dermatol* 1987;16:788–792.
3. Dungy CI. Mongolian spots, day care centers, and child abuse. *Pediatrics* 1982;69:672.

Omphalitis

Robert Hendrickson

Clinical Presentation

Initial signs of omphalitis include fluid drainage from the umbilicus and erythema of the surrounding tissues.[1] Patients may also develop fever, lethargy, and other signs of sepsis. Laboratory studies are normal early in the disease but may reveal leukocytosis and a leftward shift later in the course.[1,2]

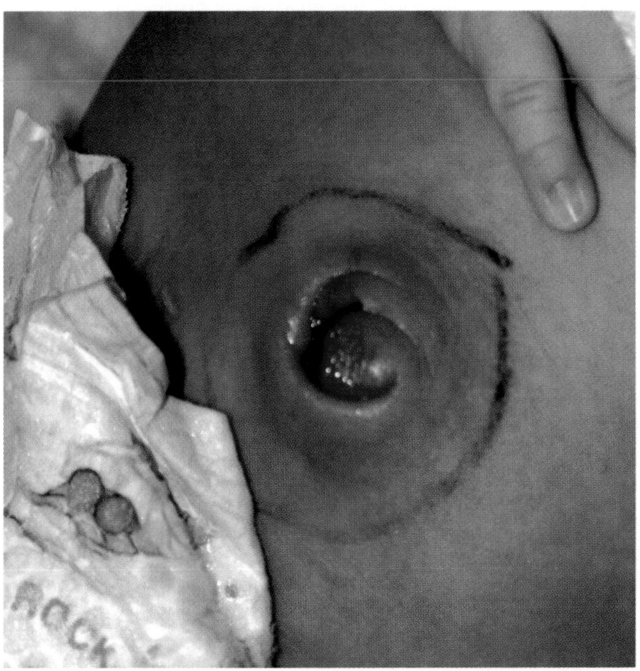

FIGURE 16–31 Erythema and fluid drainage from the umbilicus. (Courtesy of Eustacia [Jo] Su, MD.)

Pathophysiology

Omphalitis is an infection of the umbilical stump and surrounding tissues that typically occurs within the first few weeks of life.[2] After delivery, the umbilical stump undergoes necrosis and becomes colonized by bacteria. Virulent bacteria or inhibited neonatal defenses may lead to infection of the umbilicus itself, or of surrounding tissues, or both. Typical organisms include gram-negative bacteria (e.g., *Klebsiella*), streptococci, and staphylococci.[1,2]

Diagnosis

Diagnosis may be difficult early in the course of disease. Definite signs of infection include erythema encircling the umbilicus and purulent fluid drainage.

Clinical Complications

Complications include peritonitis, sepsis, and intraabdominal abscess.

Management

Patients with omphalitis require intravenous antibiotics (e.g., oxacillin and gentamicin) and admission to the hospital. Patients with minimal erythema and drainage may be closely monitored on an outpatient basis, with strict instructions to return if there is any change in behavior, fever, umbilical appearance, erythema, or drainage.[1,2]

REFERENCES

1. Mason WH, Andrews R, Ross LA, Wright HT Jr. Omphalitis in the newborn infant. *Pediatr Infect Dis J* 1989;8:521–525.
2. Faridi MM, Rattan A, Ahmad SH. Omphalitis neonatorum. *J Ind Med Assoc* 1993;91:283–285.

Electrical Cord Chewing Injury

Michael Greenberg

Clinical Presentation

Most patients with electrical cord chewing injury (ECCI) present immediately after an acute electrically induced burn injury to the lips, oral cavity, or oral commissures. Some patients present in a delayed fashion (days to weeks) after the acute electrical injury as a result of pain or symptoms related to infection or bleeding.[1-3]

Pathophysiology

The most common mechanism of electrical injury in infants and children involves chewing on, or biting through, electrical cords. As the integrity of the electrical cord is violated by moist teeth, arcing of current through the lips results in an electrical burn. These injuries may be full thickness and therefore may involve the mucosa and submucosa, as well as underlying muscles, nerves, and vascular elements. Substantial local edema may develop within hours after the injury, and in small children this may threaten airway patency. In addition, rapid eschar formation tends to occur. Eschars generally separate within 1 month after the acute injury, being replaced by granulation and potentially deforming scar tissue. Of special note is the possibility of labial artery injury. This may result in delayed and substantial bleeding, which typically occurs at the time the eschar separates and falls away.[1-3]

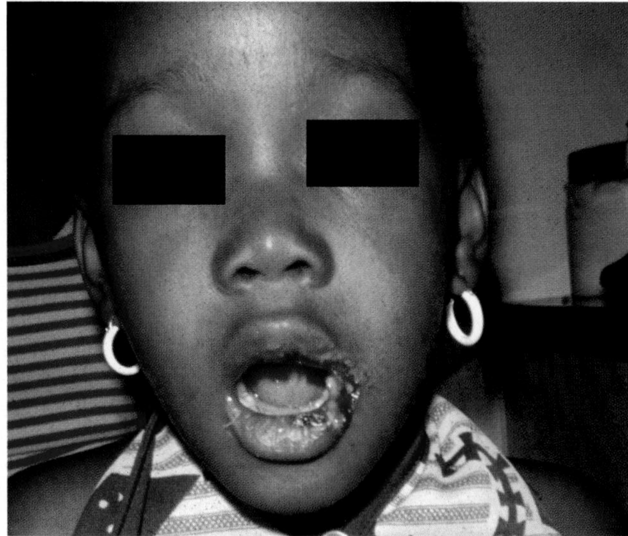

FIGURE 16–32 Lesion at the left oral commissure secondary to chewing on an electrical cord. (Courtesy of Michael Greenberg, MD.)

Diagnosis

The diagnosis of ECCI is based on clinical examination and history, as well as recognition of the typical injury pattern with tissue damage at one or both oral commissures.

Clinical Complications

Complications include airway compromise, death, delayed labial artery disruption with profuse bleeding, infection, and permanent cosmetic deformity with disorders of phonation and other oral functions.[1-3]

Management

Although ECCI may initially appear *de minimus,* it is potentially life-threatening, and many sources recommend that all patients be admitted for observation and emergency consultation with specialists in oral surgery, otolaryngology, and/or plastic surgery. However, some series report a dearth of serious complications and have prompted a re-evaluation of the admonition to admit all patients with ECCI.[3] Certainly cases involving deep injury, early edema, or questionable parental compliance require hospitalization. The use of prophylactic antibiotics and corticosteroids is controversial and should be discussed with the team of consultants before initiation. Pediatric patients with ECCI, once stable, are best transferred to specialized pediatric facilities for definitive care.

REFERENCES

1. Canady JW, Thompson SA, Bardach J. Oral commissure burns in children. *Plast Reconstr Surg* 1996;97:738–744.
2. Koumbourlis AC. Electrical injuries. *Crit Care Med* 2002;30(11 Suppl):S424–S430.
3. Zubair M, Besner GE. Pediatric electrical burns: management strategies. *Burns* 1997;23:413–420.

Toddler's Fracture

Christy Salvaggio

Clinical Presentation

Children with toddler's fracture may present acutely with refusal to bear weight on the affected leg. There may be a history of minor trauma or none at all. Frequently, the child appears otherwise well and is playful and active while not bearing weight on the affected leg. There may be point tenderness or mild swelling over the tibial shaft. There is no restricted range of motion or swelling in the hips, knees, or ankles. Restricted range of motion or fever suggests an alternative diagnosis, such as a septic joint or toxic synovitis.[1]

Pathophysiology

A toddler's fracture is a nondisplaced spiral fracture of the tibial shaft that may occur after seemingly minor trauma. Children between 1 and 5 years of age are most commonly affected. Toddler's fractures are spiral fractures that often occur secondary to a rotational force.[1]

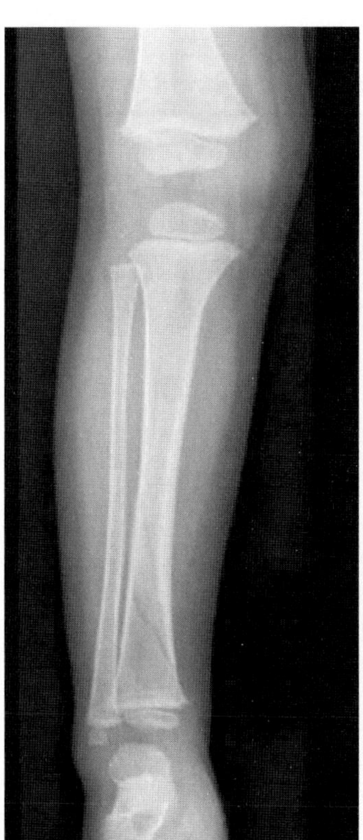

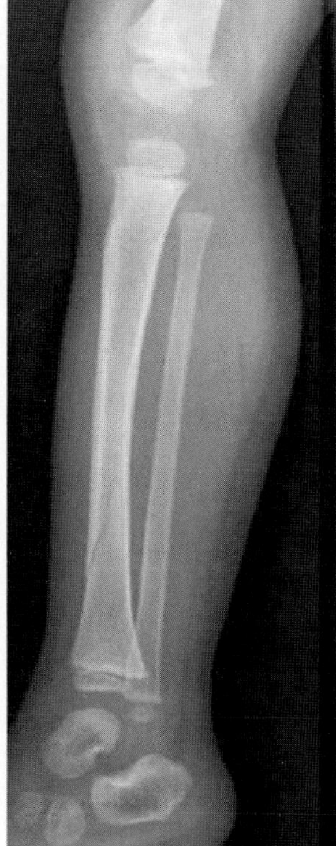

FIGURE 16–37 Toddler's fracture. (Courtesy of Mark Silverberg, MD.)

Diagnosis

A toddler's fracture should be strongly considered in any non–weight-bearing toddler or young child. The differential diagnosis includes a septic joint (most likely a septic hip), toxic synovitis, other inflammatory disorders, other occult fractures from the hip to the toes, foot blisters or foreign bodies, and neoplasms. A history of trauma or fever should be sought. The child should be examined thoroughly from the hips to the toes. The foot and toes should be examined carefully for any blisters, ulcers, cuts, or foreign bodies. Point tenderness may be present, but its absence does not rule out a toddler's fracture. If no alternative diagnosis is obvious, tibia and fibula radiographs should be obtained even in the absence of focal tenderness or swelling.[1] Radiographs may reveal a midshaft, nondisplaced tibia fracture; however, occult fractures that are not visible on initial films do occur. Consequently, if the clinical presentation strongly suggests a toddler's fracture and alternative diagnoses are unlikely, immobilization and orthopedic follow-up should be arranged despite negative radiographs.[1]

Clinical Complications

With appropriate orthopedic follow-up and casting, toddler's fractures routinely heal well without complications. Limping for several weeks after cast removal is normal; however, limping that persists beyond 4 weeks warrants further evaluation.

Management

A well-padded posterior splint should be applied from the toes to the midthigh, and the child should be kept non–weight-bearing. Orthopedic follow-up for evaluation and casting (long-leg cast for 4 weeks) should be arranged.

REFERENCES

1. Halsey MF, Finzel KC, Carrion WV, et al. Toddler's fracture: presumptive diagnosis and treatment. *J Pediatr Orthop* 2001;21: 152–156.

Intussusception

Robert Hendrickson

Clinical Presentation

Patients with intussusception typically present between 3 and 24 months of age, but they may present at virtually any age.[1] Children present with crampy, intermittent abdominal pain and may or may not have fever or signs of intestinal obstruction.

Pathophysiology

Intussusception refers to the invagination of one section of bowel into an adjacent segment, causing compression of the mesentery, edema, and increasing ischemia.[1,2] Intussusception occurs spontaneously in most cases but may occur secondary to an intestinal "lead point."[1] Lead points allow the bowel to be pulled into its distal segment; they may consist of a group of inflamed lymph nodes, Meckel's diverticulum, lymphoma, or polyp.[1]

Diagnosis

The diagnosis is based on clinical suspicion and physical, laboratory, and imaging findings. During episodes of pain, the child may curl up and raise the legs to the chest. Between painful episodes, the child may appear well or lethargic. Abdominal radiographs may show signs of obstruction, or they may appear normal. Subtle radiographic signs may include a paucity of air in the right lower quadrant or an abdominal mass representing the distal portion ("meniscus sign") of the telescoped segment.[2] A mass may be palpated in the right upper quadrant.[1] Rectal examination may reveal blood-tinged stool or, if bowel necrosis has occurred, "currant-jelly" stool.

Clinical Complications

Complications include bowel necrosis, peritonitis, sepsis, and death. Perforation may complicate therapy if barium or air enemas are used in diagnosis or therapy.

Management

Patients with evidence of bowel necrosis, peritonitis, or sepsis should be rapidly resuscitated, given broad-spectrum intravenous antibiotics, and taken for emergency surgery. In more stable patients, a complete blood count, electrolyte analysis, blood typing and cross-matching, upright abdominal radiography, and surgical consultation should be obtained. Air or barium enema may be performed to confirm the diagnosis and may be used to reduce the intussusception (effective in about 80% of cases).[1] Barium should not be used if there is suspicion of bowel perforation. If enema reduction fails, surgery is necessary for reduction. If the intussusception is reduced with enema, the patient should be monitored in the hospital for signs of intestinal necrosis and/or recurrence (1% to 3% recur). Ultrasonography may also be helpful in making the diagnosis. A "double doughnut," or bowel with bowel, may be noted, typically in the right lower quadrant.[2]

REFERENCES

1. D'Agostino J. Common abdominal emergencies in children. *Emerg Med Clin N Am* 2002;20:139–153.
2. Daneman A, Navarro O. Intussusception: part 1. A review of diagnostic approaches. *Pediatr Radiol* 2003;33:79–85.

Intussusception

Robert Hendrickson

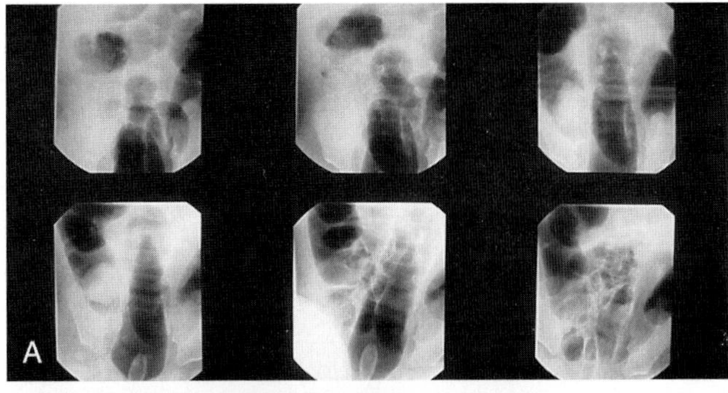

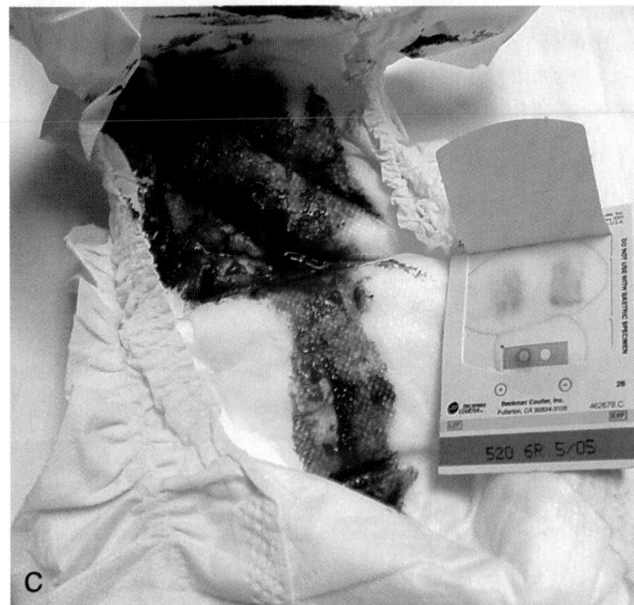

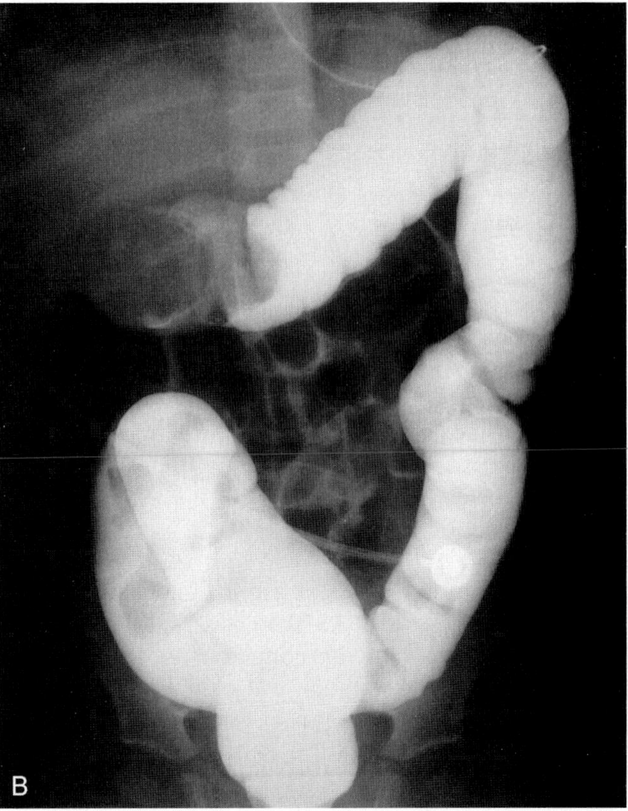

FIGURE 16–38 **A:** Air enema showing intussusception. (Courtesy of Christy Salvaggio, MD.) **B:** Barium enema showing intussusception. (Courtesy of Mark Silverberg, MD.) **C:** "Currant-jelly" stool of intussusception. (Courtesy of Christy Salvaggio, MD.)

Pyloric Stenosis

Joseph Iocono

Clinical Presentation

Newborn patients with pyloric stenosis (PS) present with progressive nonbilious vomiting. Most infants present between 3 and 8 weeks of age. There is a predilection for first-born males, and the male-to-female ratio is 4:1.

Pathophysiology

PS affects 1 of every 350 to 500 newborns. The pylorus muscle, located at the gastric outlet, becomes enlarged and thickened. This results in progressive gastric outlet obstruction. For unknown reasons, the pyloric channel hypertrophies, causing a gastric outlet obstruction. Theories abound as to the cause of the abnormal muscle growth. Impaired vagal stimuli, an infectious cause, and hormone imbalance have all been postulated.[1]

Diagnosis

A clinical diagnosis of PS is possible without radiologic studies. The diagnosis of PS should be entertained for any baby who presents with nonbilious vomiting without fever. Signs of dehydration will be present if vomiting has persisted. The abdominal examination may detect a palpable pylorus, but this must be done when the baby is calm and has an empty stomach. The clinician should gently place an open hand on the umbilicus, feel the liver edge, and guide the fingers up beneath the liver edge. Once beneath the liver, the hand is gently pushed down and swept toward the umbilicus, feeling for an "olive" beneath the extended fingers. Laboratory findings coincide with the degree of dehydration. The hallmark of PS is a hypochloremic, hypokalemic metabolic alkalosis. As dehydration worsens, paradoxic aciduria results.[1-3]

Plain abdominal radiography may show gastric distention. A barium-contrast upper gastrointestinal series shows a gastric outlet obstruction with a "shoulder sign" of the overlying pylorus. Ultrasonography is the diagnostic test of choice.[2]

Clinical Complications

Persistent vomiting may result in dehydration, hypoglycemia, electrolyte imbalances, and the aspiration of food and acid.

Management

Intravenous access should be established and the infant rehydrated as clinically indicated. Measurements of elec-

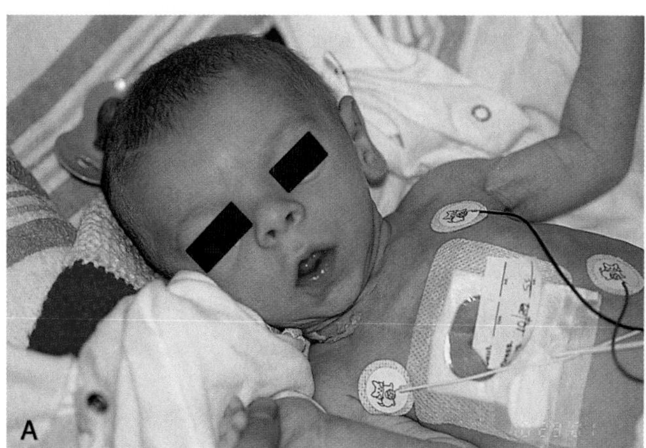

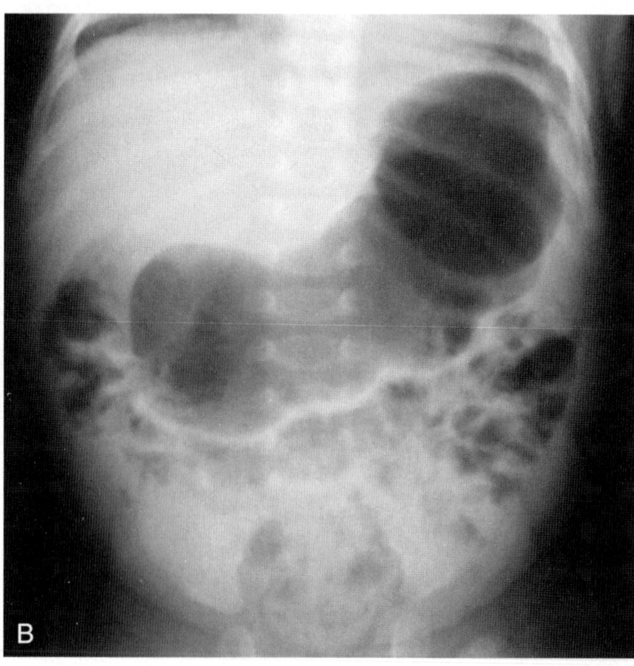

FIGURE 16–39 **A:** An infant who presented with a 6-week history of vomiting. Note the decreased subcutaneous fat over the face and the prominent skin folds of the upper and lower extremities. (From Fleisher, with permission.) **B:** A supine radiograph demonstrates a dilated gastric air bubble with the "caterpillar sign," suggesting active peristalsis. (**A** and **B**, From Fleisher, with permission.)

Pyloric Stenosis

Joseph Iocono

trolytes and glucose should be obtained. Ultrasonography is the diagnostic study of choice. For those infants evaluated with an upper gastrointestinal radiographic series, a nasogastric tube should be placed to evacuate any residual barium and prevent aspiration.[1-3] Once the diagnosis is established, prompt surgical consultation is indicated. A pyloromyotomy using open or laparoscopic techniques is the surgical procedure of choice.[3]

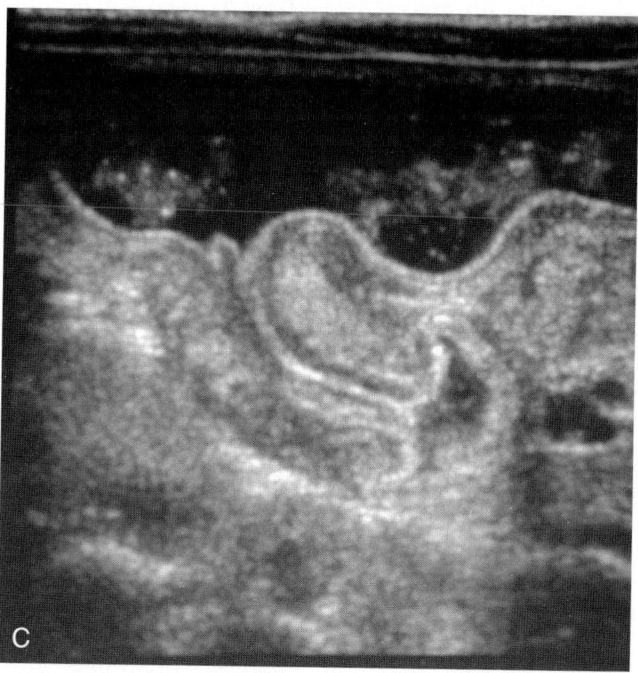

FIGURE 16–39 cont'd C: Ultrasound showing hypertrophic pylorus. (Courtesy of Robert Hendrickson, MD.)

REFERENCES

1. Letton RW Jr. Pyloric stenosis. *Pediatr Ann* 2001;30:745–750.
2. Irish MS, Pearl RH, Caty MG, Glick PL. The approach to common abdominal diagnosis in infants and children. *Pediatr Clin North Am* 1998;45:729–772.
3. Downey EC Jr. Laparoscopic pyloromyotomy. *Semin Pediatr Surg* 1998;7:220–224.

Infant Botulism

Michael Greenberg

Clinical Presentation

Patients with infant botulism (IB) range in age from 6 days to 12 months (mean, 13.7 weeks). They present with findings consistent with botulism, including descending flaccid muscular paralysis ("floppy baby"), muscle weakness (predominantly proximal), lethargy, bulbar palsies, drooling, weak cry/suck, and constipation that may precede weakness by a period of weeks.[1-3]

Pathophysiology

IB is a rare disease, with an incidence of 2 per 100,000 live births.[1-3] IB results from the ingestion of spores of *Clostridium botulinum*. The specific source for spores is unknown in most cases, but soil and honey contamination are the primary recognized sources for spores. A lack of competitive intestinal bacteria, as well as changes in bowel pH, facilitates growth of clostridial bacteria from ingested spores.[1-3] Recently weaned, breast-fed infants are at risk when variations in intestinal bacterial flora occur. Competing bacteria seem to become established rapidly in formula-fed infants, accounting for a lower incidence of disease in such infants. Replicating *C. botulinum* produces botulinum toxin, and IB is specifically associated with serotypes A and B. After systemic absorption, toxins bind to receptors on presynaptic nerve endings of cranial and peripheral nerves, resulting in blockade of acetylcholine release.[1-3]

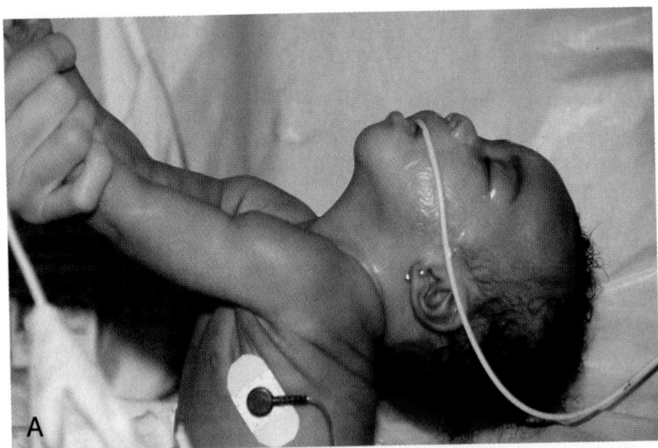

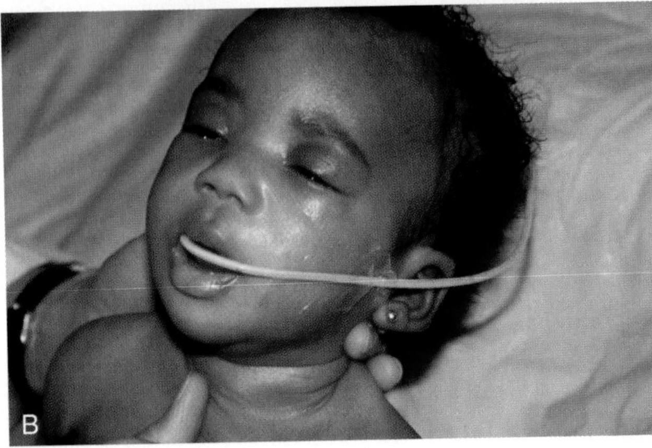

FIGURE 16–40 Infantile botulism. (From Shah, with permission.)

Diagnosis

Diagnosis is based on clinical findings and confirmed with neurophysiologic and serologic testing and by identification of the organism or toxin.

Clinical Complications

Complications include sudden catastrophic hypoxia, hypoxic encephalopathy, acute respiratory distress syndrome (ARDS), syndrome of inappropriate secretion of antidiuretic hormone (SIADH), hyponatremia, aspiration pneumonia, toxic megacolon, necrotizing enterocolitis, syndromic relapse, persistent hypotonia, deterioration with gentamicin, and severe *Clostridium difficile* infections.[1-3]

Management

IB has a limited case-fatality rate (2%), and the prognosis is favorable if it is recognized quickly and treatment is initiated promptly.[1-3] Meticulous supportive care is essential, and the early administration of intravenous human botulinum immunoglobulin (BIG) has substantially decreased hospital stays for IB patients. Fifty percent of patients require mechanical ventilation. Recovery relies on regeneration of nerve endings and motor end plates.[1-3]

REFERENCES

1. Urdaneta-Carruyo E, Suranyi A, Milano M. Infantile botulism: clinical and laboratory observations of a rare neuroparalytic disease. *J Paediatr Child Health* 2000;36:193–195.
2. Cox N, Hinkle R. Infant botulism. *Am Fam Physician* 2002;65: 1388-1392.
3. Infant botulism—New York City, 2001–2002. *MMWR Morb Mortal Wkly Rep* 2003;52:21–24.

Gastrointestinal Malrotation

Douglas Katz

Clinical Presentation

Although patients with malrotation may present at any age, 50% of the instances of volvulus develop within the first month of life, and 75% within the first year.[1] Abdominal examination may reveal distention of the abdomen with or without diffuse tenderness.[1] Blood may be evident on rectal examination if bowel necrosis is present. Abdominal radiographs may reveal stomach distention with a paucity of gas distal to the duodenum and the "double bubble sign" (distention of the stomach and proximal duodenum), because the obstruction often occurs within the middle duodenum.

Pathophysiology

By the tenth week of gestation, the midgut normally returns to the abdominal cavity and rotates around the superior mesenteric artery. Malrotation occurs when abnormal fibrous tissues (e.g., Ladd's bands) are attached to the bowel and do not allow complete rotation. The cecum remains in the right upper quadrant, and the duodenum is fixed inferiorly and to the right. The mesentery of the midgut is narrowed and is at risk for the development of acute and chronic volvulus.

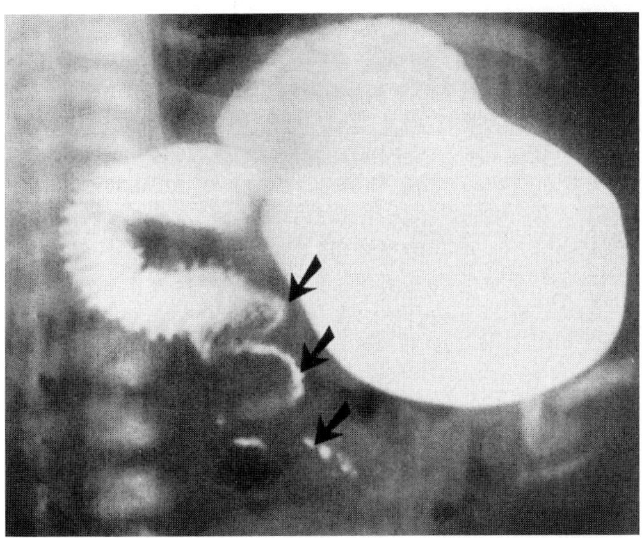

FIGURE 16–41 Barium-contrast upper gastrointestinal radiographic series demonstrates midgut volvulus in intestinal malrotation. This results in dilation of the duodenal bulb and proximal duodenum, which terminates in a cone-shaped narrowing *(upper arrow)* and a "corkscrew" pattern of the distal duodenum and proximal jejunum *(lower arrows)*. (From Yamada, with permission.)

Diagnosis

An upper gastrointestinal radiographic series most accurately demonstrates malrotation and volvulus and should be performed rapidly.[1] Findings include distention of the proximal duodenum with "corkscrewing" of the distal small bowel on the right side of the abdomen. Contrast enema and abdominal ultrasonography have also been used but are less reliable. Nonspecific laboratory studies may reveal anemia and dehydration.

Clinical Complications

Bowel ischemia may cause hypovolemia, peritonitis, bowel necrosis, shock, and death. Long-term complications include short-gut syndrome and dependence on total parenteral nutrition.[1]

Management

Patients presenting with bilious emesis should be evaluated for malrotation, volvulus, and other surgical emergencies. Initial management includes surgical consultation, volume resuscitation, and gastric decompression. For children presenting with signs and symptoms of peritonitis and imminent bowel necrosis, emergency laparotomy without confirmational imaging is occasionally indicated.[1]

During surgical correction of malrotation, the volvulus is reduced and isolated necrotic segments of bowel are resected. Ladd's bands are divided, the cecum is placed in the left upper quadrant, and an appendectomy is performed to avoid later misdiagnosis of appendicitis (the cecum is now located in the left abdomen).[1] The duodenum is freed from its abnormal attachments and placed in the right side of the abdomen. The small-bowel mesentery is incised and widened to limit the risk of volvulus.[1]

REFERENCES

1. Okada PJ, Hicks B. Neonatal surgical emergencies. *CPEM* 2002; 3:3–13.

Granuloma Annulare

Renee Turchi

Clinical Presentation

Patients with granuloma annulare (GA) present with small, firm, flesh-colored or erythematous papules or nodules in an annular distribution, with raised edges and central clearing. Classically, lesions range from 1 to 5 cm in diameter; they may be located anywhere on the body but are most commonly found in acral areas of the hand, digits, ankles, and wrist. Patients are often asymptomatic and lack systemic symptoms. Multiple, localized lesions are seen more often in children.[1–3]

There are several variants of GA, including perforating GA, which is characterized by extremity involvement with a central, crusted, or umbilicated papule; subcutaneous GA, which is common on lower extremities, the scalp, and hands with hard nodules; and generalized GA, in which diffuse papules are located over the neck and chest in patients exposed to sunlight.[1–3]

Pathophysiology

GA is a self-limited, cutaneous inflammatory disorder that is more common in children. It is characterized by papules or nodules in a ring-like configuration with beaded margins.[1–3] The cause of granuloma annulare is largely unknown. It may represent a delayed-type cell-mediated hypersensitivity reaction, or it may be related to previous trauma from sunlight and insect bites. Several studies have found GA to be present in patients with diabetes, but a direct causal relationship has not yet been substantiated.[1–3]

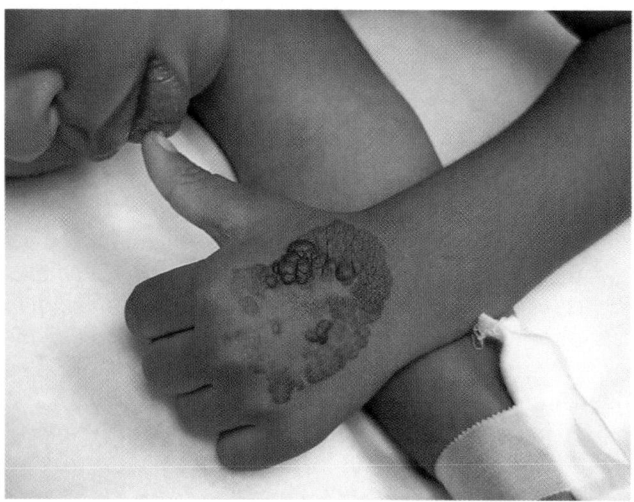

FIGURE 16–42 Granuloma annulare. (Courtesy of Christy Salvaggio, MD.)

Diagnosis

The diagnosis of GA is made from the clinical presentation. Occasionally, the lesions of GA are confused with rheumatoid nodules or tinea corporis. A negative potassium hydroxide preparation may rule out tinea corporis.[1–3]

Clinical Complications

GA is a self-limited disorder with infrequent severe complications. Rarely, fascia and tendon involvement results in sclerosis and lymphedema. Occasionally, patients have long-standing cosmetic sequelae from this disorder.[1–3]

Management

GA is usually self-limited and resolves spontaneously within months. Recurrences at the originally involved area are reported in up to 40% of patients. Although treatment with topical corticosteroids may foster prompter resolution, it is recommended that patients without generalized or disfiguring lesions be given reassurance of spontaneous remission. Because GA is associated with diabetes, some have suggested screening of patients with recurrent or recalcitrant GA for this disease, although this is not universally recommended.[1–3]

REFERENCES

1. Grogg KL, Nascimento AG. Subcutaneous granuloma annulare in childhood: clinicopathologic features in 34 cases. *Pediatrics* 2001; 107:E42.
2. Penas PF, Jones-Caballero M, Fraga J, et al. Perforating granuloma annulare. *Int J Dermatol* 1997;36:340–348.
3. Tan HH, Goh CL. Granuloma annulare: a review of 41 cases at the National Skin Centre. *Ann Acad Med Singapore* 2000;29:714–718.

Cystic Hygroma

Michael Greenberg

Clinical Presentation

Patients with cystic hygroma (CH) present in the newborn period or as young children with cystic masses of the neck, axillae, and other regions. Most cases are first identified by the parents, who detect a suspicious mass and bring the child to medical attention.[1,2]

Pathophysiology

CHs are rare, benign, congenital malformations of the lymphatic system. The cause of CH is not well understood, but some cases are associated with various chromosomal abnormalities. Some believe that CH develops if the lymphatic sacs do not connect to the central venous system in the embryonic period.[1]

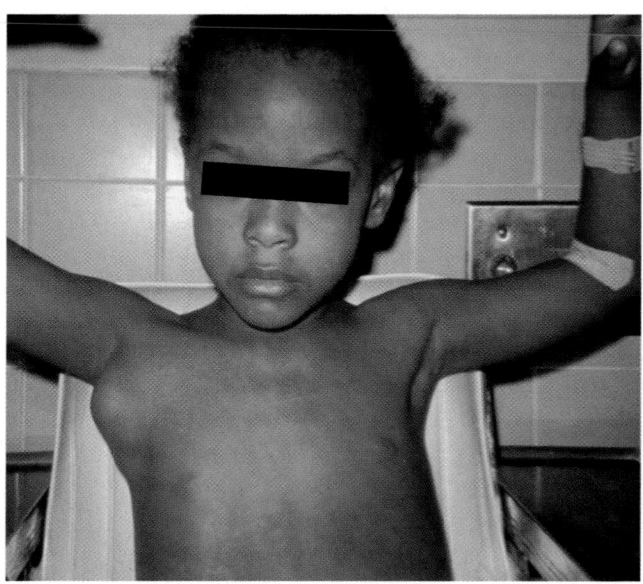

FIGURE 16–43 Axillary cystic hygroma. (Courtesy of Michael Greenberg, MD.)

Diagnosis

Boys and girls are affected equally. Fifty percent of CHs are present at birth. An additional 10% become evident by 1 year of age, and by 2 years of age, 80% of cases will have become evident. Some cases are first diagnosed in adulthood. Most CHs occur on the head and neck, but they may occur in the axillae; over the mediastinum, chest wall, or abdomen; in the inguinal area; and on the extremities. Clinically, CHs are fluctuant and lobular masses that are not attached to the skin.[1] Transillumination is the key to differentiating CH from other masses. Ultrasonography may reveal a multiloculated mass with multiple soft-tissue calcifications.[1]

Clinical Complications

Some CHs are so large as to create mechanical obstruction, depending on the location of the lesion. Other complications include reoccurrence, progressive enlargement, and infection. The surgical mortality rate has been noted to be as high as 6%.[1]

Management

Surgical resection with total excision is the treatment of choice. Some cases may respond to local injection with sclerosing agents.[1] Stable patients who are diagnosed in the emergency department should be referred to an appropriate surgeon or surgical subspecialist for evaluation at the earliest possible time.

REFERENCES

1. Wever DJ, Heeg M, Mooyaart EL. Cystic hygroma of the shoulder region: a case report. *Clin Orthop* 1997;(338):215–218.
2. Descamps P, Jourdain O, Paillet C, et al. Etiology, prognosis and management of nuchal cystic hygroma: 25 new cases and literature review. *Eur J Obstet Gynecol Reprod Biol* 1997;71:3–10.

Supernumerary Nipples

Sharon McGregor

Clinical Presentation

The clinical presentation of accessory breast tissue ranges from nipple only (polythelia), the most common form, to complete nipple, areola, and glandular breast tissue (polymastia). Accessory breast tissue may appear anywhere along the milk line, which extends from the axilla and inner upper arm to the normal nipple position, down the abdomen along the midclavicular line to the upper lateral mons and upper inner thigh. Supernumerary nipples may occur in men and women, are usually rudimentary, and may be mistaken for small moles.[1-3] Accessory glandular tissue is most common in the axilla, may enlarge during puberty, and may become tender premenstrually. It may also lactate and present as an enlarging axillary mass during pregnancy, or 2 to 5 days after delivery as a painful axillary mass.

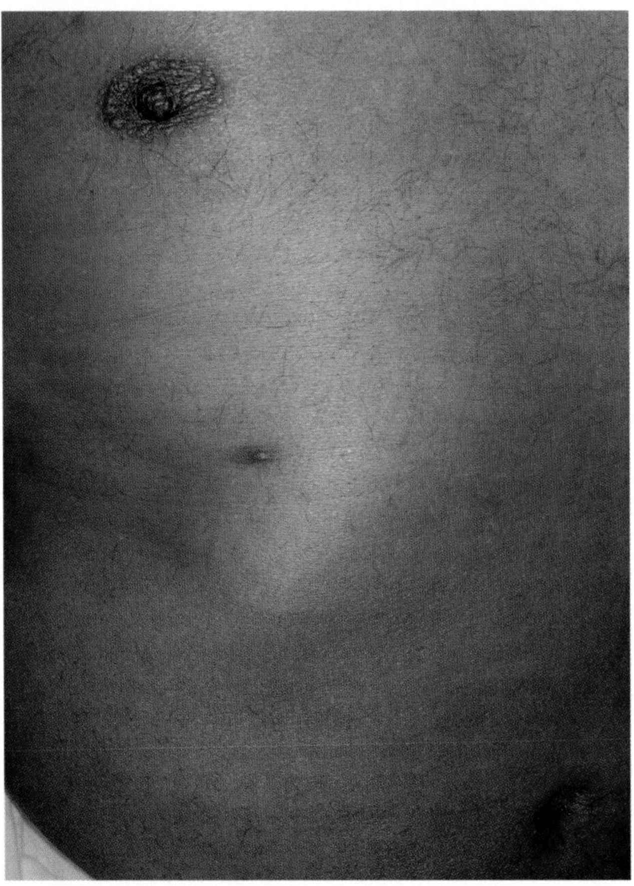

FIGURE 16–44 Supernumerary nipples. (Courtesy of Mark Silverberg, MD.)

Pathophysiology

Accessory breast tissue results from failure of the normal regression of the embryonic mammary ridges and mammary buds in all but the normal breast area. Approximately 6% of reported cases are familial (autosomal dominant with incomplete penetrance).[1-3]

Diagnosis

The diagnosis is made clinically by the presence of a nipple or other breast tissue along the mammary lines in other than the normal location.

Clinical Complications

Supernumerary nipples present only a potential cosmetic problem, not a medical one. However, accessory glandular tissue is subject to the same hormonal influences and disease processes as regular breast tissue. Although they are rare, fibroadenomas, cysts, abscess, mastitis, adenomas, and carcinoma may occur.[1-3] Reports indicate an increased incidence of renal and urinary tract abnormalities in individuals with supernumerary nipples, especially the familial variety (1% to 2% in the general population, 14% in those with nonfamilial supernumerary nipples, and 30% in those with familial supernumerary nipples).[1-3]

Management

Supernumerary nipples require no treatment but may be surgically excised if they are cosmetically unacceptable. Because of the reported association with renal anomalies, renal ultrasonography in infants and children may be indicated, especially if the supernumerary nipples are familial.[1-3]

REFERENCES

1. Brown J, Schwartz RA. Supernumerary nipples: an overview. *Cutis* 2003;71:344–346.
2. Templeman C, Hertweck SP. Breast disorders in the pediatric and adolescent patient. *Obstet Gynecol Clin North Am* 2000;27:19–34.
3. Varsano IB, Jaber L, Garty BZ, et al. Urinary tract abnormalities in children with supernumerary nipples. *Pediatrics* 1984;73:103–105.

Umbilical Hernia

Joseph A. Iocono

Clinical Presentation

An umbilical hernia usually manifests as an asymptomatic bulge emanating from the umbilicus. There is a higher incidence among infants of African-American descent.[1]

Pathophysiology

An umbilical hernia is a defect in the umbilical ring fascia (Richet's fascia) at the base of the umbilicus that allows herniation of abdominal contents.[2] The defect is covered by peritoneal lining (hernia sac) and skin.[3] The umbilical ring is open throughout gestation. It becomes progressively smaller as gestation progresses. Umbilical hernias are the result of the failure of the umbilical ring fascia to close. Most umbilical hernias are noted in the first month of life, and almost all are noted by 6 months.

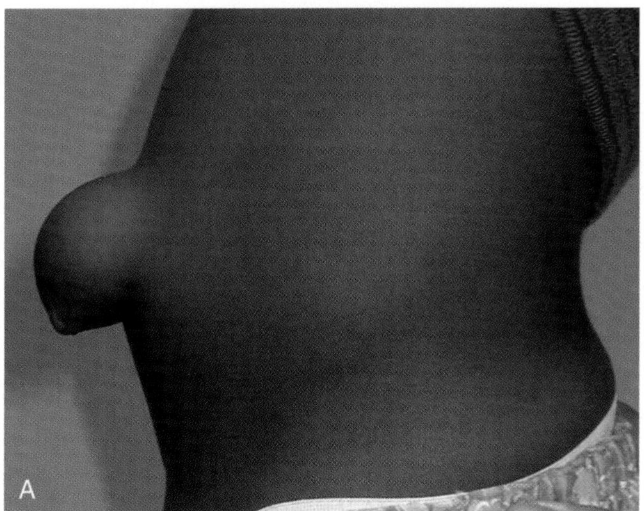

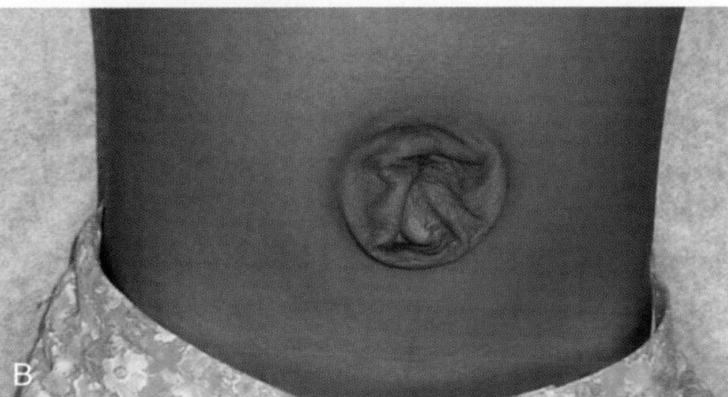

FIGURE 16–45 **A** and **B:** Large umbilical hernia defect in a 2-year-old girl. Early intervention is warranted because the fascial defect measures greater than 2 cm in diameter. (Courtesy of Joseph A. Iocono, MD.)

The majority of umbilical hernias close spontaneously without medical or surgical intervention by age 4 years. It is the size of the defect, not the amount of protrusion, that is the important factor in predicting whether the hernia will close spontaneously. Essentially all defects smaller than 1.0 cm will close by age 4 years.[1] Any defect greater than 1.5 cm will most likely need surgical correction; however, unless they are greater than 2 cm, these are observed until age 4 years as well.[3]

Diagnosis

Physical examination reveals a defect in the abdominal fascia at the level of the umbilicus. Fascial defects above the umbilicus are termed epigastric hernias and have an operative recommendation.

Clinical Complications

Umbilical hernias may incarcerate, but this is very rare. A red, swollen, tender umbilicus should trigger the suspicion of omphalitis (infection of the umbilicus) caused by the presence of a patent omphalomesenteric remnant. Both incarcerations and omphalitis are manifested by a tender mass, cellulitis, and fever. In differentiating these two conditions, the presence of either purulent or clear drainage is a sign of a patent omphalomesenteric duct. The mass should be examined carefully to see if it contains intraabdominal contents. In this scenario only, ultrasonography may be helpful in establishing the diagnosis.

Management

Symptomatic (incarcerated) hernias require prompt surgical consultation. Extremely large asymptomatic defects (greater than 2 cm), any lesion in a child older than 4 years of age, and any fascial defect above an intact umbilical ring may be referred for surgical consultation at the time of diagnosis. All other asymptomatic lesions in children younger than 4 years of age require parental reassurance that the defect will probably close spontaneously. These parents should be told to follow-up with their primary physician if the hernia is still present at age 4 years.

REFERENCES

1. Muschaweck U. Umbilical and epigastric hernia repair. *Surg Clin North Am* 2003;83:1207–1221.
2. Weber TR, Au-Fliegner M, Downard CD, Fishman SJ. Abdominal wall defects. *Curr Opin Pediatr* 2002;14:491–497.
3. Scherer LR 3rd, Grosfeld JL. Inguinal hernia and umbilical anomalies. *Pediatr Clin North Am* 1993;40:1121–1131.

Pinworm

Christy Salvaggio

Clinical Presentation

Pinworm infections usually occur in young children or institutionalized adults. Perianal itching and irritation are the most common presenting complaints, although some patients are asymptomatic and present only after pinworms are visualized on the perineum.[1,2]

Pathophysiology

Pinworm infection is caused by *Enterobius vermicularis,* a roundworm intestinal parasite. Humans are the only hosts for this parasite, and infections spread via the fecal-oral route. Swallowed eggs hatch in the duodenum, and, after maturation, adult worms migrate to the cecum. Gravid worms traverse the colon and deposit more than 10,000 eggs on the perineum. The eggs are infective within hours after deposition.[1,2]

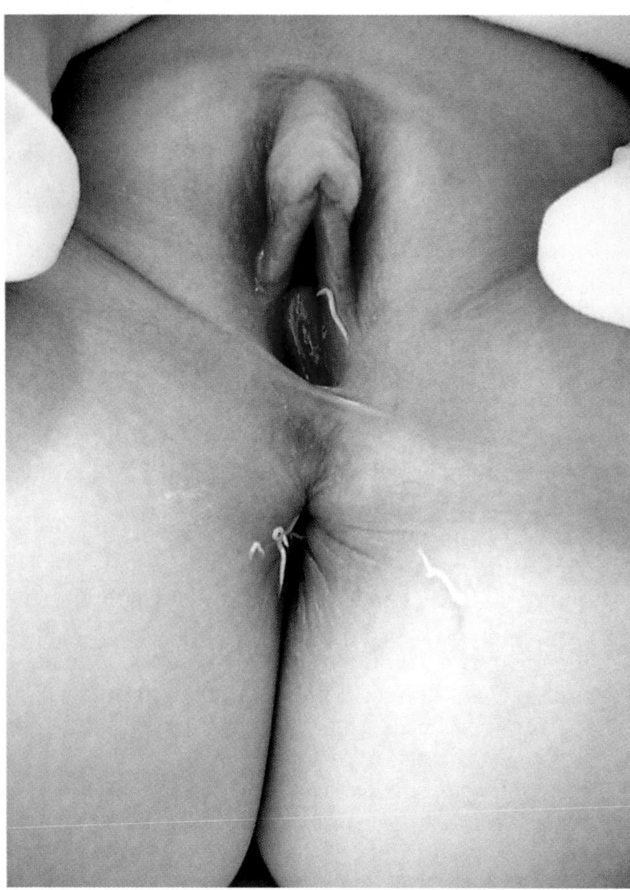

FIGURE 16–46 Pinworms on the perineum of a female infant. (Courtesy of Christy Salvaggio, MD.)

Diagnosis

Pinworms may sometimes be visualized on the perineum or on stool. If pinworms are not seen, the diagnosis may be confirmed by the cellophane tape test. At night, cellophane tape is pressed against the perianal skin and the tape is then adhered to a microscope slide. Deposited eggs can be seen on the slide with a low-power lens. The cellophane tape test detects 50% of infections after one night, and 99% of infections if the test is repeated for three nights.[1,2]

Clinical Complications

Complications include bacterial superinfection and infections of the female urogenital tract. Migrating pinworms may cause vaginitis, endometritis, or salpingitis. An association between pinworm infections and urinary tract infections in young girls has been suggested, because migrating worms are thought to carry enteric bacteria into the bladder. Although pinworms may migrate into the appendix, causal associations with appendicitis have not been substantiated.[1,2]

Management

Infections are treated with a single dose of mebendazole, albendazole, or pyrantel pamoate. Treatment should be repeated in 2 weeks. Because the eggs are resilient, the rate of reinfection is high. Bathing in the morning and washing bedding materials may reduce egg load.[1,2]

REFERENCES

1. St Georgiev V. Chemotherapy of enterobiasis (oxyuriasis). *Expert Opin Pharmacother* 2001;2:267–275.
2. Grencis RK, Cooper ES. *Enterobius, Trichuris, Capillaria,* and hookworm including *Ancylostoma caninum. Gastroenterol Clin North Am* 1996;25:579–597.

Congenital Syphilis

Christy Salvaggio

Clinical Presentation

Initial presentations of congenital syphilis (CS) include spontaneous abortion, prematurity, intrauterine growth retardation, and stillbirth; however, more than half of infected infants are asymptomatic at birth. Early-onset disease manifests before 2 years of age, with most infants diagnosed before 3 months of age. Hepatosplenomegaly is common, as are skeletal abnormalities such as osteochondritis. Skin manifestations include jaundice, petechiae, and purpura, an erythematous maculopapular rash that may include palm and sole involvement, and a bullous and highly contagious rash unique to infants, known as pemphigus syphiliticus. Highly contagious rhinitis (snuffles) may be initially mistaken for an upper respiratory tract infection until it becomes chronic and bloody from mucosal erosion. Hematologic abnormalities include thrombocytopenia, anemia, and an elevated white blood cell count. Without treatment, both symptomatic and asymptomatic infants are at risk for late-onset disease. Late-onset disease manifests after 2 years of age, and patients are no longer infectious at this time.

Pathophysiology

Vertical transmission occurs in 60% to 90% of pregnancies of untreated or inadequately treated mothers with primary or secondary syphilis. Vertical transmission rarely occurs if the woman is in the latent phase of disease. Transmission may also occur after delivery via breast milk.

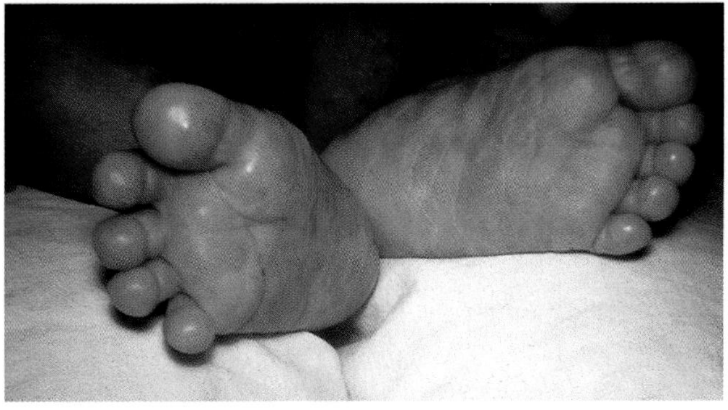

FIGURE 16–47 Congenital syphilis may exhibit a variety of manifestations, including pigmented lesions on the soles, as seen in this infant. (From Fleisher, with permission.)

Diagnosis

Hutchinson's triad of incisor defects, interstitial keratitis, and eighth nerve deafness is pathognomonic for CS. Routine prenatal testing includes maternal rapid plasma reagin (RPR) testing early in the pregnancy and again at delivery. Recently infected women may be seronegative at delivery. A high index of suspicion is needed, and symptomatic infants should be tested despite negative maternal serology results. RPR tests in newborns are unreliable, but a newborn RPR result that is two to four times higher than maternal RPR value indicates infection.

Clinical Complications

Frontal bossing, saddle nose, bilateral chronic painless knee swelling (Clutton's joints), anterior bowing of the shins (saber shins), hydrocephalus, and developmental delay are all potential late manifestations. The Jarisch-Herxheimer reaction is seen in more than 50% of infants with CS whose symptoms occur after birth. Of note, cardiovascular syphilis does not occur in CS.

Management

Treatment during pregnancy that cures the mother may not prevent CS in the child. Presumed and proven congenital infections are treated similarly. Congenital infections are treated with 10 to 14 days of aqueous penicillin G or procaine penicillin G. Benzathine penicillin G is not used because of higher failure rates. Infants with CS should be evaluated for other sexually transmitted diseases, including human immunodeficiency virus infection.[1]

REFERENCES

1. Workowski KA, Levine WC. Sexually transmitted diseases treatment guidelines—2002. *MMWR Morb Mortal Wkly Rep* 2002;51(RR-6): 1–80.

Urethral Prolapse

Michael Greenberg

Clinical Presentation

Urethral prolapse (UP) occurs almost exclusively in premenarcheal African-American girls.[1,2] However, cases of UP have occurred rarely in patients in the immediate postpartum period.[3] Patients typically present with a history of vaginal bleeding, urinary frequency, and dysuria; the lesion itself tends to be painless. Some patients present with acute urinary retention secondary to dysuria.[1-3]

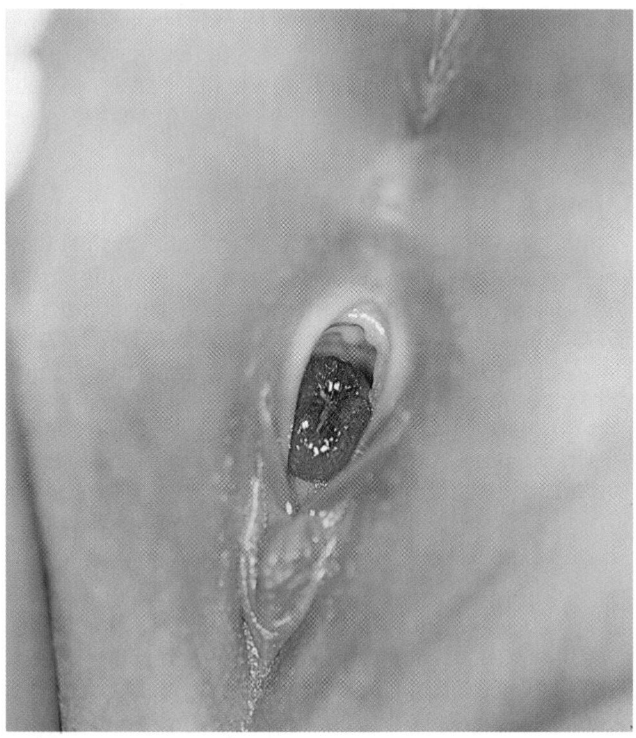

FIGURE 16–48 Urethral prolapse ("doughnut sign"). (From Fleisher, with permission.)

Pathophysiology

UP is a circumferential eversion of the urethral mucosa at the meatus.[1] The precise cause for UP is not known. However, estrogen deficiency and weak attachments between the layers of smooth muscle of the distal urethra, in association with episodic increases in intraabdominal pressure (as occurs during labor), have been postulated.[3]

Diagnosis

The diagnosis is based on recognition of the typical appearance of the prolapse, which appears as a bright-red or cyanotic and edematous mass located ventrally at the introitus. UP is frequently misdiagnosed and may be mistakenly attributed to sexual abuse or other genital trauma.[1,3]

Clinical Complications

Complications include misdiagnosis, excessive bleeding, local thrombosis, venous obstruction and strangulation, the development of gangrenous mucosa, and recurrence.

Management

Most cases resolve with conservative care, including application of topical estrogen cream, sitz baths, and reassurance. If conservative management fails, excision of the prolapsed mucosa is usually effective.

REFERENCES

1. Valerie B, Gilchrist J, Frischer R, et al. Diagnosis and treatment of urethral prolapse in children. *Pediatr Urol* 1999;54:1082–1084.
2. Cruikshank SH, Kovac SR. The functional anatomy of the urethra: role of the pubourethral ligaments. *Am J Obstet Gynecol* 1997;176: 1200–1203, 1230–1235.
3. Ketab Z, Mikines KJ. Postpartum urethral prolapse. *Acta Obstet Gynecol Scand* 2002;81:268–269.

Legg-Calvé-Perthes Disease

James Guille

Clinical Presentation

Patients with Legg-Calvé-Perthes disease (LCPD) present between the ages of 5 and 10 years. Approximately 85% of these patients are boys and present with unilateral involvement, including pain in the groin, thigh, or knee as well as a limp.[1-3]

Pathophysiology

LCPD involves idiopathic osteonecrosis of the femoral head. The cause of LCPD is unknown, but a vascular insult to the capital femoral epiphysis may be responsible. Synovitis of the hip is the first manifestation. LCPD represents a spectrum of manifestations whereby the capital femoral epiphysis undergoes four sequential stages: necrosis, fragmentation, reossification, and remodeling. Simply stated, the femoral head dies, crumbles, reforms, and reshapes.[1-3]

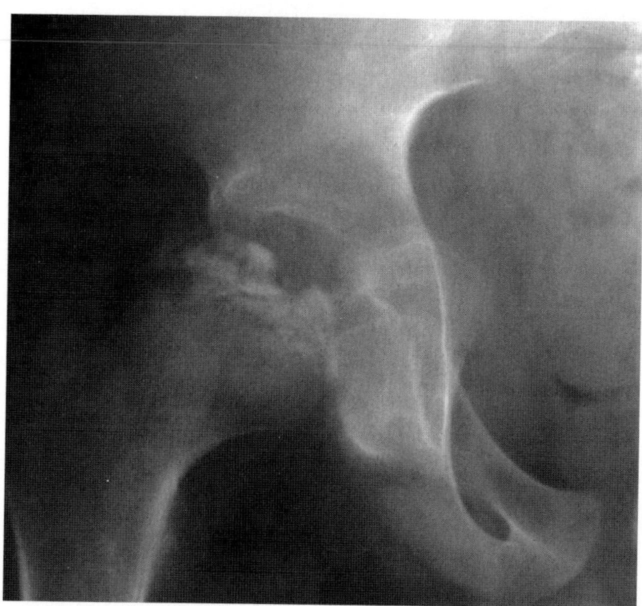

FIGURE 16–49 Osteonecrosis of the femoral head (Legg-Calvé-Perthes disease). (Courtesy of James T. Guille, MD.)

Diagnosis

The diagnosis of LCPD is made by anteroposterior radiograph of the pelvis and lateral radiographs of the hip.

Clinical Complications

LCPD rarely causes any acute clinical complications. If osteochondritis desiccans (loose body) is present, the patient may present with clicking or locking of the hip joint. If the femoral head does not resume its spherical shape during the remodeling period, the hip is at an increased risk for osteoarthritis at an earlier age. Mild limb-length discrepancy may occur late if the capital femoral physis was affected. Abductor lurch (limp) may be present if the prematurely closed capital femoral physis caused a foreshortened femoral neck with greater trochanteric overgrowth.[1-3]

Management

Pediatric orthopedic referral is warranted for any patient with suspected LCPD. Patients with LCPD are administered antiinflammatory medications during the early stages for pain. Maintenance of range of motion of the hip is of paramount importance, and referral to a physical therapist may be needed. Weight-bearing and activity are indicated as tolerated.[1-3]

REFERENCES

1. Guille JT, Lipton GE, Szoke G, et al. Legg-Calve-Perthes disease in girls: a comparison of the results with those seen in boys. *J Bone Joint Surg Am* 1998;80:1256–1263.
2. Guille JT, Lipton GE, Tsirikos AI, Bowden JR. Bilateral Legg-Calve-Perthes disease: presentation and outcome. *J Pediatr Orthop* 2002; 22:458–463.
3. Wenger DR, Ward WT, Herring JA. Legg-Calve-Perthes disease. *J Bone Joint Surg Am* 1991;73:778–788.

Tetralogy of Fallot

Madhu Hardaslamani

Clinical Presentation

Patients with tetralogy of Fallot (TOF) present at or just after birth with cyanosis and tachypnea. A systolic ejection murmur and thrill may be present. The second heart sound (S_2) is usually single. In an acyanotic infant, a systolic murmur from the ventricular septal defect (VSD) is usually audible.[1]

"Tet spells" are hypercyanotic episodes characterized by paroxysms of hyperpnea, crying, intense cyanosis, and decreased intensity of the pulmonary stenosis murmur. The mechanism underlying "tet spells" is infundibular spasm and/or decreased systemic vascular resistance with increased right-to-left shunting at the VSD, which results in decreased pulmonary blood flow. Spells usually occur in the morning after crying, feeding, or defecating, with a peak incidence between 2 and 4 months of age. "Tet spells" may result in syncope, seizure, stroke, or death.

Pathophysiology

TOF consists of a subaortic VSD, right ventricular infundibular stenosis, aortic valve positioned to override the right ventricle, and right ventricular hypertrophy.[1] Due to the presence of a large VSD, the right ventricular pressure is equal to the left ventricular and aortic pressures. The greater the pulmonary stenosis, the greater the reduction in pulmonary blood flow and the greater the increase in blood flow through the VSD to the aorta. Hence, the degree of cyanosis correlates with the degree of obstruction.[1]

Diagnosis

The diagnosis is suspected clinically and confirmed by echocardiography.

Clinical Complications

Complications include worsening cyanosis, heart failure, polycythemia, coagulopathy, endocarditis, brain abscesses, and cerebrovascular accidents secondary to paradoxical emboli.

Management

Acutely ill cyanotic neonates with a presumptive diagnosis of congenital heart disease should receive prostaglandin E_1 infusion empirically to keep the ductus arteriosus open and provide pulmonary blood flow in ductal-dependent lesions. Treatment of "tet spells" includes maneuvers to decrease right-to-left shunting and increase pulmonary blood flow. Infants are placed in the knee-chest position and administered oxygen and morphine (to reduce tachypnea). Severe attacks may require sodium bicarbonate, α-adrenergic agonists (to increase systemic vascular resistance), and/or β-adrenergic blockade. The definitive treatment is surgical repair, ideally before 3 months of age. Surgical repair involves closure of the VSD and widening of right ventricle outflow tract obstruction.[2]

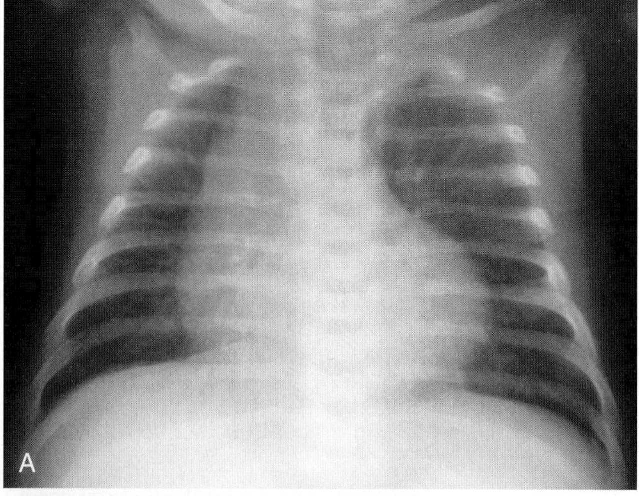

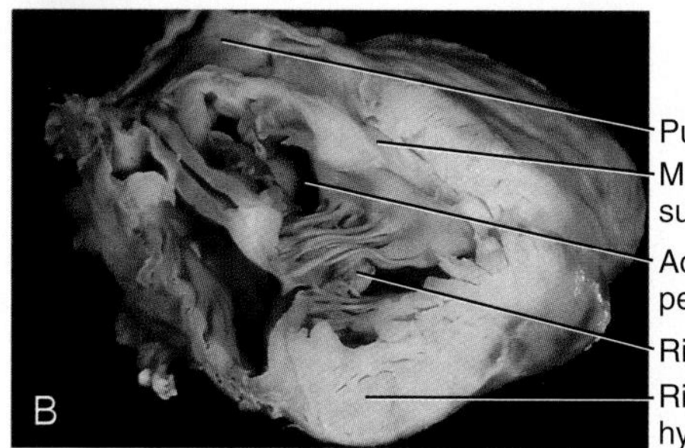

FIGURE 16–50 A: Biventricular enlargement and decreased pulmonary vascularity in a child with tetralogy of Fallot. (Courtesy of Mark Silverberg, MD.) **B:** Simulated paracoronal subcostal section of the heart with tetralogy of Fallot. A perimembranous ventricular septal defect, muscular subpulmonary obstruction as a consequence of anterocephalad deviation of the outlet septum, overriding of the aortic valve, and marked right ventricular hypertrophy are apparent. (From Hurst, with permission.)

REFERENCES

1. Waldman JD, Wernly JA. Cyanotic congenital heart disease with decreased pulmonary blood flow in children. *Pediatr Clin North Am* 1999;46:385–404.
2. Van Arsdell GS, Maharaj GS, Tom J, et al. What is the optimal age for repair of tetralogy of Fallot? *Circulation* 2000;102(19 Suppl 3):123–129.

Pediatric Cervical Spine: Normal Variants

Christy Salvaggio

Clinical Presentation

Normal pediatric cervical spine (C-spine) variants may be mistaken for pathologic conditions. The normal lordotic curvature of the C-spine is often absent in children younger than 6 years of age. A wide C1–2 interspace is also frequently seen, raising the concern of a flexion injury with posterior ligament damage. Flexion injuries are uncommon in the upper C-spine, and a wide C1–2 interspace is usually a normal pediatric variant.[1]

The predental space is wider in children than in adults (less than 5 and less than 3 mm, respectively), secondary to increased ligamentous laxity. The normal prevertebral distance is also wider in children (less than two-thirds of the width of the vertebral body between C1 and C4, and less than the width of the vertebral body below C4).

Anterior wedging of the vertebral bodies (most pronounced at C3) is indicative of incomplete ossification and not of a fracture. Anterior wedging resolves as the C-spine matures. Additionally, ossification centers and a congenital anomaly of the dens may mimic C-spine injury in children.

Pseudosubluxation (C2 on C3 or, less commonly, C3 on C4) is representative of increased upper C-spine mobility, not a hangman's fracture. Pseudosubluxation occurs in 25% of children younger than 8 years of age and may be seen up to age 16 years. A normal posterior line of Swischuk confirms the diagnosis of pseudosubluxation.

Pseudo-Jefferson fractures are a normal variant in children younger than 4 to 6 years of age, secondary to the incongruent (faster) growth of C1 compared with C2 and an element of radiolucent cartilage artifact. Pseudo-Jefferson fractures are seen in up to 90% of 2-year-olds. A computed tomogram is necessary to diagnose a true Jefferson fracture in children younger than 4 years of age.[1]

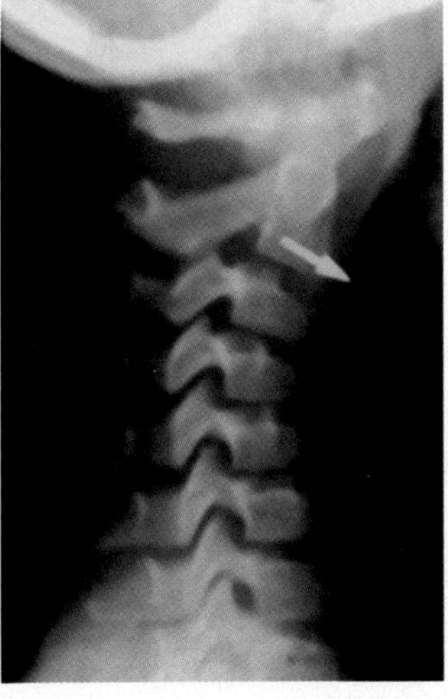

FIGURE 16–51 Pseudosubluxation. The normal alignment of the cervical spine is usually well demonstrated by a lateral radiograph. Pseudosubluxation is common in younger children, with C2 displaced forward on C3 *(yellow arrow)*. (From Staheli, with permission.)

Pathophysiology

The pediatric C-spine has increased upper C-spine mobility, in part because of the higher anatomic fulcrum. The anatomic fulcrum is at C2–3 in infants, C3–4 in children 5 years of age, and C5–6 in children older than 8 years. The increased mobility is also secondary to less developed paraspinal musculature; more horizontal apophyseal joints, which allow more anterior-posterior motion; and increased ligamentous laxity. Because of the increased upper C-spine mobility, C-spine injuries in children younger than 8 years of age are predominantly upper C-spine injuries. In contrast, adult C-spine injuries are predominantly in the lower C-spine. Importantly, the increased laxity of the pediatric C-spine is also associated with spinal cord injury without radiographic abnormality (SCIWORA).[1]

Diagnosis

Knowledge of pediatric C-spine anatomy is critical to making the correct diagnosis when distinguishing between a normal pediatric C-spine variant and true C-spine pathology.[1]

Clinical Complications

Failure to recognize these variants as normal may result in prolonged patient immobilization and unnecessary diagnostic testing.

REFERENCES

1. Kadish HA. Cervical spine evaluation in the pediatric trauma patient. *CPEM* 2001;2:41–47.

Munchausen's Syndrome by Proxy

Michael Greenberg

Clinical Presentation

Munchausen's syndrome by proxy (MSBP) is "the persistent fabrication of symptoms or actual illness in young children (usually under 8 years old) by parents, usually the mother."[1] Patients present with a wide variety of symptoms and physical findings, depending on the specific clinical deceptions at play in a given case.[1,2]

Pathophysiology

The parental psychopathology underlying MSBP is unclear. In all cases, MSBP involves a fabricated history, and at times it involves parentally inflicted injury or circumstances meant to simulate specific symptoms of disease (see Table 16–52A). Uncovering and proving MSBP is extremely difficult and often takes years. At least 10% of children victimized by MSBP die before the diagnosis is made.[1] Common symptoms that may be part of an MSBP syndrome include chronic diarrhea and vomiting, which can easily be simulated by the use of laxatives or syrup of ipecac or by other means.[1,2] In some studies, bleeding is the most common complaint or finding in MSBP.[2]

Diagnosis

The average age at diagnosis for victims of MSBP is 4 years.[2] The average length of time from onset of symptoms until diagnosis is almost 22 months.[2] In up to 30% of cases, the perpetrator has a background in health care.[2] In many cases, the perpetrators themselves have Munchausen's syndrome or some aspects of that syndrome. Victims of MSBP have often undergone multiple invasive diagnostic procedures or operative procedures (see Table 16–52B). The diagnosis of MSBP is often difficult to confirm. In *United States v White* 401 U.S. 745 (1971), the U. S. Supreme Court provided support for the use of hidden cameras placed in hospital rooms as one means of diagnostic confirmation.[3]

Clinical Complications

Complications include prolonged symptom induction, leading to injury or death.

TABLE 16–52A Documented Methods of Child Abuse in Munchausen Syndrome by Proxy

Item	Description
Fabrication of past history/current symptoms	Lying about vomiting, diarrhea, gastrointestinal bleeding, bloody stool, poor feeding, lethargy, fever, pain, seizures, apnea, bradycardia, cardiac arrest, SIDS, asthmas, headaches, psychologic/behavioral problems
Gastrointestinal bleeding or urinary tract infection	Putting blood in a stool or urine specimen
Vomiting or gastroesophageal reflux	Administering ipecac or other drugs
Diarrhea	Administering laxatives or prunes
Gastric gas/distress	Blowing air into the gastric tube
Apnea alone or leading to cardiac arrest/ SIDS-like presentation	Manual suffocation of the child
Asthma or respiratory distress	Purposeful exposure to triggers or withholding of asthma medications
Hypoglycemia	Administering insulin or withholding food from the child
Hypernatremia	Administering table salt to the child
Lethargy	Administering barbiturates, tranquilizers, or anticonvulsants to the child
Seizures	Withholding the prescribed dose of anticonvulsants, administering a medication that causes seizures as a side effect, causing a chemical imbalance such as hypoglycemia, hyponatremia, or hypernatremia
Contact dermatitis or burns	Rubbing caustic chemicals on the child's skin or placing caustic chemicals in the child's mouth
Poisoning	Administering caffeine, table salt, fingernail polish, laxatives, diuretics, an incorrect dose of prescribed medication, or any medication not prescribed to the child, such as diphenhydramine, ipecac, tranquilizers, barbiturates, anticonvulsants
Infections	Instilling foreign substances or contaminated body fluids into child's intravenous line, Foley catheter, or gastric tube to cause sepsis or HIV infection

HIV, human immunodeficiency virus; SIDS, sudden infant death syndrome.

Adapted from Thomas K. Munchausen syndrome by proxy: identification and diagnosis. *J Pediatr Nurs* 2003;18:174–180, with permission from Elsevier.

Munchausen's Syndrome by Proxy

Michael Greenberg

TABLE 16–52B Warning Signs of Munchausen Syndrome by Proxy

A child who presents with one or more medical problems that do not respond to treatment or that have an unusual, persistent, or unexplainable course
Symptoms that do not make sense
Repeated hospitalizations and extensive medical tests that fail to produce diagnosis
Physical or laboratory findings that are discrepant with the reported history or that are physically or clinically impossible
Signs and symptoms that disappear when contact between perpetrator and child is denied
Family history of similar sibling illness or unexplained sibling illness or death (e.g., SIDS)
History of unusual or numerous medical problems that have not been substantiated, raising questions about the reporter's veracity
Parent with symptoms similar to those of the child's medical problem, or with illness history that is in itself unusual
Caregiver who refuses to believe or accept a nonmedical diagnosis
Spouse who does not visit the child or has minimal contact or communication with physicians, regardless of severity of the child's illness
Victim passivity toward the perpetrator's actions
Symptoms or episodes witnessed only by the caregiver (e.g., cyanosis, apnea, "near-miss" SIDS, seizures)
Multiple resuscitations in a child who does not have cardiopulmonary abnormalities
Hospital transfers or discharge against medical advice

SIDS, sudden infant death syndrome.
Adapted from Thomas K. Munchausen syndrome by proxy: identification and diagnosis. *J Pediatr Nurs* 2003;18:174–180, with permission from Elsevier.

Management

Identification of MSBP is the essential first step to protect the victim. Once the diagnosis has been made, the child must be taken into protective custody and appropriate social and law enforcement agencies must be notified.

REFERENCES

1. de Ridder L, Hoekstra JH. Manifestations of Munchausen syndrome by proxy in pediatric gastroenterology. *J Pediatr Gastroenterol Nutr* 2000;31:208–211.
2. Sheridan MS. The deceit continues: an updated literature review of Munchausen syndrome by proxy. *Child Abuse Negl* 2003;27: 431–451.
3. Morrision CA. Cameras in hospital rooms: the Fourth Amendment to the Constitution and Munchausen syndrome by proxy. *Crit Care Nurs Q* 1999;22:65–68.

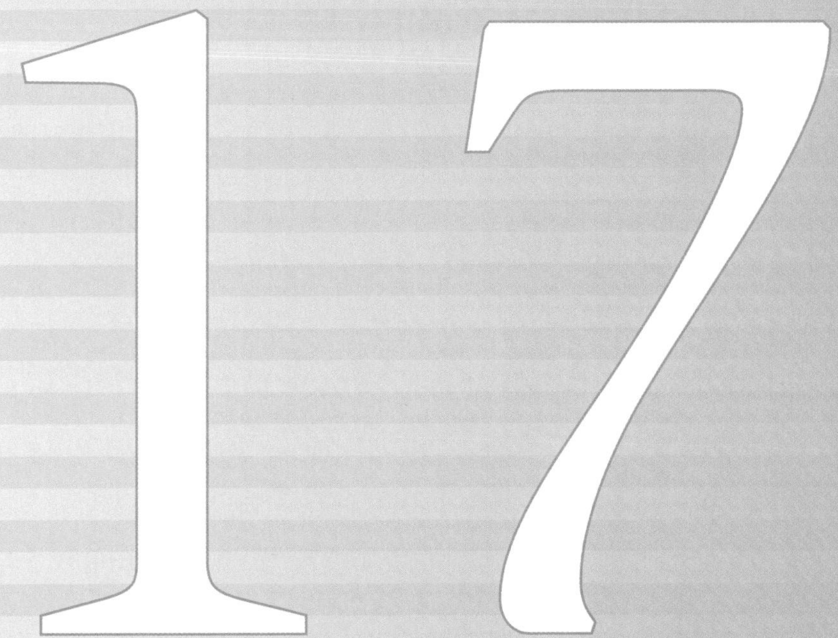

Trauma

Basilar Skull Fracture

Madelyn Garcia

Clinical Presentation

Signs and symptoms of basilar skull fracture vary depending on the area involved. Anterior fossa fractures are often accompanied by facial injury, cerebrospinal fluid (CSF) rhinorrhea, or bilateral periorbital ecchymosis.[1] Patients with middle fossa fractures present with postauricular hematoma (Battle's sign), hemotympanum, otorrhea, facial nerve palsy, vertigo, tinnitus, or hearing loss.[1] Those with posterior fossa fractures through the occipital bone may present with swallowing and airway difficulties secondary to glossopharyngeal and vagal nerve injury, or with mental status changes from associated epidural hematoma.[1]

Pathophysiology

Basilar skull fractures are associated with deceleration injuries involving head strikes on hard surfaces.[1]

Diagnosis

Basilar skull fracture should be suspected from the history and physical examination and may sometimes be visualized on plain radiographs of the skull. Computed tomography (CT) with thin cuts through the skull base is the confirmatory modality.[1-3]

Clinical Complications

Complications include CSF leakage, meningitis, and cranial nerve injuries.[1]

Management

In conjunction with advanced trauma life support (ATLS) protocols, early neurosurgical, maxillofacial, or otolaryngology consultation should be considered. Expanding hematomas need to be evacuated immediately. Orbital nerve compression may require decompression and high-dose steroids. CSF leak should be surgically closed by repair of the tear in the dura, and vascular injuries may be repaired or conservatively watched with repeat CT scanning.[1]

REFERENCES

1. Samii M, Tatagiba M. Skull base trauma: diagnosis and management. *Neurol Res* 2002;24:147–156.
2. Stone JA, Castillo M, Neelon B, Mukherji SK. Evaluation of CSF leaks: high resolution CT compared with contrast enhanced CT and radionuclide cisternography. *Am J Neuroradiol* 1999;20:706–712.
3. Dahiya R, Keller JD, Litofsky NS, et al. Temporal bone fractures: otic capsule sparing versus otic capsule violating clinical and radiographic considerations. *J Trauma* 1999:47:1079–1083.

Basilar Skull Fracture

Madelyn Garcia

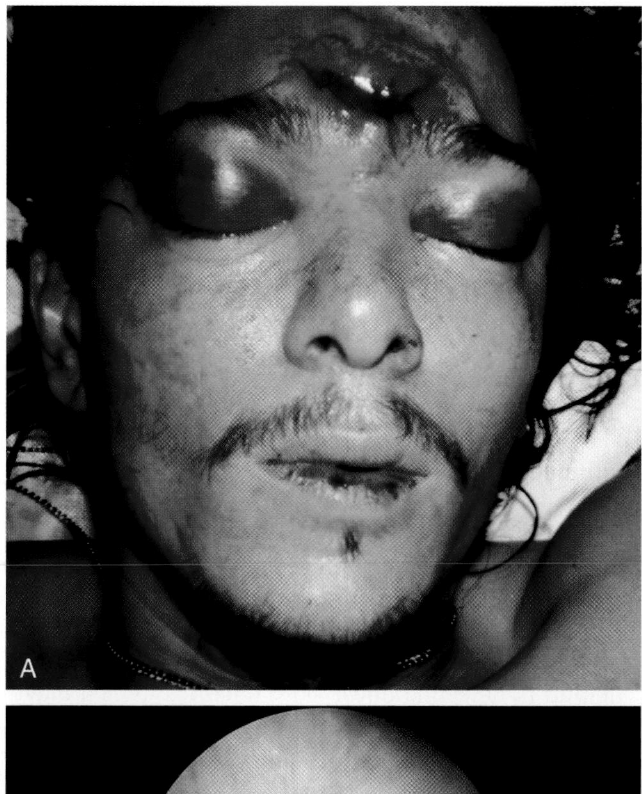

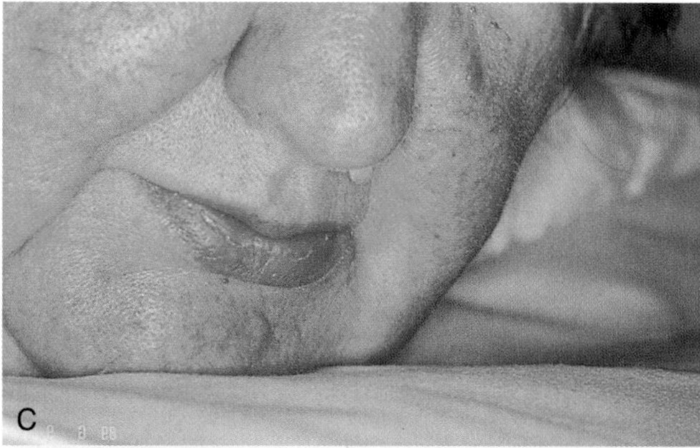

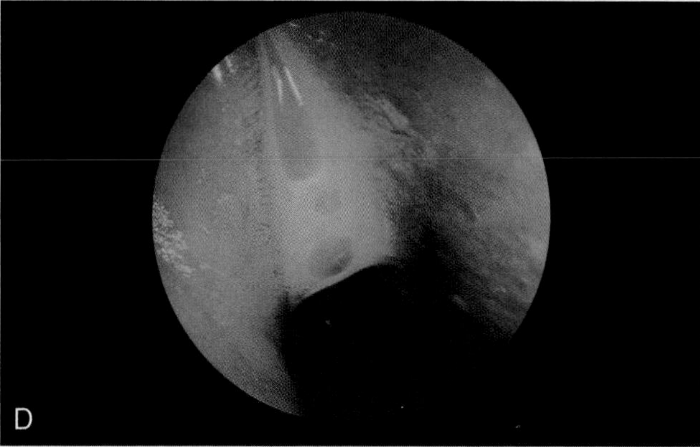

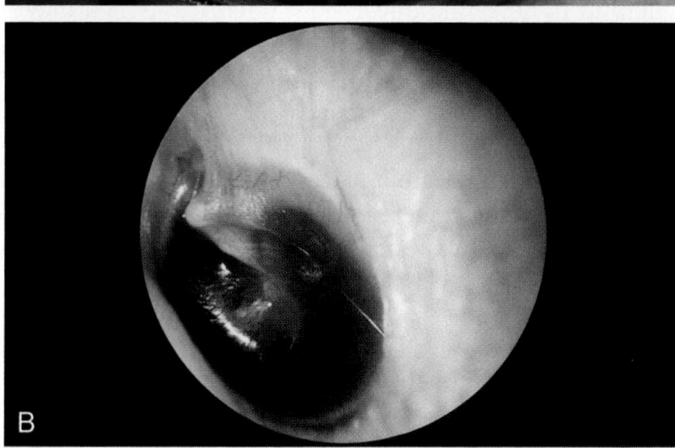

FIGURE 17–1 **A:** "Raccoon's eyes." (Courtesy of Michael Greenberg, MD.) **B:** Hemotympanum. The older, dark-brown, bloody fluid in this right middle ear has colored the tympanic membrane black. (From Benjamin, with permission.) **C:** The fluorescein test for cerebrospinal fluid (CSF) rhinorrhea. In this positive test, fluorescein-stained CSF is seen dripping from the patient's left nostril after 45 minutes. (From Benjamin, with permission.) **D:** CSF rhinorrhea. With blue light, fluorescence is induced and the CSF shines with a neon-like color. The fluorescein was followed into the sphenoethmoidal recess, close to the sphenoid sinus ostium. (From Benjamin, with permission.)

Skull Fracture

Madelyn Garcia

Clinical Presentation

Patients with skull fracture present after head trauma. Signs and symptoms vary, depending on the type of fracture and associated injuries such as intracranial hemorrhage.[1]

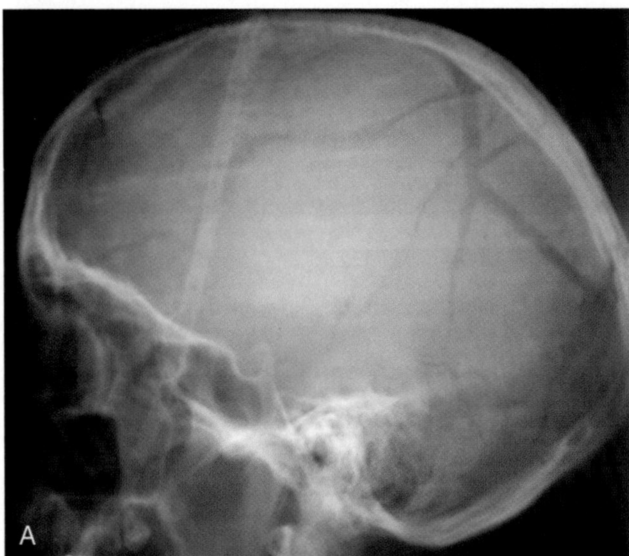

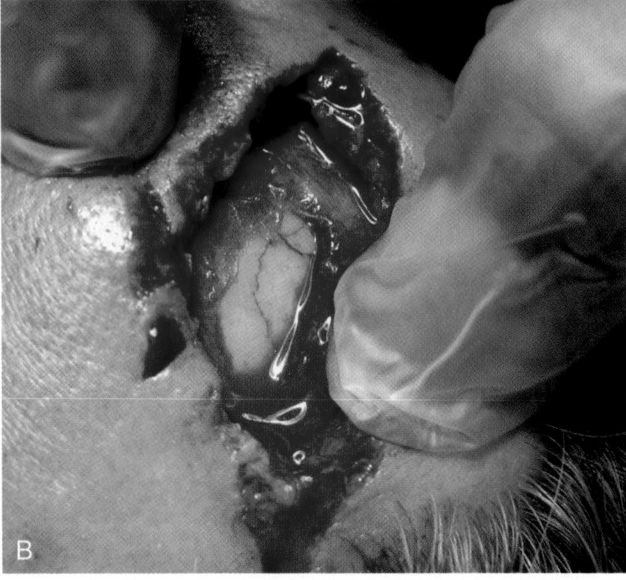

FIGURE 17–2 **A:** Radiograph showing severely comminuted skull fracture. (Courtesy of Michael Greenberg, MD.) **B:** A skull fracture is clearly visible in the base of this scalp. (Courtesy of Anthony Morocco, MD.)

Pathophysiology

Linear skull fractures go through the entire thickness of the skull and occur most often in the temporal-parietal and frontal regions. They are the most common type of skull fracture.[1] Depressed skull fractures have a bony segment that is displaced inward. These fractures are considered significant if the fragment is depressed below the inner table of the adjacent calvaria, or if the fracture overlies an important structure such as a venous sinus or the motor or sensory cortex.[1] In open skull fractures, the dura has been exposed. Open fractures can occur if a scalp laceration overlies the fracture site or if the paranasal sinuses or middle ear structures are disrupted, allowing communication between the brain and the environment.[1]

Diagnosis

Skull fractures may be suspected based on the history and physical examination, but usually radiographic confirmation is required. Computed tomographic (CT) scanning is the diagnostic modality of choice. Plain films are helpful in detecting linear skull fractures, which may be missed if they run in the same plane as the CT slices.[1]

Clinical Complications

Complications include intracranial hemorrhage, meningitis, cerebrospinal fluid leakage, abscess formation, leptomeningeal cyst, seizures, epilepsy, and future neuropsychological dysfunction.[2]

Management

It is essential to exclude underlying intracranial injury, which is up to four times more common in the presence of a skull fracture. Linear, closed skull fractures are treated symptomatically, whereas open fractures should be treated with antibiotics and tetanus toxoid.[1] Depressed skull fractures are considered "high-risk" and require close observation.[1] Intraoperative washout and fragment elevation should be considered on a case-by-case basis. Seizure prophylaxis is controversial but is recommended in the immediate postinjury period.[2] Neurosurgical consultation should be considered for all skull fractures.[1,2]

REFERENCES

1. Levine RS, Grossman RI. Head and facial trauma. *Emerg Med Clin North Am* 1985;3:447–473.
2. Annegers JF, Coan SP. The risks of epilepsy after traumatic brain injury. *Seizure* 2000;9:453–457.

Scalp Laceration

Dante Pappano

Clinical Presentation

Patients with scalp lacerations present with a history of trauma and obvious disruption of the scalp dermis and epidermis.

Pathophysiology

The scalp is a common site for lacerations, which may result from either blunt or sharp/penetrating mechanisms, or as a consequence of a bite.[1,2] The distinction is important, because lacerations caused by crushing rather than cutting forces often generate more devitalized tissue, with a higher probability of wound infection. Those lacerations caused by bites are often contaminated by bacteria and may represent the greatest risk for infection.[1]

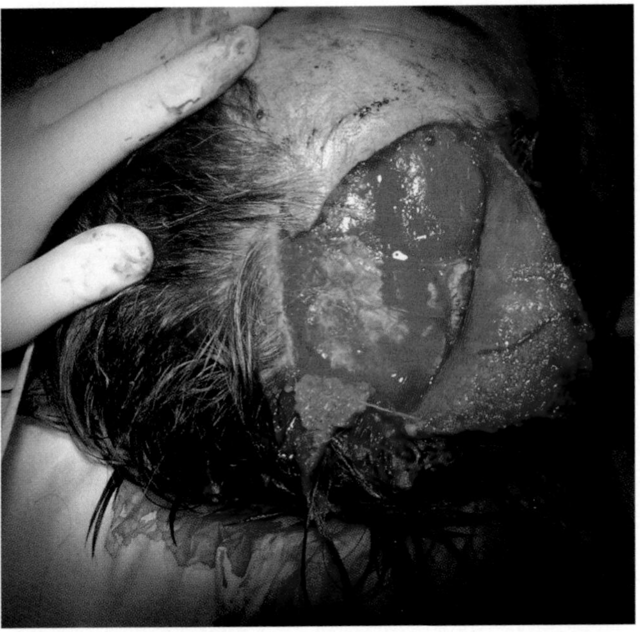

FIGURE 17–3 Complex scalp laceration with laterally based flap. (Courtesy of Andrew Liteplo, MD.)

Diagnosis

Diagnosis is based on physical findings; however, the extent of injury may not be clear until the wound area has been anesthetized, cleansed, and thoroughly inspected.[1]

Clinical Complications

Extensive hemorrhage may lead to hypotension. Wound infection, substantial scalp tissue loss, dehiscence, and poor cosmesis are potential complications. Retained foreign bodies may serve as a nidus for infection.

Management

Direct pressure to control hemorrhage is usually effective. Hemostasis may be difficult to attain due to the vascularity of the scalp. Persistent bleeding may be controlled in part by infiltration of vasoconstrictive agents and recompression of the wound. In preparing the field for closure, most authorities agree that the hair along the wound edge should be cut short but not shaved.[1,2] Once the defect is ready to be repaired, the physician must select among multiple techniques of wound closure, including standard suturing or stapling and less common alternatives such as hair tying and the hair apposition technique (HAT).[3]

REFERENCES

1. Hollander JE, Singer AJ. Laceration management. *Ann Emerg Med* 1999;34:356–367.
2. Howell JM, Morgan JA. Scalp laceration repair without prior hair removal. *Am J Emerg Med* 1988;6:7–10.
3. Hock MO, Ooi SB, Saw SM, Lim SH. A randomized controlled trial comparing the hair apposition technique with tissue glue to standard suturing in scalp lacerations (HAT Study). *Ann Emerg Med* 2002;40:19–26.

17-4

Diffuse Axonal Injury

Dante Pappano

Clinical Presentation

Diffuse axonal injury (DAI) is a form of traumatic brain injury that is characterized by immediate neurologic dysfunction with loss of consciousness and histologic evidence of axonal damage.[1] The clinical hallmark of DAI is impairment of consciousness.

Pathophysiology

DAI is caused by acceleration/deceleration forces that result in shearing injury to axons and small blood vessels.[1] Often there is associated injury related to anoxia, penetrating brain injury, intracerebral hemorrhage, or contusion. The primary axonal injury is a mechanical axotomy predominating in the brainstem, parasagittal white matter, and corpus callosum; however, secondary metabolic and neurotoxic stresses may lead to a wider area of damage.[1,2]

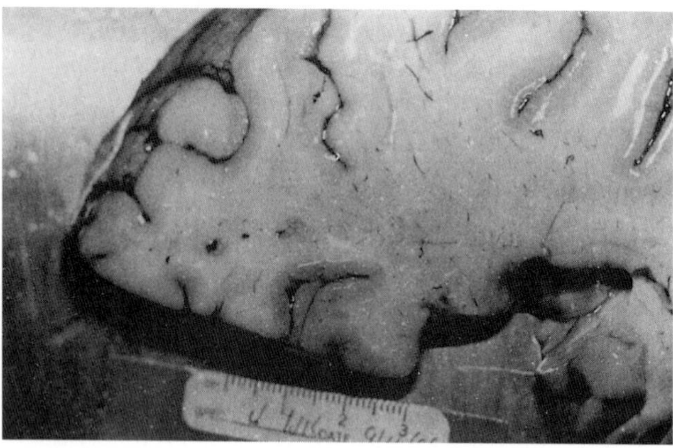

FIGURE 17–4 "Diffuse axonal injury" is a term used to describe prolonged coma occurring after head trauma that is not caused by ischemia or a mass lesion. In this autopsy specimen, small hemorrhages are seen throughout the brain and corpus callosum. (From Jones, with permission.)

Diagnosis

The diagnosis is presumptive based on clinical findings. Head computed tomography may demonstrate characteristic punctate hemorrhages but may be normal. Magnetic resonance imaging usually demonstrates acute signs of axonal shear injury.[3] Definitive pathologic confirmation is available only at autopsy.[1] In severe cases, coma may last several weeks or result in a persistent vegetative state.[1]

Clinical Complications

Death and persistent vegetative state are the most serious outcomes. Memory and cognitive impairment, balance problems, syndrome of inappropriate secretion of antidiuretic hormone (SIADH), diabetes insipidus, and hypopituitarism are also potential complications.[1]

Management

There is no specific therapy for primary axonal injury. Clinical trials with various neuroprotective agents are promising but have not yet been completed.[2] Appropriate supportive care in the emergency department should be directed at decreasing secondary injury related to hypoxia and hypotension.[2] Trauma surgery, neurosurgery, and neurology consultations usually are necessary.

REFERENCES

1. Meythaler JM, Peduzzi JD, Eleftheriou E, et al. Current concepts: diffuse axonal injury-associated traumatic brain injury. *Arch Phys Med Rehabil* 2001;82:1461–1471.
2. Bullock MR, Lyeth BG, Muizelaar JP. Current status of neuroprotection trials for traumatic brain injury: lessons from animal models and clinical studies. *Neurosurgery* 1999;45:207–217.
3. Hammoud D, Wasserman BA. Diffuse axonal injuries: pathophysiology and imaging. *Neuroimaging Clin North Am* 2002;12:205–216.

Cerebral Concussion

Dante Pappano

Clinical Presentation

Patients with cerebral concussion may appear normal or "dazed," with persistent confusion, amnesia, or overtly altered mental status.[1,2]

Pathophysiology

Concussions result from head injuries associated with acceleration or deceleration forces applied to the brain.[1] The exact mechanism of neuronal dysfunction is not clear, but mechanically induced depolarization followed by transmission abnormalities is likely.[1] Structural injury to axons and blood vessels may also occur, but this may not fully explain the brief, temporary nature of the illness.

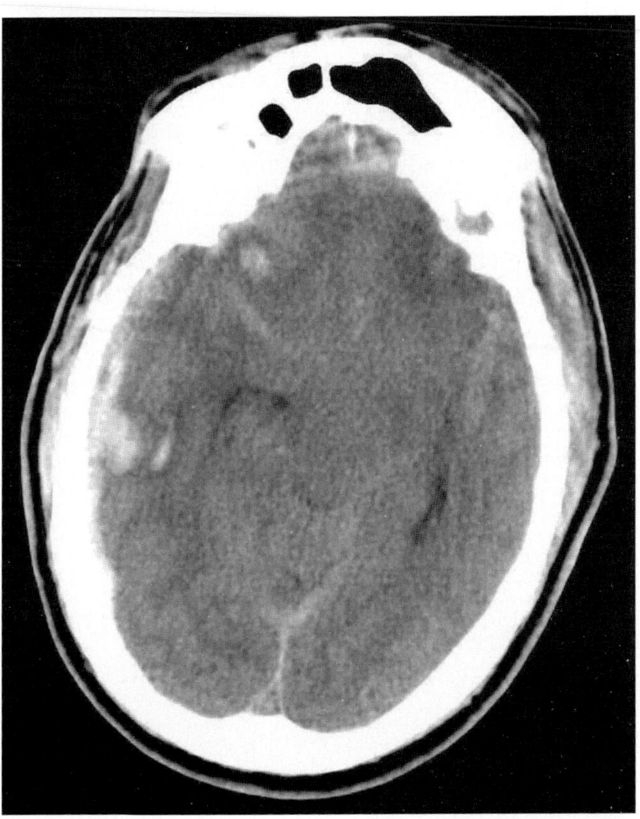

FIGURE 17–5 Computed tomogram showing evidence of intracerebral bruising. (Courtesy of Mark Silverberg, MD.)

Diagnosis

The diagnosis is made clinically, often by history alone, because there may be no physical findings. There are three grades of injury. Grade 1 concussion involves anterograde amnesia lasting less than 30 minutes, with no loss of consciousness (LOC). Grade 2 injuries involve anterograde amnesia lasting up to 24 hours or LOC lasting less than 5 minutes. Grade 3 concussion demonstrates anterograde amnesia lasting longer than 24 hours or LOC lasting longer than 5 minutes. The neurologic examination may be normal or may demonstrate impairment of memory, concentration, or balance. Focal neurologic deficits are unusual.[1,2]

Clinical Complications

Complications include intracranial bleeding, "postconcussive syndrome," seizures, or additive brain damage with multiple concussive episodes.[2]

Management

There is no specific treatment for a concussion. However, evaluation for other associated head and neck injuries is important. Additionally, if the concussion is related to sports, conservative advice regarding return to sports is necessary, because both brain and nonbrain injuries are more likely to occur when an athlete participates with less than optimal balance or concentration.[1,2]

REFERENCES

1. McCrory P, Johnston K, Mohtadi N, Meeuwisse W. Evidence-based review of sport-related concussion: basic science. *Clin J Sports Med* 2001;11:160–165.
2. Johnston K, McCrory P, Mohtadi N, Meeuwisse W. Evidence-based review of sport-related concussion: clinical science. *Clin J Sports Med* 2001;11:150–159.

Penetrating Head Injury

Michael Greenberg

Clinical Presentation

Patients with penetrating head injury (PHI) usually present with obvious penetrating injury inflicted by missiles, stab wounds, gunshots, or other penetrating objects. These injuries typically result from assaults, intentional self-harm, military- or warfare-related trauma, high-speed trauma, or industrial accidents.[1,2]

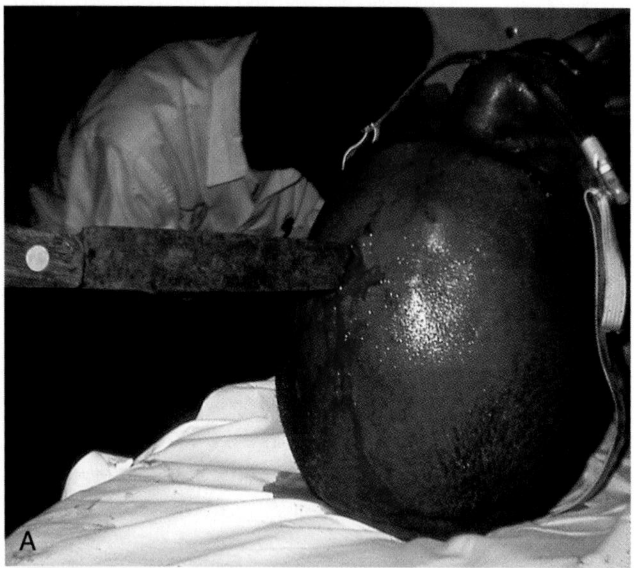

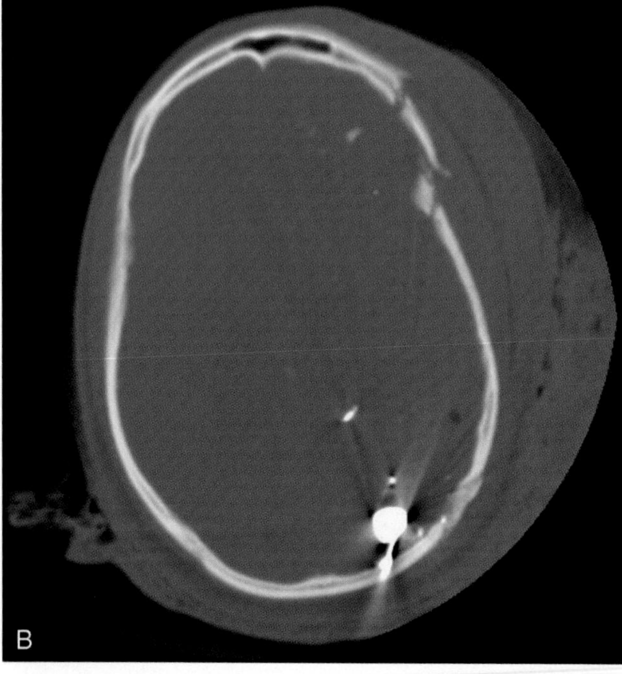

FIGURE 17–6 **A:** Stab wound to the head. (Courtesy of Michael Greenberg, MD.) **B:** Computed tomogram showing a gunshot wound to head. (Courtesy of Mark Silverberg, MD.)

Pathophysiology

The extent and nature of PHI depends on the nature and extent of the wounding mechanism.

Diagnosis

The diagnosis of PHI is based on the history and clinical examination. Various adjunctive imaging studies, including computed tomography, magnetic resonance imaging, and angiography, may be needed to define the extent of injury.

Clinical Complications

Complications range from minimal neurologic or neuropsychiatric deficits to permanent brain injury and vegetative states. Skull fractures with depression or comminution are frequent, and postinjury infection and cerebrospinal fluid leaks may also complicate any PHI.[1,2]

Management

Patients should be assessed and stabilized in accord with the principles of advanced trauma life support (ATLS). Emergency, on-site neurosurgical consultation is essential in all cases of PHI. Intravenous antibiotics and tetanus prophylaxis should be provided in all cases, while the patient is still in the emergency department.[1,2]

REFERENCES

1. Bauer M, Patzelt D. Intracranial stab injuries: case report and case study. *Forensic Sci Int* 2002;129:122–127.
2. Brain Trauma Foundation. The American Association of Neurological Surgeons. The Joint Section on Neurotrauma and Critical Care. Trauma Systems. *J Neurotrauma* 2000;17:457–462.

Le Fort Fractures

Ellen Bass

Clinical Presentation

Le Fort fractures (LFFs) are associated with substantial facial edema that may obscure the underlying facial deformities. Malocclusion is often present, with the site of premature contact of the teeth helping to pinpoint the fracture site. Additionally, patients may have numbness of the upper lip, side of the nose, or upper gingiva if the infraorbital and superior alveolar nerves are disrupted.[1] Diplopia may occasionally be present in type II or III Le Fort fractures.[2]

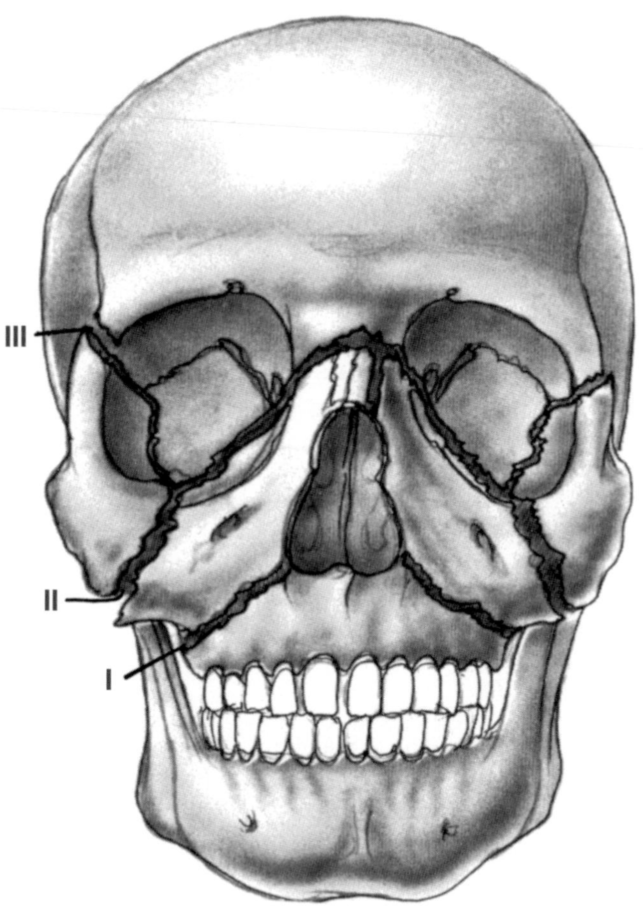

FIGURE 17–7 Le Fort fracture levels. Although these levels usually do not describe the extent or exact nature of midfacial fractures, they are still appropriately used for a general description of the injuries. (From Bailey, with permission.)

Pathophysiology

The LFFs (types I, II, and III) are a series of midface fractures named after the French army surgeon, Dr. Rene Le Fort.[2] Motor vehicle collisions, falls, and assaults are the major causes of LFFs.[1] Forceful blunt trauma to the midface is the usual mechanism of injury. A LFF type I fracture is a horizontal fracture of the maxilla above the roots of the teeth. A LFF type II fracture extends more superiorly, through the infraorbital rim and over the nasal bones. A LFF type III fracture results in a separation of the maxilla, nasoorbitoethmoid complex, and zygomas from the cranial base.[1]

Diagnosis

A mobile mandible or midface found on physical examination should raise suspicion that an LFF exists. However, facial computed tomography is the imaging modality of choice to identify these injuries.[1]

Clinical Complications

LFFs may result in severe, life-threatening hemorrhage as well as airway compromise.[1] Other associated injuries, not caused by the LFFs but often seen along with them, include cerebral contusions, intracranial hemorrhage, pulmonary infiltrates from blood aspiration, and cervical spine injuries.[1]

Management

Airway control is of paramount importance because of the amount of facial edema and bleeding.[1] All patients should receive a full trauma evaluation, and other life-threatening injuries should be investigated before the facial fractures are worked up. Consultation with an otolaryngologist or a plastic or oral surgeon is necessary, because these injuries require early operative repair with open reduction and internal fixation. Prophylactic antibiotics should be provided to cover oral and sinus-dwelling microbes.[1]

REFERENCES

1. Ellis E 3rd, Scott K. Assessment of patients with facial fractures. *Emerg Med Clin North Am* 2000;18:411–448.
2. Patterson R. The Le Fort fractures: Rene Le Fort and his work in anatomical pathology. *Can J Surg* 1991;34:183–184.

Tripod Fractures

Jason Bell and Jacob W. Ufberg

Clinical Presentation

Tripod fractures are associated with blunt-force facial trauma. Patients present with facial pain and swelling. Patients may report anesthesia over the lower eyelid, upper lip, or side of nose; pain at the injury site with opening of the jaw; or diplopia.[1]

Pathophysiology

Tripod fractures include three points of separation: a fracture of the infraorbital rim, diastasis of the zygomatic-temporal suture at the zygomatic arch, and disruption of the zygomatic-frontal suture in the lateral wall of the orbit.[1] The three fracture lines may result in a free-floating, bony fragment that resembles a tripod. The zygoma may be displaced medially, inferiorly, and posteriorly, causing a depression deformity of the lateral face. Fracture at the infraorbital foramen may transect the infraorbital nerve, producing anesthesia. The lateral canthus of the eye is attached to the zygoma, which is pulled downward as the bone is displaced inferiorly, causing vertical dystopia and diplopia. The zygoma forms the roof of the maxillary sinus; when fractured, it may tear the mucosal lining, leading to epistaxis.[2]

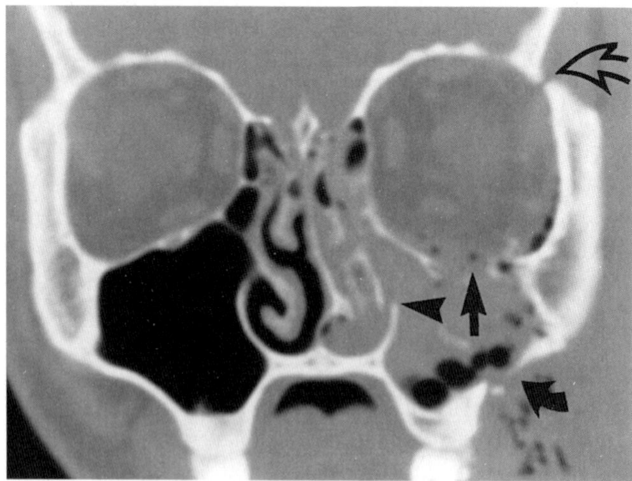

FIGURE 17–8 Comminuted, displaced fracture of the left zygomaticomaxillary complex (ZMC), as shown on coronal computed tomographic (CT) images from anterior to posterior. The CT scan shows disruption of the "friendly line" *(curved arrow),* the medial wall of the antrum *(arrowhead),* and the inferior orbital rim *(arrow),* as well as separation of the left zygomaticofrontal suture *(curved open arrow).* (From Harris and Harris, with permission.)

Diagnosis

Physical examination may reveal facial asymmetry. Other common findings include lateral subconjunctival hemorrhage, periorbital ecchymosis, vertical dystopia, and epistaxis.[2] A Water's view radiograph serves as a screening radiograph for a suspected tripod fracture, based on history and physical examination findings. Abnormalities such as interruption of the cortex and soft-tissue clouding within the maxillary sinus, representing hemorrhage, may be clues to diagnosis.[3] Patients with suspected tripod fractures should also receive axial and coronal computed tomography of the maxilla.[1]

Clinical Complications

Complications include persistent diplopia, muscle entrapment, persistent cheek anesthesia, and enophthalmos.[1-3]

Management

Patients with tripod fractures require emergency consultation and admission for surgical repair of the displaced fragments.[2]

REFERENCES

1. Ellis E 3rd, Scott K. Assessment of patients with facial fractures. *Emerg Med Clin North Am* 2000;18:411–448.
2. Hollier LH, Thornton J, Pazmino P, Stal S. The management of orbitozygomatic fractures. *Plast Reconstr Surg* 2003;111:2386–2392.
3. Keogh C, Torreggiani WC, Al-Ismail K, Munk PL. Musculoskeletal case 23: tripod fracture. *Can J Surg* 2002;45:279, 309–310.

Retrobulbar Hematoma

Ellen Bass

Clinical Presentation

Retrobulbar hematoma results from facial trauma or as a complication of orbital surgery or retrobulbar injection and usually develops within hours. However, delayed presentations up to several days have been reported.[1–3]

Pathophysiology

Retrobulbar hematoma may accompany malar, orbital floor, Le Fort II, or Le Fort III fractures and may occur after blepharoplasty.[1,2] Risk factors include perioperative and postoperative vomiting or coughing, hypertension, orbital hemangiomas, orbital scarring, coagulopathy, and the use of platelet aggregation inhibitors.[1] The major factors determining visual loss appear to be the mass effect of the retrobulbar hematoma on the optic nerve circulation and direct pressure neuropathy on the optic nerve itself.[1,2]

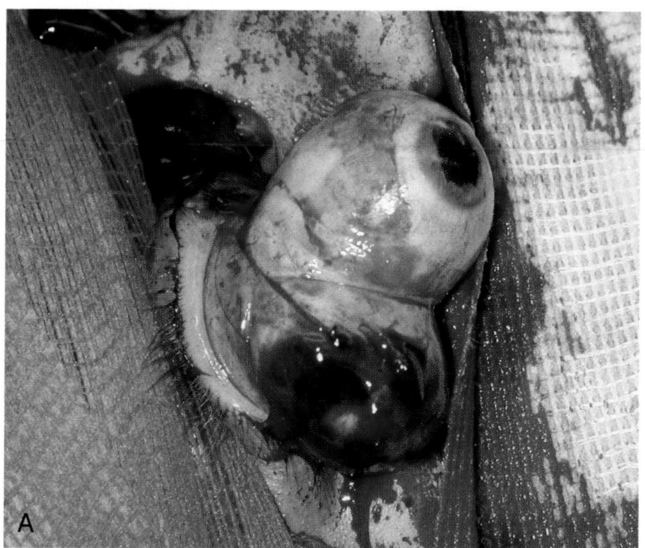

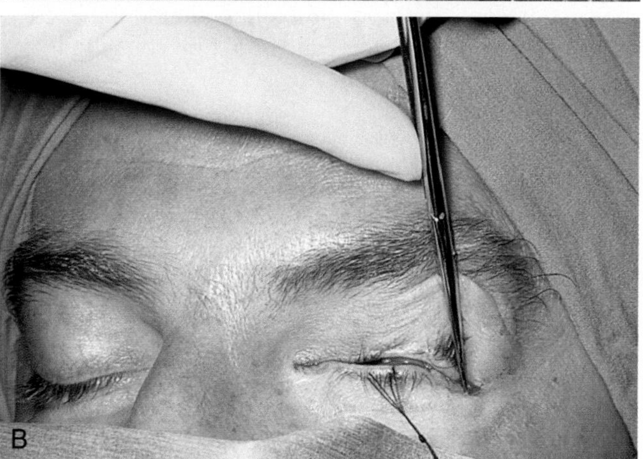

FIGURE 17–9 **A:** Gunshot wound to the head with severe proptosis due to retrobulbar hemorrhage. (Courtesy of Robert Chisolm, MD.) **B:** Lateral canthotomy. After a hemostat is placed horizontally over the lateral canthus for 1 minute, it is released, and sterile scissors are used to make a horizontal incision 1 cm toward the lateral orbital rim. (From Tasman, with permission.)

Diagnosis

Retrobulbar hematoma is diagnosed clinically and confirmed by computed tomography, ultrasonography, or magnetic resonance imaging. Early signs include painful proptosis, decreased visual acuity, and occasionally scintillating scotomas.[1,2] Late signs entail lid ecchymosis, chemosis, mydriasis, afferent pupillary defects, and ophthalmoplegia.[2,3] The funduscopic examination is often normal but may show retinal pallor.[1,2]

Clinical Complications

Permanent visual loss is the most serious complication of untreated or inadequately treated retrobulbar hematoma.[1–3]

Management

Treatment requires immediate ophthalmology consultation. In the absence of a visual deficit, medical interventions should suffice. These include ice packs, hypertension and pain control, bed rest, mannitol, acetazolamide parenteral steroids, and ocular hypotensive agents.[1,2] If visual loss is present, immediate surgical decompression by any of a variety of approaches is necessary.[1–3] In all cases, treatment should not be withheld while awaiting completion of imaging studies.[1,2]

REFERENCES

1. Wolfort FG, Vaughan TE, Wolfort SF, Nevarre DR. Retrobulbar hematoma and blepharoplasty. *Plast Reconstr Surg* 1999;104:2154–2162.
2. Ghufoor K, Sandhu G, Sutcliffe J. Delayed onset of retrobulbar haemorrhage following severe head injury: a case report and review. *Injury* 1998;29:139–141.
3. Korinth MC, Ince A, Banghard W, et al. Pterional orbita decompression in orbital hemorrhage and trauma. *J Trauma* 2002;53:73–78.

17–10

Nasal Bone Fracture

Matthew Spencer

Clinical Presentation

Patients present following trauma to the nose or face.

Pathophysiology

The nose is frequently exposed to trauma because of its central location and the fact that it protrudes from the face.[1] The nasal bones are the most commonly fractured facial bone and the third most commonly fractured bone in the body.[1] Because of the pliability of the pediatric bony architecture, children fracture their nasal bones less frequently than adults do; however, children have a higher rate of injury to the nasal septum.[2]

Diagnosis

A nasal fracture is a clinical diagnosis that can be confirmed with a plain lateral nasal radiograph of the face.[1] There may be epistaxis in addition to nasal bridge swelling, tenderness, mobility, or crepitations.[1] Patients may also have periorbital ecchymosis and swelling, and occasionally there is obvious external deviation, flattening, or broadening of the nose itself.[1] The normal average intercanthal distance is 30 to 34 mm, but this may be increased when a fracture is present.[1] Radiographs are not necessary if there is no significant deformity. The examining physician should always check for the presence of a septal hematoma, usually visible as a large purple bulge on one side of the septum. It is usually soft and easily compressed with a cotton swab, and it does not shrink after the application of vasoconstrictors.[1]

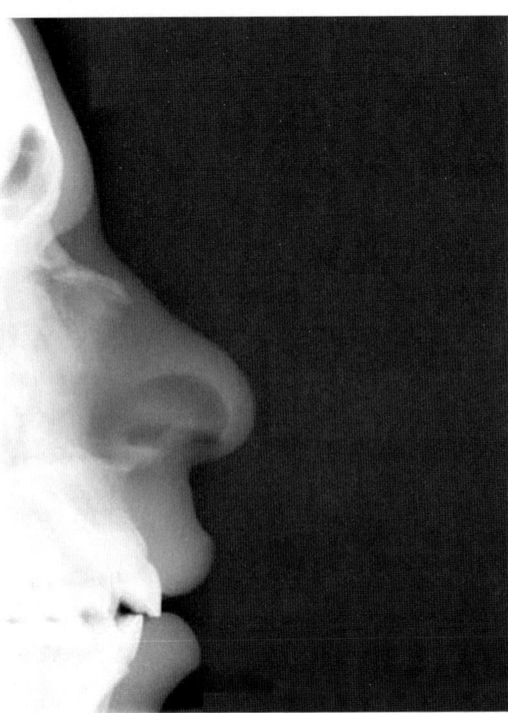

FIGURE 17–10 Minimally displaced fracture of the nasal bones. (Courtesy of Mark Silverberg, MD.)

Clinical Complications

Complications include cosmetic deformity, nasal airway obstruction, persistent epistaxis, cerebrospinal fluid rhinorrhea, and septal hematoma.[1] If left untreated, septal hematoma may lead to septal abscess formation and septal necrosis with a subsequent saddle deformity of the nose.[1]

Management

If the injury is a simple nasal fracture with minor deformity, no immediate treatment is necessary. The patient may be discharged with analgesics and told to follow-up with an otolaryngology, oral surgery, or plastic surgery specialist in 48 to 72 hours.[1] If there is a fixed nasal obstruction or severe cosmetic deformity, a subspecialty consultant should see the patient in the emergency department before discharge.[1] If cerebrospinal fluid rhinorrhea is present, empiric antibiotics should be started promptly, and a neurosurgeon should be consulted.[1]

REFERENCES

1. Ellis E 3rd, Scott K. Assessment of patients with facial fractures. *Emerg Med Clin North Am* 2000;18:411–448.
2. Koltai PJ, Rabkin D. Management of facial trauma in children. *Pediatr Clin North Am* 1996;43:1253–1275.

C1-Skull Subluxation/Dislocation

Mohamed Badawy

Clinical Presentation

Patients with subluxation/dislocation of the skull on the first cervical vertebra (C1) often have concomitant head trauma and altered mental status. Such patients should be considered to have cervical spine injury until proven otherwise. The alert patient usually complains of upper neck or occipital pain. Patients may report a broad range of neurologic deficits that may include total paralysis.

Pathophysiology

C1-skull subluxation/dislocation refers to the abnormal disruption of the occipitoatlantal articulation, which may be partial (subluxation) or complete (dislocation).[1] The occipitoatlantal junction is the transition between the cranial vault and the cervical spine. It is held together with strong ligamentous attachments. Combined hyperextension, distraction, and rotation results in either failure of the supporting ligaments or avulsion fractures of their insertions, with subsequent skull subluxation/dislocation. Children are more prone to dislocation, because of their smaller occipital condyles and the more horizontal plane of their craniocervical junction.[2]

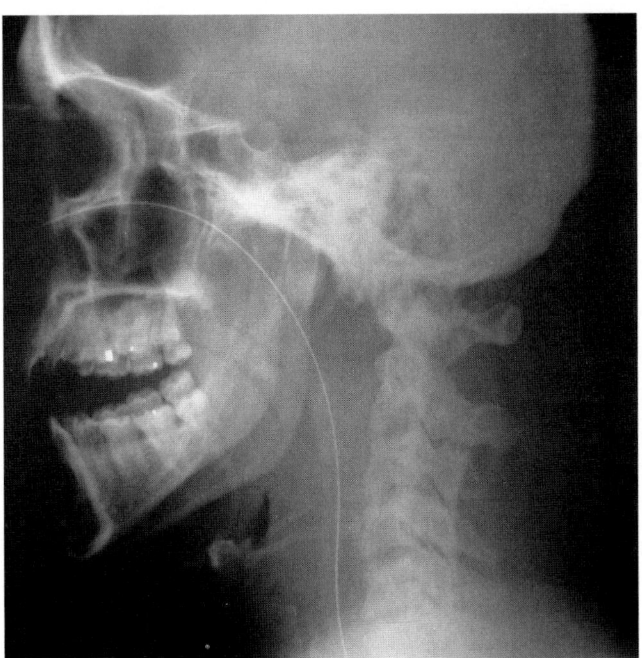

FIGURE 17–11 C1-skull subluxation/dislocation. (Courtesy of Mark Silverberg, MD.)

Diagnosis

Meticulous examination of the entire spine is necessary, with focus on the status of the deep tendon reflexes, the presence of pathologic reflexes, and cranial nerve or sensory deficits.[1] Cross-table lateral radiographs of the cervical spine should identify this injury. The "power ratio" is the ratio of the distance from the basion to the anterior edge of the posterior arch of the atlas versus the distance from the opisthion to the posterior portion of the anterior arch of the atlas.[1] This ratio is used to assess the relationship between the occiput and the atlas and should be less than 0.9.[1] A ratio of 1 or greater is considered abnormal.[1] In addition, the distance between the basion and the dens should not exceed 10 mm in children and 5 mm in adults.[1]

Clinical Complications

Victims of C1-skull subluxation/dislocation may present with fatal brainstem injuries. Survivors usually experience significant neurologic deficits of the cranial nerves, brainstem, and upper cervical spinal cord.[1,2]

Management

The treatment goals are to preserve neurologic function, reduce the subluxation/dislocation, and provide long-term spinal stability. Prehospital personnel should immobilize these patients before they are transported to the emergency department. Treatment in the hospital should focus on spinal immobilization and should involve neurosurgical or orthopedic spine consultations as quickly as possible after patient arrival. Halo vest placement and occipital cervical arthrodesis are often needed.[1]

REFERENCES

1. An HS. Cervical spine trauma. *Spine* 1998;23:2713–2729.
2. Montane I, Eismont FJ, Green BA. Traumatic occipitoatlantal dislocation. *Spine* 1991;16:112–116.

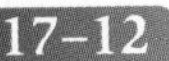

17-12

Dens Fractures

Edward Kim

Clinical Presentation

Patients with dens fractures (DFs) present after blunt trauma and hyperflexion/extension injuries, uniformly complaining of neck pain if they are awake. Patients may also report neurologic deficits such as numbness, paresthesias, or paralysis.[1]

Pathophysiology

Dens fractures account for almost 60% of all axis fractures and 10% to 18% of all cervical spine fractures.[2] They can result from acute traumatic flexion or extension. In flexion injuries, anterior displacement of the dens may occur; in extension injuries, posterior displacement is more common.[1] There are three classes of dens fractures. Type I is an avulsion of the tip of the odontoid; type II fractures obliquely traverse the body of the dens, and type III fractures extend into the body of the second cervical vertebra (C2).[1,2]

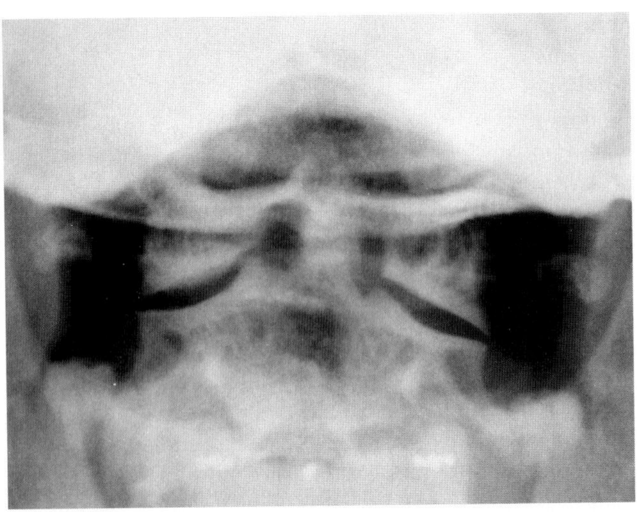

FIGURE 17–12 Type II dens fracture. (Courtesy of Mark Silverberg, MD.)

Diagnosis

The diagnosis of a dens fracture may be suspected based on the history and physical examination findings; however, conventional radiography usually is needed to confirm its presence. The open-mouth odontoid film is the favored view to diagnose most dens fractures.[1] However, helical computed tomography may be necessary if plain radiographs are inconclusive.[2]

Clinical Complications

Complications include neurologic injuries at the time of fracture and nonunion during the healing process.[1,2] Late-onset progressive myelopathy may result from nonunion.[2] Other complications include facet joint stiffness and loss of spinal alignment, both leading to cervical degenerative joint disease.[2] Skin breakdown, pin site infections, and brain abscesses are potential complications of halo vest immobilization used in the treatment of dens fractures.[2]

Management

Treatment modalities depend on the grade of the fracture. Type I dens fractures require external immobilization with a halo vest for up to 12 weeks.[1,2] Type II and III dens fractures are preferably managed nonoperatively but must be surgically corrected in cases with greater than 6 mm displacement, neurologic deficit, ventilator dependence, or nonunion after attempted nonoperative management.[2]

REFERENCES

1. An HS. Cervical spine trauma. *Spine* 1998;23:2713–2729.
2. Sasso RC. C2 dens fractures: treatment options. *J Spinal Disord* 2001;14:455–463.

Hangman's Fracture

Oren Hirsch

Clinical Presentation

Patients with hangman's fracture present with neck pain after an injury involving forced extension of the cervical spine. Inciting injuries commonly have high-energy mechanisms, such as falls, pedestrians being struck by an automobile, or high-speed motor vehicle collisions.[1] On physical examination, cervical tenderness is almost always elicited. Patients may manifest neurologic deficits, depending on the severity of vertebral displacement and the presence of other cervical spine fractures.[2]

Pathophysiology

Hangman's fracture, also known as traumatic spondylolisthesis of the axis, is a bilateral fracture of the pars interarticularis of the second cervical vertebra (C2).[1] Judicial hangings, for which this fracture is named, result in hyperextension and distraction injury.[1] However, the more common causes for this injury are motor vehicle collisions and falls, which produce the same fracture pattern through hyperextension and compression.[1] The fracture line passes through the posterior elements, more specifically between the superior and inferior articular facets of C2.[1]

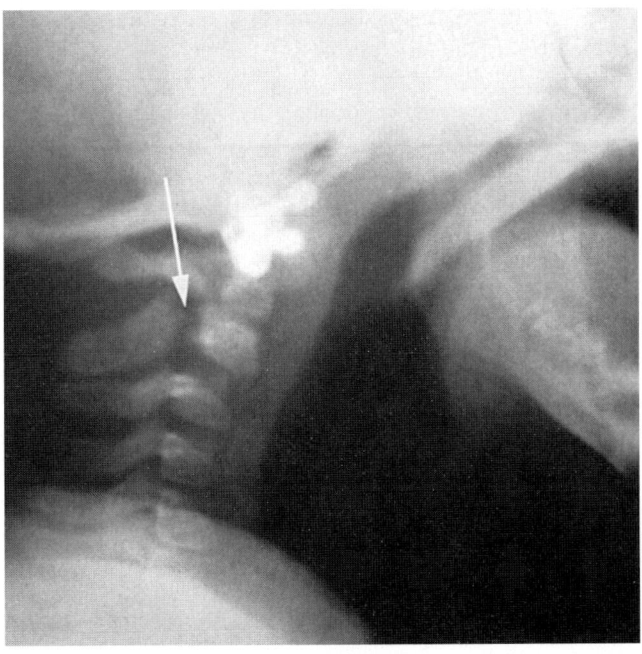

FIGURE 17–13 Hangman's fracture. A 7-week-old infant with a fracture through the posterior elements of C2 *(arrow)*. (From Sumchai A, Sternback G. Hangman's fracture in a 7-week-old infant. *Ann Emerg Med* 1991;20:87, with permission.)

Diagnosis

Plain cervical spine radiography, including lateral, anteroposterior, and odontoid views, should be obtained to confirm the diagnosis, although the lateral view is often diagnostic. Computed tomographic scanning may be helpful to delineate the precise pattern of bony injury and to visualize any possible intrusion into the spinal canal, indicating spinal cord involvement.[1,2]

Clinical Complications

Neurologic deficits secondary to concomitant intracranial injury or to spinal cord trauma may occur, particularly in cases of cervical vertebral subluxation. In addition, other cervical spine fractures may coexist and should be sought radiographically.[2]

Management

As in all patients with suspected cervical spine injuries, cervical immobilization with a rigid collar throughout the patient's emergency department course is imperative. Standard advanced trauma life support (ATLS) protocols should be followed, because hangman's fractures are often found in the setting of multisystem trauma. Individuals with hangman's fractures require emergency, on-site neurosurgical consultation. Long-term treatment includes stabilization with a rigid cervical collar or a halo immobilization device.[1] Surgical fusion usually is reserved for cases of fracture with severe angulation, disruption of the C2-C3 disk space, or failure of external immobilization to maintain fracture alignment.[1]

REFERENCES

1. Isolated fractures of the axis in adults. *Neurosurgery* 2002;50(3 Suppl):S125–S139.
2. Ryan MD, Henderson JJ. The epidemiology of fractures and fracture-dislocations of the cervical spine. *Injury* 1992;23:38–40.

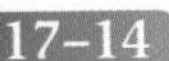
17–14

Jefferson Burst Fracture

Oren Hirsch

Clinical Presentation

Patients with Jefferson burst fractures (JBFs) present with neck pain after an injury involving axial loading of the cervical spine. Associated neurologic complaints such as focal weakness, paralysis, or paresthesias may also be present.

Pathophysiology

A JBF is a combined anterior and posterior fracture of the atlas or first cervical vertebra (C1).[1] Vertical compression forces are transmitted through the skull to the occipital condyles and onto the superior articular facets of the lateral masses of C1. The occipital condyles are downward sloping and act as a wedge to drive the ring-shaped atlas apart. Common mechanisms of injury include rollover motor vehicle collisions in which passengers are not wearing seatbelts, diving accidents, falls from height, and pedestrians being struck by motor vehicles.[1]

Diagnosis

Plain cervical spine radiography usually is adequate to confirm this diagnosis. Lateral, anteroposterior, and odontoid films should be obtained, but the open-mouth or odontoid view is the best projection to identify this fracture.[1] In the setting of a suspected or evident fracture on the plain radiograph, a computed tomographic scan is recommended to delineate the precise pattern of bony injury. Magnetic resonance imaging is currently the modality of choice for diagnosing ligamentous disruption and associated spinal instability.[2] On physical examination, cervical tenderness usually is present. Patients may manifest neurologic deficits, depending on the severity of the displacement of C1 on C2 or concomitant vertebral ligamentous injuries.[1]

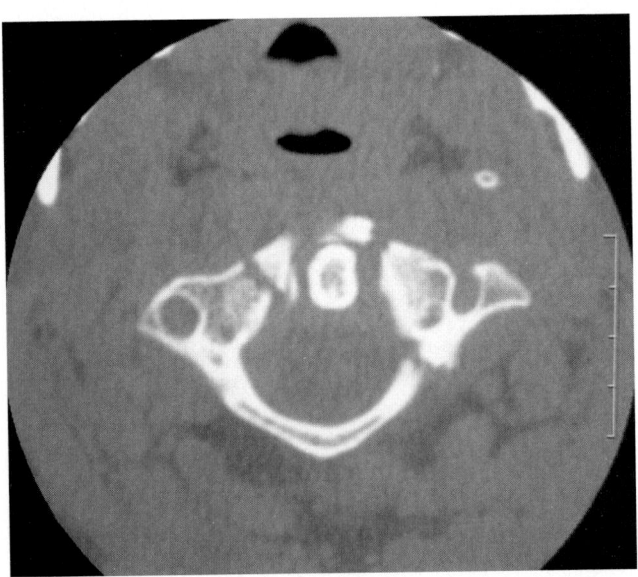

FIGURE 17–14 Computed tomogram showing vertebral "burst" fracture. (Courtesy of Mark Silverberg, MD.)

Clinical Complications

Complications include associated neurologic injuries resulting from either spinal cord trauma or concomitant intracranial injury.[2] Additional cervical spine fractures may also coexist.[2]

Management

JBFs are found in the setting of multisystem trauma. Therefore, advanced trauma life support (ATLS) protocols should be strictly followed, including cervical immobilization with a rigid collar throughout the patient's emergency department course. Individuals with JBFs require emergency neurosurgical consultation. Isolated stable Jefferson fractures should be treated with an external cervical immobilization device such as a rigid collar, suboccipital mandibular immobilizer brace, or halo ring-vest orthosis for 8 to 12 weeks. Unstable fractures with evidence of transverse atlantal ligamentous disruption should have either rigid immobilization alone with halo orthosis or surgical stabilization with vertebral fusion.[1]

REFERENCES

1. Isolated fractures of the atlas in adults. *Neurosurgery* 2002;50(3 Suppl):S120–S124.
2. Hadley MN, Dickman CA, Browner CM, Sonntag VK. Acute traumatic atlas fractures: management and long term outcome. *Neurosurgery* 1988;23:31–35.

Flexion Teardrop Fracture

Ian deSouza

Clinical Presentation

Patients with flexion teardrop fractures present after trauma with localized or generalized neck pain, paresthesia, paresis, or paralysis.[1]

Pathophysiology

A flexion teardrop fracture is a triangular fracture fragment at the anteroinferior corner of a cervical vertebral body.[1] Flexion teardrop fractures result from forceful hyperflexion and compression applied to the anterior cervical spine when the flexed head strikes an object.[2] In addition to the characteristic anteroinferior fracture, disruption of the anterior longitudinal ligament and intervertebral disk may occur. Equal and opposite posterior forces may lead to disruption of the posterior longitudinal ligament and facet joints. Posterior displacement of the vertebral body may result in compression of the anterior columns of the spinal cord and may be associated with substantial neurologic deficits.[2]

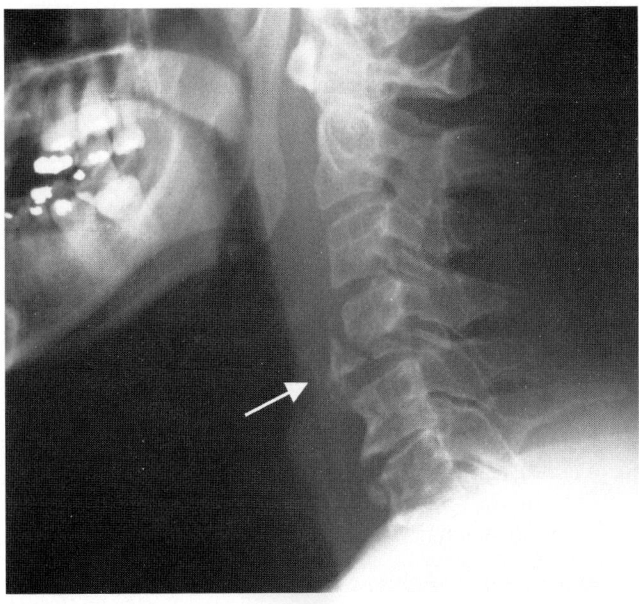

FIGURE 17–15 Anterior-inferior flexion fracture of the fourth cervical vertebra (C4). (Courtesy of Mark Silverberg, MD.)

Diagnosis

The flexion teardrop fracture usually is obvious on plain radiographs, which demonstrate the anteroinferior "teardrop" fragment, posterior displacement of the vertebral body into the spinal canal, bilateral subluxation or dislocation of the facet joints, and widening or "fanning" of the interspinous spaces.[1] Computed tomography or magnetic resonance imaging may be needed to fully define and delineate any ligamentous or spinal cord injury.[1] Physical examination may reveal tenderness on palpation of the midline of the cervical spine, as well as findings consistent with the anterior cervical cord syndrome (ACS). The ACS involves complete quadriplegia with loss of pain, temperature, and some touch sensation combined with preservation of the posterior column functions, which include position, motion, and vibratory sense.[3]

Clinical Complications

A flexion teardrop fracture often results in permanent neurologic deficits, including quadriplegia corresponding to the level of spinal injury. Death from diaphragm paralysis is possible if the injury is located high enough.[1–3]

Management

Because a flexion teardrop fracture is considered to be severely unstable, strict cervical spine immobilization is paramount.[1–3] Emergency consultation with a neurosurgeon or orthopedic surgeon for spinal cord decompression, external immobilization, and eventual spinal fusion should be initiated as quickly as possible.[2] The use of steroids in any case of spinal trauma should be considered but remains controversial.[2]

REFERENCES

1. Kim KS, Chen HH, Russel EJ, Rogers LF. Flexion teardrop fracture of the cervical spine: radiographic characteristics. *AJR Am J Roentgenol* 1989;152:319–326.
2. Petrie JG. Flexion injuries of the cervical spine. *J Bone Joint Surg Am* 1964;46;:1800–1806.
3. Schneider RC. The syndrome of acute anterior spinal cord injury. *J Neurosurg* 1955;12:95–122.

Extension Teardrop Fracture

Mohamed Badawy

Clinical Presentation

The extension teardrop fracture usually occurs in adults 40 to 70 years of age and only rarely in children.[1] If awake and alert, patients usually complain of localized neck pain and tenderness. They may present with any type of spinal cord injury, although central cord syndrome (CCS) is the most common. CCS is characterized by weakness in the arms greater than in the legs, bladder dysfunction, and varying degrees of sensory loss below the level of the lesion.[2]

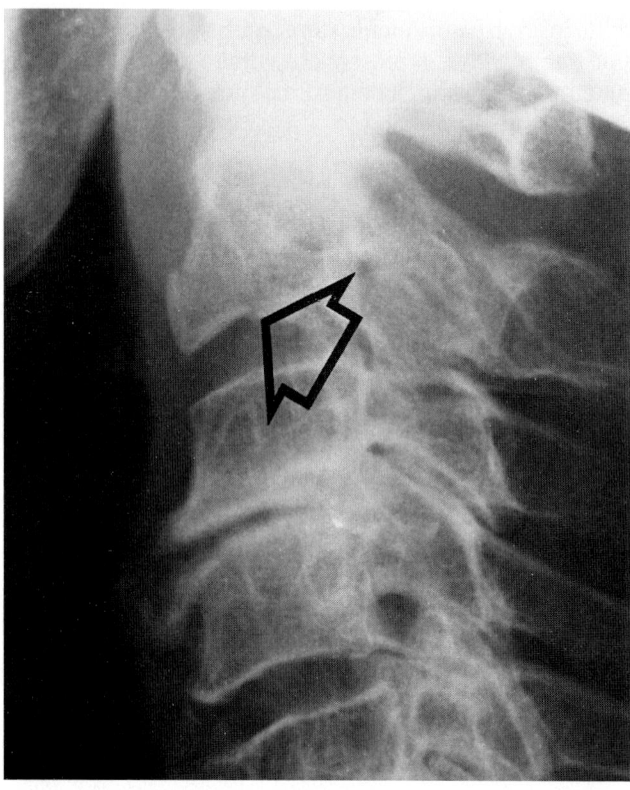

FIGURE 17–16 Extension teardrop fracture. The radiographic appearance of the classic extension teardrop fracture is an equilateral triangular avulsion fragment *(open arrow)* comprising the anteroinferior corner of the axis body. In elderly patients with osteoporosis, this fracture is associated with little or no prevertebral soft tissue swelling. (From Harris and Harris, with permission.)

Pathophysiology

An extension teardrop fracture is characterized by avulsion of the inferior portion of the anterior part of a cervical vertebral body.[1] This injury may result from a fall from heights or from high-speed trauma (e.g., motor vehicle crash). The mechanism is usually severe hyperextension of the neck. This mechanism applies tractional forces on the anterior longitudinal ligament at its insertion in the vertebral body.[1] The anterior longitudinal ligament avulses the inferior corner of the vertebral body, resulting in this characteristic fracture pattern.[1]

Diagnosis

The avulsed anteroinferior portion of the vertebral body usually is visible on the lateral view of a standard cervical spine series. However, magnetic resonance imaging may provide more information by revealing associated spinal cord and other soft-tissue injuries.[1]

Clinical Complications

An extension teardrop fracture is stable when the head is in flexion but becomes unstable as the neck is extended. This may lead to transient or persistent neurologic deficits.[1] High cervical-spine injuries may lead to death from diaphragm paralysis.

Management

Prehospital personnel should immobilize all patients with possible cervical spine injury before they are transported to the emergency department. As with all major traumatic injuries, the advanced trauma life support (ATLS) protocols should be followed. Because these neck injuries are potentially unstable, particular attention should be paid to cervical immobilization. Consultation should be sought on an emergency basis from a neurosurgery or orthopedics specialist. The use of steroids in trauma patients with neurologic deficits remains controversial.[1,2]

REFERENCES

1. Kiwerski J. Hyperextension-dislocation injuries of the cervical spine. *Injury* 1993;24:674–677.
2. Shneider RC, Thompson JM, Rebin J. The syndrome of acute central cervical spinal cord injury. *J Neurol Neurosurg Psychiatry* 1958;21:216–227.

Clay Shoveler's Fracture

Ian deSouza

Clinical Presentation

Patients with clay shoveler's fracture present with sudden onset of pain in the lower neck or between the shoulder blades that began while shoveling or lifting a heavy object.

Pathophysiology

Clay shoveler's fracture involves an avulsion of the distal portion of one or more spinous processes of the lower cervical or upper thoracic vertebrae.[1,2] The clay shoveler's fracture was named after a frequent occupational injury among untrained workers who used long-handled shovels to toss soil 10 to 15 feet while draining swampy areas in Australia.[1] Although its incidence has decreased since the advent of modern machinery, cases still occasionally arise from direct trauma in motor vehicle collisions and during sports.[1] Such fractures have also been reported to occur after simple activities such as returning a barbell to its rack after heavy lifting.[2] Fibers of the trapezius and rhomboid muscles originating from the posterior portion of the spinous processes in the lower neck vertebrae insert on the acromion, clavicle, and scapula and work to draw the scapula superomedially toward the spine. An avulsion fracture occurs when there is a sudden force on these muscles during forceful neck flexion or lifting by the arms.[1]

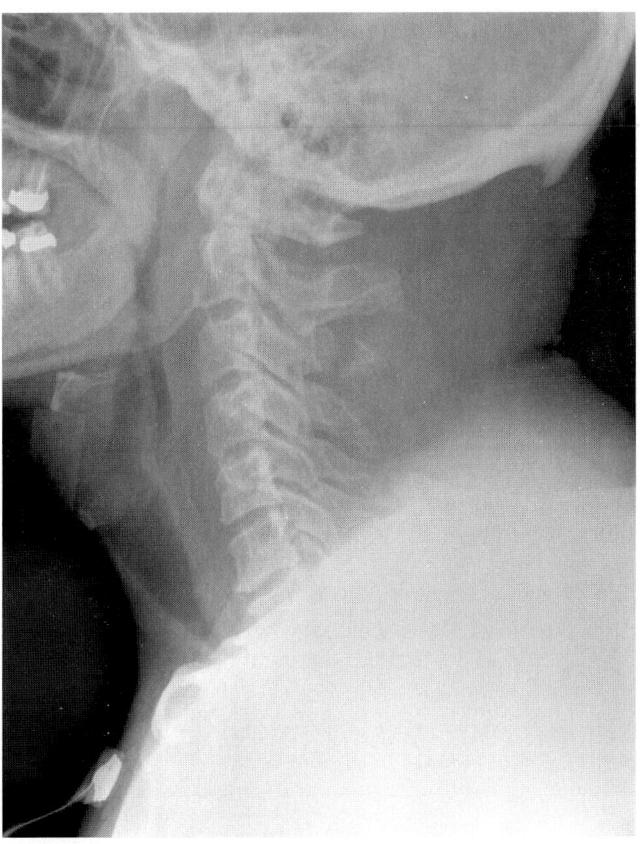

FIGURE 17–17 Second and third cervical vertebrae (C2 and C3) fractures. (Courtesy of Robert Hendrickson, MD.)

Diagnosis

The clay shoveler's fracture may be suspected based on the history and physical examination, but it is diagnosed on plain radiographs of the cervical or upper thoracic spine.[1] The anteroposterior view may reveal a "double shadow" of the spinous process, because the avulsed fragment is displaced inferiorly. Physical examination reveals tenderness to palpation of the affected spinous process, with overlying edema in some cases.[1]

Clinical Complications

Complications from these fractures are extremely rare but, when present, usually involve disability due to chronic pain or nonunion of the fracture fragments.[2]

Management

The management is conservative, because these fractures are considered to be stable. Analgesics, muscle relaxants, and referral to an orthopedist or neurosurgeon usually is all that is necessary.[1,2]

REFERENCES

1. Hakkal HG. Clay shoveler's fracture. *Am Fam Physician* 1973;81: 104–106.
2. Herrick RT. Clay-shoveler's fracture in power-lifting: a case report. *Am J Sports Med* 1981;9:29–30.

Penetrating Neck Trauma

Melissa A. Eirich

Clinical Presentation

Patients with penetrating neck trauma may present with partial or complete airway obstruction due to bleeding and edema. Because of the location of major vessels, significant bleeding may be seen. Injuries to the spinal cord, cranial nerves, brachial plexus, lung, and esophagus may also occur.[1-3]

Pathophysiology

Injuries to the anterior neck can be divided into three zones. Zone 1 injuries are located below the level of the cricoid cartilage. Zone III is above the angles of the mandible, and zone II is between zones I and III.[1]

Diagnosis

Laryngeal injuries may be apparent on physical examination, but computed tomography and bronchoscopy may be necessary to diagnose them. Suspicion of vascular injury necessitates angiography. Cervical spine radiographs should be obtained if a fracture cannot be ruled out clinically.[1-3]

Clinical Complications

Complications include laryngeal injuries, esophageal perforation, exsanguination, carotid dissection, pneumothorax, and central and peripheral neurologic deficits.[1-3]

Management

Advanced trauma life support (ATLS) protocols should be followed, but penetrating neck trauma requires special attention to airway evaluation. Zone I injuries are managed in the same manner as those caused by penetrating thoracic trauma. Zone II injuries that are symptomatic require surgical exploration with angiography. Treatment of asymptomatic zone II injuries is controversial; many surgeons explore these as well. If the wound is left unexplored and penetrated the platysma, these patients should undergo an angiogram to evaluate the neck vasculature, in addition to a bronchoscopy and esophagoscopy to evaluate the upper respiratory and gastrointestinal structures. Recent studies have shown that clinical examination alone misses only 1% of vascular injuries.[2] Zone III injuries may include vascular injury, and angiography is recommended.[3]

REFERENCES

1. Peralta R, Hurford WE. Airway trauma. *Int Anesthesiol Clin* 2000; 38:111–127.
2. Sekharan J, Dennis JW, Veldenz HC, et al. Continued experience with physical examination alone for evaluation and management of penetrating zone two neck injuries: results of 145 cases. *J Vasc Surg* 2000;32:483–489.
3. Eddy VA. Is routine arteriography mandatory for penetrating injury to zone 1 of the neck? *J Trauma* 2000;48:208–214.

Penetrating Neck Trauma

Melissa A. Eirich

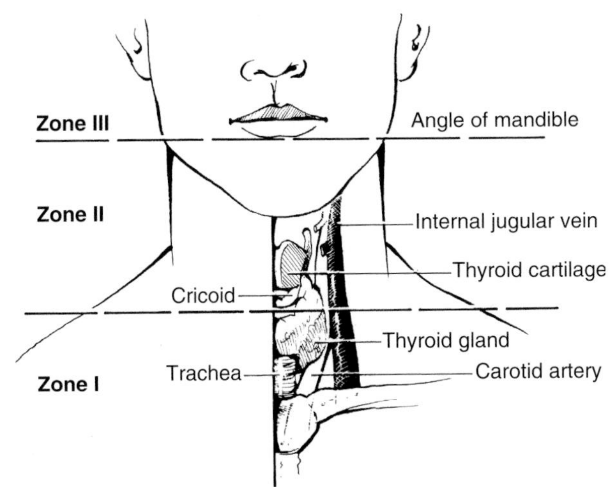

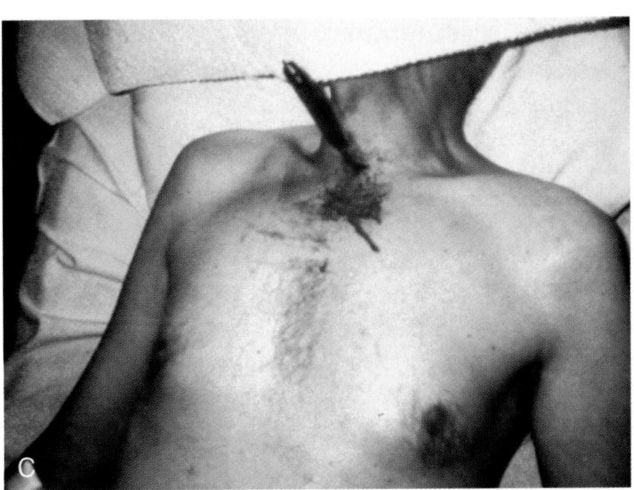

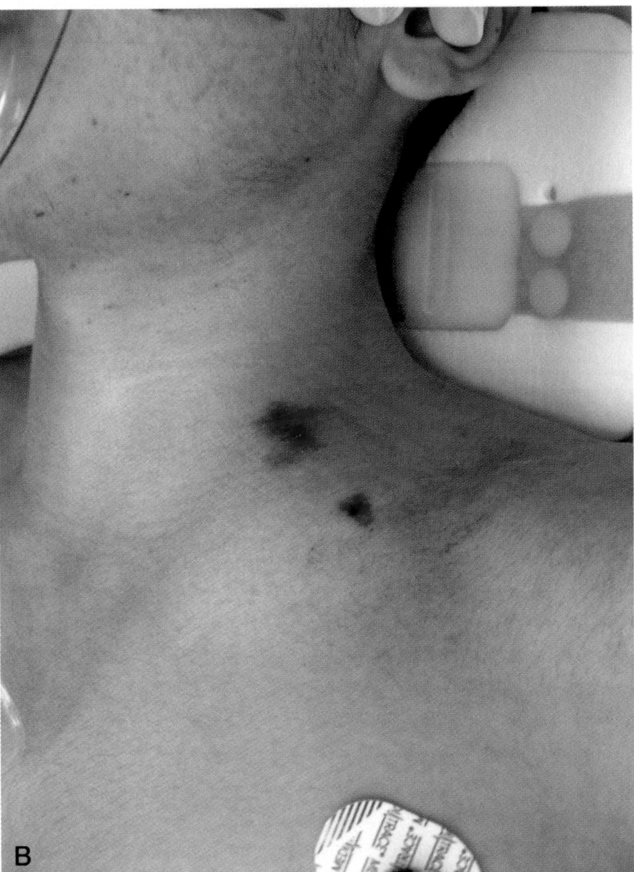

FIGURE 17–18 **A:** Anterior view of the neck. Significant structures and the zones of the neck are illustrated. (From Harwood-Nuss, with permission.) **B:** Gunshot wound in zone 1 of neck. (Courtesy of Mark Silverberg, MD.) **C:** Stab wound in zone 1 of neck. (Courtesy of Lewis J. Kaplan, MD.)

Cervical Spine Subluxation

Madelyn Garcia

Clinical Presentation

Patients with cervical spine subluxation present after a flexion injury to the neck. Common mechanisms include unrestrained motor vehicle crashes and diving accidents.

Pathophysiology

Subluxation results from an anterior flexion pattern of injury, which accounts for approximately two thirds of all neck injuries.[1] During extreme flexion, the posterior stabilizing ligaments are ruptured, and subluxation occurs with dislocation of the affected vertebrae anteriorly. In one series, subluxation without bony fracture accounted for 0.2% of cervical spine injuries.[2] Most subluxation injuries are seen in young, athletic patients, but they may certainly occur in any age group.

Diagnosis

Signs and symptoms may be nonspecific and include pain, limitation of neck movement, and muscle spasm. Pain may be referred to the neck, scapula, shoulders, or upper arms and is often accompanied by finger paresthesias or numbness.[1] In severe dislocations, the spinal cord can be injured, and patients often suffer transient neurologic symptoms that resolve before arrival at the emergency department. Definitive diagnosis is usually made on plain, three-view cervical spine series. Radiographic signs include localized kyphotic angulation of the cervical spine with or without anterior displacement (usually 1 to 3 mm) of the subluxed vertebra, altered configuration of interfaced joints, and "fanning" or widening of the spinous processes.[3] Translations of greater than 3.5 mm and angulations of greater than 11 degrees are considered unstable. Subluxation must be distinguished from the "reversal of cervical lordosis" that is seen with muscle spasm. In subluxation, the kyphosis occurs at injured levels only, whereas in muscle spasm, it is diffuse. If there is any question on plain radiographic films, computed tomography or magnetic resonance imaging should be obtained to confirm the diagnosis.[2]

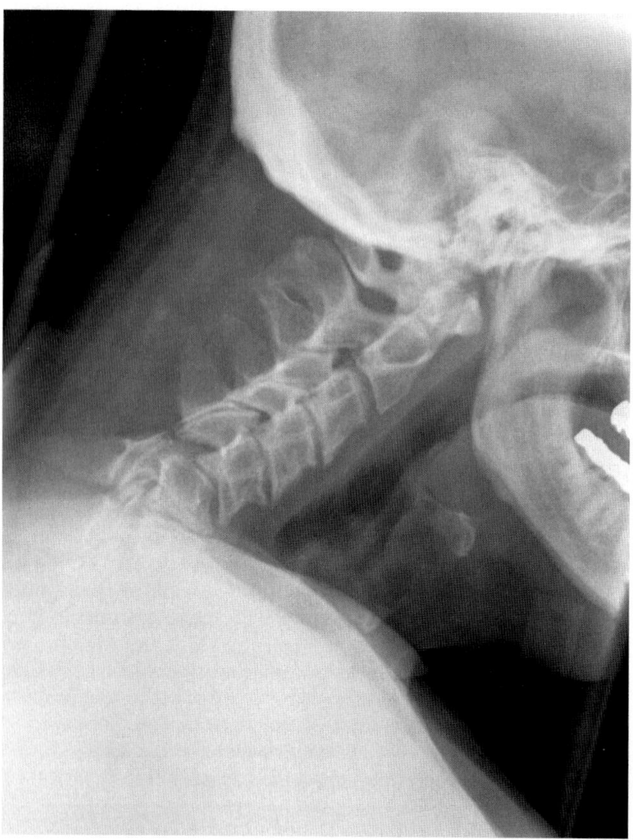

FIGURE 17–19 Subluxation of the fifth cervical vertebra (C5) on C6 with splaying of spinous processes. (Courtesy of Robert Hendrickson, MD.)

Clinical Complications

Delayed cervical spine instability resulting from incomplete ligamentous healing is the most significant complication and may lead to future spinal cord injury and disability.[3] Even with appropriate therapy, instability occurs in 20% to 50% of cases.[3]

Management

Careful spinal immobilization and orthopedic or neurosurgical consultation are essential. Most patients are treated with a cervical collar or brace for a minimum of 3 months to allow ligamentous healing, after which persistent symptoms may warrant cervical fusion or bone grafting.[1]

REFERENCES

1. Demetriades D, Charalambides K, Chahwan S, et al. Nonskeletal cervical spine injuries: epidemiology and diagnostic pitfalls. *J Trauma* 2000;48:724–727.
2. An HS. Cervical spine trauma. *Spine* 1998;23:2713–2729.
3. Green JD, Harle TS, Harris JH Jr. Anterior subluxation of the cervical spine: hyperflexion sprain. *AJNR Am J Neuroradiol* 1981;2:243–250.

Cervical Vertebral Compression Wedge Fracture

Mohamed Badawy

Clinical Presentation

Patients with wedge compression fractures usually present after head or neck trauma with localized tenderness over the injured vertebra.

Pathophysiology

A wedge compression fracture usually develops when a mild compressive force is combined with neck hyperflexion. The stability of these injuries depends on the integrity of the posterior longitudinal ligament complex. If the flexion force is more dominant than the compressive force, the posterior longitudinal complex may be disrupted with subsequent instability.[1]

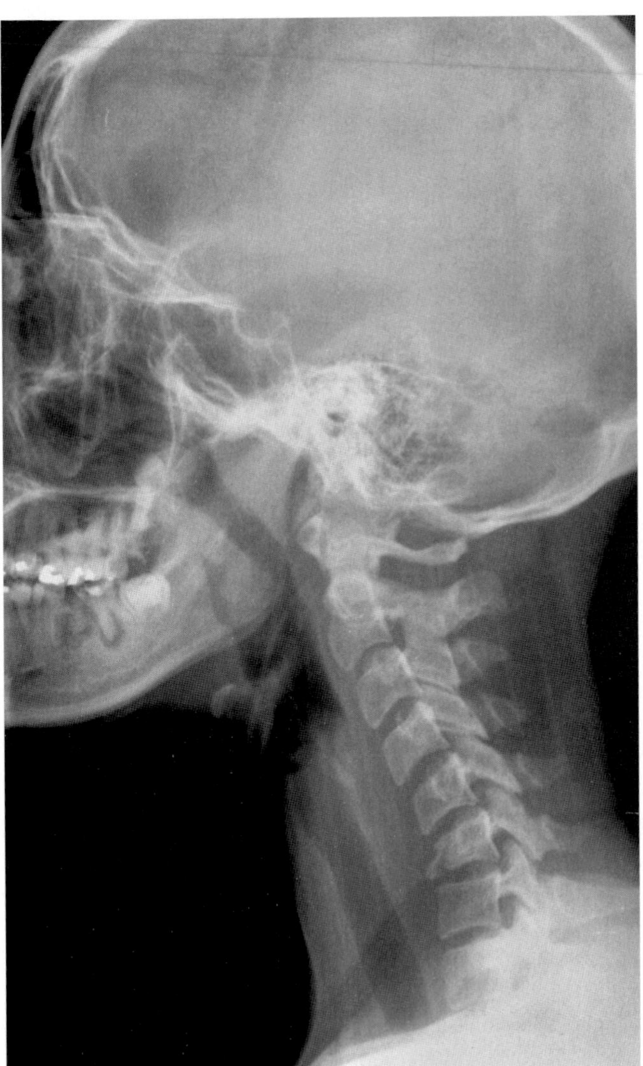

FIGURE 17–20 Sixth cervical (C6) vertebral compression fracture. (Courtesy of Robert Hendrickson, MD.)

Diagnosis

Because this fracture tends to be stable, the neurologic examination is usually normal and nonfocal.[1] A cross-table lateral radiograph of the cervical, thoracic, or lumbar regions (as required) usually identifies this injury. Buckling and loss of height of the anterior vertebral body cortex or disruption of the superior end-plate (or both) are indicative of this injury. With flexion forces of greater magnitude, the anterosuperior portion of the vertebral body may produce a separate fracture fragment.[1] Prevertebral soft-tissue swelling, if present, usually is minimal and localized to the area of the involved segment. In the anteroposterior view, the involved vertebra may be normal or may reveal decreased vertical height. The absence of a vertical fracture of the vertebral body helps to distinguish the simple wedge fracture from the vertical compression fracture caused by axial loading.[1,2]

Clinical Complications

Complications of this injury are rare because of the fracture's stability. However, if the posterior longitudinal ligament complex is disrupted, autonomic and neurologic deficits may be present.[1]

Management

As with all major traumatic injuries, advanced trauma life support (ATLS) protocols should be followed. Once the airway, breathing, and circulation have been evaluated and stabilized, the focus can be turned to the cervical spine. Treatment goals are to preserve neurologic function and to provide long-term spinal stability. In the emergency department, spinal stabilization should be maintained with a cervical collar. Consultation with a spine specialist should be obtained to coordinate further care and the need for long-term spinal immobilization.[2]

REFERENCES

1. Babcock JL. Cervical spine injuries: diagnosis and classification. *Arch Surg* 1976;111:646–651.
2. An HS. Cervical spine trauma. *Spine* 1998;23:2713–2729.

Spinal Cord Compression

Louisette Vega and Jacob Ufberg

Clinical Presentation

Pain, either localized or radicular, is the most common complaint of patients with spinal cord compression (SCC), and it usually precedes neurologic findings. Late neurologic findings, such as bladder dysfunction and ataxia, indicate a poor prognosis.[1-3] SCC should be suspected if a patient presents with back pain and a history of any of the following: (1) malignancy, (2) intravenous drug abuse, and (3) any neurologic complaint, especially bowel or bladder dysfunction.[1,2]

Pathophysiology

SCC may occur when a collection of blood, pus, or tumor tissue enters and compromises the epidural space, impinging on the spinal cord. SCC may result from external compression due to spinal stenosis, disk herniation, or vertebral fracture.

Diagnosis

The gold standard for the diagnosis of SCC has traditionally been myelography. Plain radiographs may be used to identify metastatic lesions, but they are not useful in identifying the degree of cord compromise. Computed tomographic scanning may identify bony metastases but does not clearly show the epidural space. Magnetic resonance imaging is very effective in visualizing space-occupying lesions, as well as the extent of compression, and therefore is the imaging study of choice for patients with suspected SCC.[1-3]

Clinical Complications

Complications of SCC include permanent neurologic impairment, permanent bladder and bowel dysfunction, and, in some cases, death.

Management

SCC is a bona fide emergency and must be treated as such to prevent permanent neurologic injury. Steroids may be used to reduce edema in and around the cord; however, emergency administration of radiation to reduce tumor size and consequent pressure on the cord plays an essential role in the treatment of SCC. SCC is one of only a few instances in which emergency consultation with a radiation therapist is required. Antibiotics should be started immediately for patients with infection, and neurosurgical consultation must be obtained immediately in all cases of suspected SCC.[1-3]

REFERENCES

1. Arce D, Sass P, Abul-Khoudoud H. Recognizing spinal cord emergencies. *Am Fam Physician* 2001;64:631–638.
2. Bach F, Larsen BH, Rohde K, et al. Metastatic spinal cord compression: occurrence, symptoms, clinical presentations and prognosis in 398 patients with spinal cord compression. *Acta Neurochir (Wien)* 1990;107:37–43.
3. Heimdal K, Hirschberg H, Slettebo H, et al. High incidence of serious side effects of high-dose dexamethasone treatment in patients with epidural spinal cord compression. *J Neurooncol* 1992;12:141–144.

Spinal Cord Compression

Louisette Vega and Jacob Ufberg

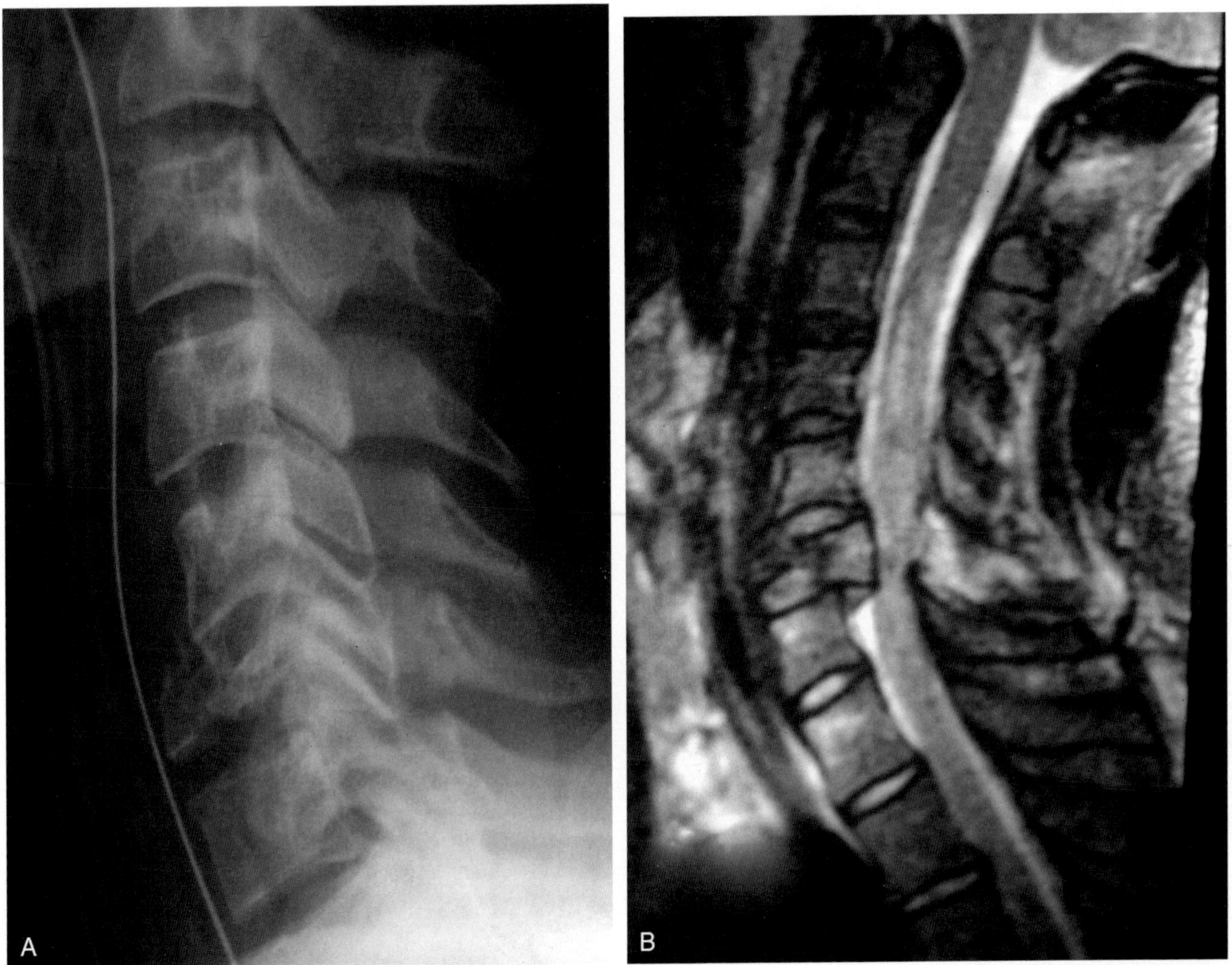

FIGURE 17–21 Spinal cord compression (SCC). **A:** A lateral plain roentgenograph revealing a stage IV flexion compression injury involving the C6 vertebral body. **B:** The magnetic resonance imaging scan reveals significant spinal cord compression (SCC) behind the retrolisthesed C5 vertebral level with evidence of spinal cord swelling superiorly up to the C3 vertebral level. (**A** and **B,** From Bucholz, with permission.)

Vertebral Compression Fractures

Louisette Vega and Jacob Ufberg

Clinical Presentation

Patients with vertebral compression fractures (VCFs) may present asymptomatically, with mild to severe back pain, or with a noticeable reduction in height.

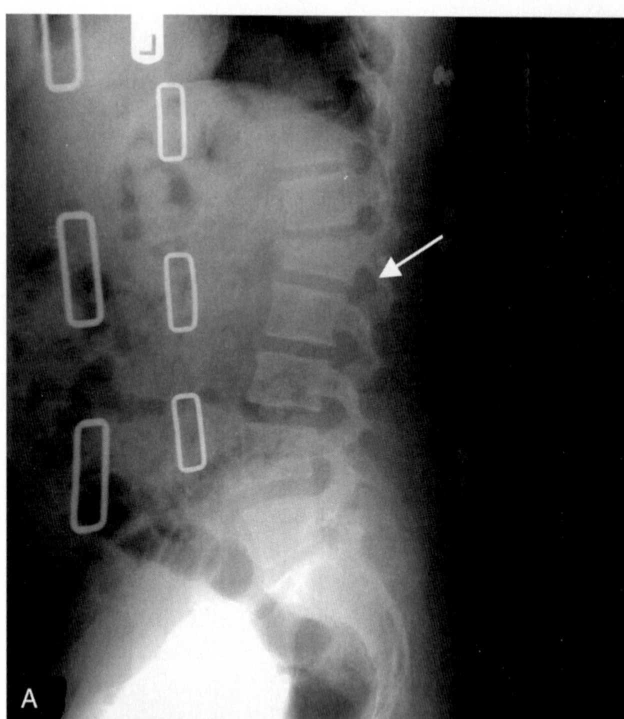

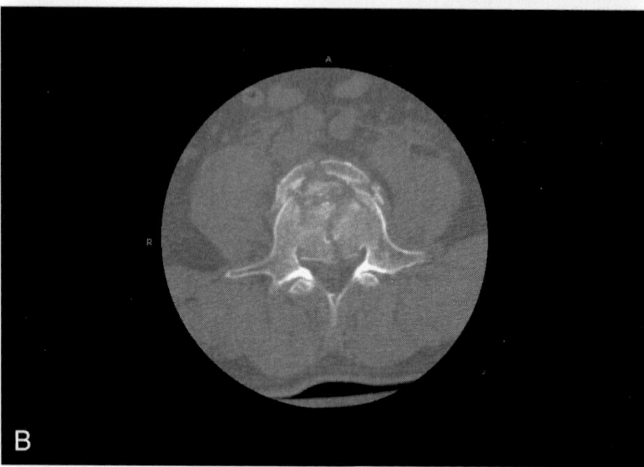

FIGURE 17–22 **A:** Compression fracture of the second lumbar vertebra (L2). (Courtesy of Mark Silverberg, MD.) **B:** Computed tomogram of L4 compression fracture. (Courtesy of Tim Lum, MD.)

Pathophysiology

Risk factors for VCF include osteoporosis and metastatic lesions to the spine. Aging Caucasian females are at risk of VCF from development of osteoporosis.[1] The most common site of injury is the thoracolumbar spine. Compression fractures may occur secondary to trauma, but occur spontaneously in up to 50% of patients.[2]

Diagnosis

The diagnosis may be suggested by the history and physical examination, but imaging confirmation is required. Magnetic resonance imaging may be used to determine the severity of the fracture and to assess the stability of the vertebral column.[1,2]

Clinical Complications

Complications include respiratory problems, autonomic neurologic dysfunction, loss of height, and psychosocial stress due to lifestyle alterations.[1,2]

Management

Traditional treatment of compression fractures includes rest, antiinflammatory agents, and analgesics. Admission to the hospital may be necessary to obtain adequate pain control. Surgical intervention usually is reserved for cases of neurologic dysfunction or refractory pain.[1,2]

REFERENCES

1. World Health Organization. Assessment of fracture risk and its application to screening for postmenopausal osteoporosis: report of a WHO Study Group. *World Health Organ Tech Rep Ser* 1994;843:1–129.
2. Myers ER, Wilson SE. Biomechanics of osteoporosis and vertebral fracture. *Spine* 1997;22:25S–31S.

Spinal Cord Injury Without Radiographic Abnormality

Mohamed Badawy

Clinical Presentation

Spinal cord injury without radiographic abnormality, known as SCIWORA, may be associated with a spectrum of clinical presentations, ranging from tingling or numbness in the extremities to substantial neurologic deficits that may include paraplegia. It is important to inquire about the mechanism of injury in addition to the presence or absence of any transient neurologic deficits after any trauma.[1,2]

Pathophysiology

The term SCIWORA was introduced by Pang and Wilberger in 1982.[1] Since then, there have been several published cases, most involving children.[1] A recent report found that SCIWORA is an uncommon disorder and, in that series, occurred only in adults.[2] Several mechanisms have been postulated to explain the development of SCIWORA, including hyperextension with inward bulging of interlaminar ligaments, reversible disk prolapse, flexion compression of the cord, and longitudinal cord traction.[1] Data suggests that spinal stenosis and intervertebral disk disease may play an important role in the development of these injuries.[2]

TABLE 17–23 Spinal Cord Injury Without Radiographic Abnormality (SCIWORA)

Approximately two thirds of cord injuries in children have no radiographic abnormalities.

SCIWORA is usually seen in children younger than 8 years of age.

Children with a history of neck injury with transient neurologic symptoms should be hospitalized.

Neurosurgical consultation is mandatory for all patients with suspected SCIWORA.

Courtesy of Michael Greenberg, MD.

Diagnosis

SCIWORA should be considered in all trauma patients with neurologic deficits (transient or persistent) or a significant mechanism of injury who are complaining of neck pain but have normal cervical spine radiographs.[1] These individuals must be further evaluated by magnetic resonance imaging to rule out soft-tissue injury.[2]

Clinical Complications

Complications of SCIWORA vary widely, ranging from transient tingling to total paralysis and even death.[1]

Management

As with all major traumatic injuries, advanced trauma life support (ATLS) protocols should be followed when assessing patients. Once airway, breathing, and circulation have been evaluated and stabilized, attention can be turned to the cervical spine. Because these neck injuries are potentially unstable, particular attention should be paid to immediate cervical immobilization, preferably in the field. However, if that has not been attended to, immobilization should be initiated immediately on presentation to the emergency department. Emergency consultation should be sought with neurosurgery and/or orthopedic specialists to provide definitive care (see Table 17–23). The use of steroids in trauma patients with neurologic deficits remains controversial.[1,2]

REFERENCES

1. Pang D, Wilberger JE Jr. Spinal cord injury without radiographic abnormalities in children. *J Neurosurg* 1982;57:114–129.
2. Hendey GW, Wolfson AB, Mower WR, Hoffman JR. Spinal cord injury without radiographic abnormality: results of the National Emergency X-Radiography Utilization Study in blunt cervical trauma. *J Trauma* 2002;53:1-4.

Blunt Chest Trauma

Bryan Gargano

Clinical Presentation

Most patients with blunt chest trauma present with chest pain or bruising after being assaulted or being involved in a motor vehicle accident. Tachycardia and tachypnea are common findings, often secondary to pain, anxiety, hypotension, or hypoxia.[1–3]

Pathophysiology

The chest is the third most likely part of the body to be injured in trauma, after the head and extremities.[2] Chest wall injuries occur in 70% of thoracic traumas, whereas in 12% of cases, organs are injured without skeletal disruption.[2] There are two primary mechanisms of blunt chest damage. Acceleration/deceleration injuries are more common and are usually a consequence of motor vehicle crashes. Compression injuries are caused by crushing, falls, and other conditions in which the impact force exceeds skeletal strength.[2]

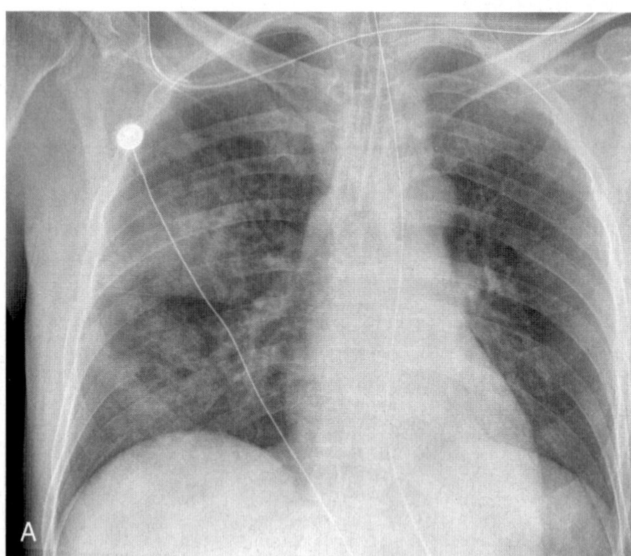

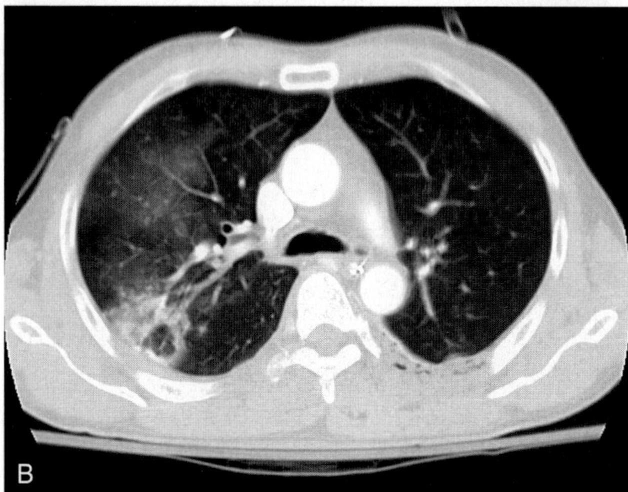

FIGURE 17–24 A: Right-sided pulmonary contusion. (Courtesy of Robert Hendrickson, MD.) **B:** Right-sided pulmonary contusion seen on computed tomogram. (**A** and **B**, Courtesy of Robert Hendrickson, MD.)

Diagnosis

Chest radiography (CXR) is the ideal screening examination in cases of suspected thoracic injury because of its availability, low cost, and safety.[2] Contrast computed tomography (CT) is four to five times more sensitive than CXR at detecting intrathoracic injuries.[2] Therefore, CT should follow the CXR if the results are abnormal or if there is suspicion of an occult injury.[2,3] Aortography is indicated for hemodynamically unstable patients who have suspicious CXR findings or mediastinal hematoma on CT.[2,3]

Clinical Complications

Blunt chest trauma may result in complications or injuries involving four anatomic structures. Chest wall injuries are most common and include muscle tears, rib fractures (including flail chest), and sternal fractures. Pulmonary injuries include parenchymal contusions, hemothorax, pneumothorax, and tracheobronchial disruption. Cardiovascular injuries can be lethal and include myocardial contusion, aortic disruption, cardiac rupture, and cardiac tamponade. Esophageal injuries may manifest in a delayed fashion as mediastinitis.[1]

Management

Blunt chest trauma frequently results in multiple thoracic injuries that need prompt surgical evaluation in the emergency department.[3] Rapid diagnosis and treatment of underlying intrathoracic injuries are essential to decrease mortality.[1]

REFERENCES

1. Greenberg MD, Rosen Carlo L. Evaluation of the patient with blunt chest trauma: an evidence based approach. *Emerg Med Clin North Am* 1999;17:41–62.
2. LoCicero J, Mattox KL. Epidemiology of chest trauma. *Surg Clin North Am* 1989;69:15–19.
3. Chan O, Hiorns M. Chest trauma. *Eur J Radiol* 1996;23:23–34.

Tension Pneumothorax

Erica McKernan

Clinical Presentation

Patients with tension pneumothorax may present with chest pain and dyspnea or in respiratory distress or arrest. Signs of a tension pneumothorax include tachypnea, tachycardia, and cyanosis with elevated jugular venous distention. Absent breath sounds and hyperresonance on the affected side may also be present. Tracheal deviation and hemodynamic compromise are hallmarks of a tension pneumothorax, which requires immediate treatment.[1,2]

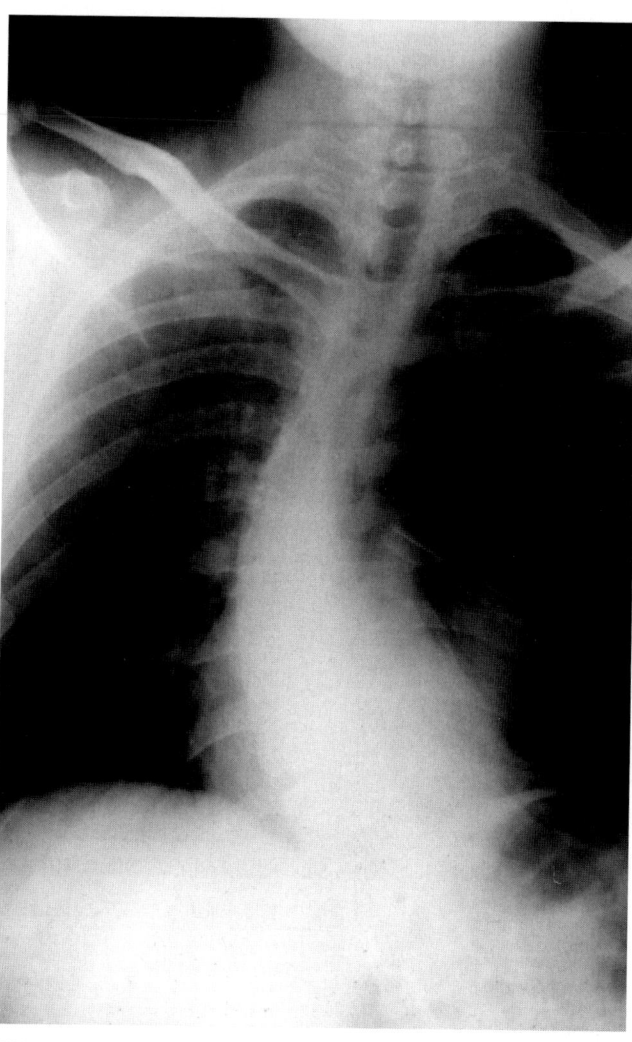

FIGURE 17–25 Left-sided tension pneumothorax with rightward shift of midline structures. (Courtesy of Michael Greenberg, MD.)

Pathophysiology

Tension pneumothorax involves a one-way valve effect that causes air to collect continually within the pleural space, displacing the mediastinal structures and compromising cardiopulmonary function.[1] The pleural cavity is a potential space between the opposing surfaces of the visceral and parietal pleurae. The visceral pleura envelopes each lung, and the parietal pleura lines the thoracic wall, diaphragm, and mediastinum. The two pleural surfaces are contiguous and maintain a resting negative pressure relative to the atmosphere, which is necessary for pulmonary expansion and passive chest wall relaxation during normal respiratory physiology.[1] When a tension pneumothorax develops, the trapped air causes collapse of the lung on the affected side and compression of the opposite lung. Decreased pulmonary compliance and increased peak airway pressures result in ineffective gas exchange.[2] Mass effect on the mediastinal structures increases intrathoracic pressures, causing decreased venous return and decreased cardiac output.[1]

Diagnosis

The diagnosis of a tension pneumothorax is a clinical one. Confirmation by chest radiography is not recommended, because immediate intervention is required.[1,2]

Clinical Complications

If a tension pneumothorax persists untreated, rapid progression to marked cardiopulmonary decompensation followed by death may occur.[1,2]

Management

Once the clinical diagnosis is suspected, needle thoracostomy should be performed. A large-bore needle should be inserted into the second intercostal space of the anterior midclavicular line. After needle decompression, definitive therapy consists of placement of a chest thoracostomy tube.[1,2]

REFERENCES

1. Ullman EA, Donley LP, Brady WJ. Pulmonary trauma: emergency department evaluation and management. *Emerg Med Clin North Am* 2003;21:291–313.
2. Domino KB. Pulmonary function and dysfunction in the traumatized patient. *Anesthesiol Clin North Am* 1996;14:59–84.

Traumatic Pneumothorax

Melissa A. Eirich

Clinical Presentation

Patients with traumatic pneumothorax complain of chest pain and shortness of breath or difficulty breathing after chest injury. Patients with tension pneumothorax may be hypotensive and may demonstrate distended neck veins and hyperresonance on the affected side, with tracheal deviation toward the opposite lung.[1]

Pathophysiology

Blunt trauma may cause pneumothorax if broken ribs puncture the lung. In penetrating trauma, the bullet or weapon causes a defect in the chest wall, letting air enter the negatively pressurized pleural space.[1]

Diagnosis

Pneumothorax should be suspected in the stable chest trauma patient and confirmed by chest radiography or computed tomography. The hypotensive or unstable trauma patient should be presumed to have a tension pneumothorax, and needle decompression or chest tube placement should be attempted immediately without obtaining a chest radiograph.[1] Plain films usually show a thin white line of the visceral pleura outlining the lung tissue with a loss of lung markings lateral to it. Up to 50% of small pneumothoraces are undetectable on chest radiographs but are found incidentally on computed tomographic scans.[1] During examination of the chest wall, wounds from penetrating trauma are easily overlooked. Lung examination reveals decreased breath sounds on the affected side.[1]

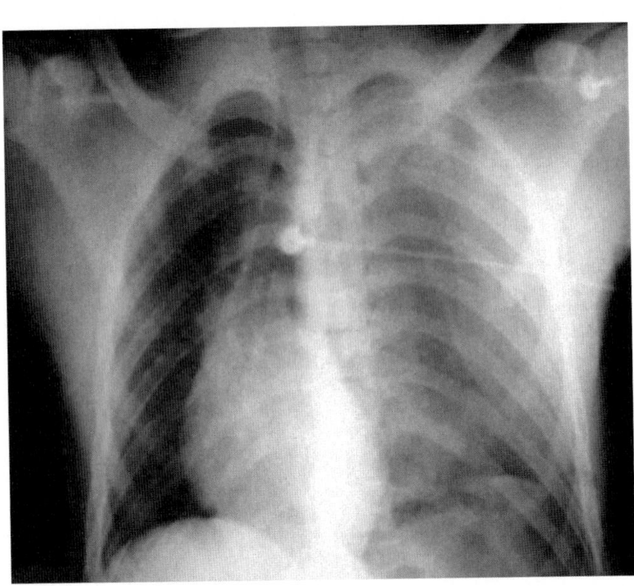

FIGURE 17–26 Left-sided tension hemopneumothorax. (Courtesy of Mark Silverberg, MD.)

Clinical Complications

Tension pneumothorax is a serious complication of pneumothorax itself and may lead to hemodynamic collapse and death if left untreated. Other complications, such as persistent pneumothorax, lung laceration, costal nerve or vessel injury, and empyema, may result from the original trauma or from inaccurate chest tube placement.[1]

Management

Traumatic pneumothoraces require the insertion of a chest tube attached to suction via an underwater seal device. Smaller chest tubes (20F) can be used for simple collapses, whereas larger tubes (35F to 40F) are necessary for a pneumothorax with associated hemothorax. Repeat chest radiographs should be obtained to confirm proper tube placement.[1]

REFERENCES

1. Neff MA, Monk JS Jr, Peters K, Nikhilesh A. Detection of occult pneumothoraces on abdominal computed tomography scans in trauma patients. *J Trauma* 2000;49:281–285.

Massive Hemothorax

Bryan Gargano

Clinical Presentation

Patients with a massive hemothorax present with acute blood loss into the chest cavity of 1,500 mL or more. Massive hemothoraces are most commonly associated with penetrating wounds involving the hilum.[1]

Pathophysiology

Sources of hemorrhage include lung parenchyma, chest wall, great vessels, and the heart.[2] Patients suffer from hypovolemic shock, collapse of the affected lung, and preload compromise.[2]

Diagnosis

Massive hemothorax may be present in a profoundly hypotensive, tachycardic patient in frank hypovolemic shock who has dullness to percussion and absent breath sounds in the affected hemithorax.[1,3] Respiratory distress, shock, and dullness on percussion along with decreased breath sounds in the affected hemithorax are suggestive.[1,3] Supine portable chest radiographic studies in patients with massive hemothorax frequently reveal an opacified lung.[1] Initial return of greater than 1,500 mL of blood after thoracostomy tube placement is diagnostic.[2]

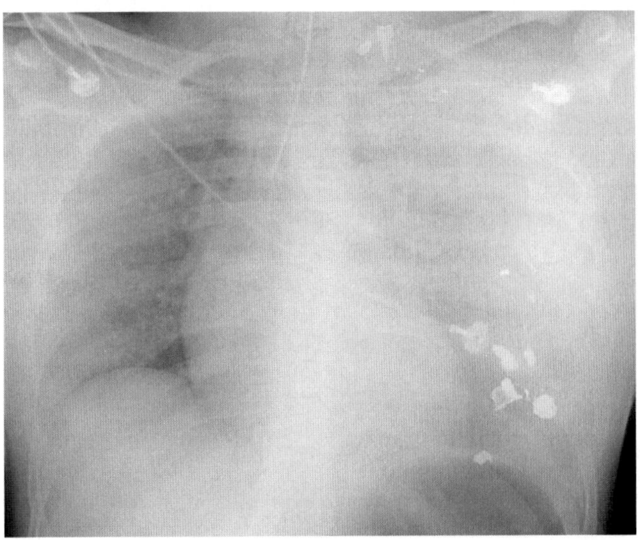

FIGURE 17–27 Gunshot wound to left chest with hemothorax. (Courtesy of Mark Silverberg, MD.)

Clinical Complications

Exsanguination into the thorax and respiratory compromise can be rapid and fatal.[1] Concomitant pneumothorax and rib fractures are frequently seen.[1,3] Associated aortic disruption or dissection and injuries to the cardiac or pulmonary arteries, are possible.[3]

Management

Advanced trauma life support (ATLS) protocols guide initial therapy.[2] Prompt intercostal drainage with a 36F or 38F thoracostomy tube, along with fluid resuscitation via two large-bore intravenous catheters, is required.[2,3] Clinical or radiographic suspicion of aortic dissection or transection should prompt consideration to delay intercostal drainage until a definitive diagnosis is established, because rapid exsanguination with drainage may occur.[3] Patients may require emergency thoracotomy if greater than 2 L of blood initially drains or there is significant hemodynamic instability.[3]

REFERENCES

1. Vukich DJ. Pneumothorax, hemothorax, and other abnormalities of the pleural space. *Emerg Med Clin North Am* 1983;1:431–448.
2. Ullman EA, Donley LP, Brady WJ. Pulmonary trauma emergency department evaluation and management. *Emerg Med Clin North Am* 2003;21:291–313.
3. Parry GW, Morgan WE, Salama FD. Management of haemothorax. *Ann R Coll Surg Engl* 1996;78:325–326.

Pericardial Tamponade

Melissa A. Eirich

Clinical Presentation

Tamponade often manifests after chest trauma, but it also may be caused by a rapidly forming effusion. Patients may report dyspnea and chest pressure or pain.[1,2]

Pathophysiology

As fluid accumulates in the pericardial sac, pressure increases and impairs diastolic venous flow, resulting in decreased cardiac output. If a pericardial effusion accumulates slowly, large volumes may be tolerated. As little as 80 mL of liquid may lead to tamponade if the fluid accumulates rapidly, as in the setting of a penetrating cardiac injury.[1]

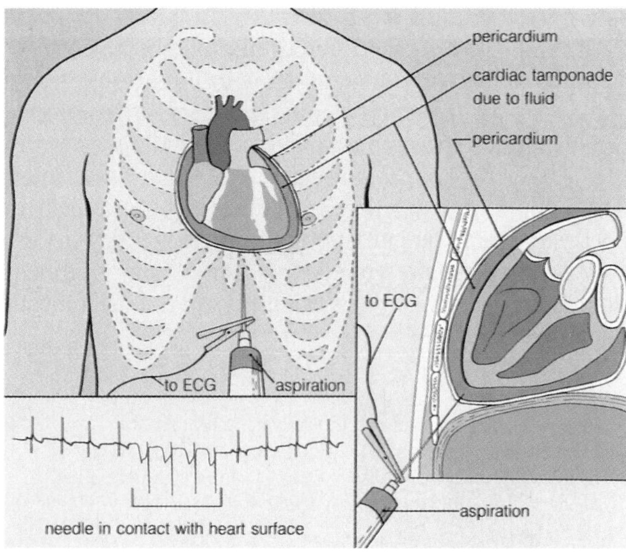

FIGURE 17–28 The subxiphoid pericardiocentesis technique. The needle is inserted to the left of the xiphoid and directed toward the midscapular area. The electrocardiogram (ECG) lead is attached to the needle. Negative deflection of the QRS complex represents contact with the heart surface. As the needle is slowly withdrawn and loses contact with the myocardium, the ECG reverts to normal. (From Hurst, with permission.)

Diagnosis

On physical examination, the patient may be tachycardic and hypotensive with distant heart sounds, a pericardial friction rub, pulsus paradoxus, and jugular venous distention.[1] Associated injuries may mask the findings of pericardial tamponade.[2] Chest radiography may show a globular heart, or the heart may appear to be normal in size and configuration. This is especially true in the setting of rapidly forming tamponade due to trauma. The electrocardiogram may show electrical alternans and low voltage, but an echocardiogram is the test of choice to diagnose a pericardial effusion.[1] Swan-Ganz catheter monitoring demonstrates equalization of the pressure within the four cardiac chambers.[1,2]

Clinical Complications

As intrapericardial pressure increases, cardiac output decreases, hypotension develops, and shock or death may ensue.[1,2]

Management

Pericardiocentesis should be performed in the emergency department if the patient does not respond to intravenous fluids or pressors. The procedure should be done under ultrasound or fluoroscopic guidance. A surgical pericardial window performed in the operating theater may be required.[1,2]

REFERENCES

1. Rozycki GS, Feliciano DV, Ochsner MG, et al. The role of ultrasound in patients with possible penetrating cardiac wounds: a prospective multicenter study. *J Trauma* 1999;46:543–551; discussion, 551–552.
2. Crawford R, Kasem H, Bleetmen A. Traumatic pericardial tamponade: relearning old lessons. *J Accid Emerg Med* 1997;14:252–254.

Pneumopericardium

Laura Spivak

Clinical Presentation

Signs and symptoms consistent with pneumopericardium include dyspnea, tachypnea, hypoxia, tachycardia, hypotension, fever, altered mental status, coarse breath sounds, hemodynamic instability, and respiratory failure.[1,2]

Pathophysiology

Barotrauma from positive-pressure ventilation may lead to alveolar rupture and subsequent air dissection at the reflection of parietal to visceral pericardium.[1] This may occur near the ostia of the pulmonary veins.[1] Pneumopericardium is more common in infants than adults, probably because of the tighter adhesion of the pericardial layers in adults.[1] Pneumopericardium has been reported in association with blunt chest trauma, spontaneous pneumothorax, sternal dehiscence after coronary artery bypass grafting, caustic ingestions, and during mechanical ventilation and continuous positive airway pressure by face mask.[1-3] Tension pneumopericardium is believed to occur when air is forced into the pericardium and is unable to escape because of the development of a one-way valve.[2] Air may arise from a contiguous tension pneumothorax, tracheal rupture, or positive-pressure ventilation.[2]

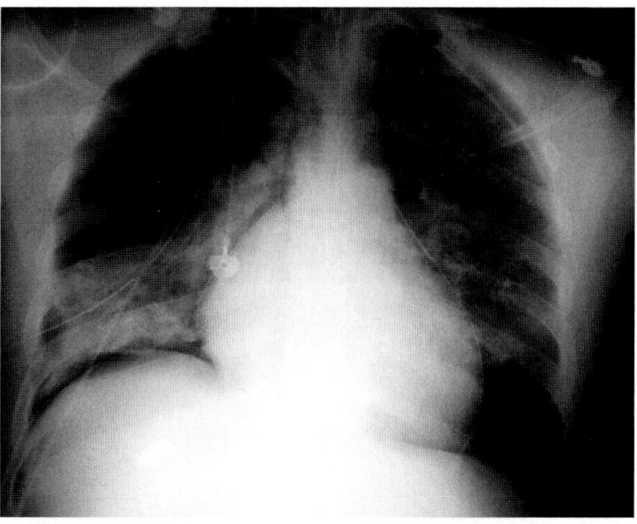

FIGURE 17–29 Pneumopericardium with pulmonary contusion and air under the diaphragm secondary to gunshot wound. (Courtesy of Mark Silverberg, MD.)

Diagnosis

Chest radiographs and computed tomography (CT) of the thorax can be used to diagnose air within the pericardial sac.[1,2] Pneumopericardium is differentiated from pneumomediastinum on a chest radiograph in three ways: the presence of a radiolucent air halo encircling the heart without extension up to the pericardial attachments; pericardial air shifting on a decubitus film; and interruption of the diaphragmatic outline.[1] CT findings suggestive of tension pneumopericardium include a decrease in the anterior-posterior heart diameter and flattening of the anterior face of the heart.[2]

Clinical Complications

Tension pneumopericardium may lead to cardiac tamponade and resultant circulatory failure.[2] Other complications include subcutaneous emphysema, pneumomediastinum, pneumothorax, and acute respiratory distress syndrome.[1]

Management

Surgical intervention is required in patients with hemodynamic instability.[1] Tension pneumopericardium requires urgent decompression.[2] Patients should be closely monitored for other complications of barotrauma.[1]

REFERENCES

1. McEachern RC, Patel RG. Pneumopericardium associated with face-mask continuous positive airway pressure. *Chest* 1997;112:1441–1443.
2. Hernandez-Luyando L, Gonzalez de las Heras E, Calvo J, et al. Posttraumatic tension pneumopericardium. *Am J Emerg Med* 1997;15:686–687.
3. Ruiz-Bailen M, Serrano-Corcoles MC, Ramos-Cuadra JA. Tracheal injury caused by ingested paraquat. *Chest* 2001;119:1956–1957.

Gunshot Wound to the Chest

Laura Rendano

Clinical Presentation

The patient with a gunshot wound (GSW) to the chest almost always gives a history of the preceding trauma, but some patients are not alert and oriented to person, place, and time, so a thorough physical examination is always important. Bullet wounds will be noted on physical examination, but it may be difficult to distinguish entrance from exit wounds.[1,2]

Pathophysiology

The muzzle velocity and bullet type, the distance of the patient from the discharged weapon, and the amount of bullet tumble and yaw all influence blast cavity formation and thus injury severity.[2] The bullet trajectory and involved organs are not always apparent on external examination, because two obvious wounds may not have been caused by the same bullet, bullets can ricochet internally, and secondary missiles may also be involved.[2]

Diagnosis

The diagnosis of GSW to the chest generally is made from the history and physical examination. However, bullets that strike the victim at unusual angles can cause atypical wounds. Additionally, small-caliber bullets can create unrecognizable wounds, and bullets that enter the body in a concealed place may be difficult to find. For all these reasons, a chest radiograph is usually necessary to confirm the diagnosis.[1,2]

Clinical Complications

Complications largely depend on the involved organ systems and consist of peripheral nerve injury, lung injury including hemothorax/pneumothorax, cardiac injury, diaphragm perforation, great vessel injury, esophageal injury, and infection.[2] Almost any GSW to the chest may be fatal.

Management

Immediate trauma surgery consultation should be obtained, and life-threatening injuries must be addressed after the advanced trauma life support (ATLS) protocols have been followed.[1] Most patients require surgical intervention.[1,2]

REFERENCES

1. Asensio JA, Stewart BM, Murray J, et al. Penetrating cardiac injuries. *Surg Clinic North Am* 1996;76:685–724.
2. Bartlett CS. Clinical update: gunshot wound ballistics. *Clin Orthop* 2003;(408):28–57.

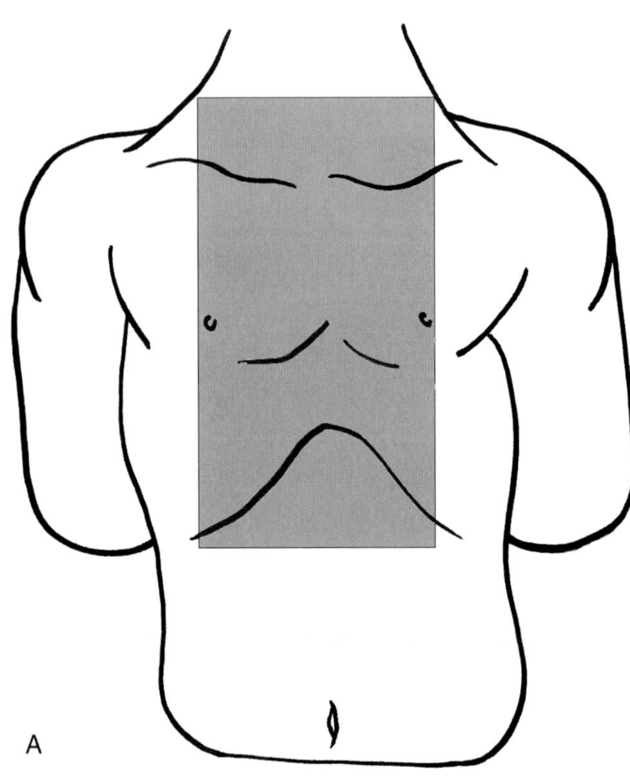

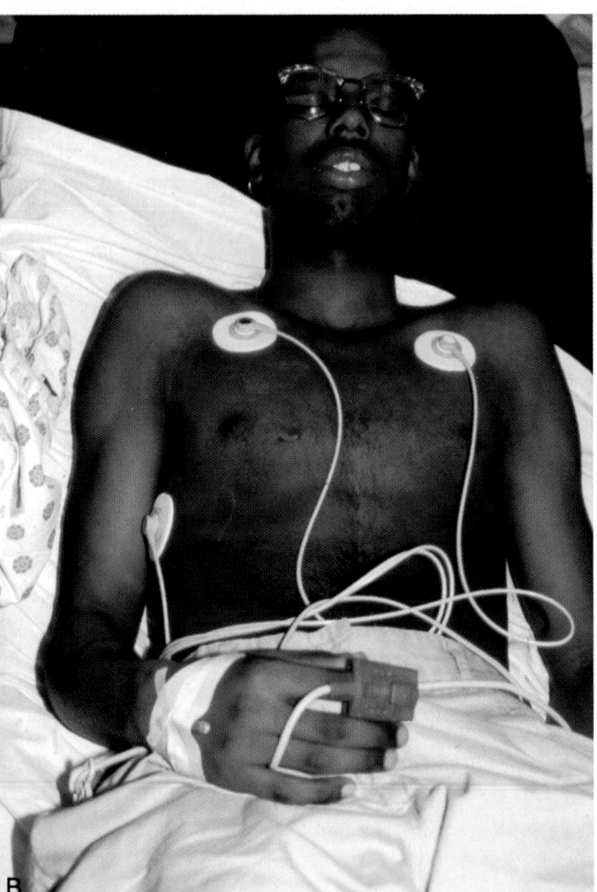

FIGURE 17–30 **A:** The box of death. Shaded area represents the danger zone for transmediastinal injury. Injuries at this site are said to be "in the box." (From Peitzman, with permission.) **B:** Gunshot wound of anterior right chest. (Copyright James R. Roberts, MD.)

Traumatic Asphyxia

Bryan Gargano

Clinical Presentation

Patients with traumatic asphyxia (TA) present with a history of thoracic or abdominal compression, massive bilateral subconjunctival hemorrhages accompanied by bluish-red to black facial discoloration, petechiae, and edema of the face, head, and neck, occasionally involving the shoulders.[1] The appearance of the face in TA is characteristic and is known as the "masque ecchymotique."[1] Discoloration may or may not involve the scalp, usually does not involve the arms or the chest below the nipple line, but may be present in the pharynx and ears.[1]

Pathophysiology

TA is a syndrome of cervicofacial cyanosis, subconjunctival hemorrhage, ecchymosis, and facial petechiae often associated with thoracic crush injuries.[2] TA results from the application of substantial force to the chest, which dramatically increases intrathoracic pressure. The increased intrathoracic pressure forces a reflux of blood through the valveless superior vena cava into the head and neck, producing capillary stasis or rupture.[3] Patients reportedly experience a fear response just before sustaining the injury and brace themselves for impact.[2,3] During this fear response, they develop increased intrathoracic and intraabdominal pressure with closure of the glottis during Valsalva. The increased intrathoracic pressure contributes to the patient's symptoms, and the increased intraabdominal pressure partially protects the intraabdominal organs from venous injury.[2,3] The most common mechanism causing TA is entrapment between an automobile or industrial piece of equipment and an immovable object.[1,4]

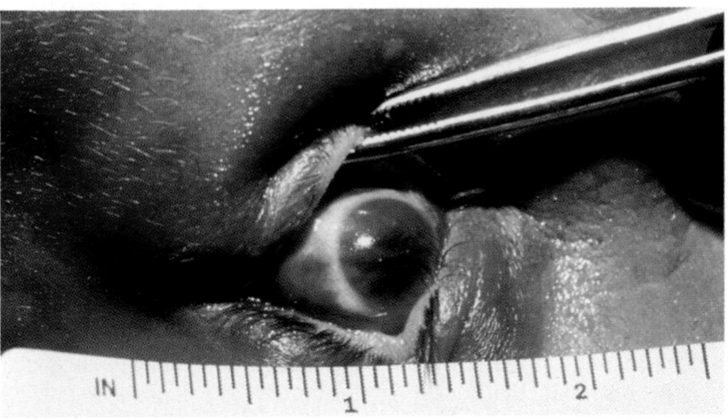

FIGURE 17–31 Subconjunctival hemorrhage and facial petechiae in an individual who died from compression asphyxia. (Courtesy of Charles Catanese, MD.)

Diagnosis

TA is diagnosed by physical examination findings of characteristic phenomena, coupled with a supporting history of compression or crush injury to the chest or abdomen.[1]

Clinical Complications

Pulmonary contusion or flail chest may complicate TA.[2] Neurologic symptoms accompany TA in about 85% of cases and may involve loss of consciousness (57%) or confusion. These symptoms are believed to be caused by transient hypoxia, not intracranial hemorrhage.[4]

Management

Advanced trauma/cardiac life support (ATLS/ACLS) protocols should be followed. Hospital admission is indicated for all patients who survive the initial TA insult.

REFERENCES

1. Fred HL, Chandler FW. Traumatic asphyxia. *Am J Med* 1960;29:508–517.
2. Lee MC, Wong SS, Chu JJ, et al. Traumatic asphyxia. *Ann Thorac Surg* 1991;51:86–88.
3. Williams JS, Minken SL, Adams JT. Traumatic asphyxia—reappraised. *Ann Surg* 1968;167:384–392.
4. Jongewaard WR, Cogbill TH, Landercasper J. Neurologic consequences of traumatic asphyxia. *J Trauma* 1992;32:28–31.

Myocardial Contusion

Bryan Gargano

Clinical Presentation

Myocardial contusion (MC) represents a spectrum of injury, with its most severe form causing hemodynamic instability.[1] Patients with less severe injury may present with palpitations, nonspecific chest pain, or no symptoms at all.[1]

Pathophysiology

A motor vehicle accident with rapid deceleration or blunt trauma from the steering wheel is a frequent mechanism of injury.[1] Direct force to the sternum compresses the heart against the spine, resulting in histologically apparent hemorrhage, edema, and necrosis of myocytes.[1] In cases of rapid deceleration, the heart continues to move forward because of its momentum and strikes the sternum, resulting in injury.[1] The right ventricle is the most common location for cardiac injury.[1] The incidence of MC in blunt thoracic trauma varies from 3% to 56%.[1]

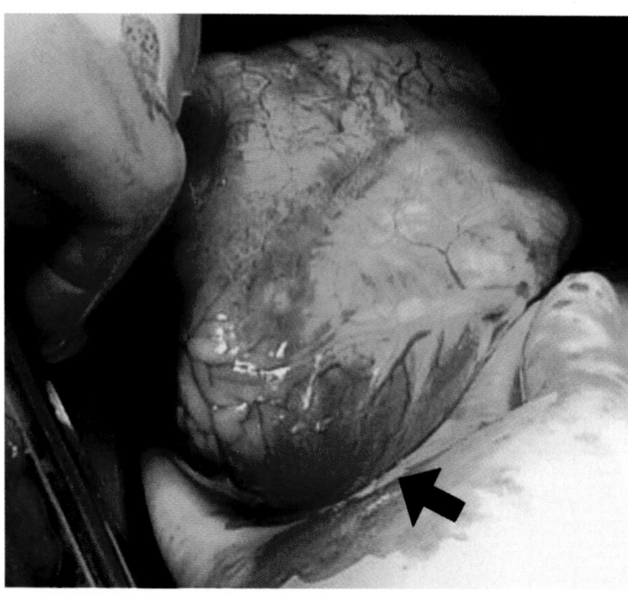

FIGURE 17–32 A small apical myocardial contusion *(arrow)*. (Courtesy of Mark Silverberg, MD.)

Diagnosis

There is no gold standard for clinical diagnosis. A high index of suspicion should be maintained based on the history and physical examination.[2] The electrocardiogram (ECG) may be normal, or it may show nonspecific abnormalities, with sinus tachycardia and atrial extrasystoles the most common tracings.[1] Echocardiography is useful in identifying wall-motion abnormalities that suggest MC.[1] Measurement of myocardial-bound creatine kinase (CK-MB) is of limited value, but troponin I and T are often elevated and are specific for myocardial injury.[1,3]

Clinical Complications

Complications from MC include structural damage to the heart or great vessels, atrial and ventricular arrhythmias, intracardiac thrombus, and coronary artery injury with acute myocardial infarction.[1]

Management

Monitoring for 24 to 48 hours in the intensive care unit is appropriate for patients with hemodynamic instability.[4] Stable patients may be monitored in the emergency department for 6 to 12 hours with a repeat troponin and ECG (at 6 to 12 hours). If the second ECG is normal, discharge may be considered; if it is not, admission is warranted.[1,4]

REFERENCES

1. Sybrandy KC, Cramer MJ, Burgersdijk C. Diagnosing cardiac contusion: old wisdom and new insights. *Heart* 2003;89:485–489.
2. Healey MA, Brown R, Fleiszer D. Blunt cardiac injury: is this diagnosis necessary? *J Trauma* 1990;30:137–146.
3. Lancey RA, Monahan TS. Correlation of clinical characteristics and outcomes with injury scoring in blunt cardiac trauma. *J Trauma* 2003;54:509–515.
4. Dubrow TJ, Mihalka J, Eisenhauer DM, et al. Myocardial contusion in the stable patient: what level of care is appropriate? *Surgery* 1989;106:267–274.

Scapular Fracture

Melissa A. Eirich

Clinical Presentation

Patients with scapular fracture present with local scapular pain, tenderness, swelling, ecchymosis, and deformity. The afflicted extremity usually is held in adduction, because abduction causes increased pain. Distal arm weakness and decreased range of motion may be caused by pain or brachial plexus injury.[1]

Pathophysiology

The scapula is a very strong bone and is anatomically well protected from trauma, making scapular fractures uncommon presentations. Scapular fractures usually are associated with major blunt or penetrating thoracic trauma. Substantial force is required to fracture the scapula, and underlying damage to the lungs, ribs, and great vessels is possible if a fracture is present.[1]

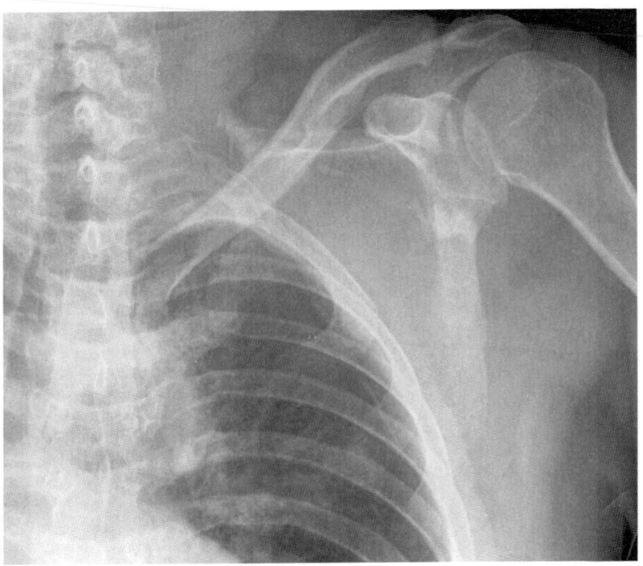

FIGURE 17–33 Scapular fracture (also note pneumothorax). (Courtesy of Gregory Schutt, MD.)

Diagnosis

The history and clinical findings may raise the physician's suspicion that a scapular fracture exists, but the diagnosis must be confirmed radiologically. These fractures are not common and may be subtle on chest radiography. In one study, scapular fractures were initially missed in 43% of patients with blunt thoracic trauma. However, 72% of the fractures were found when the chest radiograph was re-examined.[2] Traditional shoulder radiographs demonstrate the majority of scapular fractures.

Clinical Complications

Scapular fractures usually do not have any complications except occasional malunion or nonunion. Because these fractures require high-energy mechanisms, associated injuries are common and should be carefully sought.[1,2]

Management

Isolated, nondisplaced scapular fractures heal with conservative treatment (e.g., sling, ice, analgesics). Orthopedic follow-up is advised. Fractures that are displaced or have associated rotator cuff injuries may require surgical repair.[1,2]

REFERENCES

1. Cole PA. Scapula fractures. *Orthop Clin North Am* 2002;33:1–18.
2. Harris RD, Harris JH Jr. The prevalence and significance of missed scapular fractures in blunt chest trauma. *AJR Am J Roentgenol* 1988;151:747–750.

17–34

Sternal Fracture

Laura Spivak

Clinical Presentation

Indications of sternal injury after blunt anterior chest-wall trauma include complaints of sternal or substernal chest pain, sternal tenderness, ecchymoses, contusions, and deformity to palpation.[1] These fractures may be missed in patients who are unable to complain of chest pain.[1]

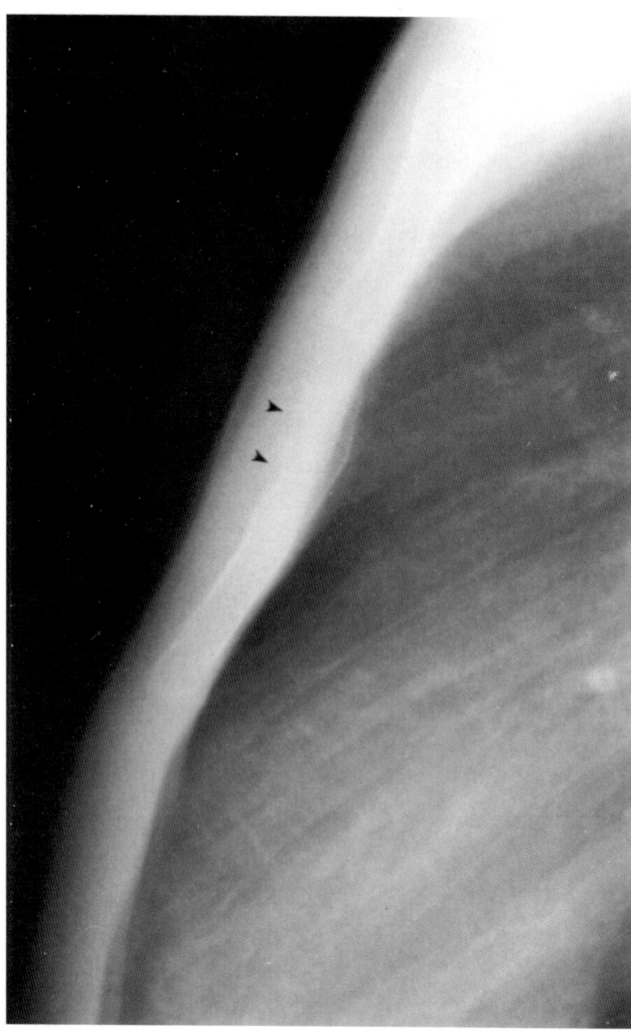

FIGURE 17–34 This patient was wrestling and suffered blunt chest trauma. The sternum is fractured *(arrows)*, and there is some presternal and retrosternal soft-tissue swelling. (From Swischuk, with permission.)

Pathophysiology

High-energy blunt trauma to the anterior chest wall, caused by impact with an over-the-shoulder seatbelt or steering wheel, can result in a sternal fracture.[1,2] Associated injuries include innominate artery avulsion, thoracic artery laceration, myocardial contusion, pneumothorax, spinal injuries, and clavicle and rib fractures.[1]

Diagnosis

A lateral chest or sternal-view radiograph is adequate to visualize fractures.[1] Thoracic computed tomography may also be used.[1] Measurement of cardiac enzymes, electrocardiography, and echocardiography are used to diagnose myocardial contusion.[1] Aortography is used for evaluation of a widened mediastinum on chest radiographs.[1,2] Sternal fractures should be sought in patients who are unable to complain of chest pain because of the severity of their injuries.[1]

Clinical Complications

Isolated sternal fractures, without evidence of a widened mediastinum, are not reliable indicators for concomitant cardiovascular injuries.[1–3] Retrosternal hematomas are seen in fractures of the body of the sternum.[2] Pain management is an important consideration.[2] Early operative reduction is sometimes performed for pain control.[2]

Management

Stable patients who have isolated sternal fractures and no evidence of other significant cardiac or respiratory complications may be safely discharged from the hospital with oral analgesics.[1,3]

REFERENCES

1. Chiu WC, D'Amelio LF, Hammond JS. Sternal fractures in blunt chest trauma: a practical algorithm for management. *Am J Emerg Med* 1997;15:252–255.
2. Rashid MA, Ortenwall P, Wikstrom T. Cardiovascular injuries associated with sternal fractures. *Eur J Surg* 2001;167:243–248.
3. Sadaba JR, Oswal D, Munsch CM. Management of isolated sternal fractures: determining the risk of blunt cardiac injury. *Ann R Coll Surg Engl* 2000;82:162–166.

Penetrating Abdominal Trauma

Laura Rendano

Clinical Presentation

Patients with penetrating abdominal trauma often present with one of three clinical scenarios: (1) near or frank cardiac arrest, (2) severe hypotension or peritonitis accompanied by tachycardia, and (3) tachypnea or hemodynamic stability with minimal to no abdominal tenderness.[1]

Pathophysiology

The mechanism and location of the penetrating injury may suggest specific injuries but should never be used to rule out pathology. Stabbing injuries usually are limited to the region below the site of entrance, but the direction and depth of penetration are often difficult to predict. Projectile wounds are more challenging to assess. The trajectory of a bullet is not immediately apparent, and internal ricochets are possible. Additionally, fragmentation with secondary missiles and cavitation injuries may occur.[2]

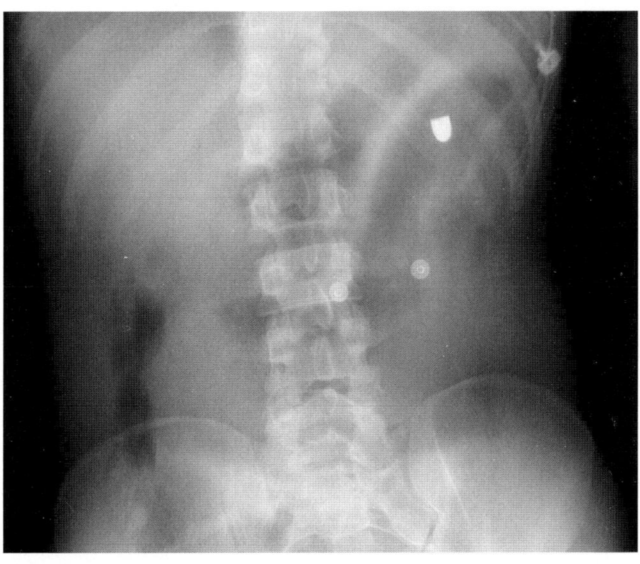

FIGURE 17–35 Gunshot wound to the abdomen. (Courtesy of Mark Silverberg, MD.)

Diagnosis

The diagnosis of penetrating abdominal trauma usually is made by history and physical examination, with the extent of injury apparent only after application of other diagnostic modalities such as computed tomography (CT), abdominal ultrasonography, or diagnostic peritoneal lavage. However, operative exploration is the gold standard to diagnose intraperitoneal injury.[1,2]

Clinical Complications

Complications include infection or abscess formation, abdominal compartmental syndrome, intraabdominal or retroperitoneal hemorrhage, and visceral edema.[3]

Management

All cases involving penetrating abdominal trauma should be managed in consultation with a trauma surgeon while following the advanced trauma life support (ATLS) protocols. Indications for operative management include failure to improve clinically after fluid resuscitation, peritoneal signs of liver or spleen lacerations, and free peritoneal fluid on CT scan or ultrasound.[1,3] Stable patients need to be monitored closely for changes in vital signs and for the development of peritoneal signs as assessed by serial abdominal examinations.[1,3] All patients with penetrating abdominal injuries should receive antibiotics and tetanus prophylaxis.[2]

REFERENCES

1. Salim A, Velmahos GC. When to operate on abdominal gunshot wounds. *Scand J Surg* 2002;91:62–66.
2. Ferrada R, Birolini D. New concepts in the management of patients with penetrating abdominal wounds. *Surg Clin North Am* 1999;79: 1331–1356.
3. Cushing BM, Clark DE, Cobean R, et al. Blunt and penetrating trauma: has anything changed? *Surg Clin North Am* 1997;77: 1321–1332.

Impalement Injuries

Sarah Jane Paris

Clinical Presentation

Any part of the body may be involved by impalement. Patients typically present in severe distress, complaining of local pain from an obviously impaled foreign body. If the object has been left in place, bleeding may be tamponaded, facilitating hemodynamic stability; if the object has been removed, rapid, life-threatening hemorrhage may develop.[1-3]

Pathophysiology

Impalement occurs when an object penetrates a part of the body and remains embedded in the patient.[1-3] Impalement occurs when an individual falls or is propelled against a fixed object, or when a mobile object is accidentally or deliberately lodged in a stationary individual. Impalements may occur in the setting of construction accidents, assaults, falls from height, motor vehicle ejections, or bow-hunting accidents.[2,3] Oropharyngeal impalements are especially common in pediatric patients.[1]

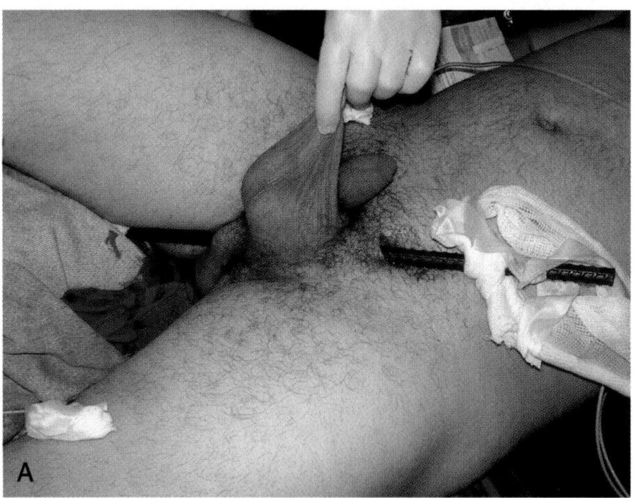

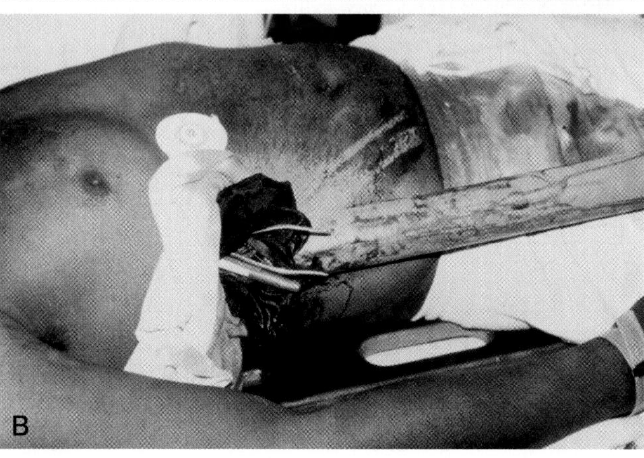

FIGURE 17–36 A: This construction worker fell from a height onto a piece of steel rebar. (Courtesy of Eric Adar, MD.) **B:** Thoracoabdominal impalement caused by high-speed trauma. (Courtesy of Lewis J. Kaplan, MD.)

Diagnosis

The diagnosis may be obvious from the history and physical examination; plain film radiographs, computed tomography, and angiography are helpful in elucidating the extent of underlying injury.[1-3]

Clinical Complications

Complications include wound infection, abscess formation, post-traumatic stress disorder, shock, exsanguination, and death.[1-3]

Management

Advanced trauma life support (ATLS) trauma resuscitation fundamentals should be followed. Tetanus status should be updated, if necessary, and treatment with prophylactic antibiotics should be started in the emergency department. Early surgical consultation is essential. Under almost all circumstances, the impaled object should be left in place during transport and emergency department evaluation. Pre-hospital personnel should stabilize the object in situ with bulky dressings. Extremely large objects may need to be cut away at the scene to facilitate transport.[1-3]

REFERENCES

1. Belfer RA, Ochsenschlager DW, Tomaski SM. Penetrating injury to the oral cavity: a case report and review of the literature. *J Emerg Med* 1995;13:331–335.
2. Eachempati SR, Barie PS, Reed RL 2nd. Survival after transabdominal impalement from a construction injury: a review of the management of impalement injuries. *J Trauma* 1999;47:864–866.
3. Kelly IP, Attwood SEA, Quilan W, Fox MJ. The management of impalement injury. *Injury* 1995;26:191–193.

Evisceration

Laura Rendano

Clinical Presentation

Evisceration is usually very easily identifiable because internal tissues such as bowel or lung are visible external to the body.[1,2] In some cases (e.g., wound dehiscence), the early stages of evisceration may not be obvious. Atypical presentations include hemodynamic instability, mental status changes, and fever.[2]

Pathophysiology

Traumatic bowel eviscerations may result from penetrating, blunt, or violent suction injuries. Pre-existing bowel disease (e.g., rectal prolapse) with a superimposed, sudden increase in intraabdominal pressure is a potential scenario.[1,3] Suction forces, such as those found in swimming pool drains, when applied to the anus, may result in a laceration along the mesenteric border of the intraperitoneal colon or rectum, causing transanal evisceration.[3] Although rare, lung parenchyma herniation has been reported as a complication of chest trauma.[1,2]

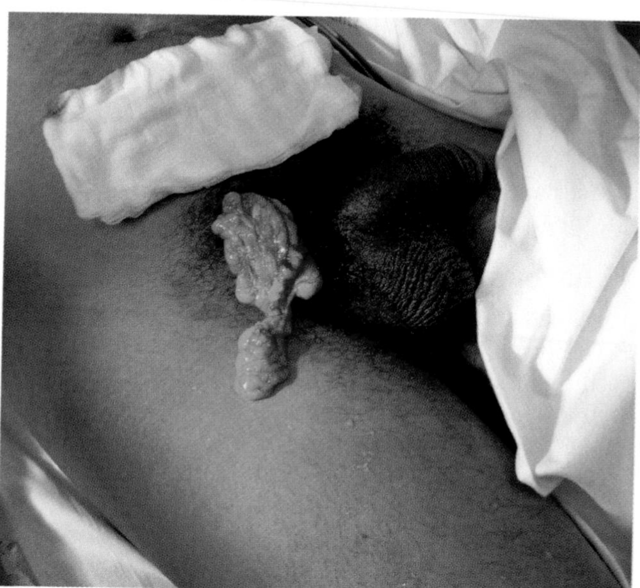

FIGURE 17–37 Abdominal stab wound with bowel evisceration. (Courtesy of Sanjay Shetty, MD.)

Diagnosis

Evisceration is a clinical diagnosis made by visualization of internal structures external to the body.

Clinical Complications

Viability of eviscerated tissue varies with length of time eviscerated, degree of contamination, and maintenance of blood flow to the externalized section. Failure to recognize bowel perforation or to properly repair fascial defects may lead to infection, abscess formation, and recurrence.[3]

Management

Advanced trauma life support (ATLS) protocols should be followed. Concomitant injuries such as organ laceration, hemothorax, pneumothorax, or cardiac tamponade must be considered. The eviscerated tissue should be wrapped in warm, saline-soaked gauze and covered with plastic to prevent further contamination, drying, and heat loss. These injuries require decontamination and reduction in the operating theater, with special attention given to repair of fascial defects.[1,2]

REFERENCES

1. Bowley DM, Boffard KD. Penetrating lung hernia with pulmonary evisceration: case report. *J Trauma* 2001;50:560–561.
2. Nagy K, Roberts R, Joseph K, et al. Evisceration after abdominal stab wounds: is laparotomy required? *J Trauma* 1999;47:622–624.
3. Rechner P, Cogbill TH. Transanal small bowel evisceration from abdominal crush injury: case report and review of the literature. *J Trauma* 2001;50:934–936.

Blunt Abdominal Trauma

George Lin

Clinical Presentation

Presenting symptoms of patients with blunt abdominal trauma vary widely, from isolated abdominal pain to shock or death.

Pathophysiology

Blunt abdominal trauma is the leading cause of morbidity and mortality due to trauma in all age groups. Intraabdominal injury usually results from compressive or deceleration forces. The spleen is the most commonly injured organ, followed by the liver and the small and large intestines.[1-3]

Diagnosis

Intraabdominal injury may be suspected based on the history and physical examination but should be confirmed with the use of other diagnostic modalities. Ultrasound has gained acceptance in most major trauma centers; it is rapid, is noninvasive, can be performed during resuscitation, and has a sensitivity of 73% to 88% and a specificity of 98% to 100%.[1,2] Computed tomography (CT) with oral and intravenous contrast is the preferred radiographic modality in stable patients with blunt abdominal trauma. It has a sensitivity of 92% to 97.6% and a specificity of 98.7%.[1,2] Diagnostic peritoneal lavage was commonly used in the past but is slowly being replaced by ultrasonography and CT because of its lack of specificity and inability to assess the retroperitoneum.[1,2] Physical examination may be unreliable in determining the extent of intraabdominal injury, especially in patients with altered level of consciousness due to hypotension or mind-altering substances.[1,3] Abdominal tenderness, abrasions, ecchymoses, and seatbelt or steering wheel marks are all signs of blunt trauma.

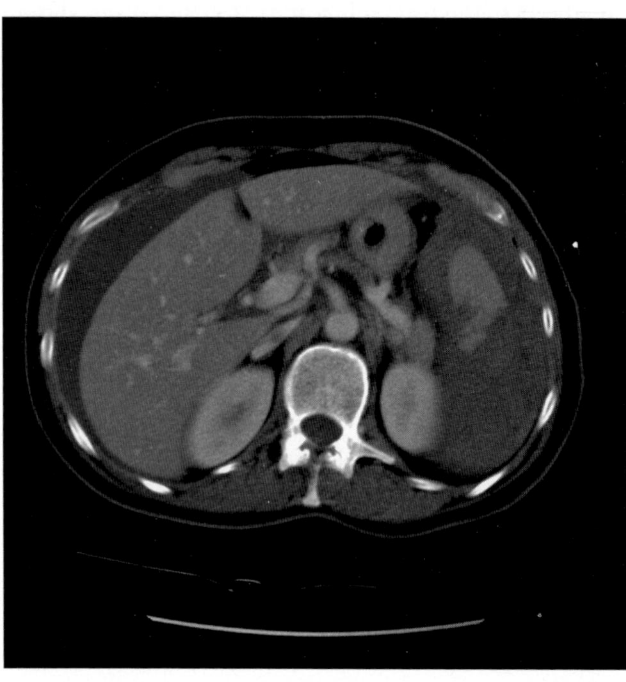

FIGURE 17–38 Peritoneal blood after blunt abdominal trauma. (Courtesy of Robert Hendrickson, MD.)

Clinical Complications

Complications of blunt abdominal trauma include solid or hollow organ injury, leading to ongoing hemorrhage, infection, organ failure, and death.[1-3]

Management

Advanced trauma life support (ATLS) protocols should be followed. All hemodynamically unstable patients need immediate resuscitation with crystalloid and blood products, as well as a trauma surgery consultation. Stable patients can be evaluated in the emergency department, with trauma consultation obtained for those patients with intraabdominal injury. Treatment depends on the severity and grade of internal injury.[1]

REFERENCES

1. Hoff WS, Holevar M, Nagy K, et al. Practice management guidelines for the evaluation of blunt abdominal trauma: the EAST Practice Management Guidelines Work Group. *J Trauma* 2002;53:602–615.
2. Brown CK, Dunn KA, Wilson K. Diagnostic evaluation of patients with blunt abdominal trauma: a decision analysis. *Acad Emerg Med* 2000;7:385–396.
3. Prall JA, Nichols JS, Brennan R, Moore EE. Early definitive abdominal evaluation in the triage of unconscious normotensive blunt abdominal trauma patients. *J Trauma* 1994;37:792–797.

Splenic Trauma

George Lin

Clinical Presentation

Patients with splenic injury after trauma may be asymptomatic, or they may present with mild left upper quadrant abdominal pain. They may be hemodynamically unstable or in traumatic arrest.[1]

Pathophysiology

The spleen is the most commonly injured intraabdominal organ in cases of blunt trauma, with mortality rates ranging from 3% to 23%.[2] Splenic injuries are classified into five grades, based on the size and length of the fracture and the presence of a vascular injury.

Diagnosis

The diagnosis of splenic injury may be suspected based on history and physical examination, with confirmation by imaging. Abdominal computed tomography (CT) with intravenous contrast is the study of choice for stable patients.[1,2] Diagnostic peritoneal lavage and ultrasonography may be useful in hemodynamically unstable individuals.[1]

Patients may have left shoulder pain referred from diaphragmatic irritation (Kehr's sign). On physical examination, there may be ecchymosis or tenderness over the lower left chest wall or left upper abdomen.[2] Rarely, patients present with a fixed area of percussed dullness in the left upper quadrant.[2]

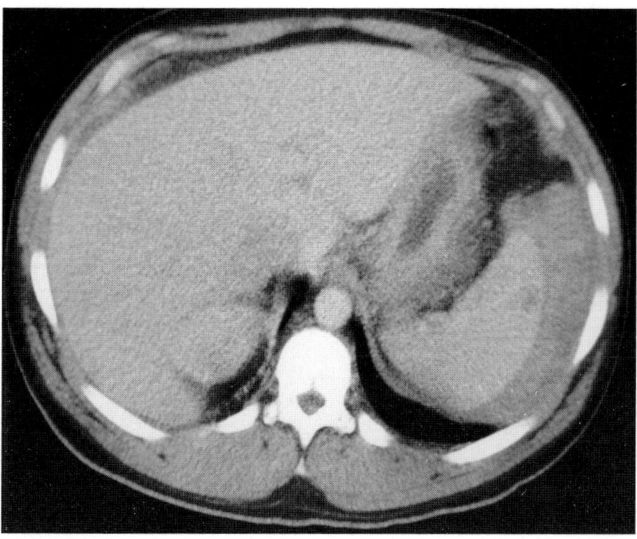

FIGURE 17–39 Splenic rupture. (Courtesy of Mark Silverberg, MD.)

Clinical Complications

Complications include splenic hematoma, massive hemorrhage, and death. Complications after splenectomy include sepsis secondary to encapsulated organisms.[2]

Management

If splenic trauma is suspected, a trauma surgeon should be promptly summoned. Splenic salvage procedures and nonoperative management, as well as the use of hemostatic agents and partial resection, have come to replace traditional splenectomy in many cases.[1,2] Nonoperative management is often recommended in cases with hemodynamic stability, minimal abdominal physical findings, no laboratory evidence of blood loss, probable low-energy trauma, isolated splenic injury on CT without associated intraabdominal injuries, and absence of hilar involvement or splenic disruption on CT.[1,2] Nonoperative management has been reported to be successful in both pediatric patients (98%) and adult patients (83%).[1,2]

REFERENCES

1. Fabian TC. What's new in trauma and critical care. *J Am Coll Surg* 2001;192:276–286.
2. Federle MP, Courcoulas AP, Powell M, et al. Blunt splenic injury in adults: clinical and CT criteria for management with emphasis on active extravasation. *Radiology* 1998;206:137–142.

Liver Fracture/Hematoma

George Lin

Clinical Presentation

Patients with liver injury may have symptoms ranging from none to hemodynamic instability, including hemorrhagic shock and traumatic cardiorespiratory arrest.[1-3]

Pathophysiology

The liver is the most frequently injured intraabdominal organ after penetrating abdominal trauma, and it is second to the spleen after blunt trauma.[2,3] Liver injuries may be classified with the use of a six-grade system based on the size and length of the hematoma or laceration and the presence of vascular injury.[2]

Diagnosis

Liver injuries may be suspected based on the history and physical examination but must be confirmed with a radiographic study or laparotomy. On physical examination, abdominal wall injuries may be grossly apparent and the patient may report abdominal tenderness or demonstrate frank peritonitis.[3] Abdominal computed tomography (CT) and ultrasonography may reveal liver injuries, and diagnostic peritoneal lavage (DPL) can be quickly performed on the unstable patient to demonstrate intraperitoneal hemorrhage, thus inferring solid-organ damage or vascular injury. Ultrasonography with or without CT is now preferred to DPL in most centers in the United States, Europe, and Japan.[2,3] Recently, DPL has also proved useful in the setting of penetrating trauma, but its role in blunt trauma is controversial.[3]

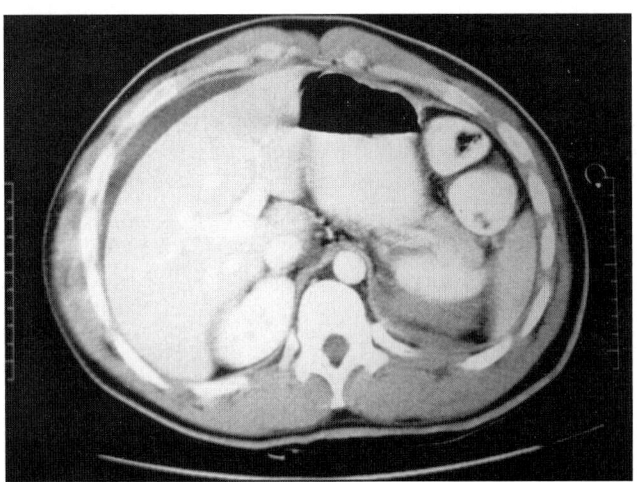

FIGURE 17–40 Hepatic hematoma. (Courtesy of Matthew Spencer, MD.)

Clinical Complications

Complications include continued hemorrhage/shock, hemobilia, bile leakage, sepsis, and transmission of viral agents from repeated blood transfusion.[2]

Management

Standard advanced trauma life support (ATLS) protocols should be followed. Early trauma surgery consultation is essential, because high-grade injuries often require surgical repair. Grade I or II injuries represent 90% of all cases and usually require minimal or no operative intervention.[1,2]

REFERENCES

1. Fabian TC. What's new in trauma and critical care. *J Am Coll Surg* 2001;192:276–286.
2. Parks RW, Chrysos E, Diamond T. Management of liver trauma. *Br J Surg* 1999;86:1121–1135.
3. Sartorelli KH, Frumiento C, Rogers FB, Osler TM. Nonoperative management of hepatic, splenic, and renal injuries in adults with multiple injuries. *J Trauma* 2000;49:56–61.

Diagnostic Peritoneal Lavage

Kelly Johnson-Arbor

Indications

Possible indications for diagnostic peritoneal lavage (DPL) include a history of abdominal trauma, physical examination findings consistent with abdominal trauma, and an unconscious patient who has physical examination findings or a mechanism that suggests abdominal trauma.[1,2] However, computed tomographic (CT) scanning of the abdomen with oral and intravenous contrast has all but taken over the role of the DPL, except in the situation in which the vital signs are too unstable for the patient to be sent for CT scanning.

Contraindications

The only absolute contraindications to DPL is the need for laparotomy.[3] Relative contraindications include pregnancy, obesity, pelvic fracture, coagulopathy, and a history of previous abdominal surgery.[1,2]

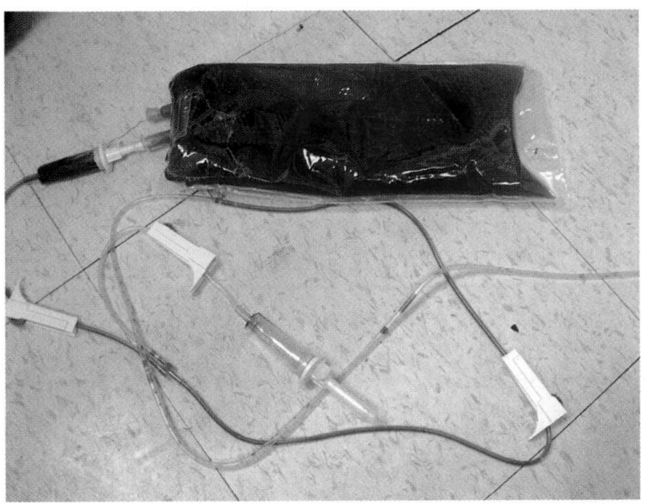

FIGURE 17–41 Positive diagnostic peritoneal lavage. (Courtesy of Mark Silverberg, MD.)

Technique

DPL can be performed "open" or "closed." In the open technique, the urinary bladder and stomach are decompressed. The abdomen is prepared and anesthetized in the infraumbilical region. A vertical midline incision is made, and blunt dissection is carried down through the peritoneum. A peritoneal dialysis catheter is then inserted into the peritoneal cavity and aspiration is performed, looking for gross blood.[1,3] If 10 mL of blood is obtained, the tap is considered positive; otherwise, 1 L of warm saline is infused through the catheter and drained back out after gentle mixing.[1] This fluid is sent to the laboratory for cell count and analysis. In the closed technique, the catheter is inserted via the Seldinger technique in the same region.[1] A DPL is considered positive if there are greater than 100,000 red blood cells or 500 white blood cells per milliliter after blunt trauma, or 50,000 red blood cells per milliliter after penetrating trauma.[1,3] Evidence of food, fibers, amylase, or bile also represents a positive DPL result.[3]

Clinical Complications

Complications include iatrogenic vascular injury, bowel perforation, peritonitis, bladder perforation, and wound infection.[1]

REFERENCES

1. American College of Surgeons Committee on Trauma. *Advanced trauma life support for doctors.* Chicago: American College of Surgeons, 1997.
2. Feied CF. Diagnostic peritoneal lavage: questions and answers. *Postgrad Med* 1989;85:40–45, 49.
3. Feliciano DV. Diagnostic modalities in abdominal trauma: peritoneal lavage, ultrasonography, computed tomography scanning, and arteriography. *Surg Clin North Am* 1991;71:241–256.

Focused Abdominal Sonography in Trauma

Kelly Johnson-Arbor

Indications

Focused abdominal sonography in trauma, known as the FAST scan, is an ultrasound procedure that is used to detect free fluid within the abdomens of trauma patients.[1]

Indications for FAST scan include all cases of suspected intraabdominal injury after trauma. It is especially useful for patients who are hemodynamically unstable or have mental status changes or spinal cord injuries, who may not appropriately be sent for computed tomographic scanning.[2] Unlike diagnostic peritoneal lavage, FAST scan can be used for patients who have had previous abdominal surgeries, are pregnant, or are coagulopathic.[3]

Contraindications

Relative contraindications to FAST scan include obesity and the presence of ascites or subcutaneous air.[3] There are no absolute contraindications.

Technique

The sonographer first looks at the right upper quadrant (Morison's pouch), the most dependent region of the abdominal cavity, to see whether fluid has collected there. Next, the left upper quadrant is scanned, to look for fluid in the subphrenic and perisplenic areas.[2,3] The final location to be scanned is the pelvis; the bladder is used as an acoustic window. The patient's bladder should be full for the examination; if it has been drained by a Foley catheter, then saline should be instilled into the bladder and the catheter clamped to facilitate the examination.[1,2] A subxiphoid view usually is added to these other views to detect a traumatic pericardial effusion.[2] If blood is found in any of these sites, there is no correlation between the location of free fluid and the actual injury.[2] Patients with a positive FAST scan should be presumed to have hemoperitoneum and should undergo abdominal surgical exploration. On the other hand, individuals with a negative FAST scan but a high clinical suspicion of injury may need additional testing, such as computed tomography.[1]

Clinical Complications

The FAST scan has no known complications, assuming that it does not delay further necessary evaluations.[3]

REFERENCES

1. McGahan JP, Richards J, Gillen M. The focused abdominal sonography for trauma scan: pearls and pitfalls. *J Ultrasound Med* 2002;21:789–800.
2. McKenney KL. Ultrasound of blunt abdominal trauma. *Radiol Clin North Am* 1999;37:879–893.
3. Nordenholz KE, Rubin MA, Gularte GG, Liang HK. Ultrasound in the evaluation and management of blunt abdominal trauma. *Ann Emerg Med* 1997;29:357–366.

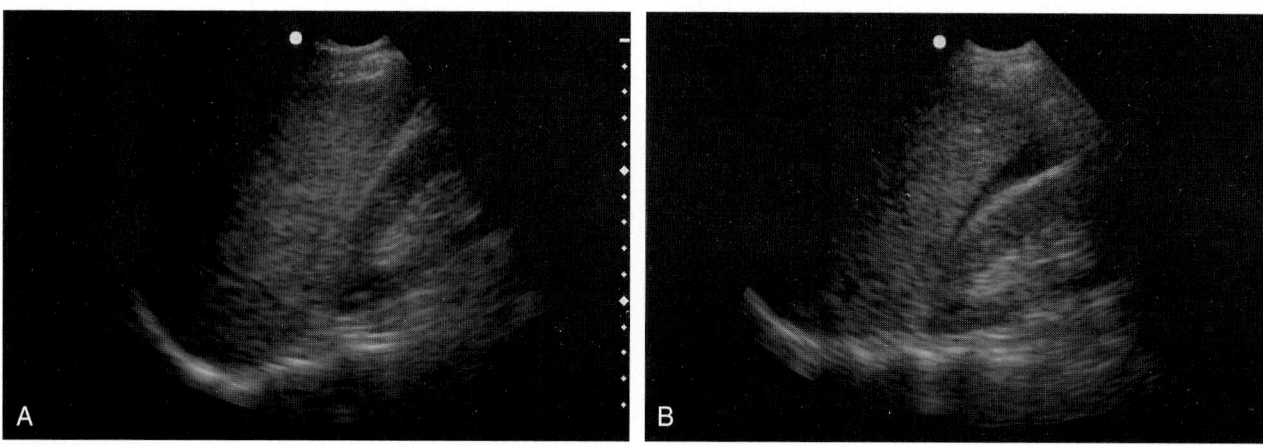

FIGURE 17–42 **A:** Normal right upper quadrant sonogram. (Courtesy of Alfredo Sabbaj, MD.) **B:** Right upper quadrant sonogram with blood in the hepatorenal space. (Courtesy of Alfredo Sabbaj, MD.)

Focused Abdominal Sonography in Trauma

Kelly Johnson-Arbor

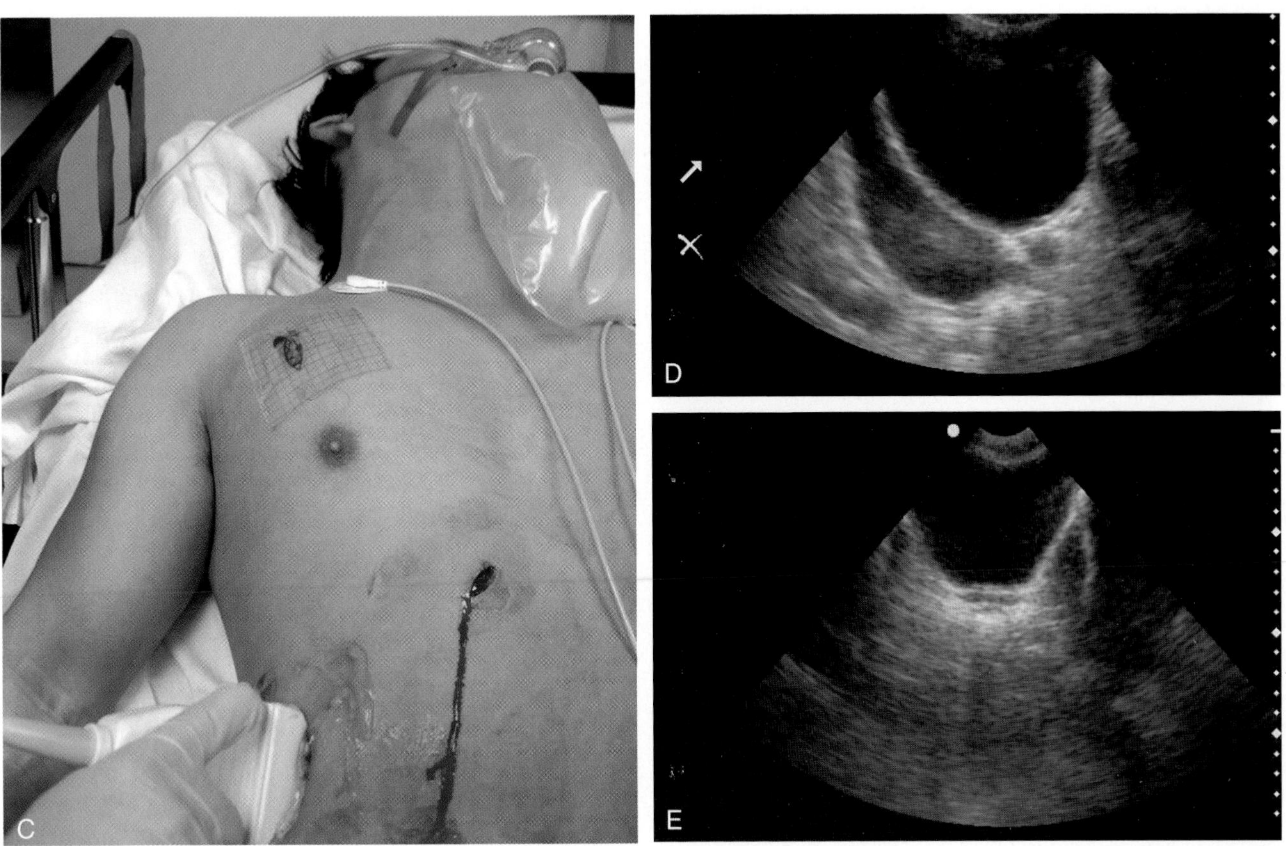

FIGURE 17–42, cont'd. **C:** A focused abdominal sonography in trauma (FAST) scan being performed in the setting of penetrating chest and abdominal trauma. (Courtesy of Mark Silverberg, MD.) **D:** Pelvic blood posterior to the bladder in a sagittal suprapubic ultrasound image. (Courtesy of Alfredo Sabbaj, MD.) **E:** The bow-tie sign: pelvic blood lateral to the bladder in the transverse suprapubic ultrasound view. (Courtesy of Alfredo Sabbaj, MD.)

Diaphragmatic Rupture

George Lin

Clinical Presentation

Presenting symptoms of diaphragmatic rupture vary depending on the size of the defect and coexisting injuries. Patients with large diaphragmatic injuries may present with shortness of breath or chest/abdominal pain, as the abdominal contents herniate into the pleural space. Others may be asymptomatic or complain of only vague abdominal discomfort.[1–3]

Pathophysiology

Diaphragmatic rupture after blunt trauma has an incidence of 1% to 3%.[2] It occurs as force applied to the abdomen increases intraperitoneal pressure. With sufficient force, the diaphragm ruptures, usually on the left side; the liver tends to protect the right hemidiaphragm by absorbing some of the energy.[2,3] Penetrating trauma usually produces small defects in the diaphragm, making large herniation less likely.[2]

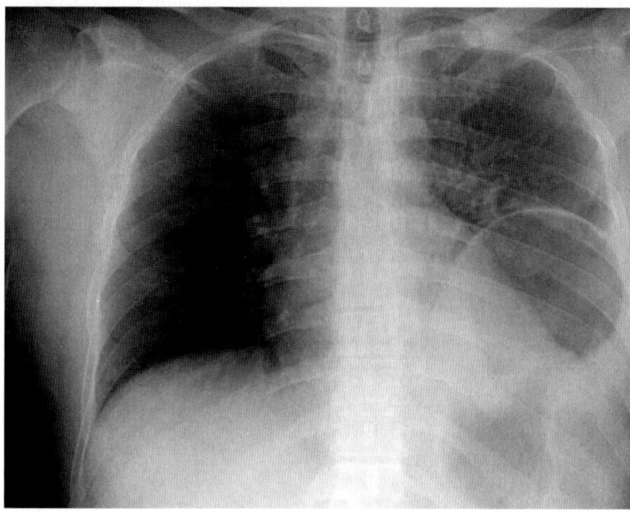

FIGURE 17–43 Rupture of left leaf of diaphragm. (Courtesy of Mark Silverberg, MD.)

Diagnosis

Physical examination is not very reliable, and clinicians must maintain a high index of suspicion in the setting of abdominal trauma.[3] Findings may include decreased breath sounds, bowel sounds in the chest, diminished bowel sounds, abdominal distention, or unstable vital signs.[2,3] Chest radiographs may reveal asymmetric hemidiaphragms, hollow abdominal viscera in the thoracic cavity, or visualization of the nasogastric tube in the thorax, but chest radiographs are often nondiagnostic.[1–3] Computed tomography may show herniated abdominal organs or omental fat in a diaphragmatic defect, but these findings are nonspecific.[1,3] Magnetic resonance imaging can provide accurate recognition of diaphragmatic defects and visceral herniation, but it may not be practical in patients with multiple trauma.[3]

Clinical Complications

Complications include viscerothorax, bowel strangulation, intestinal obstruction, and hemothorax/pneumothorax.[2,3]

Management

Advanced trauma life support (ATLS) protocols should be followed. Trauma surgery consultation is indicated for eventual surgical repair of the injured diaphragm.[2] Nasogastric tube placement allows decompression of the stomach and may help diagnose the injury.[2,3]

REFERENCES

1. Ball T, McCrory R, Smith JO, Clements JL Jr. Traumatic diaphragmatic hernia: errors in diagnosis. *AJR Am J Roentgenol* 1982;138:633–637.
2. Murray JA, Demetriades D, Cornwell EE 3rd, et al. Penetrating left thoracoabdominal trauma: the incidence and clinical presentation of diaphragm injuries. *J Trauma* 1997;43:624–626.
3. Reiff DA, McGwin G, Metzher J, et al. Identifying injuries and motor vehicle collision characteristics that together are suggestive of diaphragmatic rupture. *J Trauma* 2002;53:1139–1145.

Seatbelt Sign

Taura Blyth

Clinical Presentation

Patients with seatbelt sign (SBS) present after a motor vehicle crash with abrasions, redness, ecchymosis, and tenderness across the anterior or lateral neck, chest, or lower abdomen, corresponding to the shoulder or lap strap of their seatbelt.[1] Other associated injuries may be present.

Pathophysiology

Seatbelts are associated with specific patterns of injury when the patient's body is forcibly thrown against their restraints during a motor vehicle collision.[1] The SBS itself is a contusion or abrasion of the skin, caused by rubbing of the seatbelt or deceleration of the body it is restraining.

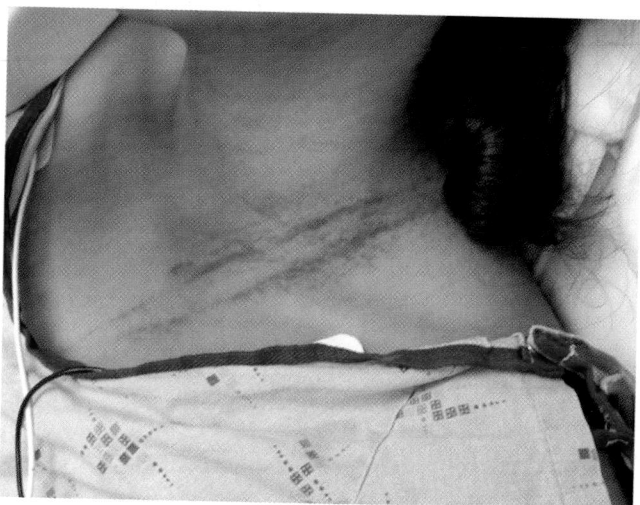

FIGURE 17–44 "Seat belt sign" seen as a patterned hematoma/abrasion of the left side of the neck. (Courtesy of Robert Hendrickson, MD.)

Diagnosis

The diagnosis of SBS is made by history and physical examination, although underlying vascular, thoracic, or intraabdominal injuries require a more extensive investigation.

Clinical Complications

Complications related to an abdominal SBS include bowel contusion or perforation, tears of the mesentery, lumbar spine fractures, diaphragmatic rupture, and, rarely, abdominal aortic dissection.[1] Injuries related to an SBS of the neck include local vascular (carotid) injury, cerebral ischemia, and cervical spine injury. These are of special concern in improperly restrained children 4 to 9 years of age.[2] Sternal and rib fractures are the most common thoracic injury related to the seatbelt.[1]

Management

Treatment should be guided by the patient's clinical condition and the presence of other injuries. Patients with severe SBS have been managed conservatively with good outcomes, whereas others with minor SBS have required laparotomy and extensive bowel resection.[1] Therefore, the severity of the mark itself does not correlate with the extent of injury. Any SBS should be used as a reminder to the physician that significant neck, chest, or abdominal pathology may exist.

REFERENCES

1. Velmahos GC, Tatevossian R, Demetriades D. The "seat belt mark" sign: a call for increased vigilance among physicians treating victims of motor vehicle accidents. *Am Surg* 1999;65:181–185.
2. Rozycki GS, Tremblay L, Feliciano DV, et al. A prospective study for the detection of vascular injury in adult and pediatric patients with cervicothoracic seat belt signs. *J Trauma* 2002;52:618–624.

17-45

Bicycle Handlebar Injuries

Gregory P. Conners

Clinical Presentation

Patients with bicycle handlebar injuries may present with pain after a fall from a bicycle; however, symptoms may be delayed as swelling and/or blood loss in the abdomen or pelvis progress. Clinical findings such as abdominal pain and tenderness, circular erythema or bruising, and abdominal wall hematoma may be present.[1-3]

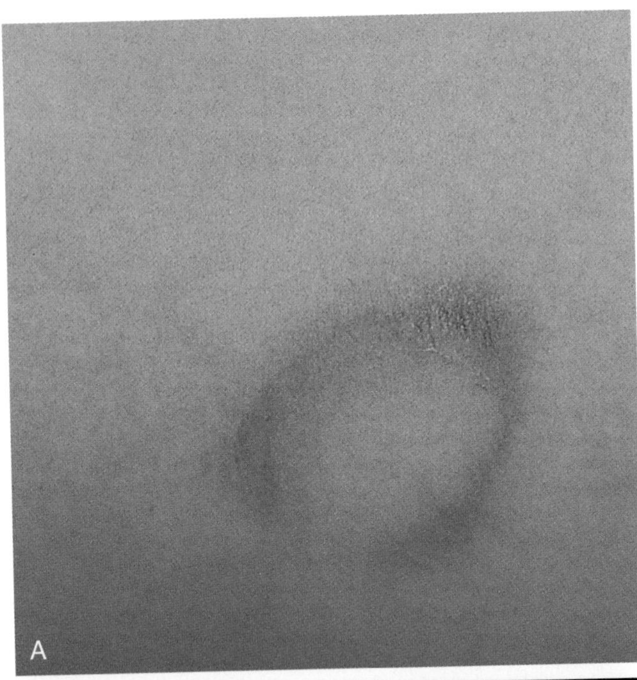

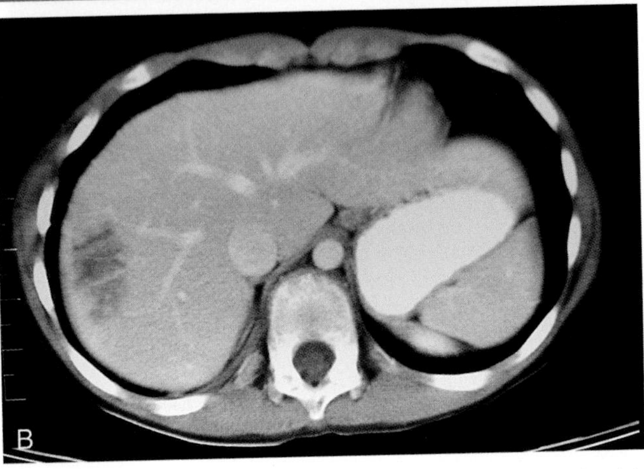

FIGURE 17-45 This 10-year-old boy fell while riding his bicycle, landing on top of the handlebars. Although he sustained only a small cutaneous bruise **(A)**, one must be concerned about an impact that is very focused in nature. In fact, the computed tomography scan **(B)** showed a significant hepatic contusion. (From Fleischer, *Atlas*, with permission.)

Pathophysiology

The bicycle's front wheel twists sharply as the rider moves forward, causing the rider's abdomen to strike the end of the handlebar. Bicycle handlebar injuries result from relatively low-energy falls, and they occur more commonly in children.[1-3]

Diagnosis

Injuries may remain occult as symptoms may develop late, and the presence of abdominal tenderness may not reliably indicate underlying injury.[1] Abdominal/pelvic computed tomographic scans and observation are frequently necessary to fully delineate or rule out serious underlying injury. Blood in the urine or abnormal levels of liver or pancreatic enzymes are also suggestive of underlying injury.[1-3]

Clinical Complications

Along with external bruising (not always present), injuries to almost all major internal organs of the abdomen and pelvis have been reported, with liver and spleen injuries being most common. Other reported injuries include abdominal wall herniation and rupture, abdominal aortic rupture, common bile duct transection, genital injury, traumatic major arterial occlusion, and death.[1-3]

Management

Once injuries have been identified, individual treatment depends on diagnosis.

REFERENCES

1. Winston FK, Shaw KN, Kreshak AA, et al. Hidden spears: handlebars as injury hazards to children. *Pediatrics* 1998;102:596–601.
2. Winston FK, Weiss HB, Nance ML, et al. Estimates of the incidence and costs associated with handlebar-related injuries in children. *Arch Pediatr Adolesc Med* 2002;156:922–928.
3. Erez I, Lazar L, Gutermacher M, Katz S. Abdominal injuries caused by bicycle handlebars. *Eur J Surg* 2001;167:331–333.

Perineal Hematoma

Timothy Lum

Clinical Presentation

Patients with perineal hematoma present complaining of pain in the perineal region after blunt or penetrating trauma.[1,2]

Pathophysiology

Because of the relatively concealed location of the perineum, it is an unusual site for injury. Perineal hematomas may occur after blunt (straddle) or penetrating trauma, after sexual assault, or in association with pelvic fractures if blood tracks down through the fascial planes.[2]

Diagnosis

A perineal hematoma can be diagnosed clinically on physical examination after a history of trauma to the region. Findings of erythema, edema, and hematoma of the perineum are concerning for urethral injury and pelvic fractures.[1] Gross hematuria or blood at the urethral meatus should raise suspicions even higher.[1] It is also imperative to explore for concomitant rectal injuries. In these patients, radiologic imaging is essential to evaluate for pelvic fractures, which may not be apparent on physical examination.[1,2] If a pelvic fracture is confirmed radiologically in a male patient with a perineal hematoma, or if there is blood at the urethral meatus, a retrograde urethrogram should be performed before a Foley catheter is placed.[1] Cystoscopy is indicated for persistent voiding difficulties or nonclearing hematuria.[1]

Clinical Complications

The worst complications of perineal trauma are uncontrolled hemorrhage, hypotension/hemorrhagic shock, and death. There may also be extension of the hematoma, urinary tract infection, dyspareunia, voiding difficulties, and associated urethral and pelvic injuries.[1,2]

Management

Advanced trauma life support (ATLS) protocols should be followed. A perineal hematoma that is associated with a penetrating vaginal laceration or difficulty obtaining hemostasis requires further exploration to ensure that the pelvic floor has not been penetrated.[2] These patients usually require operative repair.[2] Surgical (urologic or gynecologic) consultation is indicated if there are associated urethral, bladder, or renal injuries. If there are no other associated injuries, application of ice and oral analgesics may suffice. Female patients with perineal hematoma should be referred to a gynecologist for follow-up evaluation.[2]

REFERENCES

1. Brandes S, Borrelli J Jr. Pelvic fracture and associated urologic injuries. *World J Surg* 2001;25:1578–1587.
2. Dreitlein DA, Suner S, Basler J. Genitourinary trauma. *Emerg Med Clin North Am* 2001;19:569–590.

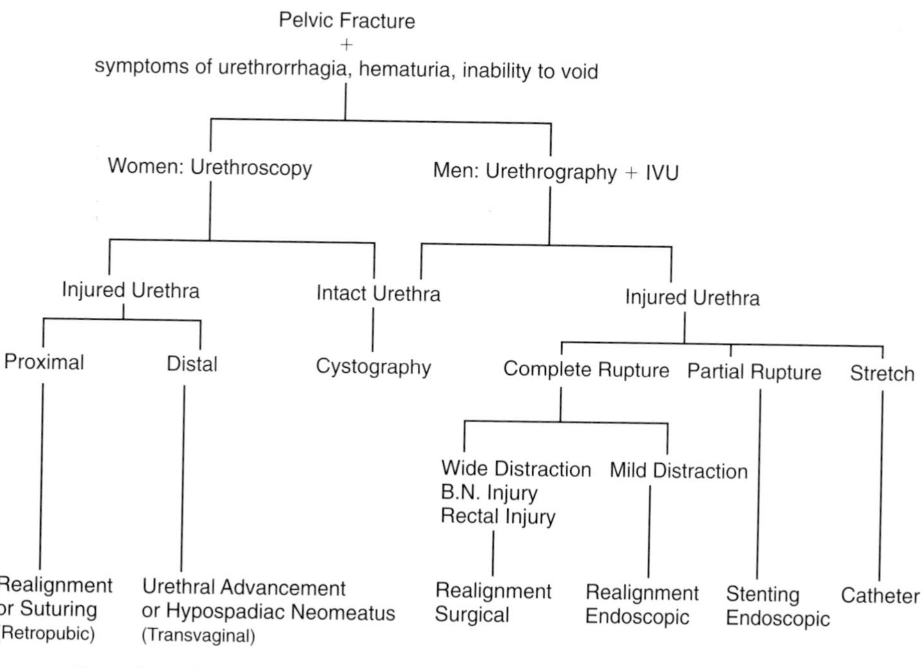

FIGURE 17–46 Treatment plan for pelvic-fracture urethral injuries. (Adapted from Koraitim MM. Pelvic fracture urethral injuries: the unresolved controversy. *J Urol* 1999;161:443–1441, used with permission.)

17–47

Urethral Rupture

Timothy Lum

Clinical Presentation

Patients with urethral rupture present after pelvic injury. Because of the short length and relative mobility of the female urethra, urethral injuries are uncommon in women. They should be suspected if the vaginal examination reveals a hematoma around the urethra or urine leakage into the vagina.[1]

Pathophysiology

Urethral injuries are generally categorized as posterior or anterior.[2] Posterior urethral injuries usually are associated with pelvic fractures, most often resulting from high-energy trauma such as a motor vehicle collision or fall from height.[2] When the pelvis fractures, shearing forces applied to the puboprostatic ligaments separate the prostate from the urogenital diaphragm and tear the bulbous urethra.[1] Pure anterior urethral disruptions usually are straddle injuries.[2]

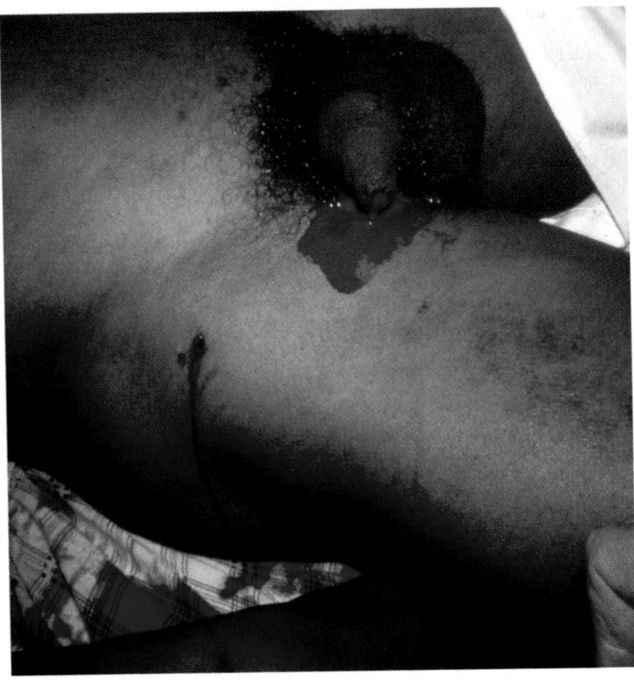

FIGURE 17–47 Gross blood seen at the urethral meatus. (Copyright James R. Roberts, MD.)

Diagnosis

Urethral rupture should be suspected if the triad of blood at the urethral meatus, inability to pass urine, and a distended bladder is present.[2] Scrotal hematoma, a characteristic butterfly-pattern bruising of the perineum, and a high-riding or "boggy" prostate are also common physical examination findings associated with pelvic fractures and urethral injuries.[2] If these signs are found, a retrograde urethrogram (RUG) should be performed before a Foley catheter is inserted, to confirm the diagnosis. In a complete posterior urethral rupture, the RUG demonstrates extensive extravasation of contrast material, both above and below the urogenital diaphragm.[1] An incomplete tear manifests as dye extravasation with partial filling of the bladder.[1] Anterior urethral injuries can be confirmed by RUG, as can injuries to the female urethra.

Clinical Complications

Infection, urethral stricture, incontinence, and impotence may complicate urethral rupture.[2]

Management

Advanced trauma life support (ATLS) protocols should be followed, with mandatory urologic consultation. Urology staff should provide adequate drainage of the bladder with a suprapubic catheter, admission for intravenous antibiotics, and surgical repair with urethral realignment if necessary.[2]

REFERENCES

1. Watnik NF, Coburn M, Goldberger M. Urologic injuries in pelvic ring disruptions. *Clin Orthop* 1996;(329):37–45.
2. Chapple CR, Png D. Contemporary management of urethral trauma and the post-traumatic stricture. *Curr Opin Urol* 1999;9:253–260.

"Open-Book" Pelvic Fracture

Timothy Lum

Clinical Presentation

Open-book pelvic fractures are caused by high-energy injuries.[1] The patient may arrive in shock with no obvious external hemorrhage.[1,2] Disruption of the symphysis pubis may cause the legs to be splayed open and the pelvis to be mobile to internal or external rotation.[1,2] Gross hematuria, blood at the urethral meatus, and ecchymosis and edema of the perineum, scrotum, or penis are also concerning findings that suggest pelvic trauma.[1,2]

Pathophysiology

An open-book pelvic fracture occurs when one or both hemipelves rotate externally due to disruption of the symphysis pubis or a vertical fracture through the pubic rami.[1] An anteroposterior compression force is applied to the pelvis that usually splits the symphysis pubis and widens the sacroiliac (SI) joint anteriorly. The ipsilateral sacrotuberous and sacrospinous ligaments often are torn. The relatively strong posterior SI ligamentous complex remains intact, giving this injury its "open-book" characteristic.[1,2]

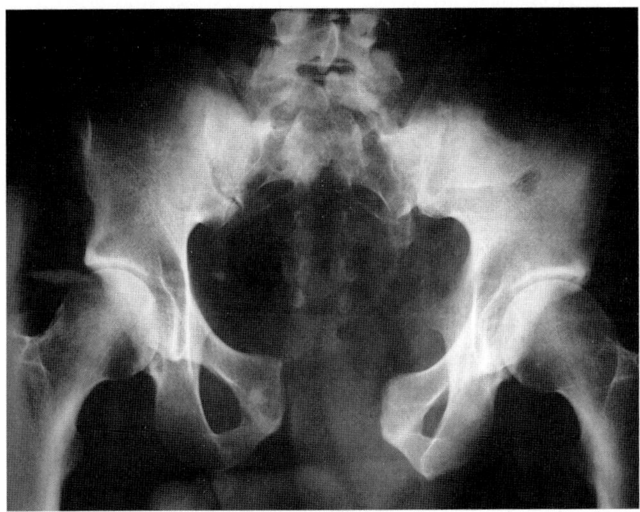

FIGURE 17–48 "Open-book" pelvic fracture. (Courtesy of Mark Silverberg, MD.)

Diagnosis

The diagnosis of this injury pattern can be suspected clinically but should be confirmed radiologically. Additional inlet and outlet pelvic films can reveal the full extent of the fracture configuration.[2] Pelvic computed tomographic scanning may give more details, but it should not delay the advanced trauma life support (ATLS) work-up.[1]

Clinical Complications

These patients often have multiple high-energy injuries and therefore have an excessive mortality rate.[2] Retroperitoneal hemorrhage and hypovolemic shock may result from tears of the sacral plexus as the pelvic bony fragments diverge. Neurologic injuries are also seen.[1]

Management

Emergently, military antishock trousers or an encircling bed sheet may be used to compress and secure the pelvic fragments from moving if orthopedic percutaneous external fixation is not immediately available. Patients with continued fluid requirements and unstable vital signs may require pelvic angiography and embolization.[1]

REFERENCES

1. Burgess AR, Eastridge BJ, Young JW, et al. Pelvic ring disruptions: effective classification system and treatment protocols. *J Trauma* 1990;30:848–856.
2. Starr AJ, Griffin DR, Reinhart CM, et al. Pelvic ring disruptions: prediction of associated injuries, transfusion requirement, pelvic arteriography, complications, and mortality. *J Orthop Trauma* 2002;16: 553–561.

Airbag Injury: Burns

Matthew Spencer

Clinical Presentation

Patients with burn injuries from deployment of an airbag may present with erythema, pain, and blistering at the involved site.[1] Chemical injuries related to airbag deployment usually affect the upper extremities or face, whereas thermal burns are generally located on the hands or forearms.[1]

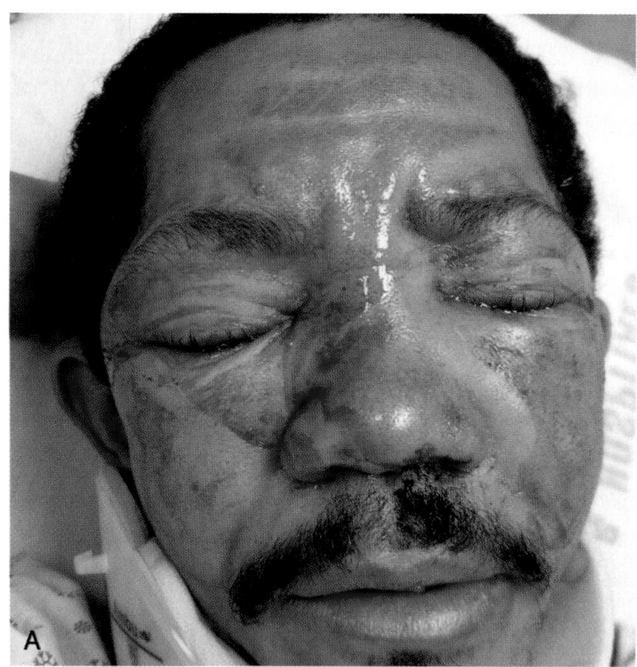

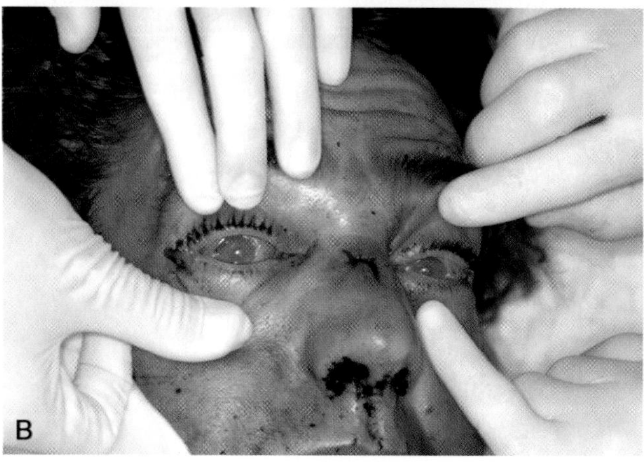

FIGURE 17–49 **A:** Facial airbag burns. (Courtesy of Mark Silverberg, MD.) **B:** Bilateral chemosis and corneal opacification resulting from deployment of an automobile airbag. (© David Effron, MD, 2004. Used with permission.)

Pathophysiology

Airbags are now standard equipment on all new automobiles in the United States.[1,2] Specific airbag-related injuries are sustained by approximately 30% of drivers in cases of airbag deployment; 7.8% of these are cutaneous burns.[1,2] During airbag deployment, sodium azide is ignited, releasing nitrogen gas, carbon dioxide, aerosolized sodium hydroxide, sodium carbonate, and metal oxides into the interior of the vehicle.[1,2] Burns may be caused by the alkaline corrosives that combine with sweat or other liquids on the skin to create a chemical injury, by direct thermal injury from superheated gases or melted clothing, or by friction from the airbag itself.[1,2]

Diagnosis

The diagnosis is made by history and physical examination.

Clinical Complications

Serious complications from dermal airbag-related burns are very unusual; most heal spontaneously without scarring.[1]

Management

Patients should be treated with standard burn therapy, including analgesics, tetanus prophylaxis, cleansing with normal saline, débridement if necessary, and topical antibiotic ointments.[1] If there is ocular involvement, copious saline irrigation and ocular pH monitoring is indicated, as well as ophthalmology consultation.[1,2]

REFERENCES

1. Ulrich D, Noah EM, Fuchs P, Pallua N. Burn injuries caused by air bag deployment. *Burns* 2001;27:196–199.
2. Baruchin AM, Jakim I, Rosenberg L, Nahlieli O. On burn injuries related to airbag deployment. *Burns* 1999;25:49–52.

Crush Injury Syndrome

Kelly Johnson-Arbor

Clinical Presentation

Crush injury syndrome (CIS) may occur in survivors of disasters such as earthquakes, mining accidents, industrial disasters, and bombings.[1,2] Patients who sustain crush injuries may initially appear asymptomatic.[1]

Pathophysiology

CIS results from direct and prolonged compression of muscle.[1] As a physical response to being crushed, the sarcolemmal membrane of the myocyte stretches, becoming more permeable.[1,2] This causes leakage of intracellular contents, including urate, phosphate, myoglobin, and potassium, leading to kidney and cardiac injury.[1,2] Increased cell membrane permeability may allow fluid shifts, leading to hemodynamic instability.[2]

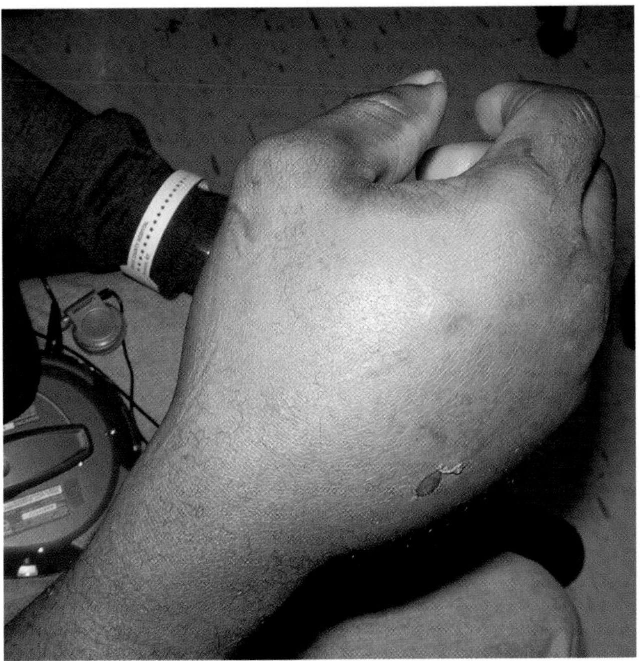

FIGURE 17-50 Crush injury of the right hand. (Courtesy of Mark Silverberg, MD.)

Diagnosis

The diagnosis is based primarily on the history and physical examination. Myoglobinuria and increased creatine kinase (CK) levels may help confirm the diagnosis.[1] Physical examination may reveal multiple ecchymoses, and edema of affected body parts may develop over time.[1] Hemodynamic instability may be present if extrication was prolonged and muscle breakdown has already progressed.[1] CK levels greater than 75,000 U/L correlate well with the development of kidney failure and with higher mortality rates.[2]

Clinical Complications

Hyperkalemia and other electrolyte imbalances, as well as malignant arrhythmias, hypotension, shock, and death may complicate CIS.[1,2] Compartmental syndromes may develop within the involved muscle groups.[1]

Management

Advanced trauma life support (ATLS) protocols should be followed. Volume resuscitation with crystalloid should be initiated before extrication.[1,2] Alkalinization of the urine (pH maintained higher than 6.5) increases the excretion of myoglobin and reduces the risk of renal failure.[1,2] Forced diuresis with large volumes of intravenous fluid and mannitol to prevent nephrotoxicity remains controversial.[1,2] Fasciotomy may be required for the treatment of compartmental syndrome.[2]

REFERENCES

1. Michaelson M. Crush injury and crush syndrome. *World J Surg* 1992;16:899–903.
2. Smith J, Greaves I. Crush injury and crush syndrome: a review. *J Trauma* 2003;54:S226–S230.

Traumatic Extremity Amputation

Michael Greenberg

Clinical Presentation

Patients with traumatic extremity amputation (TEA) present after a major traumatic event with partial or complete removal of the lower extremity, ranging from complete hemipelvic disassociation to leg, ankle, or toe amputations.

Pathophysiology

The mechanism of injury in most traumatic amputations involves extremely high kinetic energy forces applied to single or multiple extremities. These mechanisms may be associated with events such as war wounds, high-speed motor vehicle accidents, plane crashes, animal attacks, building collapses, explosions, industrial accidents, and farming accidents. TEA injuries usually are caused by major crushing or avulsing forces involving an extensive amount of tissue and leaving heavily contaminated wounds with underlying fractures that are often comminuted. These injuries tend to be conducive to life-threatening infections in the postsurgical period. Associated intrathoracic and/or intraabdominal injuries may exist and may be life-threatening in their own right.[1–3]

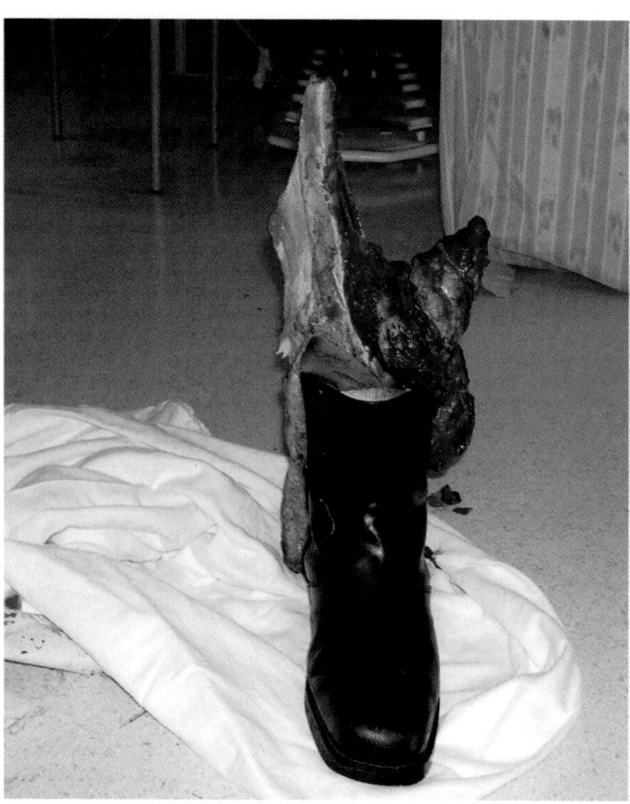

FIGURE 17–51 Traumatic lower-extremity amputation resulting from a motorcycle accident. (© Philip Mead, MD. Used with permission.)

Diagnosis

TEA injuries are straightforward and are usually obvious on examination. An understanding of the mechanism of injury requires consultation with prehospital care personnel.

Clinical Complications

Complications include inability to replant the amputated part, unsuccessful replantation, infection, hypertension, and psychological sequelae such as post-traumatic stress disorder.[1–3]

Management

All TEA injuries should be considered potentially life-threatening, and advanced trauma/cardiac life support (ATLS/ACLS) protocols must be promptly initiated. Resuscitation efforts must be aggressive, and a complete primary and secondary survey must be completed in a timely and efficient fashion. On-site surgical consultation must be obtained as quickly as possible.

Replantation and revascularization often is not indicated, especially if the forces at play resulted in major crushing or avulsing injuries involving an extensive amount of tissue and heavily contaminated wounds.[1–3] Limb shortening after replantation may create more disability than the proper use of postinjury prosthetics, although this fact may not be easily accepted by patients and families in the immediate postinjury period.[1–3]

REFERENCES

1. Tukiainen E, Suominen E, Asko-Seljavaara S. Replantation, revascularization, and reconstruction of both legs after amputations: a case report. *J Bone Joint Surg Am* 1994;76:1712–1716.
2. Dell KM, Kaplan BS. Hypertension with lower extremity traumatic amputation. *Clin Pediatr (Phila)* 2000;39:417–419.
3. Rieger H, Dietl KH. Traumatic hemipelvectomy: an update. *J Trauma* 1998;45:422–426.

Degloving Injury

Sarah Jane Paris

Clinical Presentation

Degloving injuries often result from motor vehicle collisions or industrial mishaps and often involve the upper and lower extremities, face, scalp, or male genitalia; however, any anatomic area may be affected. These injuries commonly occur in association with fractures, thoracic or abdominal trauma, or head injuries.[1,2]

Pathophysiology

Degloving injuries are caused when tangential forces are applied to the skin, causing the integument and subcutaneous tissue to be pulled away from the underlying bone, muscle, and fascia. The skin may be completely detached, leaving a large defect, or it may remain partially connected via remnants of subcutaneous tissue. Frequently, the blood vessels supplying the skin are disrupted and the avulsed skin flap is completely devitalized.[1,2]

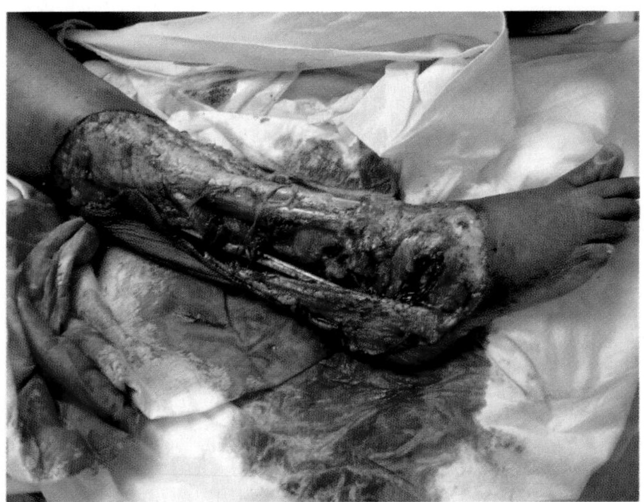

FIGURE 17–52 Extensive full-thickness skin loss. (Courtesy of Chris Doty, MD.)

Diagnosis

Diagnosis of a degloving injury should be obvious from history and simple inspection. However, these injuries may be missed if the patient is not fully undressed to facilitate complete evaluation.

Clinical Complications

Complications may include functional or cosmetic impairment. Because these injuries involve significant disruption of skin integrity and blood supply, infection is an important consideration.[1,2]

Management

Advanced trauma life support (ATLS) protocols should be followed. A trauma surgery evaluation appropriate to the mechanism of injury is warranted. The astute physician should take care not to be distracted by the dramatic nature of the degloving and fail to note other, more immediately life-threatening injuries. Radiographs may be indicated to rule out underlying fractures or retained foreign bodies.[1,2] Degloving defects almost universally require surgical repair after copious irrigation, débridement of devitalized tissues, and, in many cases, skin grafting, although some partially avulsed flaps may be reattached. Broad-spectrum antibiotics and tetanus prophylaxis should be initiated as indicated.[1,2]

REFERENCES

1. Green H, Silvani SH, Scurran BL, Karlin JM. Degloving injuries of the foot: case presentation and review of the literature. *J Am Podiatr Med Assoc* 1988;78:372–375.
2. Kudsk KA, Sheldon GF, Walton RL. Degloving injuries of the extremities and torso. *J Trauma* 1981;21:835–839.

Wringer or Mechanical Roller Injury

Matthew Spencer

Clinical Presentation

Patients with wringer injury present with varying degrees of pain, redness, swelling, and skin or tissue loss after an extremity becomes trapped within a mechanical roller device.[1] Historically, most of these injuries were caused by entrapment of the extremity within the rollers of a washing machine with an attached wringer device. However, with the advent of electric dryers, wringer injury has all but disappeared; it has been replaced by injuries from industrial machinery utilizing rollers.[1,2]

Pathophysiology

Wringer injuries are extremity traumatic injuries that usually involve the upper extremities. Wringer injuries were more common in the 1920s and have decreased in frequency as wringer washers have been slowly replaced. However, in some poorer areas, wringer washing machines are still in use.[1,2] Children were the most frequent victims of washing machine wringer injuries.[1] Thermal, compressive, and shearing injury results as the upper extremity is caught and ground by the moving rollers. A friction burn, the most common resulting injury, is usually located wherever the rollers become stuck, typically the antecubital fossa. However, the arm may be drawn into the device as far as the axillae. Burns vary in severity from mild to full-thickness.[1] Injuries can be grouped as hand/wrist, forearm/elbow, and arm/axilla but may encompass all these regions. Most injuries involve the soft tissue; however, approximately 6% of patients have underlying fractures.[2]

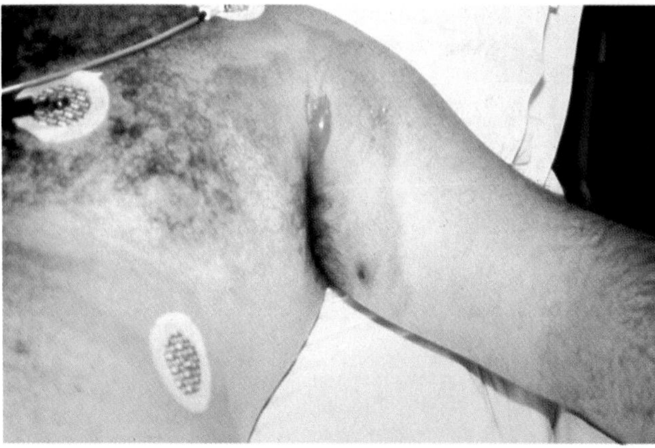

FIGURE 17–53 Axillary injury secondary to mechanical roller trauma. (Courtesy of Michael Greenberg, MD.)

Diagnosis

The diagnosis is made by history and physical examination in the applicable clinical setting.

Clinical Complications

Complications include skin loss, nerve and tendon injury, amputations, Volkman's ischemic contracture, and vascular occlusion.[1]

Management

Treatment requires adequate analgesia, appropriate wound care, tetanus prophylaxis, radiographs, reduction and splinting of any fractures, and elevation of the involved extremity.[1] Compartmental pressures should be checked regularly if a compartmental syndrome is suspected.[1] Wringer injuries should be managed in conjunction with a hand or orthopedic surgeon or burn care specialist, because skin grafting may be required. Compressive dressings have been recommended in the past but are controversial and should be applied only if the consultant agrees.[1] Nonelastic compressive dressings are preferable.[1] Although wringer injuries may appear initially to be benign, severe swelling may develop over time. Underlying injuries are easily missed. Consequently, all patients with wringer/roller injuries should be hospitalized for at least 24 hours for observation and monitoring.

REFERENCES

1. Proust AF. Special injuries of the hand. *Emerg Med Clin North Am* 1993;11:767–779.
2. Weinshel S, Greydanus W, Glicklich M. Wringer washing machine injuries: criteria for obtaining radiological studies. *J Trauma* 1986; 26:1132–1133.

Digital Ring Injury

Matthew Spencer

Clinical Presentation

Patients with digital ring injury present with pain to the involved digit after trauma. Often there is a laceration, swelling, or avulsion of tissue ranging from a simple circular abrasion to degloving to complete amputation. Burns may occur if the ring is heated, and abrasions may result if the ring is caught and rotated.[1]

Pathophysiology

A digital ring injury results from the traumatic removal of a ring from the finger.[1] These injuries take place when the patient's ring gets caught and pulled from the finger. They are categorized as follows: class I, circulation adequate with or without skeletal injury; class II, circulation inadequate, no skeletal injury; class III, circulation inadequate, fracture or joint injury present; and class IV, complete amputation.[1]

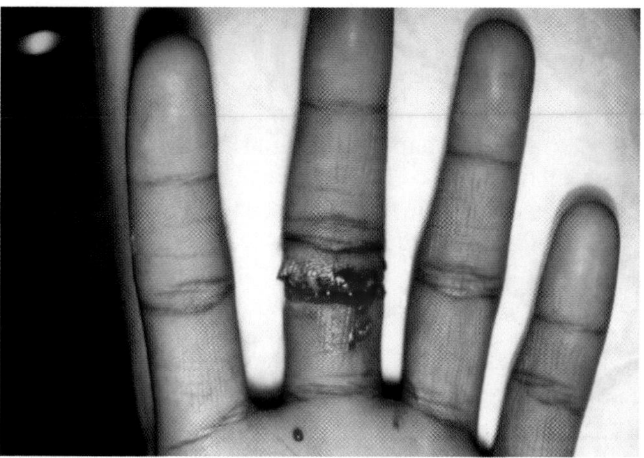

FIGURE 17–54 Injury to third digit secondary to patient's ring being caught on a metal basketball rim. (Courtesy of Michael Greenberg, MD.)

Diagnosis

The diagnosis is clinical, with the classification depending on the degree of tissue avulsion and the presence of skeletal injury.

Clinical Complications

Complications include scarring, reduced range of motion, infection, cold intolerance, reduced sensation, and impaired vascularity resulting in loss of the digit.[1]

Management

The treatment of a digital ring injury includes wound care, analgesics, antibiotics, radiographs, tetanus, and hand surgery consultation if indicated.[1] If the ring is still present, it should be removed as soon as possible, by means of a ring or wire cutter.[1]

REFERENCES

1. Kay S, Werntz J, Wolff TW. Ring avulsion injuries: classification and prognosis. *J Hand Surg Am* 1989;14:204–213.

Penetrating Hand Injury

Sarah Jane Paris

Clinical Presentation

Patients with penetrating hand injury may present with local pain, disability, and bleeding from an obvious wound. Although most patients present fairly soon after occurrence, there may be a delay in seeking medical attention in the case of certain suspicious injuries.[1,2] Some patients may be reluctant to provide an accurate history if criminal activity, abuse, or violence caused the injury.

Pathophysiology

The extent of injury is determined by the type of object involved and the degree of energy imparted at the time of injury. Blades, low-caliber missiles, and other objects usually inflict only direct damage to those tissues through which they pass. However, high-caliber missiles transmit more energy to the hand and may cause more extensive tissue injury.[2]

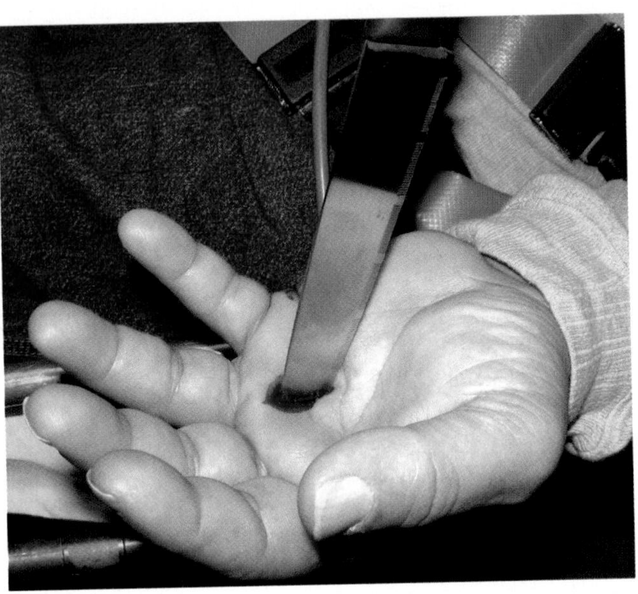

FIGURE 17–55 Penetrating hand injury. (Courtesy of Maime Caton, MD.)

Diagnosis

The diagnosis usually is evident from the history and physical examination. Radiographs may help to delineate the extent of bony injury and to identify retained foreign bodies.[1,2]

Clinical Complications

Complications include loss of function, partial or total amputation, infection, foreign body embolization, and chronic pain.[1,2]

Management

After primary stabilization of the patient, attention can be turned to the hand wound itself. These injuries require meticulous wound care, including copious irrigation, immobilization, tetanus prophylaxis, and antibiotics if indicated. In the case of more extensive structural injury or functional impairment, prompt consultation with appropriate specialists is indicated.[1,2]

REFERENCES

1. Stein F. Foreign body injuries of the hand. *Emerg Med Clin North Am* 1985;3:383–390.
2. Wilson RH. Gunshots to the hand and upper extremity. *Clin Orthop* 2003;(408):133–144.

Plantar Puncture Wound

Sarah Jane Paris

Clinical Presentation

Patients with plantar puncture wound usually report stepping on an object. Complaints may include local pain, inability to bear weight, redness, and swelling. The entry point for the wound may be difficult to appreciate.[1]

Pathophysiology

Wounds are frequently caused by nails; glass, sewing needles, wood splinters, and other objects are also reported.[1,2] If infection occurs, *Staphylococcus aureus, S. epidermidis,* and *Streptococcus* species are common. *Pseudomonas aeruginosa* is frequently implicated in osteomyelitis and is classically associated with a puncture through the sole of a tennis shoe.[1,2]

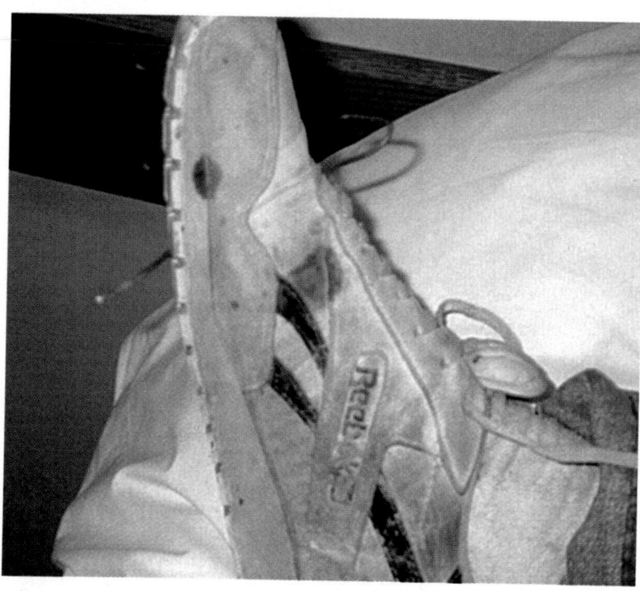

FIGURE 17–56 Penetration of the foot through a rubber-soled sneaker. (From Roberts, with permission.)

Diagnosis

Diagnosis is usually evident from history and physical examination. Signs of infection, evidence of retained foreign bodies, and neurovascular compromise must be carefully sought. Radiographs may help detect foreign bodies or bony injury and should be performed even if radiolucent objects are not suspected.[1,2]

Clinical Complications

Delays in seeking medical care are common and may lead to infection as well as other complications.[1] Approximately 10% of cases become complicated.[1,2] Complications include chronic pain, cellulitis, abscess, osteomyelitis, septic arthritis, and bursitis.[1,2]

Management

Local wound care is essential, and wound exploration is often indicated. Local anesthesia should be provided and the wound scrubbed.[1,2] Foreign bodies should be removed.[1,2] Devitalized or necrotic tissue should be débrided and fluid collections incised and drained. High-pressure irrigation should be performed, taking care not to drive contaminants deeper into the wound.[1,2] Plantar puncture wounds should never be closed primarily, because this predisposes to infection. Tetanus immunization should be updated. Although the role of prophylactic antibiotics remains controversial, secondary infections should be treated with the appropriate antibiotics.[1,2]

REFERENCES

1. Eron LJ. Targeting lurking pathogens in acute traumatic and chronic wounds. *J Emerg Med* 1999;17:189–195.
2. Brook JW. Management of pedal puncture wounds. *J Foot Ankle Surg* 1994;33:463–466.

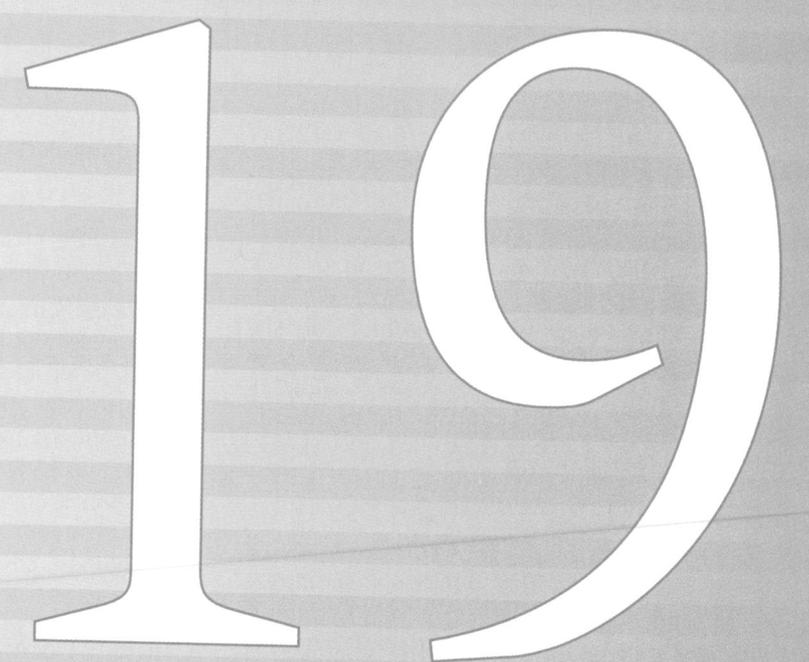

Wound Care

19–1

Cellulitis

Jay Itzkowitz

Clinical Presentation

Patients with cellulitis present with a painful, indurated area of subcutaneous/cutaneous tissue with warm and erythematous overlying skin that may be smooth or even shiny in appearance.[1] Systemic symptoms such as fever, chills, malaise, and headache may be present. If medical care is delayed, the infection may spread in the subcutaneous tissue, resulting in erythematous streaks radiating from the primary lesion.[1,2] Lymphadenitis or lymphadenopathy may be present.[1]

Pathophysiology

Staphylococcus aureus and group A β-hemolytic *Streptococcus* species are the two most common causative pathogens.[1,2] In the prevaccine era, *Haemophilus influenzae* was also routinely seen. Cellulitis usually results from local wound infection, but it may also originate from extension of underlying infections or hematogenous seeding from a distant source.[1] The primary lesion may be a puncture wound, laceration, abrasion, or insect bite, and it still may be visible at presentation.

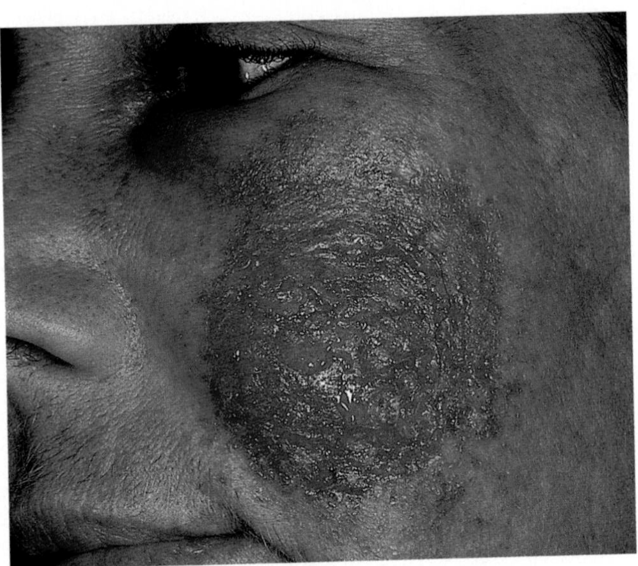

FIGURE 19–1 Cellulitis resulting from squeezing of a pimple on the cheek. (From Ostler, with permission.)

Diagnosis

Cellulitis is a clinical diagnosis. Identification of causative organisms by Gram staining or wound cultures may prove helpful for cases in which unusual microbes are suspected (e.g., immunocompromised patient, inadequate therapeutic response despite antibiotic therapy).[1] If systemic symptoms are present, blood cultures may also be positive. Laboratory testing may reveal an elevated white blood cell count. Radiographs of the area should be taken if there is a possibility of an underlying foreign body, fracture, suspicion of subcutaneous gas, or osteomyelitis.

Clinical Complications

Complications include local abscess formation, osteomyelitis, and gangrene. If left untreated, cellulitis may lead to sepsis or even death.[2]

Management

Patients who have no systemic symptoms may be treated on an outpatient basis, with the local application of moist, warm compresses every 2 hours for 10 to 15 minutes each time. Oral antibiotics may be appropriate in some cases, depending on the source of the cellulitis (e.g., cat bite), the location of the cellulitis (e.g., the area of the face draining to the cavernous sinus), and the patient's underlying medical condition (e.g., immunocompromised, diabetes mellitus).[1] Patients with signs of systemic toxicity or immunocompromise should be admitted for parenteral antibiotics. The antibiotics chosen should include empiric coverage against *S. aureus* and *Streptococcus*.[1,2]

REFERENCES

1. Bhumbra NA, McCullough SG. Skin and subcutaneous infections. *Prim Care* 2003;30:1–24.
2. Sadick NS. Current aspects of bacterial infections of the skin. *Dermatol Clin* 1997;15:341–349.

Surgical Wound Dehiscence

Michael Greenberg

Clinical Presentation

Patients with surgical wound dehiscence (SWD) may present to the emergency department (ED) after surgery with overly aggressive discharge from the hospital or after outpatient surgical procedures.[1,2] Superficial fascial dehiscence of abdominal incisions usually occurs early in the postoperative period, typically between days 3 and 7. However, patients may not recognize that separation of their wound has occurred until much later. Deep abdominal dehiscence may go unrecognized by the patient until increasing pain, fever, nausea, vomiting, or signs of local or systemic infection develop.[1,2]

Pathophysiology

Superficial wound separation usually reflects the formation of subcutaneous hematoma or seroma accumulation, as well as the development of local wound infection. True wound dehiscence involves postoperative separation of the abdominal muscular-aponeurotic layers.[2] Deep dehiscence occurs less frequently than superficial separations, but it is associated with death rates as high as 24%.[1] The type of incision (transverse versus midline) does not seem to influence the rate of dehiscence.[2]

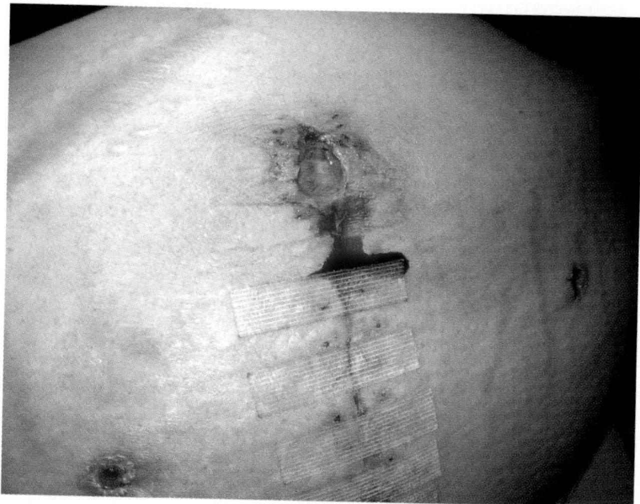

FIGURE 19–2 Surgical wound dehiscence. (Courtesy of Lorenzo Paladino, MD.)

Diagnosis

SWD usually is easily diagnosed, based on direct examination. The most frequent signs of SWD are evident in the first 72 hours after surgery and manifest with the development of serous discharge from the wound with a surrounding area of redness and tenderness.[2] Leakage of peritoneal fluid or a purulent discharge from the wound are signs of possible impending dehiscence.[2]

Clinical Complications

Failure to recognize SWD and inappropriate discharge from the emergency department (ED) may increase the death rate.[1,2] SWD increases the risk for sepsis.

Management

The operating surgeon or a surrogate should be notified as soon as possible once the stability of the patient is ensured. Most patients require hospitalization, because delayed reclosure of the disrupted wound is the preferred approach for patients with SWD.[2] In the ED, SWDs should be cleansed and covered with a moist sterile dressing. Antibiotics should be administered in the ED, in consultation with the admitting surgeon.

REFERENCES

1. Madsen G, Fischer L, Wara P. Burst abdomen: clinical features and factors influence mortality. *Dan Med Bull* 1992;39:183–185.
2. Cliby WA. Abdominal incision wound breakdown. *Clin Obstet Gynecol* 2002;45:507–517.

Human Bites

Michael Greenberg

Clinical Presentation

Patients with human bites present with obvious injury inflicted by a bite. Patients may withhold the cause of the injury if the bite wound resulted from a fight, domestic abuse, or criminal activity. Patients who have been bitten may not present acutely because of embarrassment or because of possible legal or criminal implications. Patients who delay seeking medical care may present with clinical complications. Bite wounds to pediatric patients may be indicative of child abuse.

Pathophysiology

Human bites are extraordinarily common, with a reported incidence as high as 1 human bite for every 600 pediatric emergency department visits.[1] Males are usually bitten on the hand, arm, or shoulder, whereas females are most frequently bitten on the breast, genitalia, leg, or arm.[1] The reported rate of infection for human bites varies widely. However, human bites reportedly have a higher incidence of infection than do dog or cat bites.[1] *Staphylococcus aureus* and *Streptococcus* species are the most common organisms cultured from human-bite wound infections. Anaerobes including *Eikenella, Serratia, Proteus,* and *Enterobacter* are not uncommon. Clenched-fist injuries ("fight bites") are especially prone to infection.

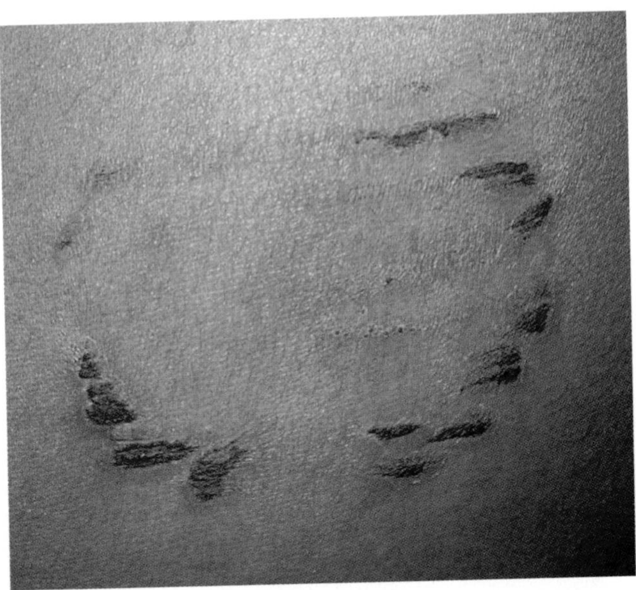

FIGURE 19–3 A 2-day-old bite on a young girl's back. (Courtesy of Mark Silverberg, MD.)

Diagnosis

Diagnosis is based on history and physical examination.

Clinical Complications

Complications may be the presenting complaint and may include deep structure injury (nerve, vessels, tendons, joints), retained teeth in the wound, spread of infectious diseases (e.g., human immunodeficiency virus, hepatitis B or C, herpes simplex, tuberculosis, tetanus, syphilis), cellulitis, lymphangitis, abscess, osteomyelitis, septic arthritis, and tenosynovitis.[1,2]

Management

Careful examination to rule out deep structure injuries is essential. Wounds should be infiltrated with local anesthetic, then scrubbed vigorously and irrigated copiously. Some wounds require surgical exploration to determine deep structure injury or retained foreign bodies. Some wounds require soft-tissue radiographic evaluation to rule out fracture or retained foreign body. Bite wounds of the hand and other sites require splinting in plaster or bulky dressings and strict elevation. Patients with probable joint violation or deep structure violation should be hospitalized and hand/plastic surgery consulted. Prophylactic antibiotics and tetanus prophylaxis should be considered in all cases. Delayed primary closure is preferred to primary closure for most bites. However, primary closure may be appropriate for some facial wounds.

REFERENCES

1. Pretty IA, Anderson GS, Sweet DJ. Human bites and the risk of human immunodeficiency virus transmission. *Am J Forensic Med Pathol* 1999;20:232–239.
2. Wenert P, Heiss J, Rinecker H, Sing A. A human bite. *Lancet* 1999; 354:572.

Dog and Cat Bites

Christy Salvaggio

Clinical Presentation

Patients with dog or cat bites may present immediately, many hours after, or days after the bite. Patients may present with lacerations, abrasions, or puncture wounds typically located on the extremities, although facial and truncal bites do occur.[1,2]

Pathophysiology

Cats inflict puncture wounds from long, thin teeth that are capable of injecting bacteria deeply into tissues or joint spaces. Dogs have broader teeth that tend to rip and crush tissue more extensively.[2] These infections are commonly polymicrobial and include *Pasteurella* species, staphylococci, streptococci, *Moraxella, Corynebacterium,* and *Neisseria.*[1]

Diagnosis

Diagnosis is made by history and physical examination. Signs of wound infection may develop within 12 hours for cat bites and 24 hours for dog bites.[1] Infection may develop in 1% to 30% of patients with dog bites and 25% to 50% of those with cat bites.[2] Wound infections typically produce erythema, edema, warmth, pain, and tenderness.

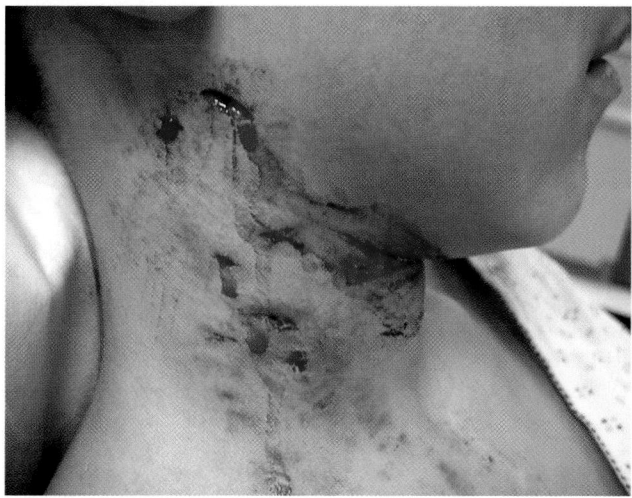

FIGURE 19–4 Dog bite to the neck. (Courtesy of Christy Salvaggio, MD.)

Clinical Complications

Complications of bites include damage to underlying structures, infection, local abscess, lymphangitis, lymphadenitis, septic arthritis, osteomyelitis, tenosynovitis, and systemic infection. In unusual circumstances, if vital anatomic structures have been violated, substantial disability and even death may result.

Management

Lacerations should be copiously irrigated. Wounds with extensive tissue damage and those with joint or tendon involvement may warrant more extensive intraoperative irrigation and débridement.[2] Primary closure of bite wounds predisposes to infection. However, primary closure may be appropriate for some facial lacerations. All bite wounds should be elevated and, if on an extremity, splinted. The role of prophylactic antibiotics in dog bites is controversial. High-risk patients (e.g., immunocompromised patients, diabetics, transplant recipients), wounds in high-risk regions (e.g., hand, foot, perineum), and wounds with extensive tissue damage warrant a 3- to 5-day course of antibiotics, such as empiric amoxicillin/clavulanate or penicillin with cephazolin, or clindamycin with ciprofloxacin.[1,2] A lower threshold for prophylaxis applies to cat bites, given their higher infection rate. Follow-up within 24 to 48 hours is essential. The need for tetanus and/or rabies prophylaxis must be addressed.

Gram stain and culture (aerobic and anaerobic) results should be obtained if appropriate, and treatment with amoxicillin/clavulanate initiated. Patients with lymphangitis, joint or tendon involvement, or systemic signs of infection should be hospitalized for intravenous antibiotic therapy, the first dose of which should be administered in the emergency department.

REFERENCES

1. Talan DA, Citron DM, Abrahamian FM, et al. Bacteriologic analysis of infected dog and cat bites. *N Engl J Med* 1999;340:85–92.
2. Capellan O, Hollander JE. Management of lacerations in the emergency department. *Emerg Med Clin North Am* 2003;21:205–231.

19–5

Lymphangitis

Michael Greenberg

Clinical Presentation

Patients with lymphangitis present with local pain, redness, red "streaks," and swelling, usually at the site of an initial rent in the skin caused by an abrasion, laceration, or bite wound. In some cases, fever and chills are present.[1,2]

Pathophysiology

Group A β-hemolytic streptococcal organisms (GABHS) are common causes of lymphangitis. These bacteria produce various fibrinolysins, as well as hyaluronidase. These chemicals facilitate the invasion of lymphatic channels and consequent rapid spread of infection. *Staphylococcus aureus, Pseudomonas* species, *Pasteurella multocida,* and *Streptococcus pneumoniae* may also be causative in some cases. In immunocompromised persons, gram-negative organisms of fungal species may cause cellulitis and resultant lymphangitis.[1,2] The most common cause for lymphangitis, on an international basis, is *Wuchereria bancrofti,* a microfilarial parasitic infection. Pediatric patients who are immunocompromised, diabetic, or receiving chronic steroid therapy may be at increased risk for the development of fulminant lymphangitis.[1,2]

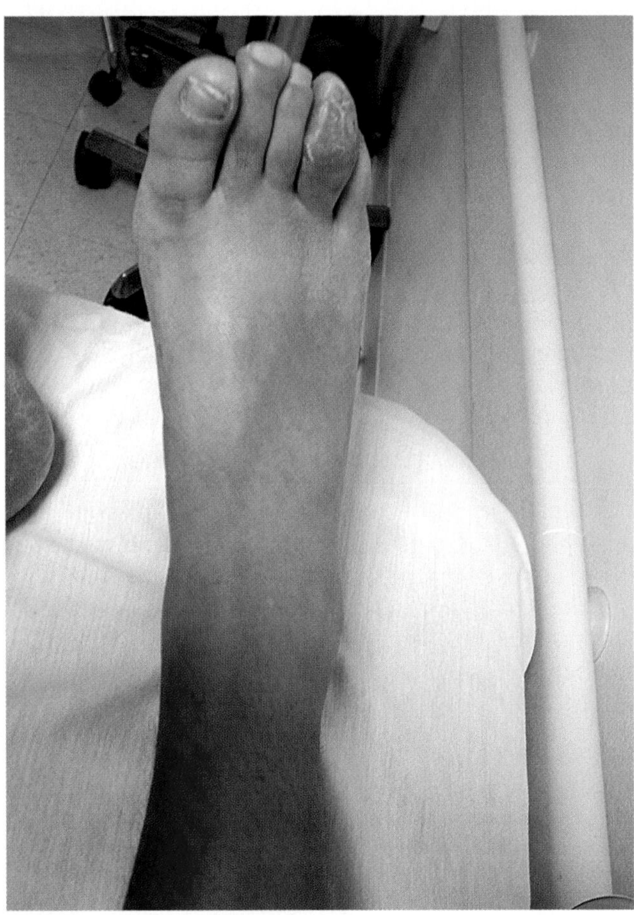

FIGURE 19–5 Lymphangitis of the dorsal right foot. (Courtesy of John Fojtik, MD.)

Diagnosis

The diagnosis is based on clinical findings, including erythematous linear streaks extending from a local skin infection or wound site toward regional lymph nodes. Tender local lymphadenopathy is common.

Clinical Complications

Complications include fulminate spread, septicemia, and death. Improper or incomplete treatment may result in cellulitis, necrosis, and local ulcer formation.[1,2]

Management

Pediatric patients who have responsible guardians and are older than 3 years of age, afebrile, and well hydrated may be successfully treated with oral antibiotic therapy as outpatients. However, careful follow-up is essential. Parenteral antibiotics and hospitalization may be indicated in cases in which patients appear ill with signs of systemic illness, or if GABHS infection is suspected. Pain control, local splinting, elevation, and the application of warm, moist compresses every 2 to 3 hours for 15 minutes are all essential.

REFERENCES

1. Brook I. Microbiology and management of human and animal bite wound infections. *Prim Care* 2003;30:25–39.
2. Ben-Amitai D, Ashkenazi S. Common bacterial skin infections in childhood. *Pediatr Ann* 1993;22:225–227, 231–233.

Puncture Wounds

Sarah Jane Paris and Michael Greenberg

Clinical Presentation

Any object may puncture human skin, resulting in damage to underlying structures or retention of foreign bodies. Patients may present acutely after injury or in a delayed fashion. Delayed presentations may be related to complications.[1-3]

Pathophysiology

Puncture wounds (PWs) are wounds with vector forces or partial forces directed to the surface of the skin at any angle. Patient presentation depends on the nature, direction, and degree of these forces. Special consideration should be given to puncture wounds that are likely to be associated with retained foreign bodies in deep soft tissue. Any PW involving the plantar surface of the foot, especially one that occurs through footwear, is at high risk for infection. *Pseudomonas* infections have been reported when PWs occur through tennis shoes.[2] *Staphylococcus aureus* and *S. epidermidis,* in addition to *Streptococcus* species, are also common infecting organisms.

Diagnosis

Diagnosis is based on history and physical examination. Radiographs may help detect foreign bodies or bony injury and should be performed even if radiolucent objects are not suspected.[1,2]

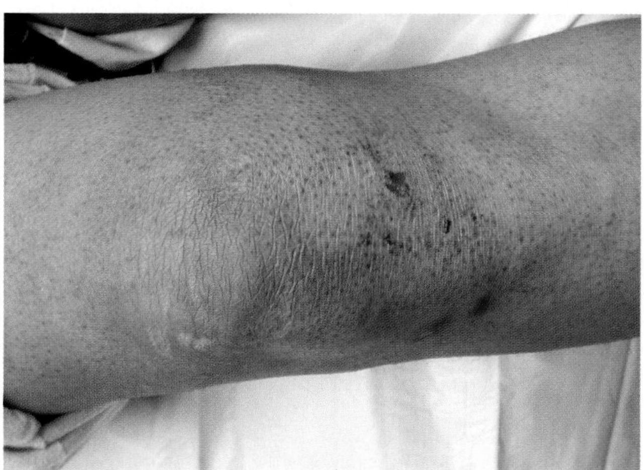

FIGURE 19–6 The small abrasion actually represented a puncture wound from a nail that penetrated into the knee joint. (Courtesy of Robert Hendrickson, MD.)

Clinical Complications

Complications may comprise the primary presenting complaint and may include deep structure injury (nerve, vessels, tendons, joints), retained foreign bodies, spread of infectious diseases, cellulitis, lymphangitis, abscess, osteomyelitis, septic arthritis, tenosynovitis, and chronic pain.[1-3]

Management

Careful examination to rule out deep structure injuries is essential. Wounds should be infiltrated with local anesthetic and then scrubbed vigorously, irrigated copiously, and débrided of devitalized tissue. Some wounds require surgical exploration to determine deep structure injury or retained foreign bodies. Radiographic imaging is required for all infected PWs and whenever there is a suspicion of retained foreign bodies.[1] PWs involving the hand and other locations require splinting in plaster or bulky dressings and strict elevation. Patents with probable joint violation or deep structure violation should be hospitalized and hand/plastic surgery consulted. Prophylactic antibiotics and tetanus prophylaxis should be considered in all cases, but extensive evidence of efficacy is lacking. Antibiotics are not a substitute for meticulous wound care.[1] Primary closure is not indicated for any PW, because it can be expected to facilitate the development of infection. Probing and "grabbing" for unseen foreign bodies is unwise, because objects may be forced into deeper tissue.[1] Tetanus immunization should be updated.

REFERENCES

1. Brook JW. Management of pedal puncture wounds. *J Foot Ankle Surg* 1994;33:463–466.
2. Graham BS, Gregory DW. *Pseudomonas aeruginosa* causing osteomyelitis after puncture wounds of the foot. *South Med J* 1984;77:1228–1230.
3. Pennycook A, Makower R, O'Donnell AM. Puncture wounds of the foot: can infective complications be avoided? *J R Soc Med* 1994; 87:581–583.

Wound Retained Foreign Bodies

James Nelson and Colleen Campbell

Clinical Presentation

In acute soft-tissue injury, retained foreign bodies (RFBs) may not produce specific symptoms or signs. Some patients complain of a sharp pain on palpation directly over a puncture wound, and some subcutaneous RFBs may be palpable.[1] Older RFBs may manifest as nonhealing wounds, cellulitis, abscess, granuloma, or osteomyelitis.[2]

Pathophysiology

Depending on the composition of the object, an inflammatory response may develop. Organic materials, notably wood, may provoke the most intense inflammatory responses.[2]

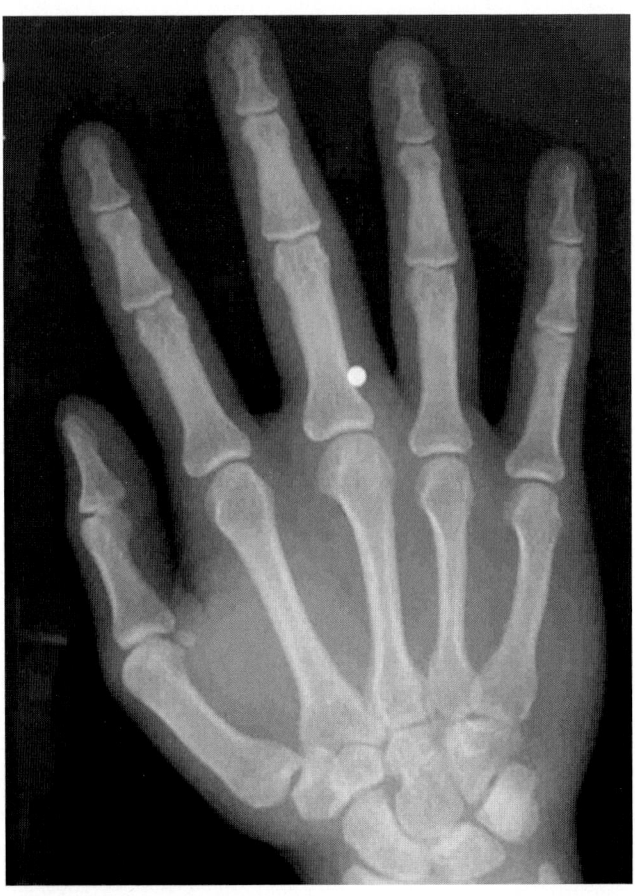

FIGURE 19–7 Metallic foreign body (a BB) retained in the soft tissue of the hand. (Courtesy of Robert Hendrickson, MD.)

Diagnosis

Wound exploration may not identify all RFBs. One study showed that 21% of wounds not accessible to inspection harbored occult foreign material, and if full exploration was possible, the incidence of occult foreign body was 7%.[2] Glass or metal fragments greater than 0.5 mm may be detected by plain radiographs. Underpenetrated soft-tissue radiographs may help visualize some foreign objects. Teeth, gravel, sand, graphite pencil, and some plastics may be visible on plain films. Computed tomography is 100% more sensitive than plain films for detection of soft-tissue RFBs.[1]

Clinical Complications

Infection, inadequate healing, and granuloma formation are common complications. Other complications include migration, damage to surrounding tissues, and thrombosis.[1]

Management

Tetanus vaccination should be updated if necessary. Puncture wounds should be explored if an RFB is suspected. This may be accomplished by extending the wound with a scalpel. Blind exploration of wounds with a hemostat can cause damage to surrounding structures.[1] Vegetative material should be removed immediately to avoid inflammation or infection. More inert material, such as glass, plastic, or nonoxidizing metals, may be removed on an elective basis.

REFERENCES

1. Capellan O, Hollander JE. Management of lacerations in the emergency department. *Emerg Med Clin North Am* 2003;21:205–231.
2. Chan C, Salam GA. Splinter removal. *Am Fam Physician* 2003;67:2557–2562.

Rabies Prophylaxis

Grant Wei

Clinical Presentation

Patients needing rabies prophylaxis may present after a bite or scratch from an animal or after direct contact with a bat.

Pathophysiology

Rabies is endemic in the United States, with several thousand animal cases annually, though only 32 cases of human rabies were reported between 1980 and 1996.[1] Rabies is transmitted in the saliva of infected mammals. The virus causes a slow, centripetal infection of the nerves, leading to a fulminate encephalitis.[1,2]

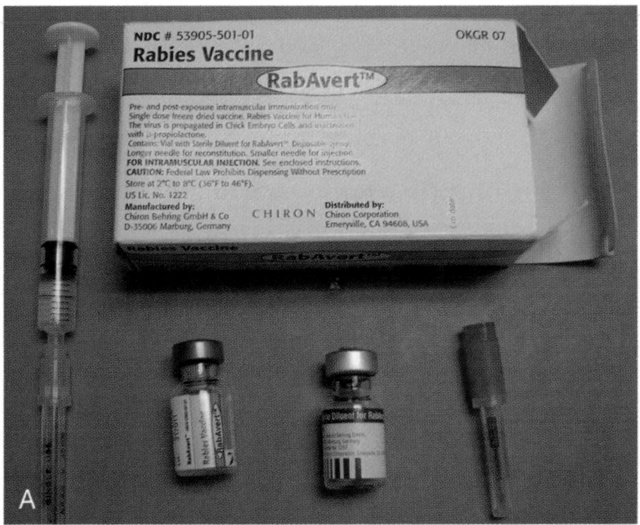

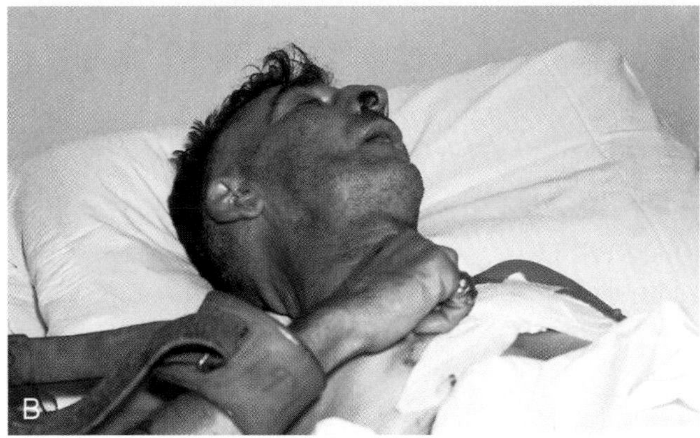

FIGURE 19–8 **A:** Five doses of this rabies vaccine are required if the offending animal cannot be observed after a bite. (Courtesy of Elzbieta Pilat, MD.) **B:** This patient with rabies presented with confusion, anxiety, hallucinations, and delirium. (Courtesy of the Centers for Disease Control and Prevention.)

Diagnosis

Patients bitten by animals known or suspected to be rabid should receive rabies prophylaxis immediately. Bites from dogs, cats, or ferrets do not require prophylaxis if the animal can be observed for 10 days. If the animal develops clinical signs of rabies, prophylaxis is then indicated. If the animal is unknown or escaped capture, local public health officials should be contacted for further guidance. Wild animals such as skunks, bats, and carnivores should be regarded as rabid unless proven by lab tests to be negative, and prophylaxis should start immediately. Rodents, lagomorphs, and livestock should be considered individually and in consultation with local public health officials with regard to prophylaxis.[2,3]

Clinical Complications

Complications of prophylaxis include local reactions at the site of vaccine injection (e.g., pain, erythema, swelling) in 30% to 70% of recipients. Systemic reactions such as headache, nausea, and myalgias occur in up to 40% of recipients. In addition, the Rabies Immune Globulin (RIG) has been associated with pain and low-grade fever. Patients may have allergic/anaphylactic reactions to either component of prophylaxis.[2]

Management

Bites and wounds should be washed and irrigated with water, soap, and povidone-iodine solution. If the patient has been previously vaccinated, RIG should not be given and the vaccine should be given on days 0 and 3. In unvaccinated patients, RIG should be injected around and into the wound, if possible; the remainder of the immune globulin should be injected intramuscularly at a site distal to the vaccine site. The vaccine should be injected intramuscularly in the deltoid area on days 0, 3, 7, 14, and 28.[2,3]

REFERENCES

1. Noah DL, Drenzek CL, Smith JS, et al. Epidemiology of human rabies in the United States, 1980 to 1996. *Ann Intern Med* 1998;128: 922–930.
2. Update on emerging infections from the Centers for Disease Control and Prevention. Update rabies postexposure prophylaxis guidelines. *Ann Emerg Med* 1999;33:590–597.
3. Moran GJ, Talan DA, Mower W, et al. Appropriateness of rabies postexposure prophylaxis treatment for animal exposures. *JAMA* 2000;284:1001–1007.

19-9

Keloid Formation

Gary M. Vilke

Clinical Presentation

Patients with keloid formation often present with a recently widened, expanding scar. A patient may already know about the diagnosis, but on occasion, the emergency physician makes the initial diagnosis.

Pathophysiology

A keloid is a region of hypertrophied, fibrous tissue that occurs after an injury and extends beyond the borders of the original wound. Keloids occur frequently in Asian, Polynesian, Indian, African, and African-American individuals. Keloids are variations of typical wound healing. In the normal wound healing process, there exists an equilibrium between anabolic and catabolic mechanisms. As the scar matures, the tensile strength of the scar improves as a result of progressive cross-linking of collagen fibers. At approximately 8 weeks, the scar usually is hyperemic, and it may be thickened, but it tends to subside gradually over months until a flat, mature scar develops. If there is an imbalance between the anabolic and catabolic phases in this healing process, more collagen is produced than is broken down, and the scar grows and hypertrophies. The excessive scar, or keloid, becomes elevated above the skin, migrates beyond the wound borders, and remains hyperemic. No specific genes have been identified in association with development of keloids.[1]

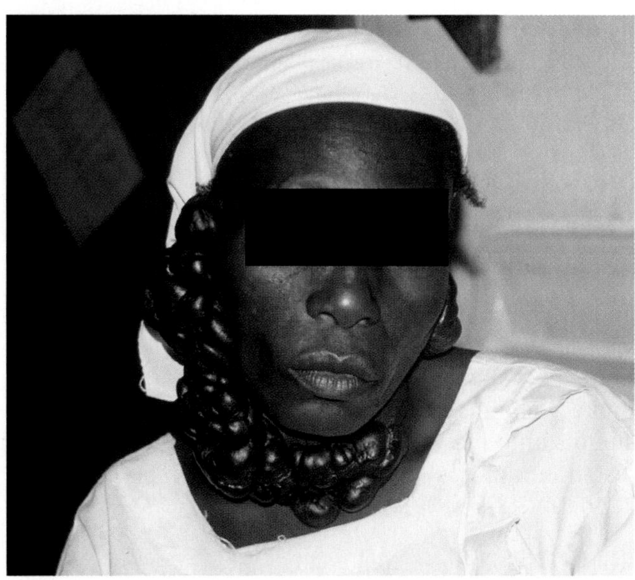

FIGURE 19–9 Exuberant keloid formation. (Courtesy of Sandra Scott, MD.)

Diagnosis

The diagnosis is clinical and is based on the history and physical examination. Keloids range in consistency from soft and doughy to hard and rubbery. Early lesions often are erythematous and become brown or brick red, then pale as they age. Keloids usually do not have hair follicles and other glands, and they typically are round or oblong with regular margins. However, some develop claw-like appearances with irregular borders.

Clinical Complications

Keloids may be painful or pruritic. Most lesions continue to grow for weeks to months, and some may grow for years. Growth usually is slow, but keloids occasionally enlarge rapidly, tripling in size within months.

Management

No specific treatment is indicated. Reassurance and patient education is usually all that is required in the emergency department. Once keloids stop growing, they usually are asymptomatic and remain stable. In the hands of a primary care physician, dermatologist, or plastic surgeon, therapeutic treatments of keloids include use of occlusive dressings, compression therapy, intralesional corticosteroid injections, cryosurgery, excision, radiation therapy, laser therapy, interferon therapy, and imiquimod cream.[1]

REFERENCES

1. Berman B, Bieley HC. Keloids. *J Am Acad Dermatol* 1995;33: 117–123.

Distal Digital Amputation

Gary M. Vilke

Clinical Presentation

A distal digital amputation (DDA) is usually self-evident, with the tip of a finger being completely or almost completely cut off.

Pathophysiology

DDA involves either the distal soft tissue of the digit without bone exposed, the distal soft tissue with bone exposed but intact, or the distal soft tissue with bone included in the amputated portion. The amputation is defined as complete if the amputated portion is completely separated from the finger, or incomplete if there is still some connecting tissue. If the amputation involves the bone of the proximal portion of the distal phalanx, the digital nerves and arteries may be compromised. With concomitant distal crush injury, venous outflow may also be affected.

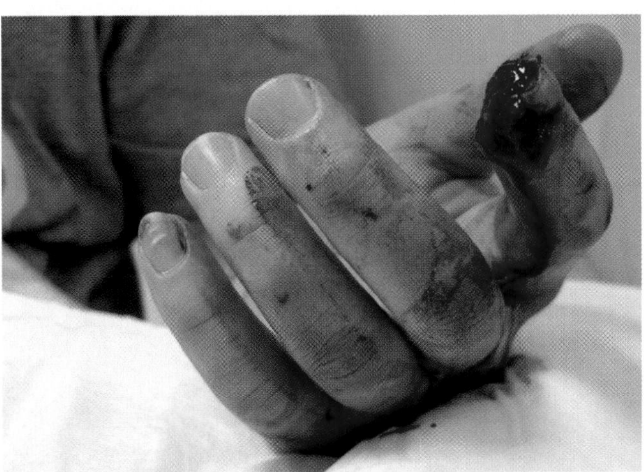

FIGURE 19–10 Full-thickness tissue loss of distal left second digit. (Courtesy of Claritza Rios, MD.)

Diagnosis

The diagnosis is based on the history and physical examination. Involvement of the distal phalanx must be determined by plain radiography, including both the involved finger and the amputated tip.

Clinical Complications

Complications include failure of the repaired tip to survive, as well as chronic cold intolerance or sensitivity changes after healing.[1]

Management

A DDA that does not involve the bone of the distal phalanx may be managed by the emergency physician.[2] A digital block for anesthesia enables copious irrigation. In most cases, conservative management is in order, and most DDAs heal with minimal shortening if they are allowed to heal by secondary intention. Microvascular surgery is not indicated for this type of injury. If the bone of the distal phalanx is exposed, it can be rongeured and closed primarily or covered and allowed to heal by secondary intention. Antibiotics usually are not indicated. However, antibiotics should be considered for excessively dirty wounds and for those with a large amount of devitalized tissue, or if the mechanism of injury involved crushing forces. Close follow-up, with a wound check in 24 to 48 hours, is optimal. Complex injuries may require consultation with a hand surgeon.[1,2]

REFERENCES

1. Fassler PR. Fingertip injuries: evaluation and treatment. *J Am Acad Orthop Surg* 1996;4:84–92.
2. Abbase EH, Tadjalli HE, Shenaq SM. Fingertip and nail bed injuries: repair techniques for optimum outcome. *Postgrad Med* 1995;98: 217–219, 223–224.

Maggots (Myiasis)

Michael Greenberg

Clinical Presentation

Patients with myiasis present with pain, pruritus, and chronic inflammation, as well as open wounds containing the larvae of flies, also known as maggots.

Pathophysiology

Maggots appear on wounds after flies lay their eggs on infected flesh. Once the larvae hatch, they burrow into and through the tissue. Maggots essentially clean the wound of rotting and devitalized tissue through the secretion of proteolytic enzymes, as well as by alkaline secretions that inhibit bacterial growth and disinfect tissue. Maggots are used medicinally for the treatment of venous stasis ulcers, diabetic foot ulcers, burns, postsurgical wounds, and decubitus ulcers, as well as tumor necrosis and necrotizing fasciitis.[1-3]

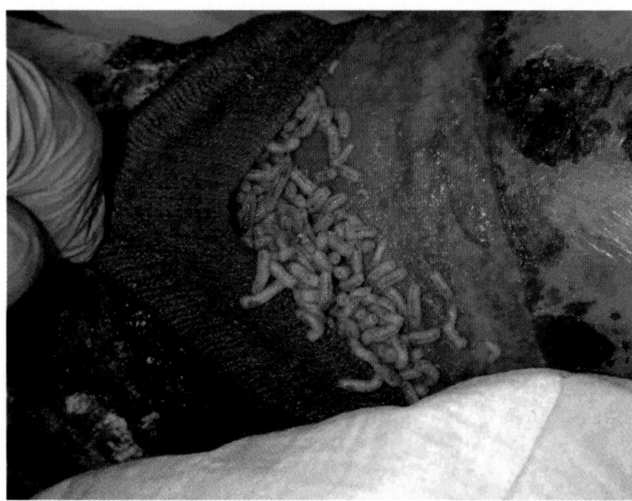

FIGURE 19-11 Wound myiasis. (Courtesy of Ralph Weiche, MD.)

Diagnosis

The presence of maggots usually is obvious on physical examination of chronic open wounds.

Clinical Complications

Pruritus and pain are frequent complications. Tetanus has been reported to result from the presence of maggots.[3]

Management

Maggots found in chronic wounds may be removed with the use of forceps and killed in formalin. Maggots that have been intentionally placed into wounds for medicinal purposes should be left in place, and the practitioner who placed the maggots should be consulted.

REFERENCES

1. Dunn C, Raghavan U, Pffleiderer AG. The use of maggots in head and neck necrotizing fasciitis. *J Laryng Otol* 2002;116:70–72.
2. Jones M, Thomas S. Larval therapy. *Nursing Standard* 2000;14: 47–51.
3. Dossey L. Maggots and leeches: when science and aesthetics collide. *Altern Ther Health Med* 2002;8:12–16, 106–107.

Eyebrow Laceration

David Wald

Clinical Presentation

Eyebrow lacerations commonly occur as a result of either blunt or penetrating trauma. Because of the underlying supraorbital ridge, injuries to the eyebrow may result from relatively minor trauma.[1]

Pathophysiology

The eyebrows consist of thickened skin on each side of the upper margin of the orbit overlying a portion of the occipitofrontalis and orbicularis oculi muscles.[1]

Diagnosis

The eye and periorbital structures should be examined to exclude an ocular injury. A systematic evaluation of the other head and neck structures should be undertaken to exclude serious injury.[1]

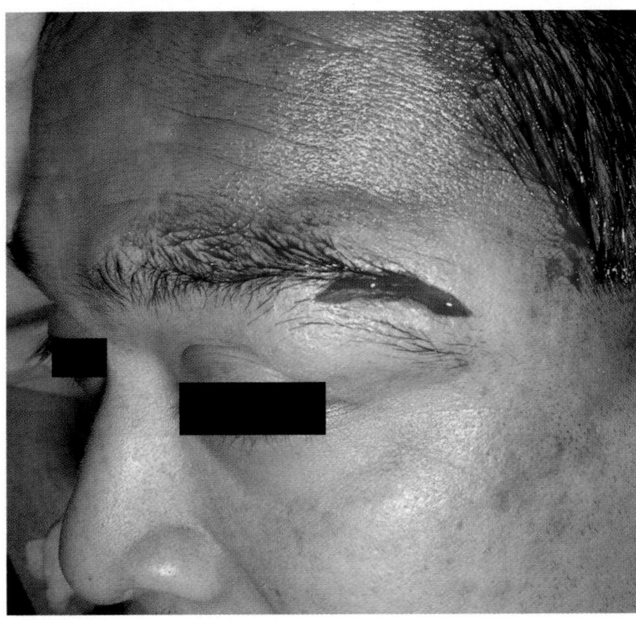

FIGURE 19–12 Simple eyebrow laceration. (Courtesy of Mark Silverberg, MD.)

Clinical Complications

Scar potential and resultant cosmetic deformity is always a concern in the repair of eyebrow lacerations. Misalignment of the eyebrow margin or extensive débridement may result in a scar that is cosmetically unacceptable.[1]

Management

Eyebrow lacerations should be irrigated and cleansed but never shaved, because proper regrowth is not predictable.[1] Linear eyebrow lacerations extending into the subcutaneous tissue may be repaired with 5-0 or 6-0 nonabsorbable suture. Deeper lacerations may require subcutaneous sutures to approximate the superficial fascia. The first sutures placed should serve to realign the eyebrow margins. As a general rule, it is not recommended to excise any eyebrow skin. However, in certain circumstances, gentile débridement of a macerated wound may be necessary. If this is undertaken, the skin excision should be performed parallel to the eyebrow hair shafts. Tetanus and rabies prophylaxis should be administered as indicated. After repair, daily wound cleaning and application of a topical antibiotic ointment is recommended. Sutures should be removed in 4 to 5 days.[1]

REFERENCES

1. Wilson JL, Kocurek K, Doty BJ. A systematic approach to laceration repair: tricks to ensure the desired cosmetic result. *Postgrad Med* 2000;107:77–83, 87–88.

19–13

Eyelid Laceration

Michael Greenberg

Clinical Presentation

Patients with eyelid lacerations present after direct trauma from falls, various blows to the face, or striking or being stuck by sharp objects.

Pathophysiology

The extent of injury depends on the mechanism of injury. Underlying globe injury is not uncommon in blunt or penetrating trauma. Adnexal structures and the internal structure of the eyelid itself may be injured as well. Injuries medial to the punctum are at high risk for damage to the canaliculus and associated drainage system.[1] Full-thickness lid injuries medial to the punctum may not be readily evident because they tend to "self-seal" into anatomic alignment.[1] This is a common occurrence with injuries from dog bites.[1] Wounds may be complex and may involve tissue loss and cosmetic deformity.

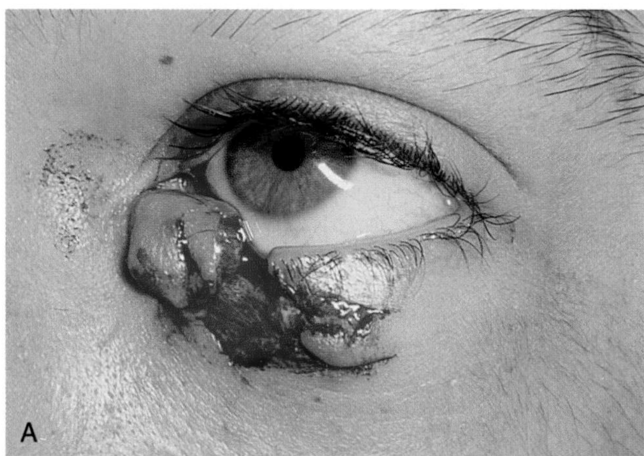

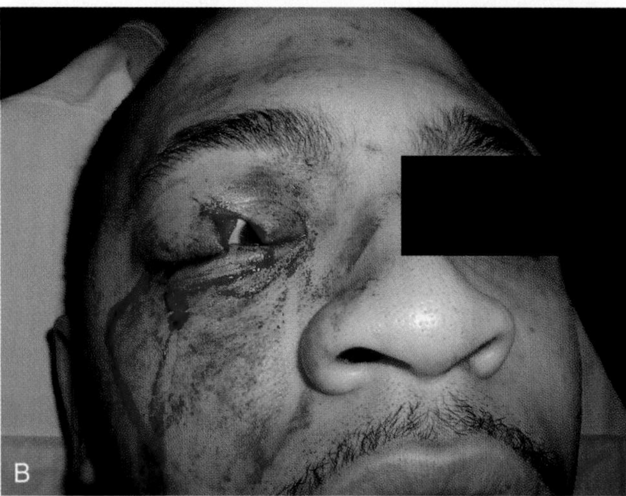

FIGURE 19–13 **A:** This 11-year-old boy fell on a shelf bracket, sustaining an irregular, full-thickness lid laceration. (From Tasman, with permission.) **B:** Laceration of the upper lid with full-thickness skin loss. (Courtesy of Rafi Israeli, MD.)

Diagnosis

The diagnosis is evident on careful examination. However, based on the variety of anatomically important structures present within the limited ocular and periocular areas, these wounds require special attention. Plain radiographs may be needed to rule out the presence of associated foreign bodies, and computed tomographic imaging may help to assess periocular injuries.

Clinical Complications

Deep lid lacerations may injure a variety of important structures, including the lacrimal sac and gland, levator muscle, canalicular system, inferior oblique muscle, and angular artery.[1] Injuries to the lid margins may lead to serious complications, including cosmetically inadequate results and entropion. Infections of eyelid lacerations are uncommon because of the excellent blood supply to the lids.[1]

Management

Eyelid wounds should be carefully cleansed and irrigated with saline solution. Visual acuity should be assessed and recorded in all cases. Tetanus prophylaxis should be ensured, and antibiotics should be considered based on the wounding mechanism, the degree of devitalized tissue present, and the patient's underlying medical conditions. Emergency repair may not be critical if the lid laceration is not complicated by associated injuries. Evaluation and repair of injured adnexal structures and lid margins requires an ophthalmologist or plastic surgeon, and patients may need to be transferred for this care. Emergency physicians should not undertake primary repair of eyelid wounds unless they are uncomplicated and the physician is absolutely certain that no associated or underlying structure injury exists.[1]

REFERENCES

1. Hartstein ME, Fink SR. Traumatic eyelid injuries. *Int Ophthalmol Clin* 2002;42:123–134.

Nasolacrimal Duct Laceration

David Wald

Clinical Presentation

Lacerations of the canalicular system or injury to the nasolacrimal duct may occur as a result of blunt or penetrating trauma. Canalicular lacerations are the most common injury to the lacrimal system. The horizontal lower limb of the inferior canaliculus is most frequently injured.[1]

Pathophysiology

Mucosal ducts (canaliculi), drain the tears from the eyes. The canalicular system is located in the medial portion of the upper and lower eye lid. The lacrimal tear-draining apparatus includes the puncta on the medial portions of the upper and lower lid, the canaliculi, the common canaliculus, the lacrimal sac, and the nasolacrimal duct. The canalicular system is vulnerable to injury because of its superficial location in the medial aspect of the eyelid.[1]

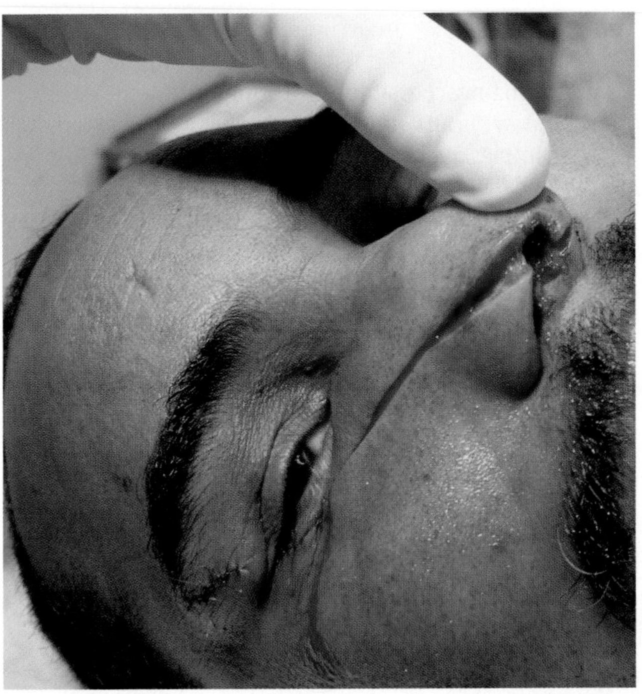

FIGURE 19–14 Nasolacrimal duct laceration should be suspected when this area of the face is injured. (Courtesy of Mark Silverberg, MD.)

Diagnosis

An eyelid laceration medial to the punctum frequently damages the lacrimal duct system.[1] Eyelid lacerations should be carefully inspected to identify injuries to the nasolacrimal duct system. Patients with eyelid lacerations should undergo careful ocular examination to exclude globe injury.[1]

Clinical Complications

If the canalicular system is not repaired properly or develops scarring, abnormal tearing may result. If the tarsal plate or levator palpebrae muscles are damaged, ptosis may develop. Eyelid asymmetry may result from injury to the eyelid, damage to the medial canthal ligament, or inadequate laceration repair.[1]

Management

Eyelid lacerations involving the lid margin usually require subspecialty consultation. Eyelid lacerations located medially to the punctum frequently involve the canaliculi or nasolacrimal duct system and require subspecialty consultation. Tetanus and rabies prophylaxis should be administered if indicated.[1]

REFERENCES

1. Baker SM, Hurwitz JJ. Management of orbital and ocular adnexal trauma. *Ophthalmol Clin North Am* 1999;12:435–455.

19–15

Parotid Duct Laceration

Steven C. Gabaeff

Clinical Presentation

Any deep laceration to the cheek or injury to the face between the tragus of the ear and the midcheek above the mandible should be evaluated for possible parotid duct laceration. The appearance of blood at the papilla suggests that the duct has been damaged and possibly lacerated. Injury to the facial nerve, parotid gland, mandible, and zygoma may also be present.[1] Injury posterior to the anterior edge of the masseter muscle usually results in simultaneous injury to the facial nerve.[1]

Pathophysiology

The parotid duct (Stensen's duct) runs along an axis from just below the tragus of the ear to the upper lip. The cross-point of a vertical axis between the lateral iris and the middle of the mandible (just lateral to the mouth), where it crosses the described horizontal axis, roughly defines the entry point of the parotid duct into the mouth.

Diagnosis

Under normal conditions, pressure on the parotid gland to the affected side should result in formation of a droplet of saliva at the papilla of the parotid duct on the buccal mucosa. This indicates that the duct is intact. Direct inspection of the buccal mucosa and the depths of any laceration may reveal the transected ends of the duct or injury to the parotid gland itself. The body of the gland can extend inferiorly into the upper neck area.

Clinical Complications

Failure to identify this injury in a timely manner, failure to document the evaluation of the injury in detail, or failure to seek consultation if any uncertainty exists can result in significant abnormalities of parotid function and subsequent litigation.

Management

Intravenous antibiotics, surgical exploration of the injured area by an ear, nose, and throat specialist, and microsurgical repair of the duct over a small polyethylene catheter using fine interrupted sutures are indicated.[1] The catheter should be left in place during healing and should remain accessible via the mouth. Any injury to the gland without injury to the duct may be repaired with a simple layered closure of the gland and skin layers, which should result in satisfactory healing. Facial nerve transections should be repaired if they are posterior to the vertical axis described.

REFERENCES

1. Lewkowicz AA, Hasson O, Nahlieli O. Traumatic injuries to the parotid gland and duct. *J Oral Maxillofac Surg* 2002;60:676–680.

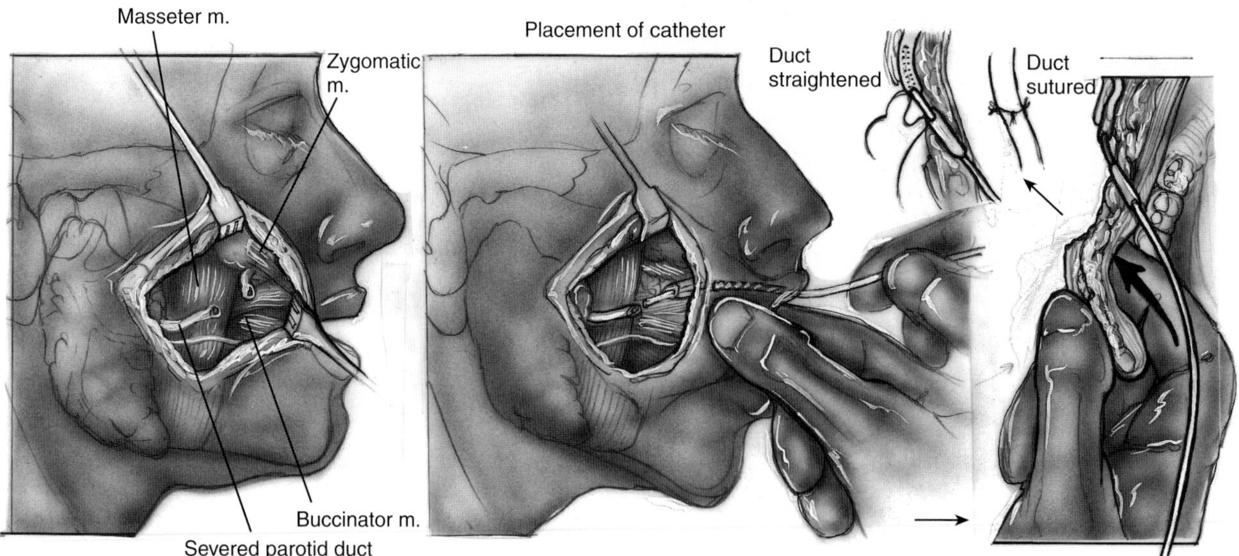

FIGURE 19–15 Repair of parotid duct. (From Bailey, with permission.)

Ear Laceration

Marc A. Hare

Clinical Presentation

Patients with lacerations of the ear usually present acutely after direct trauma.

Pathophysiology

The auricle is particularly subject to trauma because of its protrusion from the side of the head, as well as its delicate cartilaginous support and thin integument. Auricular hematomas, created by shearing forces that cause microvascular disruption, usually occur under the anterolateral perichondrium. Bite injuries are generally a combination of puncture, laceration, and avulsion and are complicated by contamination with multiple microbes.

Diagnosis

These injuries frequently are seen in conjunction with significant head trauma, and standard advanced trauma life support (ATLS) measures take first priority. Once life-threatening issues have been addressed, a detailed otologic examination is performed. Auricular hematoma manifests with swelling that may obscure the normal anatomic landmarks of the anterolateral pinna.[1]

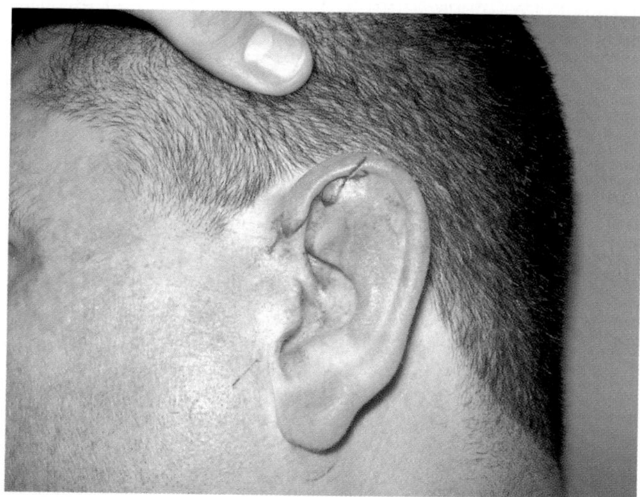

FIGURE 19–16 Laceration of the pinna. (Courtesy of Mark Silverberg, MD.)

Clinical Complications

Complications include auricular hematomas that result in a characteristic deformity known as "wrestler's ear" or "cauliflower ear."[1,2] Lacerations involving cartilage may heal with notching or other deformities and may predispose to perichondritis.

Management

Local anesthesia of the pinna may be achieved by infiltrating lidocaine along the anterior and posterior base of the pinna.[2] For auricular hematomas, the technique of complete evacuation via a small incision, suctioning, and insertion of a wick is preferred to aspiration. This should be followed by application of a formed pressure dressing. The wound should be rechecked within 48 hours, because there may be a delayed accumulation or reaccumulation of blood. Definitive evaluation by an otolaryngologist must occur before 7 to 10 days after the initial injury. Care of pinna lacerations not involving cartilage follows the same tenets as care of other soft-tissue lacerations.[1] Simple lacerations may be repaired with monofilament nylon, preferably 6-0. Suturing of cartilage should be avoided if possible.[2] If necessary, simple cartilage repairs can be done with 6-0 chromic suture or through-and-through sutures with monofilament nylon.[1,2] More complex auricular lacerations or partial avulsions should be acutely evaluated by an otolaryngologist or similar subspecialist. Total avulsions should be cleansed, and the avulsed part should be wrapped with moist gauze and stored indirectly over ice until the otolaryngologist is at the bedside. Bite wounds must be copiously irrigated and then treated according to the injury type, with the addition of antibiotics based on current recommendations for bite wounds.

REFERENCES

1. Templer J, Renner GJ. Injuries of the external ear. *Otolaryngol Clin North Am* 1990;23:1003–1018.
2. Punjabi A, Haug RH, Jordan RB. Management of injuries to the auricle. *J Oral Maxillofac Surg* 1997;55:732–739.

Lip Laceration: Vermillion Border

David Wald

Clinical Presentation

Lip lacerations occur as a result of motor vehicle accidents, altercations, animal bites, and sports-related injuries.

Pathophysiology

The external skin of the face meets the colored epithelium of the lip at the vermillion border.[1] In the upper lip, the philtrum is bordered by the philtral columns. At the lower lip, the labiomental skin crease defines the border between the lip and the chin.[1] The mucosal border distinguishes the intraoral and extraoral portions of the lip.

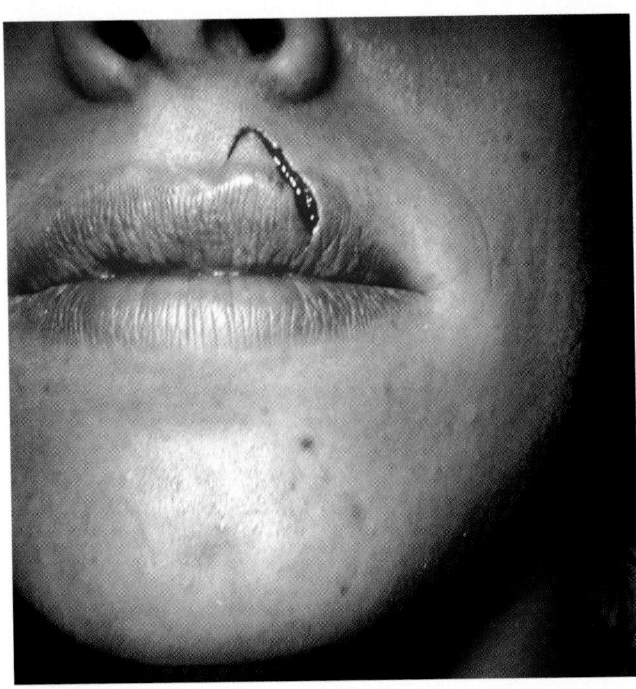

FIGURE 19–17 Vermillion border laceration. (Courtesy of Michael Greenberg, MD.)

Diagnosis

Lacerations through the vermillion border of the lip should be inspected for foreign bodies or debris. If fragments of a fractured tooth cannot be accounted for, radiographs may identify retained foreign bodies within the lip.[2] The lip should also be inspected for evidence of a through-and-through laceration. A systematic evaluation of the other head and neck structures should be undertaken to exclude serious injury.[2]

Clinical Complications

Scar potential and resultant cosmetic deformity is always a concern in the repair of lip lacerations. Misalignment of the vermillion cutaneous border by as little as 1 mm may lead to poor results. Loss of less than 25% of the lip generally permits primary closure with little deformity. Loss of more than 25% of the lip requires reconstruction by a plastic surgeon.[2] Loss of any central portion of the upper lip may require subspecialty consultation to optimize the cosmetic repair.[2]

Management

Vermillion border lacerations must be cleansed and irrigated. Local anesthesia is best administered by a regional nerve block to limit tissue distortion. An infraorbital nerve block provides adequate anesthesia for the upper lip, and a mental nerve block for the lower lip. During repair of the laceration, the first suture placed should realign the vermillion border on either side of the wound. Tetanus and rabies prophylaxis should be administered if indicated.[1,2]

REFERENCES

1. Parlin LS. Repair of lip lacerations. *Pediatr Rev* 1997;18:101–102.
2. Armstrong BD. Lacerations of the mouth. *Emerg Med Clin North Am* 2000;18:471–480.

Intraoral Laceration

Jennifer Wiler

Clinical Presentation

Wounds to the intraoral region commonly occur after facial trauma. They are also common in children who fall while holding a sharp object in their mouth.[1–3]

Pathophysiology

Puncture wounds and lacerations inside the oral cavity may damage underlying structures such as glands, ducts, nerves, and blood vessels, depending on the location of the injury. Because the carotid arteries run in close proximity to portions of the oral cavity, special attention should be paid to wounds that have the potential to damage these critical structures.[1–3]

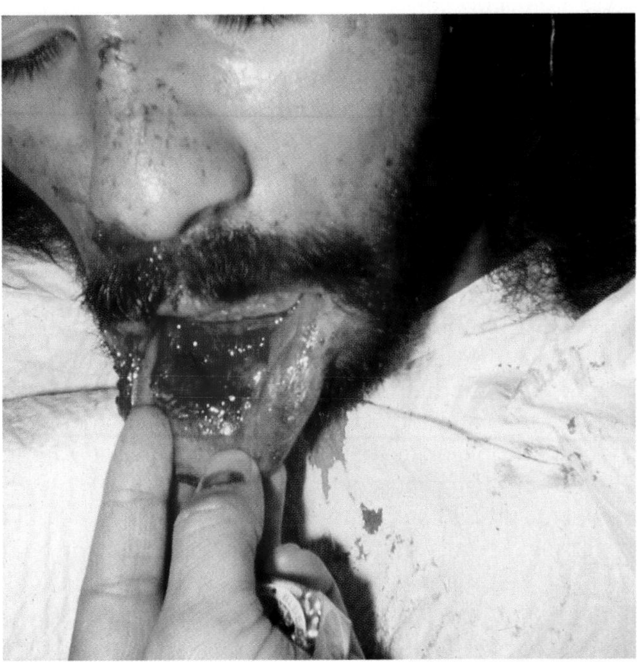

FIGURE 19–18 Laceration with mucosal disruption at the gum line. (Copyright James R. Roberts, MD.)

Diagnosis

The diagnosis is based on clinical examination. However, a careful search for broken teeth or foreign matter retained inside intraoral lacerations is necessary.

Clinical Complications

Complications include infection, uncontrolled bleeding, extension into the intraoral gland tissue, and injury to underlying neurovascular structures.

Management

Most intraoral wounds heal quickly without primary closure and may be treated with frequent warm-water mouth rinses only. Some authorities recommend closure of gaping wounds and wounds that tend to trap food materials to avoid that possibility. If closure is elected, an absorbable suture should be used to avoid extremely difficult suture removal from the oral cavity.[1–3]

REFERENCES

1. Bartholomew BJ, Poole C, Tayag EC. Unusual transoral penetrating injury of the foramen magnum: case report. *Neurosurgery* 2003;53:989–991.
2. Haug RH, Foss J. Maxillofacial injuries in the pediatric patient. *Oral Surg Oral Med Oral Pathol Oral Radiol Endod* 2000;90:126–134.
3. Gassner R, Bosch R, Tuli T, Emshoff R. Prevalence of dental trauma in 6000 patients with facial injuries: implications for prevention. *Oral Surg Oral Med Oral Pathol Oral Radiol Endod* 1999;87:27–33.

Tongue Laceration

David Wald

Clinical Presentation

Tongue lacerations may result from blunt or penetrating trauma. Patients may present with intraoral bleeding due to the extensive vascularity of the tongue.[1]

Diagnosis

The diagnosis is usually obvious after facial trauma. The oral cavity should be examined to exclude concomitant injury to the dentitia, alveolar ridge, and other intraoral structures.[1]

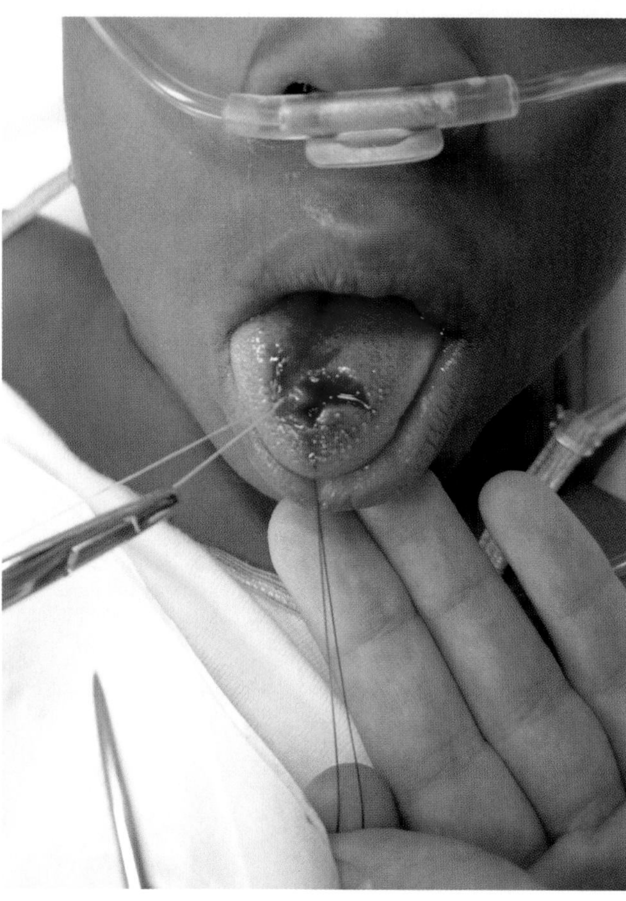

FIGURE 19–19 Tongue laceration. (Courtesy of Mark Silverberg, MD.)

Clinical Complications

The tongue is a highly vascular structure. Serious bleeding complications from tongue lacerations and associated injuries may compromise the airway.[1]

Management

Central tongue lacerations that are linear and do not widely gape open when the tongue is extended usually heal without intervention. Lacerations that continue to bleed, form flaps, involve the edge, bisect the tongue, or pass completely through the tongue margin require repair.[1] It is important to gain the patient's trust, because repair of these lacerations may prove challenging. A gauze pad soaked with 4% lidocaine solution, applied for 5 minutes, may anesthetize a small area of the tongue. For larger lacerations, anesthesia may be provided by direct infiltration of a local anesthetic with or without epinephrine, or by a lingual nerve block. The use of a bite block may help facilitate the repair and prevent injury to the physician or assistant. An assistant may gain control of the tongue with a dry gauze or by applying a towel clip to a previously anesthetized area of the tongue. Alternatively, a single suture can be placed through the anesthetized tip of the tongue. Traction can then be applied to better visualize the laceration. Lacerations usually are repaired with 4-0 or 5-0 absorbable sutures, but silk may be used. Sutures should be loosely tied and placed wide and deep to include both mucosa and muscle. Tetanus and rabies prophylaxis should be administered if indicated. A soft diet is recommended for the first 2 to 3 days after repair. Oral rinsing with a dilute peroxide solution may be helpful. Prophylactic antibiotics usually are not necessary because of the extensive vascularity of the tongue.[1]

REFERENCES

1. Armstrong BD. Lacerations of the mouth. *Emerg Med Clin North Am* 2000;18:471–480.

Superficial Thermal Burns

Craig Bates

Clinical Presentation

Superficial thermal burns (STBs), formerly known as first-degree burns, result from thermal injury involving the epidermis only. Patients present with local erythema and pain at the site of injury. However, pain may be delayed for several hours after the initial insult.[1–3]

Pathophysiology

The skin consists of epidermal and dermal layers. STBs result in epidermal damage that causes only minor disruptions in the normal functioning of the skin. Thermal damage causing STBs derives from a variety of sources, including direct contact with hot surfaces, flash burns, and solar radiation (i.e., sunburn). The erythematous appearance of STBs derives from irritation of the vascular plexus, which projects upward from the dermis into the epidermal-dermal junction.[1–3]

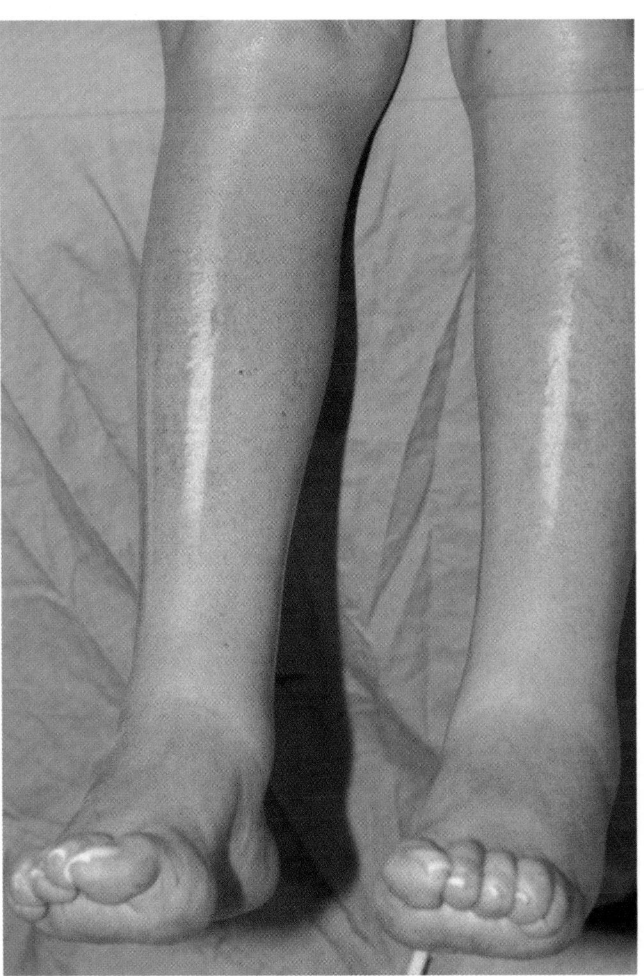

FIGURE 19–20 Superficial thermal burns. (© David Effron, MD, 2004. Used with permission.)

Diagnosis

The diagnosis is made based on historical and clinical grounds. The presence of skin changes consistent with an STB, combined with a reasonable history of thermal exposure that is typically of a limited nature, is sufficient for diagnosis. Truly superficial burns have a dry surface, with no blister formation evident. Clinicians must be mindful of the potential association between STB injury and child, spousal, or elder abuse.

Clinical Complications

STB injury is self-limited and heals over the course of 3 to 5 days. There is no risk of scarring. Secondary infection is not expected but may occur if patients manipulate, abrade, or violate the integrity of the injured tissue.

Management

Treatment entails immediate removal of the source of the burn to stop the burning process. Cooling of the area is traditionally done; however, recent research suggests that this may not change the outcome for STBs.[1] The area should be kept well moisturized, and mild analgesia should be provided. In general, a dressing is not required except for comfort considerations.

REFERENCES

1. Werner MU, Lassen B, Pedersen JL, Kehlet H. Local cooling does not prevent hyperalgesia following burn injury in humans. *Pain* 2002;98:297–303.
2. Richard R, Johnson RM. Managing superficial burn wounds. *Adv Skin Wound Care* 2002;15:246–247.
3. Palmieri TL, Greenhalgh DG. Topical treatment of pediatric patients with burns: a practical guide. *Am J Clin Dermatol* 20002;3:529–534.

Partial-Thickness Burns

Craig Bates

Clinical Presentation

Superficial partial-thickness burns (PTBs) manifest with severe pain and moderate swelling at the site of injury. Deep PTBs also manifest with severe and marked swelling, and they are characterized by areas of redness and waxy white tissue.

Pathophysiology

PTBs, formerly called second-degree burns, are divided into superficial and deep types. Superficial PTBs extend through the epidermis into the superficial layer of the dermis. Fluid-filled blisters develop within minutes after the injury. As these blisters break, exposed nerve endings make these wounds intensely painful. As a result of dermal vascular plexus injury, moderate edema develops. Deep PTBs extend to the deepest layers of the dermis. Blisters are usually absent in these injuries; however, the exposed surface of the wound tends to be moist, and edema is marked. Sensation is altered in deep PTBs.[1,2]

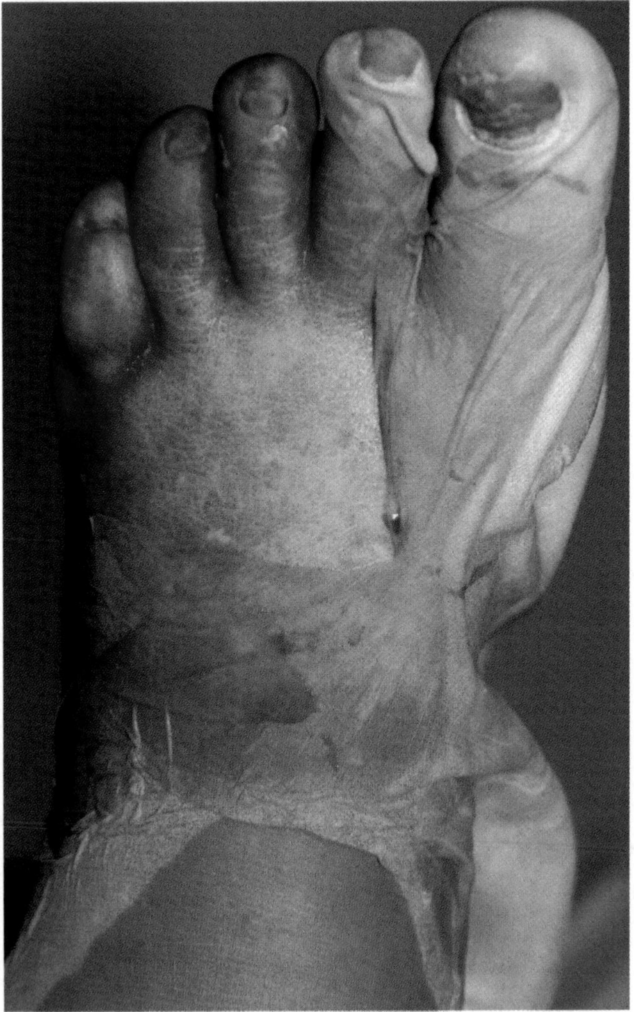

FIGURE 19–21 Partial-thickness burns. (© David Effron, MD, 2004. Used with permission.)

Diagnosis

The diagnosis is made based on historical and clinical grounds. The amount of body surface area (BSA) involved should be quantified using the "Rule of Nines" or an equivalent technique as appropriate. Another estimate is that the patient's palm (including fingers) represents about 1% of the BSA.

Clinical Complications

Complications depend on the specific circumstances of the mechanism of injury, as well as the depth and extent of injury, but may also include inhalation injury, respiratory failure, infection, and hypertrophic scar formation.[1,2]

Management

Treatment starts with immediate removal of the source of the burn, to stop the burning process. Cooling of the burned area may decrease the incidence of full-thickness burns.[1] The depth of the burn determines the specifics of treatment. Airway, breathing, and circulation (the ABCs) must be addressed. Aggressive airway management is prudent because of the risk of progressive edema. The fluid volume required for resuscitation for burns extending to more than 10% to 15% of the BSA may be guided by the Parkland formula: 2 to 4 mL/kg × %BSA, with 50% given in first 8 hours and 50% in next 16 hours from the time of the injury (not the time of presentation in the emergency department).

Admission and/or transfer to the burn unit is indicated for extremes of age; burns covering greater than 10% BSA; burns involving the hands, feet, face, airway, perineum, or major joints; medical or surgical comorbidities; inhalation injury; chemical burns; and electrical- or lightning-related burns. For those patients who will be admitted or transferred to a burn unit, a sterile moist gauze is sufficient and may easily be removed for assessment by the receiving caregivers. If the burns are extensive, dry sterile drapes should be used to avoid hypothermia. Empiric systemic antibiotics are not recommended.

For minor burns, outpatient treatment is appropriate. This consists of gentle cleaning of the area and débridement of nonintact or tense blisters and loose skin. Dressings consist of application of bacitracin ointment to the burn itself, overlying Xeroform® or similar dressing, and dry fluffy gauze to protect the area. Immunization for tetanus should be updated.[1,2]

REFERENCES

1. Nguyen NL, Gun RT, Sparnon AL, Ryan P. The importance of immediate cooling: a case series of childhood burns in Vietnam. *Burns* 2002;28:173–176.
2. Sheridan RL. Burns. *Crit Care Med* 2002;30:S500–S514.

Full-Thickness Burns

Craig Bates

Clinical Presentation

Patients with full-thickness burns (FTBs) present with burn areas that may be white, black, cherry-red, or tan.

Pathophysiology

FTBs, formerly called third-degree burns, extend through the epidermis and dermis into subcutaneous tissue with damage to bone, muscle, and interstitial tissue. Edema results from fluid and protein shifts from vascular to interstitial spaces. Immunologic responses to damaged tissue increase the risk for systemic sepsis.[1,2]

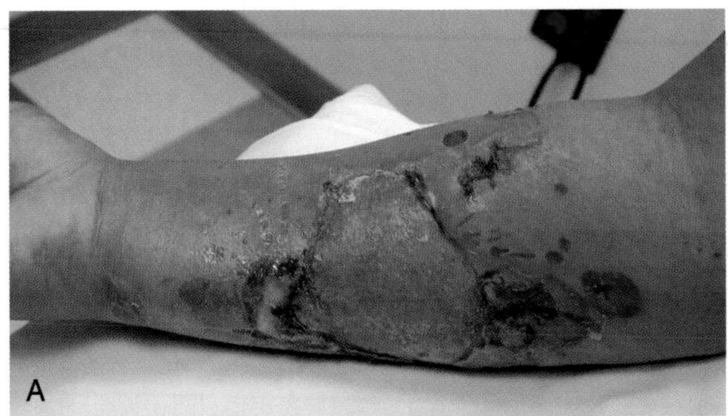

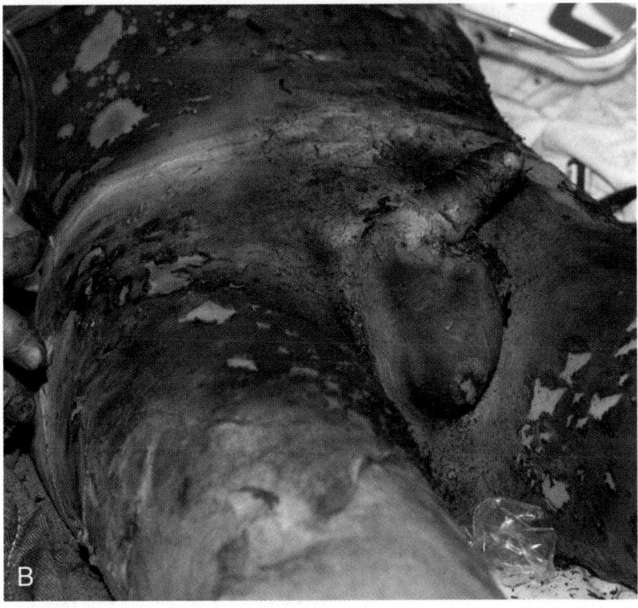

FIGURE 19–22 Full-thickness thermal burns. **A:** Forearm burn caused by boiling oil. (Courtesy of Robert Hendrickson, MD.) **B:** Extensive full-thickness thermal burns. (© Copyright David Effron, MD, 2004. Used with permission.)

Diagnosis

The diagnosis is made based on historical and clinical grounds. Burn sites appear to be dry, leathery and rigid, and pain-free due to destruction of nerve endings. Body hairs pull out easily owing to destruction of dermal appendages. The amount of body surface area (BSA) involved should be quantified using the "Rule of Nines" or an equivalent technique. Serum lactate levels and patient age have been shown to correlate with burn mortality.[1]

Clinical Complications

Complications depend on the specific circumstances of the mechanism of injury, as well as the depth and extent of injury, but may include inhalation injury, respiratory failure, infection, or hypertrophic scar formation. Extensive scarring with the need for reconstructive surgical techniques is the rule with FTBs.

Management

Circumferential burns of extremities are at risk for neurovascular compromise. Frequent assessment of neurovascular function of at-risk limbs is mandatory. Escharotomies are best performed in the operating theater; if circumstances do not allow this, than incisions down to subcutaneous tissue on the medial and lateral sides of the eschar will relieve the compromise.[1,2]

Circumferential burns of the chest wall may impede mechanical ventilation. If necessary, incisions may be made from clavicle to the 10th rib in the midclavicular line, with horizontal incisions connecting them to form a square.

Tetanus prophylaxis is indicated, because burns are tetanus-prone wounds. Aggressive treatment with narcotic analgesics and anxiolytics is indicated for FTBs; empiric systemic antibiotics are not indicated. Admission and transfer to a burn unit should be considered for all FTBs.[1,2]

REFERENCES

1. Jeng JC, Jablonski K, Bridgeman A, Jordan MH. Serum lactate, not base deficit, rapidly predicts survival after major burns. *Burns* 2002;28:161–166.
2. Stoddard FJ, Sheridan RL, Saxe GN, et al. Treatment of pain in acutely burned children. *J Burn Care Rehabil* 2002;23:135–156.

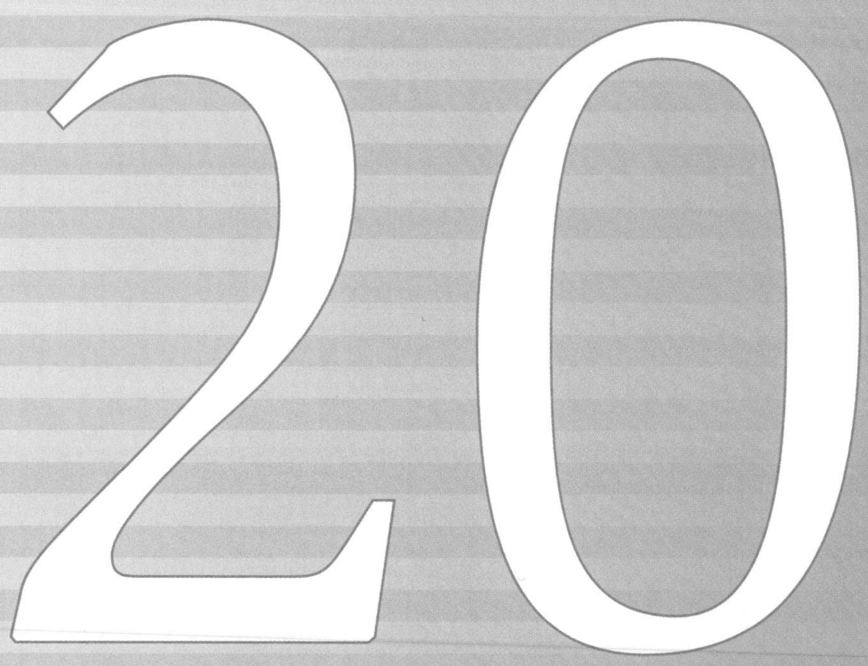

Infectious Diseases

20-1

Rocky Mountain Spotted Fever

Rakesh D. Mistry

Clinical Presentation

The clinical presentation of Rocky Mountain spotted fever (RMSF) is characterized by fever, headache, and a petechial rash. In the early phases, patients may develop high fever followed by a severe headache (85%). Between 50% and 60% of patients develop gastrointestinal symptoms.[1] Other early symptoms may include myalgias, sore throat, cough, abdominal pain, malaise, and anorexia.[1,2] Two to 3 days after onset of the illness, patients develop the characteristic rash on the ankles and wrists, initially resembling pinpoint macules. The macules quickly become petechial in nature, spread to the palms and soles, and then move centrally to involve the trunk. In severe cases, this diffuse petechial rash resembles meningococcemia. The rash may coalesce, and necrosis may follow in regions supplied by terminal arterioles. The rash is not always petechial in nature, and delayed presentation of the rash is possible. Absence of an exanthem is described in 10% of cases.[3] Other signs and symptoms that may develop during the course of RMSF include diarrhea, hepatosplenomegaly, edema, lymphadenopathy, and conjunctivitis.

Pathophysiology

The causative organism is *Rickettsia rickettsi,* an obligate, intracellular, gram-negative bacillus. The ixodid species of ticks serves as both reservoir and vector for *R. rickettsi.* The most common of these is the dog tick, *Dermacentor virabilis.* RMSF is endemic in much of North and Central America, yet, contrary to its name, the majority of cases occur in the south and Atlantic coastal regions of the United States. The bacterium is introduced into humans via a tick bite. After an incubation period of 2 to 14 days, rickettsial organisms spread via blood and lymphatics. Rickettsia then invade and proliferate in

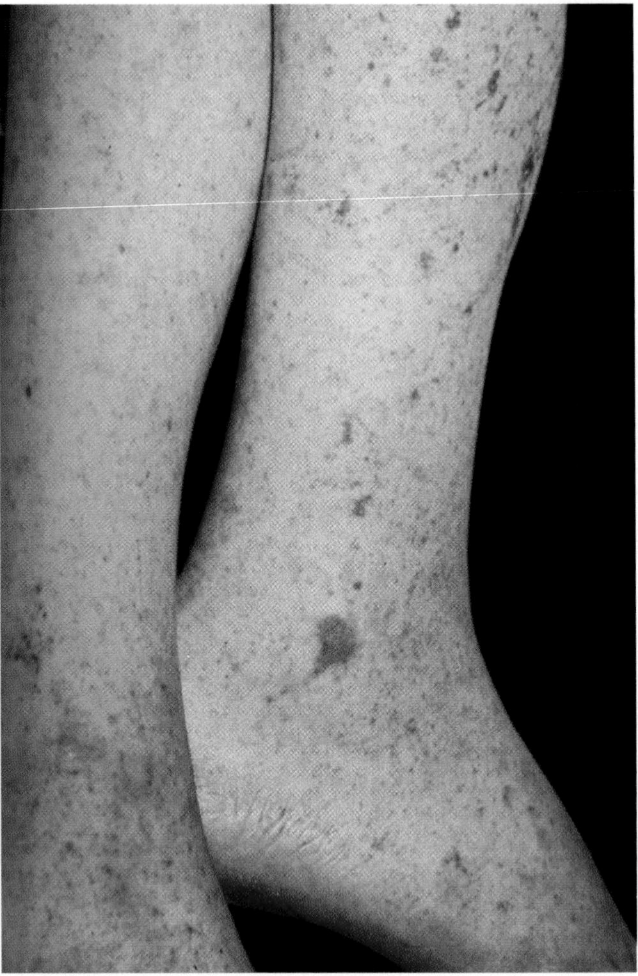

FIGURE 20–1 Rocky Mountain spotted fever. There is a generalized petechial eruption that involves the entire cutaneous surface, including the palms and soles. (From Habif, with permission.)

endothelial and mesothelial cells of blood vessels. Cell death ensues, after which the rickettsia contiguously spread and infect adjacent cells. The infection stimulates a severe inflammatory response. This widespread, systemic vasculitis is directly responsible for almost all of the symptoms of RMSF.

Diagnosis

The diagnosis is primarily clinical, because microbiologic identification of the *R. rickettsi* organism is difficult. The "classic" triad of symptoms (fever, headache, and rash) is present in fewer than 50% of patients.[1] Only 60% of patients recall being bitten by a tick.[1,2]

The indirect fluorescent antibody (IFA) test, the most widely used test for *R. rickettsi,* can detect serum immunoglobulin M or G antibody with a sensitivity of greater than 90%.[1] However, IFA serves only as a confirmatory test for RMSF, because antibody titers do not rise until late into the second week of illness, by which time resolution or death has already occurred. Alternatively, skin biopsies may be obtained for direct immunofluorescence or immunoperoxidase staining for *R. rickettsi.*

Laboratory findings may include hyponatremia, thrombocytopenia, elevated transaminases, and leukopenia or leukocytosis. Renal insufficiency, cerebrospinal fluid pleocytosis, and electrocardiographic changes may be seen. Although none of these findings are specific, their presence may be suggestive of RMSF.

Clinical Complications

Complications include encephalitis, pulmonary edema, acute respiratory distress syndrome, arrhythmias, gastrointestinal bleeding, coagulopathy, and death. Even with treatment, case-fatality rates are approximately 5%; they may be as high as 25% in untreated patients. The majority of deaths occur during the second week of illness, although fulminant cases resulting in rapid death may occur. Long-term sequelae in survivors include paraparesis, hearing loss, peripheral neuropathy, and cerebellar, vestibular, and motor dysfunction.

Management

Initial treatment of RMSF is often empiric, based on the history and physical findings. Studies have demonstrated that antibiotic therapy is most effective if instituted before the fifth day of illness. Consequently, treatment should not be withheld if RMSF is suspected. Tetracycline antibiotics remain the mainstay of treatment for RMSF. Doxycycline is the preferred agent. Doxycycline therapy usually is continued for 7 days, or 2 days after the patient becomes afebrile. Alternative treatment consists of chloramphenicol, but this drug is reserved for pregnant women, in whom doxycycline is contraindicated.

Patients with mild cases of RMSF in the early phases of illness may be treated on an outpatient basis with oral antibiotics and close follow-up. If the disease is diagnosed in the later stages, inpatient therapy and intravenous antibiotics are reasonable. Patients who appear ill or toxic, have severe vomiting, or are at risk for poor compliance should be admitted. Intensive care admission should be considered for patients with neurologic symptoms or renal insufficiency.[4]

REFERENCES

1. Sexton DJ, Kaye KS. Rocky Mountain spotted fever. *Med Clin North Am* 2002;86:351–360.
2. Thorner AR, Walker DH, Petri WA Jr. Rocky Mountain spotted fever. *Clin Infect Dis* 1998;27:1353–1360.
3. Sexton DJ, Corey GR. Rocky Mountain "spotless" and "almost spotless" fever: a wolf in sheep's clothing. *Clin Infect Dis* 1992;15:439–448.
4. Conlon PJ, Procop GW, Fowler V, et al. Predictors of prognosis and risk of acute renal failure in patients with Rocky Mountain spotted fever. *Am J Med* 1996;101:621–626.

Lyme Disease

Christopher J. Russo

Clinical Presentation

In the United States, most patients with Lyme disease (LD) present with a slowly expanding skin lesion (erythema migrans), which occurs at the site of the tick bite. Erythema migrans typically manifests after an incubation of 7 to 14 days (range, 3 to 32 days). Its classic presentation is a red, circular, macular lesion with central clearing resembling a ring or bull's-eye. Constitutional symptoms often occur in early stages of the disease and include fatigue, muscle aches, fever, headaches, and arthralgias. With dissemination, spirochetemia may result in multiple erythema migrans lesions.[1]

Neurologic manifestations in U.S. patients include symptoms of acute neuroborreliosis in approximately 15% of untreated patients; these symptoms include lymphocytic meningitis, subtle encephalitis, cranial neuropathy (unilateral or bilateral peripheral facial nerve palsy), motor or sensory radiculoneuritis, cerebellar ataxia, or myelitis. Untreated, these neurologic abnormalities typically improve or resolve within months; however, up to 5% of untreated patients develop chronic neuroborreliosis.[1] Untreated, 5% of patients demonstrate acute cardiac manifestations, including atrioventricular block and acute myopericarditis.[1] Joint involvement is common among untreated patients, with 60% reporting intermittent attacks of joint swelling and pain that often involves large joints (most commonly the knee). Swelling is generally out of proportion to pain, which is typically mild to moderate.[2]

Pathophysiology

LD, the most common tick-borne disease in the United States, is caused by the spirochete *Borrelia burgdorferi*. Currently, about 15,000 cases are reported each year.[1] Usually, prolonged tick attachment (36 hours or longer) is required for *B. burgdorferi* transmission. After infec-

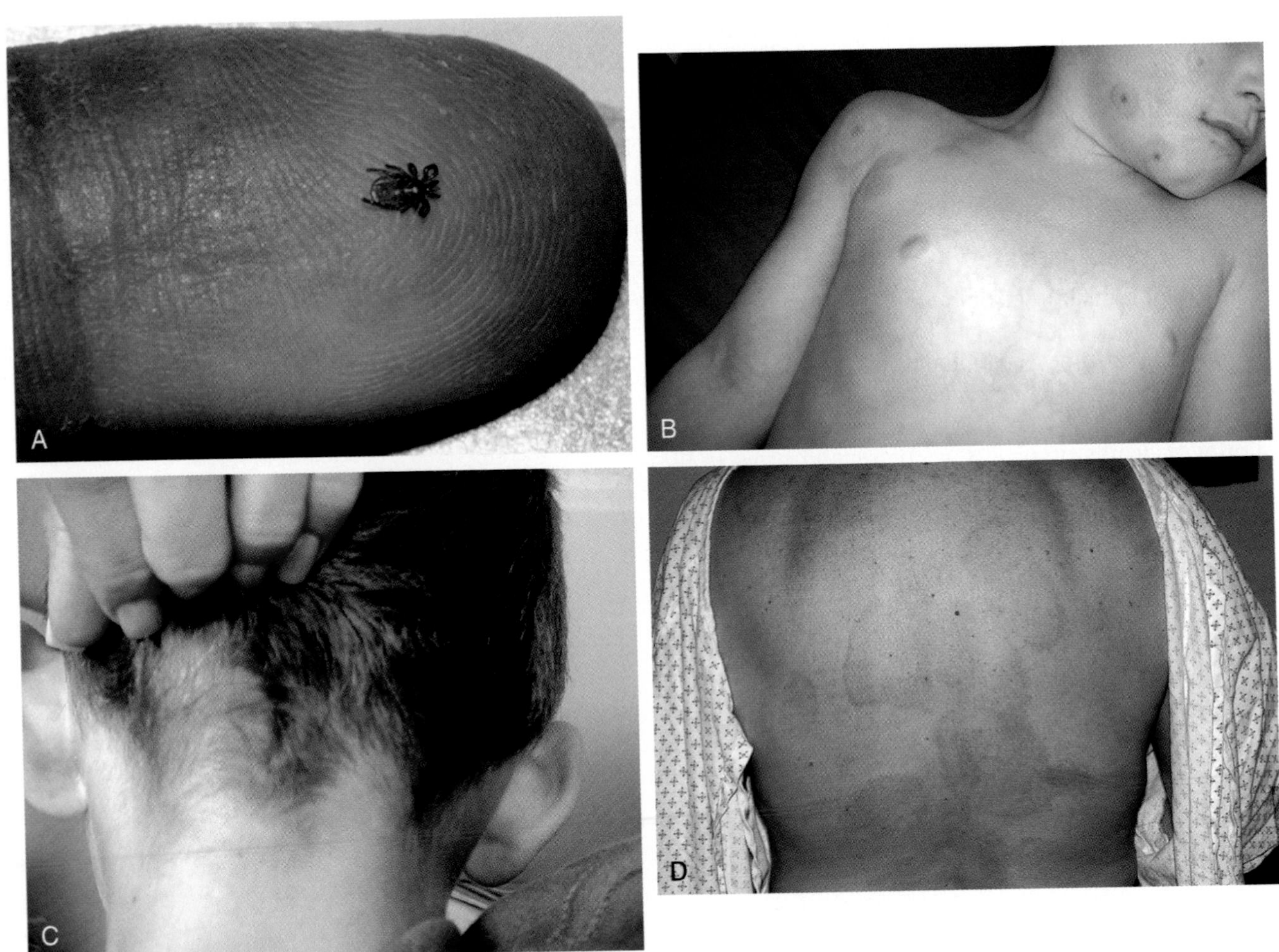

FIGURE 20–2 **A:** *Ixodes* tick. An adult tick is the size of the head of a match. (From Goodheart, with permission.) **B:** Multiple target erythema migrans lesions. (Courtesy of Alfredo Sabbaj, MD.) **C:** Target lesion of Lyme disease. (Courtesy of Christy Salvaggio, MD.) **D:** Erythema migrans lesion of Lyme disease. (From Goodheart, with permission.)

tion, spirochetes disseminate to various tissues; virulence factors influence which tissues are affected. *B. burgdorferi* remains in a constant state of antigenic flux during its life in the mammalian host, continuously triggering an inflammatory response, which may vary in severity. Chronic infection in susceptible individuals may result from this inflammatory response.[3]

Diagnosis

Positive cultures of the organism *B. burgdorferi* have been obtained only early in the course of illness, primarily from skin biopsy specimens of erythema migrans lesions. Less invasive is the "two-step" approach, which combines an enzyme-linked immunosorbent assay (ELISA) with confirmatory immunoblotting (Western blot). These tests are insensitive during the first several weeks of infection. A Lyme urine antigen test is available, but it remains unreliable and should not be used.

Clinical Complications

LD may result in chronic neurologic or rheumatologic sequelae. Patients may have recurrent episodes of arthritis, even after appropriate treatment. A small percentage of appropriately treated patients continue to have subjective symptoms (musculoskeletal pain, neurocognitive difficulties, or fatigue)—so-called "chronic Lyme disease." In a large study, however, the frequencies of these symptoms were not different from those in age-matched control subjects without LD.[1]

Management

For early localized or disseminated infection, doxycycline therapy for 14 to 21 days is recommended for all patients older than 8 years of age except pregnant women. Amoxicillin and cefuroxime axetil are accepted alternatives. For patients with neurologic abnormalities (except isolated facial nerve palsy, which is treated as described above), intravenous ceftriaxone is recommended for 2 to 4 weeks. A vaccine is available for high-risk individuals aged 15 to 70 years. Prevention of tick bites should be emphasized. After a tick bite, even in Lyme-endemic areas, neither tick analysis nor prophylactic antibiotic treatment is routinely recommended.[1–3]

REFERENCES

1. Steere AC. Lyme disease. *N Engl J Med* 2001;345:115–125.
2. Sood SK. Lyme disease. *Pediatr Infect Dis J* 1999;18:913–925.
3. Weis JJ. Host-pathogen interactions and the pathogenesis of murine Lyme disease. *Curr Opin Rheumatol* 2002;14:399–403.

Malaria

Michele Lambert

Clinical Presentation

Malaria should be considered in any patient with fever who has recently returned from, or resides in, an endemic area.[1] Although signs and symptoms may be nonspecific, the hallmark of malaria is a high, spiking, recurrent fever. Classically, the length of time between fevers may help differentiate the offending species (a 72-hour cycle for *Plasmodium malariae* and a 48-hour cycle for *Plasmodium falciparum, Plasmodium vivax,* and *Plasmodium ovale*).[2] Patients infected with *P. falciparum* may present with encephalitis. More than 90% of travelers with *P. falciparum* infection become ill within 6 weeks after travel in endemic regions.[2] Patients with *P. vivax* infection may present as long as 6 months to years after their travel.

Pathophysiology

Malaria causes between 300 and 500 million new infections annually and kills 1.5 to 2.7 million people worldwide yearly.[2,3] Four *Plasmodium* species are known to infect humans, causing two types of disease: "relapsing" (*P. vivax* and *P. ovale*) and "nonrelapsing" (*P. falciparum* and *P. malariae*). *P. falciparum* is the most common cause of malaria worldwide and is the species most likely to cause serious illness (see Table 20–3).

Diagnosis

Diagnosis is made by the examination of thick blood smears (which allows for evaluation of many cells); identification of the *Plasmodium* species and the degree of parasitemia (percentage of neutrophils containing malarial pigment) is made on thin blood smears. Blood should be obtained while the patient is febrile. If the diagnosis is highly suspected (e.g., the patient is a recent traveler to a highly endemic or hyperendemic region), negative smears should be repeated every 8 to 12 hours for a total of three smears.[2] Physical examination may reveal hepatosplenomegaly, scleral icterus, or jaundice (20% of patients). Laboratory evaluation may reveal anemia, leukopenia, or thrombocytopenia. Markers for serious infection include respiratory distress, hypoglycemia, hypotension, renal failure, and greater than 5% parasitemia.[1,2]

Clinical Complications

Cerebral malaria (altered mental status, seizures, or coma) is a complication of *P. falciparum* with a high mortality rate. Other complications include hypoglycemia, hypotension, renal failure, and severe anemia. Complications are more likely in patients with greater than 5% parasitemia, pregnant women, children, and the elderly.[1–3]

Management

Treatment depends on the species and the severity of disease. Patients with greater than 5% parasitemia or other signs of severe disease (encephalitis, end-organ involvement, shock, acidosis, or hypoglycemia) should be admitted to the intensive care unit and treated with parenteral quinidine. Other patients should be closely monitored and treated with oral medications, depending on local resistance patterns of the area in which they traveled. For all species of *Plasmodium* except chloroquine-resistant *P. falciparum* and *P. vivax,* the oral treatment of choice is chloroquine. If drug resistance is suspected, multiple medications may be needed.[1–3]

REFERENCES

1. White NJ. The treatment of malaria. *N Engl J Med* 1996;335: 800–806.
2. Suh KN, Kozarsky PE, Keystone JS. Travel medicine: evaluation of fever in the returned traveler. *Med Clin North Am* 1999;83: 997–1017.
3. Baird JK, Hoffman SL. Prevention of malaria in travelers. *Med Clin North Am* 1999;83:923–944.

Malaria

Michele Lambert

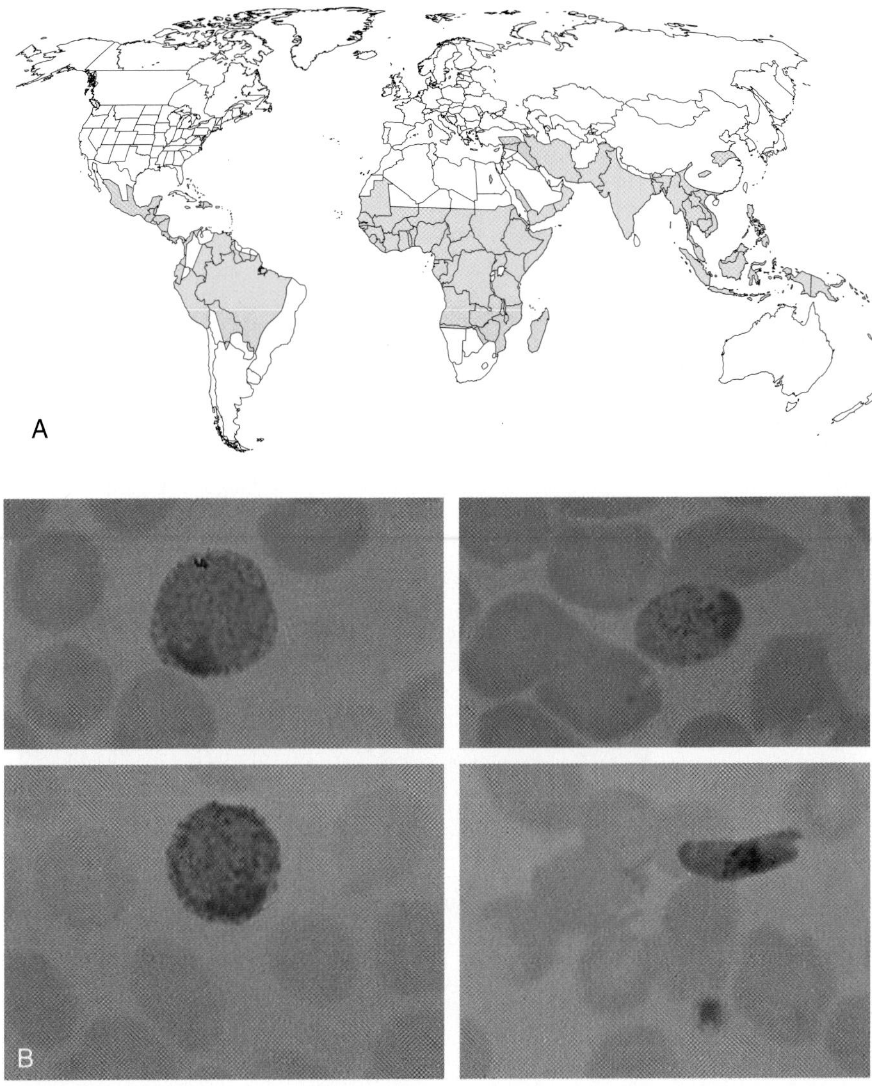

FIGURE 20–3 **A:** World distribution of malaria. Black areas indicate distribution of chloroquine-susceptible *Plasmodium falciparum* malaria, and gray areas indicate distribution of chloroquine-resistant *Plasmodium falciparum* malaria. (Modified with permission from Barat LM, Bloland PB. Drug resistance among malaria and other parasites. *Infect Dis Clin North Am* 1997;11:969–987.) **B:** Macrogametocytes of *Plasmodium vivax (top left), Plasmodium malaria (top right), Plasmodium ovale (bottom left),* and *Plasmodium falciparum (bottom right).* (From Smith JW. *Atlas of diagnostic medical parasitology: blood and tissue parasites.* Chicago: American Society of Clinical Pathologists, 1976.)

TABLE 20–3 Selected Clinical Characteristics of Four Types of Malaria

Characteristic	*Plasmodium falciparum*	*Plasmodium vivax*	*Plasmodium ovale*	*Plasmodium malariae*
Usual incubation period (d)	8–11	10–17 or longer	10–17 or longer	18–40 or longer
Severity of primary attack	Severe in nonimmune	Mild to severe	Mild	Mild
Periodicity (h)	None	48	48	72
Duration of untreated primary attack (wk)	2–3	3–8	2–3	3–24
Duration of untreated infection	6–17 mo	5–7 yr	12 mo	20+ yr
Average parasitemia (per mm^2)	≥20,000	10,000	9,000	6,000
Anemia	Frequent and severe	Mild	Mild	Mild
CNS involvement	Yes, severe	Rare	Rare	Rare
Nephritic syndrome	Rare	Rare	No	Frequent

From McClatchy, with permission.
d, days; h, hours; wk, week; mo, months; CNS, central nervous system.

Toxic Shock Syndrome

Michael Greenberg

Clinical Presentation

Patients with toxic shock syndrome (TSS) may present with malaise, chills, high fever (greater than 102° F), hypotension, mental status changes, vomiting, diarrhea, myalgias, conjunctival injection, "strawberry" tongue, and desquamation of the skin, usually involving the hands and feet.[1–3]

Pathophysiology

TSS is caused by various strains of staphylococcal and streptococcal bacteria capable of producing TSS toxins. Seventy-five percent of TSS cases involve TSS toxin-1, whereas 20% to 25% involve enterotoxin B. A small percentage of cases involve enterotoxin C.[1–3]

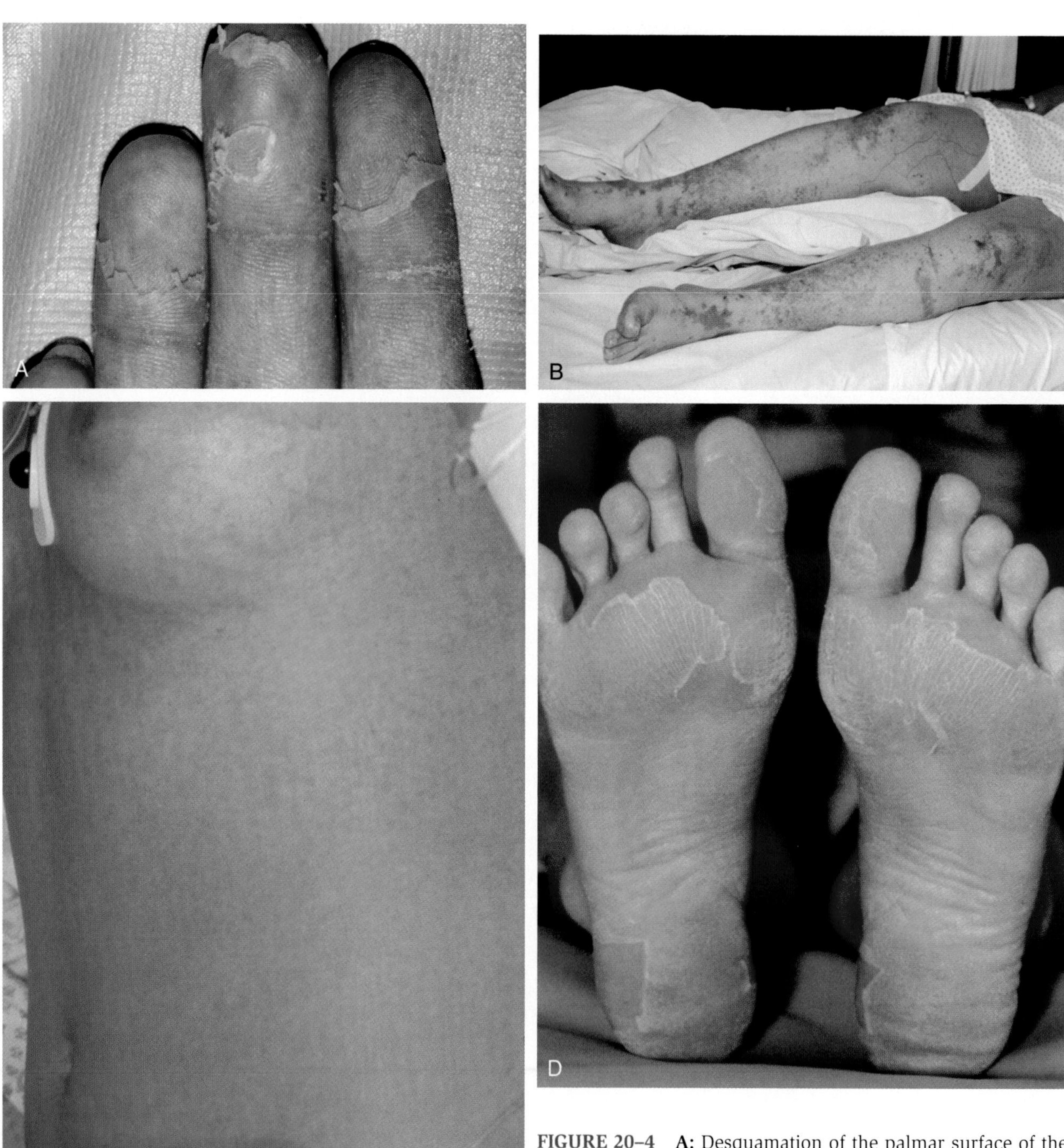

FIGURE 20–4 **A:** Desquamation of the palmar surface of the fingers. **B:** Petechiae and ecchymoses of the lower extremities. **C:** Petechiae of the trunk. **D:** Desquamation of the soles. (**A–D**, Courtesy of B. Zane Horowitz, MD.)

Toxic Shock Syndrome

Michael Greenberg

Despite the fact that the first reported cases of TSS appeared to exclusively afflict menstruating women who used tampons, recent work has shown as many as one third of cases are probably not related to menstruation.[1-3] Most cases are associated with local skin or wound infections, infected surgical wounds, or infections occurring in the postpartum period. Some cases have been associated with burns, retained nasal packing, or the use of barrier contraceptive devices.[1-3] Necrotizing fasciitis may be present in half of all TSS cases. A strong correlation exists between TSS and *Staphylococcus aureus* grown from vaginal cultures of TSS patients.[1-3] TSS occurs most often in women of childbearing age, especially teenage girls who use "hyperabsorbent" tampons.[1-3]

Diagnosis

The diagnosis of TSS is clinical and is based on the history and physical examination findings. Table 20–4 lists the current case-defining parameters for TSS.

TABLE 20–4 Case-Defining Parameters for Toxic Shock Syndrome (TSS)

Patients diagnosed as having TSS presented with shock and at least two of the following:
Acute renal insufficiency
Hematologic alterations:
Thrombocytopenia ($\leq$100,000 platelets/mm^3)
Disseminated intravascular coagulation
Hepatic injury:
Elevated aminotransferases or total bilirubin (greater than two times normal values)
Respiratory distress
Erythematous macular rash (desquamative or not desquamative)
Skin/soft-tissue necrosis

Adapted from Bernaldo De Quiros JC, Moreno S, Cercenado E, et al. Group A streptococcal bacteremia: a 10-year prospective study. *Medicine (Baltimore)* 1997;76:238–248.

Clinical Complications

Complications include septic shock, multiorgan system failure, extremity amputations, scarring, and death.[1-3]

Management

Aggressive treatment promptly initiated in the emergency department, including invasive hemodynamic monitoring and intravenous antibiotics, may be lifesaving. Usual drug regimens include clindamycin, penicillins, cephalosporins, and aminoglycoside antibiotics in combination.[1-3] In addition, emergency and extensive surgical débridement of infected areas may be lifesaving. Some cases have been successfully treated with the use of intravenous immune globulin. Patients with suspected TSS require immediate hospitalization in an intensive care setting and emergency consultation with infectious disease specialists.[1-3]

REFERENCES

1. Bisno AL, Stevens DL. Streptococcal infections of skin and soft tissues. *N Engl J Med* 1996;334:240–245.
2. Bernaldo De Quiros JC, Moreno S, et al. Group A streptococcal bacteremia: a 10-year prospective study. *Medicine (Baltimore)* 1997;76:238–248.
3. Chadwell JS, Gustafson LM, Tami TA. Toxic shock syndrome associated with frontal sinus stents. *Otolaryngol Head Neck Surg* 2001;124:573–574.

Staphylococcal Scalded Skin Syndrome

Michael Greenberg

Clinical Presentation

Patients with staphylococcal scalded skin syndrome (SSSS) present with fever and a diffuse, erythematous, tender rash of the face, trunk, and extremities. This rash rapidly develops into fluid-filled blisters that enlarge and then slough. Most cases of SSSS occur in children, but adult cases have also been reported.[1-3]

Pathophysiology

SSSS is caused by staphylococcal exfoliative toxins A (ETA) and B (ETB) that are secreted from phage II staphylococci. These toxins spread via the bloodstream.[1-3]

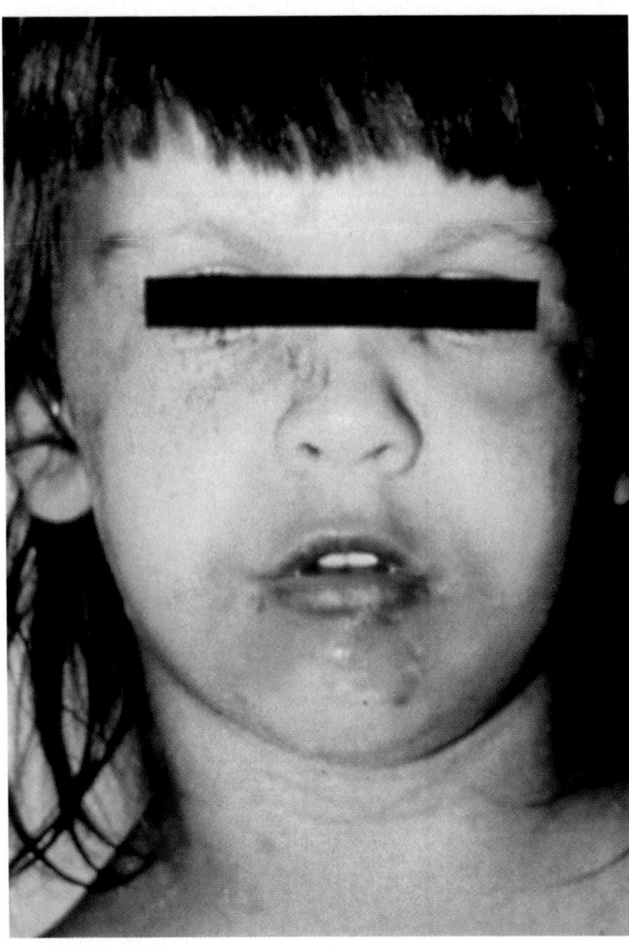

FIGURE 20-5 Staphylococcal scalded skin syndrome. Erythema is prominent on the neck and around the eyes and mouth. Crusting is also apparent in the periorificial areas. Over the chin, a bulla has ruptured, leaving a moist erosion. (From Mandell, *Essential Atlas of Infectious Diseases,* with permission.)

ETA exhibits "superantigen" characteristics, including epidermolysis and lymphocyte mitogenicity. This leads to separation of the stratum granulosum and stratum spinosum, giving rise to a positive Nikolsky's sign. Immature renal function and inefficient clearing of exotoxins may predispose neonates to SSSS. Outbreaks of SSSS in neonatal intensive care units (NICUs) are often related to the presence of medical and nursing staff who are infected or colonized with coagulase-positive *Staphylococcus aureus.* This organism may be cultured from up to 30% of NICU staff members in hospitals. Culture of blister fluid usually is not helpful.[2,3]

Diagnosis

SSSS must be considered in any infant with exfoliate dermatitis. The diagnosis is based on clinical findings. Laboratory and imaging studies are of limited help in confirming the diagnosis.

Clinical Complications

Complications include temperature instability, fluid losses, secondary skin infections, sepsis, and death.[2,3]

Management

The nares, conjunctiva, and skin around blisters of SSSS patients should be cultured. Prompt treatment with β-lactamase-resistant penicillin is usually effective. Supportive care aimed at limiting fluid and electrolyte losses is critically important. Topical antibiotics usually are not effective and therefore are not indicated.[1-3] Meticulous local wound care is essential to prevent secondary infection. The use of an incubator for infants with SSSS may help to decrease insensible fluid loss through denuded skin. All staff must adhere to strict infection control techniques, and hand washing for staff and parents is essential.[1-3]

REFERENCES

1. Prabhash K, Babu KG, Ravi S, et al. Staphylococcal scalded skin syndrome. *Lancet Infect Dis* 2003;3:442.
2. Makhoul IR, Kassis I, Hashman N, Sujov P. Staphylococcal scalded skin syndrome in a very low birth weight premature infant. *Pediatrics* 2001;108:E16.
3. Prevost G, Couppie P, Monteil H. Staphylococcal epidermolysins. *Curr Opin Infect Dis* 2003;16:71–76.

Acute Rheumatic Fever

Kyung Rhee

Clinical Presentation

Acute rheumatic fever (ARF) manifests as fever, abdominal pain, polyarthritis, carditis, erythema marginatum, and subcutaneous nodules in children between 5 and 15 years of age. Symptoms usually develop 2 to 4 weeks after an episode of acute group A β-hemolytic streptococci (GABHS) pharyngitis, although one third of patients cannot recall a recent pharyngitis. Polyarthritis (60% to 75% of cases) typically affects multiple joints (mean, six joints). The carditis is a pancarditis that may manifest with fever or only a murmur. Erythema marginatum (5%) is typically transient (present for only hours) and is found on the trunk and proximal extremities, sparing the face. Subcutaneous nodules (5%) are firm, painless nodules on extensor surfaces and bony prominences. Children may also have anemia, prolongation of the PR interval (35%), and elevation of acute phase reactants (erythrocyte sedimentation rate (ESR), C-reactive protein (CRP), and white blood cell count). Sydenham's chorea (10% to 30%) occurs 1 to 6 months after the ARF and is self-limited (usually 1 to 2 weeks, occasionally 3 to 6 months).[1,2]

Pathophysiology

ARF is a systemic inflammatory disease associated with previous pharyngeal GABHS infection.[1] ARF is the leading cause of acquired heart disease in children on a worldwide basis. ARF is an autoimmune response to proteins in the GABHS organism that are immunologically cross-reactive with human tissues (e.g., heart, joints).[1]

Diagnosis

Diagnosis is based on the Jones criteria, which include five major criteria and four minor criteria. To make the diagnosis, there must be evidence of a recent GABHS infection and the fulfillment of two major, or one major and two minor, criteria.[1,2] Evidence of recent infection usually involves rising antistreptolysin O (ASO) titers or anti-DNase B tests. A throat culture may be done at the time of ARF illness; however, it is positive in only 10% to 30% of cases. Additional laboratory findings include an elevated ESR, CRP, and leukocytosis.

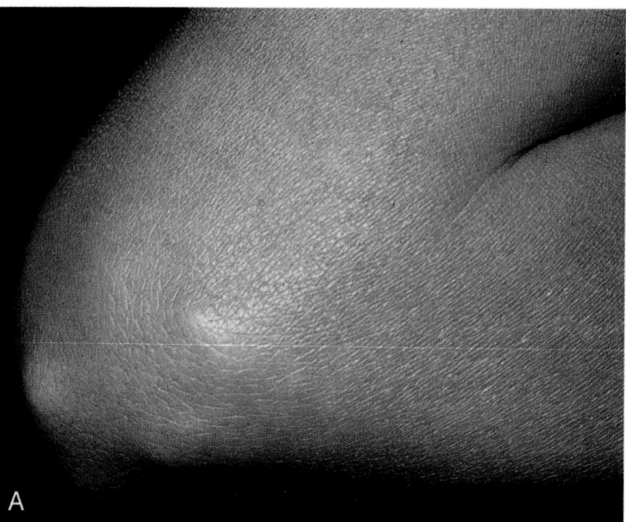

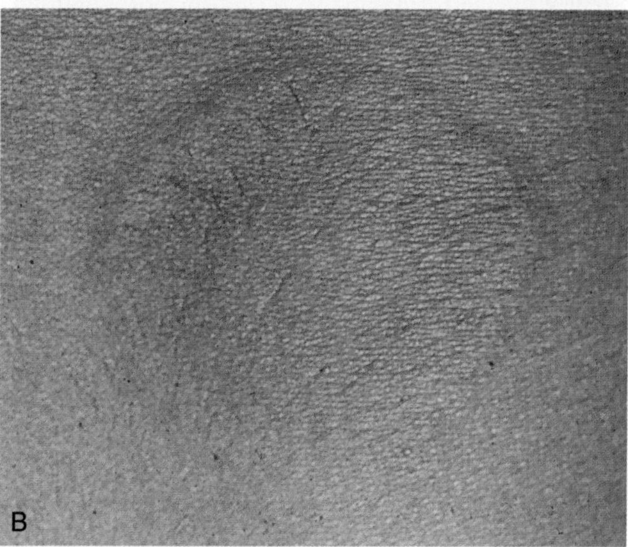

FIGURE 20–6 **A:** Subcutaneous nodules are generally associated with severe carditis. They are painless, firm, movable, measure approximately 0.5 to 2 cm, and usually are located over extensor surfaces of the joints, particularly knees, wrists, and elbows. **B:** Closer view of erythema marginatum in the same patient. (**A** and **B**, From Binotto MA, Guilherme L, Tanaka AC. Rheumatic fever. *Images Paediatr Cardiol* 2002;11:12–25.)

Clinical Complications

Complications include valvular heart disease and heart failure.

Management

Patients with ARF should be treated with oral penicillin V for 10 days or with one dose of intramuscular benzathine penicillin G (or erythromycin, if allergic to penicillin).[1] Family members should also be cultured for GABHS. Antiinflammatory agents (e.g., aspirin) may be used to treat carditis, arthritis, and chorea.[1] Glucocorticoids may be used in severe cases. Chorea is usually self-limited and does not necessarily warrant therapy. Severe cases may be treated with bed rest and anticonvulsants.

REFERENCES

1. Stollerman GH. Rheumatic fever. *Lancet* 1997;349:935–942.
2. Alsaeid K, Majeed HA. Acute rheumatic fever: diagnosis and treatment. *Pediatr Ann* 1998;27:295–300.

Tetanus

Michael Greenberg

Clinical Presentation

Tetanus is an uncommon disease in the United States but a substantial cause of death worldwide.[1,2] Patients may present after obvious injuries, including thermal burns, snakebites, otitis media, skin ulcers, gangrene, septic abortions, childbirth, intramuscular injections, surgery, and puncture wounds or other wounds contaminated with soil, manure, or rusty metal.[1,2] Up to 50% of cases occur after apparently insignificant and often clinically inapparent injuries.[1,2] Between 15% and 25% of cases are not associated with a recent wound.[1,2] The earliest symptoms of tetanus involve neck stiffness, sore throat, and difficulty opening the mouth.[1,2]

Pathophysiology

Tetanus is caused by *Clostridium tetani,* a gram-positive bacillus known to secrete two toxins, tetanospasmin and tetanolysin, under anaerobic conditions.[1,2] Tetanospasmin is responsible for causing the clinical syndrome of tetanus. Tetanospasmin is a two-chain polypeptide, the light chain of which acts presynaptically to prevent neurotransmitter release after the heavy chain facilitates entry of these molecules into cells. Tetanospasmin cleaves synaptobrevin, which is a protein required for neurotransmitter release. The incubation period ranges from 1 to 60 days (average, 7 to 10 days). Recovery from tetanus occurs as a result of toxin destruction and regrowth of axon terminals.[1,2]

Diagnosis

The diagnosis is made on the basis of index of suspicion and clinical findings alone. No specific laboratory tests rule out tetanus. Tetanus may involve a clinical triad that includes muscular rigidity, muscle spasms, and autonomic dysfunction. It affects the head and neck muscles first and then spread caudally.[1,2] Masseter spasm results in so-called "lockjaw" (trismus) and may progress to the facial muscles, causing "risus sardonicus" and difficulty swallowing. Neck muscle rigidity may cause head retractions and opisthotonus.[1,2] The differential diagnosis includes strychnine poisoning, dystonia, hypocalcemia, and hysterical conversion.[2]

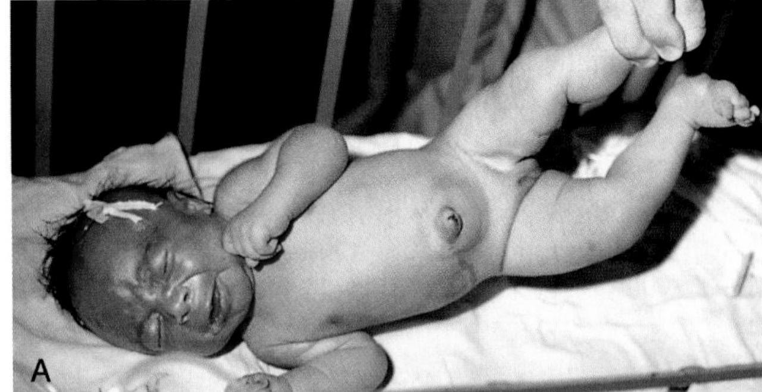

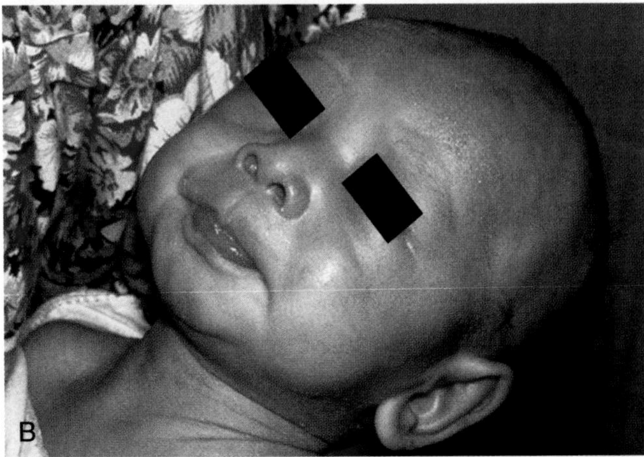

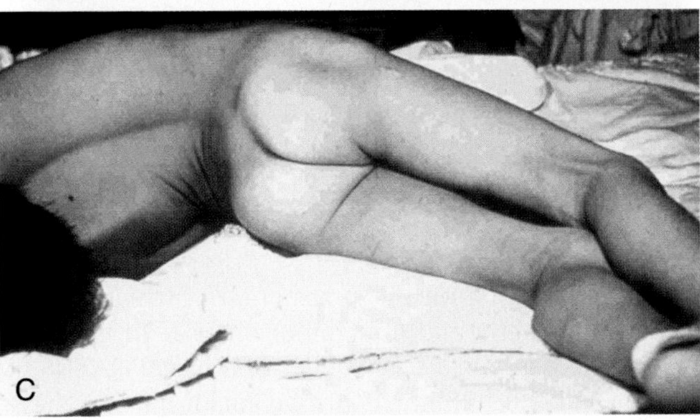

FIGURE 20–7 **A:** Neonatal tetanus at 6 days. The umbilical stump was treated with ashes. Note risus sardonicus and opisthotonus. (From Ostler, with permission.) **B:** "Lockjaw." (Courtesy of the World Health Organization.) **C:** Opisthotonus. (Courtesy of the Centers for Disease Control and Prevention.)

Clinical Complications

Potential complications are legion and may include aspiration, airway obstruction, acute respiratory distress syndrome, cardiac arrhythmias, congestive heart failure, renal failure, gastric stasis, ileus, diarrhea, gastrointestinal bleeding, thromboembolus, sepsis, multiorgan failure, vertebral fractures, and tendon avulsions during spasms.[1,2]

Management

Three concomitant modalities are employed to (1) neutralize unbound toxin by the administration of human tetanus immune globulin; (2) remove the source of infection by the use of metronidazole, erythromycin, tetracycline, chloramphenicol, or clindamycin; and (3) control rigidity, spasms, and autonomic dysfunction by the use of benzodiazepines, propofol, neuromuscular blocking agents, and/or baclofen.[1,2]

REFERENCES

1. Hsu SS, Groleau G. Tetanus in the emergency department: a current review. *J Emerg Med* 2001;20:357–365.
2. Cook TM, Protheroe RT, Handel JM. Tetanus: a review of the literature. *Br J Anaesth* 2001;87:477–487.

Botulism

Anthony Morocco

Clinical Presentation

Symptoms of botulism begin 2 hours to 8 days after exposure. Patients who develop botulism by inhalation or ingestion of toxin exhibit the same neurologic symptoms but not the gastrointestinal symptoms that may be present in the naturally occurring disease. Invariably, a descending paralysis develops, beginning with bulbar findings, including ptosis, gaze paralysis, and dilated or fixed pupils. Patients complain of blurred vision, dysarthria, dysphonia, and dysphagia. Most patients exhibit an alert mental status. Gradual decrease or loss of reflexes and respiratory muscle paralysis may occur.[1]

Pathophysiology

Botulinum toxin is a potential weapon of bioterrorism via aerosol release or food supply contamination. Botulinum toxin exists in seven serotypes, designated by the letters A through G. Types A, B, E, and, rarely, F are known to cause the natural disease. Toxin is absorbed from the gastrointestinal tract and lungs, but it does not penetrate intact skin. The lethal human oral dose is estimated to be 70 ng. The toxin prevents the release of acetylcholine by blocking the fusion of neurotransmitter-containing vesicles with the presynaptic membrane, primarily at the neuromuscular junction.[1]

Diagnosis

The diagnosis of botulism should be strongly suspected in any patient with descending paralysis and a clear sensorium. Bioterrorism should be suspected in the following circumstances: an outbreak with a common geographic area but no common food source; identification of toxin types C, D, E (without an aquatic food source) F, or G; or occurrence of a large number of cases. The mouse bioassay to confirm the diagnosis and toxin type is available through the Centers for Disease Control and Prevention (CDC). Electromyography may help to confirm the diagnosis and differentiate botulism from potential misdiagnoses, such as Guillain-Barré and Miller-Fisher syndrome.

Clinical Complications

Patients may require prolonged mechanical ventilation, resulting in complications such as nosocomial infections.[1]

Management

Treatment consists primarily of supportive care. Recovery occurs in weeks to months as new axons sprout to create new neuromuscular junctions. An equine antitoxin is available through the CDC. Antitoxin may limit progression of the disease, but it does not improve existing paralysis, so it should be administered as early as possible. This trivalent antitoxin is effective for types A, B, and E only. Secondary infections should not be treated with clindamycin or aminoglycosides, because they may worsen neuromuscular blockade.

REFERENCES

1. Arnon SS, Schecter R, Inglesby TV, et al. Botulinum toxin as a biological weapon: medical and public health management. *JAMA* 2001;285:1059–1070.

TABLE 20–8 Differential Diagnosis of Botulism

Disease	Fever	Eye signs	Ascend descend	Symmetric asymmetric	Motor sensory autonomic	Comment
Botulism	−	Yes	Descend bulbar	Symmetric	Motor > autonomic	DTR absent late, ptosis late
Guillain-Barré	+	No	Ascend bulbar	Symmetric	Motor > sensory	Abnormal CSF, DTR absent
Fisher type		Yes			Autonomic	Early, previous URI
Poliomyelitis	+	No	Ascend bulbar	Asymmetric focal	Motor	Abnormal CSF, DTR absent early
Paralytic shellfish	−	No	Ascend	Symmetric	Motor = sensory	History, onset within 30–60 min
Tick paralysis	−	No	Ascend	Symmetric	Motor > sensory	Presence of tick
Diphtheria	+	No	Ascend	Symmetric	Motor	Membrane in pharynx
Myasthenia gravis	−	Yes	Descend bulbar	Symmetric	Motor autonomic	Ptosis early, fatigue
Lead	−	No	Ascend	Symmetric	Motor	History
Arsenic	−	No	Ascend	Symmetric distal	Sensory > motor	History
Periodic familial paralysis	−	No	Ascend	Symmetric	Motor	Family history
	Does not affect muscles of respirations					

+, present; −, absent; CSF, cerebrospinal fluid; DTR, deep tendon reflexes; URI, upper respiratory infection.
Adapted from Mofenson HC, et al., eds. *PP/T News.* MMWC Poison Control Center 1989;8:139.

20–9

Hepatitis and Jaundice

Jonathan Glauser

Clinical Presentation

Patients with hepatitis or jaundice may present with a prodrome of anorexia, malaise, and low-grade fever. Dark urine and light stools may be present. Clinical jaundice requires a bilirubin concentration of 3 to 4 mg/dL. Immune complex formation may cause morbilliform rash, arthralgias, or arthritis.[1–3]

Pathophysiology

Jaundice is generally categorized as unconjugated or conjugated. Unconjugated hyperbilirubinemia may result from overproduction, as in hemolysis, or from decreased conjugation by the liver. Conjugated hyperbilirubinemia typically entails acquired liver disease, as in hepatitis, or biliary obstruction, as from a tumor or a common bile duct stone.[2]

Hepatitis A is spread by oral contact, is generally nonlethal, and does not produce a carrier state. Chronic hepatitis B virus (HBV) infection affects an estimated 1.25 million people in the United States. Hepatitis C virus (HCV) affects approximately 1.8% of the American population, causing 8,000 to 10,000 deaths annually, and is the leading cause for liver failure that necessitates transplantation. Because of their shared route of transmission, HCV infection is common among persons infected with the human immunodeficiency virus (HIV).[1] The risk of infection after a needlestick injury if the source is positive for the hepatitis B e antigen, Hb(e)Ag, is greater than 30%. In contrast, the average infection rate if the source is HCV positive is 1.8%.[2]

A variety of other viruses may cause hepatitis, including cytomegalovirus, herpes simplex, and Epstein-Barr virus.[1,2] Drugs and toxicants associated with hepatitis are listed in Table 20–9.

TABLE 20–9 Drugs and Toxicants Associated with Hepatitis

Acetaminophen
Amanita phalloides mushrooms
Halothane
Isoniazid
Lamotrigine
Lovastatin
α-Methyldopa
Nonsteroidal antiinflammatory drugs
Phenytoin
Sertraline
Terbinafine
Troglitazone

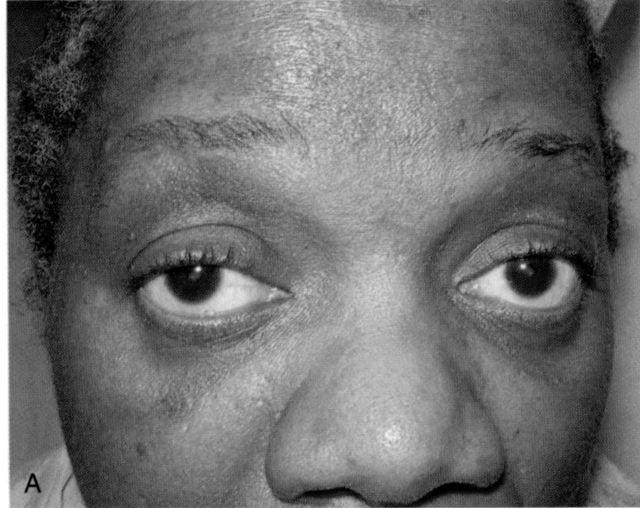

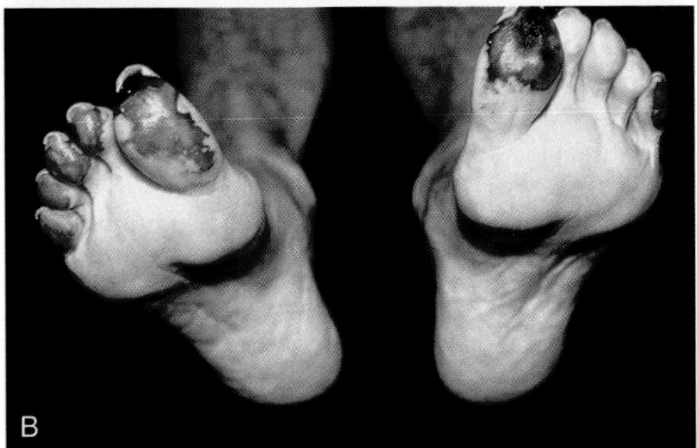

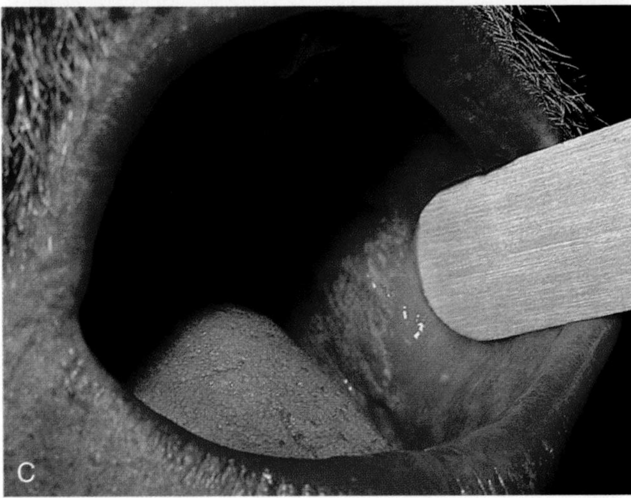

FIGURE 20–9 **A:** Icteric sclera in a patient with hepatitis C. (Courtesy of Mark Silverberg, MD.) **B:** Cryoglobulinemia produces acral vasculitic infarcts. Hepatitis C is a leading cause. (From Yamada, with permission.) **C:** Lichen planus produces lacy mucosal plaques and pruritic papules on the skin. Patients should be evaluated for hepatitis C infection. (From Yamada, with permission.)

Hepatitis and Jaundice

Jonathan Glauser

Diagnosis

Transaminase levels are elevated (more than 10 times normal). Serologic testing for hepatitis A, B, or C may yield the cause. Conjugated and unconjugated bilirubin levels may suggest whether biliary obstruction is present. Serum albumin and prothrombin time may indicate synthetic function of the liver. Computed tomography and ultrasonography are helpful in diagnosing biliary obstruction.[1-3]

Clinical Complications

Hypoglycemia, coagulopathy, portal hypertension, gastrointestinal bleeding, or encephalopathy may result from hepatic insufficiency. HBV or HCV infection may cause fulminate liver failure, chronic liver disease and cirrhosis, hepatocellular carcinoma, or death.[1-3]

Prophylaxis

Hepatitis B vaccination for high-risk adults could prevent up to 800 cases of hepatitis and 10 deaths from hepatitis per 10,000 vaccinations.[3] Hepatitis A vaccine is recommended for some travelers outside the United States and in some high-risk locations in the United States.[3]

Management

Admission and antibiotic therapy is mandatory if bacterial cholangitis is suspected. Otherwise, the decision for admission of a patient with hepatitis or jaundice depends on management of pain, hydration, vomiting, or complications of liver disease (e.g., gastrointestinal bleeding, altered mental status). Therapy for hepatitis B may include adefovir, lamivudine, or interferon alfa-2b. For HCV infection, pegylated interferon alfa-2a or -2b plus ribavirin has been used.[2,3]

REFERENCES

1. Sulkowski MS, Thomas DL. Hepatitis C in the HIV-infected person. *Ann Intern Med* 2003;138:197–207.
2. Goldmann DA. Blood-borne pathogens and nosocomial infections. *J Allergy Clin Immunol* 2002;110(2 Suppl):S21–S26.
3. Rich JD, Ching CG, Lally MA, et al. A review of the case for hepatitis B vaccination of high-risk adults. *Am J Med* 2003;114:316–318.

Necrotizing Infections

Gail Rudnitsky

Clinical Presentation

The affected area in a patient with a necrotizing infection may initially resemble cellulitis, with redness and edema at the site of infection. There is no clearcut line of demarcation or lymphangitis. As the infection progresses to necrosis, the skin turns purple or black. Hemorrhagic bullae may develop.[1-3] The subcutaneous tissues and the fascia underneath become gangrenous, and myonecrosis may develop. Bacteremia and signs of toxic shock syndrome may be present. These patients generally appear ill, with high fevers, chills, hypotension, and other constitutional symptoms. Hypotension and frank shock may develop.[1-3]

Pathophysiology

Necrotizing infections are soft-tissue infections that cause extensive local tissue damage and may lead to toxemia or death. Two common terms for these types of infections are Fournier's gangrene (localized to the perineum) and necrotizing fasciitis (deep subcutaneous infection).[1-3] Necrotizing fasciitis is frequently caused by group A β-hemolytic streptococci (GABHS), although *Staphylococcus aureus* and *Clostridium perfringens* have also been implicated.[1-3] Patients with diabetes, trauma, or immunocompromise are particularly susceptible. The organisms spread through the deep tissue above the fascia, causing thrombosis of vessels, which leads to gangrene of the subcutaneous tissues. Fishermen in warm-water areas may develop necrotizing fasciitis from *Vibrio* species. Fournier's gangrene is most commonly a polymicrobial infection, with gram-negative organisms predominating.[1-3]

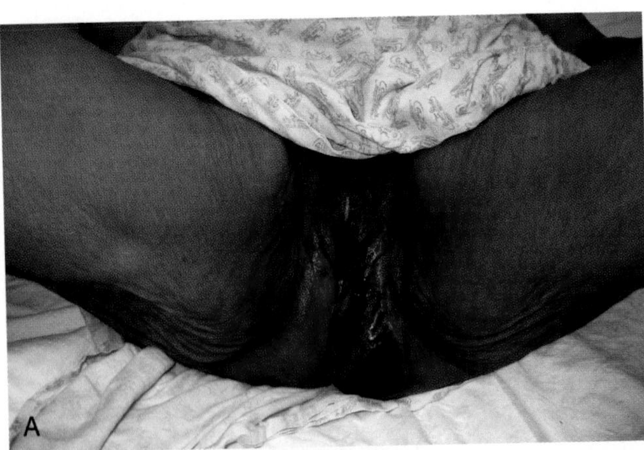

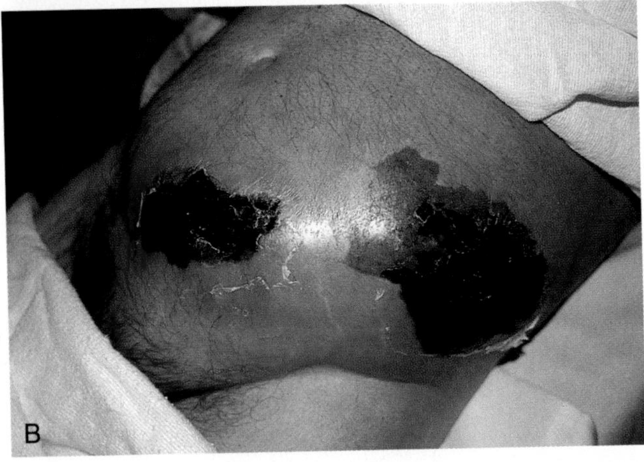

FIGURE 20–10 A: Fournier's gangrene. (Courtesy of Mark Silverberg, MD.) **B:** Necrotizing fasciitis of the anterior abdominal wall. (From Isaacs L. Necrotizing fasciitis: diagnosis and treatment. *Emerg Med News* 2002;24[8]:4, with permission.)

Diagnosis

The clinical diagnosis may be supported by diagnostic studies. Patients generally have a leukocytosis with a left shift. A Gram stain from the site of infection or from a blood culture may help identify the organism. Computed tomography and magnetic resonance imaging may be used to determine the extent of the infection.

Clinical Complications

Complications include metastatic abscesses in distant organs, septic shock, and multisystem organ failure. If left untreated, this disease has a high mortality rate.

Management

Patients with necrotizing infections should be admitted to the intensive care unit, and all necessary supportive measures should be instituted. The mainstays of treatment are high-dose antibiotics and surgical débridement. Broad-spectrum antibiotics are used until cultures and sensitivity results are obtained. Surgical débridement should include areas of thrombotic tissue to prevent further necrosis. Fasciotomy may be necessary. Hyperbaric oxygen therapy may improve the mortality rate. Intravenous immunoglobulin may be beneficial in necrotizing infections caused by GABHS.

REFERENCES

1. Trent JT, Kirsner RS. Diagnosing necrotizing fasciitis. *Adv Skin Wound Care* 2002;15:135–138.
2. Seal DV. Necrotizing fasciitis. *Curr Opin Infect Dis* 2001;14:127–132.
3. Headley AJ. Necrotizing soft tissue infections: a primary care review. *Am Fam Physician* 2003;68:323–328.

Meningococcemia

Douglas Thompson

Clinical Presentation

Patients with meningococcemia present with fever, vomiting, headache, abdominal pain, lethargy, and myalgia. The characteristic petechial rash may be subtle or absent on presentation but may progress to purpura and necrosis.[1–3] Specific signs of meningitis may not be evident.[1–3]

Pathophysiology

The spectrum of disease ranges from a self-limited illness to rapid progression to septic shock, coma, and death in as little as 12 hours. Cardiovascular collapse, change in mental status, acute respiratory distress syndrome, renal failure, hepatitis, disseminated intravascular coagulopathy (DIC), and ischemic extremities are evidence of multisystem organ dysfunction.[1–3] Massive adrenal hemorrhage in association with cardiovascular collapse is referred to as Waterhouse-Friderichsen syndrome. Arthritis occurs in a small percentage of patients.

The peak incidence occurs in late winter and early spring. Children younger than 2 years of age account for almost half of the infections, with the peak attack rate in those younger than 4 months. Individuals in crowded military barracks and college dormitories represent a much smaller peak. Those with terminal complement and properdin deficiencies are also at risk.[1–3]

Between 5% and 15% of individuals in nonendemic areas are nasopharyngeal carriers of meningococci. Serogroups B, C, and Y account for most cases of disease in the United States. Transmission occurs via small droplets in close contacts, with the development of disease usually occurring within 2 weeks after acquisition. Passive cigarette smoke and concurrent viral respiratory tract infection are risk factors for bacterial translocation across the nasopharyngeal mucosa, leading to bacteremia and release of a lipopolysaccharide endotoxin into the bloodstream. Subsequent complement activation and release of cytokines and other inflammatory mediators results in the systemic inflammatory response syndrome that is responsible for the clinical manifestations. Capillary leak, vasodilation, and myocardial dysfunction all contribute to cardiovascular collapse. The procoagulant state resulting from the inflammatory cascade leads to systemic microthrombi and petechiae, purpura, DIC, extremity ischemia, and multisystem organ dysfunction.[1–3]

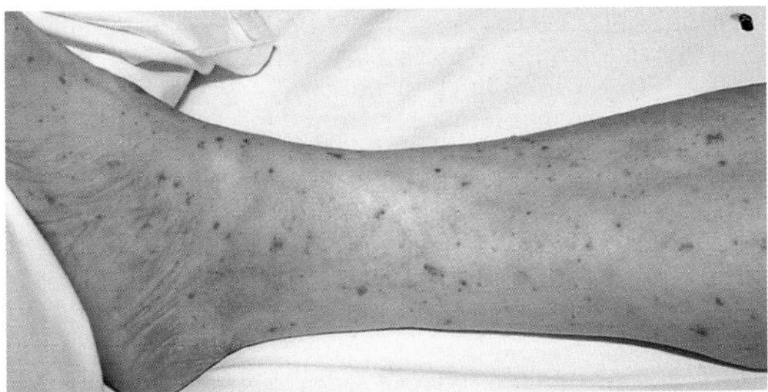

FIGURE 20–11 Petechial eruption in meningococcemia. The trunk and lower extremities are the most frequent sites of these lesions. (From Ostler, with permission.)

Diagnosis

The disease may be confirmed by culture of the blood or spinal fluid in most patients. A small percentage of diagnoses are confirmed by cultures of joint fluid or skin lesions. In some patients, the diagnosis is made on clinical grounds. Antigen testing is unreliable. Spinal fluid analysis should be performed in patients with suspected meningococcal infection who are cardiovascularly and hematologically stable.

Clinical Complications

The mortality rate ranges as high as 50%. Poor prognostic factors include the presence of petechiae for less than 12 hours, shock, absence of meningitis, a leukocyte count lower than 10,000 cells/mm^3, and an erythrocyte sedimentation rate of less than 10 mm/hour.[1,2] Between 10% and 20% of survivors experience long-term sequelae, which may include neurologic impairment, amputation of extremities, skin grafts, and renal failure.[1–3]

Management

Most experts recommend ceftriaxone or cefotaxime as first-line agents. Chloramphenicol may be used in those with anaphylactic response to penicillins. The remainder of care is supportive, with a focus on hemodynamic stability and management of DIC. Careful monitoring and support of other organ systems is important.[1–3]

Rifampin should be prescribed as chemoprophylaxis to household members, daycare center contacts, and persons exposed to the patient's oral secretions.[1–3]

REFERENCES

1. van Deuren M, Brandtzaeg P, van der Meer JW. Update on meningococcal disease with emphasis on pathogenesis and clinical management. *Clin Microbiol Rev* 2000;13:144–166.
2. Meningococcal disease prevention and control strategies for practice-based physicians. American Academy of Pediatrics. Infectious Diseases and Immunization Committee, Canadian Paediatric Society. *Pediatrics* 1996;97:404–412.
3. Prevention and control of meningococcal disease. Recommendations of the Advisory Committee on Immunization Practices (ACIP). *MMWR Morb Mortal Wkly Rep* 2000;49(RR-7):1-10.

Meningitis

Robert Hendrickson

Clinical Presentation

Patients with meningitis may present with headache (50%), neck pain/stiffness (70%), nausea/vomiting (30%), or fever (85%).[1] Presentations involving alterations in mental status, seizures, or focal neurologic deficits are not uncommon. "Atypical" presentations are frequent, and the classic signs and symptoms are uncommon in infants and the elderly.[1]

Pathophysiology

Meningitis is an infection of the meninges and cerebrospinal fluid (CSF) caused by bacteria, fungi, or viruses. Infection results from hematogenous spread or direct extension from the scalp, face, mouth, or sinuses.[2] Infectious organisms vary with age. Bacterial invasion of the meninges leads to infiltration of the CSF with white blood cells and release of inflammatory mediators. Inflammation may induce thrombosis of surface cerebral vessels or swelling of the central nervous system, leading to cerebral edema.

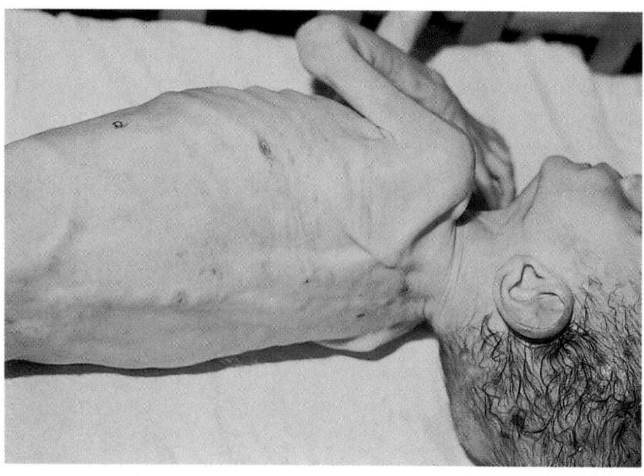

FIGURE 20-12 Meningoencephalitis (note marked opisthotonos) as a complication of chickenpox in this extremely malnourished infant seen in Central America. The patient died the day after this photograph was taken. (From Ostler, with permission.)

Diagnosis

The diagnosis is suspected clinically and confirmed by evaluation of the CSF. Clinical suspicion should be heightened by evidence of systemic infection (fever, rash) and meningeal irritation (neck pain or stiffness, headache, alteration of mental status). Kernig's and Brudzinski's signs are both specific for severe meningeal irritation, but they are not sensitive for meningitis.[1] With the patient supine and the hip flexed 90 degrees, Kernig's sign is positive if extension of the knee elicits resistance or pain in the thigh or lower back.[1] Brudzinski's sign is positive if flexion of the neck in a supine patient produces flexion of the hips.[1]

Clinical Complications

Complications include cerebral edema, cerebral thrombosis, seizures, herniation, and death. Up to 18% of healthy patients who survive meningitis experience long-term sequelae (e.g., fatigue, ataxia, dizziness, hearing loss).[1,2]

Management

Patients may require resuscitation or airway control or both. Patients with suspected bacterial meningitis should not have antibiotics delayed while waiting for imaging or lumbar puncture results (see Tables 20-12A and 20-12B).[3] Antibiotics should be selected according to the likely pathogens, based on the patient's characteristics.[3] Dexamethasone may be given before antibiotics in children older than 2 months of age with bacterial meningitis and to adults with evidence of elevated intracranial pressure or a positive Gram stain.[3] Only patients with focal neurologic deficits, alterations of mental status, immunocompromise, acquired immunodeficiency syndrome (AIDS), papilledema, or suspicion of a cerebral mass require a computed tomographic scan of the head before lumbar puncture.[2,3]

REFERENCES

1. Attia J, Hatala R, Cook DJ, Wong JG. Does this adult patient have acute meningitis? *JAMA* 1999;282:175–181.
2. Hasbun R, Abrahams J, Jekel J, Quagliarello VJ. Computed tomography of the head before lumbar puncture in adults with suspected meningitis. *N Engl J Med* 2001;345:1727–1733.
3. Quagliarello VJ, Scheld WM. Treatment of bacterial meningitis. *N Engl J Med* 1997;336:708–716.

Meningitis

Robert Hendrickson

TABLE 20–12A Initial Antimicrobial Therapy for Meningitis and Encephalitis

Predisposing Factor	Common Organisms	Therapy
0–4 weeks	*Escherichia coli*, group B strep, *Listeria monocytogenes*, *Klebsiella* spp.	Ampicillin plus cefotaxime; or ampicillin plus aminoglycoside
4–12 weeks	*E. Coli*, group B strep, *L. monocytogenes*, *Haemophilus influenzae*, *Streptococcus pneumoniae*,[e] *Neisseria meningitidis*	Ampicillin plus a third-generation cephalosporin[a]
3 months–18 years	*H. influenzae*, *N. meningitides*, *S. pneumoniae*[e]	Third-generation cephalosporin[a]; or ampicillin plus chloramphenicol
18–50 years	*S. pneumoniae*,[e] *N. meningitidis*	Third-generation cephalosporin[a] +/−ampicillin[b]
>50 years	*S. pneumoniae*,[e] *N. meningitides*, *L. monocytogenes*	Ampicillin plus a third-generation cephalosporin
Immunocompromised	*S. pneumoniae*,[e] *N. meningitides*, *L. monocytogenes*, Gram-neg. bacilli, including *Pseudomonas aeruginosa*	Vancomycin plus ampicillin plus ceftazidime[c]
	Cryptococcus neoformans, *Aspergillus mucor*	Amphotericin B and 5-Fluorocytosine
Basilar skull fracture	*S. pneumoniae*,[e] *H. influenzae*, group A β-hemolytic strep	Third-generation cephalosporin[a]
Postneurosurgery; head trauma	*Staphylococcus aureus*, *S. epidermidis*, Gram-neg. bacilli (including *P. aeruginosa*)	Vancomycin plus ceftazidime[c]
All ages	Herpes simplex	Acyclovir
	Varicella-zoster	
	Rabies	No treatment
	Rickettsial Rocky Mountain Spotted Fever	Tetracycline or chloramphenicol
	Toxoplasma gondii	Pyrimethamine[d] and sulfadiazine
	Spirochete: Leptospira	Doxycycline
	Ameba: *Naegleria fowleri*	IV and intrathecal Amphotericin B
	Mycobacterium tuberculosis	Rifampin and isoniazid and ethambutol and pyrazinamide

[a] Cefotaxime or ceftriaxone
[b] If Listeria is thought to be a likely etiological agent
[c] Add gentamicin in proven *P. aeruginosa* meningitis
[d] Folinic acid may reduce toxicity
[e] In cases in which a highly penicillin-resistant pneumococcus is suspected, vancomycin should be added
Reprinted from Schwartz, with permission.

TABLE 20–12B Cerebrospinal Fluid (CSF) Findings

Diagnosis	RBC	Mono	PMN	CSF Pressure (mmHg)	Glucose (mg/dL)	Protein (mg/dL)
Normal CSF	0	<5	0	<200	40-75	15-55
Bacterial	N	+	+ + +	+	>55	
Aseptic meningitis	N	+ +	+	+	N	+
Amebic, protozoan, fungal, tubercular	N	+ + +	+	+	<40	+
Spirochete, viral	N, +	+ +[a]	+	+	N	+
Subarachnoid hemorrhage	+ + +	+	+	+ +	N	+ +
CNS neoplasm	N	N	N	+ +	N	+ +

RBC, red blood cells; Mono, mononuclear leukocytes; CNS, central nervous system; PMN, polymorphonuclear leukocytes; N, normal; +, + +, + + +, increased. [a]A PMN reaction can be seen in this early CNS infection. This usually converts within a short time to a mononuclear majority. Reprinted from Schwartz, with permission.

Herpes Encephalitis

Gail Rudnitsky

Clinical Presentation

Neonatal herpes usually affects multiple organs, including the central nervous system (CNS). The infant may have one or more herpetic lesions on the skin, although absence of skin lesions does not rule out the diagnosis. Clinical manifestations of CNS involvement include seizures, irritability, poor feeding, temperature instability, and bulging fontanelles. In the older child or adult, herpes encephalitis (HE) should be considered in patients with fever, altered mental status, bizarre behavior, disordered thought processes, and focal neurologic findings. The exact neurologic findings depend on the area of the brain affected.[1,2]

Pathophysiology

HE usually is caused by herpes simplex virus (HSV) type 1 in the neonatal period and by HSV type 2 in the older child or adult. Neonatal herpes infection usually is acquired when the infant passes through the birth canal while the mother is actively shedding virus. The greatest risk of infection occurs if the mother has a primary herpes infection, although infection may also occur during recurrent genital herpes attacks. The virus probably reaches the CNS via hematogenous seeding.[2] In the older child or adult, the virus probably enters the brain via an intraneural route. Approximately one third of cases arise from a primary HSV infection, and the remainder from viral reactivation. Herpes may infect both neural and glial cells, resulting in widespread necrotizing encephalitis, especially in the temporal lobes.[1,2]

Diagnosis

If HE is suspected, the patient should have a lumbar puncture and a neuroimaging study (computed tomography or magnetic resonance imaging). The CSF usually shows elevated white blood cells (WBCs), red blood cells, and proteins. The WBCs are usually mononuclear. CSF samples should be sent for culture and for polymerase chain reaction (PCR) testing for herpes virus, which is both sensitive and specific. Neuroimaging may show focal disease in the temporal lobes. If culture and PCR results are both negative and herpes is still suspected, a brain biopsy may be performed.[1,2]

Clinical Complications

Untreated HE has high rates of morbidity and mortality. Even with high-dose acyclovir treatment, the neonatal mortality rate is still 29% for disseminated disease, with neurologic sequelae in 17% of survivors. In the older patient, high-dose therapy results in a 19% mortality rate, but 62% of survivors have neurologic sequelae.[1]

Management

Intravenous (IV) acyclovir is the treatment of choice for HE, regardless of the patient's age. Treatment should be continued for 14 to 21 days.[1,2]

REFERENCES

1. Whitley RJ, Gnann JW. Viral encephalitis; familiar infections and emerging pathogens. *Lancet* 2002;359:507–513.
2. Kimberlin DW. Herpes simplex virus infections of the central nervous system. *Semin Pediatr Infect Dis* 2003;14:83–89.

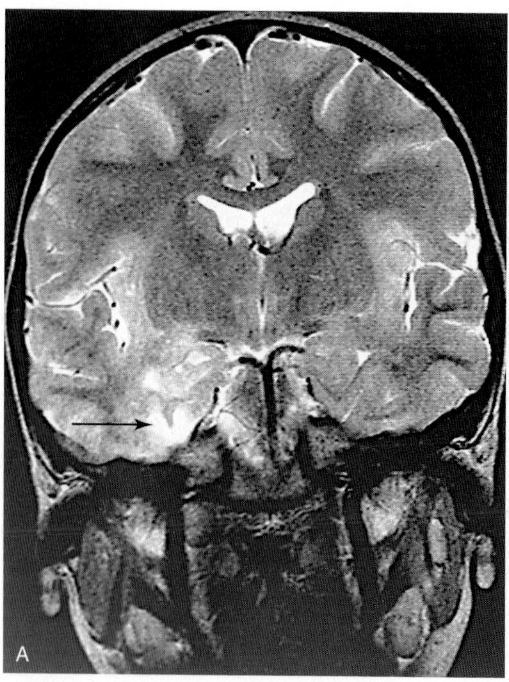

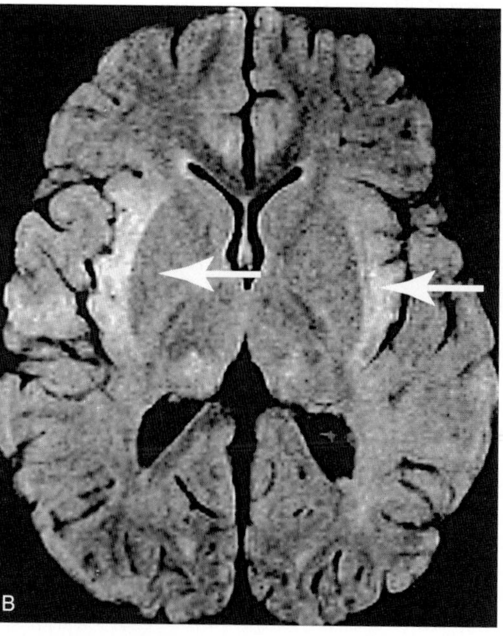

FIGURE 20–13 Coronal **(A)** and axial **(B)** T2-weighted magnetic resonance images showing multifocal areas of abnormal signal in the medial aspects of both temporal lobes *(large arrow)* and the left posterior parietal lobe *(small arrow)* in a patient with herpes simplex encephalitis. (From Fleisher, with permission.)

West Nile Virus

Kimberly Center

Clinical Presentation

Most patients infected with West Nile virus (WNV) are asymptomatic. Approximately 20% of infected people develop a nonspecific syndrome characterized by the sudden onset of fever, malaise, gastrointestinal upset, headache, myalgia, rash, and lymphadenopathy. The incubation period ranges from 3 to 14 days. WNV-related disease is generally mild, lasts 3 to 6 days, and is self-limited.[1-3]

Pathophysiology

WNV is an arbovirus in the family Flaviviridae, genus *Flavivirus;* it is most closely related to the Japanese encephalitis virus (JEV) and the St. Louis encephalitis (SLE) virus. The primary cycle of viral transmission involves birds and various mosquito species; humans are accidental, "dead-end" hosts.[1-3]

Diagnosis

Diagnostic confirmation rests on the detection of WNV immunoglobulin M (IgM) in serum or cerebrospinal fluid (CSF). The sensitivity of IgM in CSF is approximately 95%, and IgM may be detected in serum in 90% of patients within 6 days of symptom onset. Cross-reactions with other flaviviruses (JEV, SLE) may occur, and WNV IgM may persist in serum for prolonged periods, making interpretation of serology results difficult.[2,3] Laboratory findings tend to be nonspecific, and the CSF reveals lymphocytic pleocytosis and elevated protein with normal glucose. Computed tomography of the head shows no evidence of acute disease, but 33% of patients who had magnetic resonance imaging studies of the brain were found to have enhancement of the leptomeninges or the periventricular area, or both.[1-3]

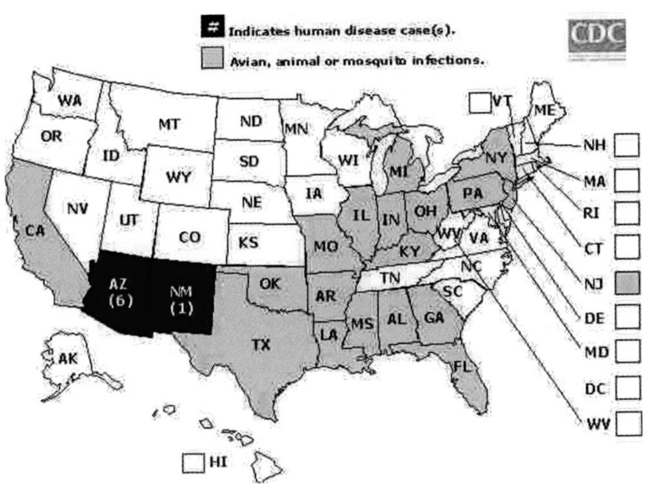

FIGURE 20-14 2004 West Nile Virus Activity in the United States (reported to Centers for Disease Control and Prevention as of June 8, 2004). From the CDC's Division of Vector-Borne Infectious Diseases (http://www.cdc.gov/ncidod/dvbid/westnile/surv&control.htm).

Clinical Complications

Although WNV illness is usually self-limited, West Nile meningoencephalitis (WNME) carries substantial morbidity and mortality. Approximately 1 in every 150 to 300 people infected with WNV develop WNME. The risk of WNME increases with advancing age. Patients with WNME typically present with predominant features of encephalitis; about 10% present with a flaccid paralysis that mimics polio.

Mortality rates for WNV infection range from 4% to 14%.[2] Risk factors for death include age greater than 50 years, presence of diabetes mellitus or immunosuppression, and severity of clinical features at presentation. Morbidity after WNME is substantial and includes persistent weakness (50% of survivors), memory loss (50%), fatigue, and depression.[1-3]

Management

Treatment is supportive. Ribavirin and interferon-alpha 2b are active in vitro, but these therapies remain unproven. Special consideration should be given to prevention of WNV infection by mosquito control and personal mosquito protection strategies.

REFERENCES

1. Nash D, Mostashari F, Fine A, et al. The outbreak of West Nile virus infection in the New York City area in 1999. *N Engl J Med* 2001; 344:1807–1814.
2. Petersen LR, Marfin AA. West Nile virus: a primer for the clinician. *Ann Intern Med* 2002;137:173–179.
3. Horga MA, Fine A. West Nile virus. *Pediatr Infect Dis J* 2001;20: 801–802.

Cutaneous Larva Migrans

Michael Greenberg

Clinical Presentation

Patients with cutaneous larva migrans (CLM) present with an erythematous and papular eruption that is intensely pruritic. After approximately 2 weeks, a red and itchy lesion may become visible along the subcutaneous route of larval migration.[1,2]

Pathophysiology

Dogs and cats may carry the hookworm *Ancylostoma braziliense*.[1,2] The larvae of this organism are found in dog and cat feces and are deposited in soil, where they may live for up to several days. Humans become infected when skin comes into contact with soil containing larvae and the larvae penetrate the epidermis. The hookworm is unable to complete its life cycle in humans, so the larvae migrate aimlessly just below the epidermis, creating a visible path.[1,2]

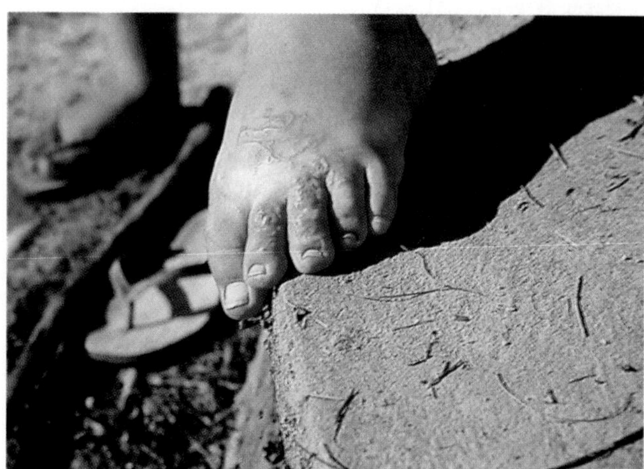

FIGURE 20–15 Cutaneous larva migrans. *Ancylostoma braziliense*, a hookworm of dogs and cats, is the most frequent but not the only cause of this syndrome. The lesions are characterized by pruritic, serpiginous tracts in which the infective-stage larvae have migrated. (From Smith JW, Ash LR, Thompson JH Jr., et al. Intestinal helminths. In: Smith JW (ed). *Atlas of diagnostic medical parasitology series*. Chicago: American Society of Clinical Pathologists, 1984.)

Diagnosis

Diagnosis is based on clinical appearance of the rash and history of possible exposure. Approximately one of every five patients exhibits eosinophilia. Biopsy is not usually necessary or recommended to make the diagnosis.[1,2]

Clinical Complications

Complications include reoccurrence, as well as superinfection in undertreated or untreated cases.

Management

CLM is usually self-limited and in most cases resolve within a few weeks. Specific therapy may not be needed. Persistent or extensive cases and those involving severe pruritus may be successfully treated with topical thiabendazole. However, oral preparations of this drug, as well as other antihelminthics such as ivermectin and albendazole may also be effective.[1]

REFERENCES

1. Caumes E. Treatment of cutaneous larva migrans and *Toxocara* infection. *Fundam Clin Pharmacol* 2003;17:213–216.
2. Kim SC, Gonzalez R, Ahmed G. Pruritic eruption on the left foot of a 36 year old woman. *Clin Infect Dis* 2003;37:448–449.

Bubonic Plague

Gail Rudnitsky

Clinical Presentation

Patients with bubonic plague present with fever, chills, and malaise 2 to 8 days after the initial bite of an infected flea. Black, necrotic, or purpuric skin lesions may develop at the bite site. Gastrointestinal symptoms (nausea, vomiting, abdominal pain) and alterations in mental status (confusion or obtundation) may occur.[1]

Pathophysiology

Bubonic plague is one of three forms of plague caused by *Yersinia pestis.* Throughout history, plague has caused pandemics, the most famous of which was the Black Plague, which killed more than 50 million people during the Middle Ages. Because of greater sanitation, there has not been a major urban plague epidemic in over 100 years, although isolated outbreaks continue to occur. Interest in plague has increased recently because of its potential to be weaponized and used as a biologic weapon.[1,2] *Y. pestis* is a gram-negative bacterium that is transmitted from an infected animal to a human via fleas. The organism infects the bite site, migrates to the regional lymph nodes, multiplies, and causes suppurative lesions called buboes.[1]

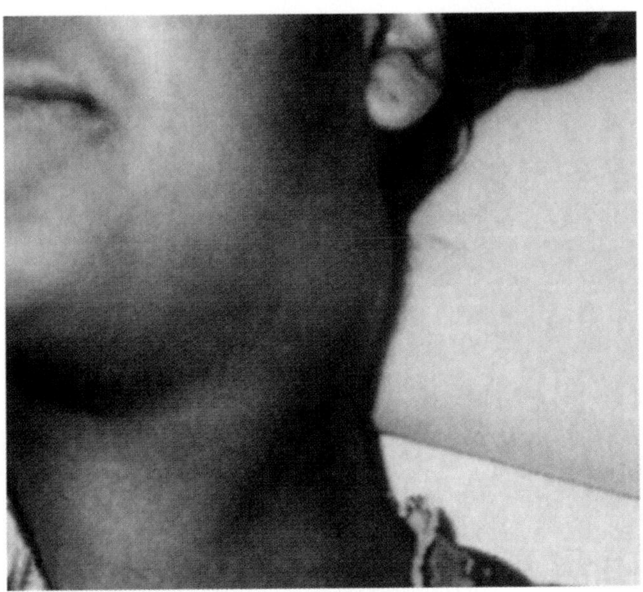

FIGURE 20–16 Cervical bubo in a patient with bubonic plague. (From Centers for Disease Control and Prevention, Division of Vector-Borne Infectious Diseases, Fort Collins, CO.)

Diagnosis

Gram or Wayson stains of lymph node aspirates, cerebrospinal fluid, or sputum show safety-pin bipolar gram-negative organisms.[1] Cultures from the aspirates, blood, or sputum may take up to 6 days to grow. A direct fluorescent antibody stain is available. Patients usually have a leukocytosis with a left shift and elevated transaminases.

Clinical Complications

Bubonic plague has a high mortality rate (50% if untreated; 5% to 15% with treatment).[2] Bacteremia, septicemia, and disseminated intravascular coagulation may develop. If the organisms seed the lungs, a secondary pneumonia may develop, with coughing and highly contagious sputum (pneumonic plague).

Management

Streptomycin is the treatment of choice. Alternative agents include gentamycin, doxycycline, chloramphenicol, and ciprofloxicin.[1] If meningitis is suspected, chloramphenicol should be used. Patients should be hospitalized, and respiratory isolation should be initiated if primary or secondary lung involvement is suspected. Hemodynamic monitoring and general supportive measures should be provided. Unprotected contacts should receive postexposure prophylaxis with doxycycline or ciprofloxacin.[1]

REFERENCES

1. Inglesby TV, Dennis DT, Henderson DA, et al. Plague as a biological weapon: medical and public health management. *JAMA* 2000;283: 2281–2290.
2. Darling RG, Catlett CL, Huebner KD, Jarrett DG. Threats in bioterrorism. I: CDC category A agents. *Emerg Med Clin North Am* 2002; 20:273–309.

Cutaneous Anthrax

Kimberly J. Center

Clinical Presentation

Fewer then 10 cases of naturally occurring cutaneous anthrax (CA) occur each year. There are three forms of human anthrax disease: cutaneous, inhalational, and gastrointestinal. All forms may progress to septicemia and meningitis. Most cases (more than 95%) are cutaneous infections, occurring in animal handlers or mill workers as a result of contact with infected animals or contaminated animal products, including hides, hair, bones, and meat.[1–3]

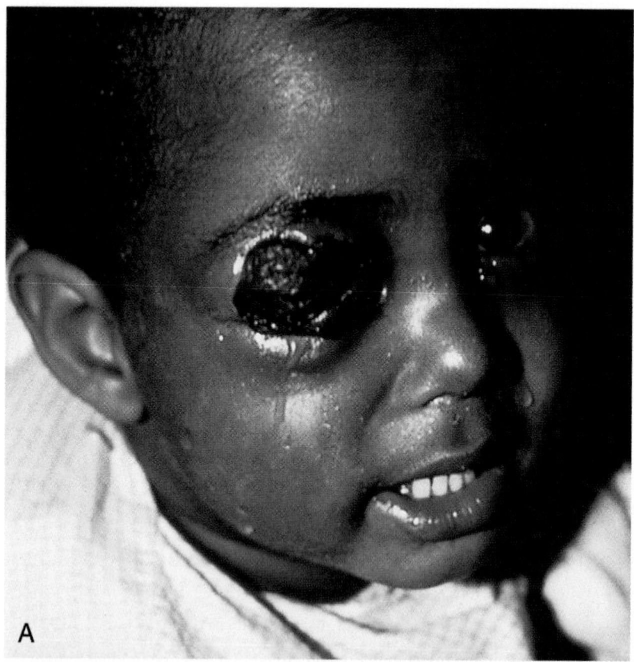

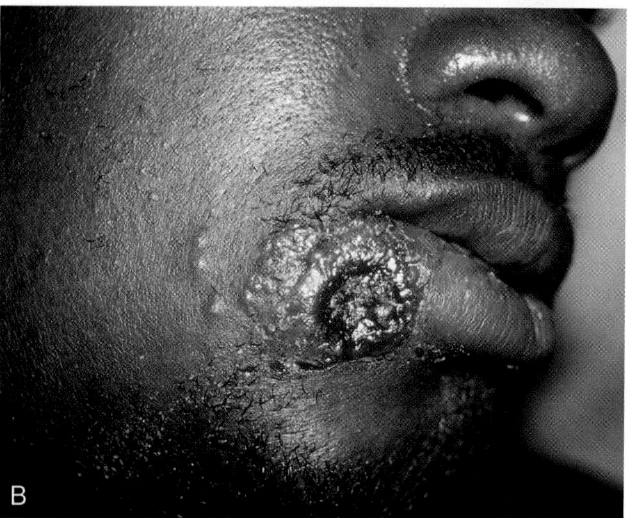

FIGURE 20–17 **A:** Anthrax of the eyelids. A black eschar is evident on both upper and lower lids. (Courtesy of Larry Schwab, MD.) (From Ostler, with permission.) **B:** Anthrax. A black eschar is evident. (Courtesy of Sandra Scott, MD.)

CA begins as a painless, occasionally pruritic, papule or vesicle at the inoculation site that enlarges and ulcerates over the course of several days to form a central black eschar. There may be edema and erythema surrounding the lesion, and local lymphadenopathy is common. The lesion may be associated with fever, malaise, and headache. Appropriately treated CA carries a mortality rate of less than 1%; if untreated, mortality may approach 20%. Discharge from cutaneous lesions is potentially infectious, and person-to-person spread is reported. Because of the rarity of naturally occurring anthrax in the United States and the recent use of anthrax as a biologic weapon, every suspected case should be reported immediately to the appropriate public health agency and to law enforcement authorities.[1–3]

Pathophysiology

CA is a zoonotic disease caused by *Bacillus anthracis,* an aerobic, gram-positive, spore-forming rod. The spores are infectious and may remain viable in soil for decades. Three distinct chemical factors influence the clinical development of CA—the antiphagocytic capsule (which allows for immune evasion), the lethal factor, and the edema factor.

Diagnosis

Laboratory diagnosis of anthrax is suspected when characteristic organisms are seen on a gram-stained specimen; the organism grows readily on routine media under standard laboratory conditions. Prior treatment with antibiotics may compromise the yield of culture.

Management

A high index of suspicion and rapid institution of appropriate therapy are critical to the outcome of CA. Penicillin is the drug of choice for naturally occurring disease.[1,3] For bioterrorism-associated anthrax, ciprofloxacin or doxycycline is recommended, pending antimicrobial susceptibility data. Several other agents have in vitro activity, including ampicillin/amoxicillin, clindamycin, rifampin, and vancomycin, which may be used in combination therapy with ciprofloxacin or doxycycline for disseminated disease. Cephalosporins and trimethoprim-sulfamethoxazole (TMP-SMX) should not be used for therapy.[1,3]

REFERENCES

1. Patt HA, Feigin RD. Diagnosis and management of suspected cases of bioterrorism: a pediatric perspective. *Pediatrics* 2002;109: 685–692.
2. Casken H, Arabaci F, Abuhandan M, et al. Cutaneous anthrax in eastern Turkey. *Cutis* 2001;67:488–492.
3. Oncu S, Oncu S, Sakarya S. Anthrax: an overview. *Med Sci Monit* 2003;9:RA276–RA283.

Cat-Scratch Disease

Kimberly J. Center

Clinical Presentation

Patients with cat-scratch disease (CSD) present with regional lymphadenopathy, usually involving the axillae, head, and neck. Most patients are between the ages of 2 to 14 years, but 20% of cases occur in adults.[1-4] Disseminated CSD accounts for roughly 1% of CSD cases and may manifest as fever of unknown origin. There is a seasonal distribution of disease, with a peak in fall-winter.

Pathophysiology

CSD is caused by *Bartonella henselae,* a gram-negative bacillus. Domestic cats are the reservoir, and more than 90% of patients with CSD have a history of recent exposure to a cat or, more commonly, a kitten. Infection is transmitted among cats primarily by the cat flea, though transmission from cat flea to human may also occur. The mechanism of human infection is not completely understood, and person-to-person infection has not been documented. The incubation period between the time of the scratch and the appearance of lymphadenopathy is 5 to 50 days, with a median of approximately 2 weeks.[1-4]

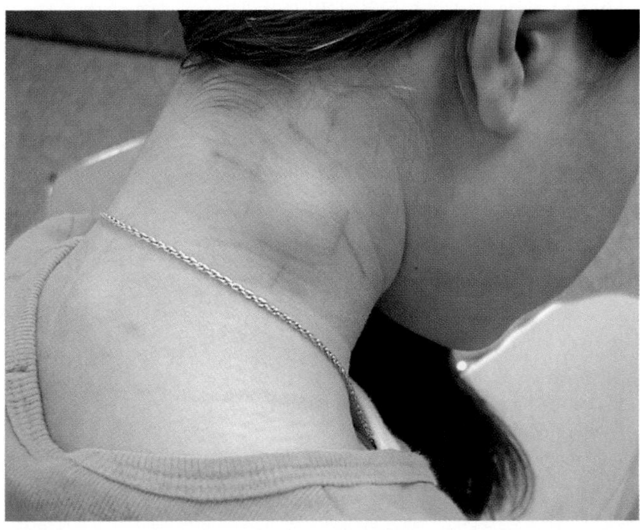

FIGURE 20–18 Posterior cervical lymphadenopathy. (Courtesy of Kim Center, MD.)

Diagnosis

Diagnosis is clinical, with verification by detection of serum antibodies to *B. henselae.*[1,4] A skin papule is often found at the inoculation site and may precede lymphadenopathy by 1 to 2 weeks. The skin overlying the affected nodes is often warm, erythematous, tender, and indurated; nodes become large and suppurate in about 25% to 30% of patients. Lymphadenopathy generally resolves spontaneously, although complete resolution may take several months. The incidence of cat-scratch encephalopathy is 0.17% to 2% of cases. The most common manifestations are seizures (46%), combativeness (39%), and coma.

Clinical Complications

Complications of CSD include disseminated disease, encephalopathy, optic neuritis, thrombotic thrombocytopenic purpura (TTP), hemolytic anemia, and osteomyelitis. CSD in immunocompromised individuals is a serious disease with significant morbidity.[1-4]

Management

CSD in healthy patients is self-limited, and management is symptomatic. Painful, suppurative nodes may require needle aspiration or incision and drainage. Antibiotics that may be useful in CSD include azithromycin, trimethoprim-sulfamethoxazole (TMP-SMX), erythromycin, doxycycline, ciprofloxacin, and gentamicin.[1-4] Antimicrobial therapy has not been shown to have any effect on the outcome of cat-scratch encephalopathy.

REFERENCES

1. Schutze GE. Diagnosis and treatment of *Bartonella henselae* infections. *Pediatr Infect Dis J* 2000;19:1185–1187.
2. Carithers HA. Cat-scratch disease. An overview based on a study of 1,200 patients. *Am J Dis Child* 1985;139:1124–1133.
3. Carithers HA, Margileth AM. Cat-scratch disease: acute encephalopathy and other neurologic manifestations. *Am J Dis Child* 1991;145:98–101.
4. Conrad DA. Treatment of cat-scratch disease. *Curr Opin Pediatr* 2001;13:56–59.

Mononucleosis

Douglas Thompson

Clinical Presentation

Patients present with sore throat, fever, malaise, and fatigue.

Pathophysiology

The most common cause of mononucleosis is Epstein-Barr virus (EBV). Transmission occurs via saliva, but transmission through blood products also occurs. Airborne transmission does not occur. Cytomegalovirus (CMV), *Toxoplasma gondii,* primary infection with human immunodeficiency virus (HIV), and lymphoreticular malignancies are other causes of mononucleosis-like syndromes.[1,2]

Diagnosis

Physical examination findings include exudative pharyngitis and lymphadenopathy. Splenomegaly occurs in 50% of patients, with hepatomegaly occurring in a smaller percentage. Maculopapular, petechial, urticarial, and erythema multiforme–like exanthems occur in a small percentage of patients. A maculopapular rash occurs in most patients treated with ampicillin and begins 5 to 10 days after the initiation of therapy. Jaundice is uncommon. Metamorphopsia, or the "Alice-in-Wonderland" phenomena, is characterized by distorted perception of size, shape, and spatial relationships. Mononucleosis caused by EBV is usually associated with a moderate leukocytosis (fewer than 20,000 cells/dL) and a lymphocytosis (greater than 5,000 cells/dL). Transaminases are two to three times the normal range. Atypical or reactive lymphocytes commonly represent more than 10% of the leukocytes.[1,2]

The presence of heterophile antibodies in patients older than 4 years of age reliably makes the diagnosis of EBV-associated mononucleosis. Testing for heterophile antibodies in patients younger than 4 years of age has poor sensitivity (20% to 50%) and should not be performed.

Clinical Complications

Complications include upper airway obstruction from lymphoid hyperplasia in Waldeyer's ring, splenic rupture, thrombocytopenia, Guillain-Barré syndrome, cranial nerve palsies, aseptic meningitis, meningoencephalitis, and transverse myelitis.

Management

Management is supportive, with a focus on comfort and hydration measures. Corticosteroids are indicated for airway obstruction. Contact sports should be avoided for at least 1 month and until any splenomegaly resolves.[1,2]

REFERENCES

1. Macsween KF, Crawford DH. Epstein-Barr virus: recent advances. *Lancet Infect Dis* 2003;3:131–140.
2. Peter J, Ray CG. Infectious mononucleosis. *Pediatr Rev* 1998;19: 276–279.

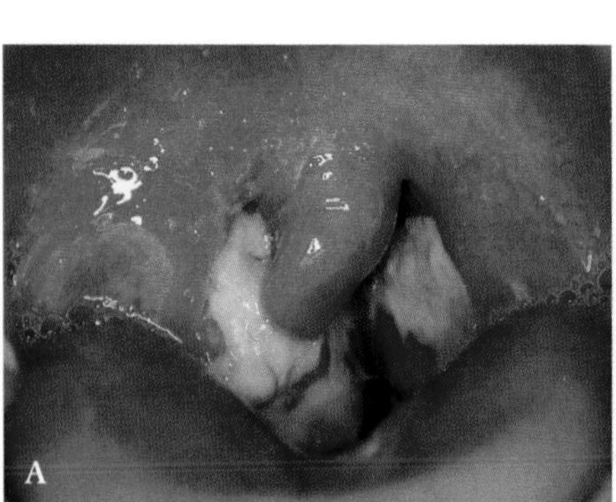

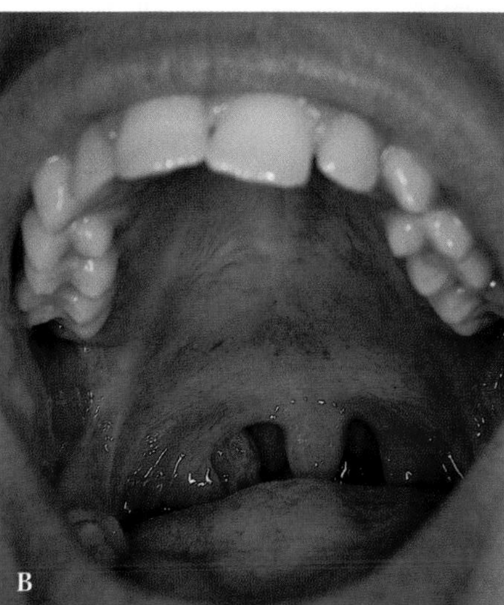

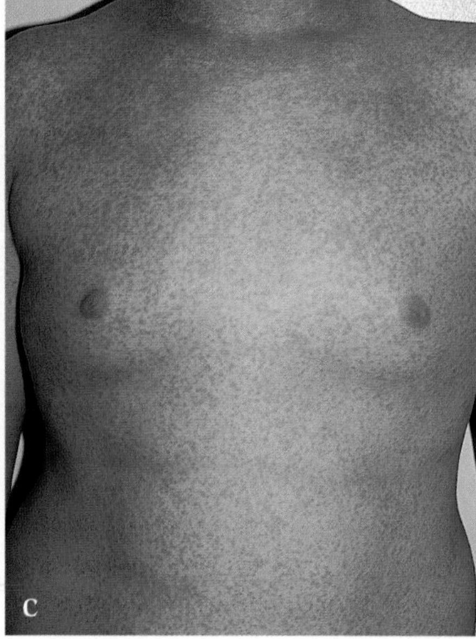

FIGURE 20–19 **A:** Infectious mononucleosis (glandular fever). These tonsils look swollen and juicy, but they are extremely hard and caused considerable discomfort in swallowing. (From Benjamin, with permission.) **B:** Petechiae at junction of hard and soft palate in a patient with infectious mononucleosis. (From Ostler, with permission.) **C:** Morbilliform rash after 5 days of ampicillin in a teenage boy with infectious mononucleosis. (From Ostler, with permission.)

Giardiasis

Robert Hendrickson

Clinical Presentation

Patients with giardiasis typically present with sudden onset of diarrhea, flatulence, cramping abdominal pain, and belching 1 to 3 weeks after exposure.[1] The diarrhea is nonbloody and contains no mucus. Occasionally, patients develop upper gastrointestinal tract symptoms, including nausea and vomiting.[1] Fever is distinctly uncommon and should direct diagnostic studies to more invasive forms of diarrhea (e.g., *Salmonella, Shigella*).[1] Laboratory and imaging evaluations usually are noncontributory. Most patients with giardiasis in endemic areas remain asymptomatic.[2] Those with an acute diarrheal illness typically have resolution of their symptoms in 2 to 4 weeks.[2] A smaller group of patients develop a more chronic, indolent infection, including mild, chronic diarrhea, malabsorption, and weight loss.[2]

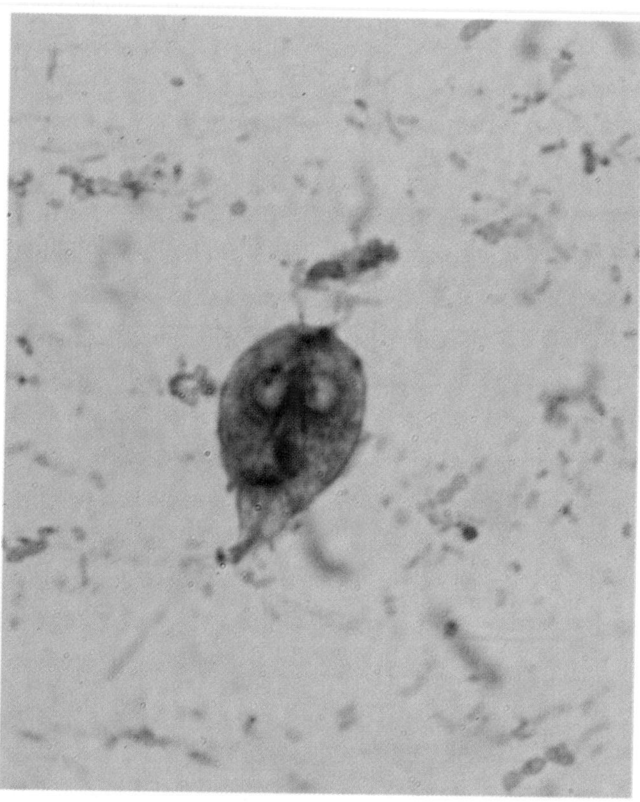

FIGURE 20–20 Trichrome stain of *Giardia lamblia* trophozoite. (Courtesy of Patrick Murray, PhD.) (From Yamada, with permission.)

Pathophysiology

Giardiasis is an infection of the small intestine caused by the protozoan *Giardia intestinalis,* also known as *Giardia lamblia.*[2] Giardia is spread through the fecal-oral route. Only a few organisms need to be ingested to produce infection. The protozoal cysts transform into trophozoites (excystation), attach to the small intestinal cells, multiply, and produce diarrhea.[2] Trophozoites that are carried to the colon by the fecal stream transform into cysts and are excreted (encystation).[2] Cysts are capable of surviving cold water for longer than 2 months, and they are able to withstand chlorinated water.

Diagnosis

The diagnosis is suspected by the typical history and confirmed by recognition of *Giardia* cysts on stool-saline wet mount (70% sensitive with one wet mount).[2] *Giardia* stool antigen tests are also available and are both sensitive (90%) and specific (90%) for the protozoan.[1]

Clinical Complications

The predominant complications of *Giardia* infection are dehydration and malabsorption.[2]

Management

Patients living in areas where reinfection is universal probably do not require treatment. Symptomatic patients in areas where reinfection is uncommon (e.g., United States) should be treated. The most common treatments involve metronidazole (more than 90% effective), quinacrine (more than 90% effective), or furazolidone (80% effective).[2] Alternative therapies include tinidazole (not available in the United States), albendazole, and paramomycin.[1]

REFERENCES

1. Nash TE. Treatment of *Giardia lamblia* infections. *Pediatr Infect Dis J* 2001;20:193–195.
2. Farthing MJ. Giardiasis. *Gastroenterol Clin North Am* 1996;25:493–515.

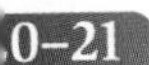

Ascariasis

Douglas Thompson

Clinical Presentation

Intestinal infection with *Ascaris lumbricoides* is frequently asymptomatic but may be associated with abdominal pain, distention, nausea, and, occasionally, diarrhea.[1] Symptoms of intestinal obstruction may occur in children with very high worm loads. Hepatobiliary and pancreatic ascariasis may manifest with symptoms of biliary colic, cholecystitis, cholangitis, pancreatitis, and hepatic abscesses. Pulmonary disease may manifest as migratory atypical pneumonia that lasts for 2 to 3 weeks (fever, cough, wheezing and respiratory distress, and hemoptysis), called Loeffler's syndrome.[1]

Pathophysiology

Ascariasis is an infection caused by the nematode, *A. lumbricoides. Ascaris* infects approximately 4 million people in the United States and 1.4 billion people worldwide.[1] Infection begins with ingestion of the *Ascaris* eggs. Larvae are produced in the duodenum when gastric secretions dissolve the eggs. After penetrating the mucosal epithelium, the larvae pass through the portal and hepatic circulation to the heart and lungs, enter the alveoli, and migrate to the hypopharynx. The larvae are swallowed and mature into adult worms in the jejunum, where they spend the remainder of their 6- to 18-month lifespan, producing eggs that are shed in the stool.[1]

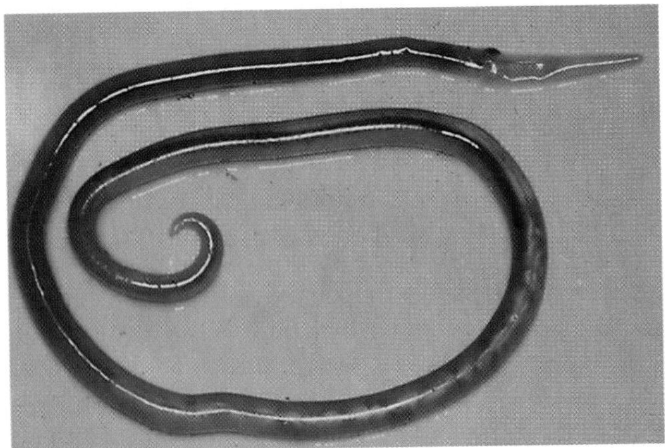

FIGURE 20–21 *Ascaris lumbricoides* adult. Adults are white or pink. Adults occasionally migrate from the gastrointestinal tract and appear in feces or in the oropharynx. *A. lumbricoides* is the only helminth that infests humans resemblng an earthworm in size and shape. (From Yamada, with permission.)

Pulmonary disease, an inflammatory response to the larvae during their migrational phase, occurs 4 to 16 days after ingestion of the eggs. This inflammatory process is more intense on reinfection. Intestinal symptoms are secondary to the physical properties of adult worms. Very high worm loads may cause partial or total bowel obstruction. Migration of worms into the hepatobiliary tree or appendix leads to obstruction of those organs. Transmural migration of adult worms leads to potentially fatal acute peritonitis and a chronic granulomatous peritonitis. Adult worms may utilize significant dietary protein and contribute to protein-energy malnutrition.

Diagnosis

During the pulmonary phase, patients may have diffuse pulmonary infiltrates and eosinophilia. Larvae may be identified on sputum samples. Ova may be identified on stool specimens 60 to 75 days after exposure (after the pulmonary phase). Adult worms may be identified when they are passed in stool or, occasionally, on abdominal radiographs or sonograms.[1]

Clinical Complications

Intestinal complications include obstruction, intussusception, bowel infarction, and perforation.[1]

Management

Treatment with mebendazole, albendazole, or pyrantel pamoate is effective. Pyrantel pamoate should be avoided if evidence of obstruction is present. Treatment of fluid and electrolyte abnormalities and surgical intervention may be necessary in complicated cases.[1]

REFERENCES

1. Valentine CC, Hoffner RJ, Henderson SO. Three common presentations of ascariasis infection in an urban emergency department. *J Emerg Med* 2001;20:135–139.

Schistosomiasis

Michael Greenberg

Clinical Presentation

Acute schistosomiasis (Katayama fever) presents with fever, urticaria, bronchospasm, headache, right upper quadrant pain, and bloody diarrhea. Tender hepatomegaly and splenomegaly are frequent findings. Respiratory symptoms are present in 70% of cases involving *Schistosoma haematobium* infection.[1,2] Chronic disease may be associated with abdominal pain and bloody diarrhea and may carry a higher risk for hepatocellular carcinoma. Central nervous system disease occurs, and patients may present with seizures (*Schistosoma japonicum*).[1]

Pathophysiology

Schistosomiasis is a parasitic disease, also called bilharziasis, that is a major health risk in developing countries.[1,2] Because of the mobility of populations, schistosomiasis may present anywhere in the world. Millions are afflicted worldwide. *Schistosoma mansoni* causes intestinal schistosomiasis and is prevalent in Africa, the Caribbean, the eastern Mediterranean, and South America. *S. japonicum/Schistosoma mekongi* causes intestinal schistosomiasis and is prevalent in Africa and the Pacific. *Schistosoma intercalatum* is found in Africa. *S. haematobium* causes urinary schistosomiasis in Africa, the eastern Mediterranean, and elsewhere.[1,2]

Infection requires skin or gastrointestinal contact with contaminated water, or it may occur as an occupational risk of workers in fishing, rice cultivation, or irrigation. Individuals then contaminate water supplies with feces or urine. Schistosome eggs in excreta open on contact with water, releasing a parasite called a miracidium. This is a motile form that must find a snail intermediate host. Once in the snail host, the miracidium divides, producing thousands of new parasites called cercariae. The cercariae are then re-excreted by the snail into water. Cercariae may penetrate human skin, obtain access to the vascular system, and thus continue their life cycle.[1,2]

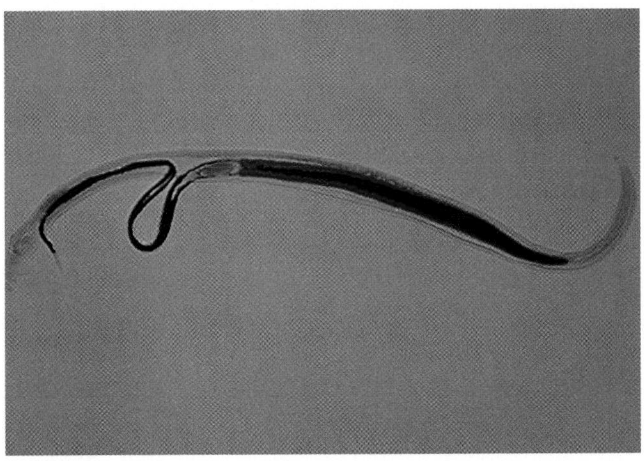

FIGURE 20–22 *Schistosoma mansoni,* adult worm pair. Pairs such as these usually reside in the mesenteric plexus in the distribution of the superior mesenteric vein (carmine stain). (From Smith JW, Ash LR, Thompson JH Jr., et al. Intestinal helminths. In: Smith JW (ed). *Atlas of diagnostic medical parasitology series.* Chicago: American Society of Clinical Pathologists, 1984.)

Diagnosis

The diagnosis should be suspected in patients who have traveled to or lived in endemic regions. Immigrants from endemic areas may remain infected for 20 to 40 years. All patients exhibit eosinophilia; definitive diagnosis depends on microscopic identification of schistosome eggs in feces or urine. In patients with clinically suspected disease but negative urine and fecal specimens, bladder or rectal biopsy may be helpful.[1]

Clinical Complications

Complications include hematuria (*S. haematobium*) and predisposition to some forms of bladder cancer. Infections in children may lead to growth retardation and anemia.[1,2]

Management

Praziquantel is effective in all forms of schistosomiasis, with virtually no side effects. Oxamniquine is used to treat intestinal schistosomiasis in Africa and South America. Metrifonate is effective for the treatment of urinary schistosomiasis.[1,2]

REFERENCES

1. Ross AG, Bartley PB, Sleigh AC, et al. Schistosomiasis. *N Engl J Med* 2002;346:1212–1220.
2. Murray HW, Pepin J, Nutman TB, et al. Recent advances: tropical medicine. *BMJ* 2000;320:490–494.

Hookworm

Michael Greenberg

Clinical Presentation

Patients with hookworm present with an itchy rash at the site where skin came into contact with contaminated soil. These symptoms reflect the penetration of the larvae through the skin, which usually results from walking barefoot.[1-3] Mild infections may cause minimal or no symptoms, whereas heavy infections often manifest with crampy abdominal pain, diarrhea, decreased appetite, and loss of weight. Some patients present simply with failure to thrive.[1-3]

Pathophysiology

The human hookworms encompass two species of roundworm, *Ancylostoma duodenale* and *Necator americanus.*[1-3] Another group of hookworms that usually infect animals may also invade humans (*Ancylostoma ceylanicum*), or may penetrate human skin resulting in cutaneous larva migrans (*Ancylostoma braziliense, Uncinaria stenocephala*).[1-3]

The life cycle of hookworms is complex, starting and ending in the human small intestine. Hookworm eggs require warm and moist soil to hatch into the larval stage. The larvae are not easily visible. Once they penetrate the skin, larvae are first transported to the lungs. They go to the mouth, are swallowed, and then travel to the small intestine. In the small intestine, the larvae develop into half-inch-long worms, attach themselves to the intestinal wall, and ingest the patient's blood. Adult worms are capable of producing large numbers of eggs that are passed into the feces. If the eggs reach soil, they hatch and develop into infective larvae within 10 days.[1-3]

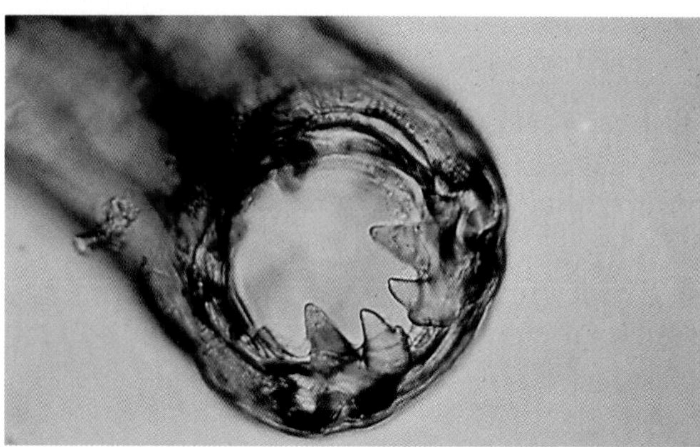

FIGURE 20–23 The characteristic buccal capsule of *Ancylostoma duodenale* has two teeth on each side of the capsule. (From Smith JW, Ash LR, Thompson JH Jr., et al. Intestinal helminths. In: Smith JW (ed). *Atlas of diagnostic medical parasitology series.* Chicago: American Society of Clinical Pathologists, 1984.)

Diagnosis

Infection is diagnosed by identifying hookworm eggs in the stool. Infection is rare in the United States; however, given the remarkable influx of immigrants, patients infected with hookworm may be expected to present to emergency departments in the United States. In some parts of the world, more than 80% of children are infected with hookworm species.[1-3]

Clinical Complications

Complications include anemia and protein deficiency related to blood loss. Pediatric growth retardation and mental retardation may occur in untreated cases. Other complications include cardiomyopathy, arrhythmias, and death.[1-3]

Management

Thiabendazole may be used topically to treat migrating larvae, and mebendazole may be used to treat intestinal infections. Mebendazole kills hookworms by blocking the worms' ability to uptake glucose and other nutrients from the host's intestinal environment. A vaccine against hookworm infection is under development.[1]

REFERENCES

1. Hotez PJ, Ghosh K, Hawdon J, et al. Vaccines for hookworm infection. *Pediatr Infect Dis* 1997;16:935–940.
2. Loukas A, Prociv P. Immune responses in hookworm infections. *Clin Microbiol Rev* 2001;14:689–703.
3. Hotez PJ, Hawdon JM, Cappello M, et al. Molecular pathobiology of hookworm infection. *Infect Agents Dis* 1995;4:71–75.

Strongyloidiasis

Michael Greenberg

Clinical Presentation

Patients with strongyloidiasis may be asymptomatic, or they may have gastrointestinal (GI), pulmonary, or cutaneous manifestations. Those presenting with GI complaints usually have abdominal crampy pain, nausea, vomiting, anorexia, and diarrhea. The sensation of "bloating" is the most common presenting GI complaint.[1] Patients with pulmonary symptoms complain of cough and shortness of breath.[1-3]

Pathophysiology

Strongyloidiasis is caused by two species of intestinal nematode, *Strongyloides stercoralis* and *Strongyloides fulleborni*. *S. stercoralis* is the more common of the two species.[1] *Strongyloides* organisms live in soil and are endemic in southeast Asia, South America, portions of Africa, and the southeastern United States.[1] Infection occurs when larval forms penetrate human skin, enter the venous circulation, and travel to the lungs. The organisms move retrograde, up the airways, and are swallowed into the GI tract. Once in the intestines, the larvae mature into adult females capable of laying eggs. Autoinfection is possible if larvae in the GI tract penetrate the intestinal mucosa and migrate to other parts of the body. Most patients who develop severe pulmonary disease are taking steroids, usually for chronic obstructive pulmonary disease.[1-3]

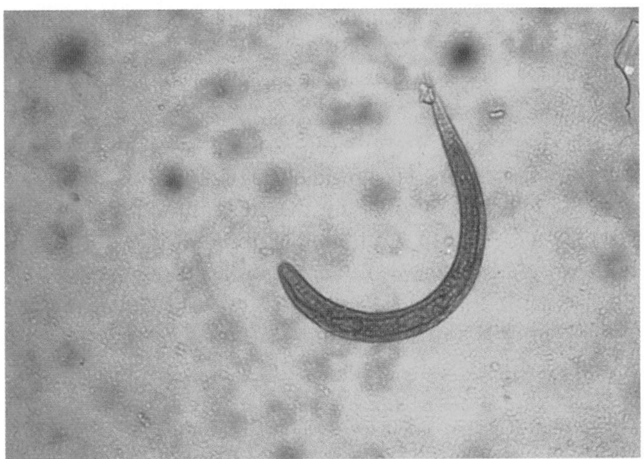

FIGURE 20–24 *Strongyloides stercoralis* rhabditiform larva, 225 by 16 mm, in the stool of a patient with epigastric pain and eosinophilia. (Courtesy of Richard L. Guerrant, MD, Charlottesville, VA.) (From Yamada, with permission.)

Diagnosis

Persons at high risk for strongyloidiasis include those with acquired immunodeficiency syndrome (AIDS), other immunocompromised individuals, those with malignancies, institutional populations, and travelers to endemic areas.[1] Strongyloidiasis is suspected based on the clinical setting in conjunction with eosinophilia, heme-positive stools, and serologic confirmation of the infection. However, microscopic examination of the stool is the most important means for diagnostic confirmation of GI disease.[1] Pulmonary disease may be associated with pulmonary infiltrates of varying description.[1]

Clinical Complications

Complications include the so-called hyperinfection syndrome, a situation in which the number of worms within the body increases dramatically, creating severe and disseminated disease with a substantial risk for death. The hyperinfection may be associated with meningitis, hemorrhagic pneumonia, hemorrhagic enteritis, and systemic gram-negative sepsis.[1-3] *S. stercoralis* is the most common cause of death related to helminth infection in the United States.[1]

Management

Strongyloidiasis is extremely difficult to treat.[1] Effective drugs include thiabendazole and ivermectin. Ivermectin is currently noted as the drug of choice by the World Health Organization.[1]

REFERENCES

1. Siddiqui AA, Berk SL. Diagnosis of *Strongyloides stercoralis* infection. *Clin Infect Dis* 2001;33:1040–1047.
2. Brennick J, Mattia A. Images in clinical medicine: *Strongyloides stercoralis* infestation. *N Engl J Med* 1996;334:1173.
3. Al Samman M, Haque S, Long JD. Strongyloidiasis colitis: a case report and review of the literature. *J Clin Gastroenterol* 1999;28:77–80.

Cysticercosis

Michael Greenberg

Clinical Presentation

Cysticercosis is of concern in the United States because of the large immigrant population from endemic regions (Africa, Mexico, and Central and South America). The clinical presentation is variable based on the location, size, and number of cysts at the time of presentation. However, most clinical manifestations are related to brain infections with *Taenia solium.*[1,2] Consequently, most patients present with symptoms of headache, change in mental status, seizures, or focal neurologic dysfunction. Patients with muscle or subcutaneous cysts may present with muscular achy pain.

Pathophysiology

Cysticercosis is caused by infection with larvae of the pork tapeworm (*T. solium*), an intestinal parasite. Humans serve as intermediate hosts when ova-containing oncospores are ingested and invade the intestines, pass into the vascular space, and spread to various body tissues (primarily brain, muscle, and subcutaneous tissue). Cysticercosis is the most common parasitic central nervous system infection in immunocompetent persons.[1]

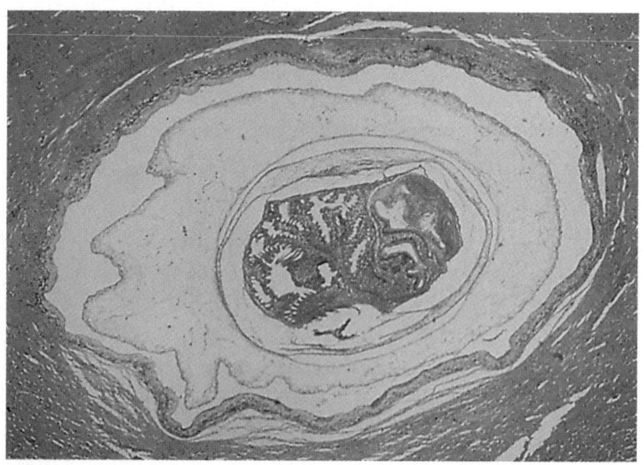

FIGURE 20–25 *Taenia solium,* cysticercosis. Tissue section (hematoxylin and eosin stain) shows cysticercus in brain tissue. The scolex region of the cysticercus is in the center. Typical hooks are evident within the inverted scolex. (From Smith JW, Ash LR, Thompson JH Jr., et al. Intestinal helminths. In: Smith JW (ed). *Atlas of diagnostic medical parasitology series.* Chicago: American Society of Clinical Pathologists, 1984.)

Diagnosis

The diagnosis is difficult because the usual presentation is nonspecific. The disease may be suspected based on the history of illness, geographic location of the patient, and physical examination findings; confirmation requires imaging. Computed tomography or magnetic resonance imaging may demonstrate multiple cystic lesions with characteristic punctate calcifications. Punctate calcified granulomata are the most common imaging finding and are seen in 15% to 20% of cases.[1,2] An enzyme-linked immunoelectrotransfer blot assay (specificity, 100%; sensitivity, 80% to 98%) for the detection of specific anticysticercal antibodies in serum is available from the Centers for Disease Control and Prevention (CDC).[1]

Clinical Complications

Complications include meningitis, encephalitis, intraventricular (cerebral) disease, spinal cord compression, and ocular disease.[1,2]

Management

A combination of therapeutic modalities is usually indicated and includes (1) larvicidal agents to kill cystic larvae; (2) corticosteroids to decrease inflammatory response; (3) anticonvulsant medications; and (4) neurosurgical intervention to debulk cystic masses, relieve obstruction, and decompress critically located cysts before initiation of drug therapy.[2]

REFERENCES

1. Ogilvie CM, Kasten P, Rovinsky D, et al. Cysticercosis of the triceps: an unusual pseudotumor. Case report and review. *Clin Orthop* 2001;(382):217–221.
2. Nash TE. Human case management and treatment of cysticercosis. *Acta Tropica* 2003;87:61–69.

Leishmaniasis

Michael Greenberg

Clinical Presentation

Leishmaniasis is an infectious parasitic disease that affects the populations of the world's poorest nations, as well as travelers to those locales. As a result of the current unprecedented ability for individual travel, this illness may potentially be seen in any emergency department worldwide. The clinical presentation depends on the specific form of the disease.[1-3]

Cutaneous leishmaniasis manifests with one or more skin lesions that develop weeks to months after an individual is bitten by infected phlebotomine sand flies. These lesions may be painful or painless, and they may or may not be associated with scab formation.[1-3] If left untreated, the sores may heal, or they may last from weeks to years, developing raised edges and a central crater. Visceral leishmaniasis manifests with fever, weight loss, enlargement of the spleen and liver, and anemia developing months to years after the initial infection.[1-3]

Pathophysiology

Leishmaniasis is endemic in most countries of South America, as well as Panama, Honduras, and various Caribbean nations. It is also endemic in Italy and Spain, throughout the Middle East, in southwest Asia, and in numerous equatorial and other African countries.[1-3] Leishmaniasis exists in three clinical forms: visceral, cutaneous, and mucocutaneous. All forms of the disease are related to human infection with protozoan parasites of the genus *Leishmania,* which are transmitted by the bite of a sand fly. Visceral leishmaniasis is an opportunistic infection in patients infected with the human immunodeficiency virus (HIV).[1-3]

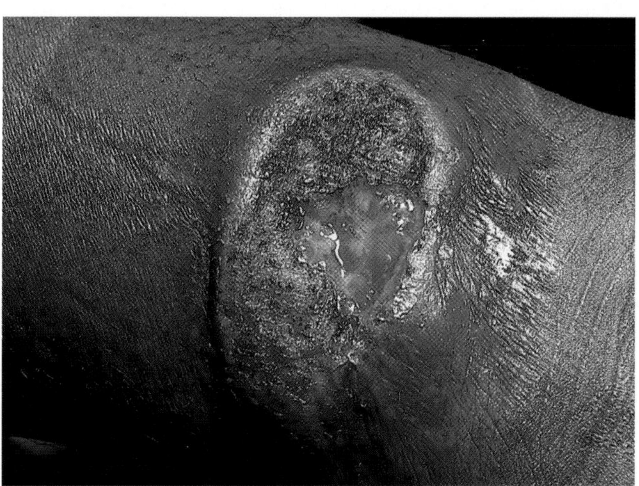

FIGURE 20–26 Cutaneous leishmaniasis, showing large ulcer with typical indurated, raised margin. (From Ostler, with permission.)

Diagnosis

A high index of suspicion must be maintained with regard to individuals who have recently traveled in endemic areas. The diagnosis of visceral leishmaniasis requires identification of the parasite in tissue preparations such as splenic, bone-marrow, or lymph-node aspirates.[1-3] However, a variety of serologic techniques are also available for diagnosis. Touch smears, exudate cultures, or lesion scrapings may be used to diagnose cutaneous and mucocutaneous disease.[1]

Clinical Complications

If untreated, symptomatic visceral leishmaniasis is often fatal.[1,2]

Management

In the past, visceral leishmaniasis was treated with antimony-containing drugs. However, many antimony-resistant strains have been reported. More recently, amphotericin B and miltefosine have been successfully used for treatment. Cutaneous disease often heals spontaneously but may be treated with paromomycin ointment, antimonials, or antifungal agents.[1-3]

REFERENCES

1. Davies CR, Kaye P, Croft SL, Sundar S. Leishmaniasis: new approaches to disease control. *BMJ* 2003;326:377–382.
2. Melby PC. Recent developments in leishmaniasis. *Curr Opin Infect Dis* 2002;15:485–490.
3. Herwaldt BL. Leishmaniasis. *Lancet* 1999;354:1191–1199.

Amebiasis

Michael Greenberg

Clinical Presentation

Patients with amebiasis may be asymptomatic, but those with colitis present with gradual onset of bloody (or heme-positive) diarrhea and abdominal pain.[1] Children may present with rectal bleeding without diarrhea. Fever is not usually reported. Pregnant women and immunocompromised individuals are at higher risk for development of amebiasis. In the United States, many cases each year involve immigrants from Mexico, Central America, or South America.[1,2]

Pathophysiology

Amebiasis is a parasitic disease caused by the organism, *Entamoeba histolytica.* It is the second leading cause of death from parasitic disease in the world.[1] Infection involves ingestion of cysts in fecally contaminated food or water.[1] These cysts pass through the gastrointestinal tract and "excyst" in the large intestines, forming motile trophozoites that may re-encyst within the colon. These cysts may then be excreted in stool, completing the life cycle.[1]

Amebic invasion into submucosal tissue is the *sine qua non* of amoebic colitis. Amebiasis involves two genetically distinct organisms: *Entamoeba dispar,* which causes no disease or mucosal invasion, and *E. histolytica,* which is the pathogenic form. *E. histolytica* causes amebic colitis and extraintestinal amebiasis.[1] Although most cases of amebiasis involve infection via ingestion of contaminated food or water, there is a high rate of infection among men who have sex with men, who transmit the infection via oral and anal sex, as well as via contaminated enema devices.[1]

Diagnosis

Diagnosis requires finding *E. histolytica* in the stool or colonic mucosa of patients with diarrhea. The most sensitive diagnostic techniques include enzyme-linked immunosorbent (ELISA) assays that identify *E. histolytica* antigens in the stool. Bowel-wall biopsy may be necessary to confirm the diagnosis in some patients. Amebic liver abscess may be visualized using sonography or computed tomography.[1,2]

Clinical Complications

Complications include the development of intraabdominal abscesses, liver abscess, brain abscess, amoebic liver abscess rupture through the diaphragm (causing empyema and fistulas), rectovaginal fistulas, perianal disease, and bacterial superinfections.[1]

Management

Current treatment recommendations include metronidazole followed by a so-called luminal agent, such as paromomycin, iodoquinol, or diloxanide furoate.[1] Asymptomatic patients may be treated with luminal agents alone. Amebic liver abscesses usually are cured with a single dose of metronidazole, and surgical drainage usually is unnecessary.[1]

REFERENCES

1. Stanley SL Jr. Amoebiasis. *Lancet* 2003;361:1025–1034.
2. Summary of notifiable diseases, United States—1994. *MMWR Morb Mortal Wkly Rep* 43(53):1–80.

Amebiasis

Michael Greenberg

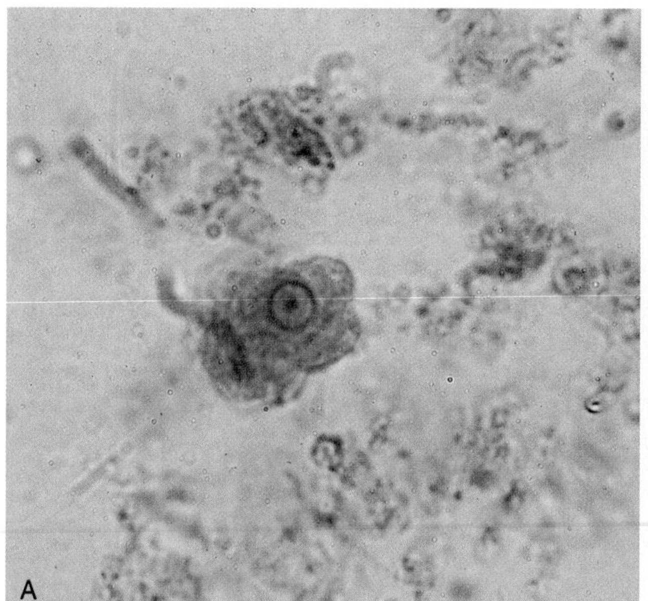

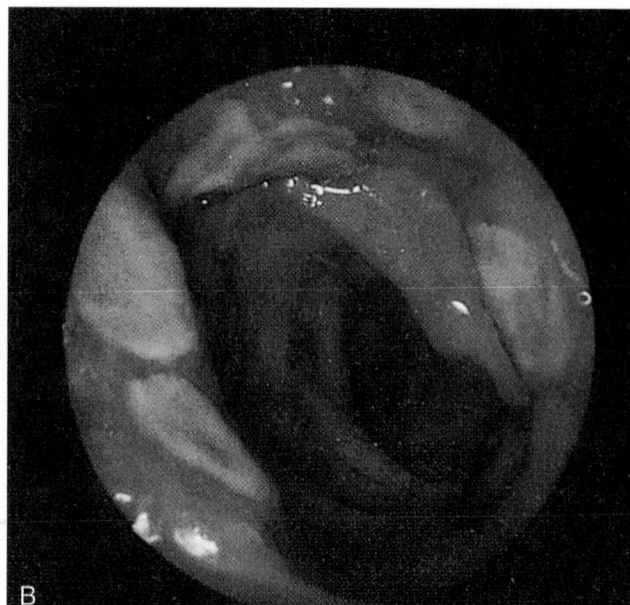

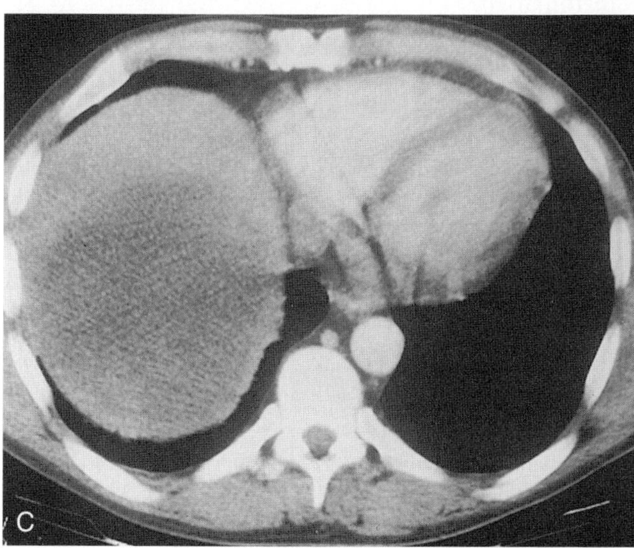

FIGURE 20–27 **A:** *Entamoeba histolytica* trophozoite in stool. This trophozoite is approximately 20 μm in diameter and has the characteristic round nucleus with a small, centrally placed karyosome. (Courtesy of Patrick Murray, PhD.) **B:** Rectosigmoidoscopic images show part of the pathologic spectrum of intestinal amoebiasis. Image shows multiple, well-defined ulcers. **C:** Computed tomographic scan of the abdomen demonstrates a large amoebic liver abscess in the right lobe of the liver. (**A–C,** From Yamada, with permission.)

20-28

Onchocerciasis

Dziwe Ntaba and Richard Hamilton

Clinical Presentation

The most common manifestation of onchocerciasis early in the course of disease is pruritus. The severity of itching varies from mild to severe. Visual changes may occur early in the course, but the classic blindness is a late finding in chronic disease.[1]

Pathophysiology

Onchocerciasis affects almost 18 million people who live or travel in Africa, Latin America, and the Arabian peninsula.[2] Larvae of the parasite *Onchocerca volvulus* enter the patient during the blood meal of an infected *Simulium* fly. Within 1 to 3 months, the parasite develops into an adult worm and migrates to dermal nodules that serve as mating centers. An adult female may release 1,300 to 1,900 offspring (microfilariae) daily for approximately 10 years.[2] The bulk of the pathology seen in onchocerciasis is attributed to the inflammatory response to dying microfilariae in the skin and eye.

Diagnosis

The most commonly used diagnostic test involves detection of microfilariae from a bloodless skin biopsy.[2] With ocular involvement, microfilariae are usually seen in the anterior chamber on slit-lamp examination.[1] An adjunctive maneuver is to have the patient sit with his or her head between the knees for 2 minutes, to allow any microfilariae in the anterior chamber to fall toward the cornea. Screening tests using the enzyme-linked immunosorbent (ELISA) method and polymerase chain reaction (PCR) are becoming more widely available.[2]

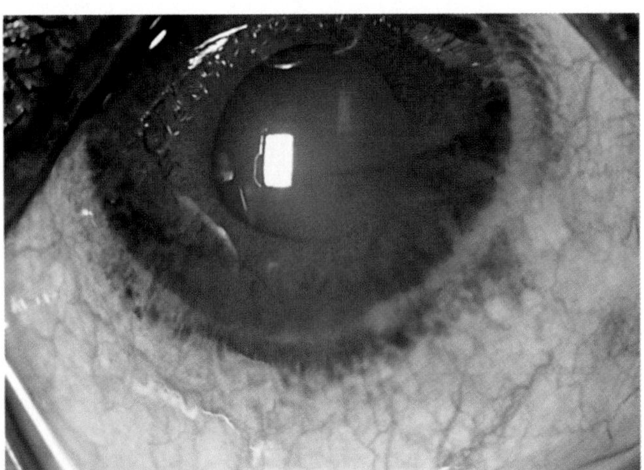

FIGURE 20–28 Onchocerciasis. Early sclerosing keratitis. (Courtesy of Mitchell Friedlaender, MD.) (From Ostler, with permission.)

Clinical Complications

Some patients may present with signs of a severe reactive dermatitis, known by the Arabic name of *sowda*. This represents an enhanced humoral and cell-mediated immune response to larval antigens and may be accompanied by inguinal lymphadenopathy or edema.[1] Elephantitis, or lymphatic filariasis, is a disfiguring complication that results from lymph stagnation secondary to lymphangitis. Some patients recently treated for onchocerciasis show a paradoxic increase in the severity of their symptoms, caused by the increased load of dying microfilariae.[2]

Management

Symptomatic control is afforded by the drug ivermectin, a single dose of which clears the skin of microfilariae for months.[2] Ivermectin does not kill the adult worm however, and therefore it is not curative. Second-line chemotherapeutic agents include antiparasitics such as suramin and diethylcarbamazine, but these are reserved for severe infections because of their potential for substantial systemic toxicity.[3]

REFERENCES

1. Malatt AE, Taylor HR. Onchocerciasis. *Infect Dis Clin North Am* 1992;6:963–977.
2. Burnham G. Onchocerciasis. *Lancet* 1998;351:1341–1346.
3. Van Laethem Y, Lopes C. Treatment of onchocerciasis. *Drugs* 1996; 52:861–869.

Scrofula

Adriana Klucar Stoudt

Clinical Presentation

Patients with scrofula present with an enlarging neck mass. Tuberculous adenitis in children manifests in the posterior triangle, whereas other forms of adenitis in children occur in the anterior triangle and the submandibular regions. In adults, the upper border of the sternocleidomastoid muscle is the most common site of adenitis. Adenopathy is usually unilateral and painless. Initially, nodes are mobile and rubbery, but they may evolve to become hard and matted with overlying erythema.

Pathophysiology

Scrofula is the cervical form of mycobacterial lymphadenitis. Causes include *Mycobacterium tuberculosis, Mycobacterium bovis,* and the atypical mycobacteria (*Mycobacterium scrofulaceum, Mycobacterium avium-intracellulare,* and *Mycobacterium kansasii*).[1] Nontuberculous mycobacteria are more frequently isolated in young children, but *M. tuberculosis* continues to predominate in older children and adolescents.[2] Scrofula is the most common extrapulmonary form of tuberculosis, and it is most likely a result of early lymphohematogenous spread.

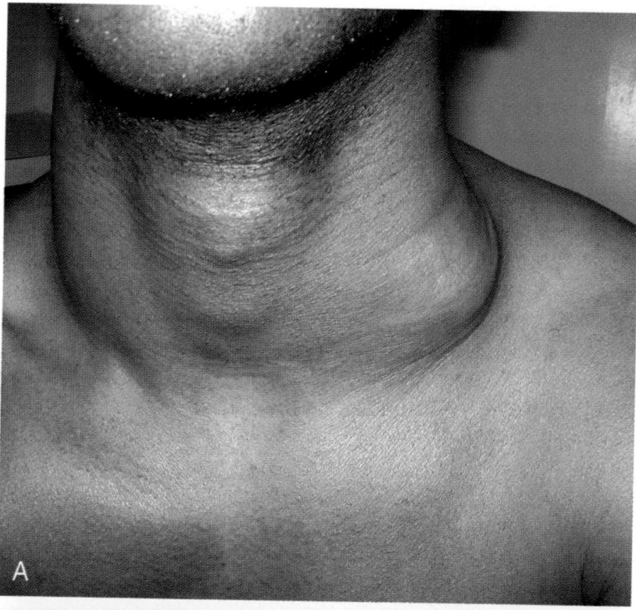

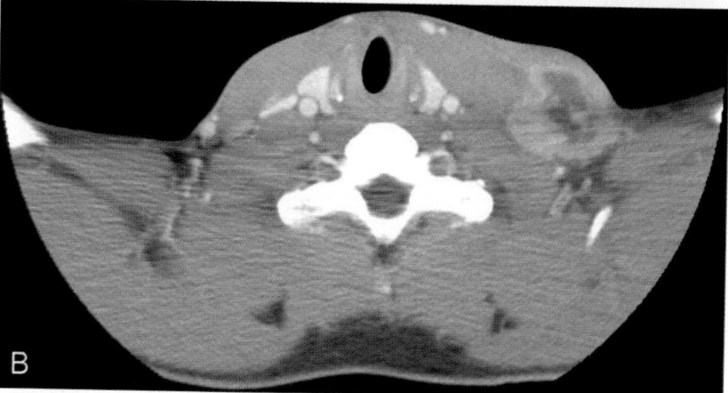

FIGURE 20–29 **A:** Tuberculous neck mass. **B:** Computed tomogram of tuberculous neck mass. (**A** and **B**, Courtesy of Boris Khodorkovsky, MD.)

Diagnosis

Mycobacterial infection must be considered in a patient with chronic, indolent adenitis that has failed to respond to standard antibiotic therapy. A strongly positive purified protein derivative (PPD) skin test is indicative of tubercular infection, and a negative PPD result essentially excludes this diagnosis. Excisional lymph node biopsy may be necessary to confirm the diagnosis.

Clinical Complications

Despite effective medical therapy, scarring and fibrosis may lead to residual adenopathy that persists for years. Excision must be performed with care; complications such as Horner's syndrome, accessory nerve palsy, and facial nerve palsy have been reported. During medical therapy, the patient may experience some transient worsening of the lymphadenopathy.

Management

Total excision of the involved nodes is the treatment of choice for nontuberculous mycobacterial adenitis. If an abscess tract is present, it should be excised together with the involved skin overlying it. Attempts should be made to close the incision primarily without a drain.

Scrofula caused by *M. tuberculosis* is best treated with antituberculosis medical therapy. Treatment consists of one of several drug regimens for 12 to 18 months; the most commonly used regimen is rifampin and isoniazid (INH). Surgical excision alone is inadequate treatment. Surgical management is usually reserved for excisional biopsy to establish the diagnosis and to remove grossly enlarged nodes, fistulous tracts, or lymph nodes that are impeding breakdown.[1]

REFERENCES

1. Shikhani AH, Hadi UM, Mufarrij AA, Zaytoun GM. Mycobacterial cervical lymphadenitis. *Ear Nose Throat J* 1989;68:660, 662–666, 668–672.
2. Bodensein L, Altman RP. Cervical lymphadenitis in infants and children. *Semin Pediatr Surg* 1994;3:134–141.
3. Lane RJ, Keane WM, Potsic WP. Pediatric infectious cervical lymphadenitis. *Otolaryngol Head Neck Surg* 1980;88:332–335.

Osteomyelitis

Michael Greenberg

Clinical Presentation

Patients with osteomyelitis present with fever, chills, local pain, and local swelling after a period or episode of bacteremia.[1–3]

Pathophysiology

Hematogenous osteomyelitis is more common in prepubertal children and elderly patients. Post-traumatic osteomyelitis occurs in patients of all ages and is the most prevalent form of this disease.[1] Normal bone is relatively resistant to infection. The development of osteomyelitis generally requires large inocula of bacteria, trauma that violates bone or produces extensive soft tissue injury, the presence of foreign bodies, or a combination of these factors. Infection may occur via direct spread from contiguous structures, by bony invasion, or via hematogenous spread.[1–3]

In children, osteomyelitis typically results from hematogenous spread after an episode of bacteremia. The most common causative organisms in these patients are *Staphylococcus aureus, Streptococcus pneumoniae,* and *Haemophilus influenza* type b.[1–3] Children with sickle cell disease are more prone to the development of osteomyelitis, and in these cases the most common organism is *Salmonella*.[4]

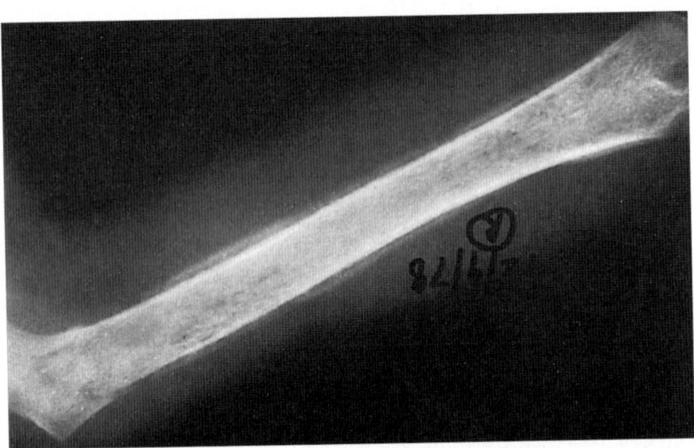

FIGURE 20–30 Radiograph showing lytic lesions and periosteal elevation with osteomyelitis. (From Fleisher, with permission.)

If clinical abnormalities persist for more than 10 days, it is generally believed that the osteomyelitis has become chronic.

Diagnosis

The diagnosis is based on clinical suspicion and confirmed with the use of various imaging techniques, including computed tomography and magnetic resonance imaging, which are capable of discerning edema, medullary destruction, periosteal reaction, and articular damages when plain radiographs remain normal. Nonetheless, plain films are necessary as part of the initial and continuing work-up.[1–3]

Clinical Complications

Complications include chronicity of infection and reoccurrence.

Management

Early antibiotic administration is crucial, and antibiotics should be started in the emergency department once the diagnosis of osteomyelitis is suspected.[1] In most cases, antibiotic therapy needs to be continued for 1 to 2 months. Some cases also require surgical intervention for débridement, decompression, revascularization, and other indications.[1] Orthopedic surgical consultation should be sought as soon as the diagnosis is suspected, and infectious disease consultation should be obtained as soon as possible.

REFERENCES

1. Lew DP, Waldvogel FA. Osteomyelitis. *N Engl J Med* 1997;336:999–1007.
2. Tsukayama DT. Pathophysiology of posttraumatic osteomyelitis. *Clin Orthop* 1999;(360):22–29.
3. Vazquez M. Osteomyelitis in children. *Curr Opin Pediatr* 2002;14:112–115.
4. Burnett MW, Bass JW, Cook BA. Etiology of osteomyelitis complicating sickle cell disease. *Pediatrics* 1998;101:296–297.

Histoplasmosis

Michael Greenberg

Clinical Presentation

Patients with histoplasmosis may present with a pulmonary syndrome including cough, malaise, shortness of breath, and difficulty breathing after inhalation of fungal spores. Patients with pulmonary histoplasmosis may also manifest erythema nodosum and erythema multiforme.[1] Some patients present with primarily skin lesions and others with disseminated disease.[1,2]

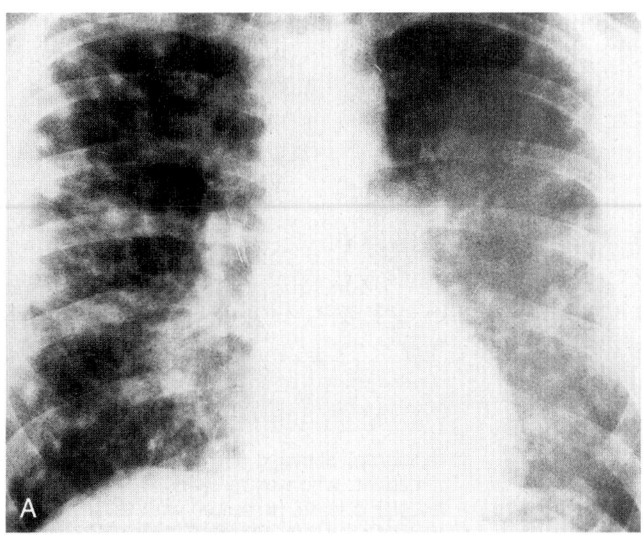

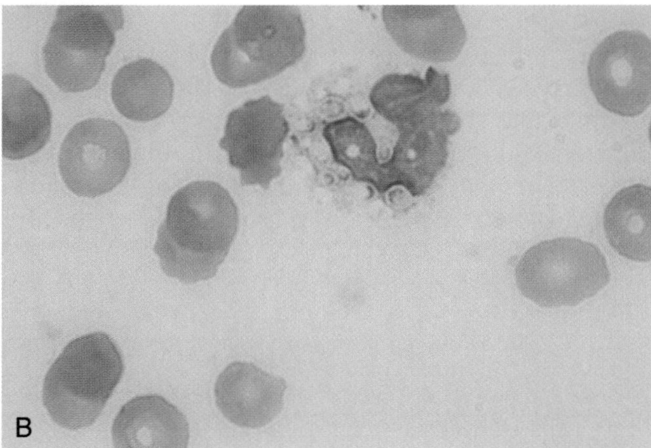

FIGURE 20–31 **A:** Chest radiograph showing diffuse, bilateral micronodular infiltrates in inhalational histoplasmosis. (From Mandell, with permission.) **B:** Small oval yeast forms within a monocyte. (From Anderson, with permission.)

Pathophysiology

The fungus *Histoplasma capsulatum* is the causative organism for histoplasmosis.[1] This organism may be found in soil as well as fecal matter from chickens, pigeons, other birds, and bats. Most North American cases of histoplasmosis have occurred in the Mississippi and Ohio river valleys.[1,2] After initial contact, the organism spreads via the bloodstream to the skin, liver, spleen, bone marrow, and lymph nodes.[1,2]

Disseminated histoplasmosis is considered to be a defining illness of acquired immunodeficiency syndrome (AIDS) and is primarily seen in immunocompromised persons. Histoplasmosis may also develop in patients with psoriasis.[1,2]

Diagnosis

The diagnosis may be suspected based on the history and clinical findings and confirmed by biopsy and staining with periodic acid–Schiff (PAS) or Gomori stain.[1] Fungal culture and complement fixation tests may also be helpful. A histoplasmin assay is available as a screening test.[1] Skin lesions occur on the trunk and upper extremities. These lesions first appear as pinkish plaques that may go on to ulcerate. Lesions of the nasal, oral, and pharyngeal areas are common.[1]

Clinical Complications

Complications include recurrent or persistent infection, bacterial superinfection, spread to the central nervous system, systemic infection, and death.[1]

Management

Intravenous amphotericin B is the treatment of choice for immunocompromised patients with histoplasmosis. These patients may also require lifelong ketoconazole therapy after initial treatment with amphotericin B.[1]

REFERENCES

1. Trent JT, Kirsner RS. Identifying and treating mycotic skin infections. *Adv Skin Wound Care* 2003;16:122–129.
2. Cohen PR, Bank DE, Silvers DN, Grossman ME. Cutaneous lesions of disseminated histoplasmosis in human deficiency virus-infected patients. *J Am Acad Dermatol* 1990;23:422–428.

Blastomycosis

Michael Greenberg

Clinical Presentation

Blastomycosis (BM) may manifest as a primary skin disorder or as a disseminated cutaneous and systemic disease, or both. Primary skin lesions may develop after local trauma to the skin in certain workers, or after the bite of an infected dog. After exposure, nodular lesions develop first on the hands and fingers, then spread proximally up the forearm and arm.[1] With time, the nodules may ulcerate. Tender and swollen axillary lymph nodes are common presenting findings.[1] Disseminated BM manifests with granulomas, crusted papules, sinus tracts, and ulcerations that may resemble various skin infections, including pyoderma gangrenosum.[1] In cases of disseminated disease, regional adenopathy does not commonly occur. BM may spread by the hematogenous route to bone, the genitourinary tract, and the central nervous system (CNS). However, the skin is clearly the most frequently affected organ.[1,2]

Pathophysiology

The fungus *Blastomyces dermatitidis* is the causative organism for North American BM.[1,2] This organism may be found in soil, pigeon droppings, and similar organic material.[1] Most cases of BM have occurred in the Great Lakes region, the southeastern coastal regions of the United States, Mexico, and Central America.[1] The male-to-female infection rate is 9:1. Agricultural workers, laborers, laboratory workers, morticians, hunters, and outdoor sports people may be at high risk for BM.[1] Up to 50% of patients with BM have malignancies associated with T-cell defects.[2]

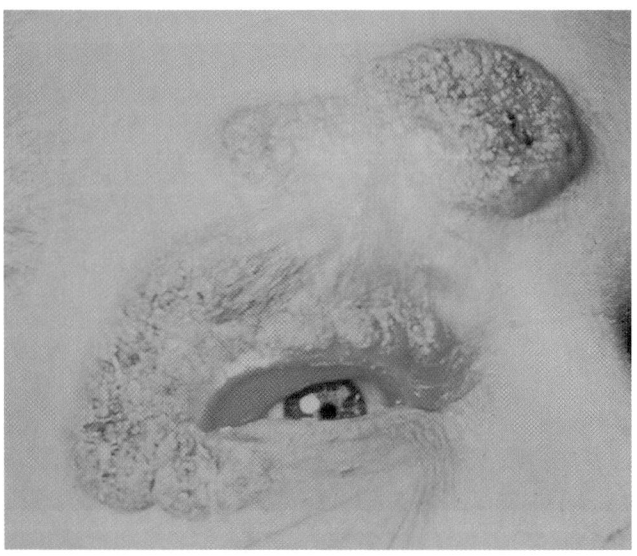

FIGURE 20–32 Blastomycosis of face and eyelid. (Courtesy of Alson E. Braley, MD.) (From Ostler, with permission.)

Diagnosis

The diagnosis may be suspected based on the history and clinical findings, and confirmed with potassium hydroxide preparation, which may reveal budding spores.[1] Other confirmatory modalities include biopsy, enzyme immunoassays, and fungal cultures. Reliable skin tests for BM are not currently available.[1]

Clinical Complications

Complications include recurrent or persistent infection, bacterial superinfection, spread to the CNS, systemic infection, and death.[1]

Management

Some cases of BM resolve spontaneously, but most patients require antifungal therapy.[1] Uncomplicated cutaneous disease may be successfully treated with oral potassium iodide. Intravenous amphotericin B is the treatment of choice for disseminated BM,[1] CNS BM, refractory primary cutaneous BM, and BM in immunocompromised patients. Itraconazole, fluconazole, and ketoconazole are other potential treatment options for disseminated BM. If BM is diagnosed in the emergency department, most patients will require hospitalization and consultation with a specialist in infectious diseases.[1,2]

REFERENCES

1. Trent JT, Kirsner RS. Identifying and treating mycotic skin infections. *Adv Skin Wound Care* 2003;16:122–129.
2. Torres HA, Rivero GA, Kontoyiannis DP. Endemic mycoses in a cancer hospital. *Medicine (Baltimore)* 2002;81:201–212.

Cryptococcosis

Michael Greenberg

Clinical Presentation

Some patients with cryptococcosis present with skin lesions, whereas others present with disseminated or systemic disease.[1,2] Skin lesions first appear on the face and neck as "painless papules or pustules,"[1] which later develop into ulcerating and purulent nodules.[1–3]

Pathophysiology

The fungus *Cryptococcus neoformans* is the causative organism for cryptococcosis.[1] This organism may be found in soil and in fecal matter from pigeons.[1] Immunocompromised persons may be at an increased risk for this disease. In fact, cryptococcosis is the most common fungal infection afflicting persons infected with human immunodeficiency virus (HIV)and individuals with acquired immunodeficiency syndrome (AIDS).[1–3]

Cryptococcal skin infection results from direct inoculation via a skin wound from an object that has been contaminated with the cryptococcal fungal organism. Primary skin infections are not common and often resolve spontaneously. However, skin infections may coexist with disseminated disease. Disseminated cryptococcal disease usually is initiated by a pulmonary infection with the fungal organism that then spreads via the bloodstream to bone, liver, kidney, prostate, and skin.[1]

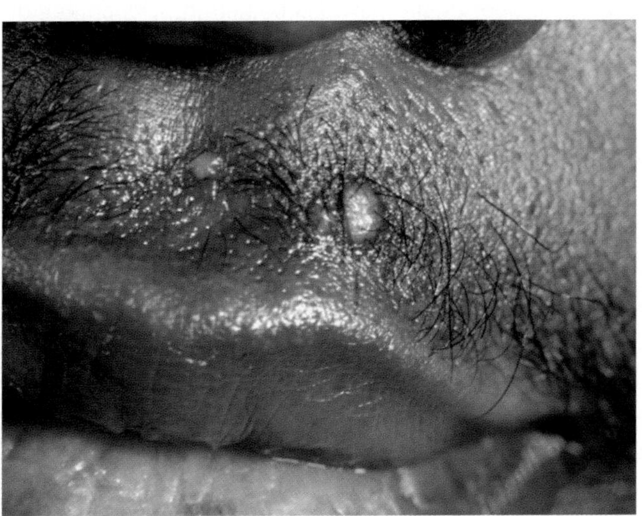

FIGURE 20–33 Disseminated cryptococcosis. Note the resemblance of these papules to those of molluscum contagiosum. (From Goodheart, with permission.)

Diagnosis

The diagnosis may be suspected based on the history and examination and confirmed by fungal culture, biopsy, or potassium hydroxide preparation of skin scrapings.[1]

Clinical Complications

Complications include recurrent or persistent infection, osteomyelitis, draining sinuses, bacterial superinfection, peritonitis, mediastinitis, spread to the central nervous system, systemic infection, and death.[1–3]

Management

IV amphotericin B is the treatment of choice for immunocompromised patients with cryptococcosis.[1] The rate of recurrence for this disease is extremely high (up to 90% of cases), and recurrence is associated with an extraordinarily high mortality rate (95% to 100%). Consequently, these patients require lifelong ketoconazole therapy after initial treatment with amphotericin B.[1]

REFERENCES

1. Trent JT, Kirsner RS. Identifying and treating mycotic skin infections. *Adv Skin Wound Care* 2003;16:122–129.
2. Kim do Y, Kim Y, Baek SY, Yoon HK. Simultaneous thoracic and abdominal presentation of disseminated cryptococcosis in two patients without HIV infection. *AJR Am J Roentgenol* 2003; 181:1055–1057.
3. Hage CA, Goldman M, Wheat LJ. Mucosal and invasive fungal infections in HIV/AIDS. *Eur J Med Res* 2002;7:236–241.

Aspergillosis

Michael Greenberg

Clinical Presentation

Patients with aspergillosis may present with symptoms related to invasive disease or allergic disease. Invasive pulmonary aspergillosis (IPA) is a life-threatening disease in immunocompromised patients. Patients with IPA present with acute onset of shortness of breath, pleuritic pain, hemoptysis, lung infiltrates, and high fever.[1-3]

Pathophysiology

Aspergillus is a ubiquitous, airborne mold that may cause disease in immunocompromised persons. IPA affects 14% of lung transplant recipients and as many as 50% of leukemia patients who become neutropenic.

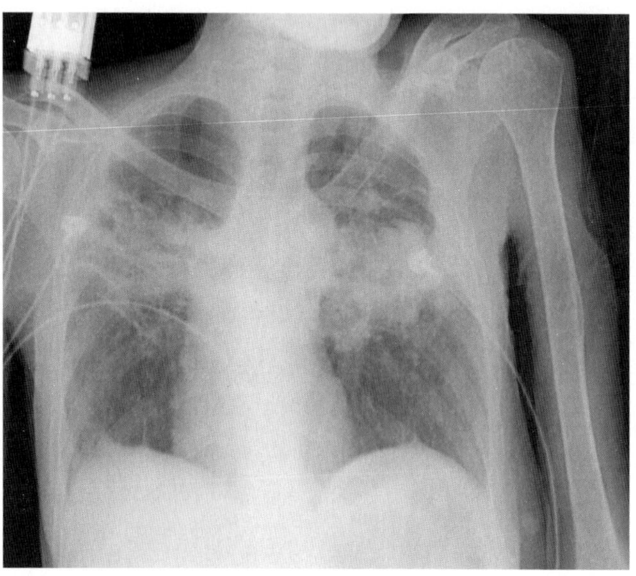

FIGURE 20–34 Bilateral pulmonary aspergillosis. (Courtesy of Mark Silverberg, MD.)

Diagnosis

The diagnosis is based on clinical suspicion in the correct clinical setting. Radiographic imaging tends to have poor specificity, and microbiologic cultures tend to lack sensitivity for this diagnosis. Advanced serologic tests such as Galactmannan antigen detection or aspergillus DNA detection may be required for confirmation. Other cases may require percutaneous or open-lung biopsy of the lung, as well as bronchoscopic specimens.[1-3]

Clinical Complications

Complications include aspergilloma formation (fungal mycelia, inflammatory cells, and debris collected in a preexisting lung cavity), invasion into pulmonary vasculature with severe hemoptysis, and death.[1-3]

Management

Intravenous amphotericin B is the treatment of choice; however, other options, such as itraconazole, voriconazole, and posaconazole, as well as newer antifungals such as caspofungin, may also be helpful. Depending on the clinical findings, surgical therapy in conjunction with antifungal medications may be indicated.[1-3]

REFERENCES

1. Patterson TF, Kirkpatrick WR, White M, et al. Invasive aspergillosis: disease spectrum, treatment practices, and outcomes. I3 Aspergillus Study Group. *Medicine (Baltimore)* 2000;79:250–260.
2. Oren I, Goldstein N. Invasive pulmonary aspergillosis. *Curr Opin Pulm Med* 2002;8:195–200.
3. Bag R. Fungal pneumonias in transplant recipients. *Curr Opin Pulm Med* 2003;9:193–198.

Mucormycosis

Robert Hendrickson

Clinical Presentation

Presenting symptoms of patients with mucormycosis vary, depending on the location of the infection: rhinocerebral—depressed mental status, cranial nerve deficits, facial edema, epistaxis, and facial necrosis; pulmonary—fever, dyspnea, and chest pain; cutaneous—skin lesions; gastrointestinal—abdominal pain and hematochezia; or central nervous system (CNS)—depressed mental status and headache.[1] Patients may be at higher risk for particular forms of the disease based on underlying conditions such as diabetes (rhinocerebral), leukemia/neutropenia (pulmonary), severe malnutrition (gastrointestinal), or intravenous drug use (central nervous system).[1]

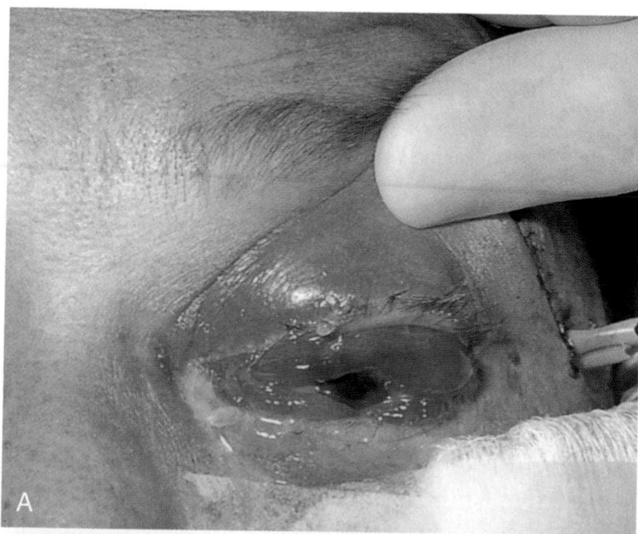

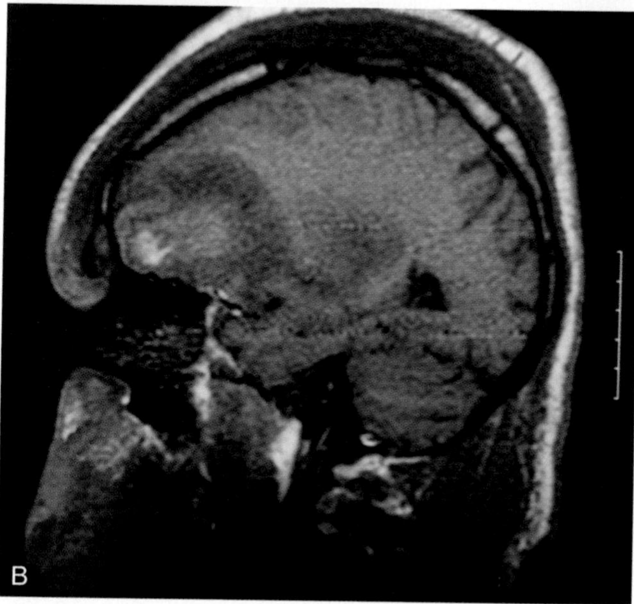

FIGURE 20–35 **A:** Periorbital erythema and edema with chemosis caused by orbital mucormycosis. (From Ostler, with permission.) **B:** Magnetic resonance image showing frontal lobe brain abscess secondary to mucormycosis. (From Hendrickson RG, Olshaker J, Duckett O. Rhinocerebral mucormycosis: a case of a rare but deadly disease. *J Emerg Med* 1999;17:641–645, with permission from Elsevier.)

Pathophysiology

Mucormycosis refers to an infection of the upper airway, gastrointestinal tract, lungs, CNS, or skin that is caused by fungi from the family Mucorales, order Mucoraceae (genera *Rhizopus, Mucor,* and *Absidia*).[1,2] In the rhinocerebral form of the disease, the fungal spores are inhaled into the upper respiratory tract. Hyphae proliferate and invade local vascular structures, leading to ischemia and necrosis of local tissue.[1,2] Spores may contaminate wounds or dressings and lead to the cutaneous form. Finally, spores may be injected during intravenous drug use and cause the CNS form of mucormycosis.[1] Most patients who develop mucormycosis have hyperglycemia and diabetes. Other risk factors include leukemia, renal disease or transplant, and treatment with deferoxamine.[2] The diagnosis should be considered in patients whose mental status does not return to normal after appropriate therapy for diabetic ketoacidosis (DKA).[2]

Diagnosis

The diagnosis may be suspected in patients with risk factors and typical symptoms, and it may be confirmed by identification of typical hyphae on a biopsy specimen of the border of a necrotic area.[1,2] Computed tomographic scan of the brain and face may reveal brain abscess, as well as sinus and bone necrosis.

Clinical Complications

Complications include facial necrosis, brain abscess, cranial nerve deficits, and death.

Management

Patients may require resuscitation and treatment for hyperglycemia or DKA. Mortality may be directly related to the time to diagnosis and treatment. Treatment includes rapid surgical débridement and therapy with amphotericin B.[2] Hyperbaric oxygen therapy may be effective; however, it should never delay surgical therapy.

REFERENCES

1. Sugar AM. Mucormycosis. *Clin Infect Dis* 1992;14(Suppl 1): S126–S129.
2. Hendrickson RG, Olshaker J, Duckett O. Rhinocerebral mucormycosis: a case of a rare, but deadly disease. *J Emerg Med* 1999;17: 641–645.

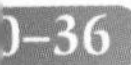

Onychomycosis

Sharon McGregor

Clinical Presentation

Patients with onychomycosis present with one or more discolored, thickened, dystrophic nail(s) with hyperkeratotic debris under the nail plate and separation of the nail plate from the nail bed (onycholysis). In distal subungual onychomycosis, the most common form in children and adults, the fungus invades between the nail plate and nail bed at the distal or lateral subungual fold, and nail changes are present distally. Proximal subungual onychomycosis manifests with color change and onycholysis beginning proximally and progressing distally. This type is more commonly seen after nail trauma or in immunocompromised individuals, and it may be a presenting sign of human immunodeficiency virus (HIV) infection.[1,2]

Pathophysiology

Onychomycosis (tinea unguium) is a fungal infection of the nail bed and/or nail plate. It is the most common nail disorder in adults, affecting up to 20% of the adult population. Fungal organisms generally invade between the nail bed and nail plate, either distally through an opening in the subungual space of the hyponychium or proximally through an opening in the cuticle. Certain individuals are at increased risk for development of onychomycosis, including the elderly and those with diabetes, compromised immune status (especially human immunodeficiency virus [HIV]/acquired immune deficience syndrome [AIDS], atopy, genetic predilection to dermatophyte infection, psoriasis, nail trauma, tinea pedis, or tinea manuum (hands). In children, Down syndrome also increases the risk.

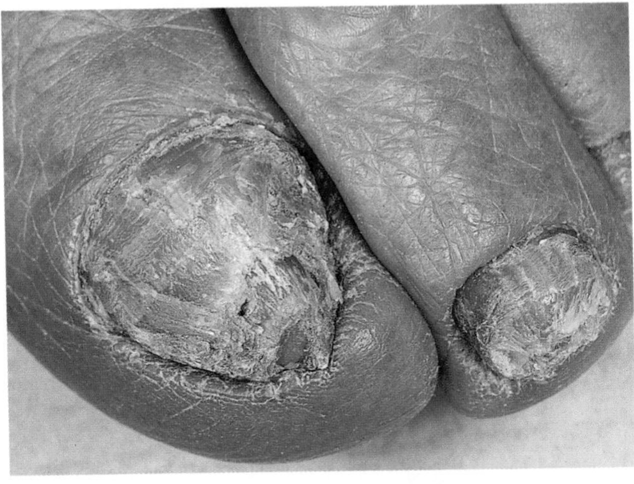

FIGURE 20–36 Nail thickening and discoloration consistent with onychomycosis. (From Ostler, with permission.)

Diagnosis

Onychomycosis is confirmed microscopically and by culture. Only 50% of cases of suspected onychomycosis are actually a fungal infection. Scrapings of subungual debris and nail clippings from the most proximal part of the involved nail should be used for potassium hydroxide preparation to microscopically confirm hyphae and for culture to verify fungal infection and determine the species.[1,2]

Clinical Complications

Onychomycosis may be a chronic and recurring infection. Complications include infections, osteomyelitis, ulcers, gangrene, and amputation.

Management

Treatment depends on the severity of the infection, the causative organism, and the presence of comorbid conditions. Useful antifungal agents include terbinafine, itraconazole, and fluconazole. Because of potential hematologic and hepatic effects, it is recommended that a baseline complete blood count and liver function tests be performed and that testing be repeated during and after the course of treatment. Topical treatment with ciclopirox 8% nail lacquer may be used in less severe cases without lunula involvement, but it is less effective (5% to 8% cure rate) than systemic therapy and requires 6 to 12 months of treatment. Nail débridement or removal of the nail may be indicated in more severe cases.[1,2]

REFERENCES

1. Gupta AK, Sibbald RG, Lynde CW, et al. Onychomycosis in children: prevalence and treatment strategies. *J Am Acad Dermatol* 1997;36:395–402.
2. Vander Straten MR, Hossain MA, Ghannoun MA. Cutaneous infections: dermatophytosis, onychomycosis, and tinea versicolor. *Infect Dis Clin North Am* 2003;17:87–112.

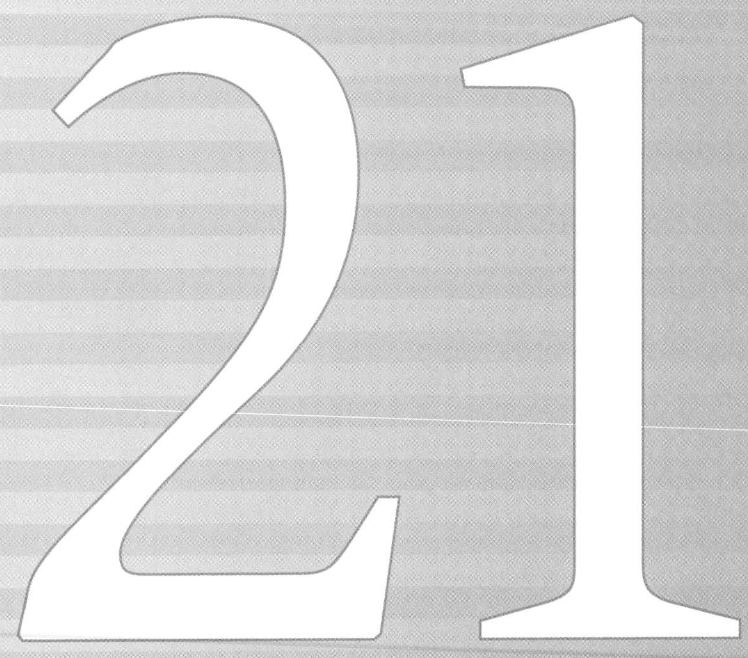

Hematologic/Oncologic

Pernicious Anemia

Robert Hendrickson

Clinical Presentation

Patients with pernicious anemia may present with symptoms of anemia (fatigue, lightheadedness, end-organ ischemia) or vitamin B_{12} deficiency (neuropathy, diarrhea). Physical examination may reveal macroglossia (large, red, smooth tongue), angular cheilitis, or "spoon nails."

Pathophysiology

Pernicious anemia is a disorder in which vitamin B_{12} deficiency anemia results from atrophic gastritis and malabsorption. It is most common in women older than 60 years of age.[1] Vitamin B_{12} is important in the growth and division of cells. Deficiency in vitamin B_{12} can lead to apoptosis of red blood cells (RBCs) and the release of immature, large reticulocytes and RBCs from the bone marrow (macrocytic anemia with numerous reticulocytes). Pernicious anemia develops secondary to destruction of gastric parietal cells due to autoantibodies and resulting malabsorption of vitamin B_{12}.[1]

Diagnosis

The diagnosis should be considered if a macrocytic anemia is discovered in a patient who has the typical characteristics of pernicious anemia (e.g., older age, female, macroglossia). Patients with pernicious anemia have decreased vitamin B_{12} concentration, normal folate concentration, and a macrocytic anemia with thrombocytopenia.[1] A Schilling test may be performed to determine whether the deficiency is the result of malabsorption.

Clinical Complications

Complications include the complications of anemia (myocardial infarction, cerebrovascular accident, syncope), as well as chronic diarrhea, peripheral neuropathy, and subacute combined degeneration of the spinal cord and cerebrum (potentially irreversible demyelination).

Management

Patients with pernicious anemia require intramuscular vitamin B_{12} supplementation monthly. Follow-up should be arranged for repeated evaluation.

REFERENCES

1. Toh BH, van Driel IR, Gleeson PA. Pernicious anemia. *N Engl J Med* 1997;337:1441–1448.

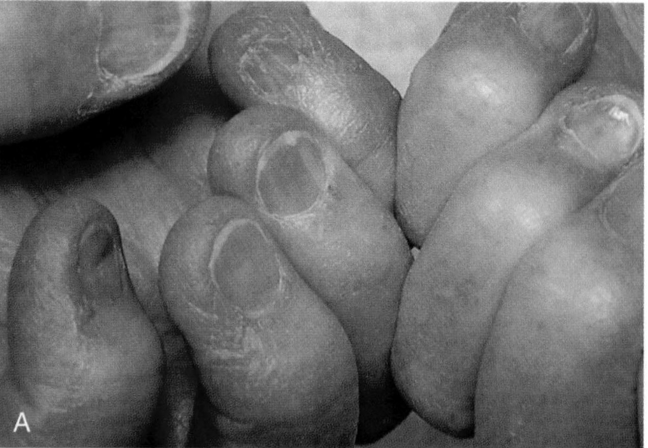

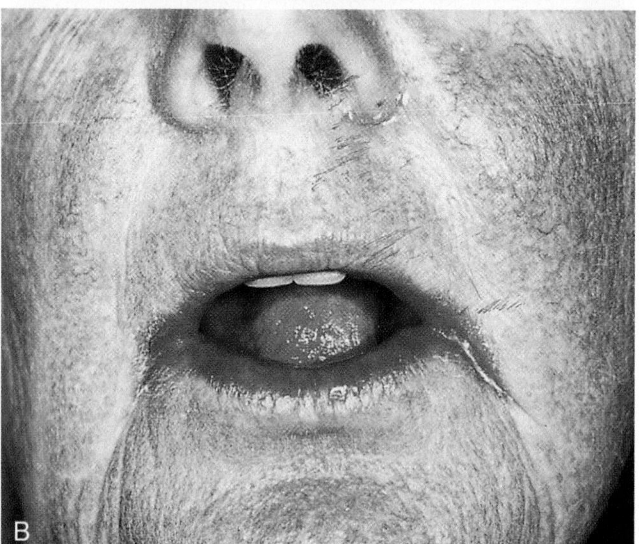

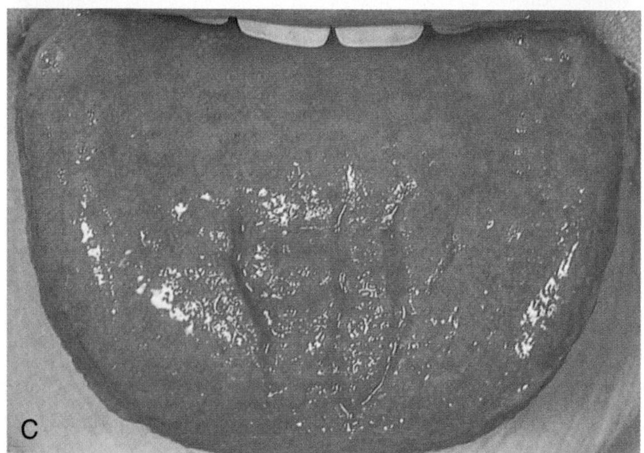

FIGURE 21–1 **A:** Koilonychia. These nail changes are characteristic of iron deficiency and consist of spooning concavity, longitudinal ridging, and brittleness. **B:** Angular cheilitis. Inflammation at the angles of the mouth is commonly associated with deficiencies of the B vitamins. **C:** A raw, fissured tongue, especially in the setting of peripheral neuropathy, should raise the suspicion of vitamin B_{12} deficiency. (**A–C** From Yamada, with permission.)

Sickle Cell Anemia

Robert Hendrickson

Clinical Presentation

The majority of patients with sickle cell anemia who present to the emergency department know that they have a diagnosis of sickle cell disease, because the clinical symptoms begin at a young age. Occasionally, patients with sickle cell variants (sickle β-thalassemia, sickle cell C disease) present in their teenage years. Patients usually are asymptomatic between sickling episodes. Stress, dehydration, trauma, hypoxia, or infection can trigger red blood cells (RBCs) to sickle and produce symptoms of end-organ ischemia. Symptoms of vaso-occlusive crisis can range from severe pain in muscles or bones to cerebrovascular accident (CVA) and pulmonary infarction (acute chest syndrome). The splenic sequestration syndrome may produce abdominal pain, anemia, and splenic rupture. Other symptoms are related to venous obstruction or ischemia and include priapism, avascular necrosis, hand-and-foot syndrome, renal papillary necrosis, and aplastic crisis (infarction of the bone marrow). Older children and adults are at risk of infection from encapsulated organisms.[1]

Pathophysiology

Sickle cell anemia is an autosomal codominant hereditary disorder of hemoglobin that produces malformation ("sickling") of RBCs. A genetic substitution in the β-globin gene produces an altered hemoglobin, HbS. HbS polymerizes on deoxygenation, resulting in a rigid, sickle-shaped, dehydrated RBC with increased affinity for the endothelial wall.[1] Sickling leads to vascular occlusion and end-organ ischemia.

Diagnosis

Most patients know their diagnosis and those of their family members; however, the diagnosis may be confirmed or clarified by hemoglobin electrophoresis.[1]

Clinical Complications

Complications include ischemia of any organ, CVA, myocardial infarction, splenic infarction, renal failure, acute chest syndrome, hemolysis, anemia, bony infarction, and sepsis from encapsulated organisms.[1]

Management

Patients with vaso-occlusive crises should be hydrated (orally or intravenously) and given adequate pain medication. Patients with pulmonary complaints or hypoxemia should receive supplemental oxygen and a chest radiograph to rule out acute chest syndrome. A complete blood count and reticulocyte count are helpful in ruling out aplastic crisis and determining the extent of anemia. For patients with fever, a search should be made for the source of infection, and cultures and antibiotic therapy should be started quickly.[1] Splenic sequestration is an emergency that requires urgent exchange transfusion and possibly splenectomy.[1] Patients with acute chest syndrome should be treated for a pulmonary infection and may require further workup and treatment for a pulmonary thrombosis. Admission should be considered for patients with central nervous system, pulmonary, or infectious crises; those who are unable to take oral fluids; and those with splenic sequestration or aplastic crisis.[1]

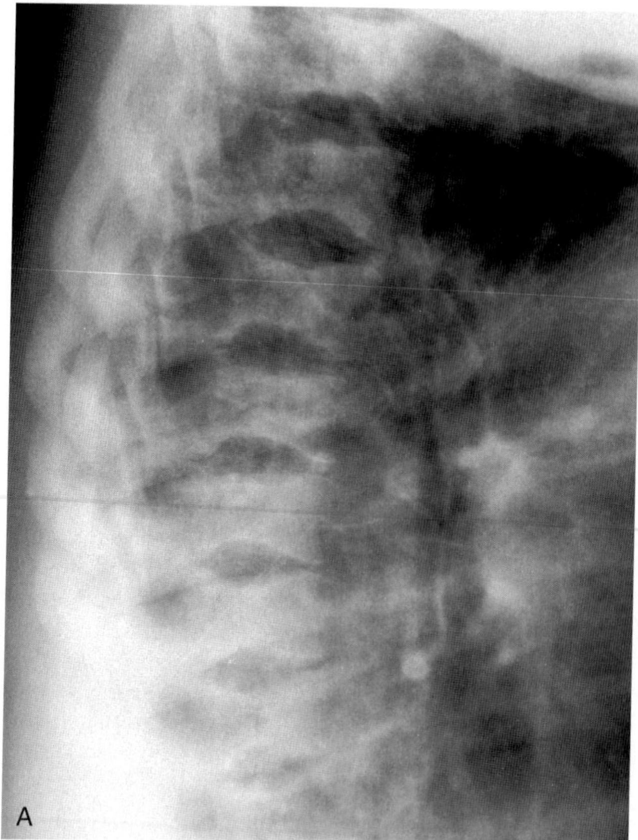

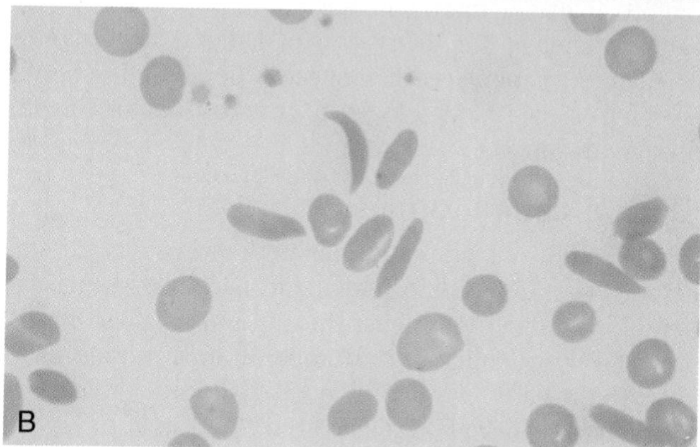

FIGURE 21–2 **A:** Fishmouth vertebrae, characteristic of long-standing sickle cell disease. (© David Effron, MD, 2004. Used with permission.) **B:** Drepanocyte (sickle cell). (From Anderson, with permission.)

REFERENCES

1. Ballas SK. Sickle cell anaemia: progress in pathogenesis and treatment. *Drugs* 2002;62:1143–1172.

The Hemophilias

Robert Hendrickson

Clinical Presentation

Patients with hemophilia present with complaints that are related to bleeding. Traumatic or atraumatic hemarthrosis and muscle bleeds are a common phenomenon and can be exceedingly painful. Other bleeding complications include central nervous system (CNS) bleeds, gastrointestinal (GI) bleeds, and exsanguinating dermal or mucosal bleeding.[1]

Pathophysiology

The hemophilias are inherited disorders of coagulation caused by deficiencies of coagulation factors. Hemophilias A, B, and C are caused by deficiencies in factors 8, 9, and 11, respectively. Hemophilia C is typically a mild disorder with minimal risk of serious bleeding.[1] Hemophilias A and B result from abnormalities in the long arm of the X chromosome. Circulating factor concentrations vary and are indirectly proportional to the severity and frequency of complications. Activated factors 8 and 9 are necessary components in the coagulation cascade and are required for amplification of activated factor 10.[1] Deficiencies in these factors prevent the stabilization of platelet clots and may lead to bleeding.[1]

Diagnosis

Severe hemophilia A or B usually manifests early in life (before 4 years of age), whereas milder forms may be diagnosed later in life. Two thirds of patients have a family history.[1] Patients with suspected hemophilia should be referred to a hematologist or primary doctor for definitive diagnosis.

Clinical Complications

Complications include exsanguinating mucosal or dermal hemorrhage, CNS hemorrhage, and GI hemorrhage. Patients with recurrent hemarthrosis and muscle bleeds may develop debilitating arthropathy and muscle atrophy.[1] In the early 1980s, only pooled plasma-derived factor replacement was available, and thousands of hemophiliacs developed human immunodeficiency virus (HIV) infection, hepatitis A, and hepatitis B from the blood supply. With the current use of recombinant factors, there is no risk of disease transmission. However, plasma-derived factors are still used, and, although there is no risk of HIV, hepatitis B, or hepatitis C transmission, there remains a risk of parvovirus and hepatitis A transmission.[1]

Management

Bleeding in a patient with hemophilia is an emergency and should be treated promptly. Patients with mild hemophilia A (or von Willebrand's disease) who present with mild bleeding (e.g., hemarthrosis) may be given desmopressin to raise the factor 8 concentration. More serious bleeding or severe underlying hemophilia may be treated with recombinant factor replacement.[1]

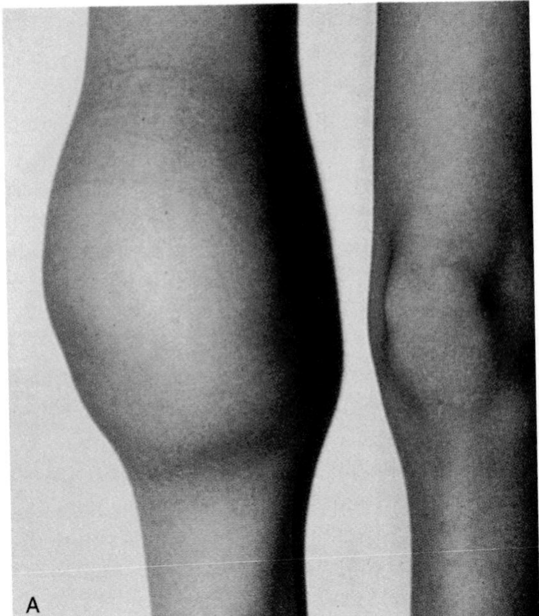

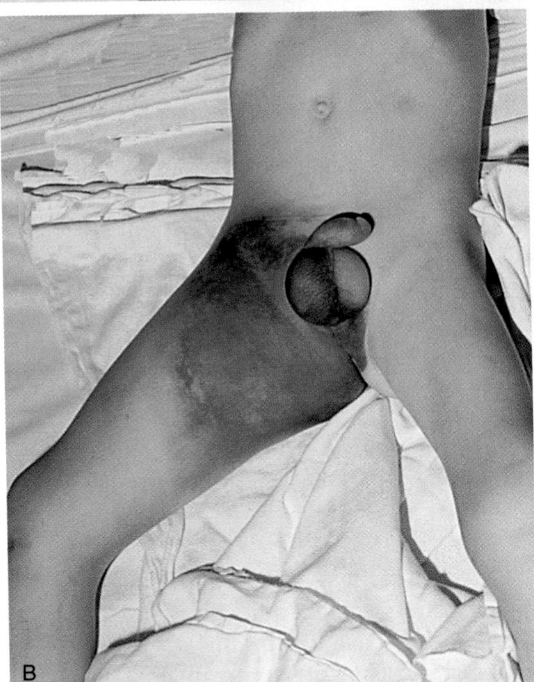

FIGURE 21–3 **A:** Hemophilic arthropathy. This figure illustrates the sequelae of recurrent joint bleeding. **B:** Large dissecting hematoma of the thigh in a patient with hemophilia A. The lesion resulted from a slight bump to the inguinal area and spread to involve the entire thigh. (**A** and **B**, from Greer, with permission.)

REFERENCES

1. Bolton-Maggs PH, Pasi KJ. Haemophilias A and B. *Lancet* 2003;361:1801–1809.

Lymphoma

Robert Hendrickson

Clinical Presentation

Patients with lymphoma may present with painless peripheral lymphadenopathy (most common), splenomegaly or abdominal mass, weight loss, night sweats, fatigue, anemia, fever, or pruritus.[1]

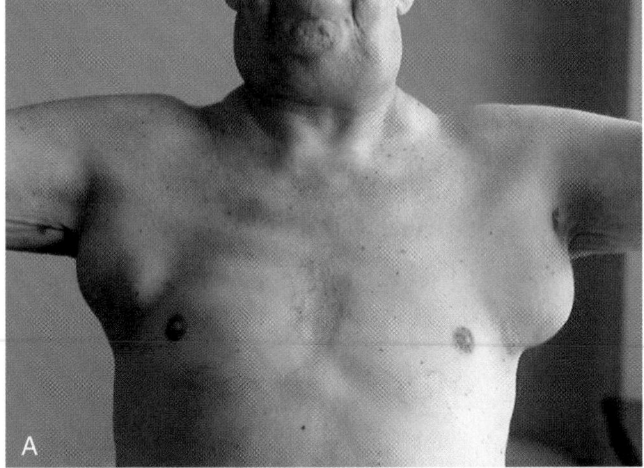

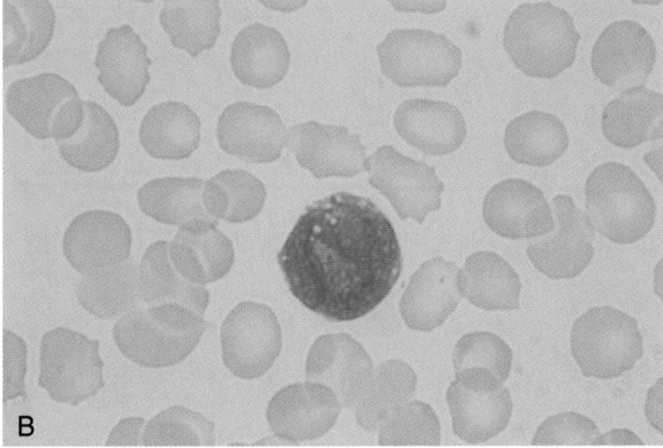

FIGURE 21–4 **A:** Malignant adenopathy of lymphoma. The nodes are larger than 2 cm in diameter, multiple, rubbery, and nontender. (From Handin, with permission.) **B:** Large follicular cell of B-cell origin (non-Hodgkin's lymphoma). (From Anderson, with permission.)

Pathophysiology

Lymphomas are a heterogenous group of idiopathic malignancies made up of lymphocytes (B and T cells) that have undergone malignant transformation. Lymphomas are usually grouped into two broad categories: Hodgkin's disease (HD) and non-Hodgkin's lymphoma (NHL). NHL includes a variety of subtypes and is the fifth most common cancer in the United States, with more than 50,000 new cases diagnosed annually.[2] The most important risk factors for NHL are primary and acquired immunosuppression. Up to 25% of patients with genetically determined immunodeficiencies develop primary B-cell lymphomas.[2] Increased risk for NHL has been noted in patients with ataxia telangiectasia, Wiskott-Aldrich syndrome, or various forms of immunodeficiency.[2]

Diagnosis

The diagnosis should be considered in patients with painless lymphadenopathy or persistent constitutional symptoms such as fever, weight loss, fatigue, or pruritus. Lymph-node enlargement may also be noted in the perihilar region on chest radiography.

Clinical Complications

The morbidity and mortality rates for lymphoma vary depending on cell type. In general, HD has a 5-year survival rate greater than 50%. NHL is rarely cured by chemotherapy, but survival longer than 5 years is possible.

Management

Treatment varies with cell type, but largely consists of chemotherapy and, occasionally, radiotherapy.[1] Consultation and close follow-up with a hematologist or oncologist is the standard of care.

REFERENCES

1. Mead GM. ABC of clinical haematology: malignant lymphomas and chronic lymphocytic leukaemia. *BMJ* 1997;314:1103–1106.
2. Baris D, Zahm SH. Epidemiology of lymphomas. *Curr Opin Oncol* 2000;12:383–394.

Multiple Myeloma

Robert Hendrickson

Clinical Presentation

Patients with multiple myeloma most commonly present with bony pain or fractures, typically in the lower back. Other common symptoms are related to renal insufficiency, anemia (fatigue, lightheadedness), hypercalcemia (weakness), infection, spinal cord compression, or hyperviscosity (blurred vision, confusion).[1]

Pathophysiology

Multiple myeloma is a plasma-cell neoplasm. The inciting cell is most likely a memory B cell located in a peripheral lymph node. The cell migrates hematogenously to the bone marrow, where a series of cell signals lead to proliferation of osteoclasts and lytic bony lesions. The myeloma produces monoclonal antibodies or light chains and decreases bone marrow production by mass effect. The resulting neutropenia leaves the patient prone to infection. The lysis of bone may lead to hypercalcemia and renal failure.[1]

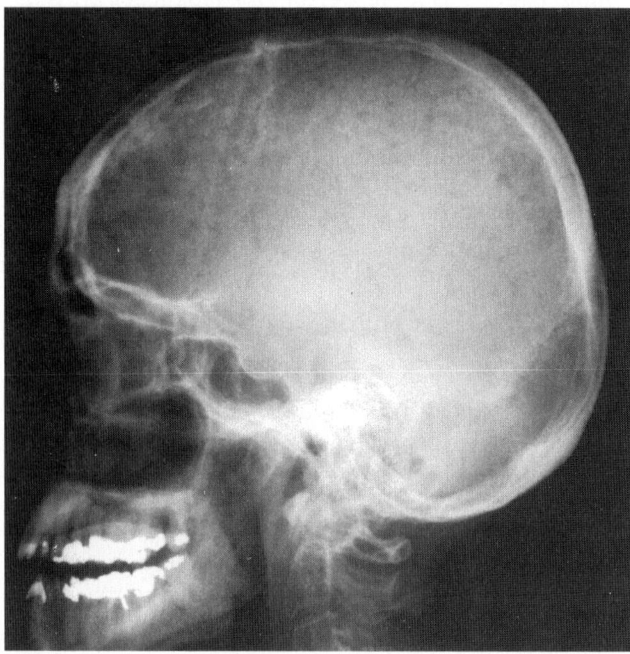

FIGURE 21–5 "Punched-out" lytic lesions of the skull associated with multiple myeloma. (From Greer, with permission.)

Diagnosis

The diagnosis should be considered in patients older than 40 years of age who have atraumatic bony pain, hypercalcemia, or anemia. Confirmation of the diagnosis in the emergency department occurs by recognition of lytic lesions on x-ray films. Bence Jones proteins may be detected by electrophoresis of the urine. A complete blood count; determination of the erythrocyte sedimentation rate; measurements of alkaline phosphatase, calcium, and uric acid; and a skeletal survey may be helpful.[1,2]

Management

Treatment of multiple myeloma should include hydration, analgesia, treatment of hypercalcemia (hydration, diuretics, bisphosphonates) if present, and treatment of any infection. Arrangements should be made with a hematologist or other specialist for further evaluation, with a possible bone marrow biopsy and chemotherapy (melphalan, cyclophosphamide, prednisolone).[1,2]

REFERENCES

1. Singer CR. ABC of clinical haematology: multiple myeloma and related conditions. *BMJ* 1997;314:960–963.
2. Bataille R, Harousseau JL. Multiple myeloma. *N Engl J Med* 1997; 336):1657–1664.

Leukemias

Robert Hendrickson

Clinical Presentation

Patients with chronic leukemias may have few symptoms, and the diagnosis may be made incidentally on routine blood work. Patients with acute leukemias may be acutely ill and may present with disorders that are related to thrombocytopenia (bruising, nose bleeds), neutropenia (infections of the mouth, throat, skin, perineum), anemia (fatigue, dyspnea), or bone pain.[1] Patients less commonly present with lymphadenopathy, splenomegaly, or mediastinal masses.[1]

Pathophysiology

Leukemia is a condition in which the bone marrow is replaced by granulocytes or lymphocytes that have undergone malignant transformation. Leukemias are divided into acute (A) and chronic (C) forms, as well as lymphoblastic (L, for lymphocytes) and myeloid (M) types; the myeloid leukemias involve eosinophils, neutrophils, monocytes, basophils, and other cells. Acute lymphoblastic leukemia (ALL) is most common in children (85% of childhood leukemias), whereas AML, CML, and CLL are more common in adults. The cause of most leukemias is not known. However, in general, they result from malignant transformation of bone marrow cells, probably under the influence of complex factors potentially involving genetic, environmental, and immune system influences. Radiation, some chemicals (e.g., benzene), and certain chemotherapy agents (e.g., etoposide, some alkylating agents) are thought to cause some kinds of leukemia, including AML.[1]

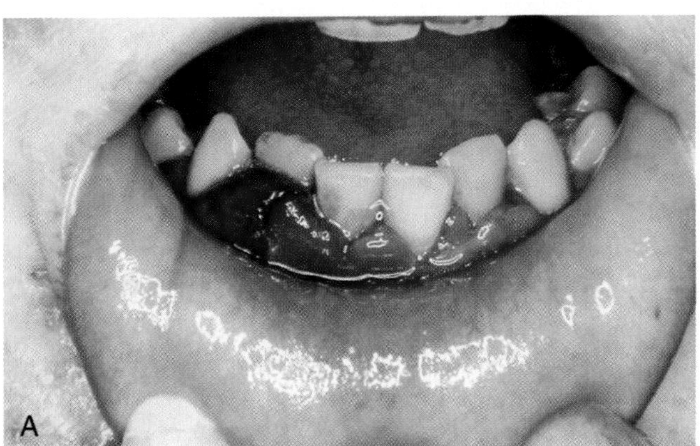

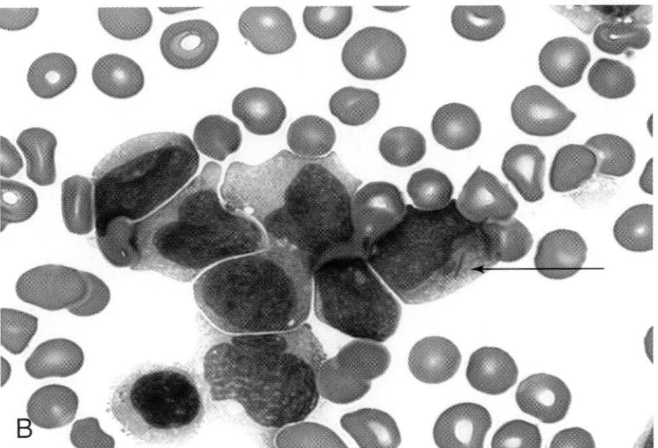

FIGURE 21-6 **A:** Gingival infiltration (leukemia). (From Benjamin, with permission.) **B:** Auer rods. (From Anderson, with permission.)

Diagnosis

The diagnosis may be suspected in patients with typical symptoms (e.g., fever, fatigue, oral infections, bleeding, bruising). Early in acute or chronic disease, a complete blood count may reveal a leukocytosis (more than 100,000 leukocytes per microliter), with irregular peripheral leukocytes or peripheral blast cells. Later in the disease, bone marrow becomes replaced, and the patient may develop neutropenia, thrombocytopenia, and anemia. Blood uric acid is elevated due to cell turnover.

Clinical Complications

Complications include neutropenic sepsis, infections, hemorrhage, and a 20% to 60% mortality rate from the disease.[1] Remission (5-yr survival) is achieved in 60% of children with ALL, 30% of adults with ALL, and 10% to 20% of people with AML.

Management

Patients with acute leukemias should be admitted and stabilized; they should be transferred to a facility that is capable of caring for them and has a hematology consultation service, if possible. Patients with chronic leukemias should have follow-up with a hematologist and may require admission for platelet transfusion, treatment of neutropenia, hydration, and psychological/social support for the patient and family. Workup and treatment require bone marrow aspiration and chemotherapy.

REFERENCES

1. Liesner RJ, Goldstone AH. ABC of clinical haematology: the acute leukaemias. *BMJ* 1997;314:733–736.

Superior Vena Cava Syndrome

Robert Hendrickson

Clinical Presentation

Patients with superior vena cava syndrome (SVCS) may present with complaints of dyspnea, headache, facial flushing, visual changes, or swelling in the face, neck, and hands.[1] Patients may report symptoms of the underlying cause of the obstruction, including tumor (weight loss, cough, history of smoking) or thrombosis (history of thromboses, intravenous catheters). Clinical signs include nonpulsatile jugular venous distention, distention of upper thoracic veins, conjunctival injection, tachypnea, and plethora and swelling of the face, hands, and neck.[1]

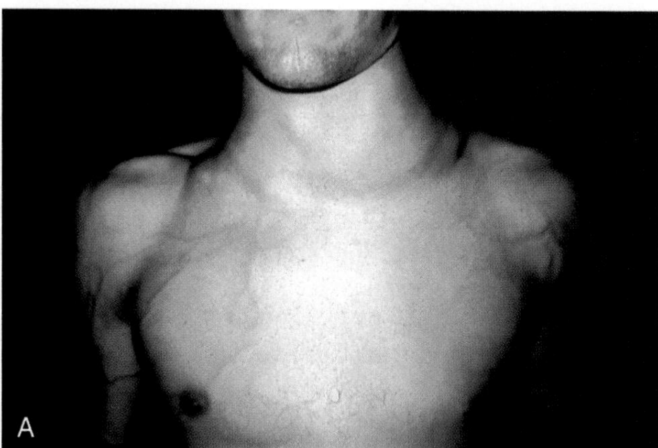

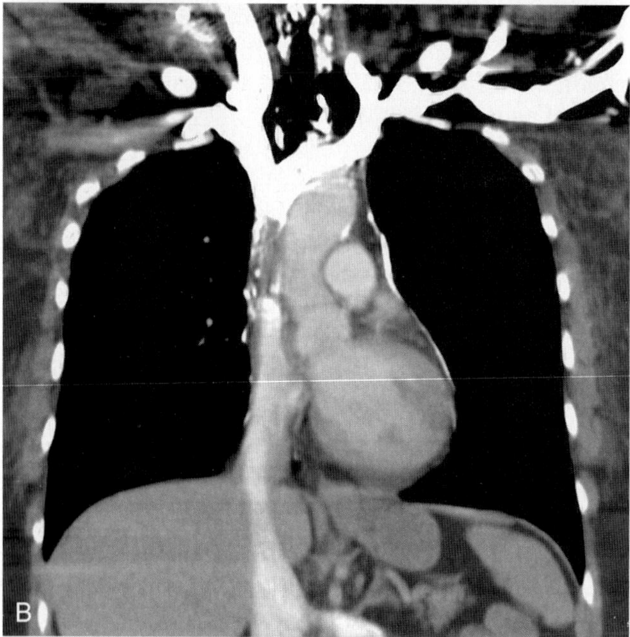

FIGURE 21–7 **A:** Venous engorgement secondary to superior vena cava obstruction. (From Handin, with permission.) **B:** Thrombosis of the superior vena cava. (Courtesy of Ralph Weiche, MD.)

Pathophysiology

SVCS is a collection of symptoms related to increased venous pressure in the head and upper extremities caused by obstruction of the superior vena cava (SVC). Obstruction of the SVC may occur via external compression or internal thrombosis. Cancer is the most common cause of SVCS, particularly bronchogenic carcinoma (65% to 80%) and lymphoma (2% to 10%).[1] Other potential causes include thoracic aneurysm, mediastinal fibrosis, and massive goiter.[1]

Diagnosis

The diagnosis of SVCS is made from the history and recognition of the typical clinical features. Chest radiography or computed tomography may reveal the cause of the obstruction.

Management

SVSC is an emergency. The cause of the obstruction must be determined as quickly as possible. If the cause is cancer and the patient has severe symptoms, emergency radiotherapy, chemotherapy, or both may be required. Radiation therapy and/or chemotherapy relieves SVCS in 60% to 77% of cases.[2] An attempt to make a cellular diagnosis via biopsy should be made before the initiation of radiation therapy. Corticosteroids may be used while awaiting definitive therapy, or if therapy is contraindicated, and may decrease the symptoms of SVCS.[1] If the cause is thrombotic, treatment modalities include anticoagulants and surgery. Stenting of the SVC relieves symptoms in up to 95% of patients with SVCS.[2]

REFERENCES

1. Falk S, Fallon M. ABC of palliative care: emergencies. *BMJ* 1997;315:1525–1528.
2. Rowell NP, Gleeson FV. Steroids, radiotherapy, chemotherapy and stents for superior vena caval obstruction in carcinoma of the bronchus: a systematic review. *Clin Oncol* 2002;14:338–351.

Thrombotic Thrombocytopenic Purpura

Robert Hendrickson

Clinical Presentation

Symptoms of thrombotic thrombocytopenic purpura (TTP) include a typical pentad of clinical features (see Tables 21–8A and 21–8B): microangiopathic hemolytic anemia, fever, neurologic symptoms (seizures, altered mental status, coma, central nervous system [CNS] abnormalities), acute renal failure, and thrombocytopenia.[1]

Pathophysiology

TTP is a disorder of microvascular thrombosis that most commonly affects young women (10 to 60 years old). TTP is produced when the body is unable to cleave unusually long multimers of von Willebrand's factor (vWF), which tend to produce platelet aggregation. vWF is produced in the endothelial cell as long multimers (strings) and is cleaved by a metalloprotease (ADAMTS 13) into smaller strings that do not produce spontaneous platelet aggregation. TTP is related to either a congenital lack of functional ADAMTS 13 or the transient production of autoantibodies to the protease (acquired TTP).[1] Diffuse endothelial thrombosis leads to hypoperfusion of the CNS and kidneys, as well as consumption of platelets and hemolytic anemia secondary to turbulent flow around thromboses.

Diagnosis

The diagnosis is made by recognition of the clinical symptoms and may be confirmed by laboratory evaluations. Anemia, reticulocytosis, thrombocytopenia, leukocytosis, and elevated concentrations of blood urea nitrogen (BUN), creatinine, and lactate dehydrogenase (LDH) are typical. Schistocytes may be visible on peripheral blood smear. Coagulation profiles are normal in TTP and may be helpful in differentiating TTP from disseminated intravascular coagulation.

Clinical Complications

Complications include renal failure, coma, seizures, anemia, cerebrovascular accident, hemorrhage, and death.[1]

Management

Platelet transfusions should be avoided, because they can exacerbate the illness.[1] Treatment includes exchange transfusion and, possibly, corticosteroids. Exchange transfusion removes the autoantibodies to ADAMTS 13 and supplies additional metalloprotease.[1] Refractory cases may be treated by splenectomy, azathioprine, vincristine, cyclophosphamide, or a combination of these therapies.

REFERENCES

1. Moake JL. Thrombotic microangiopathies. *N Engl J Med* 2002;347: 589–600.

TABLE 21–8A Incidence of Pentad Features in Patients with Thrombotic Thrombocytopenic Purpura

	Amarosi and Ultmann[a]		Ridolfi and Bell[b]	
Symptom	**No. Symptomatic/No. in Study**	**%**	**No. Symptomatic/No. in Study**	**%**
Microangiopathic hemolytic anemia	246/256	96	254/258	98
Thrombocytopenic purpura or other bleeding	241/251	96	214/258	83
Neurologic symptoms	250/271	92	218/258	84
Renal disease	191/217	88	196/258	76
Fever	237/243	98	252/258	98

From Greer, with permission.
Amorosi EL, Ultmann JE. Thrombotic thrombocytopenic purpura: report of 16 cases and review of the literature. *Medicine* 1966;45:139–159.
Ridolfi RL, Bell WR. Thrombotic thrombocytopenic purpura: report of 25 cases and review of the literature. *Medicine* 1981;60:413–428.

TABLE 21–8B Diseases Associated with Thrombotic Thrombocytopenic Purpura

Infections	Collagen vascular diseases
Human immunodeficiency virus	Pregnancy and the puerperium
Escherichia coli, Shigella	Cancer
Pancreatitis	Bone marrow transplantation
Drug treatment	
Cyclosporin A, tacrolimus (FK506)	
Antineoplastic agents	
Ticlopidine, clopidogrel	
Quinine	

From Greer, with permission.

Idiopathic Thrombocytopenic Purpura

Robert Hendrickson

Clinical Presentation

Acute idiopathic thrombocytopenic purpura (ITP) typically afflicts children 1 to 2 weeks of age after a viral illness. The disorder may last several months. Chronic ITP is more common in adults and may be permanent or intermittent.[1] Patients present with signs of thrombocytopenia, including epistaxis, hematuria, oral bleeding, or skin petechiae. Bleeding complications may occur if platelet counts decrease to less than 30,000/μL.[1] Petechial hemorrhages are typically located in dependent areas (e.g., lower extremities) and may coalesce into ecchymoses. Intracranial or gastrointestinal hemorrhage is rare but possible.[1] The peripheral blood may reveal few platelets, an increased number of megakaryocytes (i.e., megathrombocytes), and possibly leukocytosis.

Pathophysiology

ITP, also known as autoimmune thrombocytopenic purpura, is a disorder in which autoantibodies cause platelet phagocytosis, resulting in thrombocytopenia and possibly purpura and hemorrhage.[1] In some cases, autoantibody formation occurs after a viral infection; in others, an autoimmune disorder develops (3% to 16% of patients develop systemic lupus erythematosus [SLE]).[1] The antibody-coated platelets are phagocytized in the spleen, leading to a decrease in platelet survival time and thrombocytopenia.[1]

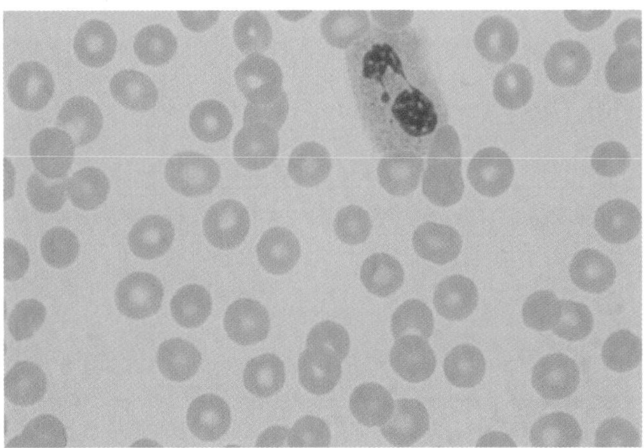

FIGURE 21–9 Thrombocytopenia. Peripheral blood smear. (From Anderson, with permission.)

Diagnosis

ITP is a diagnosis of exclusion and cannot be made in the emergency department. The patient must have evidence of thrombocytopenia or increased platelet destruction, megakaryocytes in the bone marrow, antiplatelet antibodies, no splenomegaly, and a response to typical therapy (intravenous immunoglobulin, splenectomy, or corticosteroids); in addition, other autoimmune disorders must be excluded, including SLE, human immunodeficiency virus [HIV] infection, lymphoma, thyroiditis, disseminated intravascular coagulation [DIC], and drug-induced thrombocytopenia.

Clinical Complications

Complications are related to the thrombocytopenia and include intracranial or gastrointestinal bleeding. Fifty percent of children born to mothers with ITP develop thrombocytopenia, and 1% die of intracranial bleeding.[1]

Management

In patients with thrombocytopenia or petechiae, other diseases, including meningococcemia, sepsis, and DIC, should be ruled out. ITP is a diagnosis of exclusion and requires an extensive inpatient workup. Treatment may include corticosteroids and splenectomy to reduce splenic sequestration. ITP that is refractory to these therapies may be treated with azathioprine, cyclophosphamide, danazol, and vincristine. Patients with severe thrombocytopenia (less than 10,000 platelets/μL) should receive intravenous corticosteroids, intravenous gamma globulin, platelet transfusions, and hematology consultation.[1]

REFERENCES

1. Karpatkin S. Autoimmune (idiopathic) thrombocytopenic purpura. *Lancet* 1997;349:1531–1536.

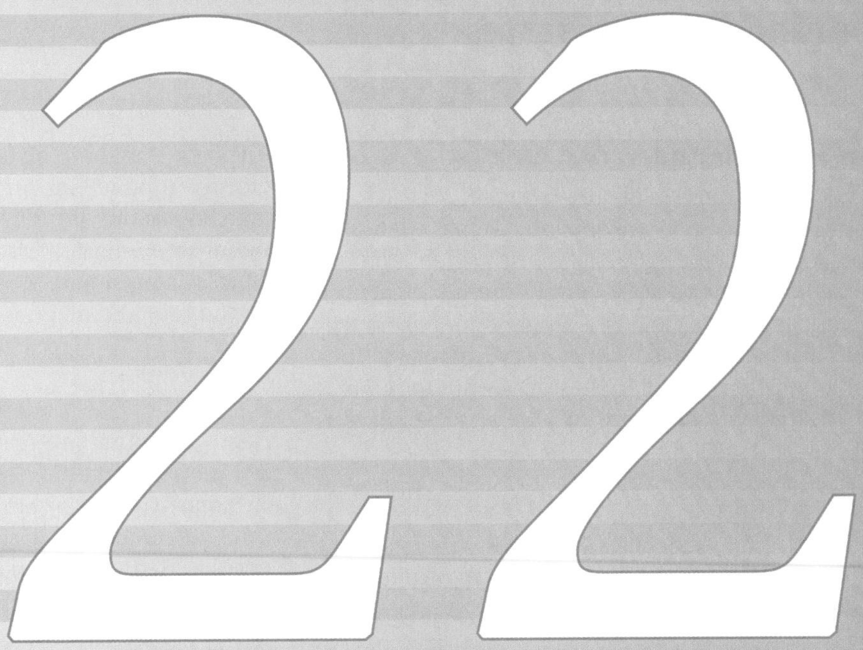

22 Endocrine

Diabetes Mellitus Types 1 and 2

Matthew Goldman

Clinical Presentation

The classic symptoms of diabetes mellitus (DM) are polyuria, polydipsia, and weight loss despite polyphagia.[1] Most cases of type 1 DM manifest acutely and are diagnosed shortly after disease onset. These patients are often metabolically unstable and progress to diabetic ketoacidosis if left untreated.[1] Type 2 DM manifests in a much more insidious manner.[1] It is important to remember that the first presentation for DM may be ketoacidosis.

Pathophysiology

In type 1 DM, pancreatic beta-islet cells are destroyed (probably via autoimmune mechanisms), resulting in rapid loss of insulin secretion. The origin of type 2 DM involves impaired insulin secretion, increased hepatic glucose production, and decreased muscle glucose uptake.[1] Screening for type 2 DM is recommended, because the onset of disease often precedes clinical diagnosis by 10 to 12 years, and 50% of patients have complications by the time the diagnosis is established.[1]

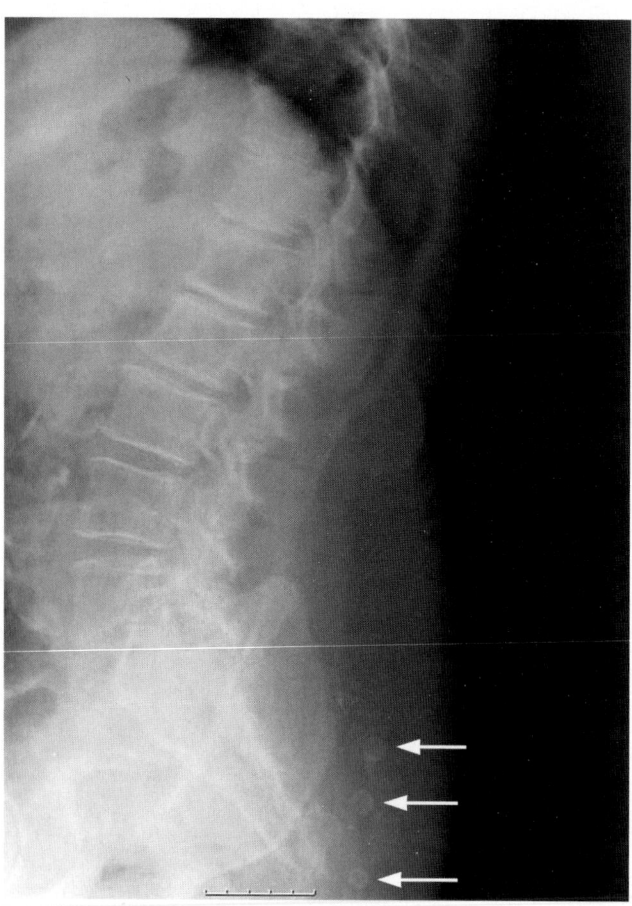

FIGURE 22–1 Injection granulomas. (Courtesy of Mark Silverberg, MD.)

Diagnosis

Diagnosis of DM is made by the finding of a random glucose concentration greater than or equal to 200 mg/dL, a fasting plasma glucose value greater than or equal to 126 mg/dL, or a 2-hour glucose value on 75-g oral glucose tolerance testing greater than or equal to 200 mg/dL.[1] This test should be repeated on a separate day for firm confirmation.[1]

Clinical Complications

Complications can be macrovascular in nature (e.g., cardiovascular plaque formation), or they may entail microvascular diseases (e.g., diabetic retinopathy, neuropathy, nephropathy).[1] Tight glycemic control is effective in controlling microvascular disease progression, but the evidence is not clear regarding macrovascular complications.[1] Diabetic retinopathy is a leading cause of blindness, diabetic nephropathy is a common cause of end-stage renal failure, and diabetic neuropathy is a chronic debilitating complication that can be quite painful.[1]

Management

Type 1 DM is treated with exogenous insulin, using a variety of preparations and injection schedules.[1] The treatment of type 2 DM ranges from diet and exercise modification to the use of an assortment of oral medications.[1] Combination regimens of oral hypoglycemic agents are recommended for patients with hard-to-control DM.[1] Type 2 diabetics may require exogenous insulin if oral medications fail to maintain euglycemia.[1]

REFERENCES

1. Weiland D, White R. Diabetes mellitus. *Clin Fam Pract* 2002;4:703.

Hyperosmolar Nonketotic Coma

Mamie Caton

Clinical Presentation

Hyperosmolar nonketotic coma manifests with severe dehydration, polydipsia, polyuria, altered mental status, tachycardia, hypotension, and weight loss.[1] Complaints mimicking neurologic diseases, including stroke, seizure, and, in very severe cases, coma, have been reported[1] (see Table 22–2).

Pathophysiology

Hyperosmolar nonketotic coma, also known as hyperglycemic hyperosmolar syndrome (HHS), is a diabetic emergency condition in which hyperglycemia and hyperosmolality result in profound dehydration.[1–3] Severe hyperglycemia leading to profound osmotic diuresis is usual.[1] Glucose-induced diuresis leads to hypovolemia and a stress-response release of the insulin counterregulatory hormones, such as growth hormone, epinephrine, and, above all, glucagon.[1] The severe hypovolemia causes a decreased glomerular filtration rate (GFR) and the inability to excrete glucose, worsening the hyperglycemia.[2] Because these patients are usually type 2 diabetics, they do make a small amount of insulin, which is enough to prevent lipolysis and diabetic ketoacidosis.[2]

Diagnosis

Diagnosis is based on the measurement of serum osmolality and the glucose level. Glucose readings are usually greater than 600 mg/dL, and the serum osmolality is greater than 320 mOsm/dL. The pH should be greater than 7.3.[1]

TABLE 22–2 Clinical Characteristics Associated with Hyperosmolar Nonketotic Coma

- Elderly
- A non-insulin-dependent patient
- Profound dehydration
- Extreme hyperglycemia (often 900 mg/dL)
- Hyperosmolality
- Absence of ketoacidosis
- Mental status changes (clouded sensorium to coma)
- Seizures

Courtesy of Mark Silverberg, MD.

Clinical Complications

The mortality associated with HHS has been divided into early (before 72 hours) and late (after 72 hours) types. Early causes of mortality include shock, sepsis, and death from the underlying cause. Late mortality is most frequently caused by a large-vessel thromboembolic event such as an infarct (cerebral or myocardial), pulmonary embolism, mesenteric vessel thrombosis, or disseminated intravascular coagulopathy.[1–3]

Management

The highest treatment priority is restoring circulatory volume. The mean total body water deficit seen in patients with HHS is approximately 9 L.[2] Although normal saline is relatively hypotonic in the HHS patient, some clinicians recommend administration of 50% normal saline until the osmolality is less than 320 Osm/dL.[1] Restoration of volume causes glucose levels to drop even in the absence of insulin, because of increased GFR. Therefore, HHS patients tend to respond quickly to insulin while fluid restoration is occurring. Potassium is the most common serious electrolyte imbalance requiring replacement. Because of the high risk of thromboembolism, prophylaxis with low-dose heparin has been recommended.[1]

REFERENCES

1. Magee MF, Bhatt BA. Management of decompensated diabetes: diabetic ketoacidosis and hyperglycemic hyperosmolar syndrome. *Crit Care Clin* 2001;17:75–106.
2. Matz R. Management of hyperosmolar hyperglycemic syndrome. *Am Fam Physician* 1999;60:1468–1476.
3. Pettigrew DC. Index of suspicion, case 2. Diagnosis: hyperglycemic nonketotic hypertonicity. *Pediatr Rev* 2001;22:169–173.

22-3

Diabetic Ketoacidosis

Mamie Caton

Clinical Presentation

Early symptoms of diabetic ketoacidosis (DKA) include those of hyperglycemia, such as polyuria, polydipsia, and fatigue.[1] Patients may develop more severe signs or symptoms, such as vomiting, tachycardia, tachypnea, Kussmaul's respirations, and hypotension, as acidosis, ketosis, and dehydration develop. The breath may have the distinct "fruity odor" of acetone. Laboratory evaluation reveals an anion gap acidosis, as well as various electrolyte abnormalities.[1,2]

Pathophysiology

DKA may be triggered by stressors such as sepsis, pancreatitis, myocardial infarction, or surgery, or it may develop in the setting of new-onset diabetes mellitus. In 2% to 10% of cases, no inciting cause can be elicited[2] (see Table 22-3A). Lack of insulin effect, due to either the absence of insulin or the loss of insulin receptor response, leads to decreased peripheral glucose utilization, resulting in serum hyperglycemia and cellular hypoglycemia. Serum hyperglycemia is further exacerbated by increases in hepatic glucogenesis and glycogenolysis. Fatty acid oxidation in the adipocytes leads to ketone production and acidosis. Hyperglycemia may lead to an osmotic diuresis and dehydration as the active reabsorption of glucose in the kidney becomes saturated.[1,2]

TABLE 22-3A The "Four I's" That Cause Diabetic Ketoacidosis

1. Ischemia (acute myocardial infarction)
2. Insulinopenia (new-onset/noncompliant)
3. Infection
4. Iatrogenic (corticosteroids)

Courtesy of Mark Silverberg, MD.

TABLE 22-3B Treatment Modalities for Diabetic Ketoacidosis

Treat underlying stressor appropriately
Correct hypoxia
Administer insulin
Rehydrate
Address electrolyte abnormalities (e.g., potassium, phosphate)

Courtesy of Mark Silverberg, MD.

Diagnosis

Diagnosis is based on serum acidosis and ketosis in the presence of elevated glucose and low bicarbonate levels. The glucose concentration is usually greater than 250 to 300 mg/dL, and the pH should be less than 7.35.[2]

Clinical Complications

Complications of DKA include thromboembolism, gastroparesis, rhabdomyolysis, seizures, coma, and death.[2] Complications of treatment may include fluid overresuscitation (cerebral edema, pulmonary edema, and acute lung injury), overcorrection of hyperglycemia (hypoglycemia), and electrolyte abnormalities (hypokalemia and hypophosphatemia).[1,2]

Management

The goals of treatment are to eliminate the cause, the ketosis, and the acidosis, and to restore circulatory volume along with electrolyte imbalances (see Table 22-3B). Glucose levels should be checked hourly and the rate of insulin adjusted accordingly. Electrolytes should be monitored at least every 2 hours during insulin infusion. If ketosis persists despite normoglycemia, the insulin drip should be continued with supplemental glucose administration to avoid hypoglycemia.[1,2]

REFERENCES

1. Rosenbauer J, Icks A, Giani G. Clinical characteristics and predictors of severe ketoacidosis at onset of type 1 DM in children in the North Rhine Westphalian region. *J Pediatr Endocrinol Metab* 2002; 15:1137–1145.
2. Magee MF, Bhatt BA. Management of decompensated diabetes. *Crit Care Clin* 2001;17:75–106.

Myxedema Coma

Jay Itzkowitz

Clinical Presentation

A history of hypothyroidism should be sought in any comatose patient with a history of hypothermia and respiratory failure. However, evidence of hypothyroidism may be minimal or absent. Most patients present with hypothermia.[1] Respiratory failure is common and is characterized by hypoxia, hypoventilation, and hypercarbia.[2] Hypotension and bradycardia are also common presentations. The patient can have a distended abdomen secondary to an ileus or ascites. As the name suggests, patients have cold, nonpitting edema of the hands and feet. Patients also present with some alteration of their mental status.

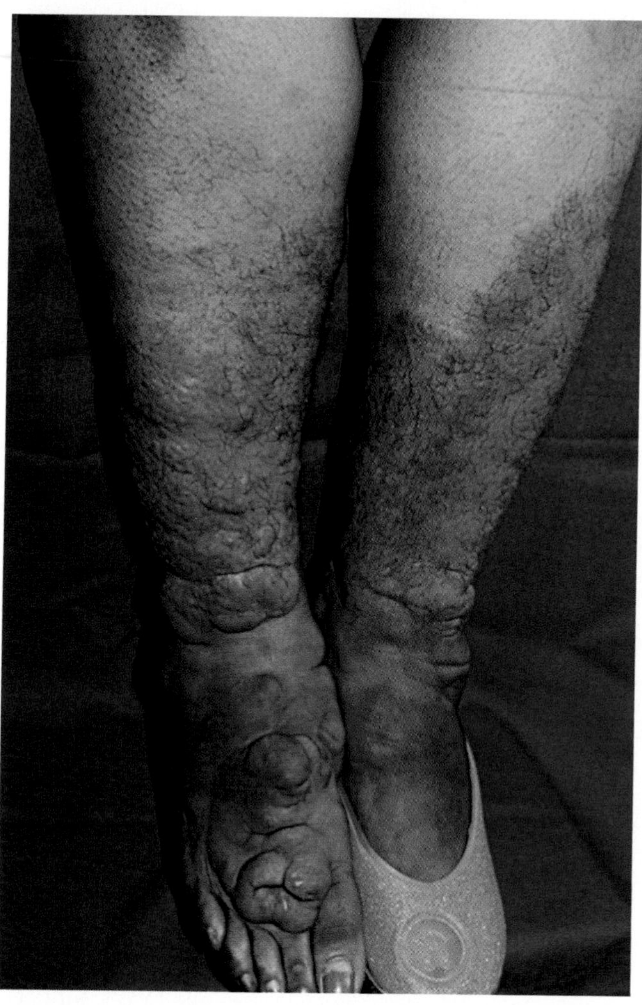

FIGURE 22–4 Pretibial myxedema lesion. Note the red-brown plaques on her shins and the dorsum of her right foot. (From Goodheart, with permission.)

Pathophysiology

The single most important factor in the evolution of hypothyroidism to myxedema coma is physiologic stress.[3] Congestive heart failure and pulmonary infections are the most common causes. Drugs (phenothiazines, narcotics, β-adrenergic blockers, lithium, and iodide), trauma, exposure to cold, infection, and hemorrhage may also be precipitants. Myxedema coma is most prevalent in elderly women and usually occurs during the winter months.[3]

Diagnosis

Although thyroid function tests are the only way to diagnose a thyroid problem with certainty and should be ordered, the results are not always available in a timely fashion. The diagnosis of myxedema coma should be entertained if an elderly patient presents with altered sensorium, hypothermia, and an array of physical and metabolic abnormalities.[1–3]

Clinical Complications

Without treatment, the major life-threatening complications of myxedema are hypotension, respiratory insufficiency, and coma.

Management

Supportive measures are essential. For the patient who presents with hypothermia, slow rewarming should be undertaken. The use of warming blankets should be avoided, because the peripheral dilatation may worsen the hypotension.[3] Electrolyte abnormalities (e.g., hyponatremia) should also be corrected. Patients who are hypoglycemic should be treated with 50% dextrose (D_{50}) in water. If an infection source is found, it should be treated with appropriate antibiotics. Treatment with thyroid hormone is the most critical aspect of therapy. Because gastrointestinal absorption is compromised in myxedema, intravenous therapy is indicated. The drug of choice is intravenous thyroxine.[3]

REFERENCES

1. Olsen CG. Myxedema coma in the elderly. *J Am Board Fam Pract* 1995;8:376–383.
2. Nicoloff JT, LoPresti JS. Myxedema coma: a form of decompensated hypothyroidism. *Endocrinol Metab Clin North Am* 1993;22:279–290.
3. Wall CR. Myxedema coma: diagnosis and treatment. *Am Fam Physician* 2000;62:2485–2490.

Hypothothyroidism

Matthew Goldman

Clinical Presentation

Hypothyroidism usually has an insidious onset, with patients commonly complaining of fatigue, cold intolerance, generalized weakness, constipation, and depression.[1]

Pathophysiology

The most common cause of hypothyroidism worldwide is iodine deficiency, but in the United States it is Hashimoto's (chronic autoimmune) thyroiditis.[1] Primary hypothyroidism results from failure of the thyroid gland to produce the thyroid hormones triiodothyronine (T_3) and thyroxine (T_4).[1] Secondary hypothyroidism results from a decrease in circulating thyroid-stimulating hormone (TSH), a hormone produced in the anterior pituitary gland that stimulates the thyroid gland to become active.[1] Tertiary hypothyroidism results from decreased thyrotropin-releasing hormone (TRH) levels secondary to hypothalamic insufficiency.[1]

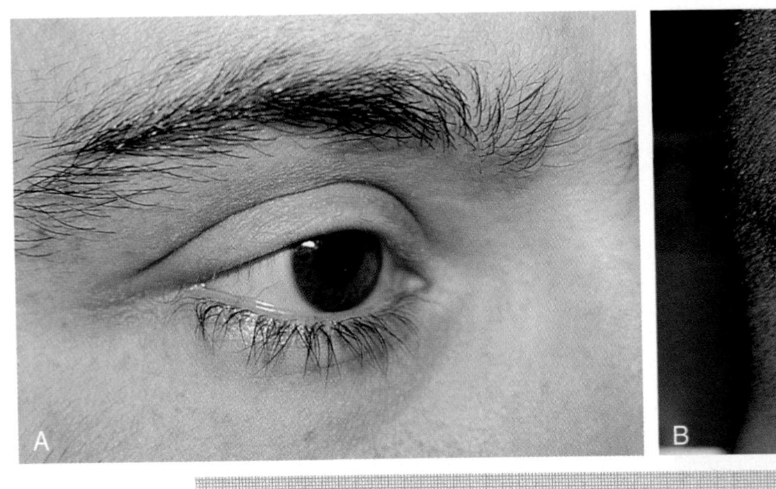

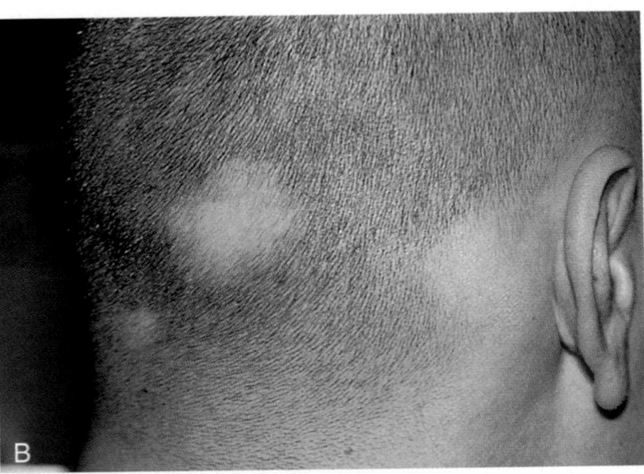

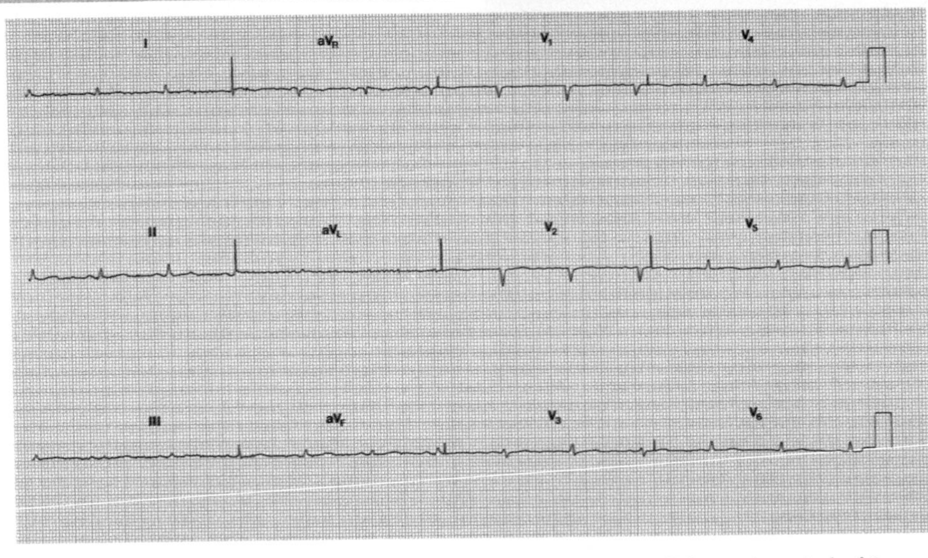

FIGURE 22-5 **A:** The patient complained of a loss of lashes from the right upper lid over a period of 2 years. There was a loss of approximately 50% of lashes from the lid, with poliosis of the remaining lashes. (From Tasman and Jaeger, with permission.) **B:** The patient's scalp shows areas of patchy alopecia and whitening of the remaining hair. (From Tasman and Jaeger, with permission.) **C:** Electrocardiographic study of a 50-year-old woman who presented with complaints of fatigue and pedal edema. (From Hurst, with permission.)

Hypothyroidism

Matthew Goldman

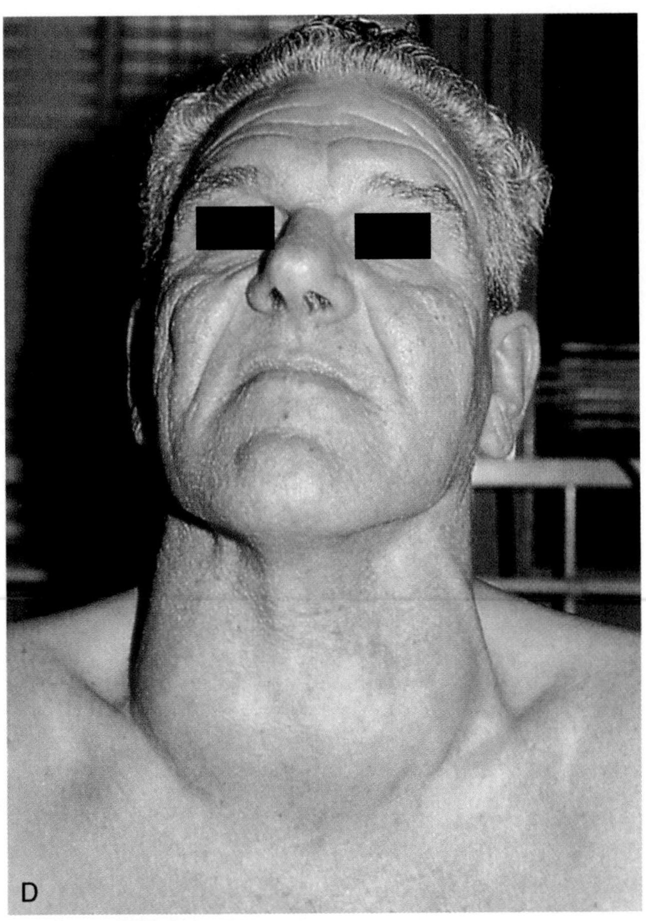

FIGURE 22–5, cont'd. D: Goiter (multinodular thyroid). This man has a massive multinodular goiter, which distorts his entire neck. He was euthyroid. (From Benjamin, with permission.)

Diagnosis

Hypothyroidism may be suspected clinically, although laboratory studies are the primary modalities used to make the diagnosis.[1] Once decreased thyroid hormone levels are confirmed, the TSH level is the most important factor to determine whether the hypothyroidism is primary or secondary. Radiographic imaging studies and tissue sampling may provide additional confirmatory information, although they generally are not needed once laboratory confirmation has been attained.[1]

Clinical Complications

Myxedema coma is the most common complication of hypothyroidism; it usually occurs during the winter months, when thermoregulatory stressors are at maximum levels.[1] Common precipitants include hypothermia, trauma, burns, surgery, strokes, sepsis, and medications. Cardinal findings are hypothermia and altered mental status, in addition to bradycardia, hypotension, hypoventilation, and hyponatremia.[1] If present, myxedema is characterized by generalized skin and soft-tissue swelling, often with associated periorbital edema, ptosis, and macroglossia.[1]

Management

Once laboratory testing has confirmed hypothyroidism, levothyroxine should be administered.[1] If the hypothyroidism is secondary to pituitary failure, glucocorticoids should also be given.[1] Serum T_4 levels usually return to normal within 1 to 2 weeks, and TSH levels normalize within an additional 4 to 6 weeks.[1]

REFERENCES

1. Wilson G. Thyroid disorders. *Clin Fam Pract* 2002;4:667.

Hyperthyroidism

Jay Itzkowitz

Clinical Presentation

Symptoms of hyperthyroidism include palpitations, nervousness, weight loss despite increased appetite, excessive sweating, hyperdefecation, and heat intolerance.[1] Women may also report a decrease in or cessation of menses.[2] Common presenting findings include atrial fibrillation, lid lag with a stare, fine tremor, muscle weakness, and unexplained tachycardia.[1]

Pathophysiology

The hypermetabolic state that is caused by excess circulation of the thyroid hormones triiodothyronine (T_3) and thyroxine (T_4).[1] Hyperthyroidism involves a disruption of the homeostatic mechanisms that normally control hormone secretion.[1] These include primary (thyroid), secondary (pituitary), and tertiary (hypothalamus) disorders. The most common cause of hyperthyroidism is Graves' disease (toxic diffuse goiter), followed by toxic multinodular goiter.[1]

Diagnosis

Patients presenting with palpable goiter, exophthalmos, and pretibial myxedema are assumed to have Graves' disease. Mild cases of hyperthyroidism are difficult to diagnose because the symptoms are vague. The most reliable screening measure of thyroid function is the thyroid stimulating hormone (TSH) concentration.[3] In patients with primary hyperthyroidism, the TSH levels are suppressed and the T_3 and T_4 levels are elevated. Patients with secondary hyperthyroidism have elevated TSH, T_3, and T_4 levels.[3]

Clinical Complications

Cardiac manifestations including high-output congestive heart failure and atrial arrhythmias may occur. Exposure keratitis can result from constant staring without blinking and lid lag. If undiagnosed or left untreated, hyperthyroidism may evolve into thyroid storm, a life-threatening condition.

Management

Mild hyperthyroidism does not require immediate treatment in the emergency department. Patients may be referred to an outpatient endocrinologist for further evaluation. Mild to moderate symptoms can be alleviated with β-adrenergic blockers. Antithyroid medication such as propylthiouracil or methimazole may also be started. Definitive therapy includes a partial or total thyroidectomy, accomplished either surgically or medically with radioactive iodine.

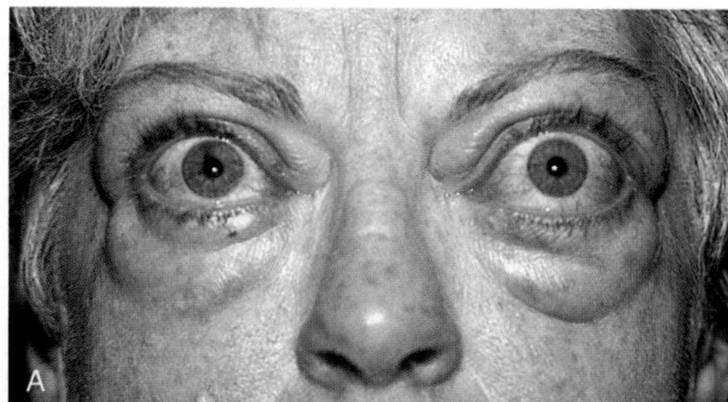

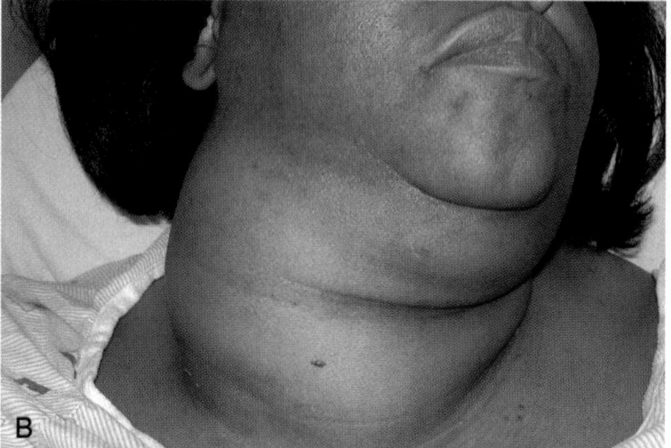

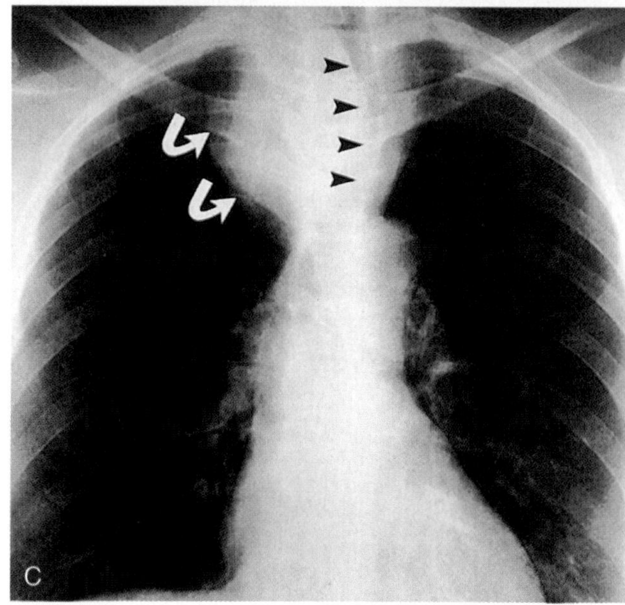

FIGURE 22–6 **A:** Thyroid-related ophthalmopathy with proptosis, lid retraction, and limited motility. (From Tasman and Jaeger, with permission.) **B:** Large goiter, mostly right-sided. (Courtesy of Mark Silverberg, MD.) **C:** Substernal goiter. A huge soft-tissue mass projects from either side of the mediastinum *(curved arrows)*. The trachea is both deviated and narrowed *(arrowheads)*. (From Ovassapian, with permission.)

REFERENCES

1. Wilson G. Thyroid disorders. *Clin Fam Pract* 2002;4:667.
2. Bryer-Ash M. Evaluation of the patient with a suspected thyroid disorder. *Obstet Gynecol Clin North Am* 2001;28:421–438.
3. de los Santos ET, Starich GH, Mazzaferri EL. Sensitivity, specificity, and cost-effectiveness of the sensitive thyrotropin in the diagnosis of thyroid disease in ambulatory patients. *Arch Intern Med* 1989;149:526–532.

Thyroid Storm

Jay Itzkowitz

Clinical Presentation

Thyroid storm (TS) manifests as severe hyperthyroidism with concomitant central nervous system hyperactivity, including anxiety, restlessness, manic behavior, and emotional lability (see Table 22–7). Patients with TS may mistakenly be thought to have a psychiatric disorder.[1,2]

Pathophysiology

TS occurs in patients with untreated or inadequately treated preexisting hyperthyroidism. A physiologic stressor such as trauma, a surgical emergency, or sepsis brings about a severe exacerbation of the disease due to stress-induced hormonal stimulation. It is more common in patients with Graves' disease.[1]

Diagnosis

The diagnosis of TS must be suspected based on clinical clues. Treatment should not be withheld while waiting for laboratory values to return. Patients may manifest all the other signs and symptoms of hyperthyroidism (e.g., tachycardia, hyperpyrexia, tremors, restlessness, vomiting, diarrhea), but they must also have altered mental status to be classified as having TS.[1,2]

TABLE 22–7 Clinical Characteristics Associated with Thyroid Storm

Usually precipitated by stressor (sepsis, surgery, acute myocardial infarction)
Mental status changes (agitation, delirium, coma)
Hyperpyrexia
Tachycardia
Diarrhea
Hyperreflexia

Courtesy of Mark Silverberg, MD.

Clinical Complications

Because of their impaired cortical function, these patients are at risk for trauma, hyperthermia, or rhabdomyolysis. They can go on to develop high-output cardiac failure, vascular collapse, and death. If left untreated, TS has a mortality rate approaching 100%.[1]

Management

Supportive therapy, including supplemental oxygen, intravenous fluids, and cooling, are essential. Peripheral effects can be minimized with a β-adrenergic blocker such as propanolol or esmolol. Antithyroid medications such as propylthiouracil or methimazole halt the production of additional triiodothyronine (T_3) and thyroxine (T_4). Propylthiouracil has the added advantage of preventing peripheral conversion of T_4 to the more potent T_3. This can also be accomplished with dexamethasone. Iodide should be given to block hormone release, but it must be given well after the antithyroid medications. Patients with TS must be admitted to an intensive care unit.[1,2]

REFERENCES

1. Wilson G. Thyroid disorders. *Clin Fam Pract* 2002;4:667.
2. Ringel MD. Management of hypothyroidism and hyperthyroidism in the intensive care unit. *Crit Care Clin* 2001;17:59–74.

Hypocalcemia

Andrew Liteplo

Clinical Presentation

Symptoms of hypocalcemia are usually neuromuscular in origin, ranging from spasms and paresthesias, to seizures, to tetany. Chvostek's or Trousseau's signs may be present. Hypotension and bradycardia may result from changes in cardiovascular smooth muscle tone.[1] Electrocardiographic findings include a prolonged QT interval that may progress to various degrees of heart block.[1]

Pathophysiology

Calcium exists in both ionized and protein-bound forms in the blood, but only the ionized form is biochemically active. Symptoms develop when the free calcium level is so low that neurons and muscles become hyperexcitable. Hypoparathyroidism is a common cause of hypocalcemia; it may occur after thyroidectomy or radiation therapy, be congenital, or be caused by tissue insensitivity to parathyroid hormone (PTH). Poor gastrointestinal absorption due to intestinal maladies or vitamin D deficiency may also be implicated, as may renal losses from kidney failure. An adequate magnesium supply is necessary for proper PTH function, so a deficiency in magnesium can also cause low calcium levels.[1]

Diagnosis

The diagnosis of hypocalcemia may be suspected from physical examination or electrocardiographic findings but must be confirmed by laboratory analysis. Because symptoms of hypocalcemia are related only to the amount of free calcium dissolved in the blood, it is important to measure ionized calcium directly; alternatively, the albumin level may be measured simultaneously, so that the ionized fraction can be calculated. Measurement of the PTH concentration may also be useful.[1,2]

Clinical Complications

Arrhythmias may develop in acute hypocalcemia. Chronic hypocalcemia may lead to coarse hair, brittle nails, poor dentition, cataracts, or skin changes.[1]

Management

Treatment of acute symptomatic hypocalcemia involves intravenous calcium replacement, identification and correction of concomitant magnesium deficiency, and calcitriol (active vitamin D) therapy. The overall clinical picture should dictate disposition, not simply the calcium level.[1,2]

REFERENCES

1. Guise TA, Mundy GR. Clinical review 69: evaluation of hypocalcemia in children and adults. *J Clin Endocrinol Metab* 1995;80: 1473–1478.
2. Kapoor M, Chan GZ: Fluid and electrolyte abnormalities. *Crit Care Clin* 2001;17:503–529.

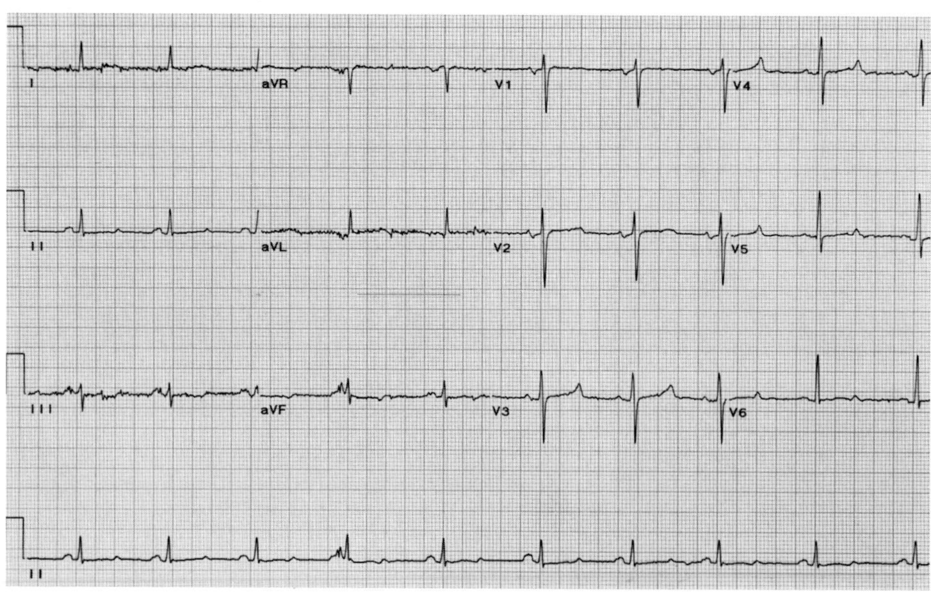

FIGURE 22–8 Electrocardiogram consistent with hypocalcemia in a 53-year-old woman who had recently undergone renal transplantation. (From Fowler, with permission.)

Hypercalcemia

Christopher I. Doty

Clinical Presentation

Hypercalcemia may manifest with nephrolithiasis, bony pain, fatigue, abdominal pain, and central nervous system disturbances.[1] This has been described as "stones, bones, groans/moans, and psychological overtones." Mild hypercalcemia and malignancy-related hypercalcemia may be asymptomatic.[2]

Pathophysiology

Bone is the major calcium storage reservoir of the body, and it is acted upon by parathyroid hormone (PTH) to increase, and by calcitonin to decrease, serum calcium levels.[1] Ninety percent of hypercalcemia cases are caused by either primary hyperparathyroidism or malignancy-related hypercalcemia. Lung and breast cancers are the most common malignancies associated with hypercalcemia.[3] Both of these tumors have been found to secrete a PTH-like hormone that acts by a mechanism similar to that of PTH[1] (see Table 22–9).

Diagnosis

A high index of suspicion in the setting of kidney stones or bony pains, in addition to a history of malignancy, should prompt the clinician to obtain a serum calcium level. Serum levels greater than 14 mg/dL are diagnostic of severe hypercalcemia, whereas levels greater than 12 mg/dL should be considered important and require treatment.[2]

TABLE 22–9 Possible Causes of Hypercalcemia

Possible Causes of Hypercalcemia
Hyperparathyroidism
Lithium use
Malignancy
Bone destruction
Parathyroid hormone–like hormone secretion
Vitamin D intoxication
Sarcoidosis
Milk-alkali syndrome

Courtesy of Mark Silverberg, MD.

Clinical Complications

Lethargy, coma, bradycardia, and ventricular arrhythmias may be associated with hypercalcemia.[2]

Management

Treatment focuses on correction of dehydration and reduction of serum calcium by increasing renal elimination and decreasing calcium release from bone. Once dehydration is corrected, continued intravascular volume expansion with saline is used to increase renal excretion of calcium. Loop diuretics are also useful to decrease renal reabsorption of calcium. Thiazide diuretics are not useful.[2] Several drugs may decrease osteoclastic calcium release from bone, including calcitonin, bisphosphonates, mithramycin, steroids, and gallium nitrate, all of which effectively decrease mobilization of calcium. Hemodialysis may be useful in severe hypercalcemia, for patients who cannot tolerate volume expansion, or if diuresis cannot be accomplished easily, such as in patients with end-stage renal disease.[3]

REFERENCES

1. Marx SJ. Hyperparathyroid and hypoparathyroid disorders. *N Engl J Med* 2000;343:1863–1875.
2. Edelson GW, Kleerekoper M. Hypercalcemic crisis. *Med Clin North Am* 1995;79:79–92.
3. Bilezikian JP. Management of acute hypercalcemia. *N Engl J Med* 1992;326:1196–1203.

Addison's Disease

Jay Itzkowitz

Clinical Presentation

Patients with Addison's disease (AD) may present with fatigability, weakness, anorexia, nausea, vomiting, weight loss, cutaneous and mucosal pigmentation, hypotension, and, at times, hypoglycemia (see Table 22–10).[1,2]

Pathophysiology

Addison's disease results from the progressive destruction of the cortex of the adrenal glands. More than 90% of the cortices must be eliminated before symptoms of adrenal insufficiency manifest. The cortex of the adrenal gland is divided into three different layers or zones—the zona glomerulosa, the zona fasciculata, and the zona reticularis—each of which is responsible for producing different classes of hormones. These three zones synthesize mineralocorticoids, glucocorticoids, and androgens, respectively. Deficiencies in any of these hormone classes may result in the clinical sequelae of Addison's disease. Destruction of the cortex may arise from chronic granulomatous diseases such as tuberculosis, or it may be infected and destroyed by *Histoplasma* or *Cryptococcus* species. The most common cause of adrenal failure and AD is idiopathic atrophy. Autoimmune mechanisms are suspected but remain unproven.[3]

Diagnosis

Diagnosis in the emergency department can be difficult, because the symptoms of AD are often vague.[1] If the patient is to be admitted and the emergency physician suspects AD, then a corticotropin (ACTH) stimulation test can be initiated. This is done by administering 250 μg of cosyntropin and monitoring the body's response by measuring cortisol and ACTH levels. Thirty to 60 minutes after administration of the cosyntropin, serum levels of cortisol and ACTH should be determined. If the cortisol level is subnormal, then either primary or secondary adrenal insufficiency can be inferred. The ACTH level differentiates between primary or secondary adrenal insufficiency: if it is high, then primary adrenal insufficiency (AD) exists; if it is normal or low, then secondary adrenal insufficiency or pituitary failure is the cause of the adrenal insufficiency.

TABLE 22–10 Clinical Characteristics Associated with Addison's Disease

- Hypotension
- Mental status changes (irritability/restlessness to coma)
- Asthenia
- Anorexia/nausea/vomiting
- Hyperpigmentation
- Hyponatremia
- Hyperkalemia

Courtesy of Mark Šilverberg, MD.

Clinical Complications

If AD is left untreated, or if the patient experiences some additional physiologic stressor, AD can develop into adrenal crisis along with circulatory collapse and eventual death.[1]

Management

Patients should receive specific hormone replacement intended to correct for both glucocorticoid and mineralocorticoid deficiencies. Hydrocortisone is the mainstay of treatment, but fludrocortisone should also be administered. All but the most minimally compromised patients require hospitalization.[1–3]

REFERENCES

1. Marik PE, Zaloga GP. Adrenal insufficiency in the critically ill: a new look at an old problem. *Chest* 2002;122:1784–1796.
2. Rosenthal FD, Davies MK, Burden AC. Malignant disease presenting as Addison's disease. *BMJ* 1978;1:1591–1592.
3. Oelkers W. Adrenal insufficiency. *N Engl J Med* 1996;335: 1206–1212.

Adrenal Crisis

Jay Itzkowitz

Clinical Presentation

Patients presenting in adrenal crisis tend to have generalized somatic complaints along with altered mental status and hypotension not responsive to repeated fluid boluses.[1,2] Hyponatremia and hyperkalemia are frequent findings.[3]

Pathophysiology

When the body encounters a physiologic stressor such as sepsis, trauma, or an acute myocardial infarction, it compensates by releasing stress hormones, including glucocorticoids. If the patient's hypothalamic-pituitary-adrenal axis has been suppressed by long-term exogenous steroid use, the body cannot produce such steroids and enters adrenal crisis.[1] A relative glucocorticoid deficit also occurs if chronic oral steroids are abruptly stopped. Additional reasons for acute adrenal failure may be adrenal hemorrhage, such as in the case of septicemia-induced Waterhouse-Friderichsen syndrome, or overanticoagulation.[1–3]

TABLE 22–11 Adrenal Crisis: Treatment Protocol

Measure levels of corticotropin (ACTH) and cortisol
Administer normal saline bolus to correct hypotension
Begin pressors if blood pressure does not respond to IV fluid
Dexamethasone 2 mg IV push
ACTH suppression test
250 μg ACTH IV push
Cortisol level 30 min later
Search for the cause of adrenal crisis
IV hydrocortisone infusion
200 mg over 24 hr, or 50 mg every 6 hr
Switch to oral glucocorticoid replacement after patient is stable

Adapted from Connery L, Coursin D. Assessment and therapy of selected endocrine disorders. *Anesthesiol Clin North Am* 2004;22:93–123.

Diagnosis

If the patient is taking prednisone chronically or has a history of Addison's disease, the diagnosis of adrenal crisis is much easier to determine. Often, however, these aspects of the history are lacking or the patient is unable to provide any history due to altered mental status. Therefore, the diagnosis of adrenal crisis should be suspected in any patient who "looks sick," is hypotensive, and does not respond to fluid resuscitation.[2,3] The corticotropin (ACTH) stimulation test can be initiated if adrenal insufficiency is suspected.

Clinical Complications

The acute, life-threatening, complicating events of adrenal crisis include hypoglycemia and hypotension. If hypotension is not corrected, myocardial and cerebral ischemia may result. Other complications include hyponatremia, hyperkalemia, lactic acidosis, and their associated problems.[3]

Management

Administration of glucocorticoids is the definitive therapy for patients in adrenal crisis (see Table 22–11). Patients with known adrenal insufficiency should receive hydrocortisone. In patients without this history, dexamethasone may be a better choice, because it does not alter the response of the ACTH stimulation test. Remember that, in contrast to hydrocortisone, dexamethasone does not have mineralocorticoid properties, so fludrocortisone should also be given.[1–3]

REFERENCES

1. Marik PE, Zaloga GP. Adrenal insufficiency in the critically ill: a new look at an old problem. *Chest* 2002;122:1784–1796.
2. Oelkers W. Adrenal insufficiency. *N Engl J Med* 1996;335: 1206–1212.
3. Leshin M. Acute adrenal insufficiency: recognition, management and prevention. *Urol Clin North Am* 1982;9:229–235.

Cushing's Syndrome

Laura Spivak

Clinical Presentation

Patients with Cushing's syndrome (CS) may have any of the following characteristics: weight gain, purple striae, acne, hirsutism, hyperglycemia, central obesity, moon facies, plethora, easy bruising, menstrual irregularity, and proximal muscle weakness.[1]

Pathophysiology

CS results from hypercortisolism arising from an endogenous or exogenous source.[1] Endogenous cortisol exposure is classified as either corticotropin (ACTH)-independent or ACTH-dependent.[1] Adrenal adenomas and carcinomas are responsible for most cases of ACTH-independent disease.[1] ACTH stimulation of the adrenal gland can result from pituitary adenomas or nonpituitary tumors.[1] Ectopic ACTH production may be seen in carcinoid tumors of the thymus or bronchus and in small cell lung carcinoma.[1]

Diagnosis

The 24-hour urinary free cortisol value is 100% sensitive and 98% specific for CS.[1] The dexamethasone suppression test, which is equally sensitive but less specific, involves administration of dexamethasone at midnight and measurement of a plasma cortisol level at 6:00 AM.[1] Plasma ACTH levels may be measured by radioimmunoassay.[1] Computed tomography of the abdomen is used to detect adrenal masses.[1] Magnetic resonance imaging, with and without gadolinium contrast, may be used to image pituitary tumors. Both modalities may be used to look for lung carcinomas or carcinoid tumors of the bronchi and thymus.[1]

Clinical Complications

Hypercortisolism may lead to hypertension, obesity, and glucose intolerance.[1] Both cognitive and psychological dysfunction are recognized complications.[2] Potentially reversible cerebral atrophy may also complicate CS.[2]

Management

The definitive treatment of CS requires surgical tumor removal as needed.[1] Agents such as mitotane, trilostane, ketoconazole, and metyrapone, which block steroid production, may be used for medical management.[1]

REFERENCES

1. Harris G. Hypertensive endocrine disorders. *Clin Family Pract* 2002;14:585.
2. Bourdeau I, Bard C, Noel B, et al. Loss of brain volume in endogenous Cushing's syndrome and its reversibility after correction of hypercortisolism. *J Clin Endocrinol Metab* 2002;87:1949–1954.

Cushing's Syndrome

Laura Spivak

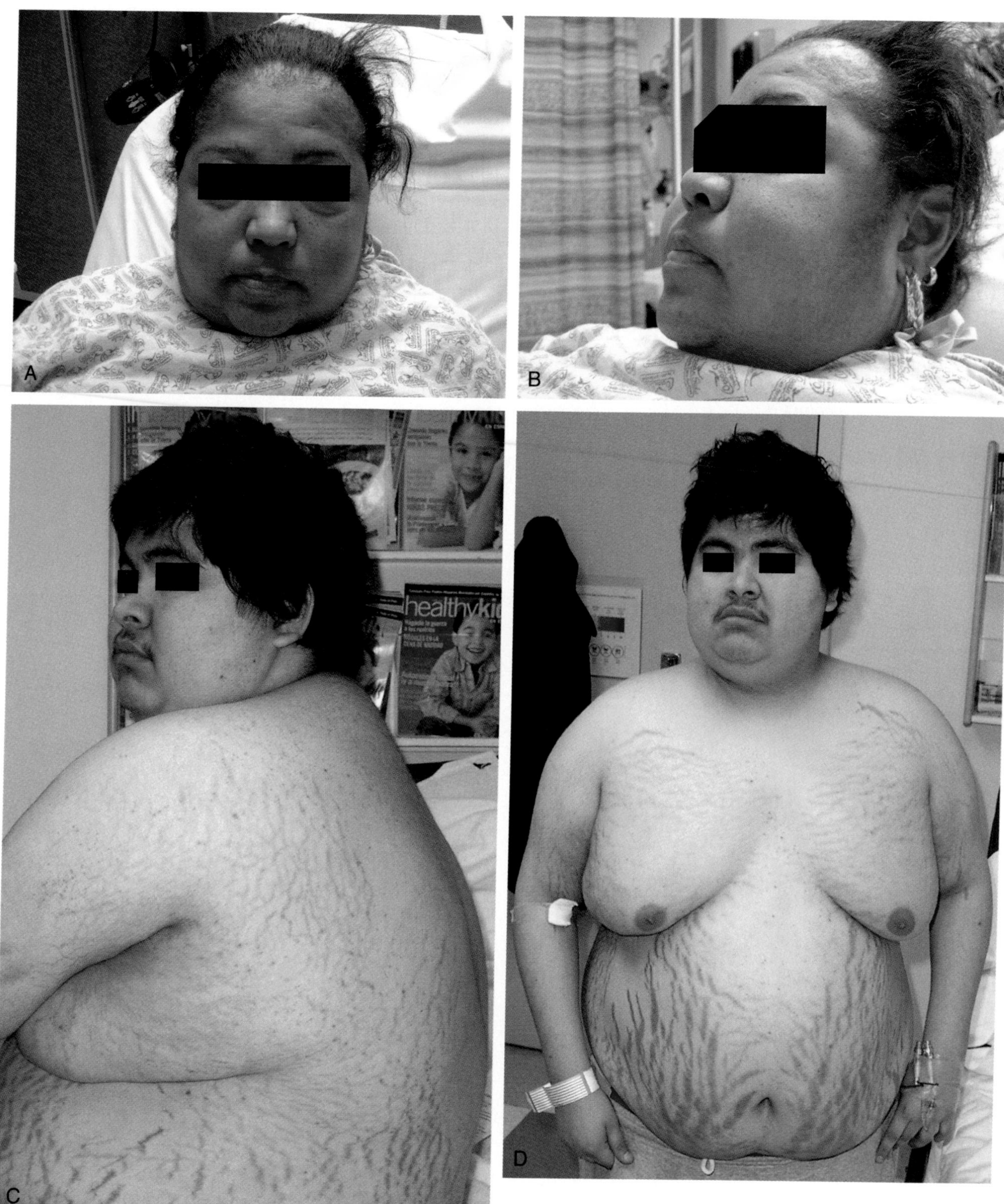

FIGURE 22–12 **A** and **B:** The typical cushingoid "moon face" associated with excessive corticosteroid use or production. (**A** and **B,** Courtesy of Mark Silverberg, MD.) **C** and **D:** The moon face, truncal obesity, buffalo hump, and purple striae seen here are all associated with Cushing's syndrome. (**C** and **D,** Courtesy of Bronson Terry, MD.)

Waterhouse-Friderichsen Syndrome

Matthew Goldman

Clinical Presentation

Children are the age group most commonly afflicted with Waterhouse-Friderichsen syndrome (WFS).[1] Symptoms are usually abrupt in onset and consist initially of nonspecific complaints such as headache, chills, fever, restlessness, apprehension, malaise, myalgias, and arthralgias.[1] Petechiae appear in 50% to 60% of cases.[1] If the disease has progressed, patients may complain of low back pain and symptoms consistent with peritonitis.[1] These patients rapidly become toxic and appear to be in septic shock, with increased cardiac output and decreased systemic vascular resistance. Hypotension in these cases is usually refractory to fluid boluses and pressor therapy.[2,3] Other clinical findings of acute adrenal insufficiency include hyponatremia, hyperkalemia, and hypoglycemia.[2,3]

Pathophysiology

WFS, or purpura fulminans, is acute hemorrhagic necrosis of the adrenal glands resulting in adrenal crisis, usually secondary to some form of septicemia.[1,3] Septicemia, often from *Neisseria meningitis* infection, leads to a coagulopathy and bilateral adrenal hemorrhage with acute adrenal failure.[1,3]

TABLE 22–13 Complications of Waterhouse-Friderichsen Syndrome

Bilateral adrenal hemorrhage/destruction
Coma
Congestive heart failure
Disseminated intravascular coagulation
Extensive intracutaneous hemorrhage
Myocarditis
Renal failure
Respiratory failure
Thrombi formation and arterial embolization
Vasomotor collapse/shock

Adapted from Agrahakar M. Waterhouse-Friderichsen syndrome and bilateral renal cortical necrosis and meningococcal sepsis. *Am J Kidney Dis* 2000;36:396–400.

Diagnosis

The diagnosis should be considered in any patient with fever, hypotension, and petechiae, especially if the hypotension is refractory to fluid boluses and pressor therapy.[2,3] A random cortisol concentration lower than 25 μg/dL further supports the diagnosis of adrenal insufficiency.[2]

Clinical Complications

Complications include adrenal destruction, circulatory collapse, shock, and death[3] (see Table 22–13).

Management

Therapy should be started as soon as the diagnosis is suspected because of the rapid progression and often devastating consequences of the disease.[1] Hypotension should be treated with aggressive hydration, and pressors and glucose should be administered if the patient is hypoglycemic.[1,2] Hydrocortisone, 100 mg intravenously as a bolus followed by an infusion of 100 to 200 mg over 24 hours, should be given.[2,3] Antibiotic therapy should also be started immediately. A third-generation cephalosporin should be used for adults and ampicillin needs to be added for infants.[1] Admission to the intensive care unit is recommended.

REFERENCES

1. Varon J, Chen K, Sternbach GL. Rupert Waterhouse and Carl Friderichsen: adrenal apoplexy. *J Emerg Med* 1998;16:643–647.
2. Marik PE, Zaloga GP. Adrenal insufficiency in the critically ill: a new look at an old problem. *Chest* 2002;122:1784–1796.
3. Ten S, New M, Maclaren N. Clinical review 130: Addison's disease 2001. *J Clin Endocrinol Metab* 2001;86:2909–2922.

Hyponatremia

Sachin J. Shah

Clinical Presentation

Patients with acute hyponatremia may present with nausea, vomiting, confusion, and muscle cramps, as well as seizures and coma in the most severe cases.[1,2]

Pathophysiology

Hyponatremia is the most commonly encountered electrolyte abnormality.[1] Sodium (Na^+) is the most dominant cation in the extracellular compartment. It is the main determinant of plasma osmolality in the body.[3] The most common scenario is hypotonic hyponatremia (see Table 22-14.). Hypotonic hyponatremia can be further characterized as hypovolemic (caused by diuretics, gastrointestinal losses, third-spacing, aldosterone deficiency), euvolemic (syndrome of inappropriate secretion of antidiuretic hormone [SIADH], other causes of increased ADH, psychogenic polydipsia), or hypervolemic (renal failure, congestive heart failure, nephritic syndrome, cirrhosis).[1-4] Patients with severe hyponatremia have mortality rates approaching 20%.[4]

TABLE 22-14 **Causes of Hyponatremia**

- Addison's disease
- Beer potomania
- Cirrhosis
- Congestive heart failure
- Drugs (thiazides, carbamazepine, chlorpropamide, cyclophosphamide, amitriptyline)
- Hyperglycemia
- Hyperhydrosis
- Iatrogenic/IV overhydration
- Hypoalbuminemia
- Hypothyroidism
- Nephrosis
- Pseudohyponatremia (Hyperlipidemia/Hyperproteinemia)
- Psychogenic polydipsia
- Reset osmostat syndrome
- Salt-losing nephropathy
- SIADH (Syndrome of Inappropriate Antidiuretic Hormone Secretion)
- Subarachnoid hemorrhage

Adapted from Fried L. Hyponatremia and hypernatremia. *Med Clin N Am* 1997;81(3):585-609. (Courtesy of Mark Silverberg, MD.)

Diagnosis

Serum levels are the most accurate determination of Na^+ levels.

Clinical Complications

Complications range from mild weakness, nausea, and vomiting to intractable seizures, coma, respiratory failure, and death. Rapid overcorrection can lead to central pontine myelinolysis (CPM), a condition associated with irreversible brain injury.[3]

Management

Treatment ranges from simple restriction of free water in patients with mild hyponatremia and no symptoms to hypertonic (3%) saline in patients exhibiting central nervous system pathology. Care must be taken not to correct too rapidly in order to avoid CPM. If rapid correction is required, hypertonic saline should be given, with frequent determinations of serum Na^+ levels.[3] Diagnosing and addressing the underlying cause is imperative to prevent subsequent episodes of hyponatremia.[3]

REFERENCES

1. Lee CT, Guo HR, Chen JB. Hyponatremia in the emergency department. *Am J Emerg Med* 2000;18:264-268.
2. Milionis HJ, Liamis GL, Elisaf MS. The hyponatremic patient: a systematic approach to laboratory diagnosis. *CMAJ* 2002;166:1056-1062.
3. Fried LF, Palevsky PM. Hyponatremia and hypernatremia. *Med Clin North Am* 1997;81:585-609.
4. Nzerue CM, Baffoe-Bonnie H, You W, et al. Predictors of outcome in hospitalized patients with severe hyponatremia. *J Natl Med Assoc* 2003;95:335-343.

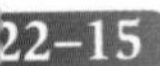

Hypernatremia

Sachin J. Shah

Clinical Presentation

Patients with hypernatremia may be asymptomatic, or they may present with seizures, altered mental status, or coma. Other signs and symptoms include ataxia, irritability, confusion, delirium, weakness, tachycardia, oliguria, or peripheral or pulmonary edema.[1] (See Table 22-15A.)

Pathophysiology

Hypernatremia usually results from dehydration. If the thirst mechanism is defective, whether through natural causes or because the patient cannot get to water even though he or she is thirsty, homeostasis is altered.[1] Patients may have diabetes insipidus from hypothalamic causes (e.g., cerebrovascular accident, infection, trauma) or nephrogenic causes (e.g., congenital causes, lithium).[2] Elderly patients are especially vulnerable because of the combination of impaired thirst receptors, barriers to fluids, and the inability of the kidneys to concentrate adequately.[1]

TABLE 22-15A Clinical Characteristics Associated with Hypernatremia

- Mental status changes
  - Confusion
  - Stupor
  - Coma
- Seizures
- Muscular weakness
- Twitching

Courtesy of Mark Silverberg, MD.

TABLE 22-15B Free Water Deficit Calculation

$$\text{Water Deficit} = \frac{Na_{actual}}{Na_{normal}} \times \frac{2}{3}\text{ Weight}$$

Courtesy of Mark Silverberg, MD.

Diagnosis

Hypernatremia is defined and diagnosed by laboratory values. Sodium (Na^+) levels greater than 145 mEq/L are considered hypernatremic.[3]

Clinical Complications

Complications of hypernatremia result from cellular effects in the brain leading to seizures and coma and from hemorrhage in the brain due to overstretching of the connecting vessels.[1] Iatrogenic hypernatremia may occur in patients who are overzealously treated with normal saline without adequate monitoring. Severe hypernatremia carries a mortality rate as high as 55%.[2]

Management

Treatment is aimed at reducing the serum Na^+ level by replenishing free water. The rate is determined by the patient's symptoms and the acuity of the hypernatremia. If the cause is volume depletion, the free-water deficit should be calculated to guide therapy. (See Table 22-15B.) The free-water deficit (FWD) is calculated from the body weight (wt) in kilograms and the plasma sodium concentration (Na^+): FWD = 0.6 × body weight × $[(Na^+/140) - 1]$. Chronic hypernatremia should be corrected at a rate of 1 to 2 mEq/L/hour until symptoms resolve. Patients in extremis can undergo rapid correction until stabilized. Free water can be given via a nasogastric tube or a percutaneous endoscopic gastrostomy tube. Dextrose 5% in water or half-normal saline may be given intravenously if necessary.[1,2]

REFERENCES

1. Kugler JP, Hustead T. Hyponatremia and hypernatremia in the elderly. *Am Fam Physician* 2000;61:3623–3630.
2. Fried LF, Palevsky PM. Hyponatremia and hypernatremia. *Med Clin North Am* 1997;81:585–609.
3. Mandal AK, Saklayen MG, Hillman NM, et al. Predictive factors for high mortality in hypernatremic patients. *Am J Emerg Med* 1997;15: 130–132.

Hypokalemia

Sachin J. Shah

Clinical Presentation

Patients with hypokalemia may be asymptomatic, or they may complain of muscle weakness, fatigue, or polyuria. Severe hypokalemia may manifest with paralysis.[1-3]

Pathophysiology

Potassium (K^+) is the largest intracellular cation in the body. Ninety-eight percent is stored intracellularly. K^+ is primarily excreted in the urine, both freely and with some regulation.[1] The kidney responds to hormones, primarily aldosterone, to also regulate K^+.[3] The vast intracellular stores can replace minor extracellular deficiencies. The earliest affected cells are usually skeletal muscle cells, followed by cardiac and central nervous system cells. (See Table 22–16.)

TABLE 22–16 Causes of Hypokalemia by Category

Excessive Renal Loss
• Acute leukemia
• Antibiotics (carbenicillin, gentamicin and amphotericin B)
• Bartter's syndrome
• Chronic metabolic alkalosis
• Gitelman's syndrome
• Increased delivery of Na^+ to collecting duct
• Increase fluid flow to distal tubule/diuresis
• Increased mineralocorticoids
• Licorice
• Liddle's syndrome
• Magnesium depletion
• Renal tubular acidosis type I and II
• Ureterosigmoidostomy
• 11b-hydroxysteroid dehydrogenase deficiency
GI Loss
• Diarrhea
• Fistula loss
• Laxative abuse
• Nasogastric tube drainage
• Vomiting
Intracellular Shifts of K^+
• Alkalosis
• Barium ingestion
• Beta-receptor stimulation
• Insulin therapy
• Thyrotoxicosis
• Vitamin B_{12} therapy
Inadequate Intake
• <40 mEQ/d

Adapted from Manal A. Hypokalemia and hyperkalemia. *Med Clin N Am* 1997;81(3):611–39; and Genneri F. Disorders of potassium hemostatis: Hypokalemia and hyperkalemia. *Crit Care Clin* 2002;18(2):273–88. (Courtesy of Mark Silverberg, MD.)

Diagnosis

Serum levels are the most accurate determination of K^+ levels. Once pseudohypokalemia, a condition in which abnormal leukocytes store K^+ and artificially lower serum levels, has been ruled out, planning for treatment can begin.[1] Certain electrocardiographic findings may also suggest hypokalemia. They include flat or inverted T waves, prominent U waves, and ST-segment depression, in addition to dysrhythmias (mostly tachycardia) and atrial and ventricular fibrillation.[2] It is also necessary to measure magnesium levels, to ensure that repletion is not undertaken in the face of hypomagnesemia, which can be futile.

Clinical Complications

Complications range from mild weakness to life-threatening dysrhythmias.

Management

Based on the clinical setting, oral or parenteral replacement of K^+ may be effective. In the severely hypokalemic patient, up to 40 mEq/L may be replaced through a central line with continuous cardiac monitoring.[1,2] Replacement of 20 mEq/hour of KCl raises the serum level by approximately 0.25 mEq/L/hour.[1-3] In patients with mild symptoms and only slightly decreased K^+ levels, oral replacement may be undertaken.

REFERENCES

1. Weiner ID, Wingo CS. Hypokalemia: consequences, causes and correction. *J Am Soc Nephrol* 1997;8:1179–1788.
2. Mandal AK. Hypokalemia and hyperkalemia. *Med Clin North Am* 1997;81:611–639.
3. Beck LH. The aging kidney: defending a delicate balance of fluid and electrolytes. *Geriatrics* 2000;55:26–28, 31–32.

Hyperkalemia

Sachin J. Shah

Clinical Presentation

Patients with hyperkalemia may be asymptomatic, or they may present with ventricular arrhythmias, complete heart block, or asystole. Patients may complain of muscle weakness or paralysis, as well as nausea, vomiting, and diarrhea.[1,2]

Pathophysiology

The normal balance of potassium (K^+) and sodium (Na^+) in the body is responsible for electrical impulses that control voluntary and involuntary functions. Rapid shifts from intracellular to extracellular stores can occur in the face of burns, trauma, or surgical stress. Acid/base imbalances, insulin deficiency, cardiac glycoside intoxication, and renal failure may cause elevations in serum K^+.[2]

Diagnosis

Serum levels are the most accurate determination of K^+ levels. An electrocardiogram (ECG) can be helpful as well. Peaked T waves represent early ECG manifestations of hyperkalemia, but they may not always appear abnormal in patients with hyperkalemia.[1–3] Hemolyzed blood specimens may lead to artificially high K^+ levels.

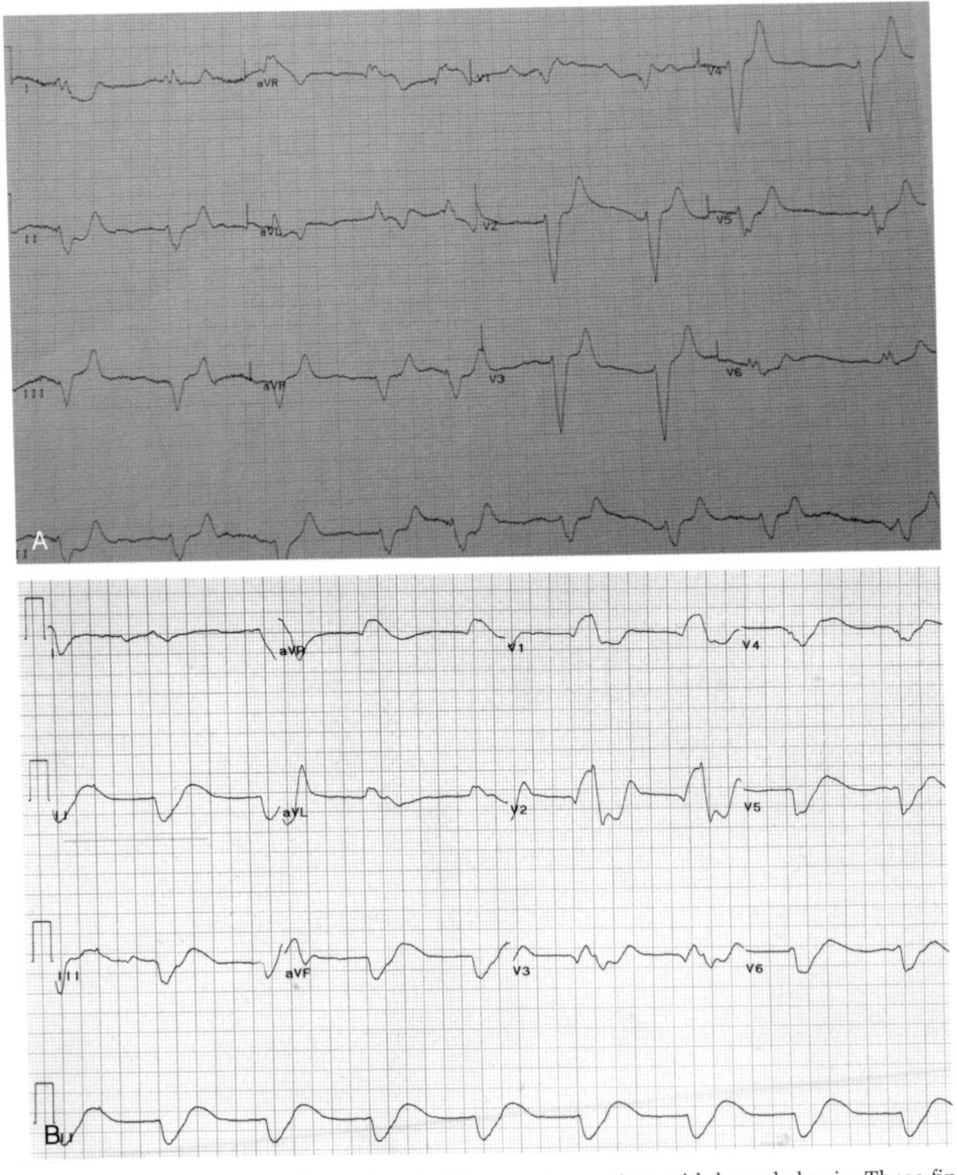

FIGURE 22–17 **A:** QRS widening, bradycardia, and peaked T waves in a patient with hyperkalemia. These findings resolved with treatment with calcium, insulin, and bicarbonate. (Courtesy of Robert Hendrickson, MD.) **B:** Near-sine wave in a patient with a serum potassium concentration of 7.2 mEq/L. Note the absence of P waves and the prolonged QRS interval. (From Fowler, with permission.)

Hyperkalemia

Sachin J. Shah

Clinical Complications

Complications range from nausea and vomiting to paralysis, dysrhythmias, heart block, and asystole.[1]

Management

Treatment depends on the level of K^+ and the underlying cause. If the K^+ concentration is between 5.5 and 6 mEq/L and there are no ECG manifestations, observation and repeat measurement may be warranted. If the patient is exhibiting signs and symptoms of hyperkalemia or there are ECG changes consistent with hyperkalemia, treatment is essential to prevent progression. In non–digoxin-toxic patients, intravenous calcium may be helpful to stabilize the cardiac cell membranes. Insulin is helpful in helping to drive K^+ into the intracellular compartment.[3] Administration of 50% dextrose (D_{50}) in water with the insulin prevents hypoglycemia. Inhaled albuterol and sodium bicarbonate may be effective in temporarily driving K^+ intracellular. Loop diuretics and sodium polystyrene sulfate (Kayexalate) may also be helpful. Hemodialysis should be considered in emergency cases.[1,2]

REFERENCES

1. Dittrich KL, Walls RM. Hyperkalemia: ECG manifestations and clinical considerations. *J Emerg Med* 1986;4: 449–455.
2. Gennari FJ. Disorders of potassium homeostasis: hypokalemia and hyperkalemia. *Crit Care Clin* 2002;18:273–288.
3. Mattu A, Brady WJ, Robinson DA. Electrocardiographic manifestations of hyperkalemia. *Am J Emerg Med* 2000;18:721–729.

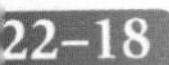

Scurvy

Jason Kitchen

Clinical Presentation

Scurvy is a disease caused by a severe deficiency in vitamin C (ascorbic acid) associated with a lack of an exogenous dietary vitamin C. Patients may present with constitutional symptoms such as fatigue, depression, irritability, and weight loss. The most common sign is follicular hyperkeratosis accompanied by perifollicular petechiae, most prominently involving the lower extremities. Other findings include bleeding, friable gums with purple discoloration, splinter hemorrhages of the nail beds, bulbar conjunctival hemorrhages, and hemarthroses.

Pathophysiology

Ascorbic acid is required for collagen synthesis and helps maintain the integrity of connective tissue and bone. Severe deficiency results in weakening of capillaries, with subsequent hemorrhage and bone defects.[1]

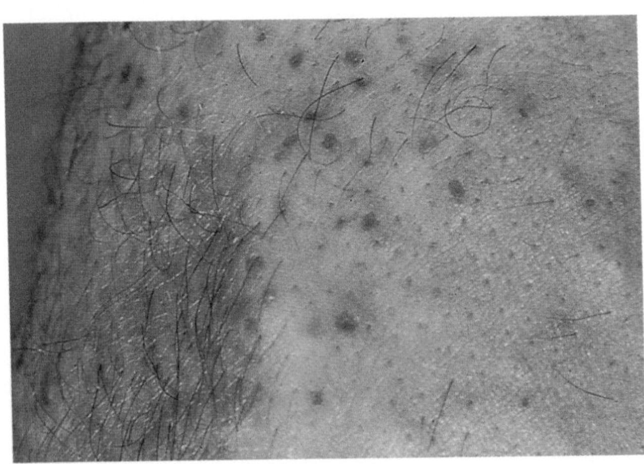

FIGURE 22–18 Scurvy in a patient with poor nutrition. Note perifollicular hemorrhage. (From Yamada, with permission.)

Diagnosis

The diagnosis of scurvy is primarily a clinical one, based on a dietary history of inadequate vitamin C intake in the context of symptoms. The combination of follicular hyperkeratosis and perifollicular hemorrhage occurs early and is pathognomonic. Anemia is a common laboratory finding, and its degree correlates with the severity and duration of the disease. Individuals with vitamin C deficiency often have concomitant folic acid deficiency, because the dietary sources tend to be the same.[1] Measurement of plasma or leukocyte ascorbic acid levels helps confirm the diagnosis but may not be necessary, because disappearance of the clinical abnormalities with vitamin C repletion uniformly establishes the diagnosis.[1]

Clinical Complications

Syncope, hypotension, shock, and sudden death have occurred, but the cause is unclear. These effects may be the result of a defect in the ability of resistance vessels to constrict in response to adrenergic stimuli.[1]

Management

Treatment with ascorbic acid needs to begin immediately, and symptoms should resolve quickly, with improvement seen even after the initial dose and complete resolution within a few weeks. Except for lost teeth, permanent damage from scurvy does not occur. In those with anemia, the hematocrit typically returns to normal within a few weeks.[1]

REFERENCES

1. Hirschmann JV, Raugi GJ. Adult scurvy. *J Am Acad Dermatol* 1999; 41:895–906.

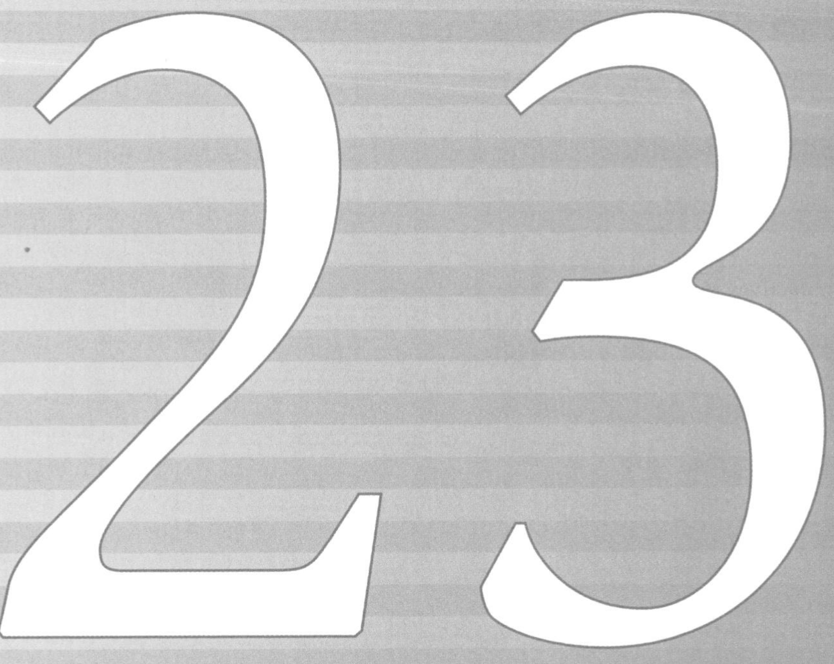

Rheumatologic

Rheumatoid Arthritis

Robert Hendrickson

Clinical Presentation

Rheumatoid arthritis (RA) affects less than 1% of the U.S. population[1] and most commonly occurs in women aged 40 to 70 years.[2] Patients may present to the emergency department (ED) without a diagnosis of RA but with new joint swelling and pain. In early RA, patients typically complain of progressive stiffness and symmetric involvement of multiple joints over a period of weeks to months. Additional symptoms may include fever, malaise, and fatigue.[2] On examination, findings of affected joints may range from minimal signs of inflammation to erythematous, tender, effusion-filled joints with limited range of motion.

Patients with an established diagnosis of RA may present with exacerbations of their disease, extraarticular symptoms, or side effects of their medications. Extraarticular symptoms include rheumatoid nodules, keratoconjunctivitis, iritis, sicca, pleural effusions, myocarditis, pericarditis, pulmonary fibrosis, cardiac valvular nodules, mononeuritis, hepatitis, anemia, leukocytosis, splenomegaly, and vasculitis.[2] Side effects of the various medications used to treat RA can be significant. They include renal failure, gastrointestinal bleeding, and cytopenias with nonsteroidal antiinflammatory drugs (NSAIDs); retinopathy with antimalarial agents; hepatitis with sulfasalazine; myelosuppression and diarrhea with gold; thrombocytopenia with D-penicillamine; infection and edema with corticosteroids; pancytopenia and hepatic fibrosis with methotrexate; pancytopenia with azathioprine; interstitial nephritis with cyclophosphamide; renal insufficiency, anemia, and hypertension with cyclosporine; and hepatitis with leflunomide.[1,3]

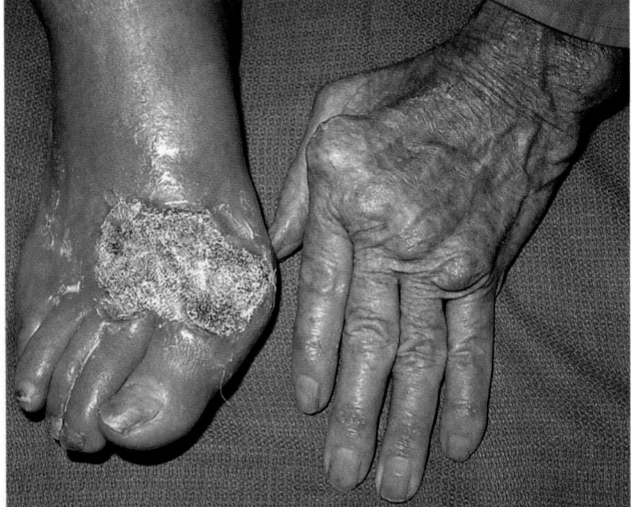

FIGURE 23–1 Felty's syndrome: rheumatoid arthritis, granulocytopenia, splenomegaly, and lower-extremity ulcers. (From Sontheimer, with permission.)

The symptoms of RA may be slowly progressive, or patients may have relatively symptom-free baseline function with intermittent exacerbations of disease.[3] During inflammatory exacerbations, laboratory markers may be present, such as elevations of the leukocyte (white blood cell [WBC]) count, erythrocyte sedimentation rate (ESR), C-reactive protein, and rheumatoid factor.

Pathophysiology

RA is an autoimmune disorder that is characterized by symmetric stiffness, swelling, and pain in peripheral joints.

The cause of RA is unknown; however, there is a genetic predisposition with variable penetrance.[2] Joint inflammation is caused by hyperplasia of synovial cells, followed by leukocyte infiltration, angiogenesis, and fibrotic destruction of cartilage and bone.[2,4]

Diagnosis

The diagnosis usually is based on typical clinical features of stiffness, swelling, and pain in peripheral (distal) joints and is confirmed with laboratory tests and biopsy of synovial tissue. Consultation with a rheumatologist or primary care physician to direct testing and arrange for close follow-up may be prudent.

Clinical Complications

Most patients experience a chronic, progressive, fluctuating course.[1] Joint inflammation and destruction causes significant morbidity. After 10 years with RA, 50% of patients are unable to work.[3] Significant complications may occur secondary to extraarticular involvement or from side effects of the medications used to treat the disease.

Management

Patients with a possible new diagnosis of RA synovitis may be treated with NSAIDs and other pain medications. They should then be thoroughly evaluated by a primary care physician or rheumatologist as soon as possible, because early initiation of additional antiinflammatory medications (e.g., corticosteroids, methotrexate) may decrease joint destruction.[1,2] Patients with an exacerbation of chronic RA may require increases in antiinflammatory medications. Extraarticular symptoms may be managed with antiinflammatory drugs and organ-specific therapy (e.g., thoracentesis for pleural effusion).

REFERENCES

1. American College of Rheumatology Subcommittee on Rheumatoid Arthritis guidelines. Guidelines for the management of rheumatoid arthritis: 2002 update. *Arthritis Rheum* 2002;46:328–346.
2. Lee DM, Weinblatt ME. Rhematoid arthritis. *Lancet* 2001;358: 903–911.
3. Brooks PM. Clinical management of rheumatoid arthritis. *Lancet* 1993;341:286–290.
4. Choy EH, Panayi GS. Cytokine pathways and joint inflammation in rheumatoid arthritis. *N Engl J Med* 2001;344:907–916.

Osteoarthritis

Robert Hendrickson

Clinical Presentation

Osteoarthritis (OA) typically causes joint pain that is exacerbated by activity and stiffness in the morning or after inactivity.[1] The joint may appear normal or have mild signs of inflammation or effusion. Systemic signs are absent. The joint is generally tender to palpation and may have bony enlargement, crepitus on movement, and limited range of motion.[1]

Pathophysiology

OA is local inflammation of the articular cartilage and subchondral bone resulting from mechanical stress.[1]

A variety of factors, including genetic, biochemical, and inflammatory factors, contribute to the destruction of synovial cartilage and inflammation of subchondral bone.[1]

Diagnosis

OA may be diagnosed by noting the typical history and physical examination.

Clinical Complications

The main complications of OA are decreases in mobility and in performance of activities of daily living.

Management

Initial treatment of OA involves nonpharmacologic therapy, including weight loss (if overweight), aerobic exercise, range-of-motion exercises, and quadriceps-strengthening exercises. Initial pharmacologic therapy for all patients with OA is acetaminophen. Nonsteroidal antiinflammatory drugs (NSAIDs) and cyclooxygenase-2 (COX-2) inhibitors may be added to acetaminophen but should not substitute for acetaminophen, because NSAIDs are no more effective and have significant side effects. Tramadol or another opioid may be used for temporary relief of pain. Other adjunctive therapies that may be efficacious are topical anesthetics (e.g., methyl salicylate, capsaicin) and glucosamine/chondroitin. Intraarticular corticosteroids may decrease pain from OA and are an excellent option in patients who are at significant risk for side effects of NSAIDs (gastrointestinal bleeding). However, intraarticular corticosteroids should not be used if there may be an infection in the joint.[1]

REFERENCES

1. Recommendations for the medical management of osteoarthritis of the hip and knee: 2000 update. American College of Rheumatology Subcommittee on Osteoarthritis Guidelines. *Arthritis Rheum* 2000; 43:1905–1915.

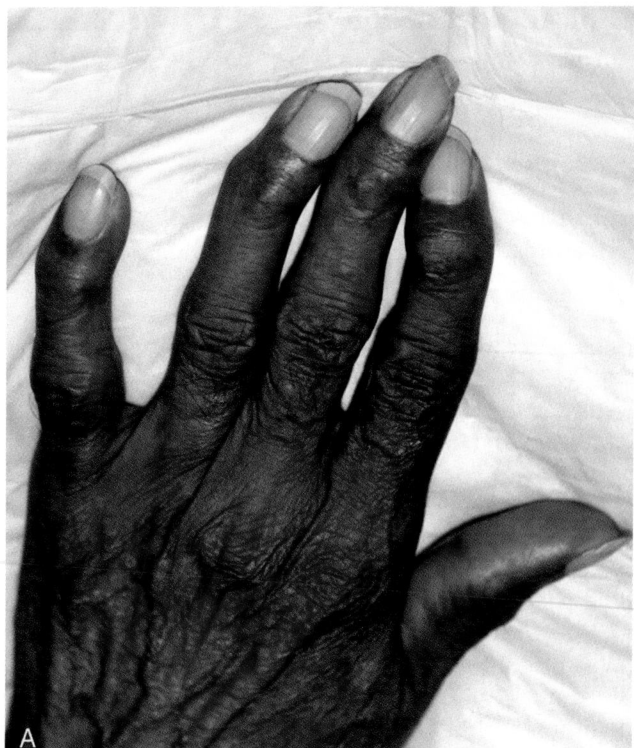

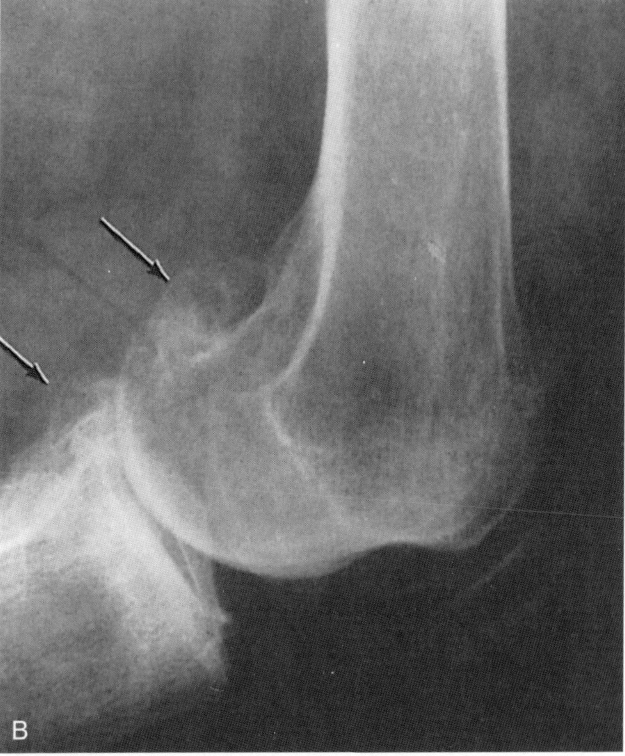

FIGURE 23–2 **A:** Moderate osteoarthritis. Note prominent Heberden's nodes. (© David Effron, MD, 2004. Used with permission.) **B:** Lateral radiograph of an osteoarthritic knee. Large osteophytes can be seen at the posterior aspects of the femur and tibia *(arrows)*. (From Koopman, with permission.)

Septic Arthritis

Robert Hendrickson

Clinical Presentation

Patients with septic arthritis (SA) typically present with an acutely painful, warm, and swollen single large joint (80% to 90% of cases).[1,2] Joints most commonly affected are those with recent manipulation (e.g., arthroscopy, surgery), prosthetic joints, and those with chronic inflammation (e.g., osteoarthritis [OA], rheumatoid arthritis [RA]).[2] SA may occasionally be polyarticular (10% to 20%) and most commonly affects the large joints, particularly the knees (50%).[2] Patients may develop fever, chills, joint effusion with swelling, redness, and tenderness of the joint space. Patients with an infection of a prosthetic joint may complain only of pain, with fever and erythema being much less common.[2]

Diagnosis

The diagnosis may be presumed in patients with typical symptoms and confirmed with arthrocentesis. Synovial fluid should be examined with Gram staining (positive in 60% to 80% of cases), cell count (white blood cell [WBC] count typically greater than 50,000 cells/hpf), differential count (predominance of polymorphonuclear neutrophils [PMNs]), crystals (to rule out crystal arthropathies, if suspected), and culture (positive in 50%).[1,2] In patients in whom gonococcal arthritis is suspected (young, healthy, sexually active adults), mucosal swabs (cervical, urethral, pharyngeal, or rectal) should be obtained for identification of *Neisseria gonorrheae.*

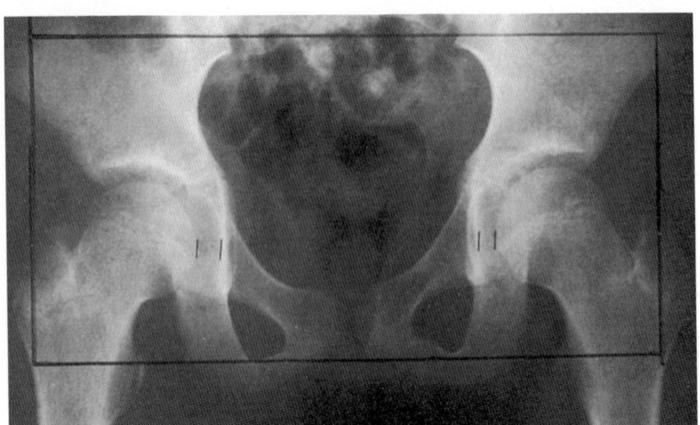

FIGURE 23–3 Septic arthritis. Note increased distance between the femoral epiphysis and acetabulum on the right, compared with the left, due to an increased volume of synovial fluid. (From the American College of Radiology Teaching Collection, with permission.)

Pathophysiology

Bacterial arthritis may be caused by hematogenous spread from an infected organ (e.g., cervix, urethra, kidney, pharynx, lung) or by direct inoculation (e.g., after surgery, puncture wound). Hematogenous spread most commonly occurs in patients with impaired immune responses (e.g., diabetes mellitus, RA, renal failure, acquired immunodeficiency syndrome) and those with damage or inflammation of the joints (OA or RA). Bacterial infection of the synovium leads to an inflammatory cascade within the joint. In 80% of the cases, the bacteria are gram-positive aerobes (*Staphylococcus aureus,* β-hemolytic streptococci, or *Streptococcus pneumoniae*), and in 20% they are gram-negative bacilli (*Escherichia coli, Haemophilus influenzae*).[1,2]

Clinical Complications

Untreated bacterial arthritis may lead to destruction of the joint space (25% to 50%), as well as systemic infection.[2]

Management

Patients with nongonococcal bacterial septic arthritis should be admitted to the hospital and treated with a parenteral dose of a third-generation cephalosporin (ceftriaxone or cefotaxime).[1] Antibiotics may be based on Gram staining of the synovial fluid if this test is rapidly available. Consultation with an orthopedist should be considered, because daily arthrocentesis or surgical débridement may be necessary. Patients with infected prostheses may require removal of the prosthetic joint after initiation of antibiotic therapy and should be cared for by an orthopedist.

REFERENCES

1. Garcia-De La Torre I. Advances in the management of septic arthritis. *Rheum Dis Clin North Am* 2003;29:61–75.
2. Goldenberg DL. Septic arthritis. *Lancet* 1998;351:197–202.

Pseudogout

Robert Hendrickson

Clinical Presentation

Pseudogout may manifest as an acute monoarticular or oligoarticular arthritis with erythema, pain, swelling, and fever. The most frequently affected joints are the knees, wrists, shoulders, and hips.[1] Calcium pyrophosphate dihydrate deposition disease (CPPD) may be asymptomatic, or it may be found in association with osteoarthritis (OA). Radiographic findings include "hook-like" osteophytes, cystic changes, and chondrocalcinosis.[1]

Pathophysiology

Pseudogout, also called CPPD, is an inflammatory arthropathy that is caused by deposition of calcium-containing crystals in joints.

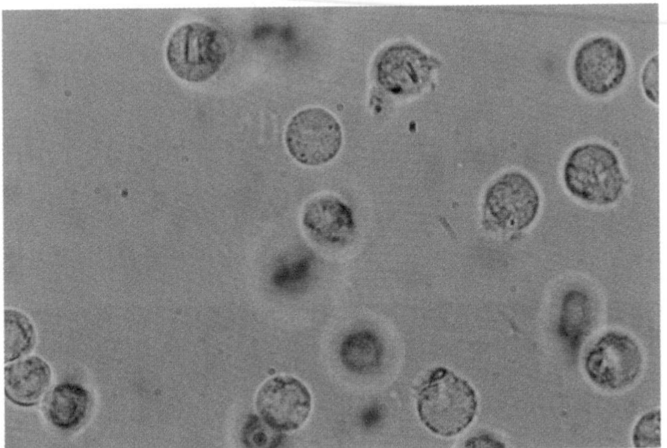

FIGURE 23–4 Synovial fluid aspirated during an acute attack of pseudogout and viewed with phase contrast microscopy shows calcium pyrophosphate dehydrate crystals within several leukocytes. (From Hunder, with permission.)

CPPD is dependent on genetic, metabolic, and endocrine influences.[1] Risk factors include older age, family history, hyperparathyroidism, hypomagnesemia, hemochromatosis, and hypophosphatemia. Synovial crystal formation leads to an inflammatory cascade, synovial hyperplasia, and collagenase production.[1]

Diagnosis

The clinical presentation may mimic that of OA, rheumatoid arthritis (RA), septic arthritis, or gout. Typical radiographic findings (e.g., chondrocalcinosis) and arthrocentesis findings may differentiate this disorder from gout and septic arthritis (SA). The synovial white blood cell (WBC) count is typically 10,000 to 20,000 cells/hpf in pseudogout, and calcium-containing crystals can be visualized by regular microscopy.[1] Crystals may be extracellular or intracellular or both, and they are weakly positively birefringent.

Clinical Complications

Complications include pain and joint destruction with limitation of function.

Management

Treatment of acute pseudogout episodes include arthrocentesis and oral nonsteroidal antiinflammatory drugs (NSAIDs).[1] Colchicine and intraarticular corticosteroids are effective but are generally reserved for patients with refractory disease. Long-term prophylactic therapy may include NSAIDs, colchicine, and oral corticosteroids.[1]

REFERENCES

1. Agudelo CA, Wise CM. Crystal-associated arthritis in the elderly. *Rheum Dis Clin North Am* 2000;26:527–546.

Gout

Robert Hendrickson

Clinical Presentation

Patients with a first gouty episode typically present with acute onset of monoarticular arthritis (85%). Sixty percent of cases involve the first metatarsal joint.[2] The joint and surrounding tissues are typically erythematous, edematous, and warm, making differentiation of gout from septic arthritis (SA) somewhat difficult. As the disease progresses, patients may present to the emergency department (ED) with polyarticular arthritis with fever and constitutional symptoms. Urate deposits located beneath the skin (tophi) may also develop, particularly on the elbows and fingers.[2] Before the age of 60 years, gout has a male predominance; however, rates of disease are equal in elderly men and women. Older patients also have more atypical presentations. Older patients are more likely to have polyarticular arthritis, arthritis of the small hand joints, and development of tophi early in their disease.[2]

Pathophysiology

Gout is a clinical syndrome of articular inflammation caused by elevated concentrations of urate (monosodium urate monohydrate), with resulting precipitation of crystals in joints.[1]

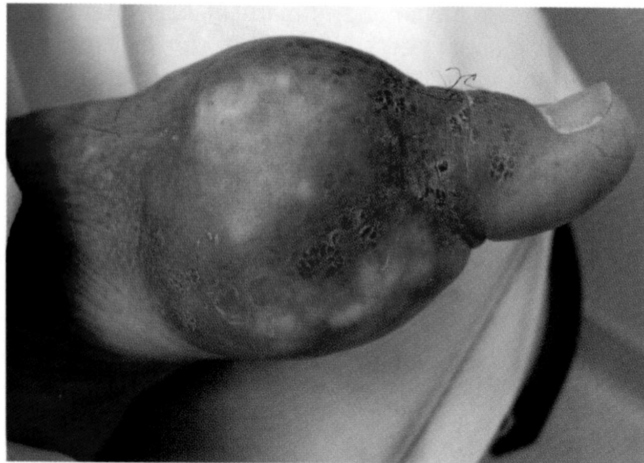

FIGURE 23–5 Severe gout of the first metatarsal joint. (Courtesy of Colleen Campbell, MD.)

The risk of developing gout is related to genetic and environmental factors and directly proportional to the serum urate concentration.[1,3] Although most people with elevated urate concentrations do not have gout, some form urate crystals within synovial cavities. These crystals are phagocytized by macrophages, initiating an inflammatory cascade that attracts more inflammatory cells to the joint and surrounding tissue.

Diagnosis

The diagnosis can be suspected with a typical clinical history (e.g., middle-aged male with acute onset of monoarticular arthritis in the first metatarsal joint without fever or lymphangitis). A definitive diagnosis of gouty arthritis may be made with the identification of urate crystals in joint fluid or tissue.[2] Urate crystals may be visible as needle-shaped crystals within white blood cells on typical microscopy, but they are best identified with a polarizing microscope (negative birefringence).[2]

Patients with gout are thought to have increased intake, overproduction and/or a decreased excretion of urate, or some combination of these.[1] Urate is a metabolic product of purine metabolism. Ingestion of foods with high purine concentrations (e.g., beer, meat, beans, peas, spinach)[1] or conditions that increase cellular turnover (e.g., cancer, inflammatory conditions) may contribute to elevated urate concentrations. Additionally, most patients with gout have decreased renal clearance of urate, secondary to renal insufficiency or use of medications that decrease excretion (e.g., loop or thiazide diuretics, pyrazinamide, didanosine, ethambutol, niacin).[1]

Clinical Complications

Gout may produce debilitating episodes of arthritis. In addition, cosmetically problematic and potentially deforming tophi may develop.

Management

Patients who present with a mild acute gouty episode may be treated with nonsteroidal antiinflammatory drugs (NSAIDs) or cyclooxygenase-2 (COX-2) inhibitors on an outpatient basis, with follow-up with their primary doctor or rheumatologist.[2,3] Although it is not necessary to perform arthrocentesis in patients with a typical history and physical examination, arthrocentesis should be considered in any patient if there is any concern for SA.

Patients with moderate episodes may require colchicine (1 mg by mouth, then 0.5 mg every 2 hours until diarrhea develops, or until a total of 8 mg has been administered). Colchicine inhibits phagocytosis of crystals by neutrophils. Colchicine is generally safe; however, bone marrow suppression, renal injury, and hepatic injury may occur, particularly in patients with renal insufficiency and in those who are given colchicine intravenously (IV).[1] Corticosteroids may be used to treat gout but probably should be selected for patients with no signs of infection on arthrocentesis.

Care should be taken to not change prophylactic gout medications without consultation with the patient's primary doctor or rheumatologist, because such changes (increases or decreases) may precipitate a gouty episode. Prophylactic medications include colchicine, NSAIDs, and corticosteroids. Patients may also be taking allopurinol, a xanthine oxidase inhibitor, which decreases the production of urate from purines. Additionally, patients may require medications that increase renal clearance of urate (e.g., probenicid, sulfinpyrazone, salicylates).[1]

REFERENCES

1. Emmerson BT. The management of gout. *N Engl J Med* 1996;334:445–451.
2. Agudelo CA, Wise CM. Crystal-associated arthritis in the elderly. *Rheum Dis Clin North Am* 2000;26:527–546.
3. Rott KT, Agudelo CA. Gout. *JAMA* 2003;289:2857–2860.

Systemic Lupus Erythematosus

Robert Hendrickson

Clinical Presentation

Patients with systemic lupus erythematosus (SLE) may present to the emergency department (ED) with their first symptoms of SLE or with lupus flares in those with established disease. Symptoms may include skin rashes—a "classic" malar rash (erythema of the nose, cheeks, and forehead), vasculitic rashes (common at the nail bed), and discoid lesions (raised erythematous plaques)—arthritis, myositis/myalgias, tenosynovitis, and fever. SLE may also cause asymptomatic lupus nephritis (proteinuria, renal failure, nephrotic syndrome), serositis (myocarditis, pericarditis, pleuritis), myocardial infarction (MI, from coronary artery vasculitis), oral ulcers, anemia, and thromobocytopenia. Central nervous system manifestations include vasculitis, cerebrovascular accident (CVA), and cerebritis (alterations of mental status, focal neurologic deficits, psychosis, and seizures).[1]

Pathophysiology

SLE is molded by genetic, endogenous, and environmental factors. Defects in suppressor T cells lead to an overabundance of B cells and the production of antibodies, including anti-DNA and antinuclear antibodies (ANA), that produce disease directly or through immune-complex formation.

Diagnosis

See Table 23-6. Antinuclear antibodies are 95% sensitive in detecting SLE, although false-positive results occur with hydralazine and procainamide use, hepatitis, subacute bacterial endocarditis (SBE), and primary biliary cirrhosis.[2] Anti-double-stranded DNA (anti-ds DNA) and anti-Smith antibodies are specific for SLE.

TABLE 23-6 Classification Criteria for Systemic Lupus Erythematosus (SLE)

At least four of the following criteria must be present for a diagnosis of SLE:
1. Malar rash (erythematous, macular or papular)
2. Discoid rash (erythematous, raised patches with keratotic scaling)
3. Photosensitivity
4. Oral ulcers (painless oral/nasal ulcers)
5. Arthritis (transient, migratory, nonerosive arthritis in more than two joints)
6. Serositis (pleuritis or pericarditis)
7. Renal disorder (proteinuria or casts)
8. Neurologic disorder (e.g., seizures, psychosis)
9. Hematologic disorder (hemolytic anemia, leukopenia, thrombocytopenia)
10. Immunologic disorder (anti-DNA or anti-Smith or antiphospholipid antibodies)
11. Antinuclear antibodies

From Petri M. Treatment of systemic lupus erythematosus: an update. *Am Fam Physician* 1998;57:2753–2760.

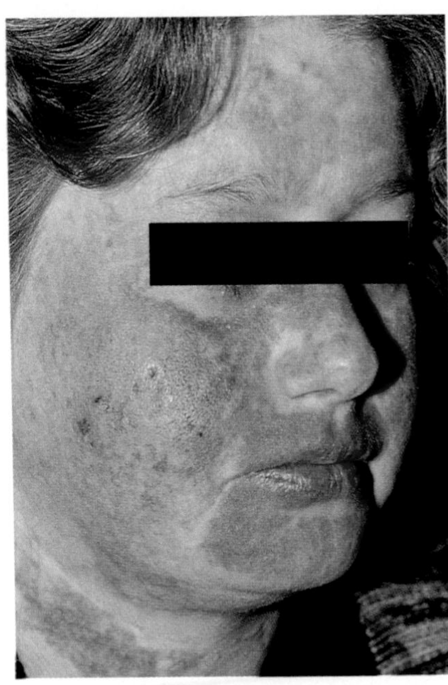

FIGURE 23-6 Localized acute cutaneous lupus erythematosus (ACLE) confined to the face and neck, as seen here, is classified under the Gilliam scheme as localized ACLE. (From Sontheimer, with permission.)

Clinical Complications

Complications include CVA, cerebritis, myocarditis/pericarditis, vasculitis, MI, renal failure, nephrotic syndrome, gastrointestinal vasculitis, hemolysis, and pulmonary fibrosis.

Management

Rheumatologic consultation or close follow-up with a qualified provider should be initiated for all patients with suspected SLE. Patients with minor inflammatory conditions, such as arthralgias or pericarditis, may be treated with nonsteroidal antiinflammatory drugs (NSAIDs) (avoid in patients with nephritis) and with corticosteroids.[1] Patients with severe chronic disease may also be treated with antimalarial agents (chloroquine, hydroxychloroquine) and immunosuppressive drugs (azathioprine, cyclophosphamide).[2]

Patients with minor conditions (e.g., monoarticular arthralgia) or minor flares of chronic SLE can often be discharged from the ED. Patients with severe conditions (e.g., renal failure, cerebritis) may require aggressive therapy, including intravenous (IV) steroids, immunosuppressive drugs, and admission to the hospital. Consultation with a rheumatologist, if possible, may be helpful in these cases.

REFERENCES

1. Mills JA. Systemic lupus erythematosus. *N Engl J Med* 1994;330: 1871–1879.
2. Petri M. Treatment of systemic lupus erythematosus: an update. *Am Fam Physician* 1998;57:2753–2760.

Discoid Lupus

Bjorn Miller

Clinical Presentation

Patients may have red, scaly, round lesions (coin lesions) on sun-exposed skin such as the face, hands, and neck. As lesions progress, the scale may thicken and become adherent, with central depigmentation. Lesions often leave scarring or alopecia once they heal. The skin lesions are typically asymptomatic, are typically 5 to 20 mm in diameter, and can produce pain or pruritis.[1,2] The lesions can last for months to years.[3]

Pathophysiology

Discoid lupus is a chronic, scarring, atrophy-producing skin disorder that produces few systemic manifestations. The disease is possibly separate from systemic lupus erythematosus (SLE), or it may be considered a nonsystemic form of SLE.

The origin of the disease is not well-understood, but it is thought that genetically predisposed individuals have an abnormal autoimmune T-cell response to some viral, hormonal, or environmental stimuli. Scaly plaques typically show follicular plugging that tends to heal with atrophy, scarring, and hyperpigmentation or hypopigmentation. Biopsy shows hyperkeratosis, follicular plugging, and atrophy of the epidermis.[3]

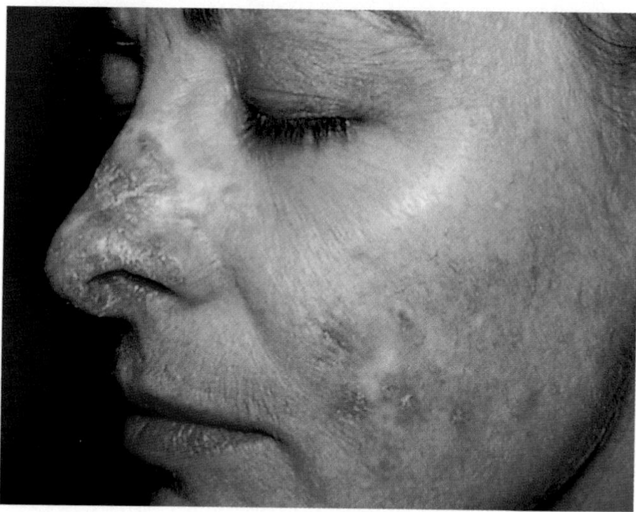

FIGURE 23–7 Chronic discoid lupus erythematosus with erythematous plaques and scarring. (From Ostler, with permission.)

Diagnosis

Discoid lupus is more common in African-Americans and typically develops in women 20 to 40 years old.[1] The diagnosis is primarily a clinical one, because few patients have serologic abnormalities (20% have positive antinuclear antibodies [ANA]). Skin biopsy of the lesions for histologic examination can help in equivocal cases. Rarely do patients have more than four of the criteria used to classify SLE.[3]

Clinical Complications

Complications are secondary to skin lesions and include alopecia (common on the scalp) and scarring. Malignant degeneration of the skin lesions is rare. Five percent of patients with discoid lupus go on to develop SLE.[2]

Management

Patients need to be instructed to avoid sun exposure and to use sunscreens with skin protection factor (SPF) of 30 whenever they are going to be outside, because ultraviolet light exacerbates the disease. Potent topical corticosteroids or steroid injections can be used directly on or in the lesions to decrease inflammation and plugging. Refractory cases can be treated with hydroxychloroquine (60% effective), dapsone, auranofin, and acitretin (retinoic acid derivative that regulates cell proliferation), which are immunomodulatory agents. Rarely do patients need to be admitted to the hospital, but they should be referred to a dermatologist and rheumatologist for follow-up.[2,3]

REFERENCES

1. Watanabe T, Tsuchida T. Classification of lupus erythematosus based upon cutaneous manifestations. *Dermatology* 1995;190: 277–283.
2. Tavadia S, Tillman D. Managing facial redness and rashes. *Practitioner* 2003;247:90–94,96–100.
3. Watson R. Cutaneous lesions in systematic lupus erythematosus. *Med Clin North Am* 1989;73:1091–1111.

Behçet's Disease

Robert Hendrickson

Clinical Presentation

Behçet's disease is rare in the United States and western Europe and more prevalent in the Middle East and Asia.[1] Patients with Behçet's disease are typically asymptomatic at baseline but develop recurrent inflammatory episodes. The most common initial presenting symptom is oral ulcers.[1] The ulcers are usually round, with an erythematous base and a yellow pseudomembrane. Most patients (70% to 90%) also develop painful genital ulcers on the penis, scrotum, or vulva.[1,2] Additional symptoms may include arthralgias and arthritis in 50% to 80% of patients and skin lesions (erythema nodosum, pseudofolliculitis) in 80%. Approximately 50% of patients develop anterior uveitis with resulting hypopyon or retinitis, with resulting hemorrhage and exudates on funduscopic examination. Multiple episodes of retinitis lead to blindness in 25% of patients.[1] Patients with a history of Behçet's disease may develop personality changes or psychiatric symptoms due to central nervous system vasculitis. Patients may develop thromboembolic events (deep venous thrombosis [DVT], thrombophlebitis, or cerebrovascular accident [CVA]) or gastrointestinal ulcerations and edema that may be difficult to differentiate from Crohn's disease.

Pathophysiology

Behçet's disease is an idiopathic inflammatory disorder that is characterized by episodic, recurrent oral ulcers, genital ulcers, uveitis, and cutaneous lesions.[1]

The cause of Behçet's disease is unknown; however, genetic factors (human leukocyte antigen [HLA] B51 allele), environmental factors, and possibly infectious factors (herpes simplex virus, hepatitis C, parvovirus) may have a role.[1] Lesions develop secondary to vasculitis and increased activity of neutrophils, lymphocytes, and cytokines.[1]

Diagnosis

Diagnosis is made clinically by noting typical recurrent oral ulcers with at least two of the following: recurrent genital ulcers, eye lesions (anterior or posterior uveitis), skin lesions (erythema nodosum, pseudofolliculitis, papullopustular lesions, or acneiform nodules), or a positive pathergy test.

Clinical Complications

Twenty-five percent of patients with Behçet's disease develop blindness secondary to recurrent retinitis. Additional complications in some cases include vasculitis, meningoencephalitis, and thromboembolic events.

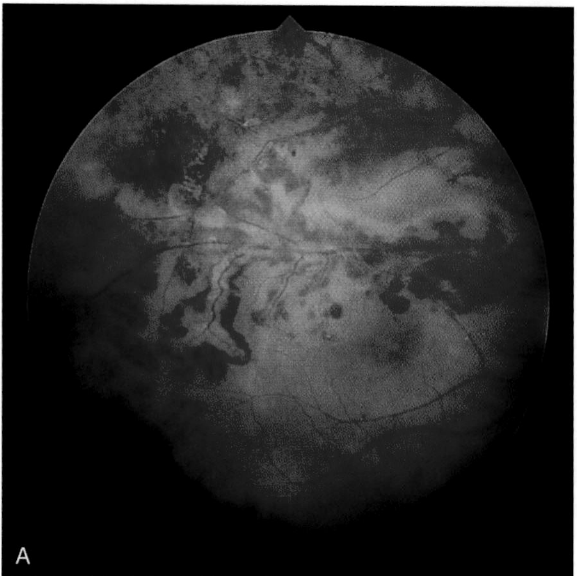

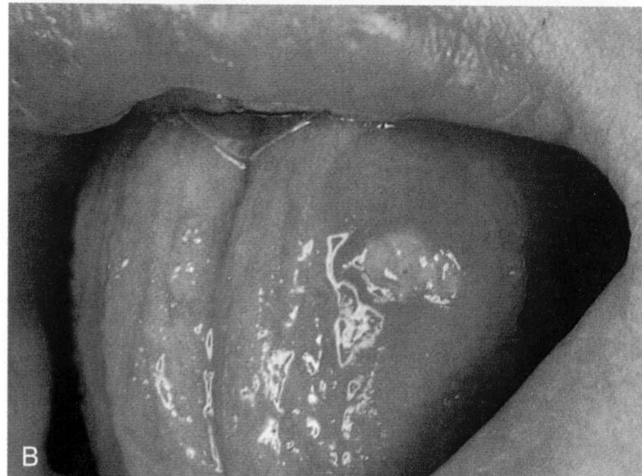

FIGURE 23–8 **A:** Acute retinal vasculitis in a patient with Behçet's syndrome. (From Tasman, with permission.) **B:** Aphthous ulcers appear as minute shallow, white ulcers along mucous membranes. Although lesions are observed in normal individuals, multiple or persistent lesions mandate exclusion of an underlying disease process such as inflammatory bowel disease or Behçet's disease. (From Yamada, with permission.)

Behçet's Disease

Robert Hendrickson

Management

The main role of the emergency physician for the patient who presents with a first episode of Behçet's disease is to rule out other diseases (herpes simplex virus, Crohn's disease, ulcerative colitis, oral apthosis) and to arrange for further evaluation and treatment by a rheumatologist or primary care physician.

Patients with meningoencephalitis should be treated with parenteral high-dose corticosteroids and admitted to the hospital. Gastrointestinal ulcerations should be treated with bowel rest, corticosteroids, and possibly sulfasalazine. Skin disorders may be treated with topical corticosteroids and oral colchicine. Arthritis may be treated with nonsteroidal antiinflammatory drugs (NSAIDs), colchicine, and possibly sulfasalazine. Care of patients with Behçet's disease and uveitis or retinitis should be coordinated with an ophthalmologist. Uveitis may be treated with mydriatics, topical corticosteroids, and colchicine. Arrangements should be made for timely follow-up with a primary care physician or rheumatologist.

REFERENCES

1. Sakane T, Takeno M, Suzuki N, Inaba G. Behçet's disease. *N Engl J Med* 1999;341:1284–1291.
2. Yazici H, Yurdakul S, Hamuryudan V. Behçet's syndrome. *Curr Opin Rheumatol* 1999;11:53–57.

Antiphospholipid Syndrome

Robert Hendrickson

Clinical Presentation

Patients with antiphospholipid (APL) syndrome may present to the emergency department (ED) with thromboembolic events including cerebrovascular accident (CVA), deep venous thrombosis (DVT), myocardial infarction (MI), or pulmonary embolism (PE). The syndrome may occur in patients with autoimmune diseases (secondary APL) or in those with no evidence of autoimmune diseases (primary APL).

Pathophysiology

APL syndrome is a syndrome of hypercoagulability that occurs secondary to the presence of circulating antibodies to phospholipids and phospholipid-binding proteins.

APL antibodies bind to phospholipids and phospholipid-binding proteins, causing activation of endothelial cells, secretion of cytokines and prostaglandins, oxidation of endothelial proteins, and interference with the coagulation cascade and platelet function.[1]

Diagnosis

The diagnosis may be considered in patients with thromboembolic events without other prominent risk factors or with multiple late spontaneous abortions. Diagnostic criteria are listed in Table 23–9; at least one clinical event and one laboratory criterion must be met.[1]

TABLE 23–9 Criteria for the Diagnosis of the Antiphospholipid (APL) Syndrome

At least one clinical criterion and one laboratory criterion must be met for the diagnosis of APL syndrome to be made:
Clinical criteria
Vascular thrombosis (arterial or venous thrombosis)
Laboratory criteria
Anticardiolipin antibodies (elevated on two or more occasions at least 6 wk apart)
Lupus anticoagulant antibodies (detected on two or more occasions at least 6 wk apart)

From Petri M. Treatment of systemic lupus erythematosus: an update. *Am Fam Physician* 1998;57:2753–2760.

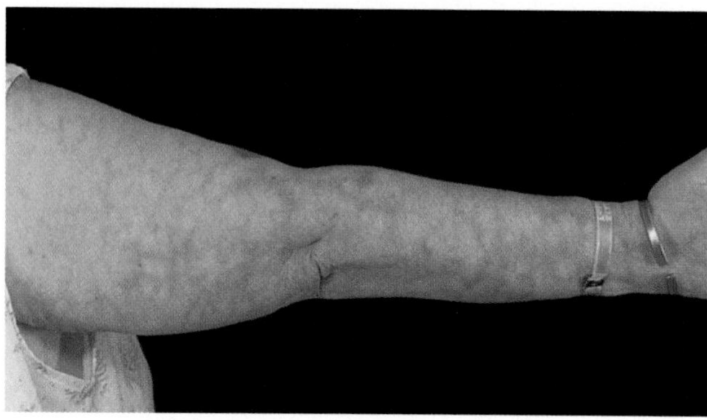

FIGURE 23–9 Prominent livedo reticularis of the arm in a woman with antiphospholipid antibodies. (From Hunder, with permission.)

Clinical Complications

Complications of APL syndrome include thromboembolic events (e.g., PE, CVA, MI, DVT), midtrimester spontaneous abortions, and fetal demise.[1,2]

Management

Patients with thromboembolic events should be treated for these events according to the underlying diagnosis (e.g., heparin for DVT). Coagulation profiles and platelet counts should be evaluated to rule out other causes of hypercoagulability (e.g., thrombocytosis). Patients who develop APL syndrome may require anticoagulation with warfarin to reduce the risk of recurrent thrombosis.[2]

REFERENCES

1. Levine JS, Branch DW, Rauch J. The antiphospholipid syndrome. *N Engl J Med* 2002;346:752–763.
2. Khamashta MA, Cuadrado MJ, Mujic F, Taub NA, Hunt BJ, Hughes GR. The management of thrombosis in the antiphospholipid-antibody syndrome. *N Engl J Med* 1995;332:993–997.

Takayasu's Arteritis

Robert Hendrickson

Clinical Presentation

The majority of patients with Takayasu's arteritis develop symptoms between 10 and 30 years of age.[1] Patients with Takayasu's arteritis may present to the emergency department (ED) with ischemic events, or signs may be noted in a patient with unrelated complaints. The disease occurs in three phases. In the initial or "prepulseless" phase, patients may develop nonspecific symptoms of inflammation (43%) such as fatigue, fever, night sweats, arthralgias, and weight loss.[1,2] Patients then develop vascular pain (typically pain along the carotid artery) and tenderness (32%). This is followed by a fibrotic stage, in which symptoms of arterial stenosis become evident.[2] Patients may develop hypertension secondary to renal artery stenosis (33%), claudication (70%), asymmetric upper-extremity blood pressures (47%), aortic regurgitation (20% to 24%), coronary vessel stenosis (6% to 16%), pulmonary stenosis/hypertension and multiple bruits (80%).[2] A small number of patients develop retinal findings consistent with carotid stenosis (e.g., neovascularization, microaneurysm, central retinal hypoperfusion).

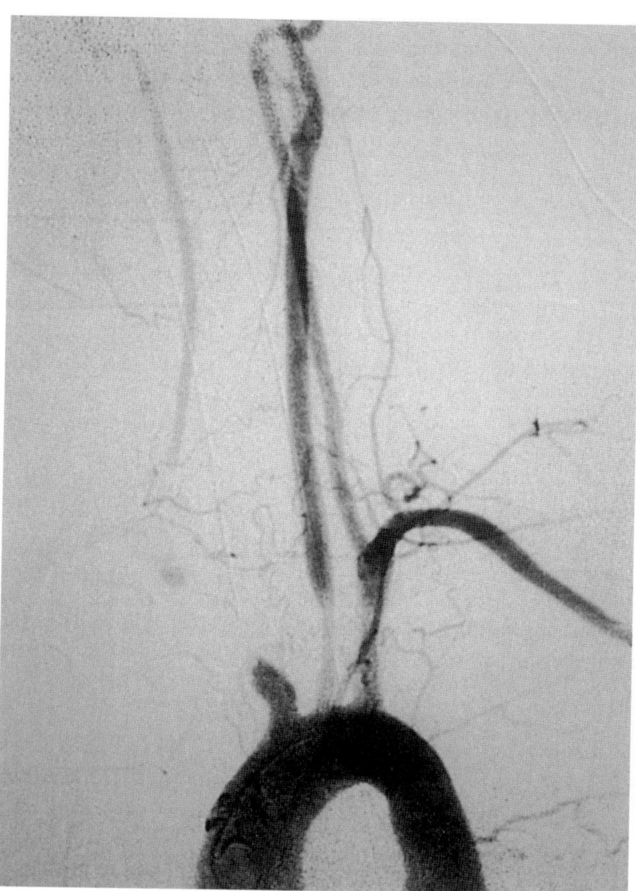

FIGURE 23–10 Angiogram of the aortic arch shows the long stenosis of the left carotid artery and the obstruction of the brachiocephalic arterial trunk. The right vertebral artery is seen after a few centimeters of total obstruction of the subclavian artery. (From Hunder, with permission.)

Pathophysiology

Takayasu's arteritis, also known as pulseless disease, is a chronic inflammatory arteritis of large blood vessels, particularly the aorta and its major branches.[1]

The cause of Takayasu's arteritis is unknown; however, genetic and infectious factors (e.g., *Mycobacterium tuberculosis,* viruses) may have a role.[1] An initial inflammatory reaction of the adventitia leads to panarteritis, followed by fibrosis, stenosis, and aneurysm formation.

Diagnosis

The diagnosis should be considered in patients with arterial stenotic symptoms, particularly in patients younger than 40 years of age. Clinical diagnosis requires at least three of the following six findings: onset of disease before 40 years of age, extremity claudication, decreased brachial artery pulse, blood pressure differential greater than 10 mm Hg, subclavian artery or aortic bruit, and typical arteriographic findings. Aortic angiography or ultrasonography of the subclavian and carotid arteries may be used to confirm the diagnosis and quantify stenosis. Laboratory evaluation, including C-reactive protein, white blood cell (WBC) count, and erythrocyte sedimentation rate, are not helpful in differentiating Takayasu's arteritis from other causes of vasculitis.

Clinical Complications

Complications of Takayasu's arteritis include cerebrovascular accident (CVA), hypertension, myocardial infarction (MI), mesenteric ischemia, claudication, necrosis of distal extremities, and blindness.

Management

Patients with Takayasu's arteritis who present with acute ischemic events should be treated with corticosteroids. Revascularization (surgery or angioplasty) should be delayed until the acute inflammatory episode has resolved. Indications for surgery include critical aortic regurgitation, critical stenosis of three or more cerebral vessels, and critical stenosis of coronary arteries. Fifty percent of patients who are treated with corticosteroids have remission of the inflammatory event. Those who do not respond to corticosteroids may be treated with methotrexate (additional 25% remission).[1]

REFERENCES

1. Johnston SL, Lock RJ, Gompels MM. Takayasu arteritis: a review. *J Clin Pathol* 2002;55:481–486.
2. Kerr GS. Takayasu's arteritis. *Rheum Dis Clin North Am* 1995;21: 1041–1058.

Temporal Arteritis

Robert Hendrickson

Clinical Presentation

Patients may present to the emergency department (ED) with complaints related to diffuse inflammation (anorexia, weight loss, fatigue, fever, arthralgias, myalgias), local inflammation (headache, scalp or temporal tenderness), or ischemia (diplopia, amaurosis fugax, blindness, jaw claudication, cerebrovascular accident [CVA]).[2] On physical examination, patients may have tenderness, redness, or swelling in the area of the temporal artery (just anterior and superior to the tragus). In addition, central pallor or retinal artery occlusion on funduscopic examination is possible.[2]

Pathophysiology

Temporal arteritis (TA) is an inflammatory vasculitis of medium to large vessels that preferentially affects cervicofacial arteries of elderly patients.[1]

The specific cause of TA has not yet been elucidated.

Diagnosis

The diagnosis must be suspected clinically and confirmed by laboratory and biopsy evaluation. Although there is no single clinical or historical finding that is highly sensitive,[2] patients may be classified as having low, medium, or high probability of TA based on history, physical examination, and erythrocyte sedimentation rate (ESR).[1] An ESR measurement should be performed for all patients with a clinical suspicion of TA. Definitive diagnosis may be made with biopsies of the temporal arteries, although even bilateral temporal artery biopsies cannot rule out the disease.[2]

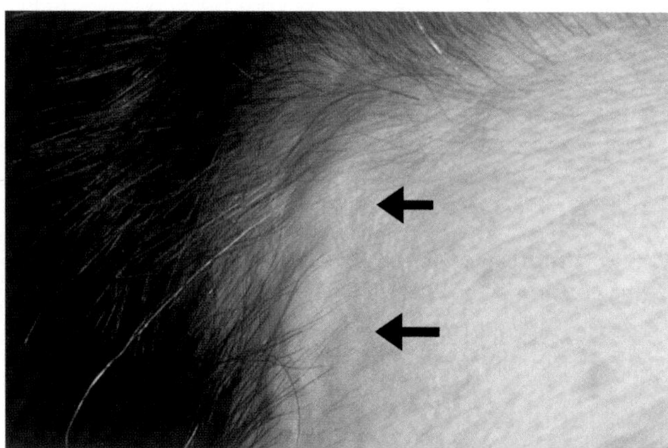

FIGURE 23–11 The right temporal artery *(arrow)* is visible and inflamed; palpation of the hard vessel is painful for the patient. (From Hunder, with permission.)

Clinical Complications

Patients with TA have no increase in mortality. However, TA may lead to permanent unilateral or bilateral visual loss.

Management

Patients with a high probability of having TA are older than 50 years, have an elevated ESR (greater than 50 mm/hour), and have at least one finding that is specific to TA (tongue or jaw claudication, visual abnormalities, or temporal artery tenderness or pain). These patients should rapidly receive intravenous (IV) corticosteroids while awaiting laboratory evaluation. Any patient with a high clinical suspicion for TA or with visual signs should be admitted to the hospital and treated with IV corticosteroids. Patients with moderate probability have a specific finding (tongue or jaw claudication, visual abnormalities, or temporal artery tenderness or pain), but are younger than 50 years of age or have a normal ESR.[1] These patients may be treated with corticosteroids, admitted to the hospital, and further evaluated with a temporal artery biopsy. Patients with low clinical suspicion and a normal ESR most likely do not have TA; they may be considered for a temporal artery biopsy or close follow-up.[1]

REFERENCES

1. Lee AG, Brazis PW. Temporal arteritis: a clinical approach. *J Am Geriatr Soc* 1999;47:1364–1370.
2. Smetana GW, Shmerling RH. Does this patient have temporal arteritis? *JAMA* 2002;287:92–101.

Polyarteritis Nodosa

Robert Hendrickson

Clinical Presentation

The typical age of onset for Polyarteritis nodosa (PAN) is 50 years, but the age ranges from the teen years to the elderly. The early manifestations of PAN include constitutional symptoms such as fever (69%), myalgias (53%), weight loss (66%), arthralgias (44%), and malaise. Later in the course of the disease, symptoms specific to the gastrointestinal tract (31%) and peripheral nerves (67%) may become evident.[1] A similar disorder sometimes grouped with PAN is microscopic polyangiitis (MPA). MPA may lead to similar symptoms, but more commonly affects the kidneys, resulting in renal failure and hypertension.[1,2]

Pathophysiology

PAN is a relatively uncommon form of vasculitis that leads to acute inflammation and fibrosis of small to medium vessels, particularly involving the gastrointestinal (GI) tract and peripheral nerves.[1,2]

TABLE 23–12 Clinical Criteria for Polyarteritis Nodosa

Patients must meet more than three of the following criteria for a diagnosis of polyarteritis nodosa:
1. Weight loss greater than 4 kg
2. Livedo reticularis
3. Testicular pain/tenderness
4. Myalgias, weakness or leg tenderness
5. Mononeuropathy or polyneuropathy
6. Diastolic blood pressure greater than 90 mm Hg
7. Elevated blood urea nitrogen or creatinine
8. Hepatitis B virus
9. Arteriographic abnormality
10. Biopsy of small- or medium-sized artery containing polymorphonuclear neutrophils (PMNs)

From Lightfoot RJ, Michel BA, Bloch DA, et al. The American College of Rheumatology 1990 criteria for the classification of polyarteritis nodosa. *Arthritis Rheum* 1990;33:1088–1093.

The etiology of PAN is unknown, and the details of the pathophysiology have not been fully elucidated.

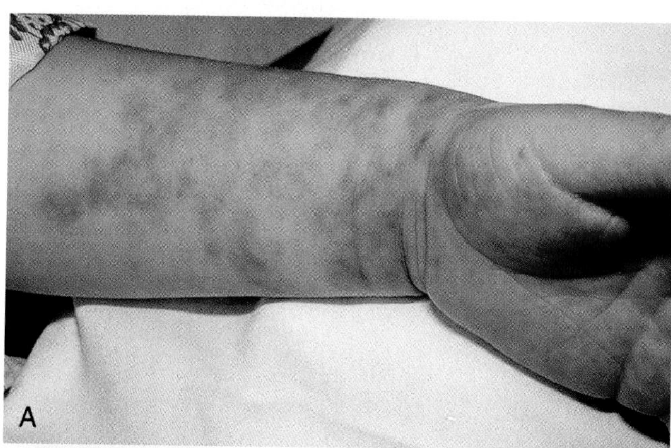

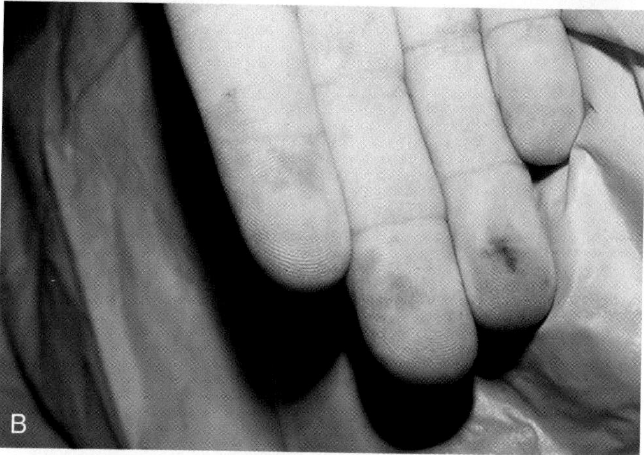

FIGURE 23–12 Polyarteritis nodosa. **A:** Livedo reticularis and tender subcutaneous nodules are characteristic. **B:** Note the necrotizing changes in multiple digits. (**A** and **B**, From Yamada, with permission.)

Diagnosis

The specific diagnostic clinical criteria for the diagnosis of PAN are listed in Table 23–12. PAN may be definitively diagnosed with a biopsy of a small- to medium-sized artery. Consultation with a rheumatologist is recommended if the clinical criteria for PAN are met. Perinuclear antineutrophil cytoplasmic antibody (p-ANCA) is typically negative in PAN, but is positive in MPA.[1,2]

Clinical Complications

PAN and MPA may lead to bowel ischemia, peripheral neuropathy, hypertension, and renal failure.[1]

Management

Initial management should be aimed at ruling out more common disorders. If the diagnosis of vasculitis / PAN is considered and the patient fits clinical criteria, a rheumatology consult may be helpful. PAN is treated with corticosteroids and, occasionally, with immunosuppressive agents.[1]

REFERENCES

1. Guillevin L, Le Thi Huong D, Godeau P, Jais P, Wechsler B. Clinical findings and prognosis of polyarteritis nodosa and Churg-Strauss angiitis: a study in 165 patients. *Br J Rheumatol* 1988;27:258–264.
2. Lightfoot RJ, Michel BA, Bloch DA, et al. The American College of Rheumatology 1990 criteria for the classification of polyarteritis nodosa. *Arthritis Rheum* 1990;33:1088–1093.

Dermatomyositis and Polymyositis

Robert Hendrickson

Clinical Presentation

These conditions affect both children and adults and are seen in approximately 5 patients per 1 million population.[1] Patients may present to the emergency department (ED) without a history of these disorders but with muscle pain and weakness or a rash. The weakness is typically proximal and symmetric and progresses over a period of weeks to months. Patients may report difficulty walking up stairs or standing from a seated position. Several typical skin manifestations may occur in dermatomyositis; heliotrope rash, Gottron's papules, poikiloderma, and periungal telangiectasias. A heliotrope rash is an erythematous rash in the periorbital area with or without periorbital edema. Gottron's papules are raised, violaceous plaques seen over bony prominences, particularly on the fingers. Poikiloderma is a rash consisting of atrophy, dyspigmentation, and telangiectasias on photoexposed skin, typically around the neck. Periungal telangiectasias may be visible to the naked eye, but they may be more easily viewed with magnification.[2]

Patients with a history of myositis may also present to the ED with exacerbations of their disease or with systemic symptoms. Systemic findings may include dysphagia (from esophageal muscle weakness; 15% to 50%), symmetric small-joint arthritis (25%), interstitial pneumonitis (15% to 30%), pericarditis or conduction defects, or calcinosis.[2] Calcinosis, or calcification of skeletal muscle, may be apparent on radiography. Calcinosis is more common in juvenile dermatomyositis than it is in adult patients.[2]

Pathophysiology

Dermatomyositis is an idiopathic autoimmune condition that produces muscular inflammation, muscle weakness, and characteristic cutaneous findings. Polymyositis is similar to dermatomyositis but lacks the skin involvement.

The cause of dermatomyositis and polymyositis is unknown, although associations with genetic, environmental, and autoimmune factors have been reported.[3]

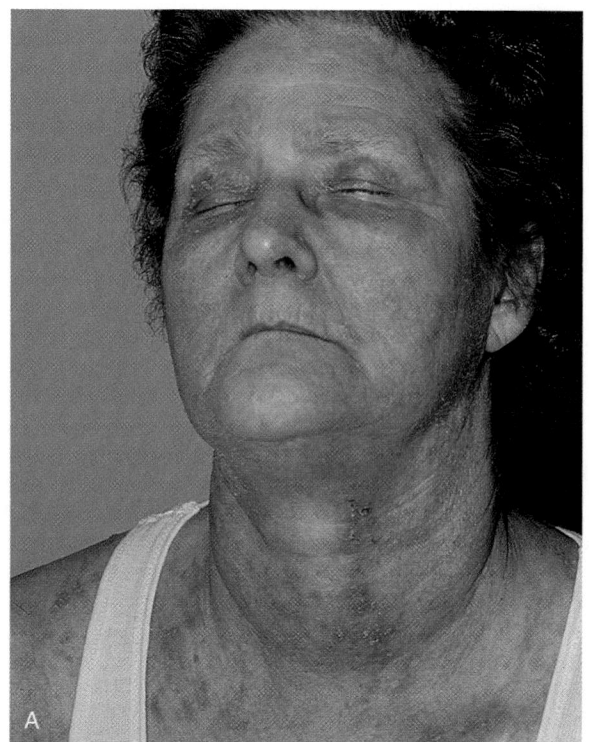

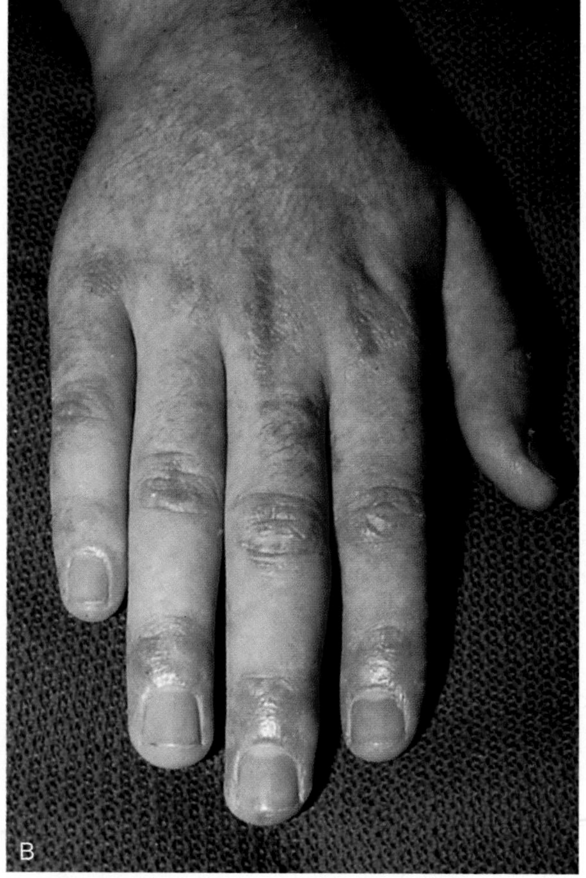

FIGURE 23–13 **A:** Classic dermatomyositis. Note the characteristic heliotrope (violaceous) periorbital erythema especially involving the upper lids. (From Sontheimer, with permission.) **B:** Dermatomyositis. Note erythematous shiny papules involving the knuckles (Gottron's sign). (From Yamada, with permission.)

Dermatomyositis and Polymyositis

Robert Hendrickson

Diagnosis

Diagnosis can be made with a typical clinical history and confirmed with laboratory analysis and muscle/skin biopsy. A classification system with significant sensitivity and specificity is listed in Table 23–13.[3] The diagnosis can be made if the patient has more than four of the nine characteristics listed. Weakness is typically in proximal muscles; patients may have difficulty standing from a seated position, or they may use their arms to stand from a prone position (Gower's sign).[3]

Clinical Complications

Complications may be related to muscle weakness (proximal muscle weakness, respiratory muscle weakness, dysphagia, dysphonia), cardiac disease (cardiomyopathy, conduction defects), pulmonary disease (pneumonitis, fibrosis), or ocular disease (iritis, optic atrophy). In addition, patients with dermatomyositis have an increased risk of age-appropriate cancer in the 3 years after their diagnosis.[3]

TABLE 23–13 Criteria for the Diagnosis of Polymyositis and Dermatomyositis

At least four of the following criteria must be present for a diagnosis of polymyositis/dermatomyositis to be made:
1. Characteristic skin lesion: Heliotrope rash Gottron's papules or keratotic, atrophic erythema Raised purple, erythematous rash on extensor surfaces
2. Proximal muscle weakness
3. Elevated creatine phosphokinase or aldolase
4. Muscle pain on grasping
5. Myogenic changes on electromyography
6. Positive anti-Jo-1 antibody test
7. Nondestructive arthritis or arthralgias
8. Systemic inflammatory signs (fever, elevated C-reactive protein or ESR)
9. Pathologic findings of inflammatory myositis

From Choy EH, Isenberg DA. Treatment of dermatomyositis and polymyositis. *Rheumatology (Oxford)* 2002;41:7–13.

Management

Patients with significant weakness or dysphagia should be admitted to the hospital for intravenous (IV) corticosteroids and observation for aspiration. Patients with new symptoms of pain or weakness should be evaluated with a thorough history and physical examination for age-appropriate malignancies (e.g., testicular cancer in young men, breast cancer in older women, colon cancer in older men). Patients with mild findings may be treated with oral corticosteroids until muscle enzyme concentrations normalize. Arrangements should be made for follow-up with a primary care physician or rheumatologist for reevaluation. Chronic, refractory disease may be treated with methotrexate, cyclosporine, azathioprine, hydroxychloroquine, or cyclophosphamide. Consultation with a rheumatologist or the patient's primary care physician may be prudent when treating an exacerbation in a patient who is taking multiple medications.

REFERENCES

1. Callen JP. Dermatomyositis. *Lancet* 2000;355:53–57.
2. Koler RA, Montemarano A. Dermatomyositis. *Am Fam Physician* 2001;64:1565–1572.
3. Choy EH, Isenberg DA. Treatment of dermatomyositis and polymyositis. *Rheumatology (Oxford)* 2002;41:7–13.

23–14

Sjögren's Syndrome

Bjorn Miller

Clinical Presentation

Patients with Sjögren's syndrome present with "sicca complex": dry eyes, dry mouth, dry skin, and dry mucous membranes, including vaginal dryness. Myalgias and arthralgias are also common.[1,2]

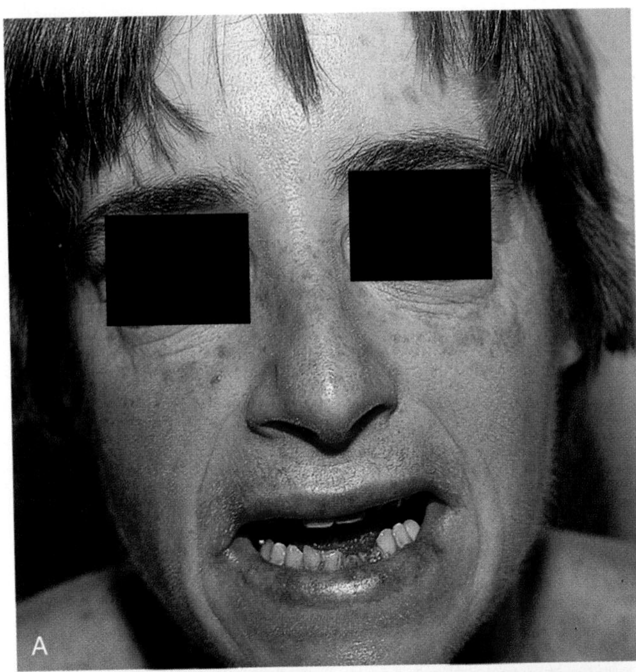

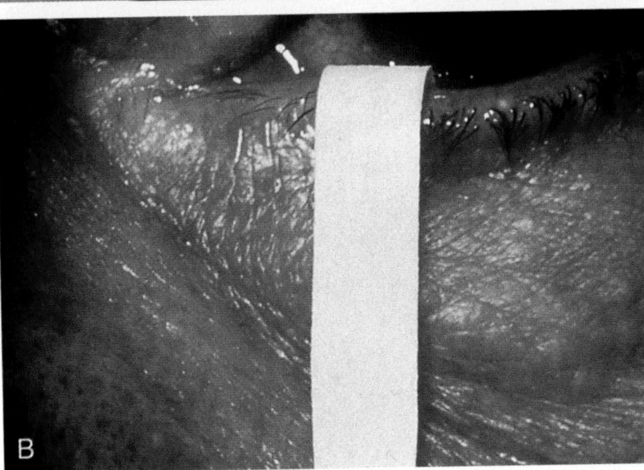

FIGURE 23–14 A: Sjögren's syndrome associated with systemic lupus erythematosus. Note dental decay caused by inadequate production of saliva. (From Ostler, with permission.) **B:** Schirmer test. In a patient with Sjögren's syndrome, a filter-paper wick is placed under the lower eyelid after application of a local anesthesic. After 5 minutes, the distance that the tears have migrated along the filter paper is measured. Healthy individuals have more than 5 mm of migration. In this patient, there are virtually no tears to migrate. (From Sontheimer, with permission.)

Pathophysiology

Sjögren's syndrome is a disease of the exocrine glands caused by immune cells attacking and destroying salivary and lacrimal glands. The exact origin of the autoimmune attack is not well-understood but possibly is related to genetic, hormonal, or viral causes.

Diagnosis

Peak incidence of disease onset is in the fourth or fifth decades of life, and there is a female preponderance. Diagnosis is made based on the clinical features of dry eyes and dry mouth and confirmed with salivary gland or lower-lip biopsy.[1] Patients have a positive antinuclear antibodies (ANA), but the more specific autoantibodies are the anti-SS-A (Ro) and anti-SS-B (La). The Schirmer test confirms the diagnosis by establishing a lack of tear film production on a test strip placed near the lower conjunctival tear sac.[1,2]

Clinical Complications

Complications may include chronic keratoconjunctivitis and corneal ulcers, dental caries, oral fissures, and dysphagia.[3] Ten percent of patients develop pseudolymphoma, and 1% develop non-Hodgkin's lymphoma.[1]

Management

Treatment is aimed at relieving symptoms of dryness with mouth gels and artificial tears. Pilocarpine and cevimeline (cholinergic agents that bind to muscarinic receptors) can increase salivary and lacrimal flow rates. Topical cyclosporine eye drops may decrease ocular inflammation and lessen symptoms. Resistant cases may be treated with hydroxychloroquine and corticosteroids to decrease systemic inflammation. Patients rarely need to be admitted to the hospital but do need prompt referral to a rheumatologist, ophthalmologist, and dentist.[1,2]

REFERENCES

1. Fox RI, Tornwall J, Maruyama T, Stern M. Evolving concepts of diagnosis, pathogenesis, and therapy of Sjögren's syndrome. *Cur Opin Rheumatol* 1998;10:446–456.
2. Gran JT. Diagnosis and definition of primary Sjögren's syndrome. *Scand J Rheumatol* 2002;31:57–59.
3. Moutsopoulos HM. Sjögren's syndrome therapy: future directions. *J Rheumatol* 1997;24[Suppl 50]:33–34.

Ankylosing Spondylitis

Bjorn Miller

Clinical Presentation

Patients with ankylosing spondylitis (AS) present with gradual onset of low back pain and tenderness over the sacroiliac joint. The pain is subtle and may be worse in the morning or after rest. The pain does improve with motion. AS most often affects the lumbar spine but can affect the thoracic or cervical spine as well.[1–3]

Pathophysiology

The cause of AS is not clear, but it is theorized that an infectious agent (*Klebsiella* spp.) in some way interacts with the HLA-B27 antigen to trigger the disease.[2]

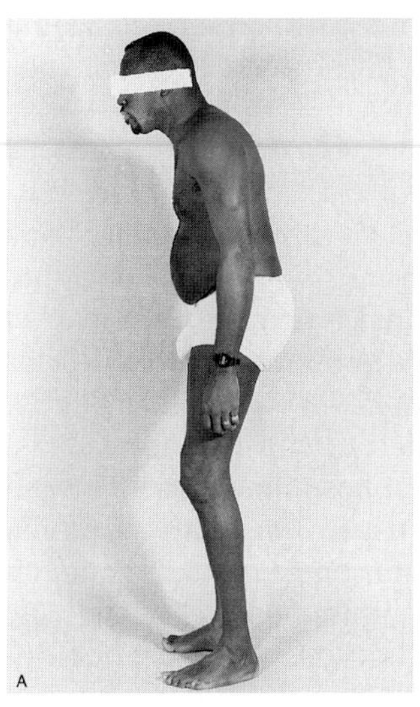

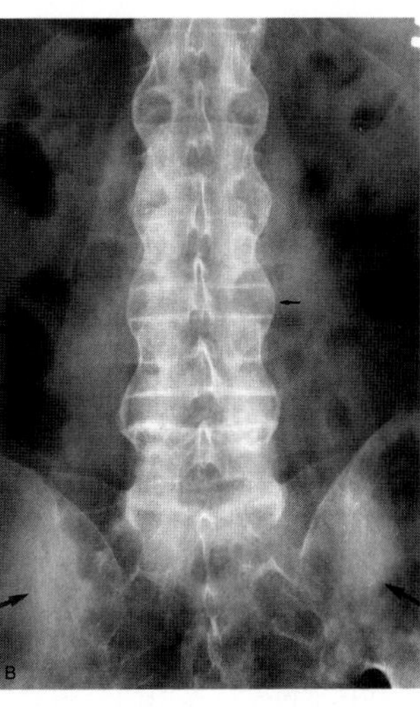

FIGURE 23–15 **A:** Typical posture of patient with advanced ankylosing spondylitis. **B:** Anteroposterior radiograph of the upper pelvis and lumber spine. Both sacroiliac joints *(large arrows)* are fused, and there are bilateral, symmetric syndesmophytes *(small arrow)*, resulting in the typical "bamboo" appearance of ankylosing spondylitis. (**A** and **B**, From Koopman, with permission.)

Diagnosis

AS affects the 15- to 30-year-old age group, with a male-to-female ratio of 3:1 and an increase in prevalence in the northern latitudes.[2] Diagnosis is made on a clinical basis and supported by radiographic studies. Between 90% and 95% of patients with AS have positive HLA-B27 antigen, but this a relatively nonspecific finding and there is no need to perform HLA-B27 type to establish the diagnosis. On radiography, patients have inflammation or fusion of their sacroiliac joint (the hallmark of AS), ossification of the anterior longitudinal ligament, and fusion of facet joints that can lead to "bamboo spine."[1,3]

Clinical Complications

Iritis and uveitis are the most common extraskeletal complications. In addition, aortitis, inflammatory bowel disease, amylodosis, pulmonary fibrosis, spinal stenosis, bony fractures, and C1–C2 subluxation may occur.[1,3]

Management

Patients with AS rarely need to be admitted to the hospital and should be referred to a primary care physician or orthopedist for further evaluation and treatment. Treatment is aimed at relieving pain, increasing mobility, and preventing spinal deformity and disability. Pain may be treated with nonsteroidal antiinflammatory drugs (NSAIDs), sulfasalazine, corticosteroids, or methotrexate.[3]

REFERENCES

1. van der Linden S, van der Heijde D. Ankylosing spondylitis: clinical features. *Rheum Dis Clin North Am* 1998;24:663–676.
2. Bakker C, Boers M, van der Linden S. Measures to assess ankylosing spondylitis: taxonomy, review, and recommendations *J Rheumatol* 1993;20:1724–1730.
3. Olivieri I, Cantini F, Salvarani C. Diagnostic and classification criteria, clinical and functional assessment, and therapeutic advancement for spondyloarthropathies *Curr Opin Rheumatol* 1997;9: 284–290.

Paget's Disease of the Bone

Robert Hendrickson

Clinical Presentation

Patients with Paget's disease may present with symptoms that relate to disordered bone matrix (pathologic fractures [8%], bony deformities), bony growth (nerve or spinal compression [1%], hearing loss [6%]), or pain in joints and bones [86%].[1]

Pathophysiology

Paget's disease of the bone, or osteitis deformans, is a disease of disordered bone growth and remodeling.

The cause of Paget's disease is not clearly understood, but theories include genetic causes (more common in North America and Europe, autosomal dominant inheritance) and viral causes (respiratory syncytial virus, paramyxovirus, measles).[2,3] Increases in osteoclast and osteoblast activity result in increased production of poor-quality, disordered bone matrix.

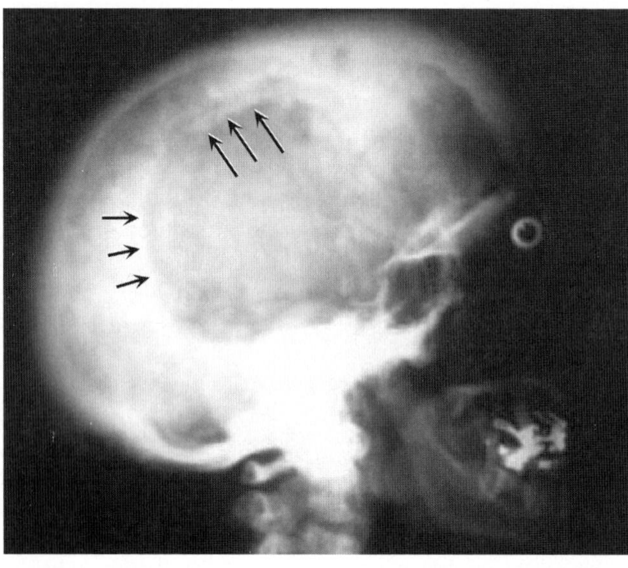

FIGURE 23–16 Lateral radiograph shows the thickened skull and osteoporosis circumscripta of both lateral temporal bones *(short arrows on the right, long arrows on the left)*. (From Koopman, with permission.)

Diagnosis

The diagnosis can be made radiographically by observation of localized enlargement of bone, typically in the pelvis, lumbar spine, skull, or long bones.[1,2] Radiographic features include "flame-shaped" lesions proximal to the distal epiphyses of long bones.[1] Serum alkaline phosphatase may be elevated in 85% of cases, but serum calcium and phosphorus levels typically are normal.[1,2]

Clinical Complications

Clinical complications are related to bony overgrowth with compression of nerves (paralysis, neurologic deficits, hearing loss), disordered bone (pathologic fractures, gross bony deformities with loss of function), destruction of joints, and pain.[2] In addition, malignant transformation may occur in 0.7% to 0.9% of patients, most commonly osteosarcoma.[3]

Management

Patients with suspected Paget's disease of the bone should be referred to a primary care physician or orthopedist for further evaluation and treatment. Pain may be treated with nonsteroidal antiinflammatory drugs (NSAIDs). Patients with acute nerve or spinal entrapment should have urgent referral with probable admission for intravenous (IV) bisphosphonate therapy and possible surgery. Treatment usually includes calcitonin and bisphosphonates (e.g., etidronate, pamidronate, alendronate), both of which inhibit osteoclast activity. Additional therapy may include plicamycin, which inhibits RNA synthesis, and gallium nitrate, which inhibits the osteoclast adenosine triphosphatase–dependent proton pump.[2,3]

REFERENCES

1. Ankrom MA, Shapiro JR. Paget's disease of bone (osteitis deformans). *J Am Geriatr Soc* 1998;46:1025–1033.
2. Delmas PD, Meunier PJ. Drug therapy: the management of Paget's disease of bone. *N Engl J Med* 1997;336:558–566.
3. Hadjipavlou AG, Gaitanis IN, Kontakis GM. Paget's disease of the bone and its management. *J Bone Joint Surg Br* 2002;84:160–169.

Scleroderma and Systemic Sclerosis

Robert Hendrickson

Clinical Presentation

The clinical presentation of systemic sclerosis is heterogenous and may range from mild, localized skin fibrosis or Raynaud's phenomenon to systemic fibrosis with renal hypertension, pulmonary fibrosis, and pulmonary hypertension.[1]

Pathophysiology

Systemic sclerosis is a connective tissue disorder that leads to fibrosis of the skin and internal organs.

Systemic sclerosis results from genetically mediated alterations in the inflammatory cascade that lead to diffuse fibrosis. Patients with systemic sclerosis develop a loss of the typical inhibitory influences of fibrosis, elevations of interleukins (IL-1, -4, and -6), and growth factors (platelet-derived growth factor, transforming growth factor-β) that lead to unregulated fibrosis of multiple organs.[1]

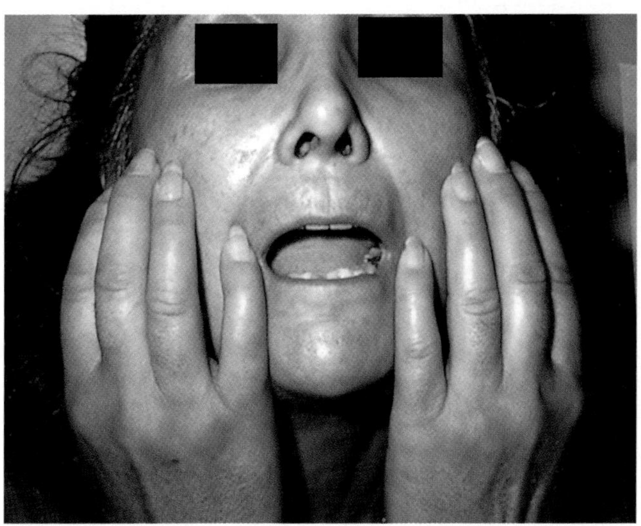

FIGURE 23–17 Acrosclerosis (note shiny, tight skin over fingers) and decreased ability to open the mouth in systemic scleroderma. (From Ostler, with permission.)

Diagnosis

The diagnosis may be made clinically by noting the typical skin findings. Eighty percent of patients with systemic sclerosis have elevated antinuclear antibodies (ANA).[2] Additional autoantibody testing may predict poor (anti-SC170) or more favorable (anti-centromere) outcomes.[2]

Clinical Complications

Complications of systemic sclerosis include pulmonary hypertension, pulmonary fibrosis, digital necrosis (secondary to Raynaud's phenomenon), renal hypertensive crisis, and progressive fibrosis of the skin.[1]

Management

Patients with new-onset systemic sclerosis may present to the emergency department (ED) with early signs of the disease (Raynaud's phenomenon, skin "tightness"). Referral to a rheumatologist or primary doctor usually is all that is necessary in these cases. Patients with a history of systemic sclerosis may be treated with a variety of immunosuppressive agents (cyclosporin, methotrexate, cyclophosphamide, azathioprine, chlorambucil) and antifibrotic agents (D-penicillamine, interferon-alpha, interferon-gamma). Patients presenting to the ED with complications of their disease may be treated symptomatically with omeprazole for reflux, prostacyclin for refractory Raynaud's phenomenon, or angiotensin-converting enzyme (ACE) inhibitors and corticosteroids for hypertensive crisis.[1]

REFERENCES

1. Systemic sclerosis: current pathogenetic concepts and future prospects for targeted therapy. *Lancet* 1996;347:1453–1458.
2. Murray KJ, Laxer RM. Scleroderma in children and adolescents. *Rheum Dis Clin North Am* 2002;28:603–624.

Raynaud's Phenomenon

Robert Hendrickson

Clinical Presentation

Raynaud's phenomenon may be primary, or it may be secondary to an autoimmune disorder (scleroderma, systemic lupus erythematosus [SLE], Sjögren's syndrome, dermatomyositis, polymyositis, or rheumatoid arthritis [RA]) or to chronic exposure to mechanical vibration (e.g., jackhammer operators).[1] Patients classically report initial acute, well-demarcated pallor of the digits that progresses to painful cyanosis and, finally, to red flushing and pain on reperfusion. Symptoms may vary, and cyanosis is somewhat rare. Patients with secondary Raynaud's phenomenon usually are older at symptom onset and have more severe symptoms and complications.[2] In addition, patients with secondary Raynaud's phenomenon more commonly have dilatation of the capillary bed at the base of the fingernails.[2] This dilatation may occasionally be visualized with the naked eye, but visualization is enhanced with the use of a lens (e.g., ophthalmoscope).

Pathophysiology

Raynaud's phenomenon is characterized by episodic vasospasm of the distal digits.

Vasospasm may occur secondary to several factors: alteration of endothelial vascular regulation (e.g., prostaglandins, cytokines, nitric oxide release), alteration of α_2-receptor response, hormonal effects (female predominance), and genetics.[1]

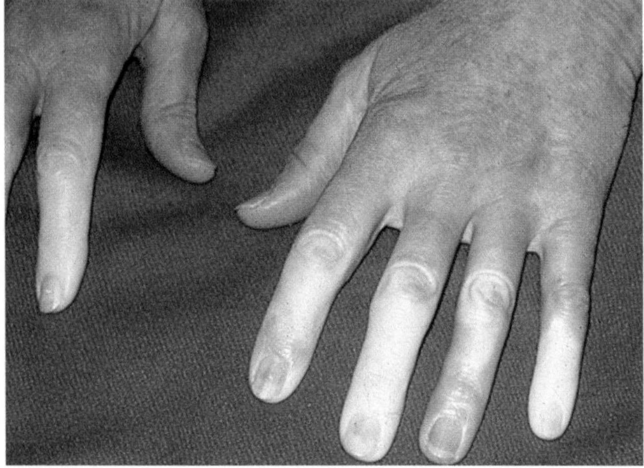

FIGURE 23–18 Raynaud's phenomenon with vasoconstriction. (From Sontheimer, with permission.)

Diagnosis

The symptoms of Raynaud's phenomenon often resolve before presentation to the emergency department (ED). The diagnosis may rely on recognition of the typical clinical features. Risk factors for Raynaud's phenomenon are female sex, family history, and residence in cold climates.[1]

Clinical Complications

Prolonged vasospasm may lead to ischemia, necrosis, and autoamputation of digits.

Management

The primary role of the emergency physician is to recognize undiagnosed autoimmune disorders or medications that may be associated with Raynaud's phenomenon. Diagnostic testing may be performed in consultation with a rheumatologist or primary care physician, and may include testing for anti-centromere antibodies (specific for primary Raynaud's phenomenon), anti-Smith antibody (SLE), anti-topoisomerase, and anti-RNA polymerase (scleroderma). Patients with elevated antinuclear antibodies (ANA) have a higher risk of progressing to a systemic inflammatory disease.[1] Patients with mild symptoms, a normal erythrocyte sedimentation rate, and normal serology findings have a low risk of developing an autoimmune disorder. Medications that are associated with Raynaud's phenomenon are bleomycin, vinblastine, polyvinyl chloride, β-blockers, clonidine, ergot alkaloids, methysergide, interferons-α and -β, and tegafur.[1,2]

Patients without active symptoms should see a rheumatologist or primary care physician as an outpatient, should avoid cold exposure and dress warmly (not just cover the hands), and should be instructed to avoid smoking, cocaine, amphetamines, β-blockers, caffeine, ergots, and decongestants.[1] Patients with active symptoms may be treated with topical nitrates, oral nifedipine, and angiotensin-converting enzyme inhibitors. Prostacyclin and iloprost infusions have been used, but their efficacy remains controversial.[1] Occasionally, vasospasm leads to thrombosis, and heparin may be necessary.

REFERENCES

1. Block JA, Sequeira W. Raynaud's phenomenon. *Lancet* 2001;357: 2042–2048.
2. Wigley FM. Raynaud's phenomenon. *N Engl J Med* 2002;347: 1001–1008.

Ehlers-Danlos Syndrome

Bjorn Miller

Clinical Presentation

Abnormal collagen results in skin hyperextensibility, with a soft and doughy feel. The skin tends to be fragile, heals poorly, and is associated with hematomas, easy bruising, and wide scars. The joints are hypermobile, leading to frequent dislocations and arthralgias. Bones are typically osteoporotic, predisposing to fractures and scoliosis. Because arteries tend to be fragile, patients are at risk for various aneurysms. Hernias, diverticula, and pes planus are rare occurrences.[1]

Pathophysiology

Ehlers-Danlos syndrome (EDS) is a group of connective tissue disorders caused by a genetic defect in collagen metabolism that results in abnormal connective tissue synthesis and structure.

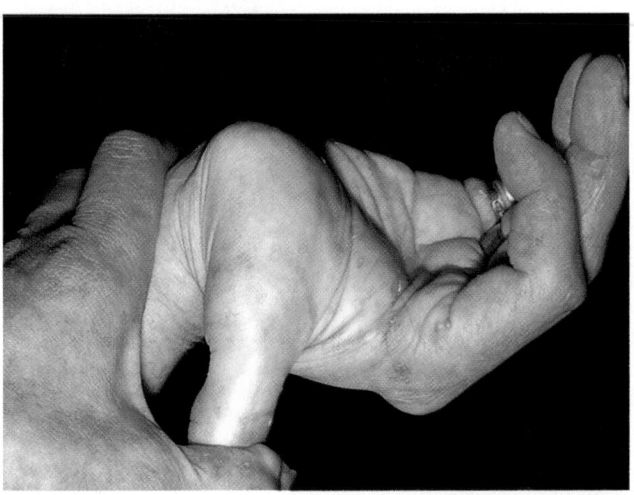

FIGURE 23-19 Ehlers-Danlos syndrome, demonstrating hyperextensible joints. (From Ostler, with permission.)

There are 10 phenotypes of EDS, but all involve abnormalities in synthesis and metabolism of collagen. Collagen is a vital constituent of connective tissue, and the abnormal connective tissue of EDS leads to defects in strength, elasticity, integrity, and healing properties of tissues.[2]

Diagnosis

The diagnosis is made on clinical grounds based on the history and physical examination of the patient.

Clinical Complications

Complications include mitral valve prolapse (MVP), premature births, bowel rupture, arterial rupture, retinal detachments, scoliosis, and dental problems.[1,2]

Management

Referral to various appropriate specialists is advisable. Few effective treatments are available. Patients should be advised to avoid heavy lifting and exercise, so as not to put additional strain on the joints. Some suggest vitamin C therapy to improve wound healing.[3]

REFERENCES

1. Grahame R. Joint hypermobility and genetic collagen disorders: are they related? *Arch Dis Child* 1999;80:188–191.
2. Mao JR, Bristow J. The Ehlers-Danlos syndrome: on beyond collagens. *J Clin Invest* 2001;107:1063–1069.
3. Beighton P, De Paepe A, Steinmann B, Tsipouras P, Wenstrup RJ. Ehlers-Danlos syndromes: revised nosology, Villefranche, 1997. *Am J Med Genet* 1998;77:31–37.

23–20

Marfan's Syndrome

Bjorn Miller

Clinical Presentation

Patients with Marfan's syndrome (MFS) typically exhibit a tall, thin stature with long limbs compared to trunk (ratio of arm span to height, greater than 1.05). MFS may include pectus excavatum (66%), scoliosis (62%), thoracic lordosis, pes planus (25%), and joint laxity. There is frequently a narrow, high-arched palate, causing crowded dentition. Heart murmurs may be found on examination secondary to valvular heart disease, such as mitral valve prolapse (MVP) or aortic regurgitation. Ocular involvement includes lens subluxation (ectopia lentis), myopia, and corneal flatness. Patients may complain of back pain secondary to dural ectasia (63%), which is a ballooning of the dural sac that most commonly affects the lumbar region.[1,2]

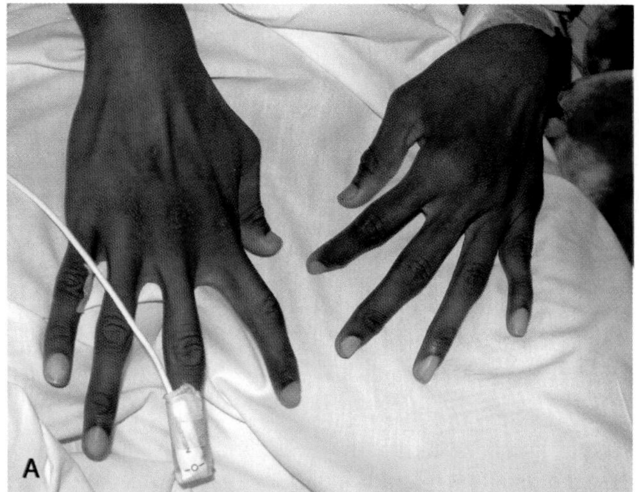

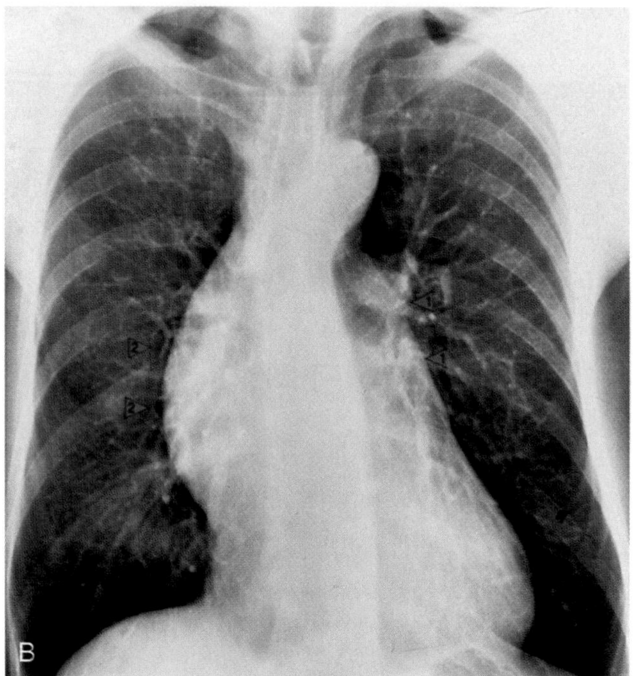

FIGURE 23–20 **A:** Arachnyldactyl digits in Marfan's syndrome. Patient presented with heart failure secondary to a 9-cm wide aortic arch. (Courtesy of Mark Silverberg, MD) **B:** Chest radiograph showing aortic root aneurysm in a 20-year-old man with Marfan's syndrome. Note the enlargement of the ascending aorta to the left *(arrows 1)* and right *(arrows 2)*, which produces a widened mediastinal image. (From Kassner, with permission.)

Pathophysiology

Patients have decreased structural integrity of connective tissue and elastin secondary to mutations (135 mutations have been identified) in the fibrillin-1 gene on chromosome 15.[1]

Diagnosis

MFS occurs in 1 in 10,000 of the U.S. population. Diagnosis is based on history and examination. Seventy-five percent of patients have an affected parent, but 15% of cases occur secondary to new sporadic mutation.[1] Chest radiography, echocardiogram, echocardiography, and eye examination are helpful adjunctive tests.

Clinical Complications

Complications include aortic dilatation (70% to 80% of cases) and subsequent aortic dissection. Between 55% and 70% of patients have MVP, possibly leading to mitral regurgitation. Fifty percent of patients develop ectopia lentis, and a few have spontaneous retinal detachment. Orthopedic complications include pes planus, scoliosis (60%), pectus excavatum, and pectus carinatum. A rare manifestation is spontaneous pneumothorax, secondary to apical blebs.[1-3]

Management

Chronic therapy for MFS may require β-blockers or calcium-channel blockers to delay aortic expansion and decrease the risk of aortic dissection.

REFERENCES

1. Giampietro PF, Raggio C, Davis JG. Marfan syndrome: orthopedic and genetic review. *Curr Opin Pediatr* 2002;14:35–41.
2. Pyeritz RE. The Marfan syndrome. *Ann Rev Med* 2000;51:481–510.
3. De Paepe A, Devereux RB, Dietz HC, Hennekam RC, Pyeritz RE. Revised diagnostic criteria for the Marfan syndrome. *Am J Med Genet* 1996;62:417–426.

SECTION IV

TOXICOLOGIC AND ENVIRONMENTAL EMERGENCIES

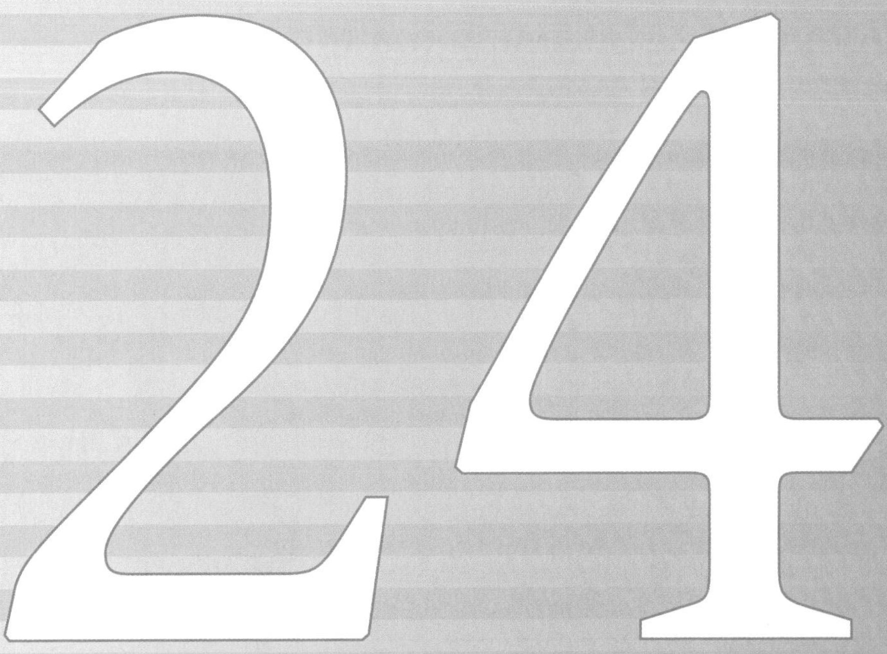

Toxicologic

24–1

Gastrointestinal Decontamination

Anthony Morocco

The appropriate use of gastrointestinal decontamination after potentially harmful ingestions remains controversial.[1–5] Modalities include single- and multi-dose activated charcoal (AC), gastric lavage, cathartics, and whole-bowel irrigation (WBI). All of these techniques have theoretical value in limiting absorption of poisons, but little or no evidence exists for improved outcomes.

Ipecac is an emetic agent used for gastric emptying. This drug is now rarely used, because its administration can cause prolonged vomiting, aspiration, and esophageal injury.[1]

Orogastric lavage involves the use of a large tube (32F to 40F in adults or 22F to 24F in children) in an attempt to retrieve intact pills or pill fragments from the stomach. The stomach is flushed with aliquots of water until a clear effluent is obtained. Potential complications include aspiration and injury to the oropharynx, esophagus, or stomach.[2]

AC adsorbs most chemicals in the gut and prevents absorption. This is considered an important treatment for most ingestions. Multi-dose AC involves repeated doses given every 2 to 4 hours. AC administration may result in vomiting and aspiration or bowel obstruction.[3,4] One dose of a cathartic, such as sorbitol, may speed the movement of substances through the gastrointestinal tract, but sorbitol should not be used alone or in multiple doses.

WBI uses polyethylene glycol electrolyte solution (PEG-ES) to cleanse the bowel of toxic agents before they are absorbed. The dose is 1 to 2 L/hour via nasogastric tube in adults, 1 L/hour in children ages 6 to 12 years, and 500 mL/hour in children ages 9 months to 6 years, given until rectal effluent is clear. WBI is used in the setting of ingestion of enteric-coated or sustained-release preparations. Nausea, vomiting, and abdominal pain may occur.[5]

REFERENCES

1. Krenzelok EP, McGuigan M, Lheur P. Position statement: ipecac syrup. *J Toxicol Clin Toxicol* 1997;35:699–709.
2. Vale JA. Position statement: gastric lavage. *J Toxicol Clin Toxicol* 1997;35:711–719.
3. Chyka PA, Seger D. Position statement: single-dose activated charcoal. *J Toxicol Clin Toxicol* 1997;35:721–741.
4. Chyka PA, Seger D. Position statement and practice guidelines on the use of multi-dose activated charcoal in the treatment of acute poisoning. *J Toxicol Clin Toxicol* 1999;37:731–751.
5. Tenenbein M. Position statement: whole bowel irrigation. *J Toxicol Clin Toxicol* 1997;35:753–762.

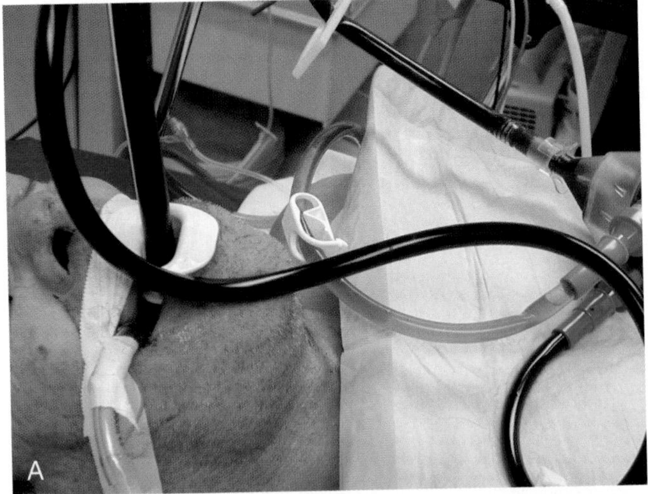

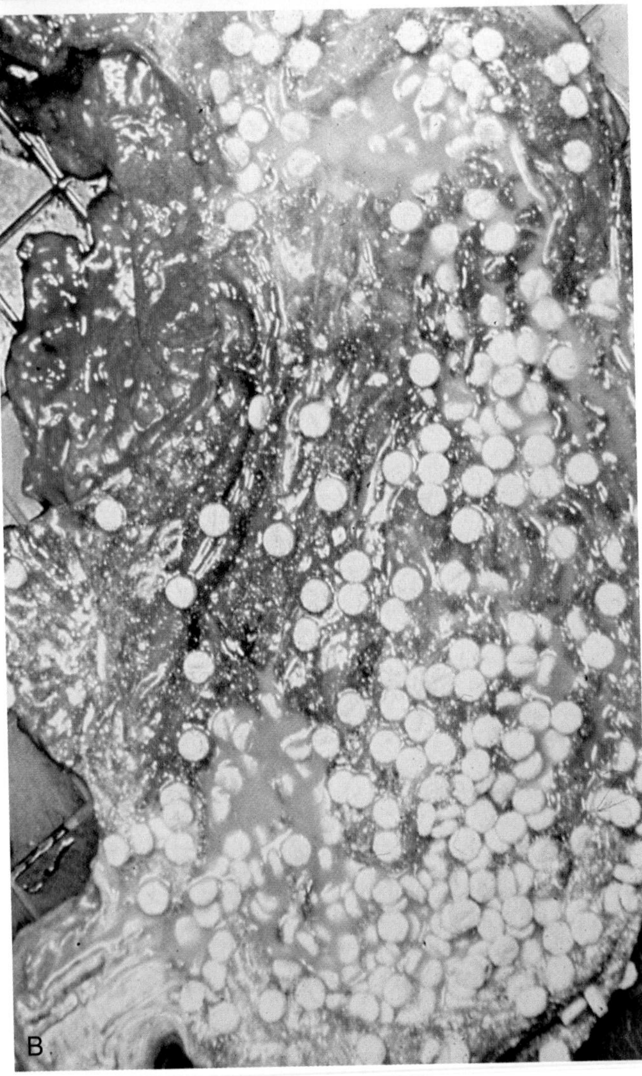

FIGURE 24–1 **A:** Gastric lavage. (Courtesy of Robert Hendrickson, MD.) **B:** Gross autopsy specimen of stomach with multiple pills adherent to the gastric wall. (Copyright James R. Roberts, MD.)

Caustic Ingestion: Alkali

Gregory Schneider

Clinical Presentation

Signs of caustic alkali ingestion include injury to the lips, oral mucosa, tongue, and pharynx. With intentional ingestions, if liquids are gulped quickly, there may be relative sparing of the oral and pharyngeal mucosa.[1]

Pathophysiology

Alkali substances cause injury by liquefaction necrosis. Ingestion of a substance with a pH of 12 or greater often involves drain cleaners, other cleansers, household bleach, Clinitest tablets, or button batteries. The extent of the injury is determined by four factors: the pH of the material, the amount ingested, solid versus liquid form, and the duration of exposure. In the first 24 to 48 hours, tissue damage is aggravated by bacterial invasion. Strictures may result 4 to 6 weeks after exposure.[2]

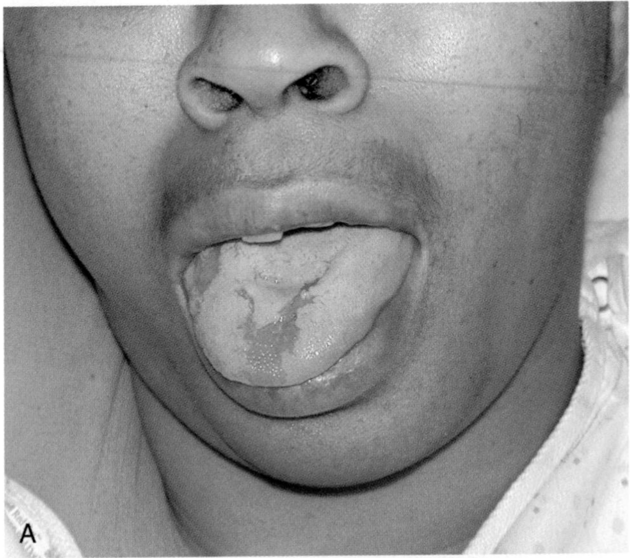

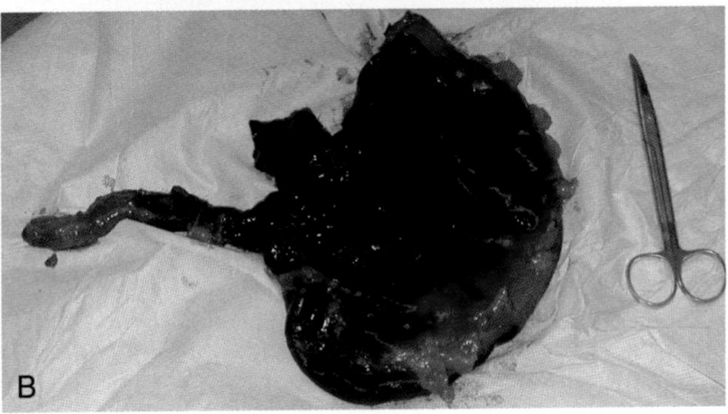

FIGURE 24–2 A: Alkaline burn of the tongue after ingestion of sodium hydroxide. (Courtesy of Robert Hendrickson, MD.) **B:** Extensive necrosis of gastrointestinal tract after ingestion of caustic liquid. (Courtesy of William Hughes, MD, and Laura Spivak, MD.)

Diagnosis

Diagnosis of alkali ingestion is made by a careful history and physical examination. It is important to determine the substance ingested, when and how much was ingested, and whether the ingestion was deliberate or accidental.[1–3]

Clinical Complications

Extensive mucosal damage leads to fever, tachypnea, tachycardia, hypotension, and shock. Perforations of the esophagus and stomach, leading to mediastinal or peritoneal abscess, sepsis, and death, have occurred. Aspiration pneumonia, burns of the epiglottis and vocal cords, and laryngeal obstruction may also occur. Long-term sequelae include esophageal stricture, vocal cord paralysis, and pyloric stenosis.[3]

Management

Dilution with milk or water should be initiated rapidly. Attempts to prevent vomiting are important to avoid reintroduction of the substance into the esophagus and oropharynx. Asymptomatic patients should be observed for 4 to 6 hours. Patients ingesting bleach have a low incidence of serious injury. Patients with refusal to swallow, nausea, vomiting, abdominal pain, drooling, coughing, dysphagia, stridor, or oral burns should be admitted to the hospital for possible endoscopy and observation.[3] Endoscopy should occur within 24 hours to determine the extent of injury and subsequent treatment. Steroid treatment remains controversial and should not be initiated until the extent of the injury is determined.[1]

REFERENCES

1. Wason S. The emergency management of caustic ingestions. *J Emerg Med* 1985;2:175–182.
2. de Jong AL, Macdonald R, Ein S, et al. Corrosive esophagitis in children: a 30-year review. *Int J Pediatr Otorhinolaryngol* 2001;57:203–211.
3. Gorman RL, Khin-Maung-Gyi MT, Klein-Schwartz W, et al. Initial symptoms as predictors of esophageal injury in alkaline corrosive ingestions. *Am J Emerg Med* 1992;10:189–194.

Caustic Ingestion: Acid

Gregory Schneider

Clinical Presentation

Patients with caustic acid ingestion complain of pain in the oropharynx, esophagus, and abdomen. Other early signs include drooling, excessive salivation, and refusal to swallow. Burns may be seen on the lips, skin, and oropharynx. The intent of the injury must be determined, because suicidal and intentional ingestions are more commonly associated with serious injury.[1]

Pathophysiology

Acids produce coagulation necrosis that tends to limit the extent of the injury by preventing penetration of the acid into the tissue. Compared with alkali ingestions, acids cause less damage to the esophagus and more damage to the stomach and small intestine.[1] Injury severity is determined by the pH and quantity of the substance, as well as the amount of time spent in the stomach. Pyloric spasm, antral mucosal edema, inflammation, and, ultimately, pyloric stricture may occur after acid ingestion.[2] Peritonitis and intestinal perforation are not uncommon.[1]

Diagnosis

Once it is determined that a corrosive ingestion has occurred, it becomes urgent to determine the extent of the injury. A complete blood count, electrolyte panel (including calcium, magnesium, and phosphate levels), upright chest radiograph (looking for perforation), arterial blood gas determination, and electrocardiography should all be performed.[1-3]

Clinical Complications

Metabolic derangements reported include metabolic acidosis, hyperkalemia, hypocalcemia, and hypomagnesemia. Disseminated intravascular coagulation after acid ingestion has been reported.[1-3]

Management

Dilution with water or milk should be initiated immediately. If perforation is suspected, a laparotomy should be performed to determine the viability of the stomach. Stable patients should be evaluated endoscopically. Hydrofluoric acid may bind calcium and magnesium, leading to serious electrolyte disorders. Aggressive repletion of calcium and magnesium should be initiated empirically.[3]

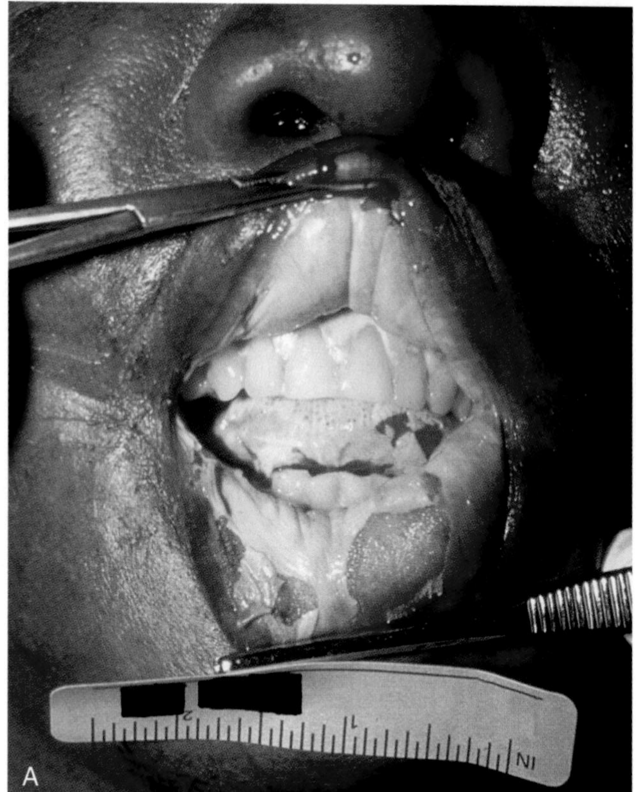

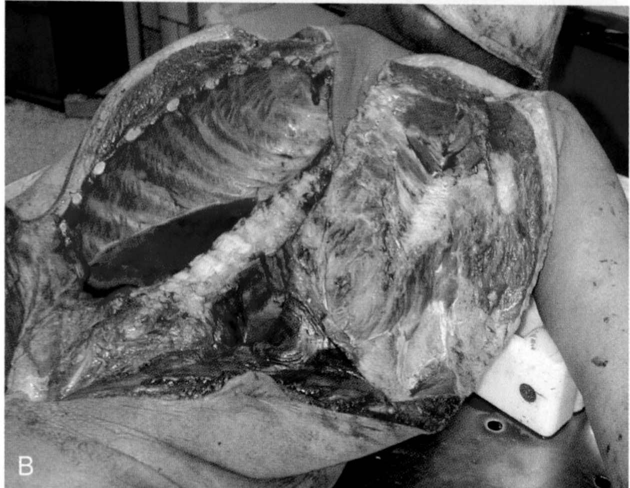

FIGURE 24–3 **A:** Postmortem oral burns in a patient who drank battery acid. **B:** Postmortem internal abdominal wall burns in a patient who drank battery acid. (**A** and **B**, Courtesy of Mark Su, MD.)

REFERENCES

1. Wason S. The emergency management of caustic ingestions. *J Emerg Med* 1985;2:175–182.
2. Gun F, Abbasoglu L, Celik A. Acute gastric perforation after acid ingestion. *J Pediatr Gastroentrol Nutr* 2002;35:360–362.
3. Yu-Jang S, Li-Hua L, Wai-Mau C, et al. Survival after a massive hydrofluoric acid ingestion with ECG changes. *Am J Emerg Med* 2001; 19:458–460.

Body Stuffing

Anthony Morocco

Clinical Presentation

The term "body stuffing" refers to the practice of hastily ingesting illicit drugs in order to dispose of evidence. In contrast to body packers, who swallow carefully packaged drugs for smuggling, body stuffers may swallow substances that are unwrapped or loosely wrapped in plastic, balloons, paper, or aluminum foil.[1,2] Consequently, these patients are at high risk for drug absorption and subsequent toxicity.

Patients typically ingest the drug when confronted by police, who subsequently bring suspects to the hospital for treatment. Patients often deny ingestion or give an inaccurate history concerning the amount ingested. Most patients are asymptomatic. If the body stuffing goes undetected by police, symptoms may occur while the patient is in jail. These symptoms may be unexplained at the time of presentation. With cocaine and other sympathomimetic agents, agitation, tachycardia, seizures, and ventricular dysrhythmias occur. Heroin results in decreased level of consciousness, miosis, and hypoventilation.

Diagnosis

The diagnosis can be difficult due to an inaccurate or absent history. Drug ingestion should be strongly suspected in any patient who is brought from jail with loss of consciousness, seizure, agitation, or cardiopulmonary arrest. Plain radiography is unlikely to show drug packets in small radiolucent packaging. Contrast-enhanced studies may be more helpful. A positive urine immunoassay drug screen may signify recent exposure to the drug but is not useful in confirming or ruling out drug-packet ingestion.

Clinical Complications

Patients may develop rapid onset of seizures, coma, and death. Symptoms may be delayed for hours after ingestion due to delayed liberation of the drug from its packaging.

Management

Patients should be given oral activated charcoal and placed on a cardiac monitor. Further management is controversial, because most patients remain asymptomatic.[1] Given the possibility of delayed toxicity and retained drug packets in the gut, whole-bowel irrigation with polyethylene glycol and admission to the intensive care unit for 24 hours of observation should be considered. Patients with symptoms of heroin ingestion should be treated with naloxone infusion. Cocaine toxicity is treated with benzodiazepines for sympathomimetic symptoms, vasodilators such as nitroprusside or phentolamine for hypertension, and, potentially, surgical retrieval of packages.[1,2]

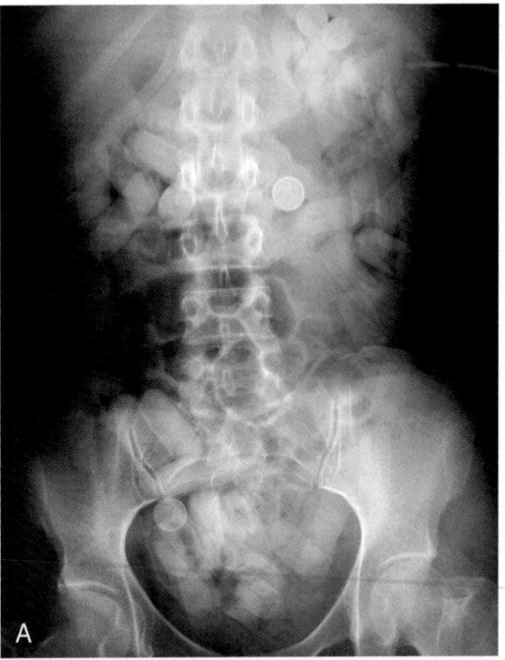

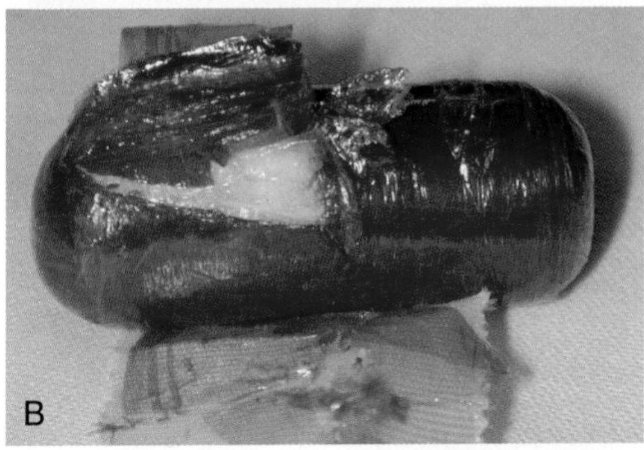

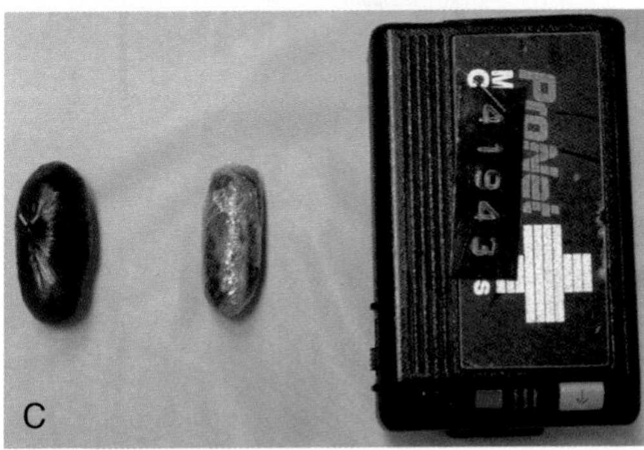

FIGURE 24–4 A: Abdominal radiograph revealing multiple packets containing cocaine. (Courtesy of Anthony Morocco, MD.) **B:** Drug packet containing cocaine. (Courtesy of Anthony Morocco, MD.) **C:** Packets containing hash. (Courtesy of Robert Hendrickson, MD.)

REFERENCES

1. June R, Aks SE, Keys N, et al. Medical outcome of cocaine bodystuffers. *J Emerg Med* 2000;18:221–224.
2. Sporer KA, Firestone J. Clinical course of crack cocaine body stuffers. *Ann Emerg Med* 1997;29:596–601.

Smoke Inhalation

Anthony Morocco

Clinical Presentation

Patients with smoke exposure may present with symptoms of mucous membrane and upper airway irritation, including burning eyes, cough, and shortness of breath, as well as signs and symptoms of lower respiratory tract injury, including dyspnea, chest pain, and hemoptysis. In severe cases, they may present with respiratory distress or apnea, loss of consciousness, and, in some cases, concomitant cutaneous burns. Hallmarks of inhalation injury include the production of soot-stained sputum and singed nasal or facial hair.[1]

Pathophysiology

Smoke inhalation is the primary cause of death for fire victims. Smoke contains a variety of chemicals, depending on the burning material. These include carbon monoxide, carbon dioxide, acrolein, cyanide, phosgene, sulfur dioxide, nitrogen oxides, particulates (soot), and other substances. Patients who sustain cutaneous burns with concomitant smoke-related injury are more likely to die.[1,2]

Smoke exposure may result in respiratory system dysfunction by direct thermal injury, neutrophil-mediated production of free radicals and inflammatory mediators, destruction of lung surfactant, bronchospasm, airway edema, bronchorrhea, and ciliary dysfunction. Harmful chemical gases act by causing asphyxiation, systemic toxicity, or direct lung injury.[1]

Diagnosis

Injury from smoke inhalation should be suspected in any patient who has been exposed to a fire in a closed space, particularly if the patient exhibits respiratory or airway-related symptoms, singed facial or nasal hair, or carbonaceous sputum. Chest radiographic findings may include patchy atelectasis and global interstitial and alveolar infiltrates. These developments may be delayed for 24 to 36 hours. Bronchoscopy, pulmonary function tests, and ventilation-perfusion scanning may help to assess the extent of lung injury. Venous blood should be obtained for carboxyhemoglobin and cyanide concentrations, and arterial blood gases may need to be assessed frequently.[1]

Clinical Complications

Acute complications include death, severe lung injury, acute respiratory distress syndrome, pneumonia, and various thermal injuries.[1] Chronic lung sequelae include reactive airway disease, bronchitis, and fibrosis.

Management

Most patients with smoke inhalation require hospitalization. Initial treatment is directed to the maintenance of a patent airway. Early endotracheal intubation should be considered for patients with potential airway injury, as evidenced by severe or progressive respiratory difficulties, significant facial or neck burns, or upper airway

Smoke Inhalation

Anthony Morocco

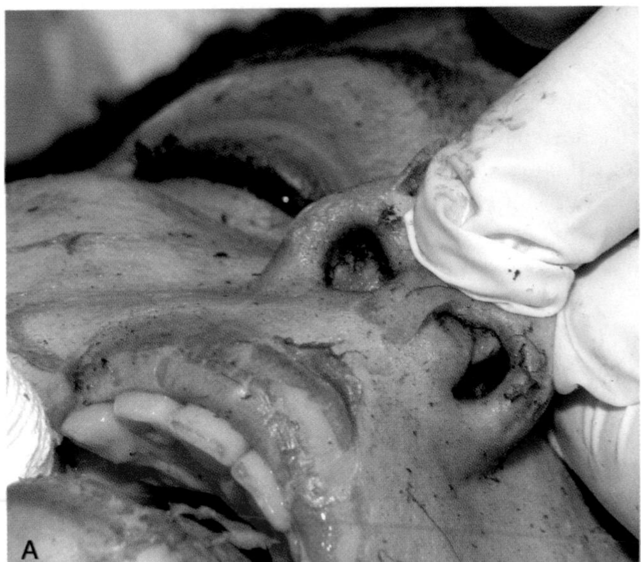

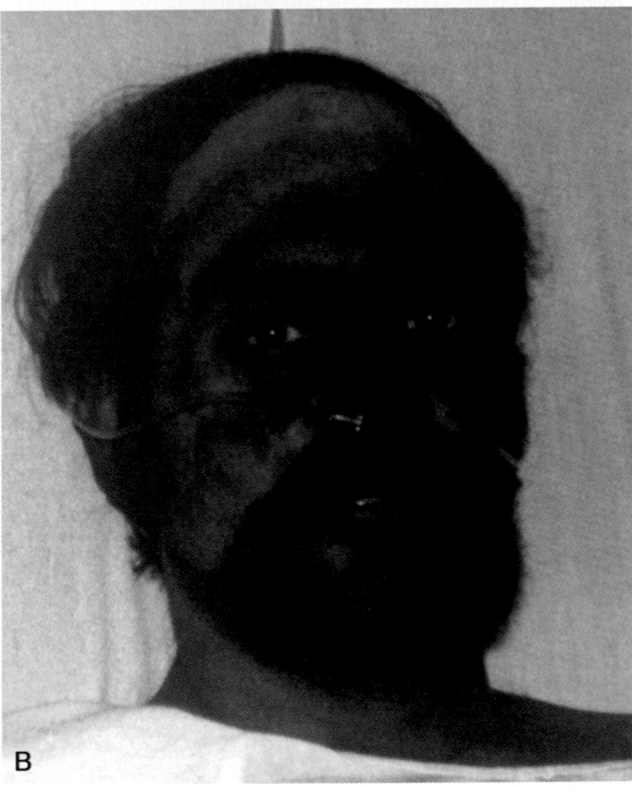

FIGURE 24–5 **A:** Singed nasal hairs. (© David Effron, MD, 2004. Used with permission.) **B:** Soot-stained face. (Courtesy of Michael Greenberg, MD.)

edema. Supportive care should include humidified oxygen, aggressive fluid resuscitation, bronchodilators, and pulmonary toilet. Prophylactic antibiotics and steroids are not indicated. Specific treatments for carbon monoxide (hyperbaric oxygen) and cyanide (nitrites, thiosulfate) may be required.[1]

REFERENCES

1. Lee-Chiong TL Jr. Smoke inhalation injury. *Postgrad Med* 1999;105: 55–62.
2. Nguyen, TT, Gilpin DA, Meyer NA, et al. Current treatment of severely burned patients. *Ann Surg* 1996;223:14–25.

24-6

Inhalant Abuse

Anthony Morocco

Clinical Presentation

Acute inhalant intoxication may appear to be similar to ethanol inebriation, with ataxia, slurred speech, and nystagmus. Chronic users may exhibit nonspecific symptoms such as headaches, dizziness, loss of appetite, and cough. Emergency care may be sought only after sudden loss of consciousness and cardiac arrest.[1]

Pathophysiology

Inhalant abuse involves the breathing of volatile substances in order to experience a euphoric effect. Methods of inhalation include breathing a product directly from its container or a surface ("sniffing" or "snorting"), from a soaked rag placed over the face ("huffing"), or from a bag filled with a volatile substance ("bagging"). Twenty percent of adolescents report having tried inhalants by eighth grade.[1] Commonly abused substances include paint thinner, airplane glue, spray paint, lighter fluid, hair spray, correction fluid, and nail polish remover. Specific substances include toluene, butane, propane, fluorocarbons, chlorinated hydrocarbons, and acetone.[1]

The mechanism of action of inhalants is unknown, but they are believed to act in the central nervous system in a manner similar to volatile anesthetic agents. Hydrocarbons are known to sensitize the myocardium to the arrhythmogenic effects of catecholamines.

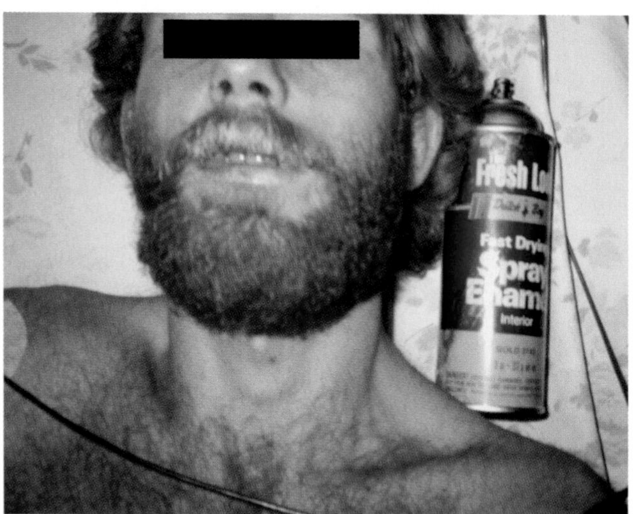

FIGURE 24-6 Gold paint on the mouth and mustache of a patient who died after huffing. (Copyright James R. Roberts, MD.)

Diagnosis

Diagnosis is based on history and may be aided by noting a chemical odor or paint stains on the patient. Inhalant abuse should be suspected in any patient, particularly an adolescent, with nonspecific complaints, neurologic dysfunction, or sudden cardiac arrest.

Clinical Complications

Sudden sniffing death syndrome may occur during inhalant use if the person is startled while intoxicated, causing a catecholamine surge that triggers a ventricular arrhythmia. Other potential complications include aspiration, accidental trauma, respiratory depression, vagal inhibition, injuries or burns due to explosion, and cold injuries. Breathing a pure inhalant gas without air can result in anoxic death. Chronic use can cause myocarditis, myocardial fibrosis, bone marrow suppression, and fetal solvent syndrome. Chronic neurotoxicity includes peripheral neuropathy, cerebellar dysfunction, and dementia, with atrophy evident on brain imaging. A withdrawal syndrome may also occur. Toluene abuse can cause lung injury, renal tubular acidosis, and renal failure.[1] Other agents with unique toxicities include methylene chloride (metabolized to carbon monoxide), carbon tetrachloride (hepatotoxicity), and nitrites (methemoglobinemia).[2]

Management

Acutely intoxicated inhalant users generally require evaluation and brief observation only. If cardiac arrhythmias occur, catecholamines should be avoided, and β-adrenergic blockers should be administered.[1,2]

REFERENCES

1. Anderson CE, Loomis GA. Recognition and prevention of inhalant abuse. *Am Fam Physician* 2003;68:869–874.
2. Lorenc JD. Inhalant abuse in the pediatric population: a persistent challenge. *Curr Opin Pediatr* 2003;15:204–209.

Hydrocarbon Pneumonitis

Anthony Morocco

Clinical Presentation

Patients with hydrocarbon pneumonitis may present with a strong odor of hydrocarbon, particularly with substances such as pine oil or gasoline. Gastrointestinal irritation with nausea, vomiting, abdominal pain, and throat pain are common. Aromatic or halogenated hydrocarbons, camphor, phenol, and pine oil may produce systemic symptoms such as central nervous system depression with ataxia, coma, seizures, and cardiac dysrhythmias. Low-viscosity hydrocarbons (e.g., gasoline, kerosene, turpentine) and the aromatic and halogenated hydrocarbons may produce respiratory symptoms that include shortness of breath, cough, and wheezing.[1]

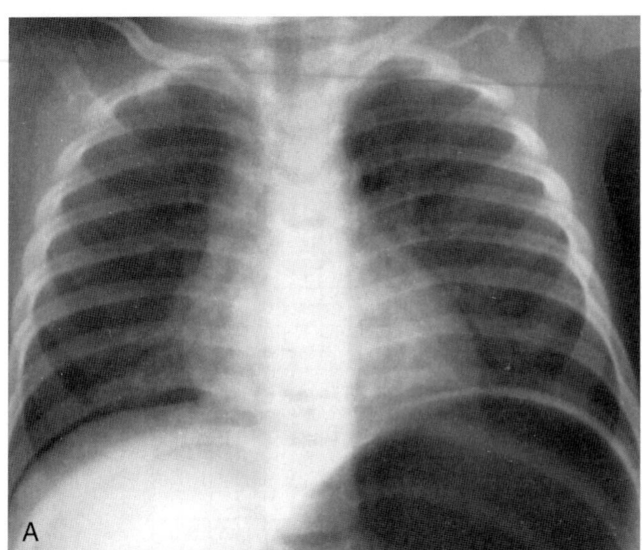

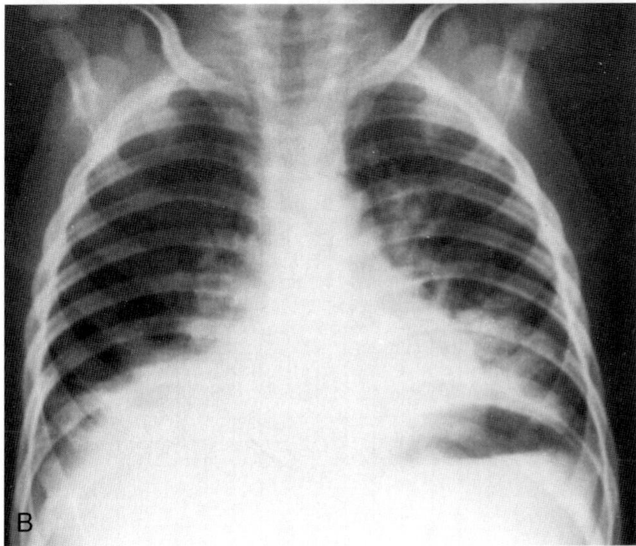

FIGURE 24–7 A: This patient aspirated red furniture polish; 2 hours after ingestion, the lungs are clear. **B:** By 12 hours after ingestion, extensive infiltrates in the lung bases are visible. (**A** and **B,** From Swischuk, with permission.)

Pathophysiology

The mechanisms of hydrocarbon effects on various body systems are unknown. Dysrhythmias may occur after ingestion of halogenated hydrocarbons, due to myocardial sensitization to catecholamines. Lung injury most likely is caused by direct cellular injury and disruption of surfactant after aspiration. Three important determinants of risk for lung injury are viscosity, surface tension, and volatility of the hydrocarbon. Lower viscosity and lower surface tension increase the risk of aspiration, whereas higher volatility increases the volume of inhalation.[1]

Diagnosis

Diagnosis is based on the history, because no confirmatory laboratory studies are readily available. Patients with aspiration may give a history of coughing, choking, or gagging after ingestion. The odor of hydrocarbon on the patient helps confirm the diagnosis. Acute lung injury may be seen on chest radiographs as diffuse infiltrates. The radiographic findings usually develop within 6 hours, but may develop up to 24 hours after hydrocarbon exposure.[1]

Clinical Complications

Lung injury may progress to acute respiratory distress syndrome, respiratory failure, and death. Sequelae may include pulmonary fibrosis and bronchiectasis.

Management

Activated charcoal should be administered only in cases of ingestion of a hydrocarbon that can have systemic toxicity. Gastric emptying by nasogastric or orogastric lavage may be considered after large ingestions, but these procedures may stimulate vomiting and lead to aspiration. Aggressive supportive care, including vasopressors and mechanical ventilation, may be necessary. Lung injury usually peaks at 72 hours after ingestion.[1]

REFERENCES

1. Welker JA, Zaloga GP. Pine oil ingestion: a common cause of poisoning. Chest 1999;116:1822–1826.

Acetaminophen

Anthony Morocco

Clinical Presentation

After acute acetaminophen, *N*-acetyl-*p*-aminophenol (APAP) overdose, patients may exhibit only mild, nonspecific symptoms such as nausea and vomiting. Diminished level of consciousness and shock may occur rarely after massive ingestions. Right upper quadrant abdominal pain and jaundice may appear 3 to 5 days after ingestion.[1]

Pathophysiology

APAP is an analgesic found in numerous over-the-counter preparations. It is the most common ingested agent in suicide attempts, and it is a common cause of fulminant hepatic failure in the United States. Unintentional overdose accounts for up to one third of APAP toxicity cases. The minimum toxic dose of APAP is considered to be at least 150 mg/kg.[1]

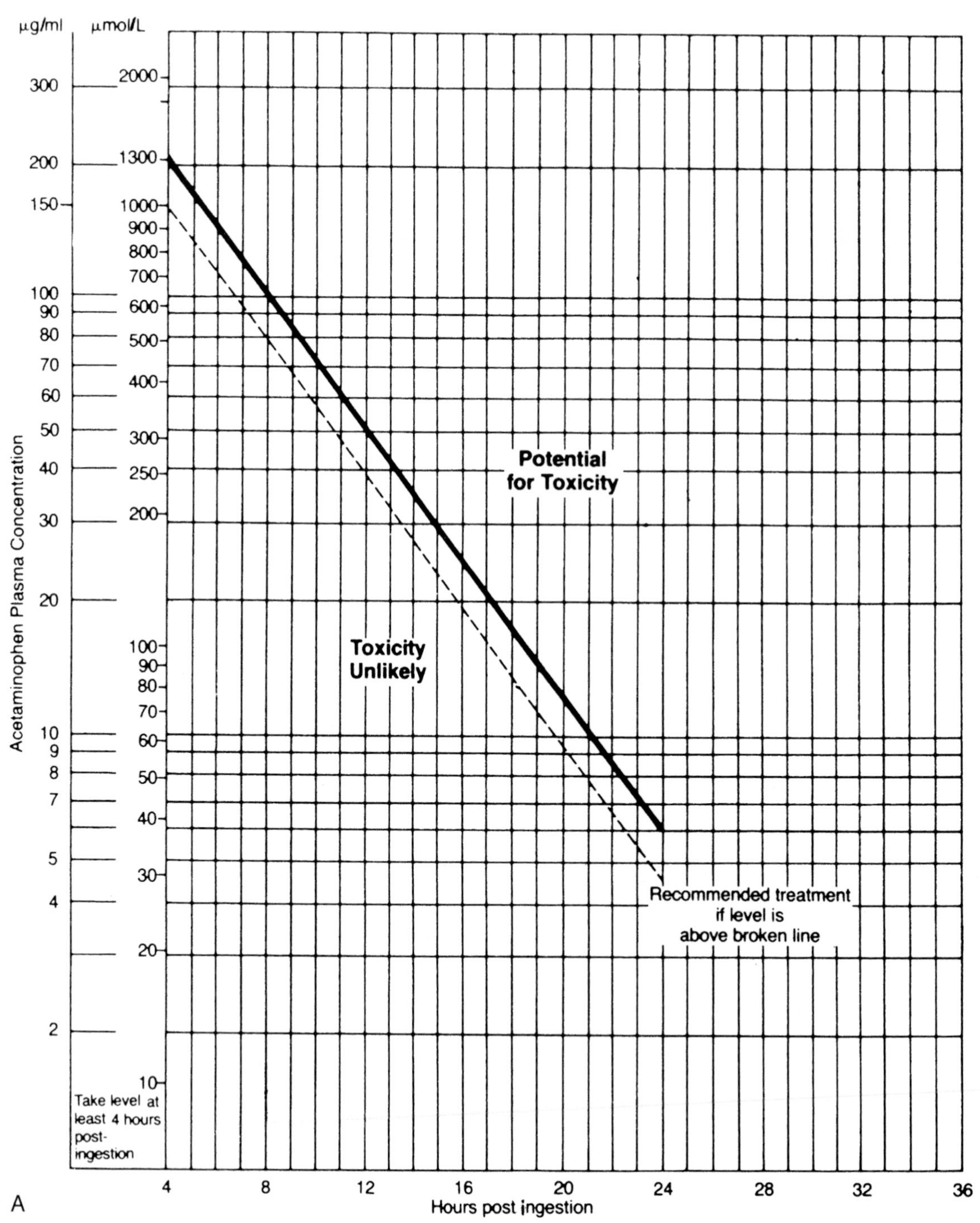

FIGURE 24–8 **A:** The modified Matthew-Rumack acetaminophen nomogram. (From Rumack, with permission.)

Acetaminophen

Anthony Morocco

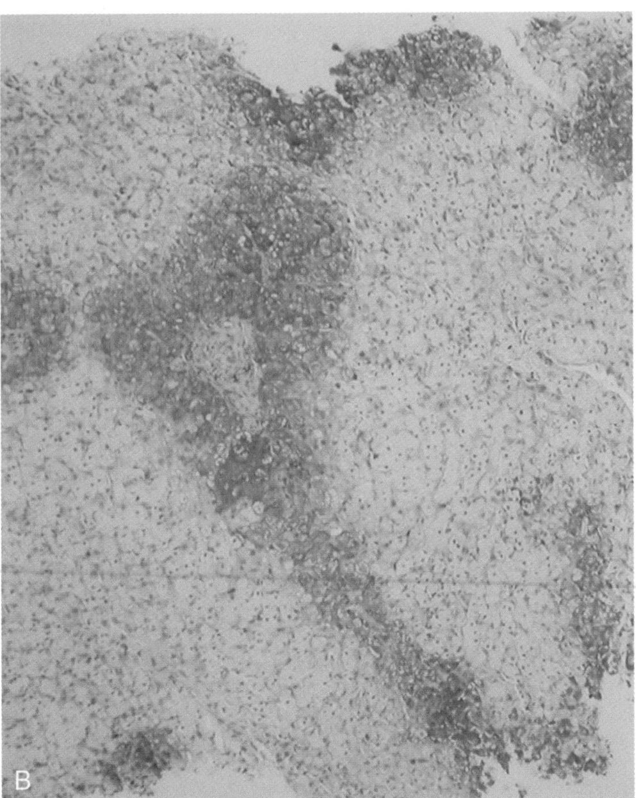

FIGURE 24–8 (cont'd) B: Centrilobular necrosis. (From Yamada, with permission.)

APAP toxicity occurs because of excessive formation by liver cytochrome P450 of a specific metabolite, *N*-acetyl-*p*-benzoquinoneimine (NAPQI). With therapeutic APAP doses, only about 5% of the administered agent is converted to NAPQI, and this fraction is quickly detoxified by glutathione and other mechanisms. However, in APAP overdose, nontoxic metabolic pathways become saturated, and more NAPQI is produced than can be bound by glutathione. NAPQI then binds and disrupts various cellular proteins, resulting in cell death and zone 3 (centrilobular) hepatic necrosis. Toxicity is more likely in patients with decreased glutathione stores (fasting, alcoholism) or increased cytochrome P450 activity (alcoholism, isoniazid).[1]

Diagnosis

APAP ingestion should be suspected in any patient with acute liver failure. All patients with a suspected oral overdose should have a serum APAP concentration measured, regardless of their history.

Clinical Complications

Without treatment, hepatic injury may be self-limited, or it may progress to fulminant hepatic necrosis, resulting in coagulopathy, hepatic encephalopathy, and death. In addition, renal failure and myocardial injury may be seen.

Management

Oral activated charcoal should be administered if it is possible to do so within 1 to 2 hours after ingestion. The APAP concentration measured 4 to 24 hours after ingestion should be plotted on the Matthew-Rumack nomogram to determine the treatment course. If the concentration is above the line, signifying possible toxicity (150 μg/mL at 4 hours after ingestion), treatment with *N*-acetylcysteine (NAC) should be instituted. NAC is usually administered orally in the United States, though many U.S. institutions and those overseas give the drug intravenously. Patients with fulminant hepatic failure should be evaluated for possible liver transplantation.[1]

REFERENCES

1. Zimmerman HJ. Acetaminophen hepatotoxicity. *Clin Liver Dis* 1998;2:523–544.

Salicylate

Anthony Morocco

Clinical Presentation

Patients with acute salicylate overdose initially develop nausea and vomiting. Tinnitus is common and progresses to decreased auditory acuity. Worsening central nervous system toxicity causes agitation, delirium, decreased level of consciousness, and seizures. Hyperthermia occurs with severe toxicity. Patients with chronic toxicity are predominantly elderly and have an insidious onset of symptoms similar to those seen in acute overdose, such as nausea, vomiting, confusion, slurred speech, and delirium.[1]

Pathophysiology

Aspirin (acetylsalicylic acid, ASA) and related salicylates (bismuth subsalicylate, methyl salicylate) can cause severe poisoning after acute or chronic overdose. These compounds are found in a wide variety of oral and topical products. Of particular concern are enteric-coated ASA preparations, which can cause a significant delay in absorption and peak blood concentrations, and oil of wintergreen, which may have a very high salicylate concentration (equivalent to 1.4 g of ASA per milliliter).[1]

Salicylates cause hyperventilation and respiratory alkalosis by stimulation of the brainstem respiratory center. Anion gap metabolic acidosis occurs from a number of mechanisms, including uncoupling of oxidative phosphorylation and ketosis secondary to increased fatty acid metabolism. Because salicylate is a weak acid, systemic acidosis increases the amount of salicylate in nonionized form. This results in enhanced entry of salicylate into the central nervous system and worsening toxicity.[1]

Diagnosis

The diagnosis is confirmed by measurement of the serum salicylate concentration. Addition of ferric chloride to urine produces a deep purple color if salicylate is present.

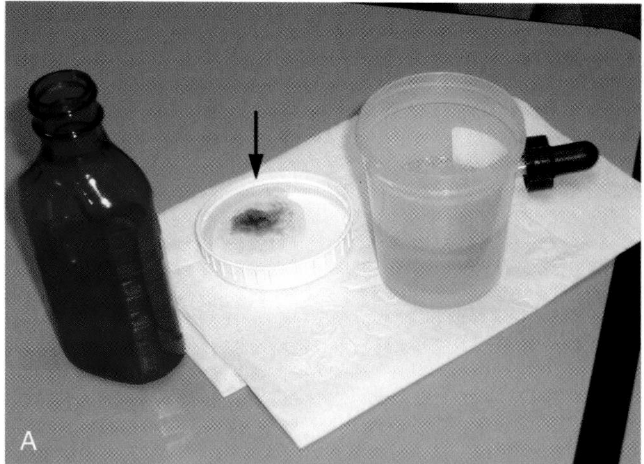

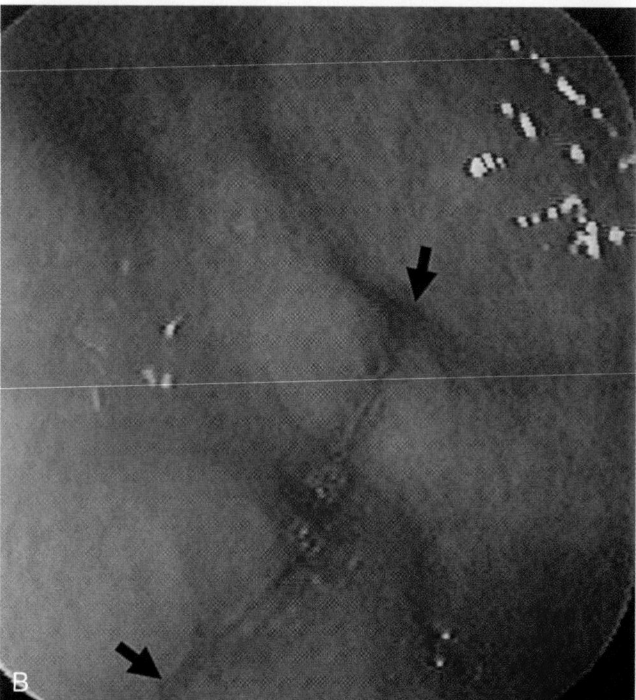

FIGURE 24–9 A: A positive ferric chloride test showing purple-brown color change in salicylate-containing urine when several drops of ferric chloride are added to a few milliliters of urine. (Courtesy of Judith Eisenberg, MD.) **B:** Characteristic of aspirin-induced linear erosion *(extending between two arrows)*. (From Yamada, with permission.)

Clinical Complications

Noncardiogenic pulmonary edema may occur after overdose. Death occurs from cerebral edema and cardiovascular collapse.[1] Reye's syndrome is a liver disorder associated with salicylate use in children.

Management

Patients should receive multidose activated charcoal to decrease absorption and enhance elimination of salicylate. Salicylate concentration and pH should be frequently measured. Whole-bowel irrigation may decrease absorption after ingestion of an enteric-coated preparation. Bicarbonate should be administered to alkalinize the serum and urine, thereby decreasing central nervous system entry and enhancing elimination in the urine by ion trapping. Hemodialysis is indicated for severe toxicity.[1]

REFERENCES

1. Dargan PI, Wallace CI, Jones AL. An evidence based flowchart to guide the management of acute salicylate (aspirin) overdose. *Emerg Med J* 2002;19:206–210.

Carbon Monoxide

Anthony Morocco

Clinical Presentation

Patients with carbon monoxide (CO) exposure may complain of a variety of nonspecific symptoms that may be mistaken for a flu-like illness. Headache is one of the most common initial complaints. Other symptoms include nausea, vomiting, malaise, drowsiness, and inability to concentrate. Increasing exposures to CO can cause confusion, shortness of breath, tachycardia, chest pain, loss of consciousness, seizures, and death.[1]

Pathophysiology

Carbon monoxide is a colorless, odorless gas that is produced during the combustion of fossil fuels. It is the most common cause of poisoning-related deaths (1,000 to 2,000 deaths per year) in the United States.[1] The most common sources of CO exposure are furnaces, automobile exhaust, charcoal fires, and gas-powered tools.[1]

CO binds to hemoglobin with a much higher affinity than oxygen, thus reducing the oxygen-carrying capacity of the blood. CO also shifts the oxyhemoglobin saturation curve leftward, resulting in a further decrease in oxygen delivery to tissues. CO acts by a number of other mechanisms, including binding to cytochrome aa_3 with resultant impairment of production of adenosine triphosphate (ATP), generation of oxygen free radicals, lipid peroxidation in the brain, and inducement of cell apoptosis.[1] An uncommon source for CO is the chemical methylene chloride, which is metabolized endogenously in humans to form CO.

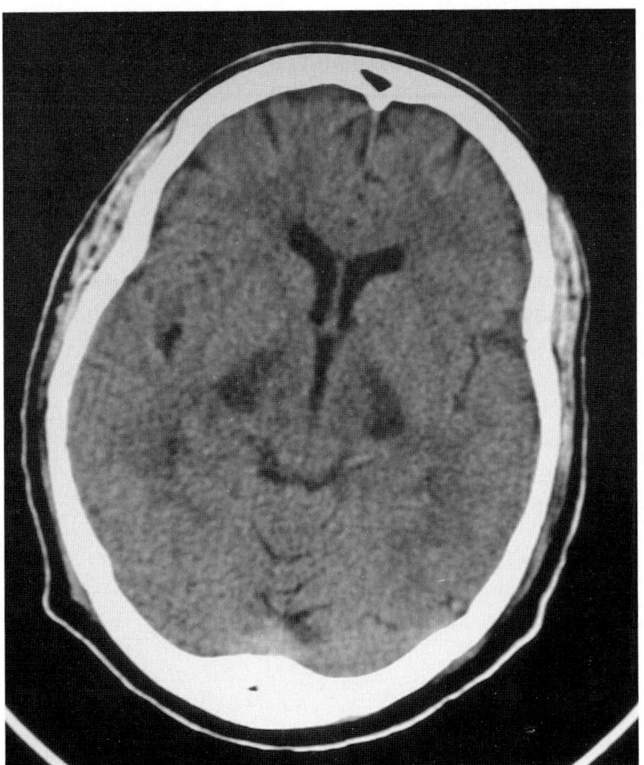

FIGURE 24–10 Bibasilar hypodensities after carbon monoxide toxicity. (Courtesy of Robert Hendrickson, MD.)

Diagnosis

The diagnosis may be made in most cases by history alone. A carboxyhemoglobin level can be measured by co-oximetry using a venous or arterial blood sample.

Clinical Complications

Patients may develop persistent and delayed neurologic sequelae after CO poisoning. In 25% and 50% of patients who either lose consciousness during exposure to CO or have a carboxyhemoglobin level greater than 25%, symptoms persist for at least 1 month.[2] Neurologic problems including ataxia, focal abnormalities, and parkinsonism may occur. Affective symptoms may include depression, sleep disturbance, personality changes, and anxiety. Neuroimaging may show abnormalities in the white matter, hippocampus, and globus pallidus.[1]

Management

Any patient with suspected toxicity should be immediately placed on high-flow supplemental oxygen to hasten CO elimination. The use of hyperbaric oxygen (HBO) to treat CO poisoning remains controversial, although recent studies provide evidence in favor of this therapy to reduce the incidence of neurologic sequelae.[2] HBO significantly increases the elimination of CO, while potentially decreasing CO-induced lipid peroxidation.[2] Suggested indications for HBO have included loss of consciousness, persistent neurologic deficits, pregnancy, and carboxyhemoglobin levels greater than 25%.

REFERENCES

1. Weaver LK. Carbon monoxide poisoning. *Crit Care Clin* 1999;15:297–317.
2. Weaver LK, Hopkins RO, Chan K, et al. Hyperbaric oxygen for acute carbon monoxide poisoning. *N Engl J Med* 2002;347:1057–1067.

Iron

Anthony Morocco

Clinical Presentation

Iron poisoning may be considered in five stages. Initially, patients develop nausea, vomiting, diarrhea, and abdominal pain and may develop gastrointestinal (GI) hemorrhage and fluid losses. The second stage is a latent phase with resolving GI symptoms that may occur 6 and 24 hours after ingestion. Severe poisonings rapidly progress to a third stage of systemic toxicity, with shock and metabolic acidosis. Stage four occurs 2 to 3 days after ingestion, when hepatic injury is evident. The final stage may occur 2 to 8 weeks after ingestion, with scarring and strictures causing gastric outlet obstruction.[1]

Pathophysiology

Available iron formulations include ferrous sulfate (28% elemental iron by weight), ferrous fumarate (33% elemental iron), ferrous gluconate (12% elemental iron), ferrous chloride (28% elemental iron), and ferrous lactate (19% elemental iron). Ingestions of greater than 20 mg/kg are considered to be clinically important and potentially harmful.[1]

Iron exerts a direct corrosive effect on GI mucosa. Formation of reactive oxygen species causes hepatic injury. Acidosis and cell injury occur by several mechanisms. Conversion of ferrous to ferric iron after absorption to release a hydrogen ion, disruption of oxidative phosphorylation, and direct myocardial toxicity and fluid losses cause hypotension, tissue hypoperfusion, and lactic acidosis.[1,2]

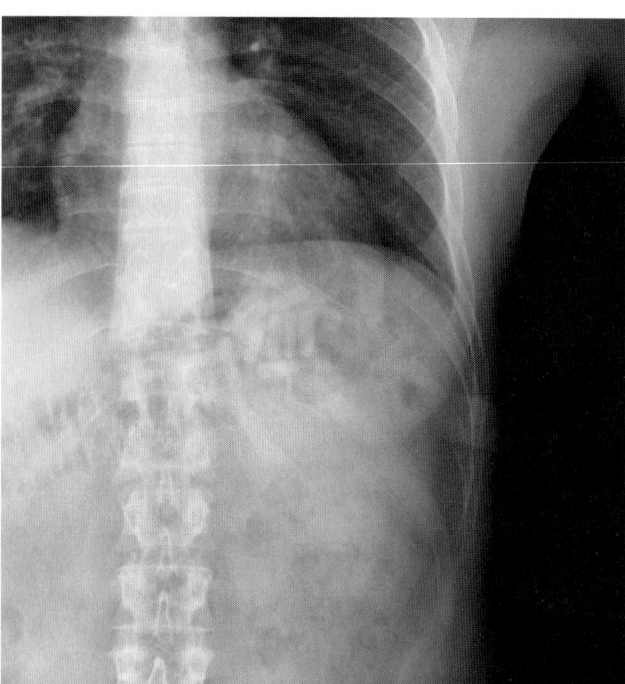

FIGURE 24–11 Multiple iron-containing tablets are seen in the left upper quadrant. (Courtesy of Mark Silverberg, MD.)

Diagnosis

Absence of symptoms within 6 hours after ingestion rules out significant toxicity. Iron-containing pills are radiopaque on abdominal radiographs, but chewable and liquid forms are rarely visible. Peak serum iron concentrations occur 2 to 6 hours after ingestion; concentrations greater than 300 μg/dL are associated with GI toxicity, greater than 500 μg/dL with systemic toxicity, and greater than 1,000 μg/dL with severe poisoning and death.[1–3]

Clinical Complications

GI injury may result in bowel edema, ulceration, necrosis, and perforation. Worsening systemic toxicity may result in seizures and coma. Hepatic injury may progress to fulminant failure. Prolonged administration of deferoxamine is associated with acute lung injury and *Yersinia enterocolitica* sepsis.[1]

Management

The emergency physician should consider gastric emptying within the first hour after ingestion and whole-bowel irrigation. Activated charcoal does not adsorb well to iron. Aggressive replacement of GI fluid losses is vital. Treatment with the iron chelator, deferoxamine, should be considered for patients with lethargy, intractable vomiting, shock, metabolic acidosis, or a serum iron concentration greater than 500 μg/dL.[1–3]

REFERENCES

1. Fine JS. Iron poisoning. *Curr Probl Pediatr* 2000;30:71–90.
2. Black J, Zenel JA. Child abuse by intentional iron poisoning presenting as shock and persistent acidosis. *Pediatrics* 2003;111:197–199.
3. Riordan M, Rylance G, Berry K. Poisoning in children 3: common medicines. *Arch Dis Child* 2002;87:400–402.

Methanol

Anthony Morocco

Clinical Presentation

Patients initially develop mild central nervous system depression, headache, and confusion. Nausea, vomiting, and abdominal pain may occur. Visual disturbances such as blurred vision, photophobia, and "snow field" vision occur after a latent period of 40 minutes to 72 hours.[1]

Pathophysiology

Methanol is a toxic alcohol that is widely used as an industrial solvent, fuel, and chemical precursor. It can be found in reformulated gasoline and in many home products such as paint thinners, windshield washer fluids, cleaning solutions, and camp-stove fuel. It is well absorbed after oral, dermal, or inhalational exposure.[1]

Methanol is converted by alcohol dehydrogenase to formaldehyde, which is quickly converted by formaldehyde dehydrogenase to formic acid. This toxic metabolite results in acidosis and inhibits cytochrome c in mitochondria. The optic disc and nerve are particularly susceptible to the latter effect. Cytochrome inhibition results in increased lactate production and exacerbates the acidosis.[1]

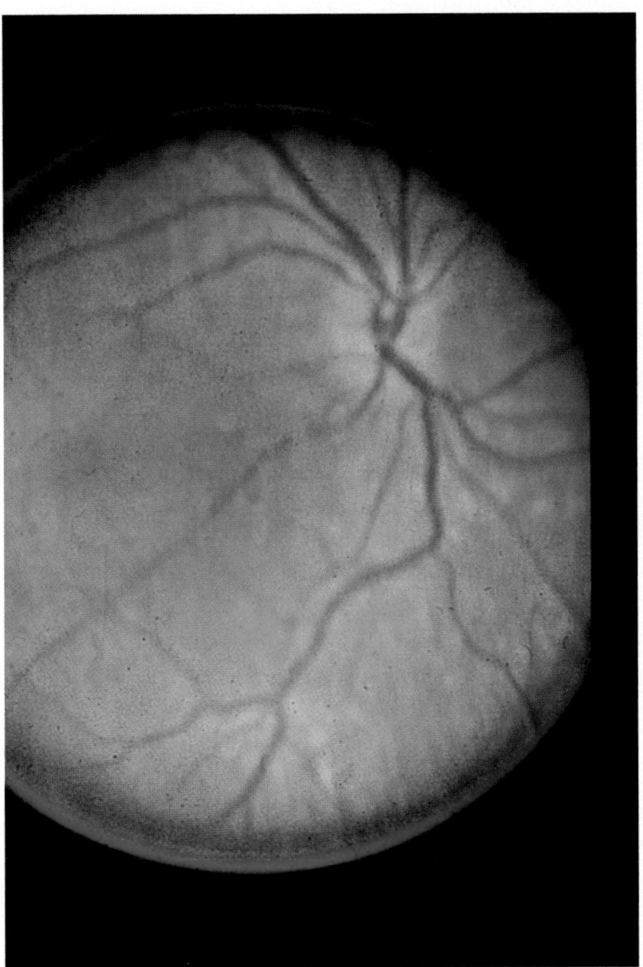

FIGURE 24–12 The right fundus of a commercial sailor who had been at sea for 3 weeks and drank methanol from the ship's compass. (From Tasman and Jaeger, with permission.)

Diagnosis

Measurement of serum methanol confirms the diagnosis. Routine laboratory testing reveals an increased osmolal gap and an anion gap metabolic acidosis. Formate levels (not readily available) and low pH correlate well with mortality. Computed tomography and magnetic resonance imaging may show cerebral edema, white-matter changes, and basal ganglia lesions. Eye examination may reveal nystagmus, decreased pupillary response, and hyperemia of the optic disc with subsequent papilledema.[1]

Clinical Complications

Permanent decreased visual acuity or blindness may occur. Serious poisonings may result in coma and seizures due to cerebral edema and brain injury occurring preferentially in the putamen. Other complications may occur, including pancreatitis, methemoglobinemia, and myoglobinuric renal failure.[1]

Management

Treatment strategy involves correction of acidosis, inhibition of formate production, and enhancement of methanol and formate clearance. General treatment indications include history of significant ingestion, osmolal gap greater than 10, pH less than 7.3, visual dysfunction, or methanol concentration greater than 20 mg/dL. Bicarbonate administration to maintain a pH greater than 7.3 decreases formate ionization and toxic effects. Ethanol and fomepizole block alcohol dehydrogenase, thus inhibiting formate production. Folinic acid or folic acid administration may enhance formate metabolism. Hemodialysis greatly enhances clearance of formate and methanol and corrects acidosis. Hemodialysis is generally recommended for methanol levels greater than 50 mg/dL, severe acidosis, visual disturbance, or other signs of severe poisoning.[1]

REFERENCES

1. Barceloux DG, Bond GR, Krenzelok EP, et al. American Academy of Clinical Toxicology practice guidelines on the treatment of methanol poisoning. *J Toxicol Clin Toxicol* 2002;40:415–446.

Ethylene Glycol

Anthony Morocco

Clinical Presentation

Patients may initially develop symptoms of inebriation, vomiting, and central nervous system depression, or they may appear relatively asymptomatic. Renal failure, acidosis, hypotension, and cerebral edema may occur and may be delayed up to 12 hours or longer.[1]

Pathophysiology

Ethylene glycol is a toxic alcohol derivative that is widely used in solvents, chemical manufacturing, and antifreeze solutions. It is sweet-tasting and well-absorbed orally, but dermal and inhalational absorptions are poor.[1]

The first step of ethylene glycol metabolism occurs when ethylene glycol is catalyzed by alcohol dehydrogenase, with further conversion to a number of toxic compounds. Accumulation of glycolic acid results in metabolic acidosis. Direct cellular toxicity and calcium oxalate crystal deposition can cause renal injury.[1]

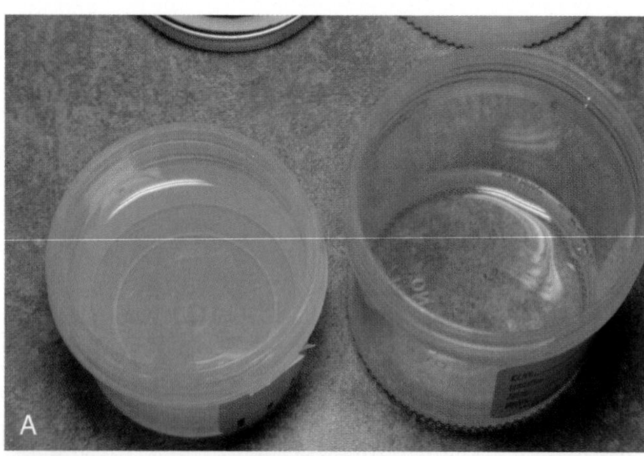

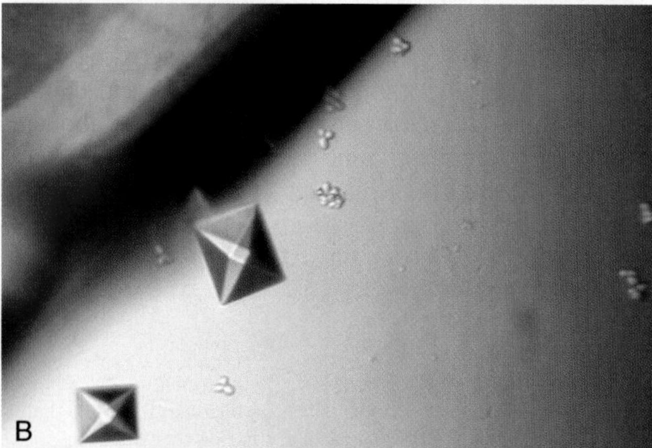

FIGURE 24–13 **A:** Fluorescence of the urine on the left under a Wood's lamp. Urine on the right is normal urine. **B:** Oxalate crystals. (**A** and **B,** Courtesy of Robert Hendrickson, MD.)

Diagnosis

Measurement of serum ethylene glycol confirms the diagnosis. Routine laboratory testing may reveal an increased osmolal gap and an anion gap metabolic acidosis. Hypocalcemia and leukocytosis may also be present. Urinalysis reveals calcium oxalate crystals in up to 50% of patients at admission. Computed tomography scans may show cerebral edema. Because antifreeze solutions often contain fluorescein, examination of urine with a Wood's lamp may reveal fluorescence and help to confirm a suspicion of ingestion.[1]

Clinical Complications

Severe poisoning can cause progressive acidosis, hypotension, congestive heart failure, acute respiratory distress syndrome, cerebral edema, seizures, coma, and death.[1] Acute tubular necrosis and oliguric renal failure develop 24 to 72 hours after ingestion and may be permanent. Bone marrow depression and cranial nerve dysfunction rarely occurs.[1]

Management

Aspiration of gastric contents should be considered if the patient presents less than 1 hour after ingestion. Treatment strategy involves correction of acidosis, inhibition of toxic metabolite production, and enhancement of ethylene glycol and toxic metabolite clearance. Ethanol and fomepizole block alcohol dehydrogenase, thus inhibiting toxic metabolite production. Indications for antidotal treatment include history of ethylene glycol ingestion, serum level greater than 20 mg/dL, osmolal gap greater than 10, pH less than 7.3, and presence of urinary oxalate crystals. Sodium bicarbonate should be administered to maintain a pH greater than 7.3. Pyridoxine, thiamine, and magnesium are cofactors for two detoxification pathways. Hemodialysis greatly enhances clearance of ethylene glycol and toxic metabolites and corrects acidosis. Hemodialysis is generally recommended for ethylene glycol levels greater than 50 mg/dL, severe acidosis, renal failure, or other signs of severe poisoning.[1]

REFERENCES

1. Barceloux DG, Krenzelok EP, Olson K, Watson W. American Academy of Clinical Toxicology practice guidelines on the treatment of ethylene glycol poisoning. *J Toxicol Clin Toxicol* 1999;37:537–560.

Isopropanol

Anthony Morocco

Clinical Presentation

Patients initially develop symptoms of inebriation, ataxia, and central nervous system depression. Cases of severe poisoning may manifest with coma. Nausea, vomiting, and abdominal pain commonly occur.[1,2]

Pathophysiology

Isopropanol (isopropyl alcohol) is a chemical that is found in many industrial and household products such as rubbing alcohol (70% isopropanol).[1] Isopropanol is well absorbed after oral, dermal, or inhalational exposure.

Because the inebriating effect of alcohol increases with the number of carbon atoms in its structure, isopropanol has twice the potency of ethanol. Isopropanol is metabolized to acetone by the enzyme alcohol dehydrogenase in the liver. The acetone also has inebriating effects. Metabolism does not produce toxic acids, as occurs with methanol and ethylene glycol exposure.[1]

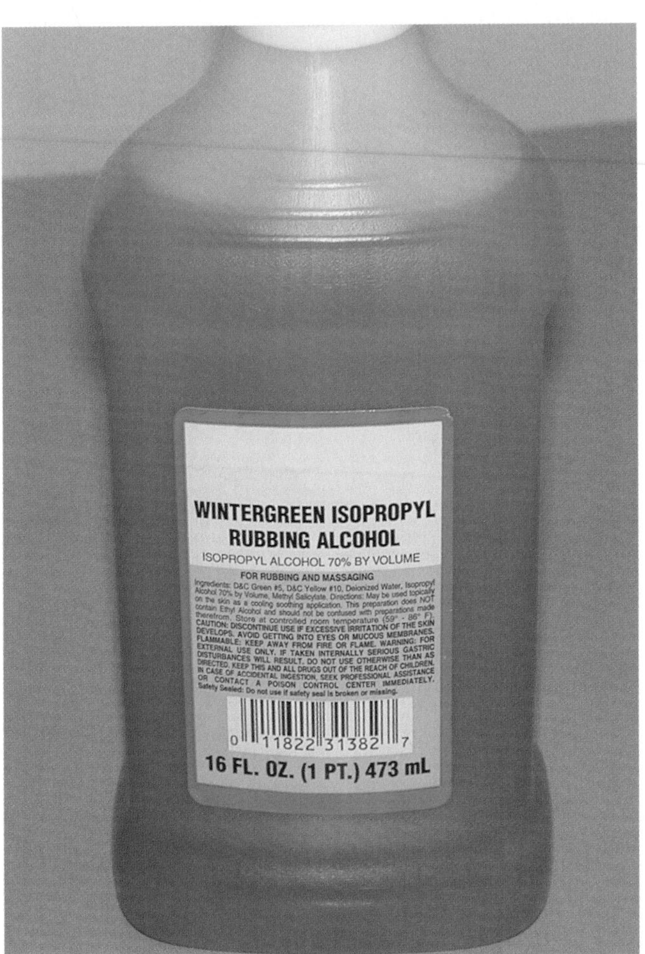

FIGURE 24–14 "Blue heaven" (isopropanol). (Courtesy of Robert Hendrickson, MD.)

Diagnosis

Measurement of serum isopropanol or acetone concentration confirms the diagnosis. Other laboratory abnormalities include an elevated osmolal gap and positive ketones on urinalysis.[3] Elevation of the anion gap and acidosis do not occur. The patient may smell strongly of acetone.

Clinical Complications

Large ingestions can cause hypotension due to vasodilation, respiratory depression, and coma. Vomiting may result in aspiration with resultant pneumonia and acute respiratory distress syndrome.[1] Hemorrhage gastritis may occur. Other reported effects include renal tubular acidosis, hemorrhagic tracheobronchitis, rhabdomyolysis, and hemolytic anemia.[1]

Management

Treatment for isopropanol intoxication is essentially the same as that for ethanol. Any complications should be treated, and supportive care should be administered until the isopropanol and acetone are eliminated by the kidneys and lungs.[1–3]

REFERENCES

1. Zaman F, Pervez A, Abreo K. Isopropyl alcohol intoxication: a diagnostic challenge. *Am J Kidney Dis* 2002;40:E12.
2. Stremski E, Hennes H. Accidental isopropanol ingestion in children. *Pediatr Emerg Care* 2000;16:238–240.
3. Church AS, Witting MD. Laboratory testing in ethanol, methanol, ethylene glycol, and isopropanol toxicities. *J Emerg Med* 1997;15: 687–692.

Lead

Anthony Morocco

Clinical Presentation

Acute ingestion of large doses of lead may result in altered mental status reflective of encephalopathy within hours. Chronic lead toxicity may have a more subtle presentation, with anorexia as one of the earliest symptoms. Other symptoms may include nausea, vomiting, intermittent abdominal pain, constipation, irritability, distractibility, impulsiveness, encephalopathy, headache, tremor, fatigue, arthralgias, and anemia.

Pathophysiology

Lead is a heavy metal that commonly causes toxicity, particularly in children. Common sources of lead intoxication include ingestion of residue and chips of lead-based paint, occupational exposure, environmental contamination by leaded gasoline and industrial fallout, use of cookware with glazes containing lead oxide (greta), retained bullets, and folk remedies containing greta and azarcon (lead tetroxide).[1]

Lead may be absorbed by dermal exposure, ingestion, or inhalation. Children absorb more of an ingested lead dose (up to 50%) than adults do (10%).[1] Lead causes toxicity by binding and inhibiting the function of many enzymes (e.g., those involved in heme synthesis).[2]

Diagnosis

The blood lead concentration should be measured in all suspected cases. Laboratory studies may reveal a microcytic, hypochromic anemia and basophilic stippling of red blood cells on peripheral blood smear. Long-bone radiographs in children may reveal opacities at metaphyses ("lead lines") due to abnormal bone growth (not lead deposition). Radiography may reveal unabsorbed lead in the gut.[1]

Clinical Complications

Acute, large lead ingestions may result in hemolysis and hepatorenal failure. Chronic exposure may result in cognitive deficits in some children and hypertension, peripheral neuropathy (i.e., wrist drop), and renal insufficiency in some adults. Patients with high lead concentrations may develop encephalopathy, seizures, and cerebral edema. Lead is teratogenic and may be associated with preterm delivery, low birth weight, and developmental delay.[1]

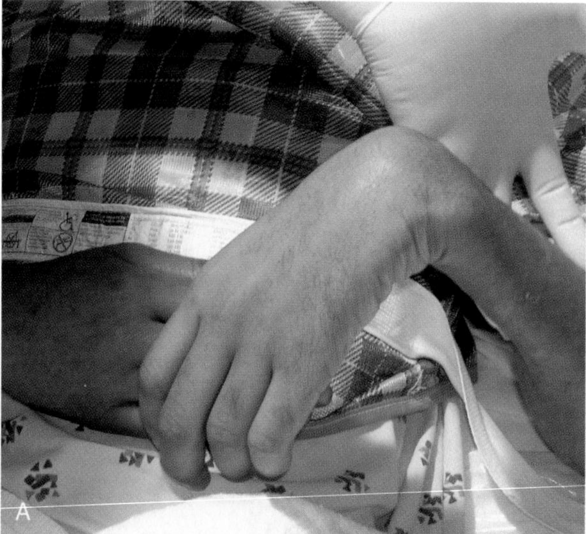

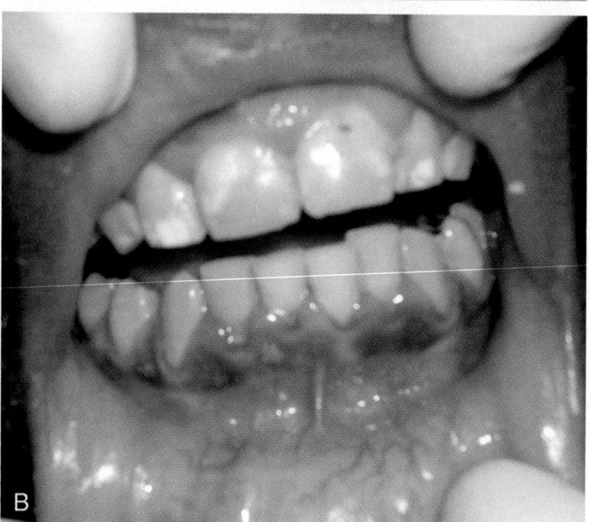

FIGURE 24–15 **A:** Wrist drop in a patient with elevated blood lead levels. (Courtesy of Rachel Haroz, MD.) **B:** The gingival discoloration represents "lead lines" in this man who presented with chronic lead intoxication from a bullet retained in his neck due to a gunshot wound 20 years previously. (Courtesy of Judith Eisenberg, MD, Rachel Haroz, MD, and Greg Schneider, MD.)

Management

Gastric lavage and whole-bowel irrigation should be considered if lead remains in the gut. Symptomatic patients should receive chelation therapy, but the concentration at which to chelate an asymptomatic child (generally recommended at 45 μg/dL) is controversial. Levels greater than 70 μg/dL or significant symptoms may necessitate hospitalization and aggressive chelation. Oral succimer (DMSA) may be used in patients without serious gastrointestinal toxicity. Ethylenediaminetetraacetic acid (EDTA) and dimercaprol (BAL) are parenteral chelators and may be used in cases of encephalopathy, highly elevated blood lead concentration (greater than 70 μg/dL in children or 100 μg/dL in adults), or severe gastrointestinal symptoms.[1] BAL and EDTA can have substantial side effects, including hypertension, renal failure, and anaphylaxis; they should be used with caution.

REFERENCES

1. Graeme KA, Pollack CV Jr. Heavy metal toxicity, part II: lead and metal fume fever. *J Emerg Med* 1998;16:171–177.
2. Markowitz M. Lead poisoning. *Pediatr Rev* 2000;21:327–335.

Retained Bullets

Anthony Morocco

Clinical Presentation

Patients may present with symptoms of lead toxicity days to years after the initial injury. Complaints may include nausea, constipation, irritability, headache, and insomnia.[1]

Pathophysiology

Lead bullets and lead-containing fragments often remain in the body after survival from gunshot injuries. In this setting, lead may subsequently be absorbed into the systemic circulation, representing a source for potential toxicity.[2]

Lead fragments are generally isolated from the surrounding tissue by the formation of a fibrous capsule, and most patients consequently do not develop lead toxicity. However, contact with joint spaces, synovial tissue or membranes, cerebrospinal fluid, or vascularized cystic structures may result in dissolution of lead-containing fragments and substantial lead absorption. The relatively acidic pH, in conjunction with hyaluronic acid in synovial fluid, contributes to this effect. Absorption is more pronounced in joints with increased mobility or weight bearing, and in individuals with chronic inflammatory conditions such as arthritis. Retained shrapnel, fragmented bullets, and buckshot have higher surface areas of exposed lead and therefore may be associated with increased lead absorption. Prolonged time of exposure may also increase lead absorption.[1,2]

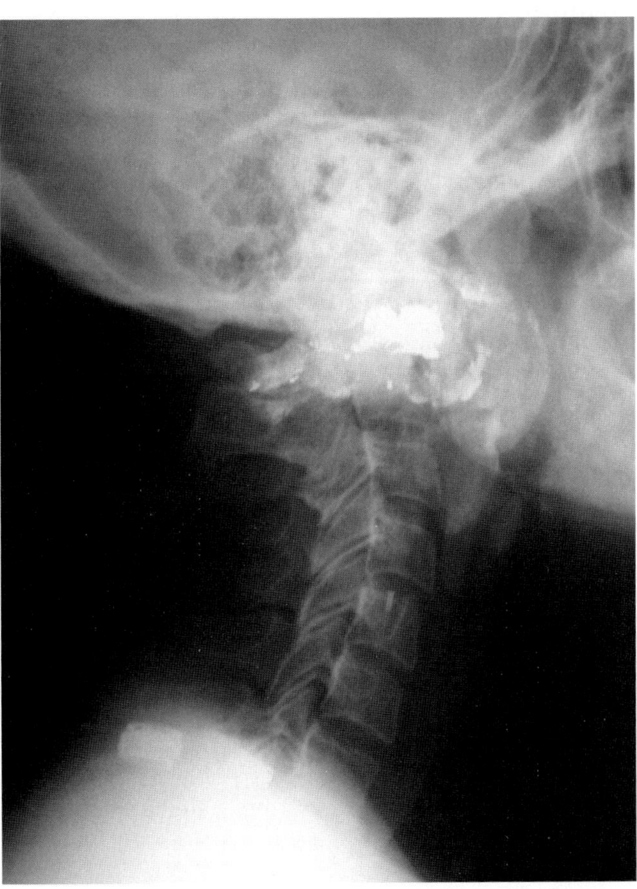

FIGURE 24–16 Retained bullets that are in contact with synovial, peritoneal, or cerebrospinal fluid may produce elevations in serum lead concentration many years after the injury. (Courtesy of Robert Hendrickson, MD.)

Diagnosis

The potential for lead toxicity can be assessed by measuring the blood lead concentration (BLC). Plain radiography and computed tomographic scanning may help to assess the precise location of lead fragments and aid in removal strategies. Microcytic, hypochromic anemia and basophilic stippling of red blood cells may be evident on peripheral blood smear.[1]

Clinical Complications

Chronic lead exposure results in lead sequestration in bone. Systemic illness (e.g., sepsis, thyrotoxicosis), surgery, or pregnancy increases bone turnover and releases lead from bony stores.[1] Elevated BLCs may be associated with the development of cerebral edema, encephalopathy, and seizures. Chronic lead toxicity may be associated with the development of hypertension, peripheral neuropathy, and renal insufficiency in some patients.[1,2]

Management

Strong consideration should be given to surgical removal of lead-containing fragments, especially if they are in contact with joint spaces or cerebrospinal fluid. Symptomatic patients may require chelation with parenteral dimercaprol (BAL) and ethylenediaminetetraacetic acid (EDTA), with or without oral succimer (DMSA). If lead fragments are not amenable to surgical removal, management can be problematic, and careful and frequent monitoring of BLCs is required.

REFERENCES

1. McQuirter JL, Rothenberg SJ, Dinkins GA, et al. The effects of retained lead bullets on body lead burden. *J Trauma* 2001;50:892–899.
2. Farrell SE, Vandevander P, Schoffstall JM, et al. Blood lead levels in emergency department patients with retained lead bullets and shrapnel. *Acad Emerg Med* 1999;6:208–212.

Arsenic

Anthony Morocco

Clinical Presentation

Within minutes to hours after acute arsenic ingestion, patients may develop nausea, vomiting, abdominal pain, and profuse watery diarrhea. Cardiovascular effects may include hypotension, endothelial damage, pulmonary edema, prolonged QT interval on electrocardiography, and dysrhythmias. Severe cases may manifest with delirium and seizures.[1] Chronic arsenic poisoning may manifest with encephalopathy, peripheral neuropathies, and dermatitis. Chronic skin lesions may include abnormal pigmentation and hyperkeratosis, particularly on the palms and soles. The hallmark of arsine gas exposure is hemolysis, and patients who survive long enough to reach the emergency department may present with various sequelae of hemolysis.[1,2]

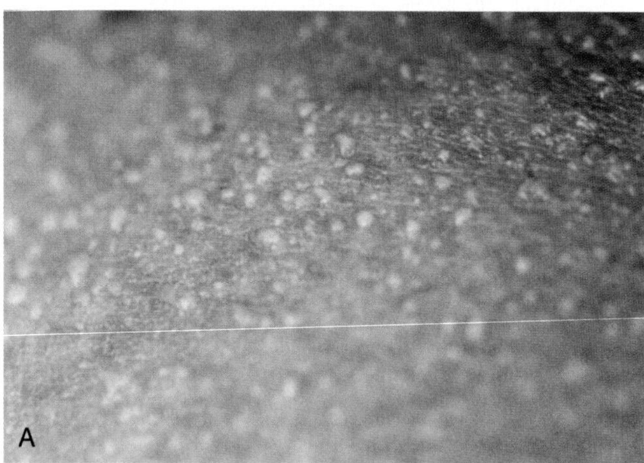

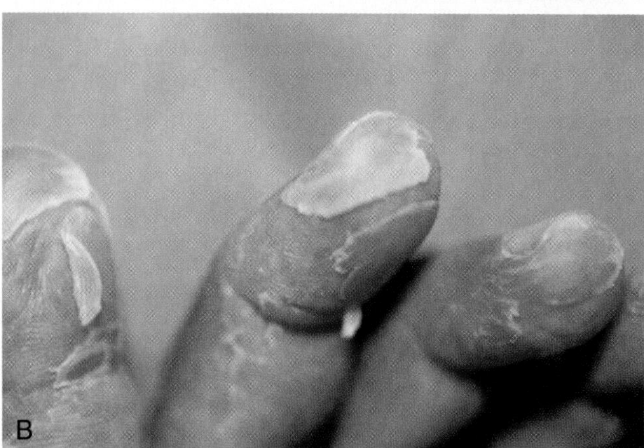

FIGURE 24–17 **A:** A group of pustules measuring 1 to 3 mm in diameter is seen on erythematous skin on the abdomen. **B:** Lamellar desquamation and hyperkeratosis are evident on the fingers. (**A** and **B,** From Bartolomé B, Córdoba S, Nieto S, et al. Acute arsenic poisoning: clinical and histopathologic features. *Br J Dermatol* 1999;141:1106–1109, with permission.)

Pathophysiology

Arsenic exists in several forms: elemental arsenic, organic arsenic, inorganic arsenate (trivalent), inorganic arsenite (pentavalent), and arsine gas. Arsenic is commonly found in the environment (soil and ground water). It is used in some medicines (arsenic trioxide for leukemia), pesticides, chemical warfare agents (lewisite), semiconductor manufacturing (arsine), and wood preservatives and has a myriad of industrial uses.[1] Seafood contains predominantly nonharmful organic arsenic compounds.[1,2]

Arsenic compounds may be absorbed by oral, dermal, or inhalational routes. Arsenic binds to sulfhydryl groups, thereby interfering with a number of enzymes and structural proteins. Arsenate substitutes for phosphate and uncouples oxidative phosphorylation. Arsine binds to red blood cells and causes hemolysis.[1,2]

Diagnosis

The odor of garlic may be noted on or about the patient. Arsenic in the gastrointestinal tract may be radiopaque. Peripheral blood smears may show basophilic stippling or rouleaux formation.[1] Urinary arsenic should be measured, preferably in a 24-hour specimen collected in acid-free containers. Special laboratory techniques can differentiate organic from inorganic forms of arsenic.[2]

Clinical Complications

Complications of acute arsenic poisoning include seizures, coma, peripheral neuropathy, cardiac arrhythmia, severe fluid loss, shock, liver injury, acute respiratory distress syndrome, pancytopenia, seizures, coma, and death. Complications of chronic arsenic exposure include basal cell and squamous cell carcinoma and lung cancer. Severe anemia and renal failure can complicate arsine gas exposure.[1,2]

Management

Aggressive supportive care is essential. Whole-bowel irrigation may help clear any arsenic that remains in the gastrointestinal tract. Acute toxicity may be treated with intramuscular dimercaprol (BAL), a chelating agent. Chronic or subacute toxicity may be treated with the oral chelator succimer (DMSA). Chelation usually is not effective for arsine poisoning.[1,2]

REFERENCES

1. Graeme KA, Pollack CV Jr. Heavy metal toxicity, part 1: arsenic and mercury. *J Emerg Med* 1998;16:45–56.
2. Ratnaike RN. Acute and chronic arsenic toxicity. *Postgrad Med J* 2003;79:391–396.

Mercury

Anthony Morocco

Clinical Presentation

Manifestations of toxicity vary, depending on the type of mercury and the route of exposure. Exposure to elemental mercury may cause fever, cough, shortness of breath, vomiting, diarrhea, and weakness. Ingested mercury salts may cause severe gastrointestinal irritation. Acrodynia ("pink disease") is a hypersensitivity syndrome of rash and neurologic symptoms that usually is seen in children exposed to mercury salts.[1] Elemental and inorganic mercury can cause subacute or chronic mercury toxicity. Patients may be upset at presentation, with loose teeth, renal dysfunction, intention tremor, and personality changes such as shyness (erethism), depression, and fatigue (neurasthenia). The short-chain organic compounds methylmercury and dimethylmercury cause acute dermatitis and gastrointestinal injury, with severe neurologic dysfunction developing over days to weeks.

Pathophysiology

Mercury is a heavy metal that may exist in an elemental, inorganic salt, or organic form.[1] Elemental mercury is widely available and may be found in some scientific instruments, thermostats, thermometers, and dental amalgams. Mercury salts may be found in some disc batteries, disinfectants, and various industrial processes. Organic mercury may be encountered in laboratories, pesticides, and wood preservatives.

Elemental mercury is best absorbed by inhalation; absorption in a normal gastrointestinal tract is negligible. Organic mercury and mercury salts may be absorbed orally or dermally. Mercury binds to sulfhydryl, phosphoryl, and other groups, causing disruption of enzymes and structural proteins and resultant tissue damage.[1]

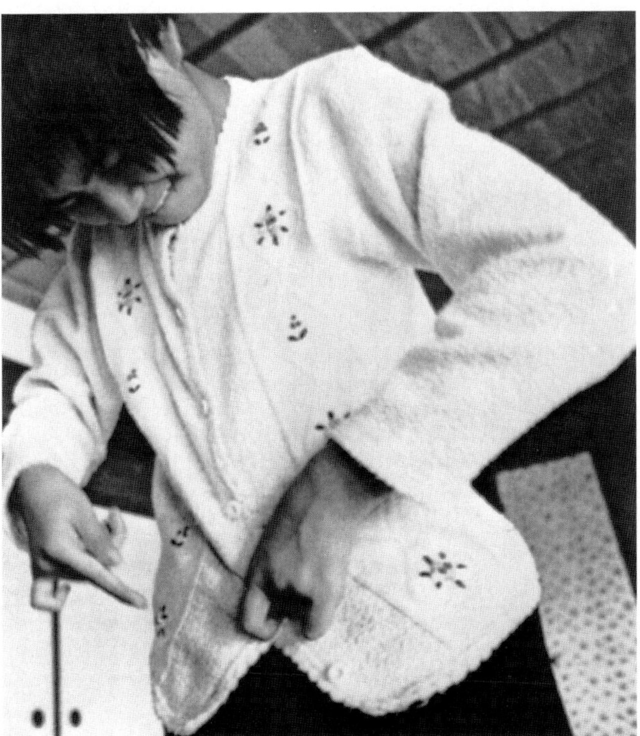

FIGURE 24–18 Minamata victim: severe ataxia of upper limb displayed by buttoning. (From Putnam JJ. Quicksilver and slow death. *Natl Geog* 1972;142:507, with permission.)

Diagnosis

The diagnosis may be confirmed by measurement of blood mercury concentration (acute toxicity) or a 24-hour urine mercury concentration (chronic toxicity), or both.[1]

Clinical Complications

Intravenous administration of mercury reportedly may cause pulmonary emboli, and subcutaneous injection may cause aseptic abscesses and granulomas.[2] Acute mercury inhalation can result in respiratory failure and death. Mercuric salt ingestion can cause renal failure. Shock and death may occur from hemorrhagic gastroenteritis and fluid loss. Under certain circumstances, exposure to organic mercury, particularly dimethylmercury, has caused progressive, irreversible, and sometimes fatal central nervous system damage.[3]

Management

Acute mercury intoxication should be treated with intramuscular dimercaprol (BAL). BAL may not be useful in methylmercury toxicity, because it may increase blood concentrations.[1] Succimer (DMSA) may be used if patients can tolerate an oral agent.[1]

REFERENCES

1. Graeme KA, Pollack CV Jr. Heavy metal toxicity, part 1: arsenic and mercury. *J Emerg Med* 1998;16:45–56.
2. Ruha AM, Tanen DA, Suchard JR, et al. Combined ingestion and subcutaneous injection of elemental mercury. *J Emerg Med* 2001;20:39–42.
3. Nierenberg DW, Nordgren RE, Chang MB, et al. Delayed cerebellar disease and death after accidental exposure to dimethylmercury. *N Engl J Med* 1998;338:1672–1676.

24–19

Thallium

Anthony Morocco

Clinical Presentation

Symptoms develop hours to days after exposure. The classic presentation of thallium toxicity is the combination of alopecia and a painful, ascending peripheral neuropathy. The neuropathy begins in the lower extremities 2 to 5 days after exposure, and patients may experience severe pain with light touch. Central nervous system involvement results in a variety of problems, including ataxia, delirium, psychosis, sleep disturbance, optic neuropathy, and cranial nerve dysfunction. Alopecia begins approximately 10 days after exposure; it may be complete or may spare axillary and facial hair. Other signs and symptoms include nausea, vomiting, constipation, abdominal pain, tachycardia, hypertension, palmar erythema, anhydrosis, and Mee's lines.[1]

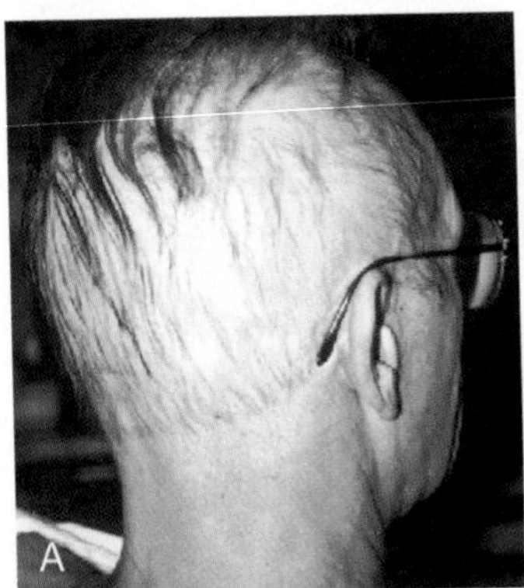

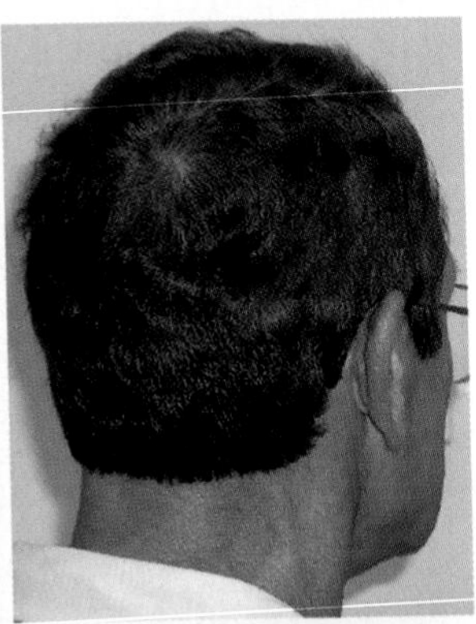

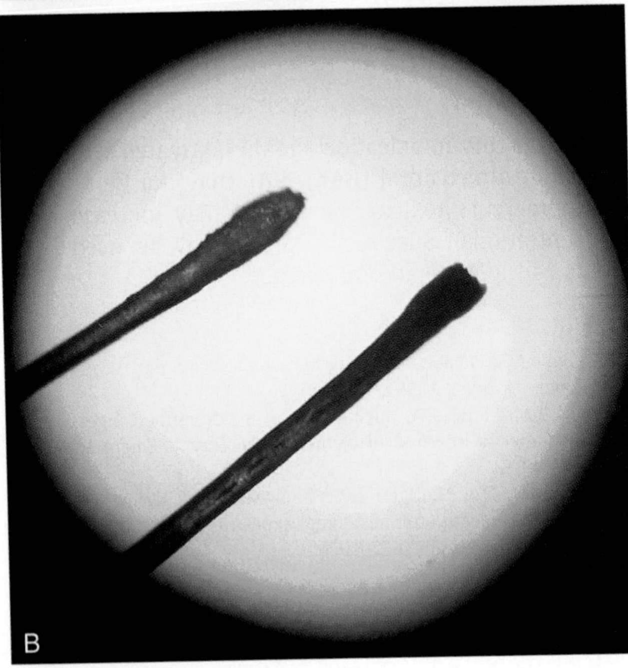

FIGURE 24–19 **A:** On the left is a patient with thallium-induced alopecia. On the right is the same patient 6 months later. **B:** Blackened hair root on the right compared with normal hair on the left. (**A** and **B** reprinted from Rusyniak with permission.)

Pathophysiology

Thallium is a metal that may be found in its elemental form or as a salt. Although elemental thallium is usually harmless, the thallous (Tl^{+1}) and thallic (Tl^{+3}) salts are potentially harmful. Thallium salts such as thallium sulfate have been used in depilatories, antimicrobial agents, and rodenticide agents. The use of thallium salts as rodenticides was banned in the United States in 1975 but persists elsewhere.[1]

Thallium salts are well absorbed by oral, dermal, and inhalational routes. Thallium inhibits a number of potassium-dependent enzymes and disrupts Krebs cycle enzymes, sodium-potassium adenosine triphosphatase (Na^+/K^+-ATPase), mitochondrial enzymes, and others. Cells of the central and peripheral nervous system are particularly affected, resulting in numerous lesions, including axonopathy.

Diagnosis

Thallium poisoning should be strongly suspected in any patient with alopecia and peripheral neuropathy. The metal can be seen under a microscope as black deposits in hair roots in 95% of patients, in several bands if multiple exposures have occurred. Abdominal radiography may reveal metallic material in the gastrointestinal tract. Laboratory confirmation of thallium toxicity involves measurement in a 24-hour urine collection.

Clinical Complications

Patients with severe toxicity progressively worsen over days, ultimately to coma, respiratory paralysis, and death.

Management

Multidose activated charcoal decreases thallium absorption and enhances elimination. Whole-bowel irrigation should be considered, especially if thallium remains in the gastrointestinal tract. Prussian blue (ferric hexacyanoferrate) should be administered as soon as possible, because it binds thallium and enhances elimination.[1,2] Prussian blue may not be readily available, but substantial supplies are maintained by the Radiation Emergency Assistance Center Training Site (REAC/TS) in Oak Ridge, Tennessee (telephone, 1-865-576-1005). Practitioners may contact REAC/TS for guidance in obtaining this antidote. Charcoal hemoperfusion with or without hemodialysis may be beneficial.

REFERENCES

1. Galvan-Arzate S, Santamaria A. Thallium toxicity. *Toxicol Lett* 1998; 99:1–13.
2. Hoffman RS. Thallium poisoning during pregnancy: a case report and comprehensive literature review. *J Toxicol Clin Toxicol* 2000;38:767–775.

Methemoglobinemia

Anthony Morocco

Clinical Presentation

Patients with chronic methemoglobinemia may be asymptomatic despite large fractions of methemoglobin. Patients with acute methemoglobinemia, as occurs after exposure to a medication, may present with signs and symptoms of hypoxemia. Patients may develop dyspnea, tachycardia, cyanosis, and nausea as the methemoglobin fraction rises to 30% or more of total hemoglobin. As the methemoglobin fraction rises to greater than 50%, symptoms worsen, mental status may become altered, and hypotension may develop.[1]

Pathophysiology

Normal hemoglobin is converted to methemoglobin when its iron atom is oxidized from the ferrous (Fe^{2+}) to the ferric (Fe^{3+}) state, which renders it unable to bind oxygen. Chronic methemoglobinemia results from an enzyme deficiency and inherited abnormal forms of hemoglobin, although a small amount of methemoglobin is present in all individuals. Large concentrations of methemoglobin may be produced on exposure to oxidizing agents such as nitrates, nitrites, local anesthetics, chlorates, naphthalene, phenazopyridine, and dapsone.[1] Methemoglobinemia may also occur in young infants with diarrhea, dehydration, and acidosis.[1]

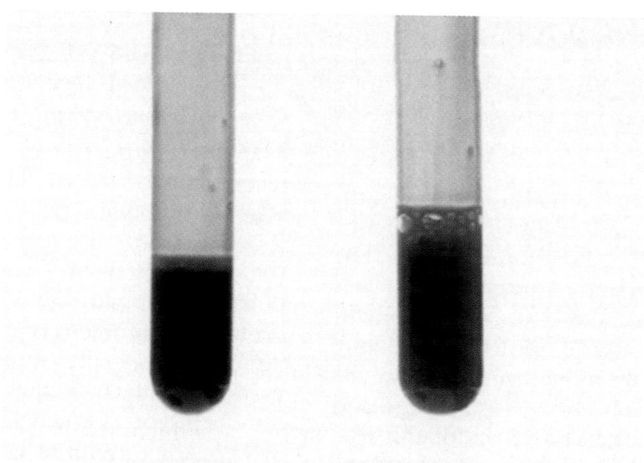

FIGURE 24–20 Chocolate-brown blood on left (methemoglobinemia) and normal blood on right. (From Donnelly R. Methemoglobinemia. *N Engl J Med* 2000;343:337. © 2000 Massachusetts Medical Society. All rights reserved.)

Diagnosis

The blood from affected patients appears dark brown in color. The methemoglobin concentration can be measured directly by a co-oximeter. Pulse oximetry is unreliable when methemoglobin is present and reveals a "saturation gap." The partial pressure of oxygen (pO_2) on an arterial blood gas measurement is elevated, and therefore the saturation, which is calculated from the pO_2, is falsely elevated. The bedside pulse oximeter may overestimate the arterial hemoglobin oxygen saturation because it falsely reads methemoglobin as oxygenated hemoglobin. For this reason, patients with methemoglobinemia rarely have bedside pulse oximeter readings lower than 85%.[1]

Clinical Complications

A methemoglobin fraction greater than 70% is reported to be lethal. Other complications include cardiac dysrhythmias, hypotension, hemolysis, and renal failure.[1]

Management

Treatment is indicated for symptomatic patients with greater than 20% methemoglobin and for asymptomatic patients with greater than 30% methemoglobin.[1] Methylene blue, 1 to 2 mg/kg, is given by slow intravenous infusion. This agent accelerates the natural conversion of methemoglobin to hemoglobin. Methylene blue is contraindicated in patients with glucose-6-phosphate dehydrogenase (G6PD) deficiency. Multiple courses of treatment may be needed, particularly after overdose from drugs with a long half-life, such as dapsone.[1]

REFERENCES

1. Rehman HU. Methemoglobinemia. *West J Med* 2001;175:193–196.

Hydrogen Sulfide

Anthony Morocco

Clinical Presentation

The clinical presentation depends on the concentration of hydrogen sulfide (H_2S) and duration of exposure. H_2S is known as a "knockdown" gas, because exposure to high concentrations is capable of causing loss of consciousness within seconds. With low-dose exposure, patients report smelling the gas, but olfactory paralysis develops quickly, and those exposed to high concentrations may not perceive the smell. Initial symptoms during exposure may include irritation of eyes and mucous membranes. Respiratory irritation may be associated with chest tightness, shortness of breath, and cough. Patients may exhibit central nervous system effects such as dizziness, headache, confusion, decreased level of consciousness, and seizures.[1]

TABLE 24–21 Physiologic Effects of Human Exposure to Hydrogen Sulfide

Concentration (ppm)	Physiologic effect
0.02	Odor threshold
0.13	Detectable, minimum perceptible odor
0.77	Faint, weak odor, readily perceptible
3–5	Offensive, moderately intense odor
10	Obvious and unpleasant odor, threshold limit value-time weighted average, "sore eyes"
20	Maximum allowable concentration for daily 8-h exposure
20–30	Strong and intense odor but not intolerable
50	Conjunctival irritation is first noticeable
50–100	Mild irritation to the respiratory tract and especially to the eyes after 1 h of exposure
100	Loss of smell in 3–15 min, may sting eyes and throat, olfactory fatigue level
150	Olfactory nerve paralysis
~ 200	Less intense odor, olfactory paralysis
250	Prolonged exposure may cause pulmonary edema
300–500	Pulmonary edema, imminent threat to life
500	In 0.5–1.0 h causes excitement, headache, dizziness, and staggering followed by unconsciousness and respiratory failure
500–1000	Acts primarily as a systemic poison causing unconsciousness and death through respiratory paralysis
700	Unconscious quickly, death results if not rescued promptly
5000	Imminent death

ppm, parts per million.
From Dart, with permission. Adapted from Beauchamp RD Jr., Bus JS, Popp JA, et al. *CRC Crit Rev Toxicol* 1984;13:40.

Pathophysiology

Hydrogen sulfide is a colorless, irritant gas with a strong sulfurous or "rotten-egg" smell. It is produced by the decay of organic waste, and it is used or produced during a number of industrial processes. H_2S is produced naturally by bacterial action in sewers, swamps, manure pits, septic tanks, and active volcanic areas. It is also produced on-site at many petroleum refineries, paper mills, and chemical processing plants. Because H_2S is heavier than air, it settles and accumulates in low-lying areas.[1] H_2S is second only to carbon monoxide as a toxicologic cause of death in the workplace.[2]

H_2S impairs oxygen utilization by inhibiting mitochondrial cytochrome oxidase aa_3.[1]

Diagnosis

Diagnosis is based on the history; incidents typically occur in closed spaces and involve multiple victims, including rescuers. Laboratory testing may reveal a lactic acidosis and elevated venous blood oxygen content, signifying impairment of oxygen utilization.[1]

Clinical Complications

Death occurs within minutes during exposure to high concentrations. In some survivors, persistent neurologic sequelae have reportedly included spasticity, tremor, and persistent vegetative stare. Brain imaging may reveal basal ganglia lesions. Noncardiogenic pulmonary edema has been reported.[1]

Management

Aggressive supportive care is essential. Hyperbaric oxygen therapy may be beneficial if readily available. The administration of sodium nitrite has also been recommended to induce methemoglobin, which binds H_2S with greater affinity than the cytochrome enzymes do. Both therapies should be considered for severe toxicity, though data on efficacy in human poisoning are lacking.[1]

REFERENCES

1. Snyder JW, Safir EF, Summerville GP, et al. Occupational fatality and persistent neurological sequelae after mass exposure to hydrogen sulfide. *Am J Emerg Med* 1995;13:199–203.
2. Fuller DC, Suruda AJ. Occupationally related hydrogen sulfide deaths in the United States from 1984 to 1994. *J Occup Environ Med* 2000;9:939–942.

Cyclic Antidepressants

Anthony Morocco

Clinical Presentation

Patients may complain of various side effects during cyclic antidepressants (CA) therapy, including dry mouth, sedation, orthostatic hypotension, blurred vision, constipation, and weight gain.[1] In overdose, patients may develop agitation, delirium, and myoclonus, followed by depressed level of consciousness, seizure, dysrhythmias (sinus tachycardia or ventricular tachycardia), and refractory hypotension.[2] Amoxapine is associated with significantly higher risk for seizure than other CAs. Anticholinergic effects such as hyperthermia, dry skin, and urinary retention commonly occur.

Pathophysiology

The cyclic antidepressants include the tricyclics (amitriptyline, nortriptyline, doxepin, amoxapine) and the tetracyclics (maprotiline). These agents are useful in the treatment of depression, obsessive-compulsive disorder, chronic pain syndromes, and other disorders, but they can be very dangerous in the overdose setting.[1]

The antidepressant action of the CAs is believed to result from blockade of the reuptake of serotonin and norepinephrine. CAs also antagonize muscarinic cholinergic receptors. Sedation and hypotension result from histamine (H_1) and α_1-adrenergic receptor blockade, respectively. Individual agents differ in the relative strength of these effects.[1] CAs block influx of sodium through fast channels in the myocardium (class I anti-arrhythmic effect), resulting in cardiotoxicity.[1]

Diagnosis

Diagnosis is based on the history and the signs and symptoms. Cardiac dysfunction includes tachycardia, QRS and QT_c prolongation, and a terminal R wave in lead aVR. QRS duration may be used to predict toxicity: a duration longer than 100 msec is predictive of increased risk of seizures, and longer than 160 msec is predictive of increased risk of dysrhythmias. CA levels are not reliable and do not correlate with toxicity due to significant protein binding. Rapid qualitative immunoassay screens can detect the presence of CAs, but there are several potential causes of false-positive results (e.g., diphenhydramine, cyclobenzaprine, quetiapine).

Clinical Complications

Mean time to death after overdose is 5.4 hours.[1] Seizures may result in abrupt worsening of cardiovascular status. Pulmonary edema, acute respiratory distress syndrome, aspiration pneumonitis, infection, and bowel ischemia may occur.

Management

Gastric lavage should be considered within the first 1 to 2 hours, and activated charcoal should be administered. Sodium bicarbonate should be given as a bolus and drip if the QRS duration exceeds 100 msec. Hypertonic saline may also be beneficial for CA cardiotoxicity.[2] Hypotension may be treated with fluid boluses and α-adrenergic agonists (e.g., norepinephrine).

REFERENCES

1. Sarko J. Antidepressants, old and new. *Emerg Med Clin North Am* 2000;18:637–654.
2. McCabe JL, Cobaugh DJ, Menegazzi JJ, et al. Experimental tricyclic antidepressant toxicity: a randomized controlled comparison of hypertonic saline solution, sodium bicarbonate, and hyperventilation. *Ann Emerg Med* 1998;32:329–333.

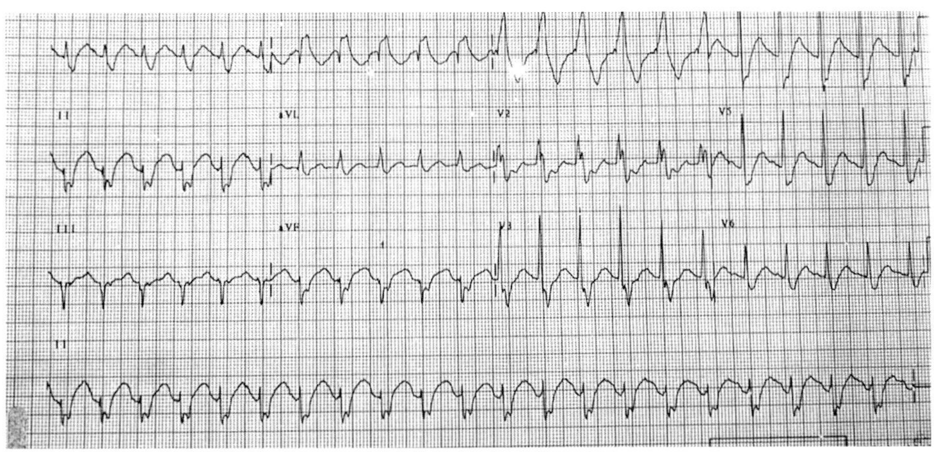

FIGURE 24–22 QRS widening and rightward deviation of the terminal 30-msec segment in aVR. (Courtesy of Anthony Morocco, MD.)

Cardiac Glycosides

Anthony Morocco

Clinical Presentation

Patients with acute cardiac glycoside toxicity present with nausea, vomiting, abdominal pain, lethargy, and confusion. The onset may be minutes to hours after ingestion. Chronic toxicity manifests similarly but with more subtle symptoms. Patients may exhibit delirium, disorientation, and visual disturbances such as blurring, chromatopsia (abnormal colors), and xanthopsia (yellow halos). Both acute and chronic toxicity can result in significant cardiac disturbances. The most common arrhythmia is ventricular ectopy, and bidirectional ventricular tachycardia is almost pathognomonic. Other rhythms of atrial or ventricular automaticity with depressed atrioventricular (AV) conduction may be seen.[1]

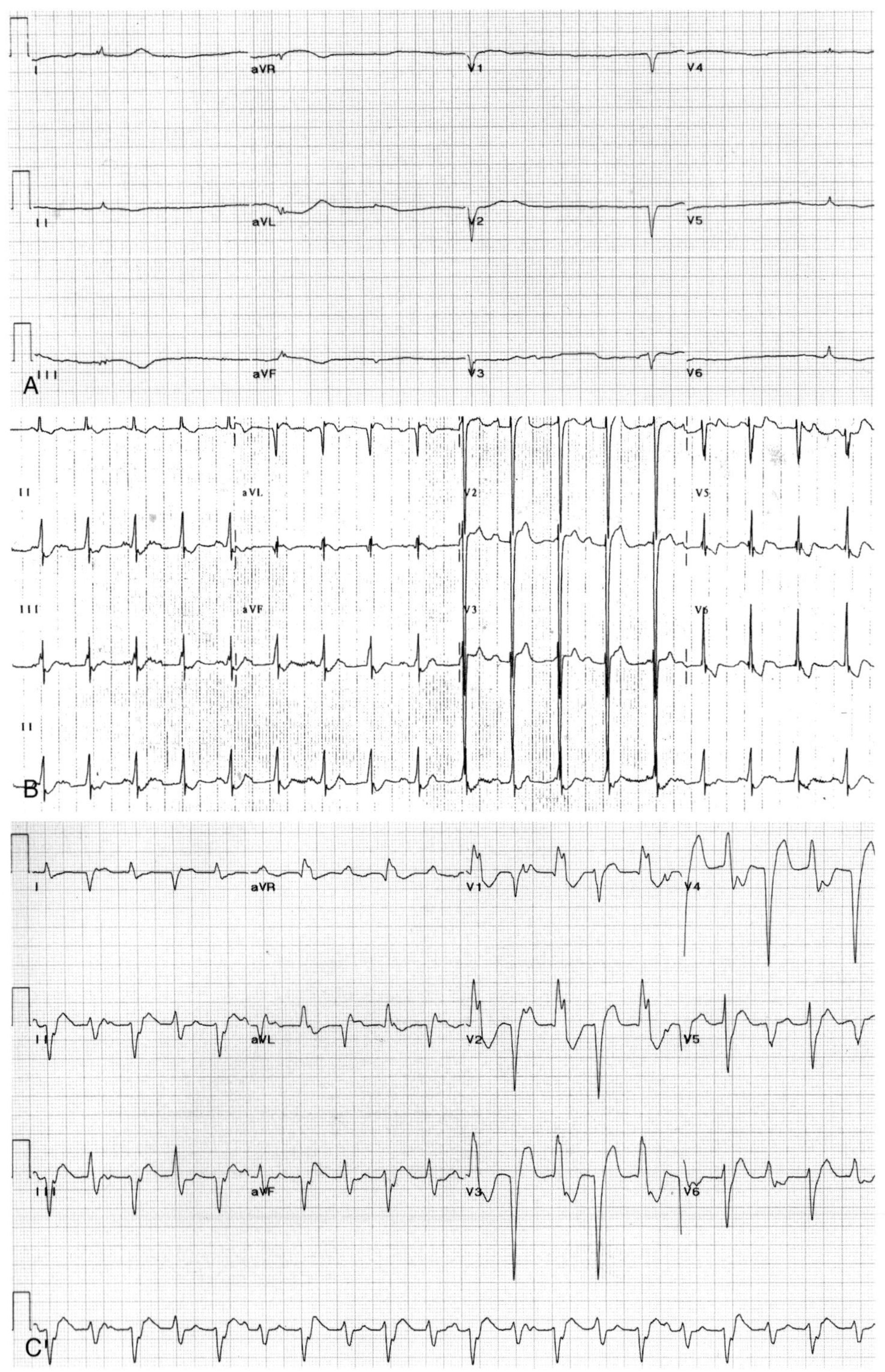

FIGURE 24–23 **A:** Bradycardic junctional rhythm secondary to digoxin toxicity. (From Fowler, with permission.) **B:** Paroxysmal atrial tachycardia with block. (From Fowler, with permission.) **C:** Bidirectional ventricular tachycardia. (From Fowler, with permission.)

Cardiac Glycosides

Anthony Morocco

Pathophysiology

The cardiac glycosides are a group of pharmaceuticals and plant and animal compounds with similar structures and effects on the cardiovascular system. Digoxin (derived from the foxglove plant) and digitoxin are the best-known chemicals of this class.[1] Several other plants contain cardiac glycosides, including oleander, squill, lily of the valley, and henbane.[2] An animal source is the secretions of *Bufo* toad species.[1]

Cardiac glycosides inhibit sodium-potassium adenosine triphosphatase (Na^+/K^+-ATPase), resulting in increased intracellular calcium and enhanced contraction of cardiac muscle cells. This effect also causes enhanced automaticity. Action on vagal fibers increases parasympathetic input to the heart, depressing sinoatrial (SA) and AV nodal conduction.[1]

Diagnosis

The serum digoxin concentration should be measured at least 6 hours after ingestion, to account for the tissue-distribution phase of the drug. Various cardiac glycosides may cross-react with the assays.[1,2] In acute toxicity, the serum potassium concentration may be elevated; concentrations greater than 5.5 mEq/L may be predictive of death in some cases.[1]

Clinical Complications

Death may occur due to ventricular arrhythmias.

Management

The treatment of choice for digoxin poisoning is the use of digoxin-specific antibody fragments. The antibodies also cross-react with other cardiac glycosides.[2] Indications for use include serious arrhythmias, potassium concentration greater than 5.0 mEq/L, serum digoxin concentration greater than 15 ng/mL at any time or greater than 10 ng/L at 6 hours after ingestion, and ingestion of 10 mg in an adult or 4 mg in a child.[1]

REFERENCES

1. Hack JB, Lewin NA. Cardiac glycosides. In: Goldfrank LR, Flomenbaum NE, Lewin NA, et al., eds. *Goldfrank's toxicologic emergencies*, 7th ed. New York, McGraw-Hill, 2002, pp 724–734.
2. Eddleston M, Rajapakse S, Rajakanthan K, et al. Anti-digoxin Fab fragments in cardiotoxicity induced by ingestion of yellow oleander: a randomised controlled trial. *Lancet* 2000;355:967–972.

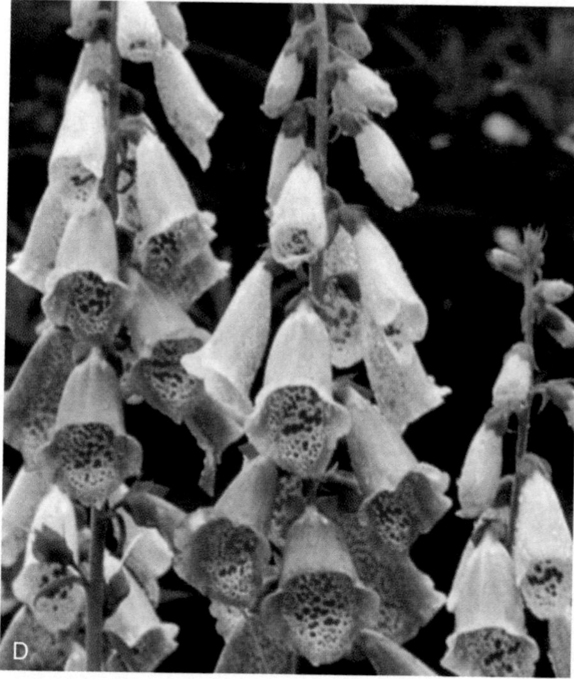

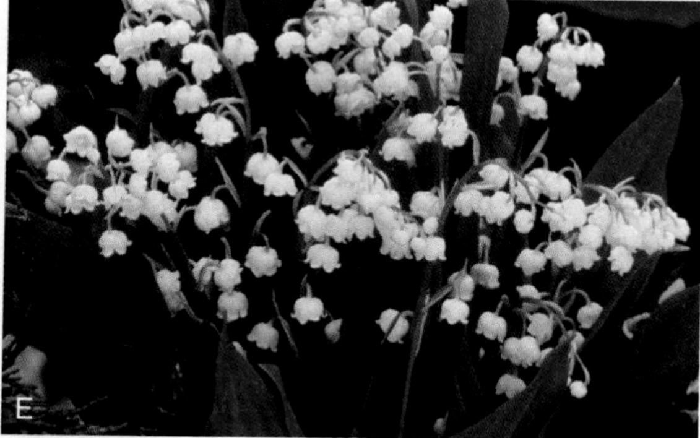

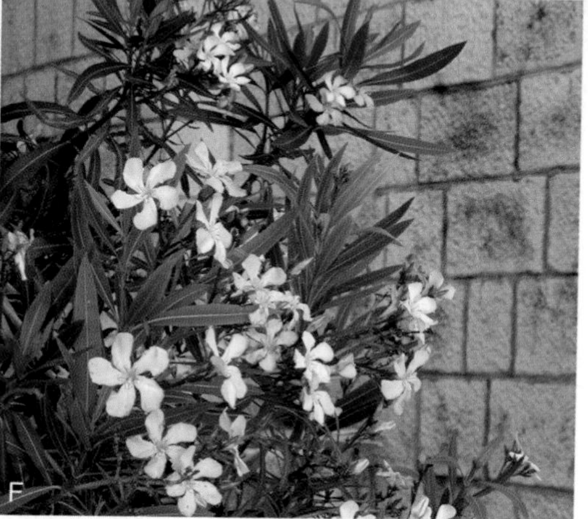

FIGURE 24–23, cont'd. D: Digitalis (foxglove). (Courtesy of Robert H. Poppenga, DVM, PhD.) **E:** Lily-of-the-valley. (Courtesy of Robert H. Poppenga, DVM, PhD.) **F:** Nerium oleander. (Courtesy of Robert H. Poppenga, DVM, PhD.)

Niacin Toxicity

Michael Greenberg

Clinical Presentation

Patients who take niacin, a B vitamin sometimes used to treat dyslipidemia, may present with a syndrome of acute vasodilatation/flushing manifested by intense, diffuse itching in conjunction with an erythematous, warm rash, as well as nausea and headache within 30 minutes after niacin ingestion. Other patients may present with subacute hepatitis after longer-term use of niacin.

Pathophysiology

The flushing and hepatotoxicity—associated with immediate-release (IR) and sustained-release (SR) niacin, respectively—are directly related to the dissolution rates and metabolic profiles for the various formulations of niacin. Niacin goes through hepatic first-pass metabolism via two separate pathways, a conjugative pathway and an amidation pathway. Glycine conjugates such as nicotinuric acid are formed by the conjugative pathway. These compounds have been associated with vasodilatation and flushing. The conjugative pathway is a low-affinity, high-capacity pathway that is used only after the amidation pathway becomes saturated. The amidation pathway results in the formation of nicotinamide and pyrimidine metabolites. These compounds have been associated with hepatotoxicity occurring with some SR niacin formulations. The amidation pathway is high-affinity and low-capacity. After amidation has been saturated, niacin is metabolized exclusively by conjugation.

As a result of rapid dissolution and absorption, IR niacin saturates the amidation pathway, resulting in the metabolism by the conjugative pathway. This results in flushing. SR niacin releases the drug more slowly, so it is mostly metabolized by the amidation pathway. As a result, a relatively greater amount of metabolites associated with hepatotoxicity are generated.

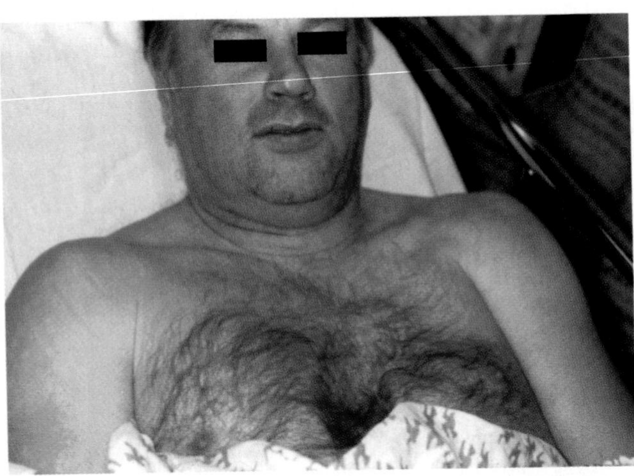

FIGURE 24–24 Flushing from niacin reaction. (Copyright James R. Roberts, MD.)

Diagnosis

The diagnosis of niacin-related flushing is based on the history and finding of the characteristic rash. The syndrome of hepatotoxicity is diagnosed based on clinical findings and liver function test abnormalities.

Clinical Complications

Complications of therapeutic niacin use include diarrhea, abdominal pain, hyperuricemia, gout, hyperglycemia, and acanthosis nigricans.

Management

The vasodilatation syndrome is usually self-limited. Tolerance regarding vasodilatation may develop over time. The syndrome may be treated with aspirin or other nonsteroidal antiinflammatory drugs (NSAIDs). Patients taking therapeutic niacin should be counseled to take the drug with food and to avoid concurrent spicy foods, hot beverages, and hot showers in temporal proximity to ingesting the drug.

REFERENCES

1. Pieper JA. Overview of niacin formulations: differences in pharmacokinetics, efficacy, and safety. *Am J Health Syst Pharm* 2003;60(13 Suppl 2):S9–S14.
2. Wolf R, Orion E, Matz H, et al. Miscellaneous treatments: II. Niacin and heparin: unapproved uses, dosages or indications. *Clin Dermatol* 2002;20:547–557.
3. Miller M. Niacin as a component of combination therapy for dyslipidemia. *Clin Proc* 2003;78:735–742.

Red Man Syndrome

Michael Greenberg

Clinical Presentation

Patients with red man syndrome (RMS) present with a red rash involving the face, neck, and torso within minutes after receiving the glycoprotein antibiotic vancomycin. The eruption may be associated with pruritus, and in severe cases patients may experience hypotension, shock, angioedema, difficulty breathing, and urticaria.[1–3]

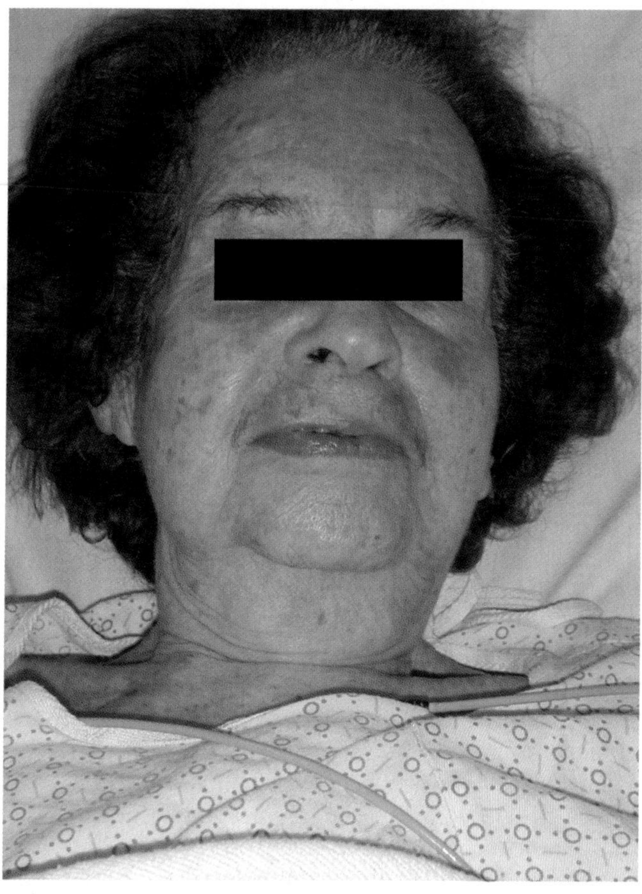

FIGURE 24–25 Red man syndrome. (Courtesy of Anthony Morocco, MD.)

Pathophysiology

The incidence of RMS in healthy volunteers is as high as 90% and represents an anaphylactoid reaction as opposed to a true allergic reaction.[3] RMS usually manifests with the first dose of vancomycin an individual receives. Subsequent doses usually, but not always, result in lesser reactions. RMS is usually associated with rapid intravenous vancomycin administration and is probably a histamine-mediated phenomenon.

Diagnosis

The diagnosis is based on the history of receiving vancomycin in close temporality to development of the typical erythematous rash and associated findings.

Clinical Complications

Complications include reoccurrence, severe exfoliative dermatitis, and cardiovascular collapse.

Management

RMS may be anticipated and minimized by pretreating with antihistamines and by administering the drug slowly and in multiple, small doses. Once RMS develops, vancomycin should be discontinued; it should be reinstated with extreme caution and with antihistamine pretreatment.

REFERENCES

1. Lobel EZ, Korelitz BI, Warman JI. Red man syndrome and infliximab. *J Clin Gastroenterol* 2003;36:186.
2. Renz CL, Thurn JD, Finn HA, et al. Oral antihistamines reduce the side effects from rapid vancomycin infusion. *Anesth Analg* 1998;87: 681–685.
3. Khurana C, de Belder MA. Red man syndrome after vancomycin: potential cross-reactivity with teicoplanin. *Postgrad Med J* 1999;75: 41–43.

Acute Dystonia

Anthony Morocco

Clinical Presentation

In 95% of cases, symptoms occur within 96 hours after medication exposure or an increase in medication dose.[1,2] Patients present with muscle spasms and abnormal postures of the head and neck, including grimacing, oculogyric crisis, blepharospasm, involuntary mouth opening, dysarthria, trismus, and torticollis.[1,2] Mild symptoms may include spasms of small muscle groups (fingers or hands) or an isolated sensation of spasm in the throat. More severe reactions may affect large muscle groups (opisthotonos, tortipelvis) and may produce profuse diaphoresis and anxiety.[1,2] Movement may exacerbate symptoms.

Pathophysiology

Acute dystonia is a movement disorder, usually affecting the head and neck, that occurs after use of dopamine-receptor–blocking drugs. Antipsychotics, antiemetics, and antidepressants are commonly associated with the disorder, and several other drug classes have been occasionally implicated. Risk factors for development of medication-induced acute dystonia include male sex (relative risk [RR], 2.0), young age (RR, 2 to 3 for age 10 to 19 years compared with 30 to 39 years), recent cocaine use (RR, 3 to 4), previous episode of acute dystonia (RR, 6), dehydration, and hypocalcemia.[1]

The precise mechanism of acute dystonia is unknown. It is likely that blockade of dopamine (D_2) receptors is important in the pathogenesis. Opposing hypotheses implicate both dopamine understimulation due to receptor blockade and overstimulation due to a compensatory increase in dopaminergic activity after receptor blockade.[2] Among antipsychotic drugs, a higher ratio of dopamine- to acetylcholine-receptor–blocking effect correlates with risk of acute dystonia.[1]

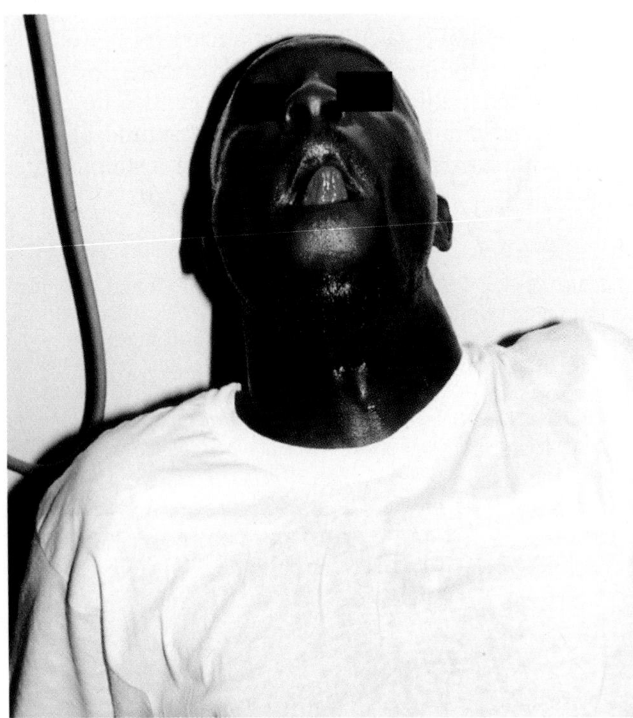

FIGURE 24–26 Note characteristic head and neck posture and associated diaphoresis. (Copyright James R. Roberts, MD.)

Diagnosis

Diagnosis is based on symptoms and recent use of medication associated with dystonia. Acute dystonia should be differentiated from chronic conditions, such as tardive dyskinesia, that occur after months or years of treatment. The differential diagnosis includes hypocalcemia, temporal epilepsy, and conversion reactions.[1]

Clinical Complications

Life-threatening symptoms may theoretically occur if dystonia manifests as laryngospasm with stridor.[1]

Management

Rapid relief of symptoms usually occurs with parenteral administration of an anticholinergic drug, such as diphenhydramine, benztropine, or biperiden. Benzodiazepines may also be beneficial to relieve anxiety and muscular symptoms that do not respond to anticholinergic treatment. Oral anticholinergic drugs should be continued for 4 to 7 days to prevent recurrence of the symptoms.[1]

REFERENCES

1. van Harten PN, Hoek HW, Kahn RS. Acute dystonia induced by drug treatment. *BMJ* 1999;319:623–626.
2. Diederich NJ, Goetz CG. Drug-induced movement disorders. *Neurol Clin* 1998;16:125–139.

Jimson Weed

Anthony Morocco

Clinical Presentation

Symptoms occur 30 to 60 minutes after ingestion. Patients present with a classic anticholinergic toxidrome. Signs and symptoms include dilated pupils, dry skin and mucous membranes, slurred speech, blurred vision, hyperthermia, tachycardia, red and hot skin, and urinary retention. Central nervous system effects range from confusion, hallucinations, and agitation to seizures and coma.[1]

Pathophysiology

Jimson weed, *Datura stramonium,* is commonly abused for its hallucinogenic effects. It is most often ingested as tea made from the seeds. It is a member of the nightshade family and is also known as thorn apple, angel's trumpet, and Jamestown weed.[1]

D. stramonium contains atropine, hyoscyamine, and scopolamine. All three antagonize the effect of acetylcholine at the muscarinic receptor. These postsynaptic receptors are found in the brain, at postganglionic sites in the parasympathetic nervous system, and in the sympathetic system at postganglionic receptors for sweat glands. All the clinical signs and symptoms are related to this anticholinergic effect. The seeds of the plant have the highest concentration of atropine, with up to 0.1 mg per seed.[1]

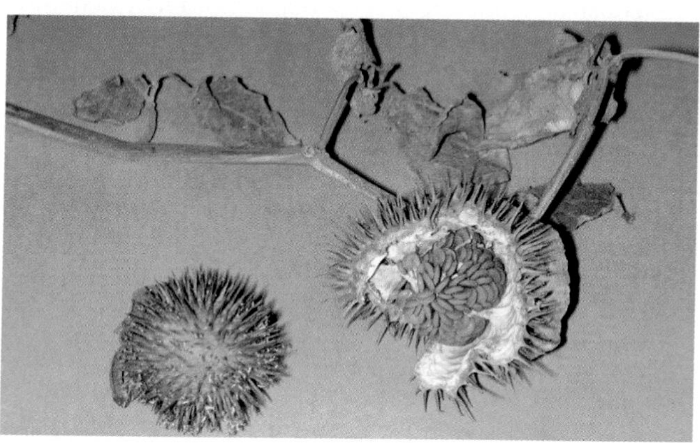

FIGURE 24–27 *Datura stramonium* (jimson weed). (Courtesy of Robert Hendrickson, MD.)

Diagnosis

There is no readily available diagnostic test, so the diagnosis must be made based on the presentation. *D. stramonium* intoxication should be suspected in any patient with anticholinergic toxicity, particularly if several patients present simultaneously. Such clusters of cases often occur among teenagers.

Clinical Complications

Large doses of an anticholinergic agent may result in hyperthermia, seizures, coma, and death. The lethal dose of atropine is about 10 mg.[1]

Management

Patients with mild to moderate symptoms require only general supportive care, including benzodiazepines for sedation. Symptoms may last 24 to 48 hours. Patients with severe agitation may be treated with physostigmine, an acetylcholinesterase inhibitor that increases acetylcholine levels at the synaptic junction to overcome the muscarinic antagonism. Physostigmine should be administered in a dose of 1 to 2 mg by slow intravenous injection over at least 5 minutes. Rapid administration can cause bradycardia and seizures.[1]

REFERENCES

1. Centers for Disease Control and Prevention. Jimson weed poisoning—Texas, New York, and California, 1994. *Morb Mortal Wkly Rep MMWR* 1995;44:41–44.

Poison Hemlock

Anthony Morocco

Clinical Presentation

Patients present with a cholinergic toxidrome: salivation, lacrimation, urination, vomiting, diarrhea, bronchospasm, and miosis. Vital signs may demonstrate bradycardia or tachycardia and hypertension. Weakness, muscle fasciculations, seizures, and coma also occur.[1]

Pathophysiology

Poison hemlock, *Conium maculatum*, is commonly found along roadways throughout the United States and southern Canada. The plant may grow to 10 feet in height, and it is similar in appearance to parsley, Queen Anne's lace, or water hemlock. Misidentification as wild carrot has resulted in accidental poison hemlock ingestion.[2]

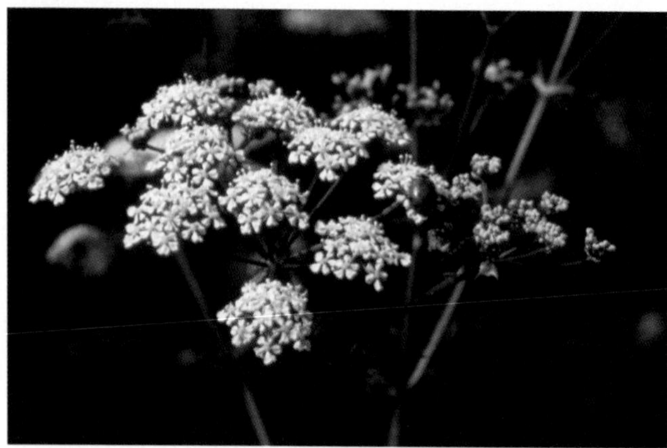

FIGURE 24-28 *Conium maculatum* (poison hemlock). (Courtesy of Robert H. Poppenga, DVM, PhD.)

Poison hemlock contains the toxin coniine, which is similar to nicotine. The highest concentration of the toxin is in the roots and seeds. Stimulation of ganglionic nicotinic receptors causes parasympathetic and sympathetic stimulation consistent with a cholinergic toxidrome. Coma and seizures result from central nervous system cholinergic stimulation. Coniine also acts as a depolarizing neuromuscular blocker.[1]

Diagnosis

Diagnosis is based on clinical presentation and history of foraging for edible plants. Creatine phosphokinase and renal function should be monitored.

Clinical Complications

Death and rhabdomyolysis with resultant renal failure have been reported.[1]

Management

There is no specific antidote, although treatment with atropine decreases the muscarinic symptoms (vomiting, bronchospasm, and other secretory symptoms). Activated charcoal may limit absorption of the toxin. Asymptomatic patients should be observed for at least 4 hours after ingestion. Supportive care should include intravenous fluid, airway management, and control of seizures with benzodiazepines. Urine should be alkalinized if rhabdomyolysis occurs.[1,2]

REFERENCES

1. Furbee B, Wermuth M. Life-threatening plant poisoning. *Crit Care Clin* 1997;13:849–888.
2. Frank BS, Michelson WB, Panter KE, et al. Ingestion of poison hemlock (*Conium maculatum*). *West J Med* 1995;163:573–574.

Water Hemlock

Anthony Morocco

Clinical Presentation

Patients may develop nausea, vomiting, abdominal pain, salivation, mydriasis, flushing, and diaphoresis 15 to 90 minutes after ingestion.[1] Increased bronchial secretions and respiratory distress may ensue. Multiple seizures commonly occur and may begin within 1 hour after ingestion.[1,2]

Pathophysiology

Water hemlock, *Cicuta maculata,* is in the same family as carrots, parsley, and parsnip. It is found growing in or near lakes, streams, and marshes in the eastern United States and Canada. The plant may be mistaken for nontoxic plants, such as cow parsnip and Queen Anne's lace, because of their similar appearance and odor of fresh carrots or turnips. Related toxic plants are *Cicuta douglasii,* the western water hemlock, found in the western United States, and *Oenanthe crocata,* the hemlock water dropwort, found in Europe.[2] Other common names for water hemlock are false parsley, poison parsnip, beaver poison, children's bane, and death-of-man.[1]

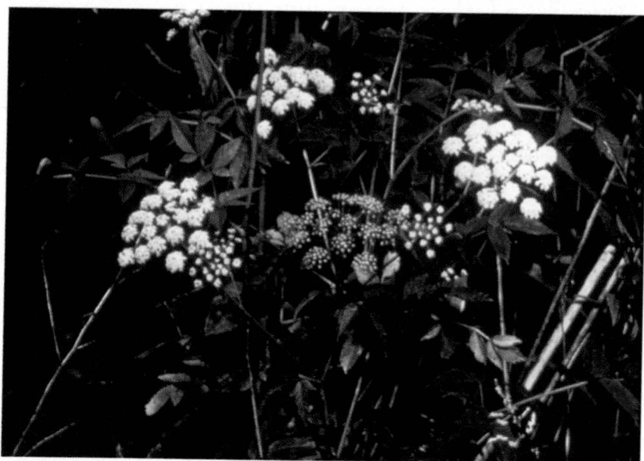

FIGURE 24–29 *Cicuta maculata* (water hemlock). (Courtesy of Robert H. Poppenga, DVM, PhD.)

Cicutoxin, found in highest concentration in the plant's roots, is responsible for the toxicity. The toxin is absorbed orally and dermally. The mechanism of action is unclear but may involve γ-aminobutyric acid (GABA) antagonism.[1]

Diagnosis

Diagnosis is based on clinical presentation and history of foraging for edible plants. Creatine phosphokinase and renal function should be monitored.

Clinical Complications

Rhabdomyolysis with resultant renal failure, hypotension, bradycardia, and severe metabolic acidosis have been reported.[1,2] Status epilepticus and death frequently occur. The mortality rate for water hemlock is reported to be 30%; *O. crocata* ingestion resulted in 70% mortality in one series.[1,2] Death in an adult may occur after ingestion of 2 to 3 cm of root, and death of a child after using a whistle made from the plant's stem has been reported.[2]

Management

There is no specific antidote. Activated charcoal may limit absorption of the toxin. Asymptomatic patients should be observed for at least 4 to 6 hours after ingestion. Supportive care should include intravenous fluid, airway management, and control of seizures with benzodiazepines. Urine should be alkalinized if rhabdomyolysis occurs.[1,2]

REFERENCES

1. Water hemlock poisoning—Maine, 1992. *Morb Mortal Wkly Rep MMWR* 1994;43:229–231.
2. Furbee B, Wermuth M. Life-threatening plant poisoning. *Crit Care Clin* 1997;13:849–888.

Pokeweed

Anthony Morocco

Clinical Presentation

Patients commonly present with nausea, oral burning, abdominal pain, vomiting, and diarrhea 15 minutes to 6 hours after ingestion. Neurologic symptoms such as visual disturbance, weakness, and seizures may occur.[1]

Pathophysiology

Pokeweed, *Phytolacca americana,* is a toxic plant that is native to the eastern United States. It is known by many other common names, including inkberry, poke, pigeonberry, and crowberry. The plant can grow to several feet in height. It produces long clusters of green-white flowers and dark purple berries. Young leaves of the plant are commonly eaten after being prepared by cooking in boiling water, discarding of the liquid, and boiling again. The leaves have been canned and sold as "poke salet." The plant has also been used as an herbal remedy for a number of conditions. Improper preparation, consumption of the berries, or misidentification of the plant often results in toxicity.[1]

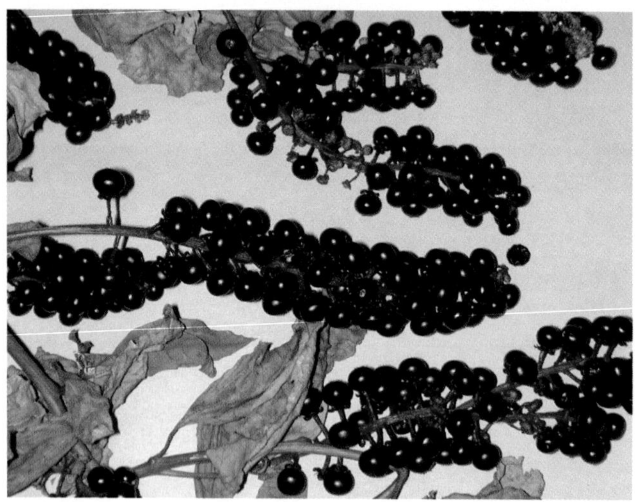

FIGURE 24–30 *Phytolacca americana* (pokeweed). (Courtesy of Robert Hendrickson, MD.)

All parts of the plant contain saponin glycosides, phytolaccigenin, phytolaccin, and phytolaccatoxin, which are direct irritants of the skin and mucous membranes. A glycoprotein known as pokeweed mitogen stimulates lymphocyte proliferation.[1]

Diagnosis

Diagnosis is primarily based on the history of plant ingestion. Children may report eating the purple berries. Evidence of lymphocytosis on complete blood count may be helpful.[1]

Clinical Complications

Gastrointestinal bleeding and significant volume depletion may occur with severe gastroenteritis. Deaths have reportedly occurred in children.[1]

Management

Activated charcoal should be administered for recent ingestion, although severe vomiting may limit oral intake. There is no specific treatment other than supportive care, primarily intravenous fluid and antiemetics. Symptoms generally resolve in 24 to 48 hours. The lymphocytosis may last for 2 weeks but requires no treatment.[1]

REFERENCES

1. Shoff WH, Shepherd SM. Plant poisoning: berries. In: Ford MD, Delaney KA, Ling LJ, Erickson T, eds. *Clinical toxicology.* Philadelphia, WB Saunders, 2001, pp 990–1001.

Betel Nut

Anthony Morocco

Clinical Presentation

Users report a mild stimulant and euphoric effect. A small drop in blood pressure and tachycardia occurs. Miosis or mydriasis may be present. Chronic users are noted to have red-stained teeth and oral mucosa, with fissures at the corners of the mouth (betel chewer's perlèche). First-time users of a large dose develop dizziness, flushing, diaphoresis, and vomiting, similar to the symptoms caused by tobacco toxicity.[1]

Pathophysiology

An estimated 600 million people, mostly in India, east Asia, and the western Pacific, chew betel nut daily. The nut grows on the betel or areca palm tree, *Areca catechu*. Betel is chewed after it has been combined with various ingredients into a "quid." The type of betel used and the substances in the quid vary by geographic region. To prepare the quid, the shell of the nut is opened, and the inner meat is used. It may be combined with lime, wrapped in the leaf of the betel pepper (*Piper betel*), and placed in the mouth. Other ingredients may be added to the quid, most commonly tobacco and catechu gum (the sap of the tree *Acacia nilotica*), as well as nutmeg, cardamom, anise, clove, and cinnamon.[1]

Betel contains arecoline and arecaidine, which are central and peripheral cholinergic agonists at nicotinic and muscarinic receptors. The betel pepper leaf also contains psychoactive compounds, including the cocaine-like cadinene. Lime, pepper leaf, and catechu are used to stimulate salivation, enhance the release of the betel alkaloids, and add to the euphoric effects.[1] A large dose of betel nut could cause severe cholinergic toxicity, with symptoms described by the mnemonic SLUDGE: **s**alivation, **l**acrimation, **u**rinary incontinence, **d**iarrhea, **g**astrointestinal upset, and **e**mesis.

Diagnosis

The diagnosis of betel nut use may be ascertained by history and physical examination.

Clinical Complications

Complications include pulmonary edema, bronchoconstriction, and death. Chronic, heavy use may cause oral leukoplakia and oral submucosal fibrosis. Betel is associated with oropharyngeal squamous cell carcinoma and is believed to act synergistically with tobacco in causing cancer. Betel nut is also associated with increased risk of asthma due to cholinergic-induced bronchoconstriction. Other consequences of heavy use include transient psychosis, extrapyramidal symptoms in patients taking neuroleptics, and milk-alkali syndrome (because of the lime). Betel use causes dependence and withdrawal symptoms similar to those of nicotine.[1]

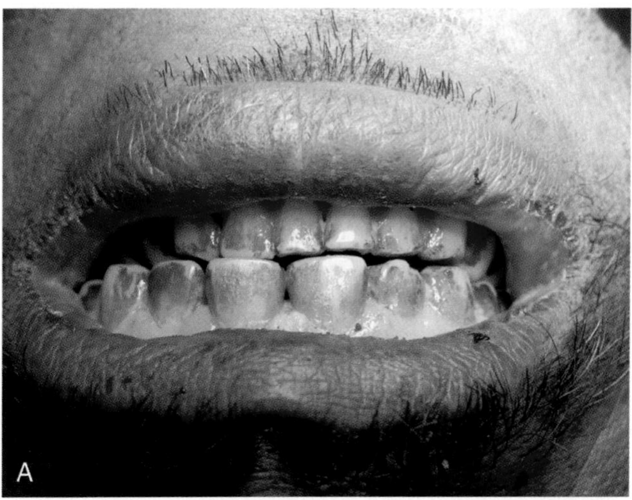

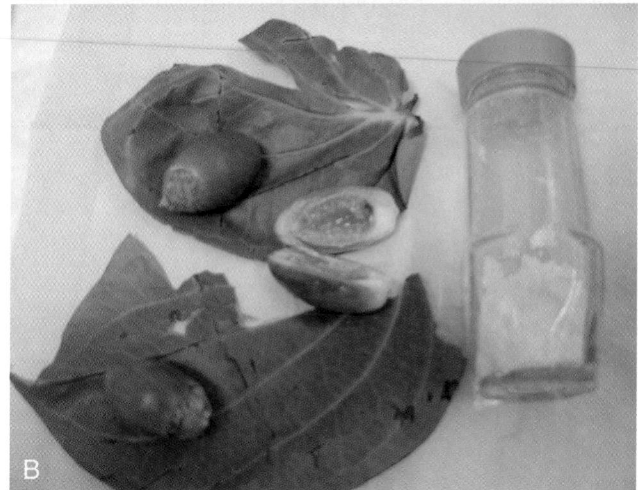

FIGURE 24–31 **A:** Intraoral and tooth staining from betel nut. **B:** Betel nut paraphernalia. (**A** and **B,** Courtesy of Anthony Morocco, MD.)

Management

The acute effects of betel nut are short-lived, but patients with severe cholinergic symptoms may be treated with atropine.[1]

REFERENCES

1. Nelson BS, Heischober B. Betel nut: a common drug used by naturalized citizens from India, Far East Asia, and the South Pacific Islands. *Ann Emerg Med* 1999;34:238–243.

Kava

Anthony Morocco

Clinical Presentation

Kava consumption may cause mild euphoria and relaxation, along with mild gastrointestinal upset, difficulty with visual accommodation, and allergic skin reactions. High doses may cause ataxia and muscle weakness.[1,2] Chronic ingestion of high doses results in kava dermopathy. Patients may develop facial edema, scleral injection, and skin changes that include yellow discoloration and scaly lesions on the palms, soles, forearms, shins, and back.[1] Patients with kava-related hepatitis present with nausea, vomiting, and jaundice.[2]

Pathophysiology

Kava, *Piper methysticum,* is an herb indigenous to Polynesia. It is also known as kava kava, ava, awa, intoxicating pepper, and yagona. It is consumed as a beverage made from the pulverized root and is used in native South Pacific cultures for ceremonies and recreation.[1,2] Kava is also available in commercial herbal formulations as dried root or liquid extract with standardized kava lactone concentrations.[1]

Kava may possess anxiolytic, sedative, muscle-relaxant, analgesic, and local anesthetic effects.[1,2] The active ingredients are believed to be the kava lactones, such as methysticin, kawain, and dihydrokawain. Potential mechanisms of action include activity at γ-aminobutyric acid and benzodiazepine receptors, dopamine antagonism, and monoamine oxidase inhibition. The mechanisms of kava dermopathy and hepatitis are unknown.[1,2]

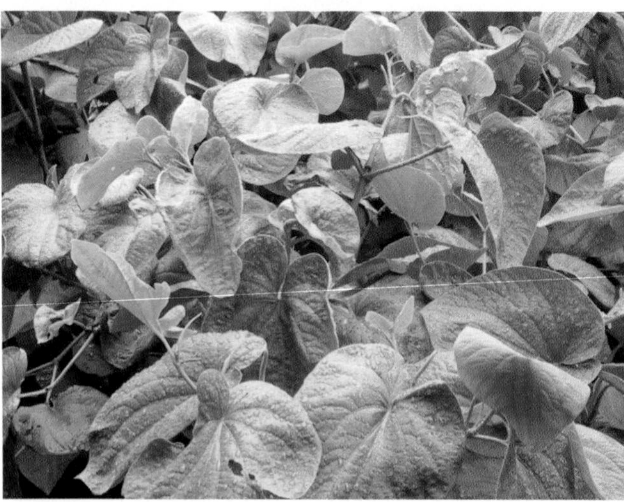

FIGURE 24–32 *Piper methysticum* (kava) is an evergreen shrub with heart-shaped leaves and jointed stems that grows predominantly in the Pacific Islands. (With permission from H. C. "Skip" Bittenbender, PhD, and the Farmer's Bookshelf, College of Tropical Agriculture and Human Resources, University of Hawaii at Manoa [http://www.CTAHR.Hawaii.edu/fb/].)

Diagnosis

Workup of kava-induced hepatotoxicity should rule out other possible causes, such as viruses and other toxic substances.

Clinical Complications

Hepatotoxicity can progress to hepatic failure and death or liver transplantation.

Management

Side effects, including dermopathy, resolve after discontinuation of use. Hepatitis should be treated with aggressive supportive therapy and evaluation for liver transplantation.

REFERENCES

1. Pepping J. Kava: *Piper methysticum. Am J Health Syst Pharm* 1999; 56:957–960.
2. Humberston CL, Akhtar J, Krenzelok EP. Acute hepatitis induced by kava kava. *J Toxicol Clin Toxicol* 2003;41:109–113.

Khat

Anthony Morocco

Clinical Presentation

Khat users report effects similar to those of amphetamines, including enhanced alertness, increased energy, and euphoria. Less desirable effects of anxiety, irritability, and insomnia also occur. After the drug effects subside, patients develop a depressive phase, with lethargy and drug craving.[1]

Pathophysiology

Khat is the common name for the plant *Catha edulis.* Its leaves are chewed commonly during social gatherings in east and central Africa and the Arabian peninsula. Khat is also popular in the United States and elsewhere among immigrants from the plant's native areas. Fresh leaves are preferred, because the plant's stimulant effect diminishes after drying.[1]

The active ingredient in khat is the amine cathinone, which causes release of catecholamines. The synthetic drug methcathinone is similar in structure. Other active substances in khat include cathine and norephedrine.[1]

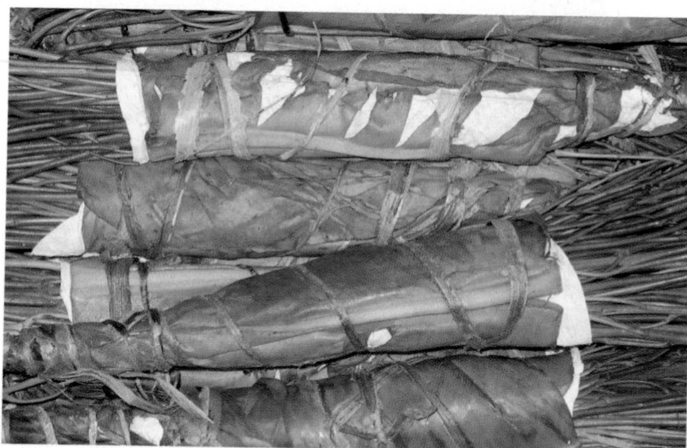

FIGURE 24–33 Khat. (Courtesy of Glenn Everett. Khat wrapped in banana leaves and smuggled in a suitcase. *Microgram Bulletin* 2002;35:237.)

Diagnosis

Readily available drug screens do not test for cathinone.

Clinical Complications

Hyperthermia occurs, although khat users generally do not seem to experience the severe sympathomimetic toxicity that occurs with amphetamine use. Reported adverse effects from chronic use are esophageal cancer, hypertension, coronary vasospasm, myocardial infarction, psychosis, and cognitive impairment.[1]

Management

Agitated patients should be treated with reassurance and benzodiazepines. Hyperthermia should be rapidly corrected.[1]

REFERENCES

1. Carvalho F. The toxicological potential of khat. *J Ethnopharmacol* 2003;87:1–2.

Cocaine

Anthony Morocco

Clinical Presentation

Onset of drug action is within seconds after smoking or injection, and less than 3 minutes after insufflation. Users may report intense euphoria and enhanced wakefulness. Patients may present with signs of sympathetic stimulation, including tachycardia, hypertension, diaphoresis, mydriasis, restlessness, and agitated delirium. In addition, chest pain after cocaine use is a common reason for emergency department presentation.[2]

Pathophysiology

Cocaine is an alkaloid derived from the coca plant, *Erythroxylon coca*. In addition to its widespread illicit use, the drug is used medicinally for its local anesthetic and vasoconstrictive properties. Cocaine may be used in the hydrochloride or base forms. The hydrochloride is readily soluble in water and is taken by injection or insufflation. Cocaine base, or freebase, is made from the hydrochloride form and is more stable when heated. "Crack" (named for the "popping" sound made during heating) is a commonly smoked form of cocaine base.[1]

Cocaine acts within the central nervous system to block the reuptake of catecholamines at the synaptic cleft. This effect is particularly important in dopaminergic areas that mediate euphoria and drug craving. The local anesthetic effect is produced by blockade of neuronal fast-sodium channels. Cocaine's sodium-channel blockade in the myocardium mimics the effects of class I antidysrhythmic agents. The drug also causes a prothrombotic effect through its action on platelets and coagulation factors. Cocaine has pharmacologically active metabolites, including the potent cocaethylene, which is produced in the presence of ethanol.

Diagnosis

Many commonly available and widely used immunoassay drug screens detect the cocaine metabolite benzoylecgonine in the urine for several days (typically 2 to 3 days) after drug use.[1]

Clinical Complications

Large doses of cocaine can produce myocardial depression, seizures, and death. Other complications include hypertensive emergencies, severe hyperthermia, rhabdomyolysis, renal failure, cerebrovascular accident, myocardial infarction, chest pain, gastrointestinal ischemia, placental abruption, and aortic dissection.[1,2]

Management

Benzodiazepines should be used for patients with agitation and other signs of sympathomimetic excess. Hyperthermic patients should be aggressively cooled. Bicarbonate therapy may be instituted in cases of rhabdomyolysis. β-Adrenergic blockers should not be used in cocaine-toxic patients, because an increase in blood pressure may occur due to the remaining "unopposed" α-adrenergic effect.

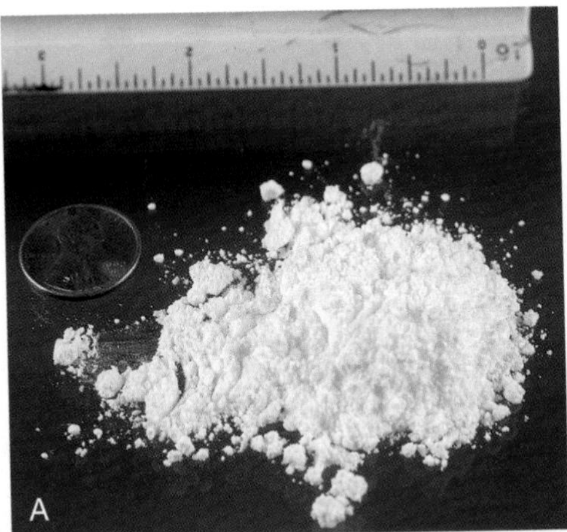

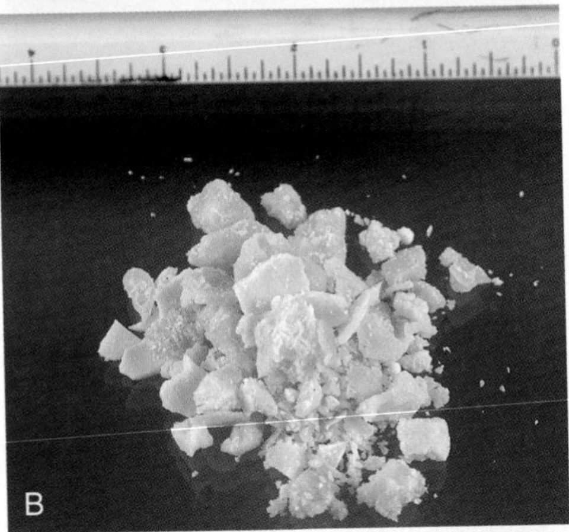

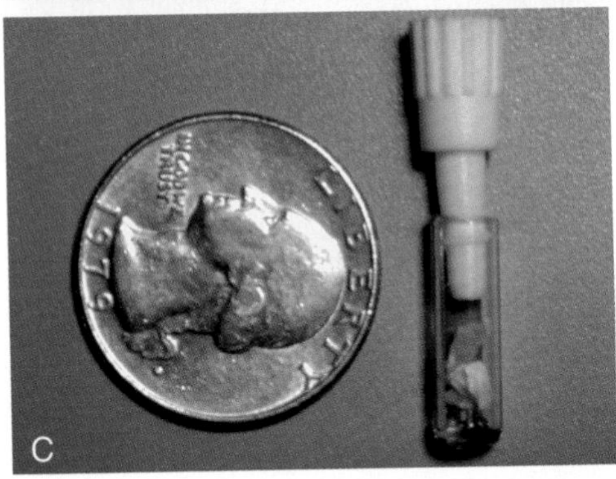

FIGURE 24–34 **A:** Cocaine powder. (Used with permission from the U.S. Drug Enforcement Administration.) **B:** Crack. (Used with permission from the U.S. Drug Enforcement Administration.) **C:** Crack vial. (Courtesy of Robert Hendrickson, MD.)

REFERENCES

1. Shanti CM, Lucas CE. Cocaine and the critical care challenge. *Crit Care Med* 2003;31:1851–1859.
2. Erwin MB, Deliargyria EN. Cocaine-associated chest pain. *Am J Med Sci* 2002;324:37–44.

Heroin

Anthony Morocco

Clinical Presentation

Heroin users may report a rapid euphoria or "rush," particularly after intravenous administration.[1] Other clinical effects include respiratory depression, sedation, analgesia, miosis, and delayed gastrointestinal motility.[1]

Pathophysiology

Heroin, diacetylmorphine, is a synthetic opioid that may be used by injection, insufflation, or smoking. Heroin is sold as the hydrochloride salt (a white powder) or in the base form (a brown or black substance referred to as "black tar heroin"). Black tar heroin has been associated with the development of wound botulism in some cases.[2]

Heroin is highly lipid soluble and rapidly crosses the blood-brain barrier. In the central nervous system, the drug is converted to 6-monoacetylmorphine. Heroin and its active metabolites are agonists at the μ-, κ-, and δ-opioid receptors, which account for the drug's clinical effects.[2]

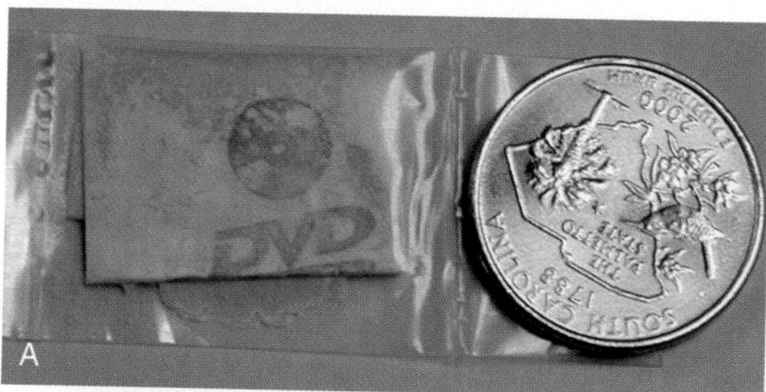

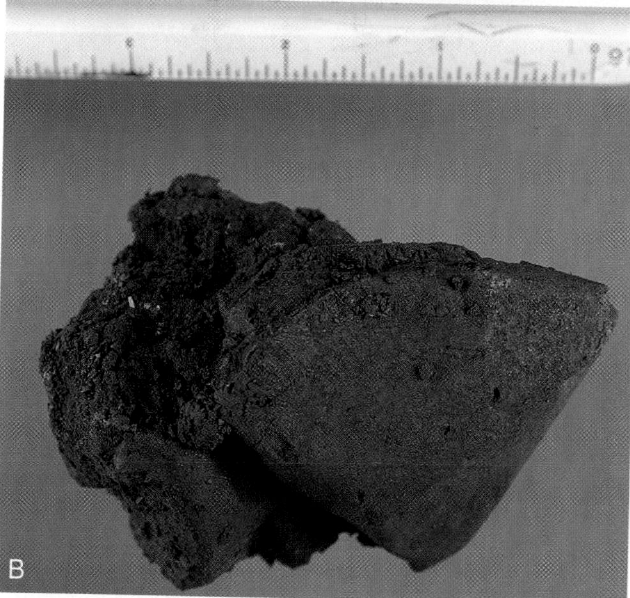

FIGURE 24–35 **A:** Heroin packet. Note "branding" of this heroin as "DVD." (Courtesy of Robert Hendrickson, MD.) **B:** Black tar heroin. (Used with permission from the U.S. Drug Enforcement Administration.)

Diagnosis

Diagnosis of heroin intoxication is clinical, with the classic triad of altered level of consciousness, hypoventilation, and miosis. Identification of injection sites, or "track marks," may aid the diagnosis. Urine immunoassay drug screens are positive for the presence of an opiate.

Clinical Complications

Overdose of heroin can result in death due to hypoventilation. Aspiration and noncardiogenic pulmonary edema may also occur. Intravenous users commonly develop infectious complications, including abscesses, wound botulism, endocarditis, and human immunodeficiency virus infection. The heroin may be "cut" with substances such as talc that cause tissue injury after injection. Exposure to the pyrolysate of heroin ("chasing the dragon") has been associated with the development of vacuolar leukoencephalopathy in some cases.[3]

Management

Heroin users may require medical intervention for hypoventilation. These patients should be ventilated by bag-valve-mask while naloxone is administered by intravenous, subcutaneous, intramuscular, or endotracheal routes, with an initial dose of 0.2 to 0.4 mg. A second dose of 2 mg should be administered after 5 minutes if there is an inadequate response. Endotracheal intubation should be reserved for cases of inadequate ventilation, poor oxygenation despite adequate ventilation, or continued hypoventilation after naloxone.[2] Patients who look well after awakening should be observed for relapse and signs of noncardiogenic pulmonary edema in the emergency department for at least 2 to 3 hours.[1] Intravenous heroin users who present with fever require evaluation for infections such as endocarditis.

REFERENCES

1. Sporer KA. Acute heroin overdose. *Ann Intern Med* 1999;130: 584–590.
2. Mitchell PA, Pons PT. Wound botulism associated with black tar heroin and lower extremity cellulites. *J Emerg Med* 2001;20: 371–375.
3. Kriegstein AR, Shungu DC, Millar WS, et al. Leukoencephalopathy and raised brain lactate from heroin vapor inhalation ("chasing the dragon"). *Neurology* 1999;53:1765–1773.

Marijuana

Anthony Morocco

Clinical Presentation

The effects of marijuana peak 10 to 30 minutes after smoking and last 1 to 4 hours. Users report a number of effects, including euphoria, perceptual alterations, and relaxation. Attention, memory, and motor skills are impaired. One notable physiologic effect is an increase in heart rate, by up to 50%.[1] Other effects include increased appetite, tremor, conjunctival injection, urinary retention, and decreased intraocular pressure. Those seeking medical attention after marijuana use are usually suffering from anxiety reactions, a common side effect of the drug.

Pathophysiology

Marijuana consists of the dried leaves and flowering tops of the *Cannabis sativa* plant. The most common method of use is by smoking in the form of a cigarette (joint) or hollowed cigar (blunt) or with the use of a water pipe. The drug may be mixed with tobacco or other illicit drugs such as phencyclidine (PCP). Marijuana may also be ingested. Another form of cannabis, hashish, is the dried resin of the plant.[1]

The primary active ingredient of marijuana is δ-9-tetrahydrocannabinol (THC).[1] This compound may be present in concentrations of 0.5% to 5% in marijuana, and up to 20% in hashish. The precise mechanisms of action of the drug are unknown, but specific cannabinoid receptors and an endogenous ligand, anandamide, are found in the human brain.[1]

Diagnosis

Patients presenting with marijuana-related complaints usually will admit to using the drug. Common urine drug screen immunoassays detect cannabinoids.

Clinical Complications

Large doses of marijuana can produce severe anxiety and transient psychosis. Pneumomediastinum and pneumothorax can occur due to lung overdistension while smoking. A number of adverse effects may result from long-term heavy use. A decline in respiratory function, which is additive with concurrent tobacco use, results from heavy smoking. Tolerance, subtle cognitive impairments, and a syndrome of dependence occur.[1] Death due to marijuana toxicity has not been reported.

Management

Specific treatment is usually unnecessary for marijuana intoxication, but the presence of coingestants may complicate the clinical course.

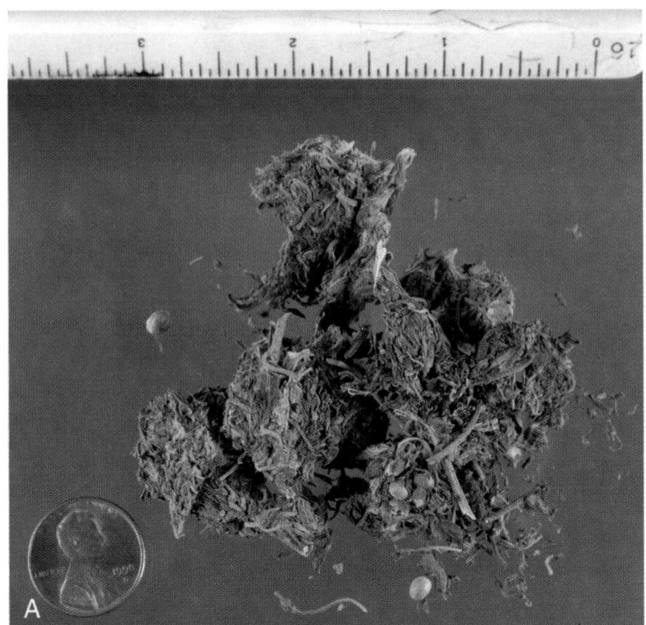

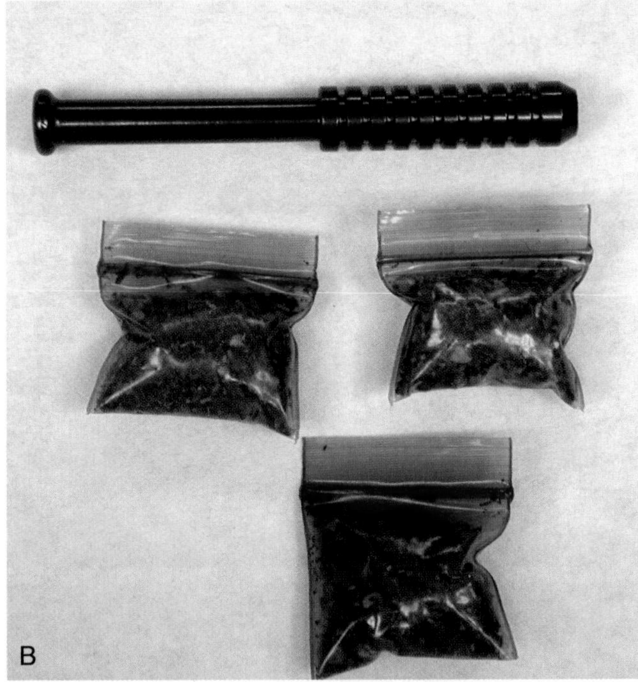

FIGURE 24–36 **A:** Marijuana. (Used with permission from the U.S. Drug Enforcement Administration.) **B:** Marijuana baggies and a bat. (Courtesy of Robert Hendrickson, MD.)

REFERENCES

1. Hall W, Solowij N. Adverse effects of cannabis. *Lancet* 1998;352:1611–1616.

Amphetamines

Anthony Morocco

Clinical Presentation

Amphetamine use may be associated with increased alertness, euphoria, aggression, decreased appetite, and altered self-esteem. Clinical signs of sympathomimetic stimulation are prominent, including tachycardia, hypertension, mydriasis, diaphoresis, and hyperthermia. Patients complain of anxiety, irritability, insomnia, chest pain, and heart palpitations.[1]

Pathophysiology

"Amphetamine" is the common name for α-methylphenylethylamine, and it is also used in reference to numerous analogues, such as methamphetamine and ephedrine, that are closely related in structure and effect. Amphetamines are used for treatment of narcolepsy, obesity, and attention-deficit hyperactivity disorder.[1–3] Methamphetamine is a commonly abused illicit drug that is smoked, ingested, or injected. Street names for methamphetamine include "ice," "crystal," and "crank."[1]

Amphetamines act by causing the release of dopamine and norepinephrine from the presynaptic terminals, while inhibiting the reuptake of catecholamines. Small differences in the basic amphetamine structure confer varying properties, such as enhanced serotonin release with 3,4-methylenedioxymethamphetamine (MDMA, "ecstasy"). Methamphetamine possesses a prolonged half-life and greater central nervous system penetration than amphetamine.[1]

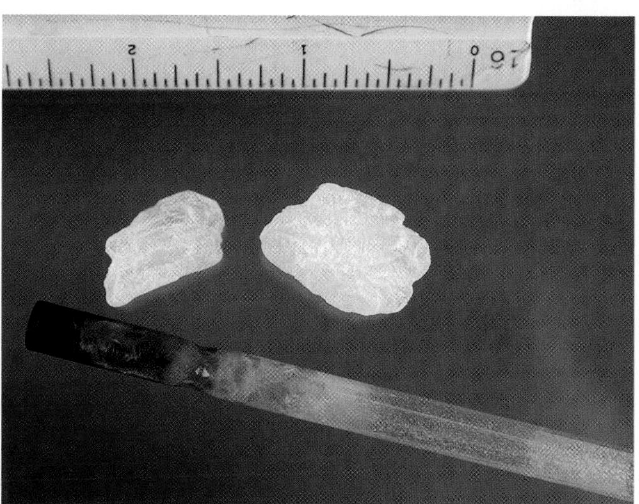

FIGURE 24–37 Crystal "meth." (Used with permission from the U.S. Drug Enforcement Administration.)

Diagnosis

Usually, the diagnosis of amphetamine toxicity is made based on a history of use of the drug in conjunction with clinical findings consistent with the sympathomimetic toxidrome. Urine drug immunoassays detect amphetamine but may not cross-react with so-called designer amphetamines such as MDMA.[1]

Clinical Complications

Patients may develop various psychiatric symptoms, including paranoia, emotional lability, delirium, or psychosis. These symptoms are usually associated with long-term use. Other complications include myocardial infarction, arrhythmia, valvular disease, cardiomyopathy, aortic dissection, seizure, vasculitis, intracranial hemorrhage, rhabdomyolysis, renal failure, hyperthermia, and pulmonary hypertension.[1,2] Intravenous users commonly develop infectious complications, including abscesses, endocarditis, and human immunodeficiency virus infection.[1]

Management

Severe amphetamine toxicity requires aggressive supportive care, including airway control, cooling, and sedation. Benzodiazepines are the drug of choice for seizures and for control of agitation and delirium. Hypertension improves with adequate sedation, but severe cases may require phentolamine or nitroprusside. Creatine phosphokinase and renal function should be monitored. Sodium bicarbonate therapy, to alkalinize the urine, is indicated if rhabdomyolysis occurs.

REFERENCES

1. Albertson TE, Derlet RW, Van Hoozen BE. Methamphetamine and the expanding complications of amphetamines. *West J Med* 1999;170:214–219.
2. Chaudhuri C, Salahudeen AK. Massive intracerebral hemorrhage in an amphetamine addict. *Am J Med Sci* 1999;317:350–352.
3. Morgan JP. Amphetamine and methamphetamine during the 1990s. *Pediatr Rev* 1992;13:330–333.

Ecstasy and Related Drugs

Anthony Morocco

Clinical Presentation

3,4-methylenedioxymethamphetamine (MDMA) users report increased energy, euphoria, sexual arousal, extraversion, and closeness to others.[1] Undesirable side effects include jaw clenching, bruxism, muscle tension, insomnia, nausea, dry mouth, hyperactivity, depersonalization, anxiety, agitation, and delirium. Within 2 days after MDMA use, patients report feeling muscle aches, anxiety, depression, and fatigue.[1,2]

Pathophysiology

Ecstasy, or MDMA, is a synthetic amphetamine derivative that has become a popular recreational drug over the past decade, often associated with "club" drugs and "rave" parties.[1-3] A number of related compounds are sometimes referred to interchangeably with MDMA, including methylenedioxyamphetamine (MDA, "love drug") and 3,4-methylenedioxyethamphetamine (MDEA, "eve"). Ecstasy pills may contain all three of these compounds, as well as ephedrine at times.[1] The usual dose of 50 to 150 mg of MDMA is taken in pill form, though it may be insufflated or used intravenously.

MDMA acts by increasing the release of monoamine neurotransmitters and blocking the reuptake of serotonin and dopamine. In addition to stimulant effects similar to those of amphetamine, the drug possesses hallucinogenic properties.

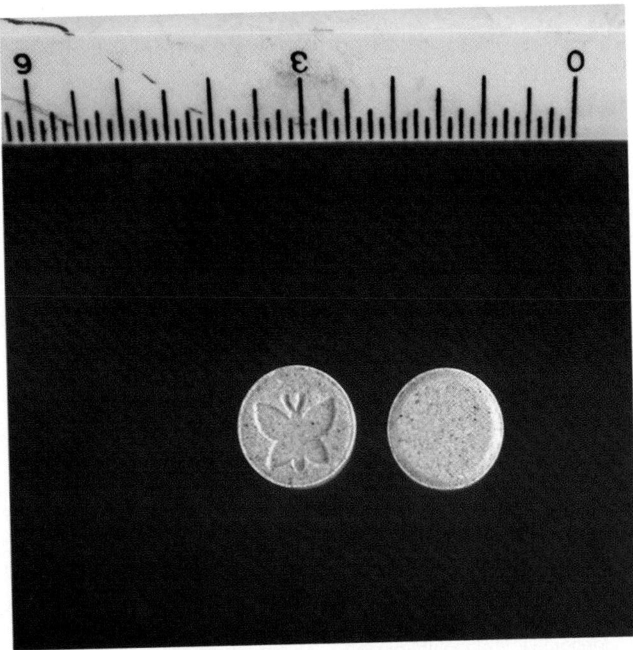

FIGURE 24–38 Tablets of 3,4-methylenedioxymethamphetamine (MDMA), or "ecstasy." (Used with permission from the U.S. Drug Enforcement Administration.)

Diagnosis

MDMA assay is not usually included in routine drug screens, and it may or may not react with amphetamine immunoassays, depending on the assay, the dose taken, and the time since ingestion.[1]

Clinical Complications

Acute toxicity has reportedly caused hepatitis with jaundice, hypertension, intracranial hemorrhage, cardiac arrhythmias, brain death, and liver failure.[1-3] The combination of MDMA-induced syndrome of inappropriate secretion of antidiuretic hormone (SIADH), vigorous physical activity (e.g., dancing), profuse sweating, and excessive intake of water may result in hyponatremia, cerebral edema, seizures, hyperthermia, rhabdomyolysis, liver injury, disseminated intravascular coagulation, and death.[1,2] Long-term use may be associated with neurotoxicity, resulting in decreased serotonergic activity in the brain, impaired memory and decision-making, greater impulsivity, panic attacks, paranoia, and depression.[1-3]

Management

Severely hyperthermic patients must be rapidly cooled within 30 to 60 minutes after presentation. Benzodiazepines may also be useful to provide sedation as needed, and dantrolene sodium has been recommended for patients with hyperthermia.[1-3]

REFERENCES

1. Kalant H. The pharmacology and toxicology of "ecstasy" (MDMA) and related drugs. *CMAJ* 2001;165:917–928.
2. Greene SL, Dargan PI, O'Connor N, et al. Multiple toxicity from 3,4-methylenedioxymethamphetamine ("ecstasy"). *Am J Emerg Med* 2003;21:121–124.
3. Caballero F, Lopez-Navidad A, Cotorruelo J, et al. Ecstasy-induced brain death and acute hepatocellular failure: multiorgan donor and liver transplantation. *Transplantation* 2002;74:532–537.

Gamma Hydroxybutyric Acid

Anthony Morocco

Clinical Presentation

γ-Hydroxybutyric acid (GHB) is used recreationally for its hypnotic and euphoric effects. Ataxia, somnolence, and nystagmus are seen in conscious patients. Intoxicated patients usually present for medical care because of significant central nervous system (CNS) depression. Unique features of GHB intoxication are the abrupt awakening and periods of agitation interspersed with coma and apnea. Myoclonic jerks may be mistaken for seizure activity. Vomiting occurs in 14% to 44% of patients.

Pathophysiology

GHB is used in the treatment of narcolepsy. It is also a common drug of abuse, along with its prodrugs γ-butyrolactone (GBL) and 1,4-butanediol. These agents are associated with "rave" parties and nightclubs, where they are sold in liquid form in small vials. The three drugs are sold interchangeably, with specific common street names: Liquid X, Grievous Bodily Harm, and Georgia Homeboy for GHB; Blue Nitro, Renewtrient, and Revivarent for GBL; and Pine Needle Extract and Serenity for 1,4-butanediol.[1,2]

GHB is found naturally in the brain, and there is a GHB-specific receptor. The drug also binds the γ-aminobutyric acid ($GABA_B$) receptor. Stimulation of these receptors by GHB, or an increase in GABA concentrations, may be responsible for GHB-induced CNS depression. The drug may also act through effects on acetylcholine, serotonin, and opioids. Another reported effect is enhanced growth hormone release, which accounts for its use by bodybuilders.[1,2]

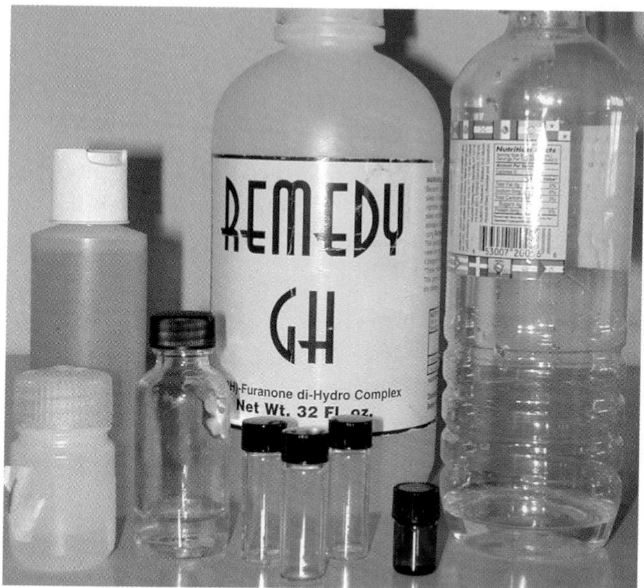

FIGURE 24–39 Various bottles used to carry, and in some cases to disguise, GHB. (Courtesy of Robert Hendrickson, MD.)

Diagnosis

Diagnosis is based on a history and clinical appearance. Laboratory testing is rarely available to confirm the diagnosis, because the drug is rapidly eliminated (usually within 6 hours) and requires special techniques (gas chromatography/mass spectrometry) for detection. Common immunoassay urine drug screens can be used to rule out intoxication by other substances.

Clinical Complications

Seizures, cerebral anoxia, and death can occur secondary to apnea or after vomiting and aspiration. Uncommonly, bradycardia and hypotension may occur.[1,2]

Management

Patients usually regain consciousness 2 to 6 hours after presentation.[1,2] Airway management (including endotracheal intubation) may be necessary for ventilation and protection against aspiration, but patients can often be quickly extubated and discharged without hospital admission. Sudden awakenings during attempts at endotracheal intubation have been reported, so even patients who appear comatose may need an induction agent before this procedure is undertaken.[1,2]

REFERENCES

1. Mason PE, Kerns WP 2nd. Gamma hydroxybutyric acid (GHB) intoxication. *Acad Emerg Med* 2002;9:730–739.
2. Tancredi DN, Shannon MW. Case records of the Massachusetts General Hospital: weekly clinicopathological exercises. Case 30-2003: a 21-year-old man with sudden alteration of mental status. *N Engl J Med* 2003;349:1267–1275.

Lysergic Acid Diethylamide

Anthony Morocco

Clinical Presentation

Lysergic acid diethylamide (LSD)-intoxicated patients demonstrate distortions in time perception, sensory alterations, and thought disorders. Hallucinations and various visual distortions commonly occur. Patients may describe synesthesia, which is a blending of sensations that can result in hearing colors and visualizing sounds. Despite these symptoms, patients are usually alert and able to give a history of use of the drug. Signs of sympathetic stimulation, such as tachycardia, tachypnea, diaphoresis, and mydriasis, are common. Some patients appear extremely anxious due to the dysphoria involved in a "bad trip."[1]

Pathophysiology

LSD is a potent hallucinogen. It is a synthetic compound related to another hallucinogenic, lysergamide, which is found in the morning glory seed. The drug is most often impregnated on sheets of blotter paper and ingested, but it may also be found in powder, liquid, pill, and other forms.

The structure of the drug is similar to that of serotonin, and the hallucinogenic potency of LSD and other psychedelic agents is related to their affinity for the serotonin 5-HT_2 receptor.[2]

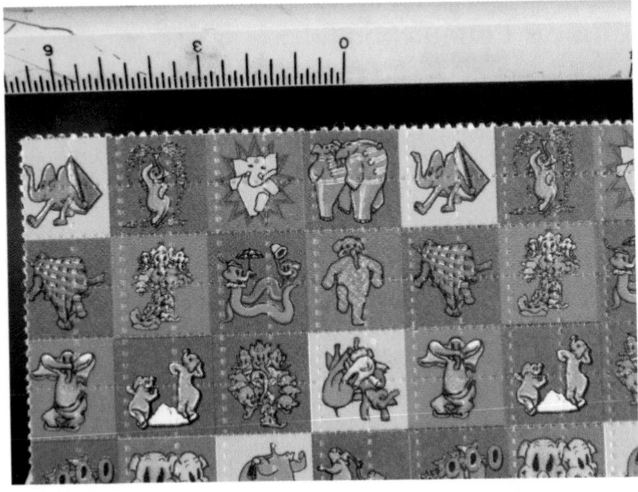

FIGURE 24–40 Lysergic acid diethylamide (LSD) on blotter paper. (Used with permission from the U.S. Drug Enforcement Administration.)

Diagnosis

Diagnosis is based on the patient's history of drug use and clinical appearance. Laboratory testing is rarely available to confirm the diagnosis, because the drug is present in minute quantities, making it difficult to detect.

Clinical Complications

The most significant acute complication is the dysphoria and severe anxiety that may result from frightening hallucinations and depersonalization. The nature and causes of long-term side effects are open to debate. Extended episodes of psychosis are probably related to underlying psychiatric disease. Hallucinogen persisting perception disorder (HPPD), or "flashbacks," consists of brief perceptual disturbances that may occur for several years after drug use.

Management

Most patients can be placed in a quiet area and reassured for several hours while the drug effect subsides. Severe anxiety may require physical restraint and administration of a parenteral benzodiazepine. There is no effective treatment for HPPD.

REFERENCES

1. Schwartz RH. LSD: its rise, fall, and renewed popularity among high school students. *Pediatr Clin North Am* 1995;42:403–413.
2. Aghajanian GK. Serotonin and the action of LSD in the brain. *Psychiatr Ann* 1994;24:137–141.

Phencyclidine

Anthony Morocco

Clinical Presentation

Phencyclidine (PCP) intoxication can have a wide variety of clinical effects. The drug causes a dissociative state, resulting in detachment from the environment and disordered thoughts. Patients may be alert and oriented (45%), violent (35%), catatonic (12%), and even unconscious (11%). PCP can cause psychosis that is clinically indistinguishable from schizophrenia. The most common physical examination findings are hypertension (57%), nystagmus (57%), and tachycardia (30%). The nystagmus may be horizontal, vertical, and rotatory. Other findings include increased muscle tone (5%), tachypnea (4%), profuse diaphoresis (4%), hyperthermia (3%), hypersalivation (2%), urinary retention (2%), and dystonia (2%). Laboratory abnormalities may include elevated creatine kinase, blood urea nitrogen, creatinine, and hepatic transaminases, as well as leukocytosis and hypoglycemia.[2]

Pathophysiology

PCP is a dissociative anesthetic that is sold illicitly in many forms. The drug is commonly dissolved in an organic solvent and sold as "embalming fluid." Street terms such as "wet," "fry," "illy," "water," "dipping," and many others refer to tobacco or marijuana cigarettes soaked in a PCP-containing solution.[1]

PCP is similar in structure and effects to ketamine and several analogues such as thienylcyclohexylpiperidine (TCP), phenylcyclohexylpyrrolidine (PHP), and phenylcyclohexylethylamine (PCE). The most important effect is believed to be noncompetitive antagonism of the excitatory neurotransmitter glutamate at the *N*-methyl-D-aspartate (NMDA) receptor. Higher doses inhibit the reuptake of norepinephrine, serotonin, and dopamine, and stimulate σ-receptors.[3] Though PCP is often dissolved in organic solvents such as formalin, the solvents are not believed to contribute to the clinical effects.

Diagnosis

Most widely available urine immunoassay drug screen panels test for the presence of PCP and can confirm the diagnosis. Patients frequently admit to use of various street forms of the drug, and they may be unaware that the effects of the "embalming fluid" were caused by PCP.

Clinical Complications

Rhabdomyolysis with resultant renal failure has been reported. A persistent psychosis may occur, particularly in patients who have taken large doses of the drug and in those with an underlying psychiatric disorder. Violent PCP-intoxicated patients may suffer serious traumatic injuries.

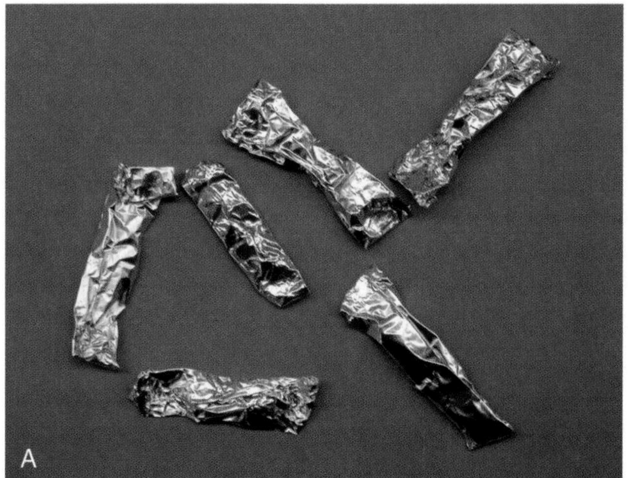

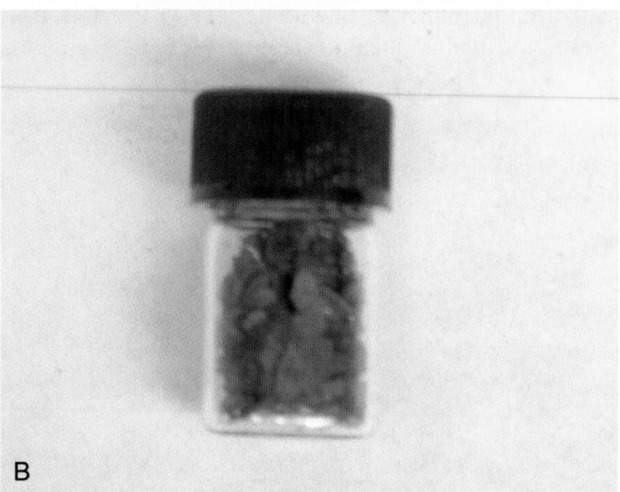

FIGURE 24–41 **A:** Packages of phencyclidine (PCP). (Used with permission from the U.S. Drug Enforcement Administration.) **B:** PCP may also be added to marijuana and smoked. (Courtesy of Robert Hendrickson, MD.)

Management

Treatment depends on the degree of agitation and the presence of any medical complications or traumatic injury. Many patients can simply be placed in a quiet environment for a few hours. Severe agitation requires physical restraint and treatment with a parenteral benzodiazepine. Multidose activated charcoal can enhance elimination of the drug. Consultation with psychiatry is necessary for any patient with prolonged psychosis.

REFERENCES

1. Holland JA, Nelson L, Ravikumar PR, et al. Embalming fluid-soaked marijuana: new high or new guise for PCP? *J Psychoactive Drugs* 1998;30:215–219.
2. McCarron MM, Schulze BW, Thompson GA, et al. Acute phencyclidine intoxication: incidence of clinical findings in 1,000 cases. *Ann Emerg Med* 1981;10:237–242.
3. Javitt DC, Zukin SR. Recent advances in the phencyclidine model of schizophrenia. *Am J Psychiatry* 1991;148:1301–1308.

Ketamine

Anthony Morocco

Clinical Presentation

The drug produces rapid effects that last 30 to 45 minutes. Users describe the dissociative effects as an "out-of-body" or "floating" sensation, often referred to as a "k-hole" or "k-hold."[1,2] Alterations of perception similar to those of schizophrenia occur, as well as hallucinations, illusions, and vivid dreams. Patients may appear withdrawn, anxious, or agitated. Signs and symptoms of intoxication may include psychomotor retardation, nystagmus, mydriasis, tachycardia, hypertension, vomiting, palpitations, slurred speech, delirium, repetitive behaviors, bizarre movements, ataxia, and dystonia.[1,2]

Pathophysiology

Ketamine is a dissociative anesthetic that is similar in structure and effect to phencyclidine (PCP). It is used commonly in human and veterinary medical practice.

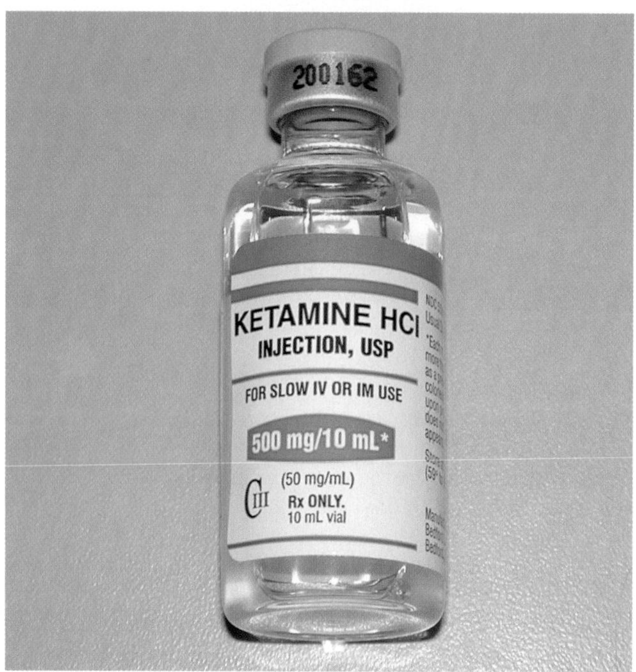

FIGURE 24–42 Ketamine is frequently stolen from pharmacies or veterinarians and used as the liquid, shown here, or converted to powder. (Courtesy of Robert Hendrickson, MD.)

Ketamine is considered a "club" drug, owing to its use at nightclubs and rave parties. Street terms for the drug include "K," "special K," and "vitamin K." Pharmaceutical ketamine is supplied as a solution, which users often heat to obtain the crystal. Methods of use include insufflation, ingestion, smoking, and injection.[1]

Ketamine is believed to act primarily by antagonism of the excitatory neurotransmitter glutamate at the *N*-methyl-D-aspartate (NMDA) receptor. The drug has a number of other neurotransmitter effects, including inhibition of reuptake of norepinephrine, dopamine, and serotonin. Metabolism produces the active compound norketamine.[1]

Diagnosis

The diagnosis usually is clinical, because assays for ketamine are not readily available. The drug may produce a false-positive result on some phencyclidine immunoassays.

Clinical Complications

Respiratory depression, apnea, pulmonary edema, and death may rarely occur. Patients are also at risk for aspiration and rhabdomyolysis. Users may have flashbacks and memory problems.[1]

Management

Patients generally require no treatment other than placement in a quiet environment, although supportive care, including mechanical ventilation, may occasionally be necessary. Benzodiazepines should be administered for the treatment of agitation.

REFERENCES

1. Graeme KA. New drugs of abuse. *Emerg Med Clin North Am* 2000; 18:625–636.
2. Freese TE, Miotto K, Reback CJ. The effects and consequences of selected club drugs. *J Subst Abuse Treat* 2002;23:151–156.

Mushrooms Containing Psilocybin

Anthony Morocco

Clinical Presentation

Symptoms develop 15 to 30 minutes after ingestion. Patients develop a clinical syndrome similar to that of other hallucinogens such as lysergic acid diethylamide (LSD), with distortions in time perception, sensory alterations, and thought disorder. They may appear anxious and dysphoric. Signs of sympathetic stimulation, such as tachycardia, tachypnea, diaphoresis, and mydriasis, are common.[1,2]

Pathophysiology

Mushrooms containing the hallucinogen psilocybin include *Psilocybe* species (*P. caerulescens, P. cubensis*) and members of several other genera, including *Conocybe, Panaeolus, Gymnopilus,* and *Psathyrella*. The *Psilocybe* mushrooms often grow on manure and turn blue or green when cut.[1,2]

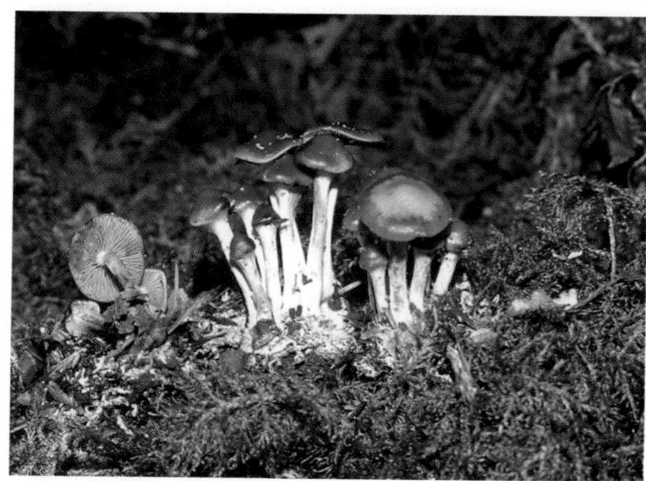

FIGURE 24–43 *Psilocybe stuntzii.* (Courtesy of Judy Roger, MD.)

The toxin psilocybin and its metabolite psilocin are similar in structure to serotonin. The hallucinogenic properties of these compounds and other psychedelic agents is related to their effect at the serotonin 5-HT_2 receptor.[1,2]

Diagnosis

Diagnosis may often be made from the clinical appearance and history, because patients often admit to hallucinogenic mushroom use. There are no readily available assays for the toxin, but routine drugs-of-abuse screens may aid in ruling out other forms of intoxication. If the patient can produce a specimen of the implicated mushroom, identification by a mycologist may also be useful.[1,2]

Clinical Complications

Most patients recover from intoxication uneventfully in about 2 to 6 hours, but some patients may develop severe anxiety. Rarely, renal failure, seizures, and myocardial infarction have been reported.[1,2]

Management

As with most hallucinogen intoxications, most patients require only a quiet room and reassurance until the effects subside. Activated charcoal may decrease absorption of the toxin. A parenteral benzodiazepine should be administered for severe anxiety or agitation.[1,2]

REFERENCES

1. Goldfrank LR. Mushrooms. In: Goldfrank LR, Flomenbaum NE, Lewin NA, et al., eds. *Goldfrank's toxicologic emergencies,* 7th ed. New York, McGraw-Hill, 2002, pp 1115–1128.
2. Badham ER. Ethnobotany of psilocybin mushrooms, especially *Psilocybin cubensis. J Ethnopharmacol* 1984;10:249–254.

Mushrooms Containing Cyclopeptides

Anthony Morocco

Clinical Presentation

Patients present with gastroenteritis at least 6 to 12 hours after mushroom ingestion. The diarrhea is described as profuse and cholera-like, with accompanying abdominal pain, vomiting, and dehydration. Signs of liver and other organ toxicities appear after 24 to 48 hours.[1,2]

Pathophysiology

The cyclopeptides are toxins that are contained in at least 35 species of mushrooms worldwide. These include *Amanita* (*A. phalloides, A. verna, A. virosa*), *Galerina* (*G. autumnalis, G. marginata, G. venenata*), and *Lepiota* (*L. helveola, L. josserandi, L. brunneo-incarnata*).[1,2]

The clinically important cyclopeptides are the amatoxins, including α-, β-, and γ-amanitin. They are heat stable, are rapidly absorbed from the gastrointestinal tract, and undergo enterohepatic recirculation. The amanitins prevent the transcription of DNA by inhibiting RNA polymerase II. This results in toxic effects on the gastrointestinal mucosa, liver, and kidneys. The liver toxicity results in an injury pattern of centrilobular necrosis; acute tubular necrosis and hyaline casts are seen in the kidneys.[1,2]

Diagnosis

Amatoxin poisoning should be suspected in any patient who develops gastroenteritis 6 hours or more after a mushroom meal. Abnormal liver function tests are an ominous sign. Amatoxins can be detected in urine and feces, but testing is not readily available. If the patient can produce a specimen of the implicated mushroom, identification by a mycologist may be useful.[1,2]

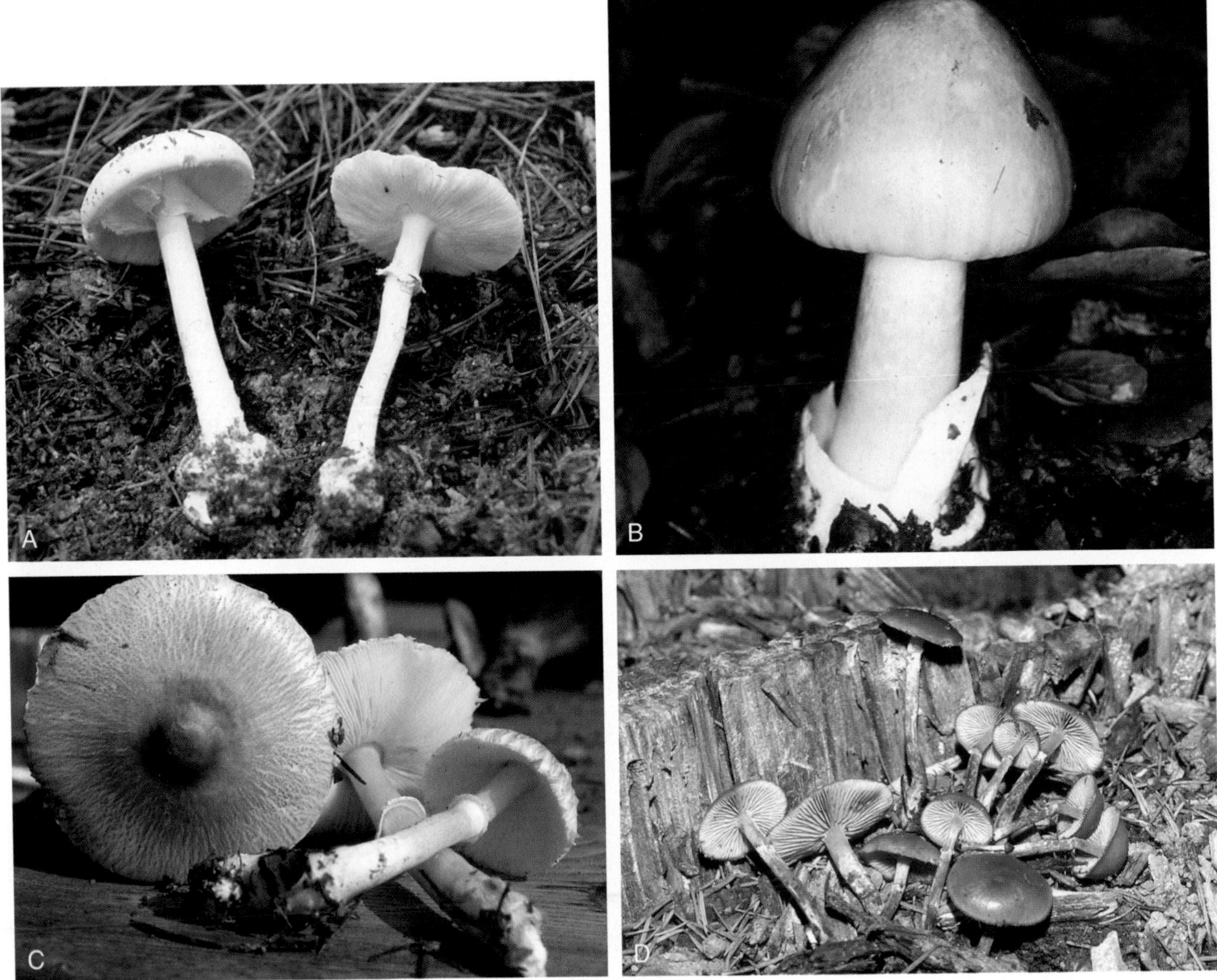

FIGURE 24–44 **A:** *Amanita ocreata.* (Courtesy of Judy Roger, MD.) **B:** *Amanita phalloides.* (Courtesy of Judy Roger, MD.) **C:** *Lepiota rubrotincta.* (Copyright Dick Bishop, MD.) **D:** *Galerina autumnalis.* (Courtesy of Judy Roger, MD.)

Mushrooms Containing Cyclopeptides

Anthony Morocco

Clinical Complications

Patients may develop fulminant hepatic failure, coagulopathy, hepatorenal syndrome, and cerebral edema. The mortality rate is 20% to 30%, and death occurs 4 to 7 days after the mushroom ingestion. The cyclopeptides account for 90% of mushroom-related deaths. Significant endocrine dysfunction involving glucose, calcium, and thyroid hormone regulation has been reported, as well as neuropathy after ingestion of some *Lepiota* spp.[1,2]

Management

Multidose activated charcoal and intravenous fluids should be administered. Complications of hepatic failure should be treated with vitamin K and fresh-frozen plasma for coagulopathy and lactulose and neomycin for hepatic encephalopathy. Mannitol may decrease intracranial pressure. Hemodialysis, hemoperfusion, plasma exchange, or a combination of the three enhances elimination, whereas forced diuresis does not. A number of therapeutic agents have been suggested to decrease the effects of amatoxins. High-dose penicillin or ceftazidime may decrease liver injury by an unknown mechanism. Thioctic acid is an antioxidant that may lessen free radical–mediated damage. Silibinin may decrease α-amanitin entry into hepatocytes. However, there is no truly effective antidote, and liver transplantation may ultimately be necessary.[1,2]

REFERENCES

1. Goldfrank LR. Mushrooms. In: Goldfrank LR, Flomenbaum NE, Lewin NA, et al., eds. *Goldfrank's toxicologic emergencies,* 7th ed. New York, McGraw-Hill, 2002, pp 1115–1128.
2. Enjabert F, Rapior S, Nougier-Soule J, et al. Treatment of amatoxin poisoning: 20-year retrospective analysis. *J Toxicol Clin Toxicol* 2002;40:715–757.

Mushrooms Containing Gyromitrin

Anthony Morocco

Clinical Presentation

Five to 10 hours after ingestion of the mushrooms, patients develop gastroenteritis, muscle cramps, dizziness, and decreased coordination. Less commonly, signs of severe liver and central nervous system dysfunction occur, including jaundice, altered mental status, and seizures.[1,2]

Pathophysiology

Gyromitra esculenta, known as the "false morel," and other mushrooms such as *Gyromitra californica* and *Gyromitra brunnea* contain the toxin gyromitrin.[1,2]

This compound is broken down to monomethylhydrazine, which binds pyridoxine (vitamin B_6) and consequently decreases the formation of the inhibitory neurotransmitter γ-aminobutyric acid (GABA). Decreased GABA in the brain leads to seizures. A free-radical metabolite may be responsible for the hepatotoxicity.[1,2]

Diagnosis

Diagnosis is made based on the history of mushroom ingestion and the clinical presentation, particularly the presence of seizures. Patients may report eating mushrooms that they thought were true morels, *Morchella esculenta,* when they mistakenly ate the false morel. There are no readily available assays for the toxin. If the patient can produce a specimen of the implicated mushroom, identification by a mycologist may be useful.[1,2]

Clinical Complications

Severely affected patients may develop status epilepticus and coma. *Gyromitra* poisoning is also known to cause hepatic necrosis and hepatorenal syndrome. Death rates have been estimated to be as high as 35%.[1,2]

Management

Parenteral pyridoxine therapy increases GABA production. It should be administered to patients with central nervous system toxicity, particularly seizures. There is no effective treatment for the hepatotoxicity other than supportive care. Activated charcoal may limit systemic absorption of the toxin.[1,2]

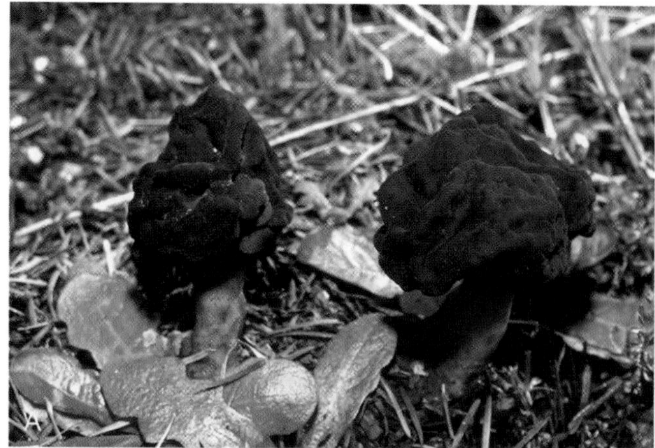

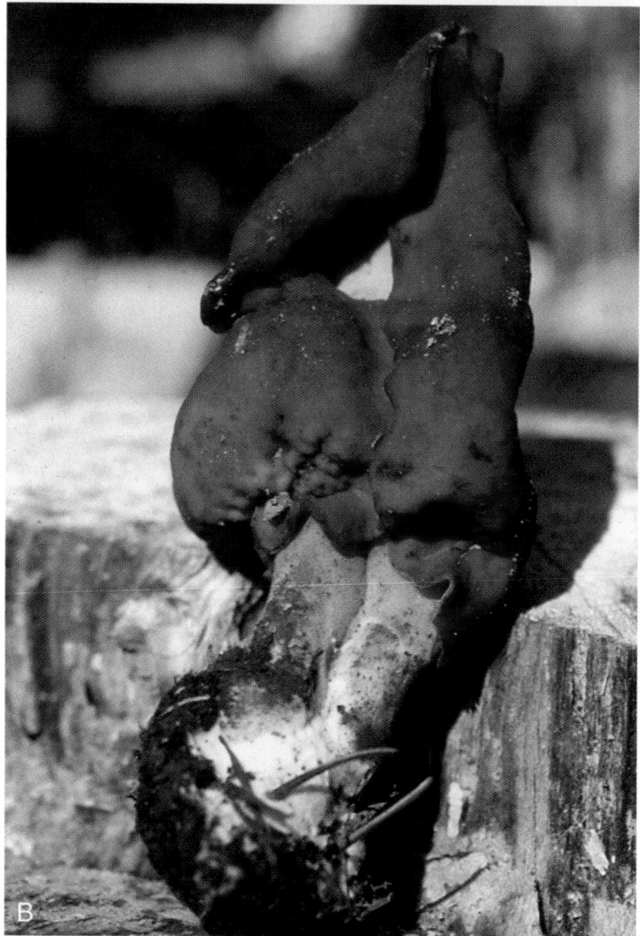

FIGURE 24-45 **A:** *Gyrometra esculenta.* (Courtesy of Judy Roger, MD.) **B:** *Helvella infula.* (Courtesy of Dick Bishop, MD.)

REFERENCES

1. Goldfrank LR. Mushrooms. In: Goldfrank LR, Flomenbaum NE, Lewin NA, et al., eds. *Goldfrank's toxicologic emergencies,* 7th ed. New York, McGraw-Hill, 2002, pp 1115–1128.
2. Michelot D, Toth B. Poisoning by *Gyromitra esculenta:* a review. *J Appl Toxicol* 1991;11:235–243.

Mushrooms Containing Muscarine

Anthony Morocco

Clinical Presentation

Patients develop symptoms consistent with a cholinergic toxidrome within 30 minutes to 2 hours after ingestion. These include the classic SLUDGE syndrome of **s**alivation, **l**acrimation, **u**rination, **d**iarrhea, **g**astric upset, and **e**mesis, as well as miosis, diaphoresis, bradycardia, bronchospasm, and bronchorrhea. No central nervous system cholinergic effects are seen.[1]

Pathophysiology

Several species of *Clitocybe* (*C. dealbata,* or "sweater"), *Inocybe* (*I. lacera, I. geophylla*), and *Omphalotus* ("jack o'lantern") mushrooms contain muscarine and cause a cholinergic toxidrome on ingestion. Much smaller amounts of muscarine are contained in *Amanita muscaria* and *Amanita pantherina* (both are discussed in the section on mushrooms containing isoxazole derivatives).[1]

These mushrooms contain muscarine, which is similar in structure to acetylcholine and directly stimulates cholinergic muscarinic receptors. The muscarinic receptors are postsynaptic and postganglionic for parasympathetic nerves and the sympathetic innervation of sweat glands. Muscarine does not affect central nervous system cholinergic neurons because it does not cross the blood-brain barrier.[1]

Diagnosis

Diagnosis is made by recognition of the SLUDGE syndrome in a patient with a history of recent mushroom ingestion. If the patient can produce a specimen of the implicated mushroom, identification by a mycologist may also be useful. There are no readily available assays for muscarine.[1]

Clinical Complications

Symptoms are generally mild and self-limited, with resolution in several hours. Severe symptoms can cause respiratory compromise, bradydysrhythmia, and volume depletion.[1]

Management

Aggressive treatment usually is not required. Intravenous fluids, antiemetics, and inhaled β_2-adrenergic agonists may be helpful. For severe symptoms, the muscarinic receptor antagonist atropine may be given and titrated to effect.[1]

REFERENCES

1. Goldfrank LR. Mushrooms. In: Goldfrank LR, Flomenbaum NE, Lewin NA, et al., eds. *Goldfrank's toxicologic emergencies,* 7th ed. New York, McGraw-Hill, 2002, pp 1115–1128.

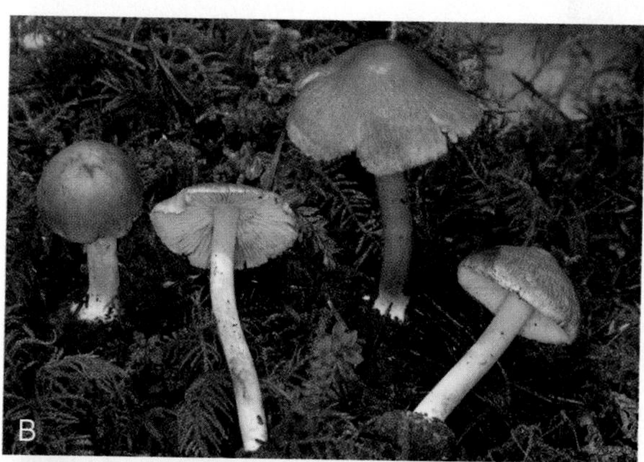

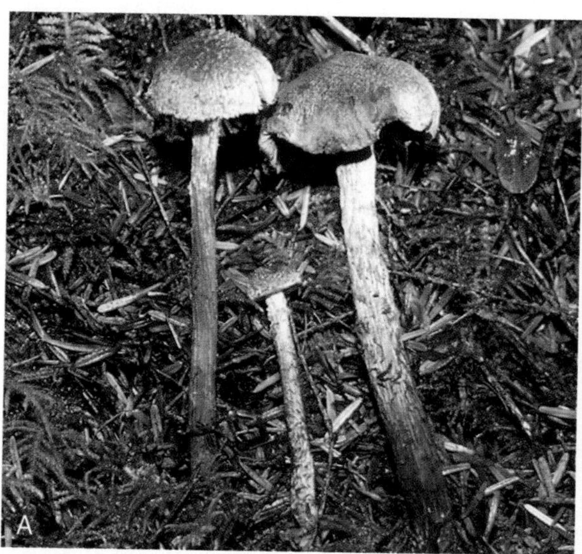

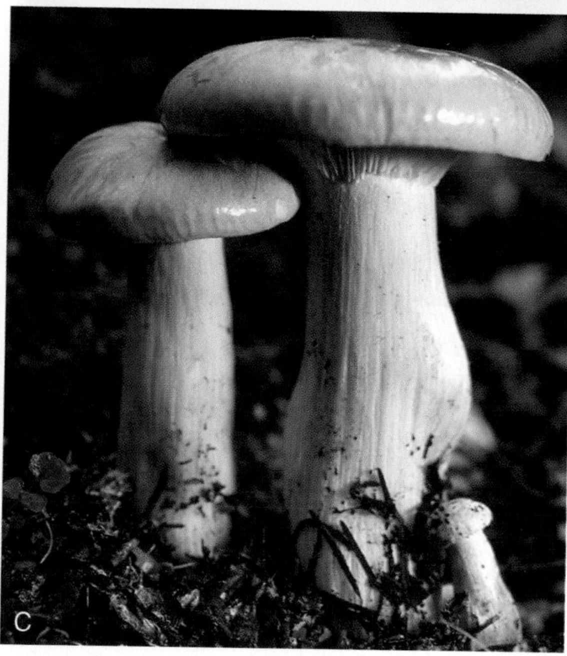

FIGURE 24–46 **A:** *Inocybe calamistrata.* **B:** *Inocybe olympiana.* **C:** *Clitocybe nebularis.* (**A–C,** Copyright Judy Roger, MD.)

Mushrooms Containing Coprine

Anthony Morocco

Clinical Presentation

Symptoms occur 30 minutes to 2 hours after ingestion and in combination with alcohol consumption. Patients develop symptoms similar to the disulfiram-ethanol effect, including nausea, vomiting, skin flushing, headache, tachycardia, and palpitations. This effect may continue up to 72 hours after mushroom ingestion.[1,2]

Pathophysiology

Several *Coprinus* mushrooms contain the toxin coprine. They are referred to as "inky caps," because the gills dissolve into a dark liquid after harvesting.[1,2]

The toxin coprine is metabolized to 1-aminocyclopropanol. This substance inhibits the enzyme aldehyde dehydrogenase, which catalyzes the breakdown of acetaldehyde in the second step of ethanol metabolism. If ethanol is then ingested, it is metabolized by alcohol dehydrogenase to acetaldehyde, and there is an accumulation of the acetaldehyde intermediate, which causes the clinical symptoms.[1,2]

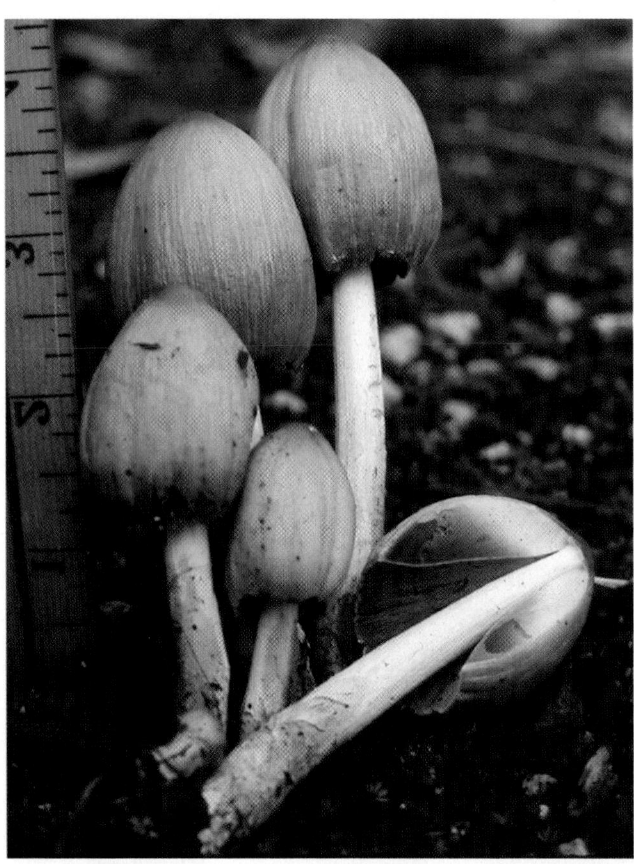

FIGURE 24–47 *Coprinus atramentarius.* (Courtesy of Judy Roger, MD.)

Diagnosis

Diagnosis is made from the clinical presentation in combination with recent mushroom and alcohol ingestion. Given the potential delay in symptoms, the mushroom ingestion may be overlooked as a potential source of the illness. Patients may give a history of eating a mushroom that they thought was the nontoxic *Coprinus comatus.* There are no readily available laboratory assays for the toxin. If the patient can produce a specimen of the implicated mushroom, identification by a mycologist may be useful.[1,2]

Clinical Complications

Hypotension, significant volume depletion, and death may rarely occur.[1,2]

Management

No specific treatment is indicated other than supportive care, because symptoms typically resolve within several hours after alcohol abstinence. Intravenous fluid should be given in cases of hypotension or dehydration, and antiemetics may decrease vomiting. A vasopressor agent may be necessary for refractory hypotension. Cutaneous flushing may improve with antihistamine therapy. Treatment with fomepizole, an alcohol dehydrogenase inhibitor, has been used in cases of the disulfiram-alcohol reaction to halt the formation of aldehyde.[1,2]

REFERENCES

1. Goldfrank LR. Mushrooms. In: Goldfrank LR, Flomenbaum NE, Lewin NA, et al., eds. *Goldfrank's toxicologic emergencies,* 7th ed. New York, McGraw-Hill, 2002, pp 1115–1128.
2. Michelot D. Poisoning by *Coprinus atramentarius. Nat Toxins* 1992; 1:73–80.

Mushrooms Containing Isoxazole Derivatives

Anthony Morocco

Clinical Presentation

Effects occur 15 to 30 minutes after ingestion, and patients may present with a variety of signs and symptoms. Hallucinations, ataxia, dizziness, and delirium may occur. Anticholinergic symptoms such as urinary retention have also been reported.[1-3]

Pathophysiology

Several mushrooms of the genus *Amanita,* including *A. muscaria, A. pantherina,* and *A. gemmata,* contain isoxazole-derivative neurotoxins. These mushrooms often have a large red cap that has made them the stereotypical cartoon mushroom, as in "Alice in Wonderland" and "The Smurfs."[1-3]

The isoxazole derivatives, ibotenic acid and its metabolite muscimol, are responsible for most clinical effects. Ibotenic acid is structurally similar to the inhibitory neurotransmitter γ-aminobutyric acid (GABA), whereas muscimol is similar to the excitatory neurotransmitter, glutamic acid. Despite its name, *A. muscaria* contains relatively little muscarine compared with *Clitocybe* and *Inocybe* species, though the anticholinergic symptoms may still occur.[1-3]

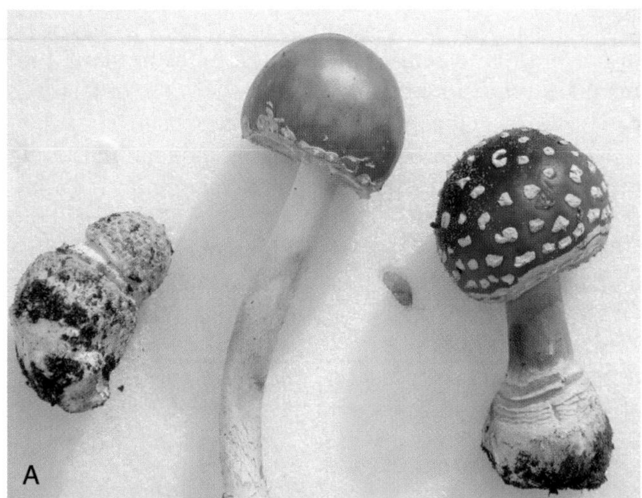

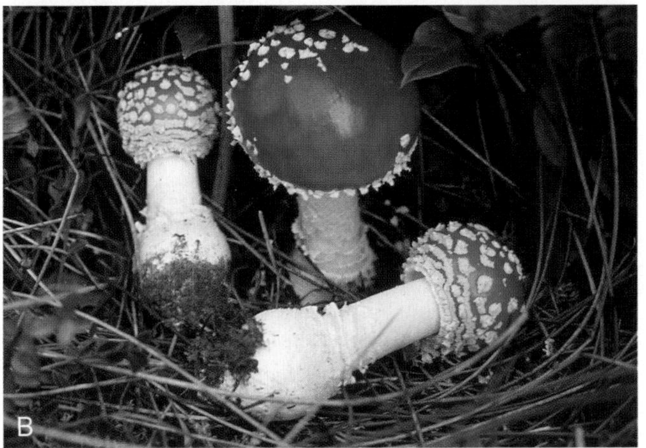

FIGURE 24–48 **A:** *Amanita muscaria.* (Courtesy of Robert Hendrickson, MD.) **B:** *Amanita muscaria.* (Courtesy of Judy Roger, MD.)

Diagnosis

Many times the diagnosis can be made from the clinical appearance and history, because patients often admit to hallucinogenic mushroom use. There are no readily available assays for the toxin, but routine drugs-of-abuse screens may aid in ruling out other forms of intoxication. If the patient can produce a specimen of the implicated mushroom, identification by a mycologist may also be useful.[1-3]

Clinical Complications

Most patients recover from intoxication uneventfully in about 2 to 6 hours, but some patients develop severe anxiety. Children are more likely to develop significant neurologic symptoms such as myoclonus and seizures.[1-3]

Management

General supportive therapy is all that is required for the majority of patients. Patients with severe agitation or seizures should be treated with a parenteral benzodiazepine.[1-3]

REFERENCES

1. Goldfrank LR. Mushrooms. In: Goldfrank LR, Flomenbaum NE, Lewin NA, et al., eds. *Goldfrank's toxicologic emergencies,* 7th ed. New York, McGraw-Hill, 2002, pp 1115–1128.
2. Williams SR, Davis DP, Williams SR. *Amanita muscaria. J Emerg Med* 1999;17:739.
3. Benjamin DR. Mushroom poisoning in infants and children: the *Amanita pantherina/muscaria* group. *J Toxicol Clin Toxicol* 1992;30:13–22.

Mushrooms Causing Renal Toxicity

Anthony Morocco

Clinical Presentation

The usual onset of symptoms from *Cortinarius* intoxication occurs 2 to 3 days after ingestion. Patients experience nausea, vomiting, abdominal pain, headache, chills, dry mouth, and polyuria or oliguria. In the limited number of reported *Amanita smithiana* cases, all from the northwestern United States, symptoms of gastroenteritis, malaise, and dizziness occurred 1 to 12 hours after ingestion. These symptoms may persist until the development of oliguria or anuria (within 2 to 4 days).[1-3]

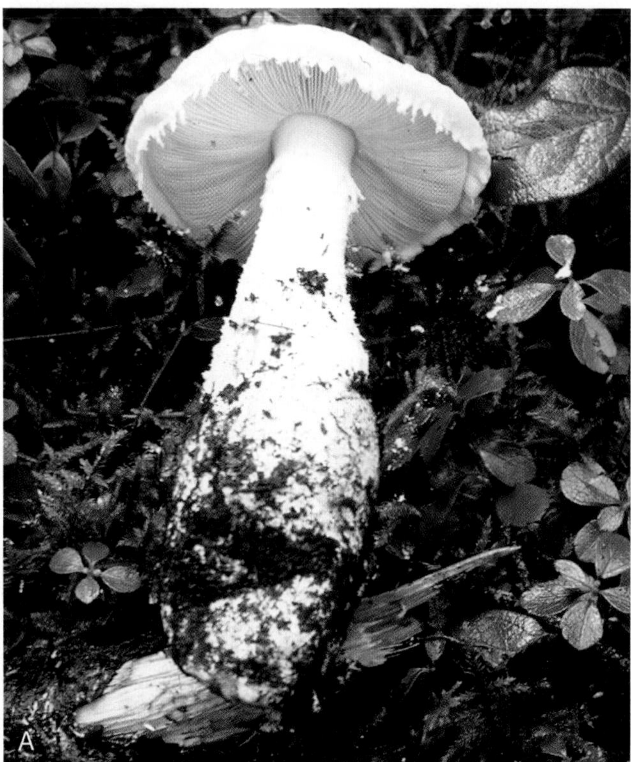

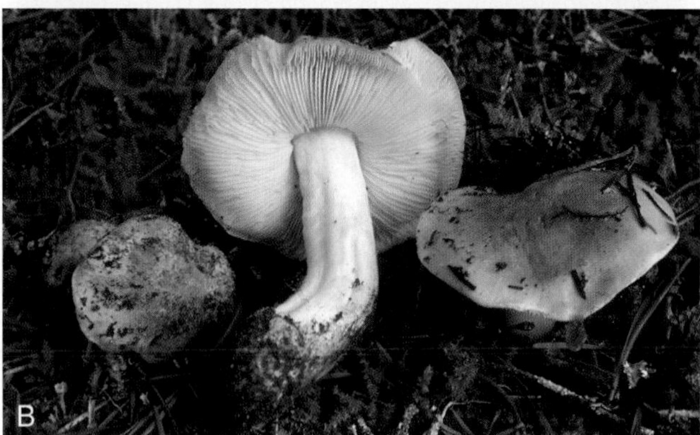

FIGURE 24-49 **A:** *Amanita smithiana.* **B:** *Tricholoma flavovirens.* (**A** and **B,** Copyright Dick Bishop, MD.)

Pathophysiology

Mushrooms causing primarily renal toxicity include several *Cortinarius* species (*C. orellanus, C. speciosissimus, C. rainierensis*) and *A. smithiana.*[1-3]

Cortinarius spp. contain the renal toxin orellanine. The toxin may act by generation of superoxide radicals in a manner similar to the herbicides paraquat and diquat. The renal tubular epithelium is damaged, resulting in interstitial nephritis and fibrosis. *A. smithiana* contains the renal toxins allenic norleucine and chlorocrotylglycine.[1-3]

Diagnosis

The delay in onset of symptoms can make the diagnosis of *Cortinarius* toxicity challenging. Clinicians should remember to include mushroom toxicity in the differential diagnosis of acute renal failure. It has been suggested that early gastrointestinal symptoms indicate poisoning by a mildly toxic mushroom, but *A. smithiana* is an important exception to this rule. Patients may report consuming mushrooms that they thought were the edible and similar-appearing pine mushrooms or matsutake (*Tricholoma magnivalere).* If the patient can produce a specimen of the implicated mushroom, identification by a mycologist may be useful. There are no readily available assays for any of the implicated toxins.[1-3]

Clinical Complications

Cortinarius intoxication results in renal failure in 30% to 45% of patients. One third will require chronic hemodialysis or renal transplantation. Hepatotoxicity is possible. *A. smithiana* can also cause renal failure, resulting in the need for hemodialysis, but in all reported cases function was recovered after 1 month. Patients may also develop significant volume depletion due to severe gastroenteritis.[1-3]

Management

No specific treatment is indicated for *Cortinarius* intoxication other than supportive care, including hemodialysis if necessary. Patients with suspected *A. smithiana* intoxication should be given activated charcoal if presenting with early gastrointestinal complaints. Hemodialysis or charcoal hemoperfusion has been suggested as a means to enhance elimination of the toxins.[1-3]

REFERENCES

1. Goldfrank LR. Mushrooms. In: Goldfrank LR, Flomenbaum NE, Lewin NA, et al., eds. *Goldfrank's toxicologic emergencies,* 7th ed. New York, McGraw-Hill, 2002, pp 1115–1128.
2. Danel VC, Saviuc PF, Garon D. Main features of *Cortinarius* spp. poisoning: a literature review. *Toxicon* 2001;39:1053–1060.
3. Leathem AM, Purssel RA, Chan VR, Kroeger PD. Renal failure caused by mushroom poisoning. *J Toxicol Clin Toxicol* 1997;35: 67–75.

Mushrooms Causing Isolated Gastrointestinal Toxicity

Anthony Morocco

Clinical Presentation

Symptoms occur within 1 to 2 hours after ingestion. Patients experience nausea, vomiting, diarrhea, and abdominal pain and cramping.[1]

Pathophysiology

A large group of mushrooms are known to cause rapid-onset gastroenteritis. Examples include *Chlorophyllum molybdites, Boletes* spp., *Lactarius* spp., and many others.[1]

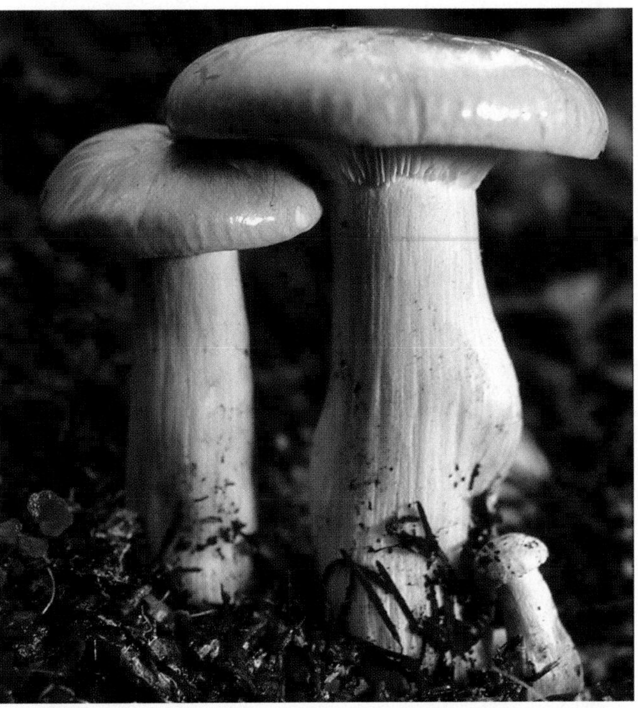

FIGURE 24–50 *Clitocybe nebularis* may produce gastrointestinal symptoms. (Courtesy of Judy Roger, MD.)

The nature of the various toxins and mechanisms of action are unknown.[1]

Diagnosis

Diagnosis may often be made from the clinical appearance and history of mushroom ingestion. Symptoms may be mistaken for those of a bacterial food-borne illness. Early onset of gastroenteritis, compared with delayed onset, suggests poisoning by one of the less dangerous mushroom species; however, this should not be considered the rule. The patient may have eaten a mixture of several types of mushrooms, and there are mushrooms such as *Amanita smithiana* that cause early-onset gastroenteritis followed by more serious toxicity. If the patient can produce a specimen of the implicated mushroom, identification by a mycologist may be useful.[1]

Clinical Complications

Symptoms are usually self-limited, resolving within 24 hours in most cases. However, severe gastroenteritis leading to volume depletion, hypovolemia, and death has been reported on rare occasions. More severe toxicity could occur if other toxic species were coingested.[1]

Management

No specific treatment other than supportive care is indicated. Patients may require antiemetics and intravenous fluids. Aggressive volume replacement may be necessary in severe cases.[1]

REFERENCES

1. Goldfrank LR. Mushrooms. In: Goldfrank LR, Flomenbaum NE, Lewin NA, et al., eds. *Goldfrank's toxicologic emergencies,* 7th ed. New York, McGraw-Hill, 2002, pp 1115–1128.

Drug Eruptions

Anthony Morocco

Clinical Presentation

The most common drug eruptions are morbilliform or maculopapular rashes. Many drugs can cause such reactions, which are generalized and symmetric, usually sparing the face, palms, and soles. Other symptoms may include fever, facial edema, pruritus, and exfoliative dermatitis. The cause of these reactions is unknown, but they resolve on discontinuation of the offending drug. Fixed drug eruptions recur at the same sites with repeat exposure to the causative drug. The lesions are elevated, circumscribed, and red or dusky in appearance, and they resolve after discontinuation of the drug. Commonly affected areas include the genitalia and the face. Medications commonly associated with this type of reaction are tetracyclines, sulfonamides, and barbiturates. Immunoglobulin E (IgE)–mediated immune reactions occur after sensitization, most commonly to β-lactam antibiotics. Urticaria, erythema, pruritus, angioedema, and anaphylaxis may occur. Many drugs, such as opioids, salicylates, and radiocontrast media, can cause similar symptoms by directly inducing degranulation of mast cells and basophils by nonimmunologic mechanisms. Pemphigus reactions (associated with penicillamine, rifampin, and captopril) occur due to development of Immunoglobulin G (IgG) antibodies against keratinocytes, resulting in bullae and mucosal erosions. Serum sickness–like reactions are caused by immune complexes and consist of fever, arthralgias, and urticaria. Other eruptions may be vasculitic, lichenoid, or acneiform.[1]

Pathophysiology

A drug eruption is any cutaneous reaction that is caused by a drug. There is a multitude of possible potential reactions, including immunologically mediated and nonallergic reactions. Drugs most likely to cause reactions include antibiotics, nonsteroidal antiinflammatory drugs (NSAIDs), anticonvulsants, and many cardiovascular agents.[1] Drug eruptions may be dose-dependent or idiosyncratic. Possible contributing factors include photosensitivity, hypersensitivity, overdose, drug accumulation, specific pharmacologic side effects, drug-drug interactions, individual differences in metabolism, and the Jarisch-Herxheimer reaction. Previous allergy to a drug increases the risk of future reactions to unrelated drugs (risk increases from 1.2% to 14%). An immunocompromised condition (e.g., acquired immunodeficiency syndrome) substantially increases the risk of drug reaction.[1]

Diagnosis

The diagnosis can be difficult, because drug eruptions produce lesions similar to those observed in other diverse medical conditions. Skin biopsy and skin allergy testing may be used to confirm the diagnosis.[1]

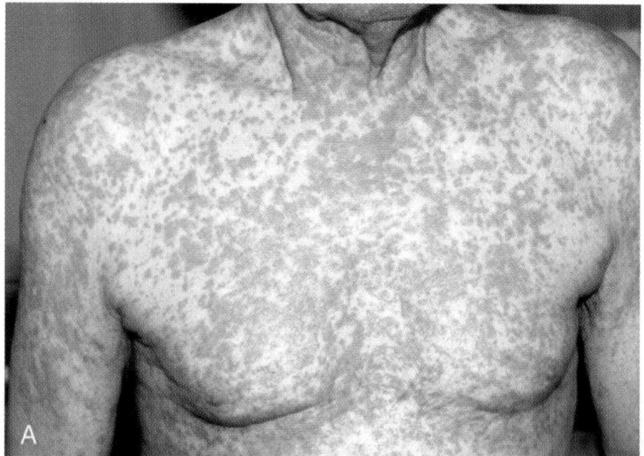

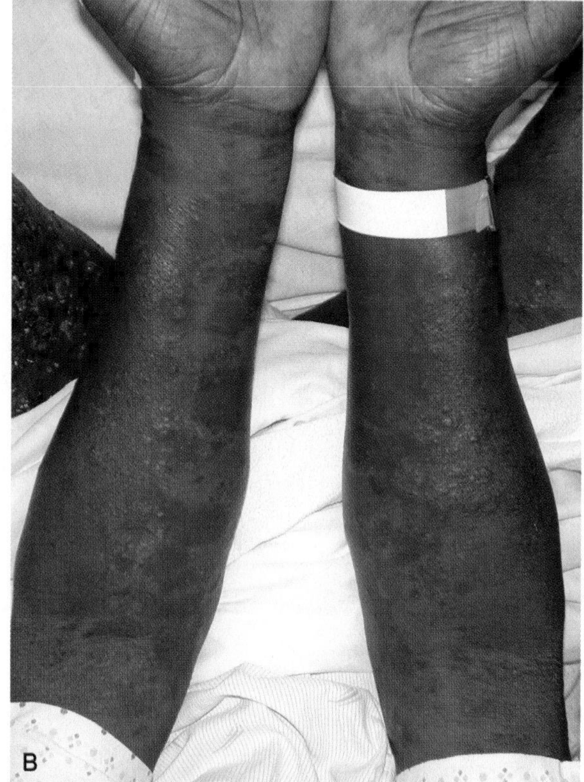

FIGURE 24–51 **A:** Exanthematous ampicillin reaction. (From Goodheart, with permission.) **B:** Drug eruption. (Courtesy of Anthony Morocco, MD.)

Clinical Complications

Severe reactions, such as Stevens-Johnson syndrome and toxic epidermal necrolysis, can be fatal.[1]

Management

The offending drug should be discontinued in most cases. Corticosteroids may be beneficial for severe reactions.[1]

REFERENCES

1. Beltrani VS. Cutaneous manifestations of adverse drug reactions. *Immunol Allergy Clin North Am* 198;18:866–895.

Drug-Induced Photosensitivity

Anthony Morocco

Clinical Presentation

Phototoxic reactions are of three varieties: (1) rapid erythema within 30 minutes after sunlight exposure with burning and itching, lasting 1 to 2 days; (2) shorter-duration rapid reaction with development of wheals and burning; (3) the most severe form, which develops 1 to 2 days after sunlight exposure and results in erythema, edema, and hyperpigmentation. Photoallergic reactions result in papulovesicular rash and pruritus 1 to 14 days after sunlight exposure.[1] Unlike phototoxic reactions, photoallergic reactions require previous exposure to the sensitizer and can spread to non–sun-exposed areas.[2]

Pathophysiology

Drugs cause two types of photosensitivity reactions, phototoxic and photoallergic. Numerous drug classes may cause these reactions, including diuretics, nonsteroidal antiinflammatory drugs (NSAIDs), antimicrobials, antipsychotics, tricyclic antidepressants, sulfonylureas, anticonvulsants, porphyrins, and others.[1] Some drugs rarely cause reactions, whereas others, such as amiodarone, cause photosensitivity in more than 50% of patients.[2] A number of ingredients of topical agents can also cause photosensitization, including retinoids, essential oils, dyes, and preservatives.[1] The phototoxic effect is sometimes used therapeutically for malignancies and skin conditions such as psoriasis.

Photosensitizing drugs are chromophores because they absorb ultraviolet (UV) and/or visible light. Absorbed energy results in the formation of free radicals or in transfer of energy that generates reactive oxygen species or alteration of various biomolecules. Stable photoproducts may form that can damage cells distant to the skin. The end results are direct cellular damage and generation of inflammatory mediators, which cause further injury. Photoallergic reactions result from the formation of a photoantigen that causes both immediate and delayed hypersensitivity reactions.[1]

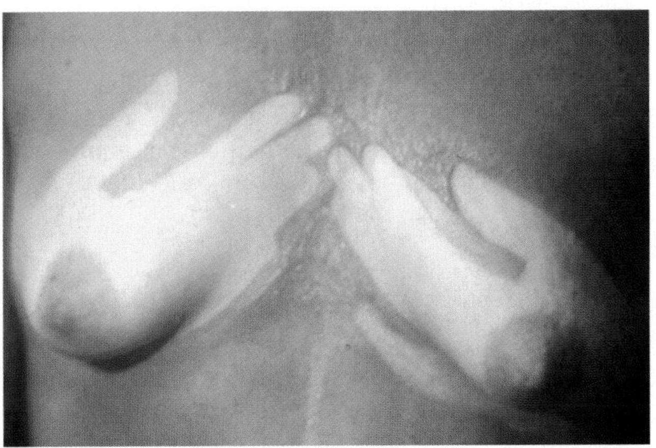

FIGURE 24–52 Drug photosensitivity eruption. Erythematous (exaggerated sunburn) reaction in an individual who was taking demeclocycline (Declomycin) and fell asleep on the beach. (From Goodheart, with permission.)

Diagnosis

Diagnosis is based on the appearance of rash in sun-exposed areas. Testing with an artificial UV light source (photopatch testing) may reproduce the rash and confirm the diagnosis.[1]

Clinical Complications

Hyperpigmentation may be prominent and may last for months. Photo-onycholysis and pseudoporphyria (formation of large bullae with easy bruising) are rare. Chronic photodermatitis (known as persistent light reaction) that continues after withdrawal of the photosensitizer may occur.[2]

Management

Specific treatment is not needed, because reactions are self-limited. Antihistamines may reduce itching, and corticosteroids may be indicated for severe reactions. Patients must be counseled to be vigilant against sun exposure during therapy with a photosensitizing drug.[1]

REFERENCES

1. Moore DE. Drug-induced cutaneous photosensitivity: incidence, mechanism, prevention and management. *Drug Saf* 2002;25:345–372.
2. Gould JW, Mercurio MG, Elmets CA. Cutaneous photosensitivity diseases induced by exogenous agents. *J Am Acad Dermatol* 1995;33:551–573.

Purple Glove Syndrome

Michael Greenberg

Clinical Presentation

Patients with purple glove syndrome (PGS) develop edema, discoloration, and moderate to severe pain distal to the site of intravenous administration of phenytoin.[1–3]

Diagnosis

The diagnosis is based on typical clinical findings in light of intercurrent or recent intravenous phenytoin administration. The syndrome is characterized by pain out of proportion to what might be expected in association with routine intravenous infiltrations.[1]

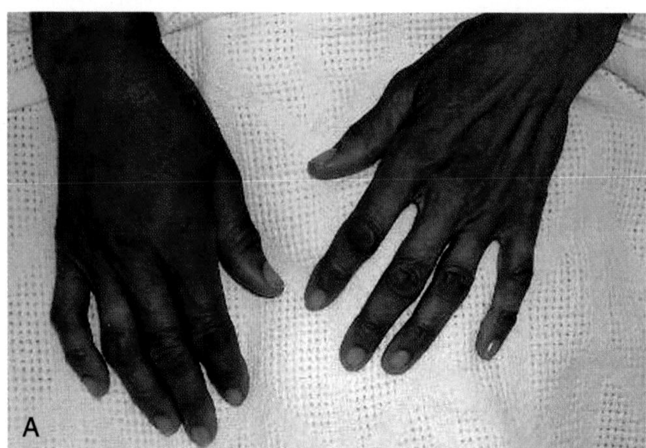

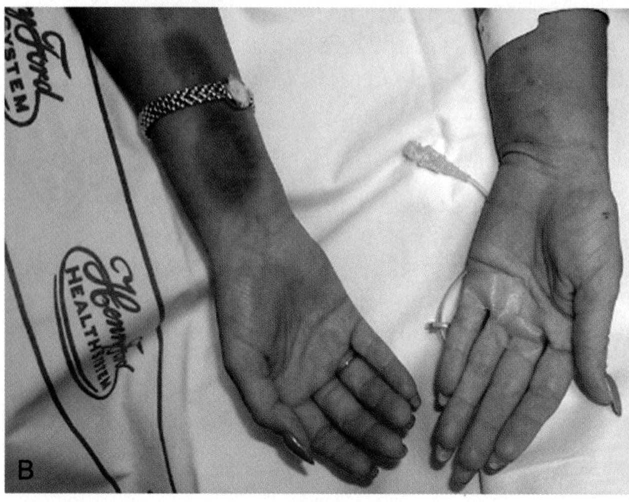

FIGURE 24–53 **A** and **B:** Skin discoloration characteristic of purple glove syndrome. (From Burneo JG, Anandan JV, Barkley GL. A prospective study of the incidence of the purple glove syndrome. *Epilepsia* 2001;42:1156–1159.)

Pathophysiology

PGS is a local adverse reaction to phenytoin. PGS occurs in three stages. First, a pale blue or dark purple discoloration appears at and around the intravenous site within 2 to 12 hours after phenytoin administration. During the ensuing 12 to 16 hours, edema develops and the discoloration spreads. The third and final stage involves healing and resolution of the discoloration.[1–3]

The precise cause of PGS is not known. Most authors attribute the syndrome to local effects of phenytoin, which is a weak acid carried in an alkaline vehicle along with ethanol and propylene glycol, all of which make for a highly tissue-irritating solution. However, this theory was called into question with the identification of a case of PGS associated with oral administration of phenytoin.[2] In addition, infiltration of the drug is not part and parcel of PGS; however, PGS may be related to the rate of phenytoin administration.[1,3]

Clinical Complications

Complications and long-term sequelae have not been reported.

Management

Treatment requires immediate discontinuation of the drug. Generally, local care with elevation, warm compresses, and administration of nonsteroidal antiinflammatory drugs for pain is adequate to treat PGS.

REFERENCES

1. Burneo J, Anandan J, Barkley G. A prospective study of the incidence of the purple glove syndrome. *Epilepsia* 2001;42:1156–1159.
2. Yoshilawa H, Abe T, Oda Y. Purple glove syndrome caused by oral administration of phenytoin. *J Child Neurol* 2000;15:762.
3. O'Brien T, Cascino G. Incidence and clinical consequence of the purple glove syndrome in patients receiving intravenous phenytoin. *Neurology* 1998;51:1034–1039.

Carotenoderma

Michael Greenberg

Clinical Presentation

Patients with carotenoderma present with orange-yellow discoloration of the skin that does not involve the sclera or oral mucosa.[1-3]

Pathophysiology

The volitional and chronic intake of very large quantities of β-carotene results in elevated plasma carotene levels. An orange-yellow pigmentation of the skin, known as carotenoderma (often incorrectly termed "hypercarotonemia"), may develop as a result of deposition of carotene in the stratum corneum, which has a special affinity for carotene based on its high lipid content.[1]

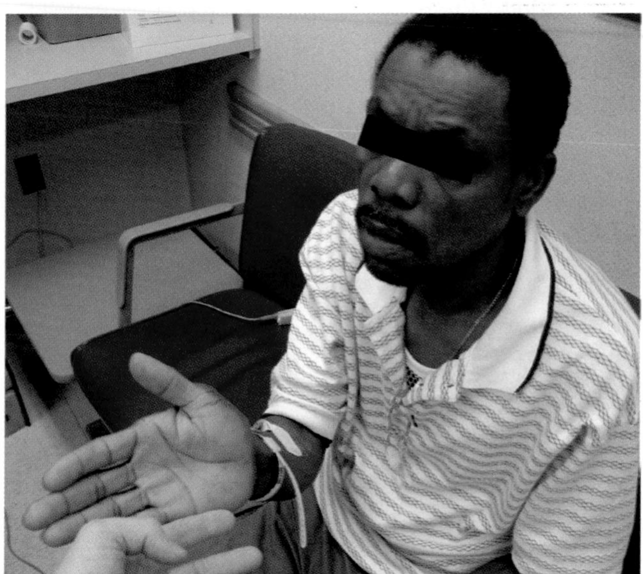

FIGURE 24–54 Orange pigmentation of the hands secondary to excessive chronic β-carotene ingestion. (Courtesy of Wayne Satz, MD.)

Carotenoderma is clinically innocuous and completely reversible on cessation of β-carotene intake. It is important to recognize that abnormal plasma levels of vitamin A and clinical signs of hypervitaminosis A do not result from the excessive consumption of β-carotene.[1] A variety of causes have been identified for carotenoderma, including nutritional supplements, eggs, fruits, vegetables, and certain metabolic conditions such as hypothyroidism, diabetes mellitus, pregnancy, anorexia, and familial carotenemia.[1]

Carotenoderma develops approximately 1 to 2 months after the patient begins to ingest excessive amounts of β-carotene. This correlates with serum β-carotene levels in excess of 250 μg/dL.[1]

Diagnosis

Carotenoderma is often seen in children and may sometimes be confused with jaundice. The skin discoloration associated with carotenoderma may be differentiated from jaundice in that the sclera and oral mucosa are not involved in benign carotenoderma.

Clinical Complications

Carotenoderma-related skin findings are benign, and no associated complications have been reported.

Management

Specific therapy is not indicated. Carotenoderma is reversible on cessation of excessive β-carotene intake.[1-3]

REFERENCES

1. Maharshak N, Shapiro J, Trau H. Carotenoderma: a review of the current literature. *Int J Dermatol* 2003;42:178–181.
2. Russel RM. The vitamin A spectrum: from deficiency to toxicity. *Am J Clin Nutr* 2000;71:878–884.
3. Omaye ST, Krinsky NI, Kagan VE, et al. Beta-carotene: friend or foe? *Fundam Appl Toxicol* 1997;40:163–174.

Heparin-Induced Thrombocytopenia

Anthony Morocco

Clinical Presentation

In heparin-induced thrombocytopenia, patients have a transient reduction in platelet count on the first day of therapy but remain asymptomatic. With heparin-associated thrombocytopenia, thrombocytopenia occurs 5 to 15 days after administration of heparin. Patients with a recent heparin exposure (less than 100 days) may develop thrombocytopenia on day 1 of re-exposure.[1] Acute systemic reactions (fever, chills) may also occur with heparin bolus. Petechiae and bleeding rarely occur, despite the low platelet count. Instead, thrombosis occurs in approximately 20% of HIT patients. The most common sites of thrombosis are the deep veins of the lower extremities. Patients may present with lower-extremity pain or edema consistent with deep venous thrombosis, or chest pain and shortness of breath due to pulmonary embolism. Other possible areas of thrombosis are the upper extremities, cerebral veins and dural sinus, and adrenal veins. Arterial thromboses manifesting as stroke or symptoms of local ischemia (e.g., bowel, kidney, spinal cord, extremities) occur less commonly.[2] Skin involvement includes lesions at heparin injection sites, erythematous plaques, and worsening of coumarin necrosis.[1]

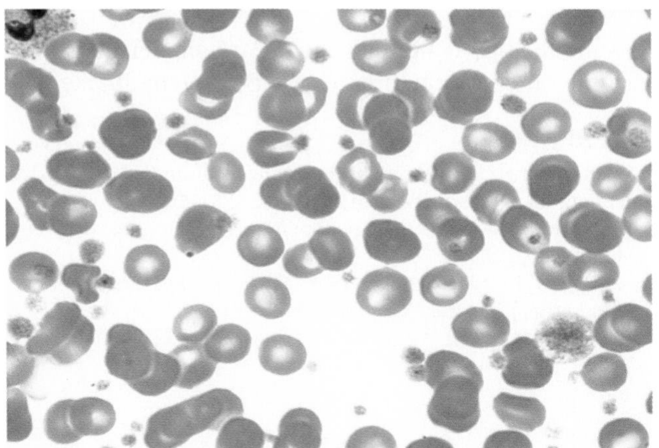

FIGURE 24–55 Peripheral blood smear consistent with heparin-induced thrombocytopenia. (From Anderson, with permission.)

Pathophysiology

Heparin-induced thrombocytopenia is an immune-mediated reaction that occurs in up to 5% of patients receiving heparin and may result in serious thrombotic complications. HIT should not be confused with heparin-associated thrombocytopenia, a non–immune-mediated process sometimes called HIT I.[1,2] The term HIT is commonly used only in reference to HIT II, also called HIT-associated thrombosis or white clot syndrome.[1] HIT is 8 to 10 times less likely with low-molecular-weight heparin (LMWH) than with unfractionated heparin (UFH), and HIT is less likely with porcine than bovine UFH.

Platelet factor 4 (PF4) binds to heparin, resulting in the formation of antibodies to this complex. The heparin-PF4 antibody then attaches to and activates platelets. The antibodies and PF4 also bind endogenous heparin on endothelial cells, resulting in injury and further activation of clotting.[1]

Diagnosis

Diagnosis is based on the detection of HIT antibodies in combination with the clinical syndrome.[2]

Clinical Complications

Complications include death due to pulmonary embolism and ischemic injury, such as bowel necrosis and gangrenous limbs.[2]

Management

Heparin therapy should be immediately discontinued, and treatment with alternative anticoagulants such as argatroban, danaparoid, or lepirudin should be instituted. Long-term anticoagulation with warfarin may also be required. Future therapy with UFH or LMWH is contraindicated.[2]

REFERENCES

1. Warkentin TE. Heparin-induced thrombocytopenia: pathogenesis and management. *Br J Haematol* 2003;121:535–555.
2. Goor Y, Goor O, Eldor A. Heparin-induced thrombocytopenia with thrombotic sequelae: a review. *Autoimmun Rev* 2002;1:183–189.

Autoinjector Injury

Anthony Morocco

Clinical Presentation

Patients most often inadvertently inject the unit into a finger. Epinephrine injection into a digit can cause pain, numbness, edema, and pallor. Systemic signs and symptoms may be present, including tachycardia, hypertension, tremor, and diaphoresis.[1] Blood flow to the affected area should be evaluated by assessing capillary refill. A pulse oximeter may be useful in demonstrating arterial flow in a digit.[2] After atropine injection, patients present with tachycardia, dry mucous membranes, blurry vision, and mydriasis.

Pathophysiology

Autoinjectors are spring-loaded syringes designed for emergency prehospital administration of medications. Epinephrine autoinjectors are used for the prehospital treatment of acute anaphylaxis, and atropine autoinjectors are included in kits for treatment of nerve agent casualties. The EpiPen® and EpiPen Jr.® are available in the United States, and contain 0.3 mg and 0.15 mg of epinephrine, respectively. These devices are designed to inject only 0.3 mL of the 2 mL in the syringe. For proper use of an autoinjector, the patient grasps it with a fist, removes the activator cap, and jabs the unit into the anterolateral thigh.

Epinephrine stimulates α- and β-adrenergic receptors, resulting in local vasoconstriction, vasospasm, and systemic sympathetic stimulation. Atropine antagonizes the effect of acetylcholine at muscarinic receptors.

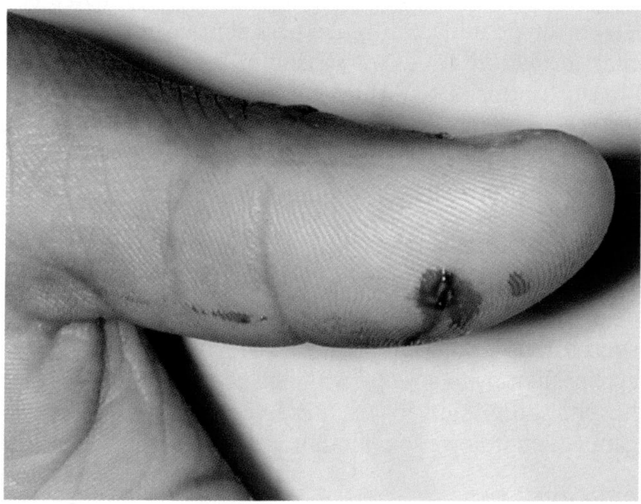

FIGURE 24–56 Needle from an Epi-Pen® device retained in the soft tissue of the thumb. Note pallor of the digit. (Courtesy of Robert Hendrickson, MD.)

Diagnosis

The diagnosis is made by history and physical examination. No laboratory tests are necessary.

Clinical Complications

Prolonged ischemia may result in tissue necrosis.

Management

The use of topical nitroglycerin paste to treat epinephrine injection has been recommended to induce vasodilation and restoration of perfusion in an affected digit, but this treatment is not likely to be effective. Phentolamine, an α-adrenergic receptor antagonist, is the recommended treatment for patients with definite ischemia after epinephrine injection. Up to 10 mL of a 1 mg/mL solution of phentolamine is injected into the ischemic tissue or at the base of the finger near the digital arteries.[1] Terbutaline may be used in a similar manner (1 mg in 10 mL) if phentolamine is unavailable.[2] The symptoms after atropine injection are self-limited and require no treatment.

REFERENCES

1. McCauley WA, Gerace RV, Scilley C. Treatment of accidental digital injection of epinephrine. *Ann Emerg Med* 1991;20:665–668.
2. Stier PA, Bogner MD, Webster K, et al. Use of subcutaneous terbutaline to reverse peripheral ischemia. *Am J Emerg Med* 1999;17:91–94.

Warfarin-Induced Skin Necrosis

Michael Greenberg

Clinical Presentation

Patients with warfarin-induced skin necrosis (WISN) present with paresthesias, sensations of pressure, or localized skin discomfort; these patients typically are obese, perimenopausal, middle-aged women who have received warfarin for thromboembolic disease. WISN usually is associated with large doses of warfarin. Most patients present between day 3 and day 6 of therapy. Late-onset WISN may manifest as late as 15 years after therapy.[1-3]

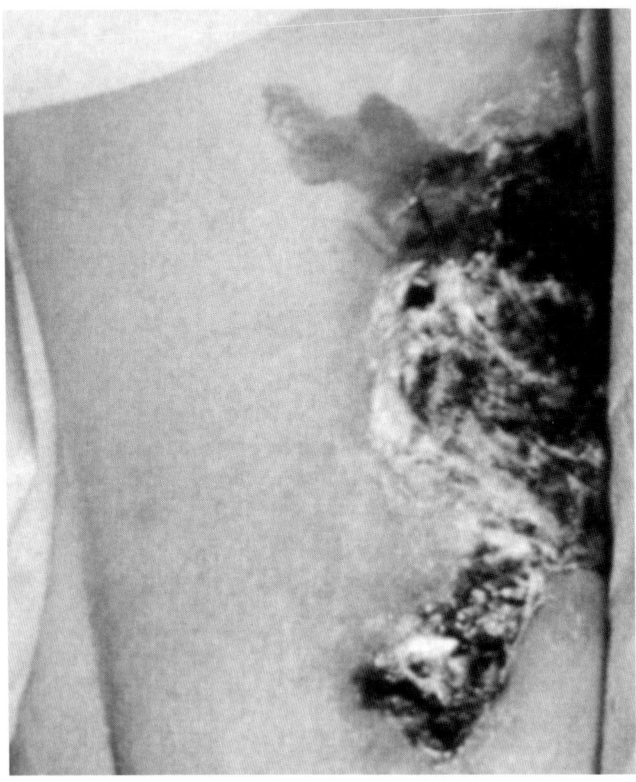

FIGURE 24–57 Warfarin-induced skin necrosis. An initial area of tenderness over the right calf became erythematous and indurated and then evolved into overt skin necrosis as shown. (From Greer, with permission.)

Pathophysiology

WISN involves widespread thrombosis with microvascular injury and fibrin deposition in the postcapillary venules and small veins. Lack of vascular or perivascular inflammation and absence of arteriolar thrombosis are distinctive features. The cause of WISN is not certain; however, protein C deficiency, protein S deficiency, factor VII deficiency, hypersensitivity, direct toxic effect of warfarin, and other mechanisms have all been proposed.[1-3]

The specific pathogenesis of WISN may involve rapid declines in factor VII and protein C levels after the initiation of warfarin. Other hypercoagulable conditions (protein S deficiency, antithrombin deficiency, and lupus) have also been associated with WISN.[1-3]

Diagnosis

The diagnosis requires a high index of clinical suspicion. Initially, these lesions may be erythematous or hemorrhagic and tend to be painful and well demarcated. Hemorrhagic bullae, full-thickness skin necrosis, and eschar formation are characteristic of the late stages. The breasts, buttocks, and thighs are the most common sites for WISN in women. The penile skin may be involved in men. The trunk, extremities, and face may also be involved in some cases.[1-3]

Management

The progression of WISN may be ameliorated with high-dose vitamin K or with heparin anticoagulation. Some success has also been achieved with the use of prostacyclin therapy. Patients with suspected WISN require hospital admission to an intensive care unit and emergency hematology consultation.[1-3]

REFERENCES

1. Essex DW, Wynn SS, Jin DK. Late-onset warfarin-induced skin necrosis: case report and review of the literature. *Am J Hematol* 1998;57:233–237.
2. Gelwix TJ, Beeson MS. Warfarin-induced skin necrosis. *Am J Emerg Med* 1998;16:541–543.
3. Gallerani M, Manfredini R, Moratelli S. Non-haemorrhagic adverse reactions of oral anticoagulant therapy. *Int J Cardiol* 1995;49:1–7.

Serum Sickness

Michael Greenberg

Clinical Presentation

Patients with serum sickness (SS) present with fever and adenopathy as well as arthralgias, rashes, nausea, vomiting, diarrhea, and malaise. Many cases are associated with proteinuria. SS usually manifests within days to 3 weeks after exposure to one or more inciting antigens.[1]

Pathophysiology

SS is mediated by tissue deposition of immune complexes and activation of complement; and usually is associated with administration of, or exposure to, foreign proteins. Various drugs also are associated with the development of SS reactions, including allopurinol, arsenicals, barbiturates, angiotensin-converting enzyme inhibitors, cephalosporins, and penicillins. In addition, SS may be associated with exposure to various heterologous sera such as those used in the prophylaxis and treatment of botulism, diphtheria, and snake and spider bites. Desensitizing allergens, various blood products, animal and insect venoms, and various vaccines may also be causative.[1]

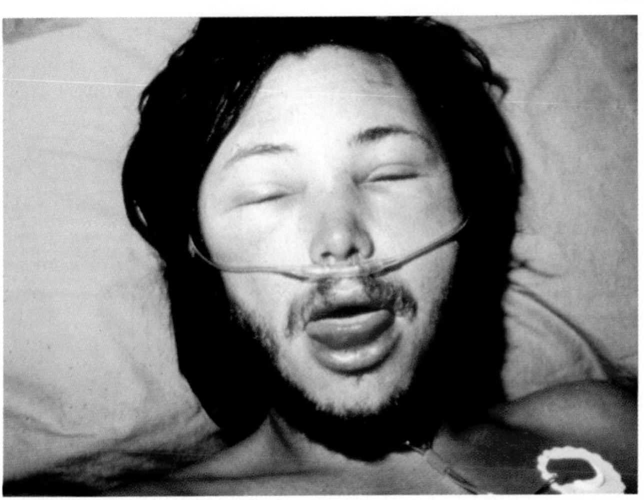

FIGURE 24–58 Swelling of the face and tongue caused by serum sickness after administration of crotalid antivenom. (Courtesy of Scott Phillips, MD.)

Diagnosis

The diagnosis is based on finding typical physical manifestations, including fever, urticaria, adenopathy, arthritis/arthralgias, peripheral edema, and renal, cardiovascular, or pulmonary manifestations. Renal problems may include proteinuria, hematuria, and oliguria, and cardiovascular manifestations may include myocarditis, pericarditis, or both. Neurologic problems may include peripheral neuropathies, optic neuritis, and cranial nerve dysfunction. Some cases may involve encephalopathy.[1]

Clinical Complications

Complications include vasculitis, various neuropathies, glomerulonephritis, anaphylaxis with or without shock, and death.[1]

Management

Treatment involves supportive care and removal of the inciting antigens if possible. In addition, therapy with corticosteroids, antihistamines, and antipyretics may be indicated. Hospitalization may be needed for moderate and severe cases, whereas mild cases may, at times, be managed on an outpatient basis.

REFERENCES

1. Roujeau JC, Stern RS. Severe adverse cutaneous reactions to drugs. *N Engl J Med* 1994;331:1272–1285.

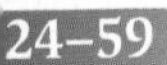

Argyria

Michael Greenberg

Clinical Presentation

Patients with argyria present with diffuse, silver-grey skin discoloration.[1,2]

Pathophysiology

Dermal deposits of silver-albumin compounds result in irreversible skin discoloration. Argyria has historically been related to occupational exposures to silver compounds. It may also be related to the use of silver-containing pharmaceuticals or herbal preparations.[1] The silver deposits associated with argyria are not allergenic and have not been reported to cause systemic disease.[2]

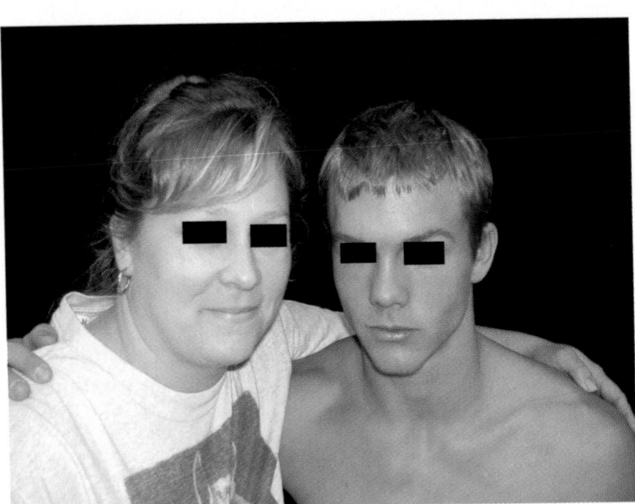

FIGURE 24–59 Note the slate grey skin discoloration of the young man on the right, in contrast to the normal skin color of the woman on the left. (Courtesy of Scott C. Wickless, DO, Tor Shwayder, MD, Davide Iacobelli, MD, and Susan Smolinske, PharmD.)

Diagnosis

The diagnosis is clinical and rests on the finding of a slate-grey, diffuse skin discoloration, including mucosal surfaces and the sclera.

Clinical Complications

Complications are limited to the cosmetic problems engendered by the obvious and profound skin discoloration. Some degree of psychosocial dysfunction may result from embarrassment and concern regarding the permanency of the condition.[1,2]

Management

Argyria is irreversible, and the discoloration is not amenable to treatment.

REFERENCES

1. Tomi NS, Kranke B, Aberer W. A silver man. *Lancet* 2004;363:532.
2. White JM, Powell AM, Brady K, et al. Severe generalized argyria secondary to ingestion of colloidal silver protein. *Clin Exp Dermatol* 2003;28:254–256.

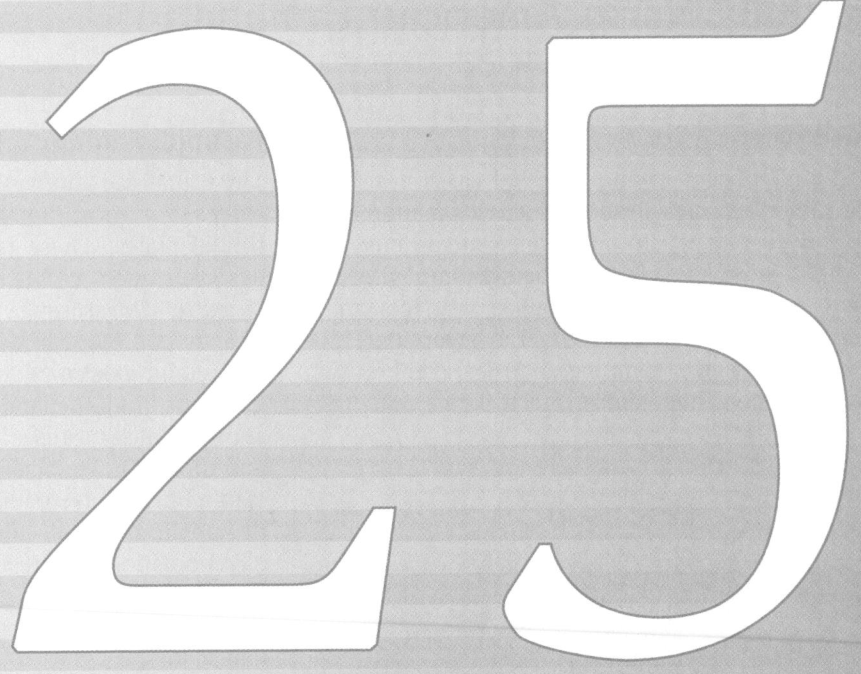

Environmental

Snake Bite: North American Crotalid

Anthony Morocco

Clinical Presentation

Dry bites, which occur in up to 20% of cases, result in no significant symptoms. After true envenomation, patients quickly develop pain and edema at the envenomation site. Edema spreads from the bite site, with development of ecchymoses and bullae. Patients may exhibit a variety of systemic signs and symptoms, including anxiety, nausea, vomiting, diarrhea, diaphoresis, dyspnea, confusion, hypotension, tachycardia, and fasciculations.[1]

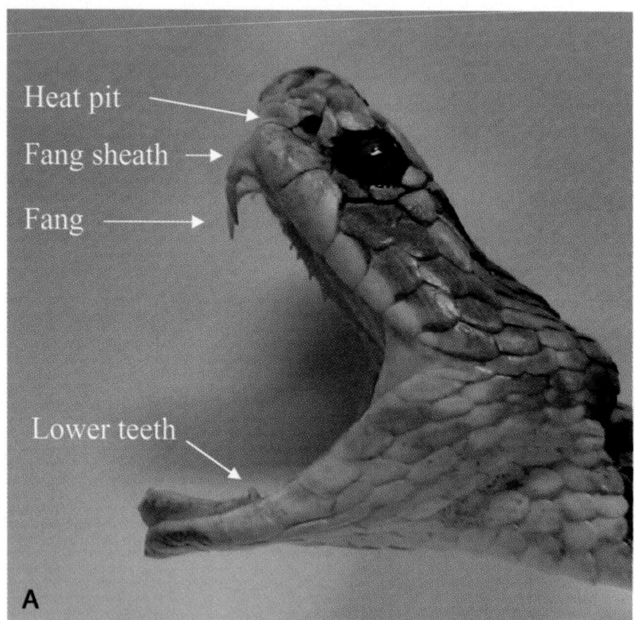

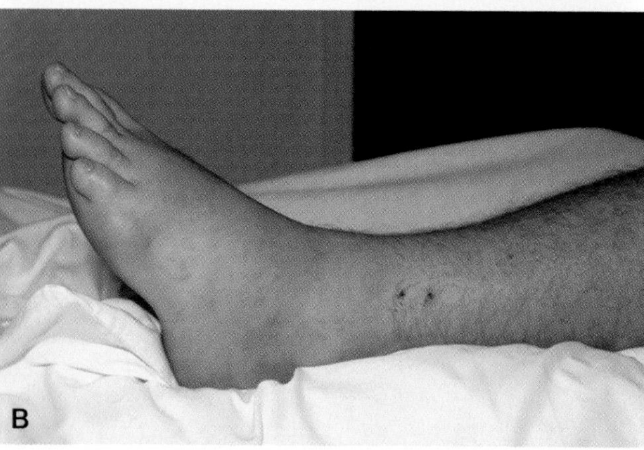

FIGURE 25–1 **A:** Crotaline head. (Rocky Mountain Poison Center, Dean Olsen. Used with permission.) **B:** Left-foot bite showing classic bite marks and presence of faint ecchymosis distal to the lateral malleolus. (From Dart, with permission.)

Pathophysiology

The Crotalidae family of snakes, known as pit vipers, includes the most important venomous snakes in the United States. These include the genera *Crotalus* (rattlesnakes such as Eastern and Western diamondback), *Sistrurus* (Massasauga and pigmy rattlesnakes), and *Agkistrodon* (copperhead and cottonmouth).[1]

Crotalid venom contains a multitude of cytotoxic ingredients. Endothelial damage by polypeptides and metalloproteinases causes tissue edema and ecchymoses, and thrombin-like glycoproteins cause production of unstable fibrin clots, leading to hypofibrinogenemia, fibrin degradation, and bleeding. Platelets are consumed at the envenomation site, resulting in thrombocytopenia. The Mojave rattlesnake is unique among crotalids, because its venom contains a neurotoxin that causes neuromuscular blockade.[1]

Diagnosis

The diagnosis of envenomation is made with an appropriate history and typical physical examination findings. Laboratory tests should include creatine phosphokinase (CPK), creatinine, hemoglobin, platelets, prothrombin time (PT), partial thromboplastin time (PTT), fibrinogen, and fibrin degradation products.[1]

Clinical Complications

Rhabdomyolysis can occur, with subsequent myoglobin-induced renal failure. Bites to the face can result in edema and airway compromise. Other complications include hypovolemic shock, anaphylaxis, seizures, and multiorgan system failure. Acute reactions and serum sickness can complicate antivenom administration.[1]

Management

Immobilization of the affected area and rapid transport to a hospital are the most important field interventions. Devices such as a venom extractor may be of some benefit. A sheep-derived Fab fragment antivenom is available and is indicated for significant progression of signs and symptoms or evidence of coagulopathy. Aggressive supportive care and airway management are indicated. Heparin and blood products are not useful in treating crotalid venom-induced thrombocytopenia and disseminated intravascular coagulation (DIC)–like syndromes. Surgical débridement or fasciotomy is rarely necessary.[1]

REFERENCES

1. Walter FG, Bilden EF, Gibly RL. Envenomations. *Crit Care Clin* 1999;15:353–386.

Snake Bite: North American Coral Snake

Anthony Morocco

Clinical Presentation

Little or no local reaction may be noted, even with significant envenomation, although patients may complain of mild swelling or paresthesias at the bite site. Symptom onset may be delayed by 13 hours or longer. The Eastern and Texas coral snakes produce more significant neurotoxicity than the Arizona species does. Reported symptoms from one series of Eastern coral snake bites included paresthesias (35%), vomiting (25%), weakness (15%), diplopia (10%), dyspnea (10%), diaphoresis (10%), muscle pain (10%), fasciculations (5%) and confusion (5%).[1] Cranial nerve dysfunction, including dysarthria and hypersalivation, may also occur.

Pathophysiology

Coral snakes are neurotoxic members of the Elapidae family found in the United States and Mexico; they include the Western *(Micruroides euryoxanthus)*, the Arizona *(M. euryoxanthus euryoxanthus)*, the Eastern *(Micrurus fulvius)*, and the Texas (*M. fulvius tenere)* coral snakes, as well as several Mexican *Micrurus* species. The coral snakes are known for their bright coloring, which consists of red, yellow, and black bands. In the United States, the saying, "red on yellow, kill a fellow; red on black, venom lack" differentiates the dangerous coral snakes from harmless varieties.[2]

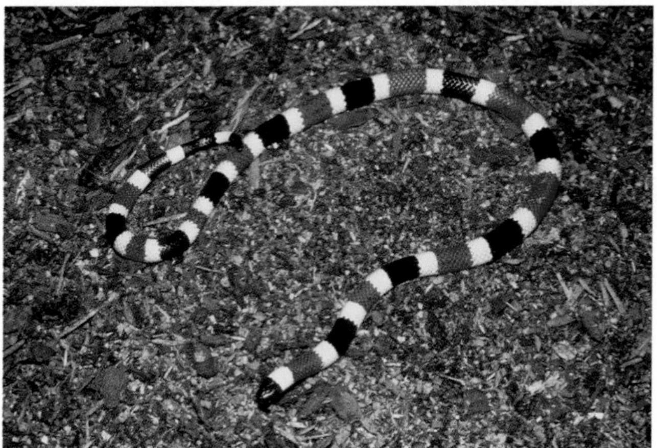

FIGURE 25–2 Western coral snake. North American identification is aided by the mnemonic, "red on yellow, kill a fellow; red on black, venom lack." (© Dr. Julian White)

Coral snakes have small, fixed, grooved fangs; they cause significant envenomation by holding on to the victim. The venom contains neurotoxic peptides that bind to the postsynaptic acetylcholine receptor of the neuromuscular junction.[1,2]

Clinical Complications

Death from respiratory failure within as little as 4 hours after envenomation has been reported. Seizures have also been reported, most commonly in children. Antivenom treatment may result in anaphylaxis, anaphylactic reactions, or serum sickness.

Management

Application of a compression bandage and immobilization of the affected area immediately after a bite may slow the lymphatic spread of the venom. Aggressive supportive care, including airway management, is indicated. All patients with suspected coral snake bites should be admitted and observed for at least 24 hours. An equine-derived *M. fulvius* antivenom is available in the United States and is effective for the Eastern and Texas coral snakes, but not the Arizona coral snake. The initial dose is three to six vials. A *Micrurus* species antivenom is also produced in Mexico. Antivenom treatment is indicated for any patient with a known coral snake bite. Treatment may be much less effective if delayed until after symptom onset.[1]

REFERENCES

1. Walter FG, Bilden EF, Gibly RL. Envenomations. *Crit Care Clin* 1999;15:353–386.
2. Gomez HF, Dart RC. Clinical toxicology of snakebite in North America. In: Meier J, White J, eds. *Handbook of clinical toxicology of animal venoms and poisons.* Boca Raton, FL: CRC Press, 1995:619–644.

Snake Bite: Elapids

Anthony Morocco

Clinical Presentation

No significant envenomation occurs in up to 80% of bites by elapids such as the Australian death adder. Elapids such as the taipan and the krait are known for their neurotoxic effects; local pain, edema, and tissue necrosis can be a significant effect of the bites of many species, including cobras. In general, systemic symptoms include nausea, vomiting, abdominal pain, headache, and dizziness. Neurologic manifestations usually begin with ptosis and diplopia, and then dysarthria, with subsequent generalized muscle weakness and respiratory failure.[1,2]

Pathophysiology

The Elapidae family is a group of snakes found in the Americas, Africa, Asia, and Australia. The Elapids include several of the most toxic snakes known, including all of the highly poisonous terrestrial snakes of Australia and other deadly varieties such as cobras and mambas. A few of the notable genera are *Pseudonaja* (brown snakes), *Pseudechis* (black snakes), *Acanthophis* (death adders), and *Oxyuranus* (taipans) in Australia; *Micrurus* (coral snakes) in the Americas; *Naja* and other cobras and *Dendroaspis* (mambas) in Africa; and *Bungarus* (kraits—the cobras, including *Ophiophagus hannah*, the king cobra) and *Calliophis* (coral snakes) in Asia.[1,2]

Elapid venom varies among species but generally contains substances that result in neurotoxicity, cytotoxicity, and hematotoxicity. Elapids are best known for the neurotoxic components of their venom; these include α-toxins and phospholipases A_2, which cause paralysis by acting presynaptically and postsynaptically at the neuromuscular junction. Mamba venom contains unique toxins that block neuronal potassium channels (dendrotoxins) and inhibit cholinesterases (fasciculins).[1,2]

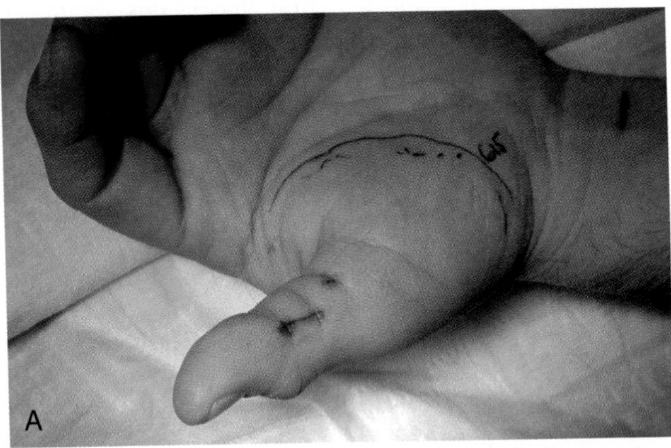

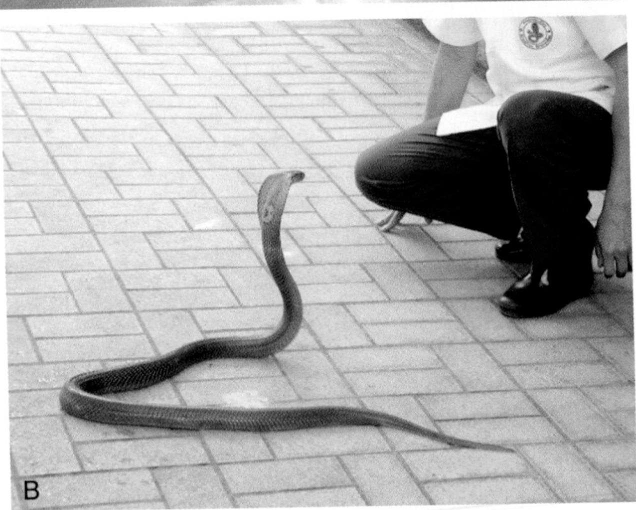

FIGURE 25–3 **A:** Elapid bite on thumb. (Courtesy of Anthony Morocco, MD.) **B:** Elapid species include the monocellate cobra, seen here. (Courtesy of Michael Greenberg, MD.)

Diagnosis

In Australia, a detection kit is available to identify venom from either the wound site or urine.[1,2]

Clinical Complications

Bites to the face can result in edema and airway compromise. Unconsciousness and seizures can occur in less than 60 minutes after severe envenomations. Other potential complications include hemolysis, renal failure, compartment syndrome, shock, anaphylaxis, and death. Acute reactions and serum sickness can complicate antivenom administration.[1,2]

Management

Initial first aid includes immobilization of the affected area and transport to a hospital. Aggressive supportive care and airway management are indicated. Various antivenoms are available, mostly horse-derived and varying by geographical area, that may be effective against one or several species of elapids and members of other snake families.[1,2]

REFERENCES

1. White J. Clinical toxicology of snakebite in Australia and New Guinea. In: Meier J, White J, eds. *Handbook of clinical toxicology of animal venoms and poisons.* Boca Raton, FL: CRC Press, 1995:595–617.
2. Warrell DA. Clinical toxicology of snakebite in Asia. In: Meier J, White J, eds. *Handbook of clinical toxicology of animal venoms and poisons.* Boca Raton, FL: CRC Press, 1995:493–594.

Snake Bite: Vipers

Anthony Morocco

Clinical Presentation

After envenomation, substantial local effects may develop within minutes to hours. Severe local edema, ecchymoses, bullae formation, tissue necrosis, and regional lymphadenopathy occur. The most severe signs and symptoms occur after *Bitis* species and *Echis* species bites. Tissue injury may spread from the bite site to involve an entire limb and part of the torso. Patients may also develop widespread hemorrhage and ecchymoses. Systemic symptoms may include nausea, vomiting, diarrhea, abdominal pain, hyperventilation, dizziness, and chest tightness. A few species can cause mild neurotoxic effects such as ptosis and other cranial nerve abnormalities.[1,2]

Pathophysiology

The vipers, family Viperidae (or subfamily Viperinae), are a group of medically important snakes found in Europe, Africa, and Asia. A few of the notable species are *Vipera berus* (adder), *Vipera aspis* (asp), and *Vipera ammodytes* (long-nosed viper) in Europe; *Bitis* species (e.g., *Bitis arietans,* the puff adder), *Echis* species (saw-scaled or carpet vipers), and many others in Africa and the Middle East; and *Daboia russelii* (Russel's viper) as well as *Echis* and *Vipera* species in Asia. These snakes inhabit a wide variety of forest, mountain, and desert areas.[1,2]

Vipers inject their venom through long, hollow, folding fangs. The venom contains a number of ingredients, including hyaluronidase, histamine, myotoxins, fibrinogenases, kallikrein-like glycoproteins, clotting-factor activators, neurotoxins, and many others. Direct cytotoxicity, platelet destruction, and coagulation-factor consumption occur.[1,2]

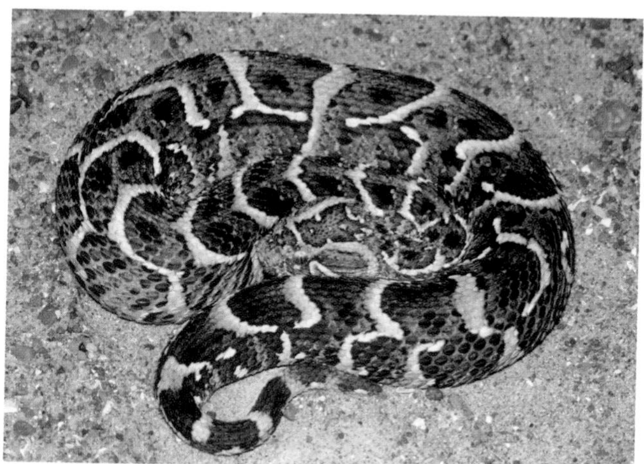

FIGURE 25–4 Puff Adder (*Bitis arietans*). (©Julian White, MD, 2004. Used with permission.)

Diagnosis

Laboratory tests should include creatine phosphokinase (CPK), creatinine, hemoglobin, platelets, prothrombin time (PT), partial thromboplastin time (PTT), fibrinogen, and fibrin degradation products.

Clinical Complications

Massive third-spacing of fluids and hemorrhage due to coagulopathy can result in shock. Bites to the face can result in edema and airway compromise. Other potential complications include hemolysis, renal failure, compartment syndrome, myocardial injury, pulmonary edema, anaphylaxis, and death. Acute reactions and serum sickness can complicate antivenom administration.[1,2]

Management

Initial first aid includes immobilization of the affected area and transport to a hospital. Aggressive supportive care and airway management are indicated. Various antivenoms are available, mostly horse-derived and varying by geographical area, that may be effective against one or several species of vipers as well as members of other snake families. Surgical débridement or fasciotomy is rarely necessary.[1,2]

REFERENCES

1. Warrel DA. Clinical toxicology of snakebite in Africa and the Middle East/Arabian Peninsula. In: Meier J, White J, eds. *Handbook of clinical toxicology of animal venoms and poisons.* Boca Raton, FL: CRC Press, 1995:433–492.
2. Meier J, Stocker KF. Biology and importance of venomous snakes of medical importance and the composition of snake venoms. In: Meier J, White J, eds. *Handbook of clinical toxicology of animal venoms and poisons.* Boca Raton, FL: CRC Press, 1995:367–412.

Snake Bite: Sea Snakes

Anthony Morocco

Clinical Presentation

Patients may present with a dry bite, which results in no symptoms, in 80% of cases. The bite is usually painless, and no local symptoms occur even with significant envenomation. Symptom onset occurs in 30 minutes to 3 hours, starting with myalgias, dizziness, weakness, nausea, vomiting, and dry mouth. The myalgias may progress to severe pain and myolysis. Up to 60 hours after envenomation, patients may develop ptosis, dysarthria, and diminished deep tendon reflexes.[1]

Pathophysiology

Sea snakes are all members of the family Hydrophiidae; they are found near shores or reefs in the tropical waters of the western Pacific and Indian Oceans. Sea snakes are not aggressive, and most bites are sustained by traditional fisherman who inadvertently capture or step on a snake.[1]

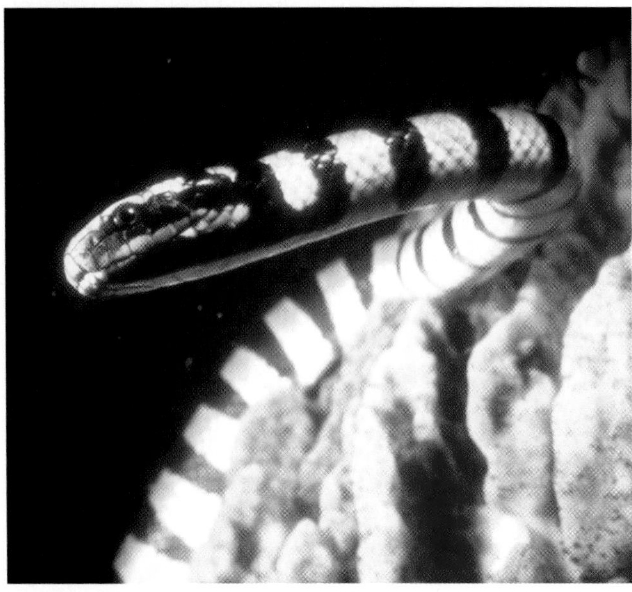

FIGURE 25–5 Sea snakes contain potent venoms. Any case involving systemic envenomation by a sea snake requires treatment with antivenom. (©Robert Yin, 2004. Used with permission.)

The venom is injected through small, hollow fangs. Unlike most land snakes, the sea snake often holds its bite onto the victim for a prolonged period. The venom contains myotoxins and neurotoxins. The myotoxins are similar to those of crotalid species and cause hyaline necrosis. The neurotoxins bind to the postsynaptic acetylcholine receptor at the neuromuscular junction. Hematotoxicity does not occur.[1]

Clinical Complications

The combination of vomiting and glossopharyngeal muscle impairment may result in aspiration of gastric contents. Myoglobinuric renal failure occurs due to rhabdomyolysis. Deaths may occur from respiratory muscle paralysis.[1]

Management

Application of a compression bandage and immobilization of the affected area immediately after a bite may slow the lymphatic spread of the venom. Aggressive supportive care, including airway management, is indicated. Creatine kinase (CK), urine myoglobin, blood urea nitrogen (BUN), and creatinine concentrations should be monitored while administering intravenous fluids to maintain good urine output. Sea snake antivenom is indicated if systemic signs and symptoms of envenomation are present.[1]

REFERENCES

1. White J. Clinical toxicology of sea snakebites. In: Meier J, White J, eds. *Handbook of clinical toxicology of animal venoms and poisons.* Boca Raton, FL: CRC Press, 1995:159–170.

Scorpion Envenomation

Anthony Morocco

Clinical Presentation

Initial symptoms include local pain, pruritus, and hyperesthesia. Mild local erythema and edema may be evident. Systemic signs and symptoms arise within 5 to 30 minutes and may include restlessness, photophobia, dysphagia, diaphoresis, vomiting, diarrhea, dyspnea, cough, lacrimation, salivation, bronchorrhea, muscle spasms and fasciculations, and hypertension or hypotension.[2] After *Centruroides exilicauda* envenomation, tapping on the envenomation site may elicit pain, even in the absence of other local findings. Young children may exhibit agitation, flailing, and roving eye movements.[1,2]

Pathophysiology

The Scorpiones class of arachnids are all venomous, but fewer than 50 species are considered to be medically important. These include *Tityus* (Central and South America and the West Indies), *Centruroides* (southwestern United States, Central and South America), *Leiurus* (Middle East), *Buthus* (North Africa, Middle East, southern France and Spain), *Androctonus* (North Africa and Middle East), *Bothotus* (India), and *Parabuthus* (southern Africa). These creatures typically are nocturnal, and they are often encountered hiding in dark areas such as shoes or piles of blankets or clothing. *Centruroides exilicauda* (bark scorpion) is the most important species in the United States.[1,2]

The scorpion's tail ends in the bulbous telson, which contains the venom gland and a sharp stinger called the aculeus. Scorpion venoms differ among species but generally contain peptides that affect neuronal and muscle sodium, potassium, and ryanodine-sensitive calcium channels. The venoms also cause release of catecholamines.[1,2]

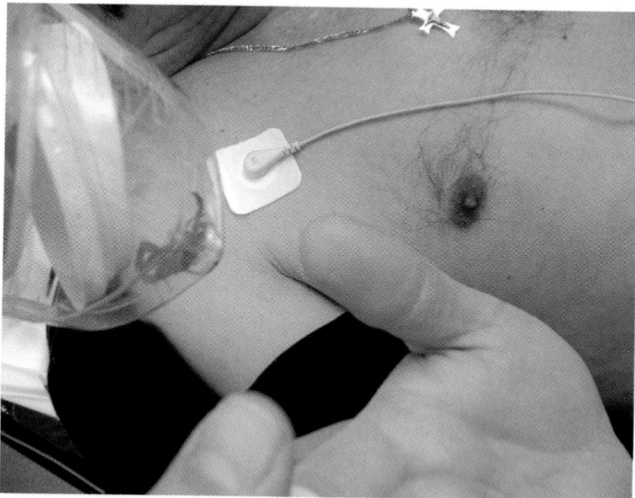

FIGURE 25–6 The scorpion in the jar stung this man's thumb, causing intense pain and pruritus. (Courtesy of Robert Hendrickson, MD.)

Clinical Complications

Severe or fatal effects such as respiratory depression or arrest, shock, pulmonary edema, heart failure, seizures, and coma may occur. Children and the elderly are more severely affected. Other reported complications include pancreatitis, hyperglycemia, allergic reactions, and spontaneous abortion. Serum sickness can occur after antivenom therapy.[2]

Management

Although antivenoms are available for several species of scorpion, most patients have mild symptoms that can be managed with application of ice and administration of analgesics. Aggressive supportive care and antivenom administration are indicated for severe envenomations. Benzodiazepines may be useful for agitated patients.[2]

REFERENCES

1. Walter FG, Bilden EF, Gibly RL. Envenomations. *Crit Care Clin* 1999;15:353–386.
2. Gibly R, Williams M, Walter F, McNally J, Conroy C, Berg RA. Continuous intravenous midazolam infusion for *Centruroides exilicauda* scorpion envenomation. *Ann Emerg Med* 1999;34:620–625.

Widow Spider Envenomation

Anthony Morocco

Clinical Presentation

The initial bite usually causes little or no pain. After 5 to 60 minutes, more severe pain occurs, which may spread to include the regional lymph nodes. Local edema, warmth, and sweating may occur. The local symptoms may be brief and give way to systemic effects (latrodectism) up to 12 or more hours later, particularly after *Latrodectus mactans* envenomation. Generalized, severe, cramping pain may occur, with abdominal symptoms mimicking those of an acute abdomen. Regional diaphoresis may occur at or distant to the bite site. Hypertension is a common finding; other common symptoms include nausea, vomiting, diarrhea, weakness, psychosis, and headache. The term "facies latrodectismica" refers to the facial grimace, trismus, periorbital edema, and diaphoresis associated with *L. mactans* envenomation.[1,2]

Pathophysiology

The widow spiders, of the genus *Latrodectus,* cause a clinical syndrome known as latrodectism. These spiders can be found worldwide. Five species are found in the United States, including the black widow spider (*Latrodectus mactans*). Other important species include the brown widow (*Latrodectus geometricus*) and the redback (*Latrodectus hasseltii*). The spiders are often found along metal fence lines and in outhouse toilets, sheds, and crop fields. Species such as the black widow are known for their distinctive red hourglass mark on the ventral abdomen.[1,2]

Venom is injected through the paired, hollow fangs. The major toxic component is the neurotoxic protein α-latrotoxin. This substance causes excessive calcium-mediated release of multiple neurotransmitters.[1,2]

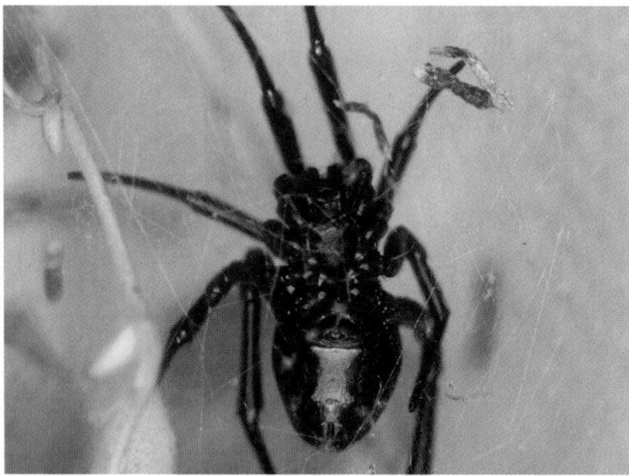

FIGURE 25–7 Black widow spider (*Latrodectus mactans*). (Courtesy of William Banner, MD.)

Diagnosis

Diagnosis is based on the patient's history and clinical appearance. However, the initial bite may go unnoticed, and symptoms such as abdominal pain may be mistaken for those of an acute intraabdominal process. No specific laboratory tests are available to confirm the diagnosis.[1,2]

Clinical Complications

Death is rare but may occur as a result of complications of severe hypertension, cardiotoxicity, or renal failure. Patients at higher risk for serious complications include infants, the elderly, pregnant women, and those with comorbidities.[1,2]

Management

Treatment of mild to moderate symptoms consists of local ice packs and administration of nonsteroidal antiinflammatory drugs (NSAIDs) or opioids for pain control. Benzodiazepines are helpful to control the painful muscle spasms and to decrease anxiety. Symptoms usually resolve in 24 to 48 hours but may be more prolonged in severe cases. Treatments with calcium and methocarbamol were advocated in the past but are no longer recommended. Horse serum antivenom is available and is highly efficacious in resolving symptoms of severe latrodectism. It is recommended in cases of severe hypertension, intractable pain, or pregnancy. As with any horse-derived antivenom, severe allergic reactions are possible. The antivenom is made using *L. mactans,* but is likely to be useful for all *Latrodectus* species.[1,2]

REFERENCES

1. Clark RF. The safety and efficacy of antivenin *Latrodectus mactans. J Toxicol Clin Toxicol* 2001;39:125–127.
2. White J, Cardoso JL, Fan HW. Clinical toxicology of spider bites. In: Meier J, White J, eds. *Handbook of clinical toxicology of animal venoms and poisons.* Boca Raton, FL: CRC Press, 1995:259–329.

Necrotic Arachnidism

Anthony Morocco

Clinical Presentation

The brown recluse bite is often painless, with development of vesicles, bullae, and erythema after 1 to 3 hours. Pruritus and pain begin as the wound becomes hemorrhagic and erythematous, and the "red, white, and blue sign" appears. The erythema may be wider on the dependent side of the wound, because the venom is pulled inferiorly by gravity. At 24 to 72 hours, the wound becomes pale, edematous, and well demarcated. At this stage, systemic symptoms, which include nausea, vomiting, malaise, and myalgias, may occur. Over the next several weeks, the wound may enlarge, with necrosis and eschar formation. Several other spider species can cause a similar progression of symptoms. The hobo spider can cause a severe headache lasting up to 1 week, with reports of associated hallucinations and paresthesias. The bite of the jumping spider is sharply painful.[1]

Pathophysiology

The term *necrotic arachnidism* refers to wounds resulting from envenomation by various spiders. The brown recluse (*Loxosceles reclusa*) in the southeastern United States, the hobo spider (*Tegenaria agrestis*) in the northwestern United States, the jumping spider (*Phiddipus audax*) in the southern United States, and other species have been implicated.[1]

Loxosceles venom contains a phospholipase known as sphingomyelinase D. This substance causes activation of neutrophils and platelets, with resulting tissue injury, necrosis, and thrombosis.[1]

Diagnosis

Accurate diagnosis may be difficult, and wounds from diverse causes are often wrongly attributed to the brown recluse. There is no readily available test to confirm the diagnosis.[1]

Clinical Complications

Ulcers can take months to heal. Severe systemic reactions, including hemolysis, disseminated intravascular coagulation (DIC), and death, may rarely occur after brown recluse envenomation.[1]

Management

Treatment includes rest, ice, and elevation of the envenomated area. Antibiotic prophylaxis may be helpful for ulcerated lesions.[1] Steroids, hyperbaric oxygen, and dapsone have not been shown to be beneficial after *Loxosceles* envenomation.[1] Surgical excision, if considered, should be delayed for 6 to 10 weeks, until the eschar has stabilized.[1]

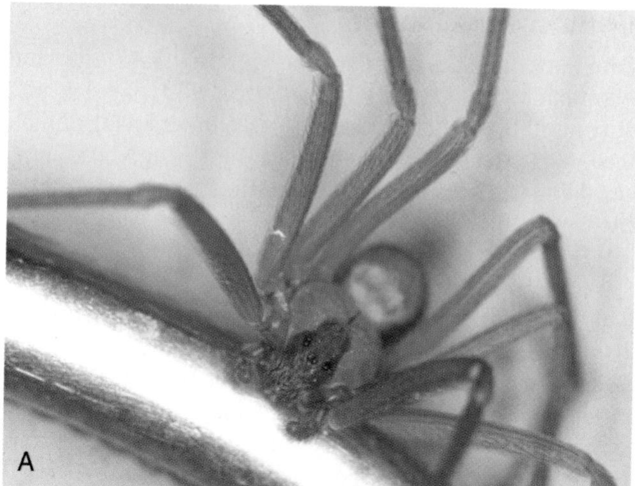

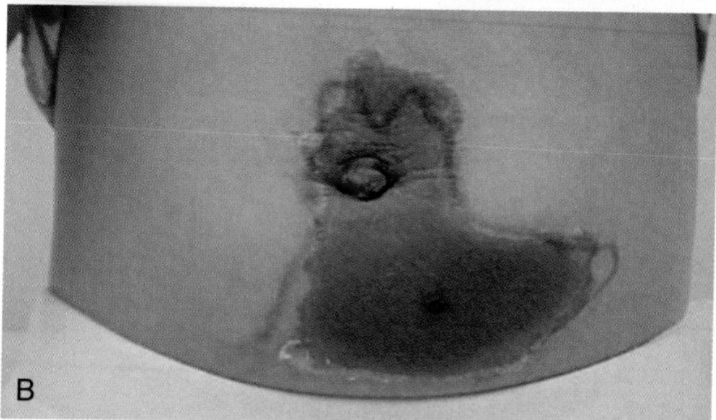

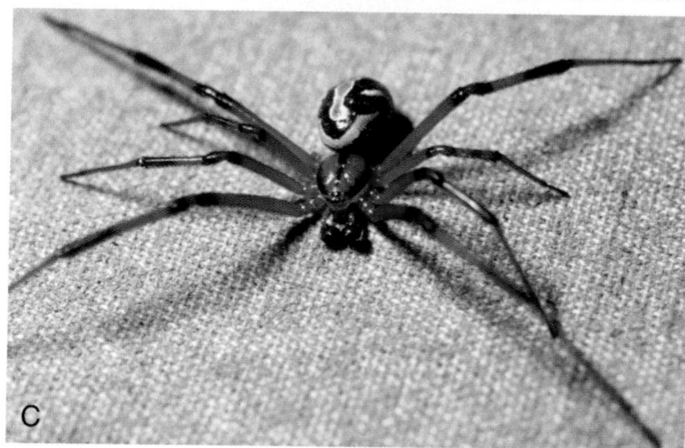

FIGURE 25–8 **A:** Brown recluse spider. **B:** Skin lesion from a brown recluse bite. **C:** Hobo spider. (**A–C,** Courtesy of William Banner, MD.)

REFERENCES

1. Sams HH, Dunnick CA, Smith ML, King LE. Necrotic arachnidism. *J Am Acad Dermatol* 2001;44:561–573.

Portuguese Man-of-War Envenomation

Anthony Morocco

Clinical Presentation

Patients complain of immediate intense pain after envenomation. Elliptical wheals form, with papules and surrounding erythema along the area of tentacle contact. Systemic effects such as nausea, vomiting, headache, myalgias, and respiratory and cardiac compromise may be seen.[1]

Pathophysiology

The *Physalia* species are of the phylum Coelenterata (Cnidaria), but they are not true jellyfish of the class Scyphozoa. Instead, they are members of the Hydrozoa class. These stinging creatures consist of a colony of symbiotic organisms that are specialized to perform various tasks, such as reproduction and digestion. The organisms form a blue, air-filled float called the pneumophore, with dangling tentacles up to several feet in length. The two common species are *Physalia utriculus,* called the "bluebottle," which is found in the Pacific Ocean, and the larger *Physalia physalis,* called the "Portuguese man-of-war," which is found in the Atlantic Ocean. The latter common name refers to the pneumophore, which is similar in appearance to old Portuguese war helmets. The *Physalia* are often found in large swarms that may wash ashore during the heavy onshore winds of strong tropical storms.[1]

The precise toxic components of *Physalia* venom are unclear. It appears to contain dermonecrotic, myotoxic, hemolytic, and cardiotoxic components, as well as vasoactive amines. The venom is delivered by nematocysts, which are cells that contain a harpoon and syringe-like stinging apparatus. The cells discharge after being triggered by mechanical or chemical stimulation. Thousands of nematocysts may be present on one tentacle.[1]

Diagnosis

Patients may give a history of contact with the easily recognizable blue *Physalia*. However, the patient may not have seen the pneumophore, because stinging can occur after contact with the end of a long tentacle or fragments of tentacle suspended in the water. In these cases, diagnosis is based on the patient's clinical presentation and history of potential exposure. There are no specific diagnostic tests.[1]

Clinical Complications

P. physalis (but probably not *P. utriculus*) is associated with severe envenomation and systemic toxicity. Deaths due to cardiovascular collapse and respiratory failure have been reported.[1]

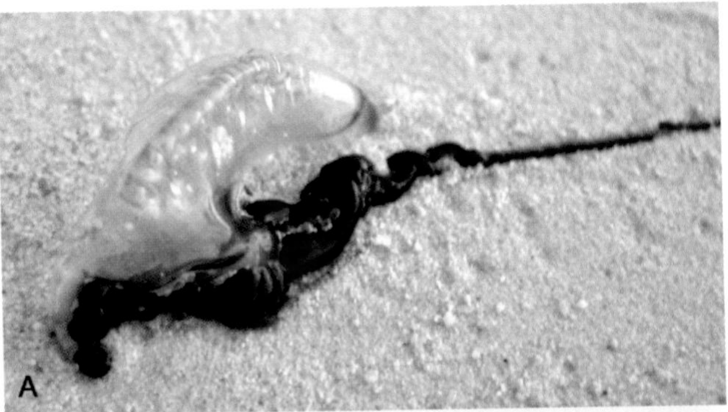

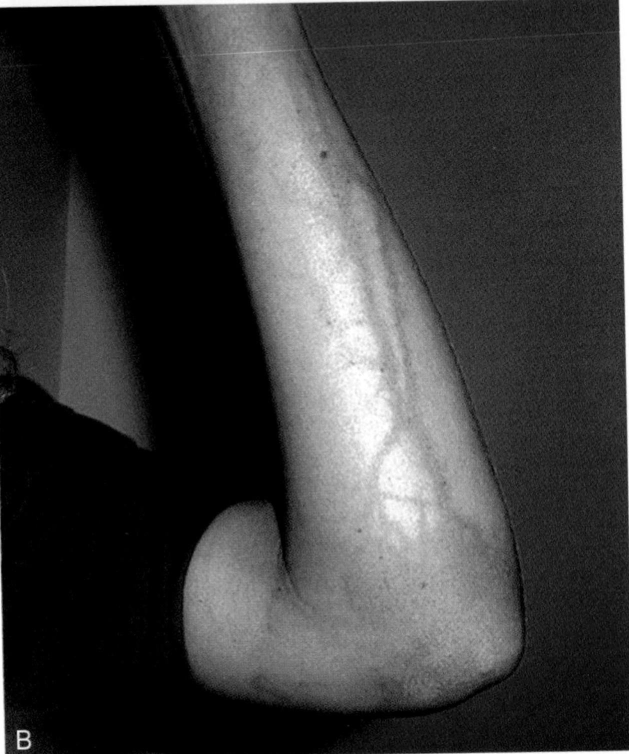

FIGURE 25–9 A: Man-of-war. (Courtesy of Anthony Morocco, MD.) **B:** Portuguese man-of-war sting. Note the linear lesions. (From Goodheart, with permission.)

Management

There is conflicting evidence regarding the effect of acetic acid on any undischarged *Physalia* nematocysts, so this common treatment should probably be avoided. Any remaining nematocysts should be rinsed off with seawater. Local pain should be treated with opioids and ice packs. Supportive care alone is indicated for severe reactions, because no antivenom is available.[1]

REFERENCES

1. Williamson J, Burnett J. Clinical toxicology of marine coelenterate injuries. In: Meier J, White J, eds. *Handbook of clinical toxicology of animal venoms and poisons.* Boca Raton, FL: CRC Press, 1995: 89–115.

Box Jellyfish Envenomation

Anthony Morocco

Clinical Presentation

Patients develop a spectrum of effects after envenomation by *C. fleckeri*, ranging from mild local effects to rapid cardiovascular collapse and death. Severe local pain, linear tentacle marks, vesiculation, and edema, followed by dermatonecrosis, may occur. Fragments of tentacle may be seen on the skin.[1,2]

Pathophysiology

The box jellyfish, *Chironex fleckeri*, is found in the waters of northern Australia, with higher numbers present in the summer months. The stinging tentacles may reach 60 m in length and can be fatal to humans. This organism has often been called "the world's most venomous animal."[1,2]

The precise toxic components of *C. fleckeri* venom are unclear. It appears to contain dermonecrotic, myotoxic, hemolytic, and cardiotoxic components. The venom is delivered by nematocysts, which are cells that contain a harpoon and syringe-like stinging apparatus. The cells discharge after being triggered by mechanical or chemical stimulation. Thousands of nematocysts may be present on one tentacle.[1,2]

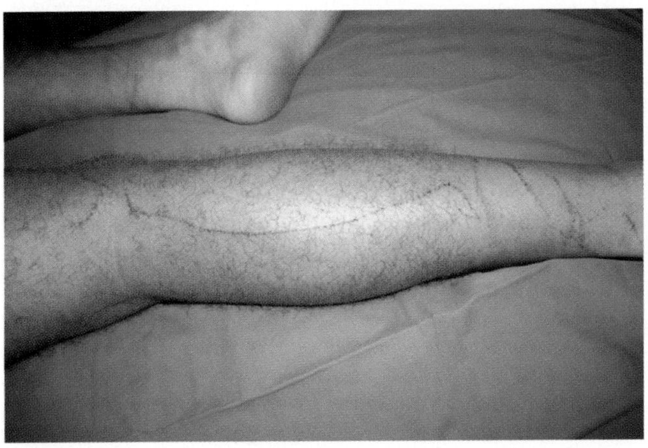

FIGURE 25–10 Stings from box jellyfish (*Chironex fleckeri*). (Image taken in Darwin, Northern Territory, Australia, 2000, by Geoff Isbister, MD, University of Newcastle, Newcastle Mater Hospital, Newcastle, Australia). (From Fleisher, Baskin, and Ludwig, with permission.)

Diagnosis

The organism is transparent and extremely difficult to see in the water; therefore, the diagnosis is based on the patient's clinical presentation and history of potential exposure. There are no specific diagnostic tests.[1,2]

Clinical Complications

Sixty-seven deaths have been reported after *C. fleckeri* envenomation. In addition to rapid cardiovascular collapse, hypotension, autonomic dysfunction, and vasospasm may occur. However, despite the reputation for lethality, most stings result in mild symptoms. A delayed hypersensitivity reaction occurs at the site of envenomation in 50% of cases.[1,2]

Management

Initial first aid should include application of acetic acid to prevent the firing of any remaining nematocysts. Pressure-immobilization bandaging has been advocated but is not likely to be beneficial, and may result in additional nematocyst discharge. In severe cases, patients may require rapid cardiopulmonary resuscitation (CPR). Local pain should be treated with opioids and ice packs. A sheep-derived antivenom is available. Indications for antivenom administration include severe pain unrelieved by opioids, cardiorespiratory decompensation, and cardiac arrest.[1,2]

REFERENCES

1. Bailey PM, Little M, Jelinek GA, Wilce JA. Jellyfish envenoming syndromes: unknown toxic mechanisms and unproven therapies. *Med J Aust* 2003;178:34–37.
2. O'Reilly GM, Isbister GK, Lawrie PM, Treston GT, Currie BJ. Prospective study of jellyfish stings from tropical Australia, including the major box jellyfish *Chironex fleckeri*. *Med J Aust* 2001;175: 652-655.

Blue-Ringed Octopus Envenomation

Anthony Morocco

Clinical Presentation

The initial bite causes minor bleeding and little or no pain. A significant number of bites are "dry" and produce no further symptoms. Envenomated victims develop perioral paresthesia or numbness that spreads to the tongue and face, followed by diffuse muscle weakness. Difficulty with speech, swallowing, and breathing may occur.[1,2]

Pathophysiology

The blue-ringed octopus is the only octopus capable of causing significant human toxicity. It is found in the waters of Australia and the Indo-Pacific, with *Hapalochlaena maculosa* in the south and *Hapalochlaena lunulata* in the north. The characteristic blue rings appear when the animal is distressed. Most bites occur when an octopus is removed from the water and handled.[1,2]

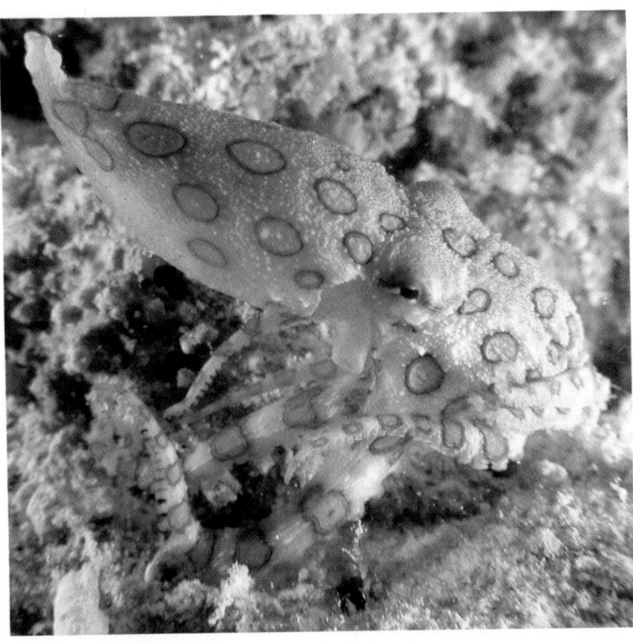

FIGURE 25–11 The blue-ringed octopus (*Hapalochlaena* spp.) can inject a neurotoxin, which the animal stores in modified venom glands. (©Robert Yin, 2004. Used with permission.)

Tetrodotoxin, a toxin found in many marine organisms and amphibians, is responsible for the clinical symptoms. It is produced in the salivary glands and is introduced into the victim during a bite from the animal's beak. The toxin binds to and blocks voltage-gated sodium channels, blocking the inward sodium current responsible for nerve conduction.[1,2]

Diagnosis

The patient or a witness may report a history of octopus exposure, but the diagnosis can be difficult if the bite is initially unrecognized or the responsible organism is not seen. No laboratory tests are readily available to confirm the diagnosis.[1,2]

Clinical Complications

Muscle paralysis may lead to death from respiratory failure. Cardiotoxicity, including hypotension, bradycardia, and asystole, may also occur.[1,2]

Management

There is no specific antidote for tetrodotoxin. Treatment consists of supportive care, including mechanical ventilation, until the effects of the toxin subside over a few hours to several days. Paralyzed patients require sedation, because they may be fully conscious. Acetylcholinesterase inhibitors, such as neostigmine, have been advocated to reverse the paralysis but are of unproven benefit. Patients who are asymptomatic after a suspected bite should be observed for any signs of toxin effects for at least 6 hours.[1,2]

REFERENCES

1. Walker DG. Survival after severe envenomation by the blue-ringed octopus (*Hapalochlaena maculosa*). Med J Aust 1983;2:663–665.
2. White J. Clinical toxicology of blue ringed octopus bites. In: Meier J, White J, eds. *Handbook of clinical toxicology of animal venoms and poisons.* Boca Raton, FL: CRC Press, 1995:171–175.

Stonefish Envenomation

Anthony Morocco

Clinical Presentation

Envenomation by a stonefish often causes a profound degree of pain. Symptom onset is immediate, and the pain increases in severity over the next several hours. Edema, erythema, and ecchymosis occur at the wound site and may spread. Syncope, hypotension, nausea, and vomiting may occur due to effects of the toxin or to pain. Severe systemic reactions may include dysrhythmias, coma, pulmonary edema, and cardiovascular collapse.[1,2]

Pathophysiology

The stonefish belongs to the Scorpaenidae family of venomous fish, which includes the lionfish and zebrafish. The three species of stonefish, *Synanceia horrida, Synanceia trachynis,* and *Synanceia verrucosa,* are found in shallow tropical waters.[1,2]

Venom is produced in paired glands located along the 13 dorsal spines. Disturbance of the fish causes erection of the spines, which results in puncture of the offending body part and the expelling of venom into the wound. The venom contains the heat-labile verrucotoxin (*S. verrucosa*), stonustoxin (*S. horrida*), and trachynilysin (*S. trachynis*). These toxins exhibit myotoxic, cytolytic, neurotoxic, and cardiotoxic effects. Cardiovascular toxicity and severe pain may be mediated by effects at adrenergic, muscarinic, and bradykinin receptors.[1,2]

Diagnosis

Diagnosis is based on the clinical presentation of severe pain and systemic symptoms after aquatic envenomation. Patients often do not see the offending stonefish because of its camouflage; therefore, the cause of the symptoms may be unclear.[1,2]

Clinical Complications

Death has been reported after rapid cardiovascular collapse. Retained foreign material in the wound is common and may be a nidus for infection.[1,2]

Management

Rapid and effective pain relief is a priority. Soaking in water of 110° to 115° F may inactivate the heat-labile toxin. Severe pain should be treated with parenteral opioids, with local or regional anesthesia, or both. The wound should be explored to locate any retained foreign material. A horse-derived antivenom is available and may be administered in cases of severe systemic symptoms or refractory pain.[1,2]

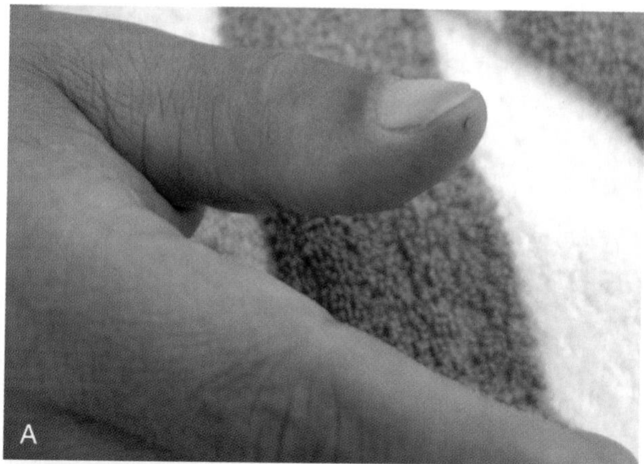

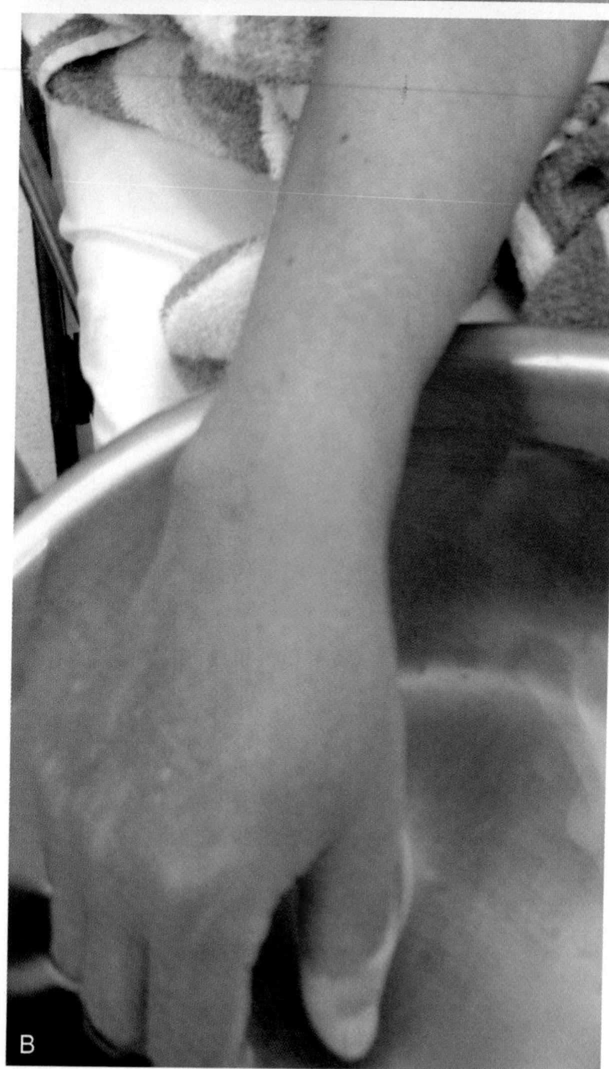

FIGURE 25–12 **A:** Stonefish stings are characterized by immediate and severe pain, swelling, and erythema. **B:** Note proximal progression of swelling and redness. (**A** and **B**, Courtesy of Anthony Morocco, MD.)

REFERENCES

1. Williamson J. Clinical toxicology of venomous Scorpaenidae and other selected fish stings. In: Meier J, White J, eds. *Handbook of clinical toxicology of animal venoms and poisons.* Boca Raton, FL: CRC Press, 1995:141–158.
2. Church JE, Hodgson WC. Dose-dependent cardiovascular and neuromuscular effects of stonefish (*Synanceia trachynis*) venom. *Toxicon* 2000;38:391–407.

25–13

Crown-of-Thorns Envenomation

Anthony Morocco

Clinical Presentation

Patients experience severe pain that lasts for a few hours after envenomation. Erythema and edema develop at the wound site. Nausea and vomiting may occur.[1]

Pathophysiology

The crown-of-thorns, *Acanthaster planci,* is the only starfish capable of human envenomation. These creatures measure up to 40 cm in diameter and are found on Indo-Pacific reefs, where they feed on coral. They are not aggressive, and envenomation occurs after accidental contact or handling.[1]

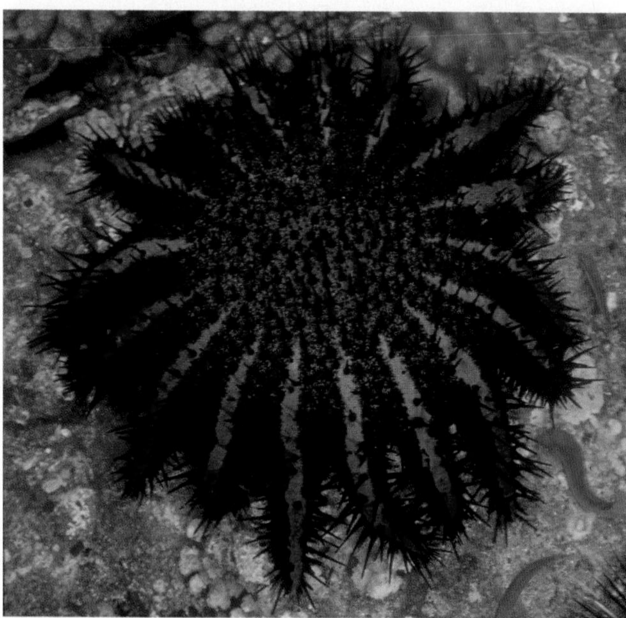

FIGURE 25–13 Crown-of-thorns (*Asteroidea planci*), a stinging sea star that causes generally minor injuries. (©Robert Yin, 2004. Used with permission.)

Each of the 7 to 23 arms of *A. planci* contains numerous sharp spines, each of which is covered by integument that contains venom glands. The spines penetrate deep into the skin and may break off and become embedded. The venom contains a mixture of toxins, including phospholipase A_2.[1]

Diagnosis

Patients usually give a history of crown-of-thorns contact, although injury often occurs after the patient steps on an unseen creature.[1]

Clinical Complications

Retained spines can cause prolonged inflammatory reactions or infection. Rarely, cardiovascular effects occur.[1]

Management

Retained spines should be removed carefully. Basic wound care and analgesia usually are all that is necessary. No antivenom exists for this envenomation.[1]

REFERENCES

1. Mebs D. Clinical toxicology of sea urchin and starfish injuries. In: Meier J, White J, eds. *Handbook of clinical toxicology of animal venoms and poisons.* Boca Raton, FL: CRC Press, 1995:129–134.

Lionfish Envenomation

Michael Greenberg

Clinical Presentation

Patients stung by *Pterois volitans,* the lionfish, present with severe pain at the site of the sting that extends the entire length of the affected extremity.[1] Divers in tropical or warm-water environments are at special risk for being stung by lionfish. However, individuals who keep these fish as pets in aquaria are also at risk.[1,2]

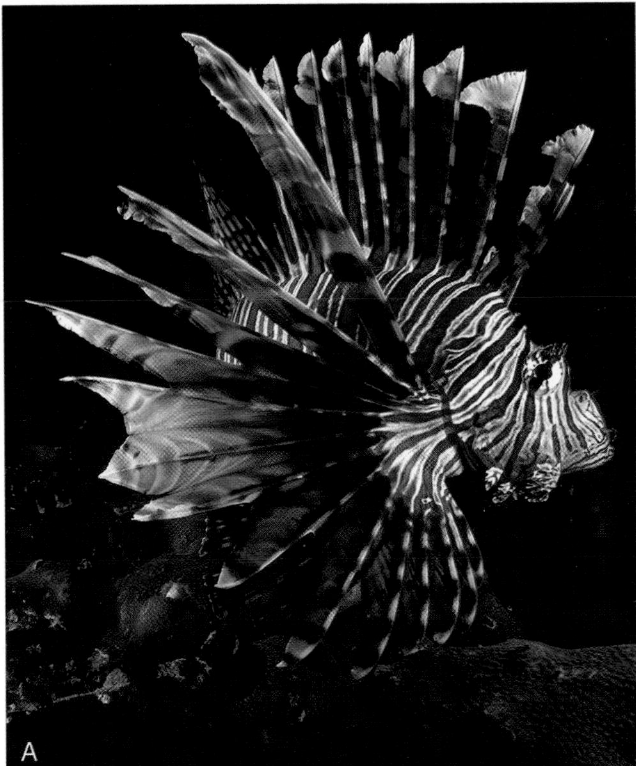

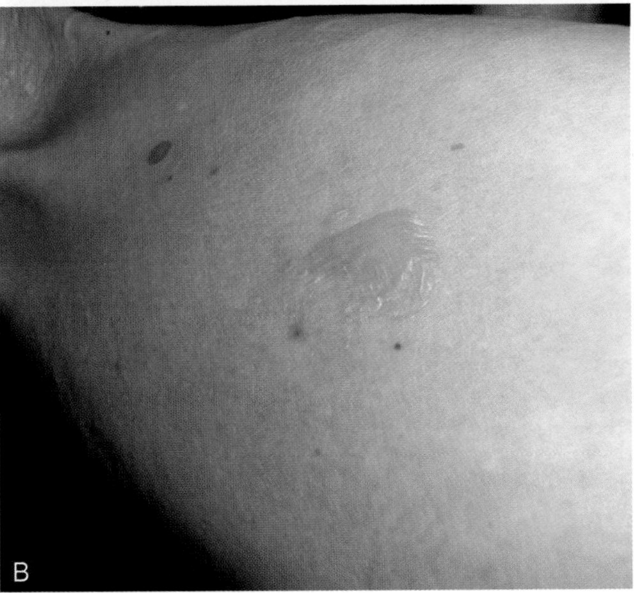

FIGURE 25–14 **A:** Lionfish (*Pterois volitans*). **B:** Lionfish sting, second day. (©Robert Yin, 2004. Used with permission.)

Pathophysiology

Lionfish have spines with attached paired venom glands. The venom is injected into the skin via a puncture wound inflicted by one or more spines. Spines have been reported to break off in the skin.[1,2] Envenomations are graded based on clinical findings. Grade I injuries are characterized by redness, bruising, and dusky cyanosis at the wound site. Grade II envenomations are characterized by vesicle formation. Necrosis characterizes Grade III injuries.[2]

Diagnosis

Lionfish envenomation is diagnosed based on a history of contact associated with the development of severe pain at the site of contact.

Clinical Complications

In rare cases, signs of systemic envenomation may occur, including abdominal pain, vomiting, convulsions, hypotension, hypertension, limb paralysis, respiratory compromise, cardiac arrhythmias, myocardial ischemia, heart failure, and pulmonary edema.[1,2]

Management

Lionfish venom is probably heat-labile, so therapy includes immersion in hot water for 1 to 2 hours, or until the pain subsides.[1,2] Parenteral analgesia may be required for pain control in some cases. Various other modalities have been proposed, but none have been scientifically proven to be effective. Foreign bodies, including lionfish spines, should be removed, and blisters and necrotic tissue should be débrided under sterile conditions. Antibiotics are not indicated in the absence of obvious infection.

REFERENCES

1. Garyfallou GT, Madden JF. Lionfish envenomation. *Ann Emerg Med* 1996;28:456–457.
2. Vetrano SJ, Lebowitz JB, Marcus S. Lionfish envenomation. *J Emerg Med* 2002;23:379–382.

25–15

Sea Nettle Envenomation

Anthony Morocco

Clinical Presentation

Patients complain of immediate, intense pain after envenomation. Erythema and edema of affected areas may also occur.[1]

Pathophysiology

"Sea nettle" is the common name for the *Chrysaora* species of jellyfish. These stinging creatures are from the class Scyphozoa, or true jellyfish. They occur worldwide, with the well-known North American sea nettle, *Chrysaora quinquecirrha,* occurring in summertime swarms in the Chesapeake Bay.[1]

The venom is delivered by nematocysts, which are cells that contain a harpoon and syringe-like stinging apparatus. The cells discharge after being triggered by mechanical or chemical stimulation. Thousands of nematocysts may be present on one tentacle. The venom contains a number of ill-defined toxins that are cytotoxic.[1]

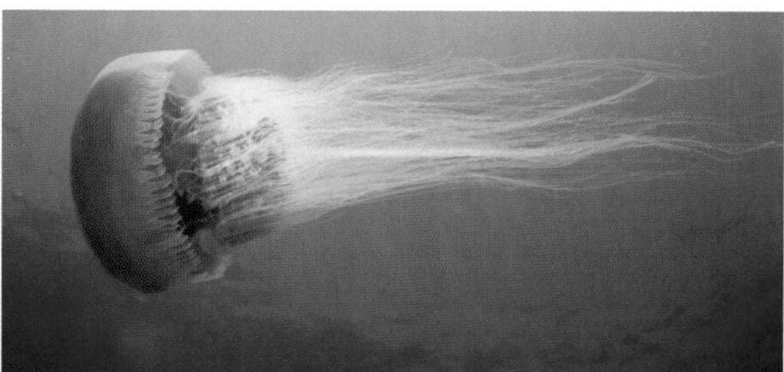

FIGURE 25–15 Sea nettle (*Chrysaora* spp.) are abundant in North American waters. They cause painful stings as well as severe reactions. (©Robert Yin, 2004. Used with permission.)

Diagnosis

Diagnosis is based on the patient's clinical presentation and history of potential exposure. There are no specific diagnostic tests.[1]

Clinical Complications

Severe complications are very unlikely after envenomation by *Chrysaora,* although severe allergic reactions may occur.[1]

Management

Application of a slurry of sodium bicarbonate to inhibit the firing of any remaining nematocysts has been advocated for *Chrysaora* victims, but the efficacy of this treatment is unproven. The general recommendation of topical vinegar after a jellyfish sting is also of unknown benefit for *Chrysaora* species, and it has been suggested that this treatment may actually cause further nematocyst firing. Local pain should be treated with opioids and ice packs. No antivenom is available.[1]

REFERENCES

1. Williamson J, Burnett J. Clinical toxicology of marine coelenterate injuries. In: Meier J, White J, eds. *Handbook of clinical toxicology of animal venoms and poisons.* Boca Raton, FL: CRC Press, 1995: 89–115.

Sea Urchin Injury

Anthony Morocco

Clinical Presentation

Patients commonly present for removal of retained spines in the skin. However, patients with aquatic envenomations may present with a painful wound of unknown origin. Specific species may produce unique symptoms. Victims of *Diadema* species complain of burning pain and discomfort that may last for weeks. Leather urchins can cause severe pain followed by local numbness. *Toxopneustes* species can cause pain and facial muscle paralysis.[1]

Pathophysiology

Sea urchins are members of the phylum Echinodermata, class Echinodermata. Related echinoderms include sea stars and sea cucumbers. Sea urchins are covered by calcareous (calcium carbonate) plates, from which spines and pedicellariae protrude. These animals are slow-moving, nocturnal, and nonaggressive, but the spines cause injury when stepped on or inadvertently contacted by swimmers and divers. Sea urchins are found throughout the world, in both shallow and deep waters.[1]

The spines of some sea urchin species contain venom. The long, hollow spines of *Diadema* species contain a venomous blue liquid, whereas the spines of leather urchins have a venom sac at the tip. The calcareous spines penetrate skin and become fragmented. Pedicellariae are smaller and are used to seize prey and inject venom. These organs cannot penetrate human skin, except in a few species (i.e., *Toxopneustes*). The venoms remain poorly characterized.[1]

Diagnosis

Diagnosis is usually obvious from the appearance of numerous spines in the skin. Radiographic studies may be required to detect spines in these cases.[1]

Clinical Complications

Chronic granulomatous skin lesions may occur at the puncture site.[2]

Management

Severe pain usually resolves quickly without treatment. Immersion of the affected part in hot water is not useful for sea urchin injuries. Tetanus prophylaxis should be administered. Spines should be removed, if possible, particularly if penetration into a joint space has occurred.[1]

REFERENCES

1. Mebs D. Clinical toxicology of sea urchin and starfish injuries. In: Meier J, White J, eds. *Handbook of clinical toxicology of animal venoms and poisons.* Boca Raton, FL: CRC Press, 1995:129–133.
2. De la Torre C, Toribio J. Sea urchin granuloma: histologic profile. A pathologic study of 50 biopsies. *Am Fam Physician* 2003;68: 869–874.

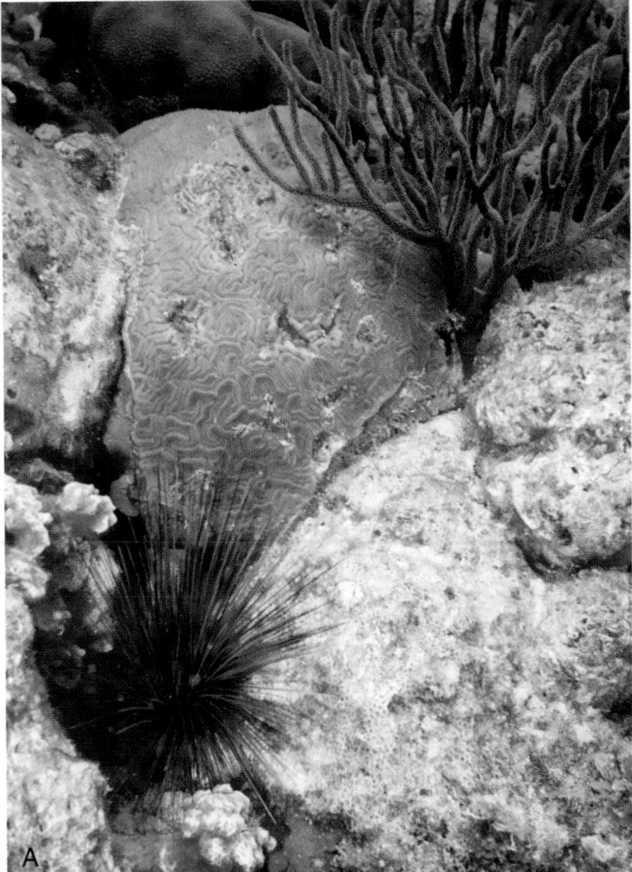

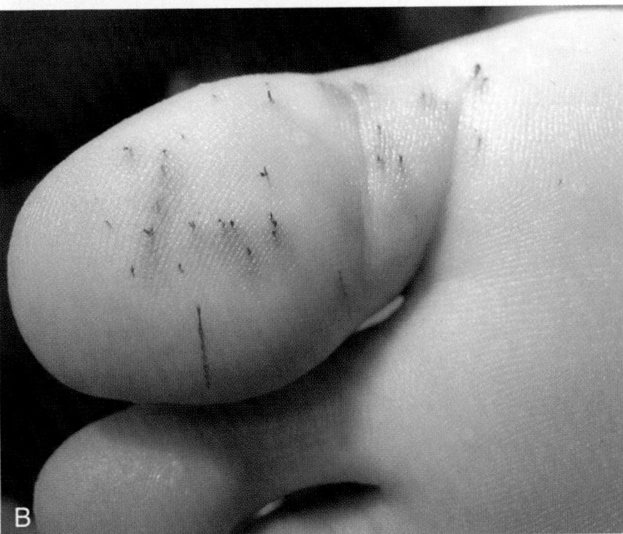

FIGURE 25–16 **A:** Sea urchins (Echinoidea) are found worldwide but are most common in tropical waters. (Courtesy of Mark Silverberg, MD.) **B:** Sea urchin spines embedded in patient's foot. Note associated swelling and redness. (Courtesy of Anthony Morocco, MD.)

Hymenoptera: Fire Ant Sting

Anthony Morocco

Clinical Presentation

Patients complain of immediate and severe burning (hence the name "fire ant") and itching at the site of envenomation. An initial erythematous appearance evolves into a necrotic, sterile pustule within 8 to 10 hours. Late cutaneous reactions occur as pruritic, indurated lesions in previously sensitized individuals. Allergic reactions may manifest as severe local reactions or as systemic reactions such as urticaria, chest tightness, nausea, vomiting, diarrhea, dizziness, anxiety, and weakness. Patients with anaphylaxis may become hypotensive, cyanotic, and unconscious.[1]

Pathophysiology

The order Hymenoptera contains a variety of stinging insects, including wasps, bees, and ants. Among ants, the most significant stingers are the *Solenopsis* species, or fire ants, with *Solenopsis invicta* being most common. These creatures originated in South America but now infest large areas of the southern United States. The ants live in large colonies and attack in swarms if their nest is disturbed.[1]

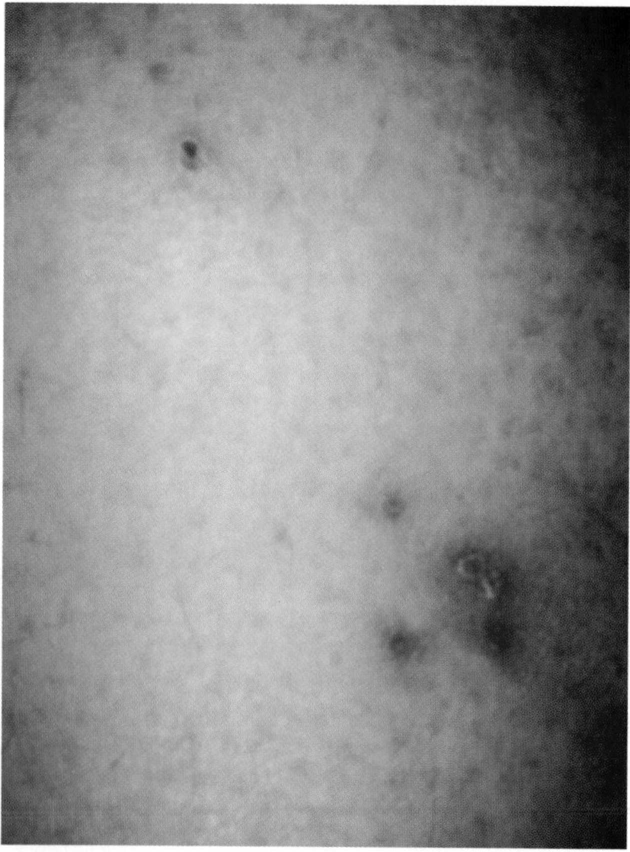

FIGURE 25–17 A fire ant attaches its jaws to the skin and creates a typical small circle of stings in rapid succession, as seen here on the lower calf area. (From Dockery and Crawford, with permission.)

Fire ants use their stinger apparatus (a modified ovipositor) to pierce the skin and inject venom. Some ant species cannot sting, but instead bite and excrete venom into the wound. Fire ants swarm over the victim and sting almost simultaneously. The venom differs from that of other hymenopterans in that it consists mostly of cytotoxic alkaloids, with a small percentage of peptides and enzymes. Between 17% and 56% of individuals stung by fire ants become sensitized, and between 0.6% to 6% of patients develop anaphylaxis after repeat envenomation.[1]

Diagnosis

Diagnosis is usually obvious from the history, but hymenoptera envenomation should be considered in any patient who has symptoms consistent with anaphylaxis.

Clinical Complications

Death can occur due to airway compromise or shock. Other complications include secondary infection of skin lesions, nephrotic syndrome, neuropathy, cerebrovascular accidents, and seizures.[1]

Management

Mild reactions may be treated with antihistamines only. Severe reactions should be treated with intravenous fluid, parenteral epinephrine, and corticosteroids, along with aggressive airway management. Any patient with a large local reaction or a systemic reaction should be given an epinephrine autoinjector in case of future stings. The pustules usually heal in 2 to 3 weeks and should be left intact to decrease the risk of secondary infection.[1]

REFERENCES

1. deShazo RD, Williams DF, Moak ES. Fire ant attacks on residents in health care facilities: a report of two cases. *Ann Intern Med* 1999; 131:424–429.

Hymenoptera: Bee and Wasp Stings

Anthony Morocco

Clinical Presentation

Patients may present solely with local symptoms of pain, erythema, and edema lasting a few days. Allergic responses may manifest as severe local reactions or as systemic reactions such as urticaria, chest tightness, nausea, vomiting, diarrhea, dizziness, anxiety, and weakness. Patients with anaphylaxis may become hypotensive, cyanotic, and unconscious.[1,2]

Pathophysiology

The order Hymenoptera contains various stinging insects, including wasps, bees, and ants. The wasps, family Vespidae, include yellowjackets and hornets. The family Apidae includes bumble bees and honey bees. The most dangerous member of this family is the aggressive "killer bee," a Brazilian hybrid of the African honeybee.[1,2]

The hymenopteran stinging apparatus, the ovipositor, is present only in the female. The barbed stinger pierces the victim to inject venom. Hymenopteran venoms are complex mixtures that contain histamine, dopamine, serotonin, melittin, kinins, phospholipases (potential allergens), and other enzymes. These substances can cause local pain, inflammation, tissue injury, and a type I, immunoglobulin E–mediated allergic reaction.[1]

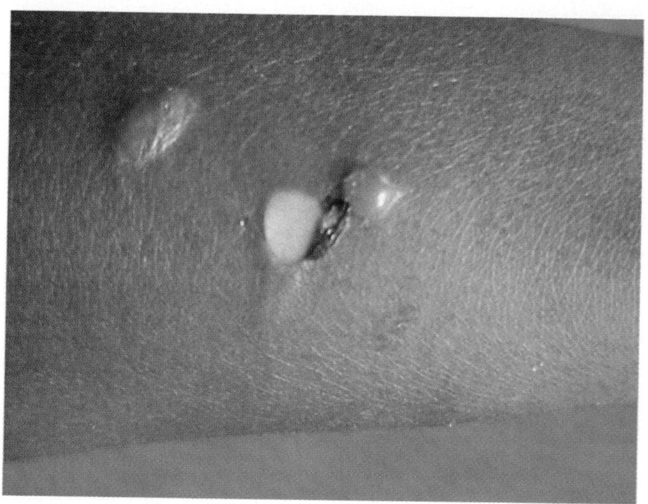

FIGURE 25–18 Vesicular reaction to bee sting. (Courtesy of Christy Salvaggio, MD.)

Diagnosis

Diagnosis is usually obvious from the history, but hymenoptera envenomation should be considered in any patient who has symptoms consistent with anaphylaxis.[1,2]

Clinical Complications

Death may occur due to airway compromise or shock. Two thirds of hymenoptera-related deaths occur after only one sting, with the majority of patients being older than 40 years of age and location of the sting most commonly on the head or neck. Unusual complications include serum sickness, vasculitis, glomerulonephritis, and coagulopathy.[2]

Management

A retained stinger should be manually scraped off. Mild reactions may be treated with antihistamines only. Severe reactions should be treated with intravenous fluid, parenteral epinephrine, and corticosteroids, along with aggressive airway management. Any patient with a large local reaction or a systemic reaction should receive an epinephrine autoinjector in case of future stings.[1,2]

REFERENCES

1. Meier J. Biology and distribution of hymenopterans of medical importance, their venom apparatus and venom composition. In: Meier J, White J, eds. *Handbook of clinical toxicology of animal venoms and poisons.* Boca Raton, FL: CRC Press, 1995:331–348.
2. Mosbech H. Clinical toxicology of hymenopteran stings. In: Meier J, White J, eds. *Handbook of clinical toxicology of animal venoms and poisons.* Boca Raton, FL: CRC Press, 1995:349–359.

Stingray Injury

Anthony Morocco

Clinical Presentation

Patients usually present with stingray injuries to the lower extremities, because the usual cause of attack is inadvertently stepping on the animal. Wounds may be deep punctures or lacerations and may develop a blue-grey color. Patients complain of pain that increases in severity for 30 to 90 minutes after injury. Systemic symptoms such as nausea, vomiting, diarrhea, muscle cramps, excessive salivation, and lightheadedness may occur.[1]

Pathophysiology

Rays are bottom-dwelling aquatic creatures; like sharks, they have a cartilaginous skeleton. Stingrays encompass six families of rays capable of envenomating humans. They are found worldwide, including the east, west, and Gulf coasts of the United States. They dwell in shallow, warm water, and some species can reach 2 m in diameter.[1]

Stingrays have one or more serrated spines of up to 30 cm in length on the dorsum of the tail. The animal flicks the tail forward in a defensive reflex. The bony spines are covered by integument with venom-producing glandular tissue on the grooved underside.[1] The integument or the spine itself may break off and remain in the wound. Injuries are caused by traumatic injury (stab wound) and envenomation.[1]

Diagnosis

The diagnosis should be obvious from the history and appearance of the injury, although the patient may not have seen the stingray.[1]

Clinical Complications

Local tissue necrosis, loss of consciousness, seizures, and cardiovascular collapse may occur with severe envenomations. Death can occur after penetrating injury to the chest or major vessels, or from wound infections.[1]

Management

The affected area should be soaked in 110° to 120° F water, because the toxin is heat-labile and this treatment may diminish the pain.[1] Local or regional anesthesia may be considered for control of severe pain. Wounds should be irrigated and carefully explored for retained foreign body. Surgical débridement and repair of tendon injuries may be indicated for severe wounds. Tetanus immunization should be updated, if necessary. Use of prophylactic antibiotics is controversial, but, if given, they should cover skin flora and *Vibrio* species (trimethoprim-sulfamethoxazole [TMP–SMX], ciprofloxacin, tetracycline).[1]

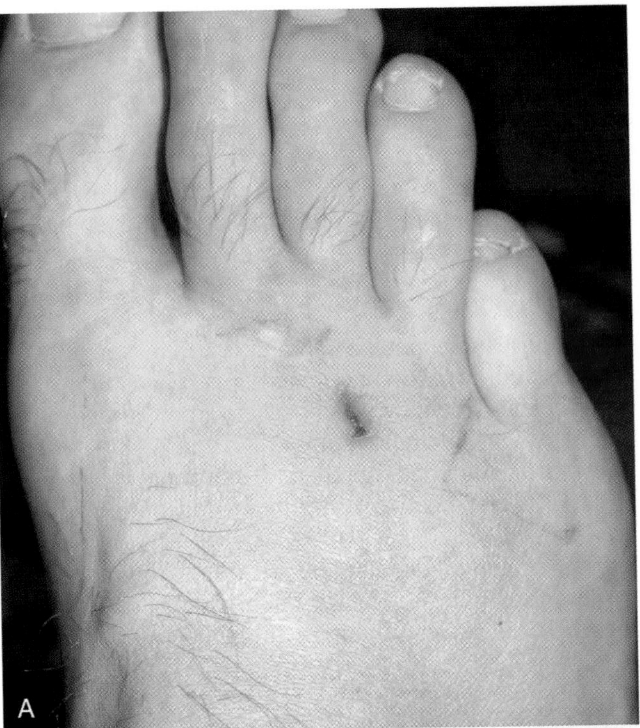

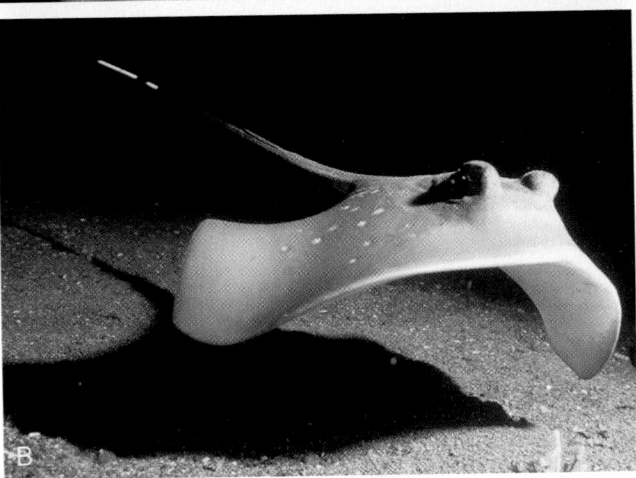

FIGURE 25–19 A: Most stingray injuries involve the lower extremity and result from stepping on the ray in shallow water. (Courtesy of Paul C. Johnston, MD.) **B:** The stinging apparatus is located in the tail. (©Robert Yin, 2004. Used with permission.)

REFERENCES

1. Meyer PK. Stingray injuries. *Wilderness Environ Med* 1997;8:24–28.

Gila Monster Bite

Anthony Morocco

Clinical Presentation

Envenomated patients complain of immediate and intense pain that peaks after 30 to 60 minutes and may last for several hours. Patients may also complain of dizziness and weakness. The bite site may contain small puncture wounds and may appear edematous and cyanotic.[1]

Pathophysiology

Gila monsters are the only venomous lizards. The two species, *Heloderma suspectum* and *Heloderma horridum,* can be up to 1 m in length and are found in the southwestern United States and Mexico. Bites usually occur on the hand, after the animal is provoked.[1]

Heloderma have paired venom glands in the mouth, with ducts that open at the base of grooved teeth. The animal forcefully bites and holds on to the victim, allowing time for the venom to mix with saliva and enter the wounds. The venom, which is lethal to small animals, contains several toxins, including gilatoxin, a number of enzymes such as hyaluronidase and kallikreins, the peptides helodermin and helospectin, and helothermine.[1]

Clinical Complications

The major systemic symptom is hypotension, and death has been very rarely reported. There is no occurrence of neurotoxicity or coagulopathy.[1]

Management

The first task often is to remove the animal from the victim. The strong jaws may need to be pried open, at the risk of worsening the wound. General wound care and immobilization of the limb are indicated, and the possibility of retained tooth fragments should be ruled out. Opioids should be administered for pain relief. There is no specific antidote. Hypotension should be treated with intravenous fluids and vasopressors, if needed.[1]

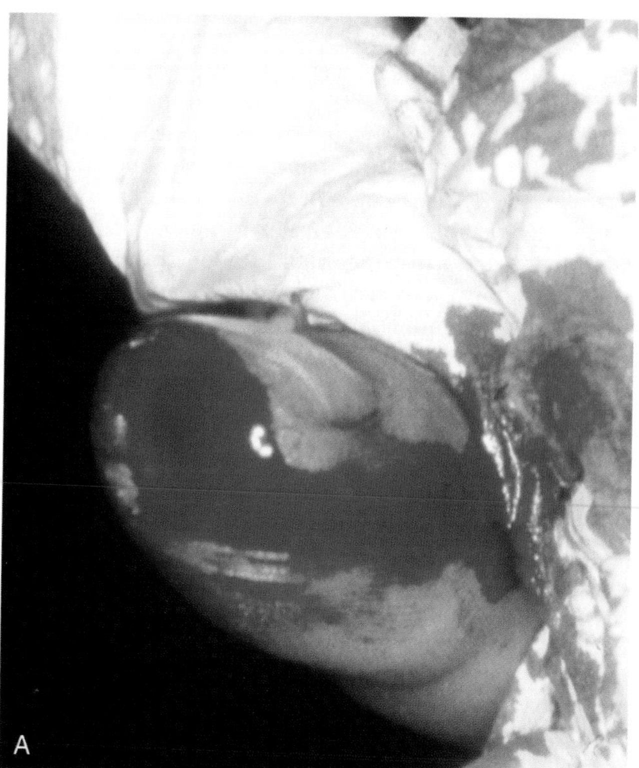

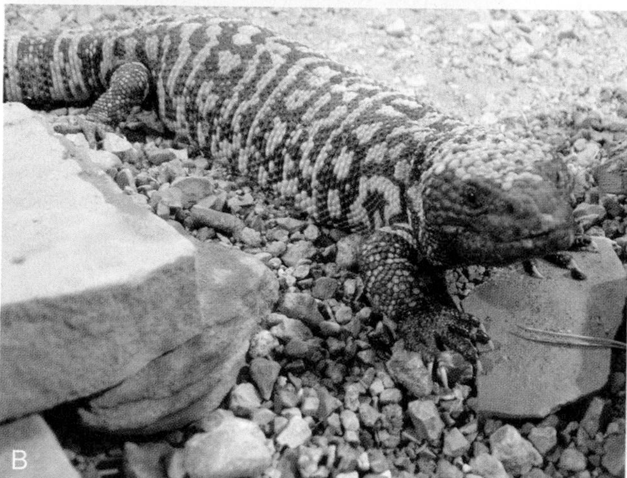

FIGURE 25–20 **A:** Bite inflicted by pet Gila monster (Courtesy of Michael Greenberg, MD). **B:** Gila monster (*Heloderma suspectus*). (Hogle Zoo, Salt Lake City, UT. Used with permission.)

REFERENCES

1. Mebs D. Clinical toxicology of Helodermatidae lizard bites. In: Meier J, White J, eds. *Handbook of clinical toxicology of animal venoms and poisons.* Boca Raton, FL: CRC Press, 1995:361–366.

Seabather's Eruption

Anthony Morocco

Clinical Presentation

Patients present with intensely pruritic lesions that are vesicular and maculopapular in appearance. Skin covered by swimwear is affected, particularly areas of tight fit, such as under waistband, straps, and breasts. Scattered lesions may also occur in skin areas that are subject to friction, such as in flexor regions, in the axillae, on the chest in surfers, and under swimming caps and fins. Individuals wearing well-covering suits or T-shirts while swimming may develop a rash over large areas. Symptoms begin 4 to 24 hours after ocean water contact. Patients may also develop low-grade fever, chills, headache, malaise, vomiting, conjunctivitis, and urethritis.[1]

Pathophysiology

Seabather's eruption, known colloquially as "sea lice," is a self-limited dermatitis that occurs in swimmers and divers. The condition occurs commonly in the Caribbean between March and August, with the highest incidence in May. Outbreaks of seabather's eruption occur intermittently; in 1992, more than 10,000 cases were reported in south Florida.[1]

Seabather's eruption is caused by cnidarian (jellyfish) larvae. Most outbreaks are attributed to the larvae of the thimble jellyfish, *Linuche unguiculata,* found in tropical waters of the Americas and in the Indo-Pacific.[1] These larvae are 0.5 mm long and are trapped as water flows through bathing suits. The larvae discharge nematocysts when disturbed, similar to adult cnidarians. The dermatitis is believed to be primarily an allergic response. Patients with previous outbreaks may feel an immediate mild stinging sensation when reexposed to the larvae.

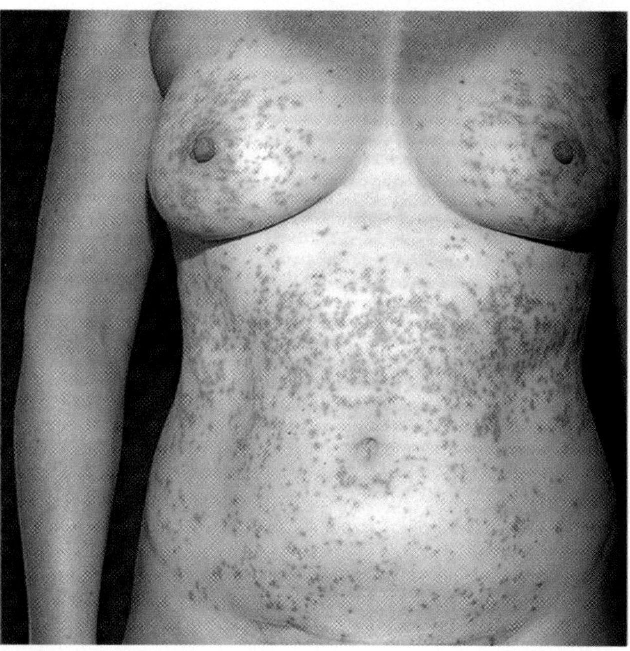

FIGURE 25–21 Seabather's eruption. Nematocyst-bearing larvae become trapped under the bathing suit, producing an intensely itchy and painful papular eruption. (From Habif, with permission.)

Diagnosis

Diagnosis is based on the history and location of skin lesions.

Clinical Complications

Vesicular eruptions may recur in affected areas for up to 1 year. Secondary bacterial infection of skin lesions may occur.

Management

Symptoms are generally self-limited and last only several days. Antihistamines can be used to control itching, and topical or systemic corticosteroids may be beneficial.

REFERENCES

1. Tomchik RS, Russell MT, Szmant AM, Black NA. Clinical perspectives on seabather's eruption, also known as "sea lice." *JAMA* 1993;269:1669–1672.

Toxicodendron Dermatitis

Anthony Morocco

Clinical Presentation

Symptoms appear within 24 to 48 hours after contact with the plant. Patients develop erythema, followed by papules, vesicles, and bullae. Skin lesions often appear in a linear distribution (lines of plant contact) and are accompanied by severe pruritus. Significant edema occurs if the face, neck, or genitals are affected. After exposure to smoke from burning toxicodendron plants, patients may complain of eye or airway irritation.[1]

Pathophysiology

Several *Toxicodendron* species are commonly responsible for allergic contact dermatitis (sometimes called rhus dermatitis) in the United States. These include *Toxicodendron radicans* and *Toxicodendron rydbergii* (poison ivy), *Toxicodendron diversilobum* (western poison oak), *Toxicodendron quercifolium* and *Toxicodendron toxicarium* (eastern poison oak), and *Toxicodendron vernix* (poison sumac). Symptoms may occur after contact with any part of the plant, with an object such as clothing or shoes that has contacted a plant, or with smoke from a burning plant. Between 50% and 70% of the population is sensitized to toxicodendron. Poison ivy and poison oak are known for their appearance with groups of three leaves.[1]

All parts of the plants (leaves, stems, roots) contain urushiol, an oleoresin containing a mixture of compounds that act as potent sensitizers. Patients develop a delayed hypersensitivity reaction after repeat contact.[1]

Diagnosis

Patients with an itchy rash should be questioned about outdoor activities and potential plant exposures.

Clinical Complications

Secondary bacterial infection of lesions, particularly after skin breakdown due to intense itching, may occur. Erythema multiforme occurs rarely.[1]

Management

Usually, no treatment is needed, because lesions resolve spontaneously in 1 to 2 weeks. Cool compresses or topical lotions such as calamine may provide some relief from itching. Oral antihistamines also help relieve symptoms. For severe cases, systemic steroids may be beneficial. Prednisone may be given for 2 to 3 weeks, starting with a dose of 1 mg/kg and tapering slowly. Shorter courses, such as those given in methylprednisolone dose packs, may result in severe rebound dermatitis. Attention should be given to prevention, particularly in the outdoor workplace. Lotions are available that are designed to act as barrier protection. If contact with a plant does occur, the resin must be washed off within 10 minutes to prevent dermatitis. Exposed clothing should be carefully removed and washed, because urushiol can stay active for years.[1]

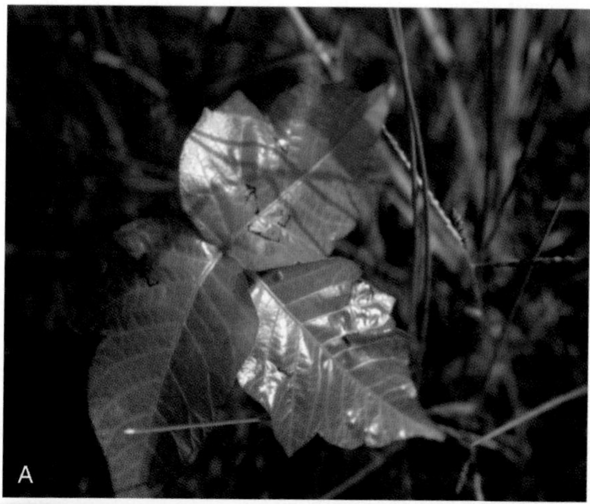

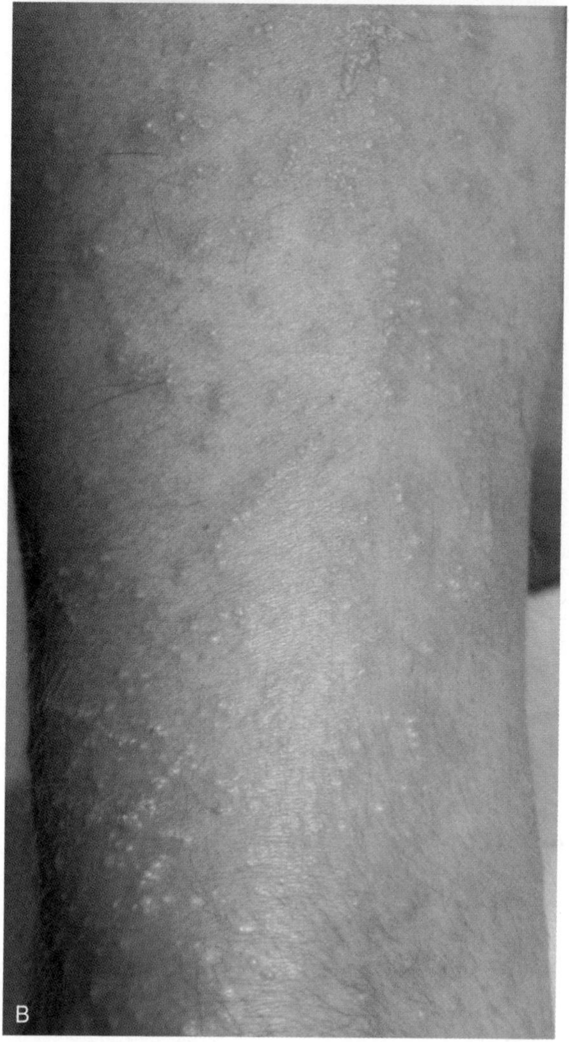

FIGURE 25–22 A: Poison ivy (*Rhus toxicodendron*). (Courtesy of Robert H. Poppenga, DVM, PhD.) **B:** Toxicodendron dermatitis. (©David Effron, MD, 2004. Used with permission.)

REFERENCES

1. Lee NP, Arriola ER. Poison ivy, oak, and sumac dermatitis. *West J Med* 1999;171:354–355.

Tick Bite and Removal

Anthony Morocco

Clinical Presentation

Tick bites are often asymptomatic, and patients may present with a desire for tick removal or a request for antibiotic prophylaxis. Patients with tick paralysis may present, 2 to 7 days after tick attachment, with weakness starting in the lower extremities and ataxia.[1,2]

Pathophysiology

Ticks are arthropods that feed on the blood of mammals. Various tick species are responsible for the transmission of numerous infectious diseases, including Lyme disease, Rocky Mountain spotted fever, ehrlichiosis, tularemia, Colorado tick fever, and babesiosis. Several species of ticks are associated with envenomation and development of tick paralysis.[1,2]

The tick burrows into the patient's skin and releases saliva while feeding on blood. The saliva may contain infectious organisms or neurotoxins. The longer the time of attachment of the tick, the more likely there will be infection transmission or development of paralysis. The tick paralysis toxins are poorly characterized but may act presynaptically at the neuromuscular junction.[1]

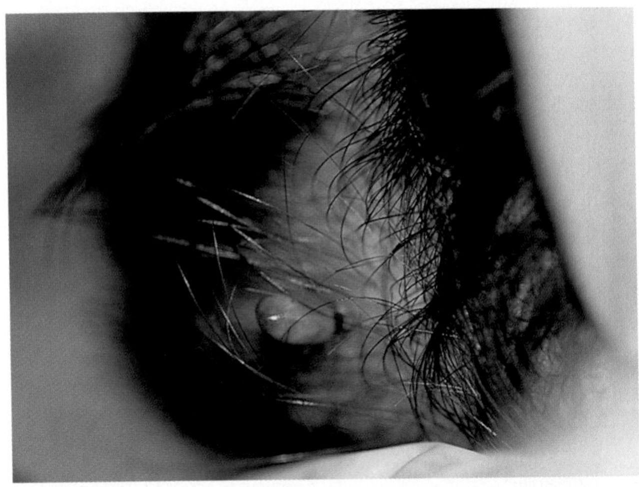

FIGURE 25–23 Tick bite. Typical appearance of engorged tick. (From Fleisher, Baskin, and Ludwig, with permission.)

Clinical Complications

The various infectious diseases have a variety of potential complications. Tick paralysis can cause death due to respiratory depression. Any tick-bite site can develop a secondary bacterial infection or granuloma.[1,2]

Management

Any tick found attached to the skin should be removed as quickly as possible. The preferred technique for removal is to grasp the tick with forceps, as close to the skin as possible, and gently pull with steady, upward and outward pressure. Care should be taken to avoid squeezing the tick or being exposed to the saliva. The skin should be examined closely for any remaining mouth parts. Application of heat or irritants to the tick before removal is not recommended; however, application of viscous lidocaine for 10 minutes to the bite site may facilitate removal. Antibiotic prophylaxis for Lyme disease should be considered, based on several factors including the geographic area and the duration of tick attachment. The symptoms of tick paralysis resolve within hours to days after tick removal.[2]

REFERENCES

1. White J. Clinical toxicology of tick bites. In: Meier J, White J, eds. *Handbook of clinical toxicology of animal venoms and poisons.* Boca Raton, FL: CRC Press, 1995:191–203.
2. Diekema DS, Reuter DG. Arthropod bites and stings. *CPEM* 2001;2: 155–167.

Scombroid Toxicity

Anthony Morocco

Clinical Presentation

Symptoms occur within about 1 hour after eating fish, and there can be marked variability in symptoms among patients who have consumed the same fish meal. Patients present with flushing and a urticarial, pruritic rash located primarily on the face, neck, and upper chest. Gastrointestinal symptoms include crampy pain, vomiting, and diarrhea. Other symptoms include headache, perioral tingling and burning, diaphoresis, and heart palpitations.[1,2]

Pathophysiology

Scombroid fish poisoning is probably the most common fish-related toxicity. It occurs after consumption of fish from the family Scombridae (e.g., mackerel, tuna). Fish from several other families are also capable of causing this syndrome. These include Scomberosocidae (bonito, saury), mahimahi, sardines, bluefish, salmon, amberjack, anchovies, and herring. The terms *histamine poisoning* or *histamine fish poisoning* have been suggested as more accurate descriptions of "scombroid," because of the variety of implicated fish.[1,2]

The cause of scombroid poisoning is presumed to be the presence in the fish of high concentrations of histamine and other biologically active amines (e.g., putrescine, cadaverine), which develop when enterobacterial histidine decarboxylase converts histidine to amines. This process is the result of contamination of fish meat during evisceration and poor refrigeration. The existence of another scombroid toxin and endogenous release or decreased detoxification of histamine have also been postulated.[1]

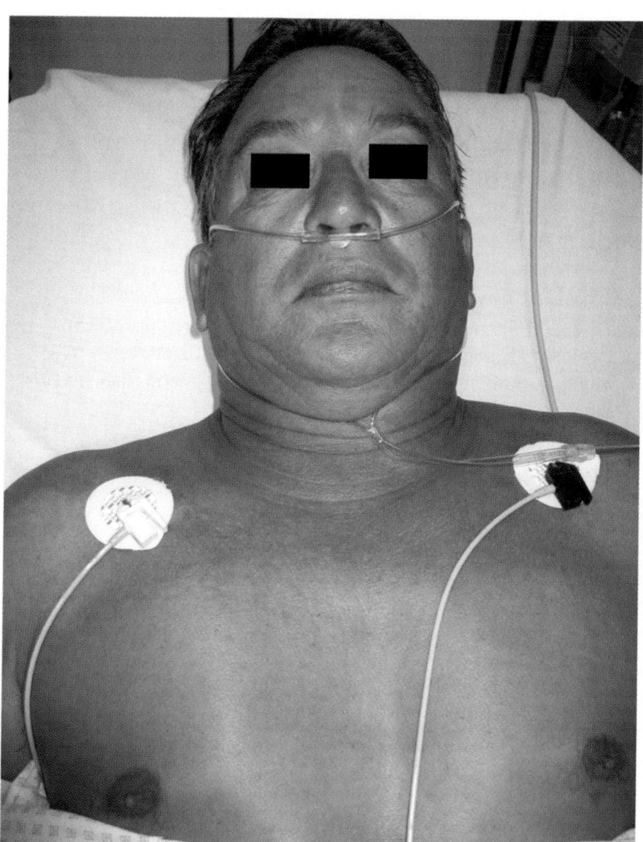

FIGURE 25–24 Intense facial and chest erythema in scombroid toxicity. (Courtesy of Anthony Morocco, MD.)

Diagnosis

Diagnosis is made on clinical grounds alone, so scombroid poisoning may be mistaken for an allergic reaction. A history of eating causative fish, multiple victims from the same meal, and the presence of an unusually peppery taste to the fish increase confidence in the diagnosis.[1]

Clinical Complications

Serious symptoms such as hypotension and bronchospasm rarely occur, but there is the potential for life-threatening reactions in patients with preexisting cardiac or respiratory disease.[1,2]

Management

Symptoms are self-limited and typically last 8 to 12 hours, although persistence for several days is possible. Histamine blockers (H_1 and H_2) are used for symptomatic relief. Activated charcoal may be considered in severe cases, to decrease toxin absorption. Corticosteroids are not beneficial and may prolong symptoms. Hypotension and respiratory compromise require aggressive treatment with intravenous fluids and adrenergic agents, as well as general adherence to advanced cardiac life support (ACLS) principles.[1]

REFERENCES

1. Hall M. Something fishy: six patients with an unusual cause of food poisoning! *Emerg Med (Fremantle)* 2003;15:293–295.
2. Becker K, Southwick K, Reardon J, Berg K, MacCormack JN. Histamine poisoning associated with eating tuna burgers. *JAMA* 2001;285:1327–1330.

Ciguatera Toxicity

Robert Hendrickson

Clinical Presentation

Patients present with nausea, vomiting, and diarrhea beginning within 12 hours after eating fish. Systemic symptoms develop within 72 hours after ingestion and may include diverse neurologic symptoms (perioral paresthesias, dysesthesias of the hands and genitals, reversal of cold/hot sensation), musculoskeletal symptoms (myalgias, arthralgias), and dermatologic symptoms (sweating, intense pruritus).

Pathophysiology

Ciguatera toxicity is a food-borne illness associated with the ingestion of reef-dwelling fish that contain ciguatoxin.[1] Ciguatoxin is a heat-stable, colorless, odorless, and tasteless toxin produced by the dinoflagellate *Gambierdiscus toxicus,* which is found on coral reef algae.[1,2] Small reef fish eat the algae, larger reef fish eat the smaller fish, and the toxin is thus concentrated vertically up the food chain. High-risk fish include large (more than 3 kg) reef fish such as barracuda, mackerel, jacks, sea bass, red snapper, and grouper.[1,2]

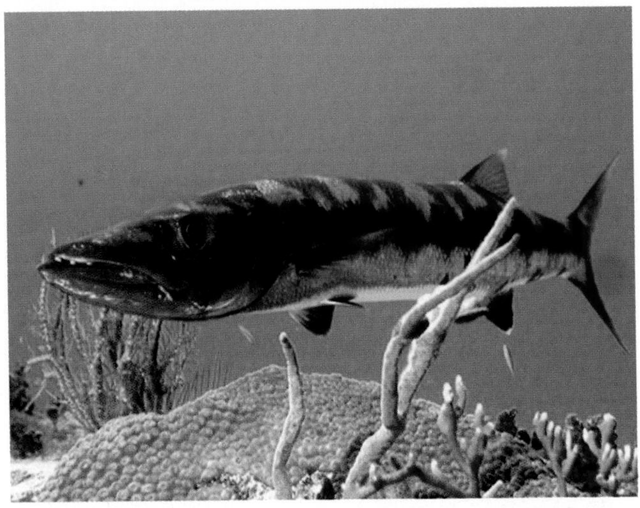

FIGURE 25–25 Ciguatera may result from eating large reef-dwelling fish, such as barracuda. (Courtesy of Mark Silverberg, MD.)

Diagnosis

The diagnosis of ciguatera-related illness is largely clinical. Specific symptoms that are relatively unique for ciguatera include the reversal of hot/cold sensation (e.g., the patient reports a hot sensation when touched by an ice cube), and a variety of orolingual sensations (such as the sensation that the teeth are loose, or that noncarbonated drinks are carbonated). Although cases involving severe toxicity are not common, patients may develop autonomic instability, coma, seizures, respiratory failure, and paralysis.[1,2] Various laboratory techniques exist to test both fish and serum, but they are not readily available in most health care settings.[2]

Clinical Complications

Complications include the persistence of symptoms (days to months), cardiovascular collapse, and relapse of symptoms. Symptoms may relapse after exposure to ethanol or to another fish meal (including nonciguatoxic fish).[1] Symptoms related to ciguatera exposure have reportedly been transmitted from person to person via sexual contact.[1]

Management

Most patients simply require pain control, antihistamines for pruritus, and fluid hydration. However, patients *in extremis* often require intensive supportive care, including airway control and resuscitation. Mannitol has been reported to resolve neurologic symptoms, through unclear mechanisms.[1,2]

REFERENCES

1. Ting JY, Brown AF. Ciguatera poisoning: a global issue with common management problems. *Eur J Emerg Med* 2001;8:295–300.
2. Mines D, Stahmer S, Shepherd SM. Poisonings: food, fish, shellfish. *Emerg Med Clin North Am* 1997;15:157–177.

Hypothermia

Anthony Morocco

Clinical Presentation

Patients develop variable findings as body temperature declines. With mild hypothermia, shivering, tachycardia, cyanosis, clumsiness, and dysarthria are evident. Shivering ceases with moderate hypothermia, and patients become confused or delirious. Blood pressure decreases, and muscle rigidity is noted. As the body temperature falls below 29° C, mental status deteriorates to coma with absent deep tendon reflexes, the heart rate decreases, and breathing ceases.[1]

Pathophysiology

Hypothermia is defined as a body temperature lower than 35° C. It is classified as mild (31° to 35° C), moderate (29° to 31° C), or severe (less than 29° C). Several factors may predispose to the development of hypothermia, including homelessness, cold-weather sporting activities, mental illness, intoxication, immersion, trauma, burns, sepsis, hypoglycemia, hypothyroidism, hypothalamic injury, and malnutrition.[1]

With mild hypothermia, the body attempts to warm itself through increased metabolic rate, shivering, and peripheral vasoconstriction. As the temperature drops, there are decreases in metabolic rate, central nervous system activity, and nerve and cardiac conduction, and cardiac output become impaired.[1]

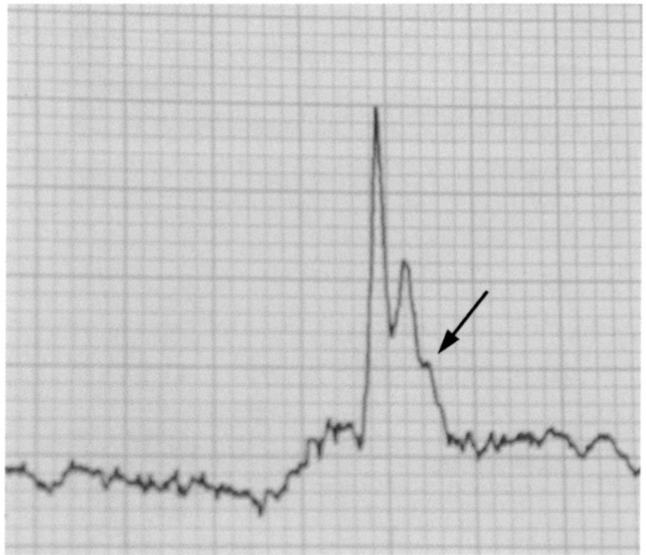

FIGURE 25–26 Osborne wave of hypothermia. Note the fluctuating baseline secondary to shivering. (Courtesy of Robert Hendrickson, MD.)

Diagnosis

Hypothermia may be misdiagnosed. Low-reading thermometers may be required to obtain accurate temperatures. The electrocardiogram (ECG) may show the pathognomonic J wave (Osborne wave) or arrhythmias such as atrial fibrillation with slow ventricular response.[1]

Clinical Complications

Myocardial irritability leads to dysrhythmias that may be triggered by the simple act of moving the patient.[1]

Management

Passive rewarming, suitable for only the mildest cases, consists of removing wet clothing and applying blankets. External rewarming is best accomplished with the use of warm forced air, pumped through a semiclosed cover placed over the patient. Other external warming methods, such as water immersion or heating blankets, may be impractical and can cause skin burns. External warming may not be effective if peripheral blood flow is compromised. For moderate or severe cases, core rewarming is preferred. Techniques include (in order of increasing effectiveness) warm intravenous fluid; heat and humidified air; warm fluid lavage of the bladder, stomach, colon, peritoneum, and pleural space; mediastinal irrigation after thoracotomy; and extracorporal blood warming. Defibrillation may be less successful in the hypothermic patient, so if initial attempts fail, repeat attempts should be delayed until temperature increases to 28° to 32° C.[1]

REFERENCES

1. Corneli HM. Hot topics in cold medicine: controversies in accidental hypothermia. *Clin Pediatr Emerg Med* 2001;2:179–191.

Frostbite

Anthony Morocco

Clinical Presentation

Ninety percent of cases involve the hands and feet; the cheeks, ears, nose, and penis are also commonly affected. Presenting symptoms include numbness and clumsiness of the affected area. Rewarming can cause intense, throbbing pain. The injury may be divided into four degrees, based on the appearance after rewarming: first-degree injury, with a central, pale area and surrounding erythema; second-degree injury, with blisters surrounded by erythema and edema; third-degree injury, with hemorrhagic blisters and eschar formation, and fourth-degree injury, with necrosis and tissue loss.[1,2]

Pathophysiology

Populations at risk for frostbite include homeless persons, alcoholics, military personnel, hikers, skiers, climbers, and those with psychiatric illness.[1,2]

Initially, freezing causes formation of extracellular ice crystals, with resultant cell membrane damage and intracellular dehydration. Further injury occurs on formation of intracellular ice. As blood vessels alternately vasoconstrict and vasodilate, damaging cycles of freezing and thawing occur. The other major mechanism of injury is progressive dermal ischemia, which is related to release of inflammatory mediators, neutrophil adhesion, endothelial damage, edema, and thrombosis.

Diagnosis

Techniques such as technetium scintigraphy, magnetic resonance imaging, and magnetic resonance angiography have been suggested to help determine the anatomic boundaries of viable tissue. However, these methods have not proved effective in the early postthaw period.

Clinical Complications

Severe injuries can result in large areas of necrosis and eventual amputation. Years after the initial injury, the affected area may continue to have hyperhydrosis, cold sensitivity, chronic pain, and sensory loss.[1] Other sequelae include rhabdomyolysis and renal failure, growth plate injury, osteoarthritis, and heterotopic calcification.

Management

First aid in the field should involve avoidance of trauma and delay in thawing until definitive rewarming is possible. Rewarming should be done in a warm-water bath at 40° to 42° C. The affected area should be elevated to limit edema. Nonhemorrhagic blisters should be débrided, because they contain high levels of inflammatory mediators.[1] Tetanus prophylaxis should be administered. Ibuprofen and aloe vera have been advocated for systemic and topical thromboxane inhibition. The timing of surgical débridement is controversial, as are experimental treatments such as dextran, anticoagulation, thrombolysis, hyperbaric oxygen, vasodilators, and sympathectomy.[1]

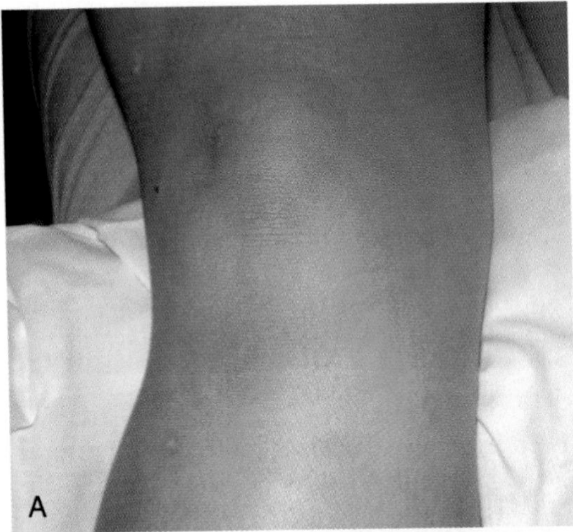

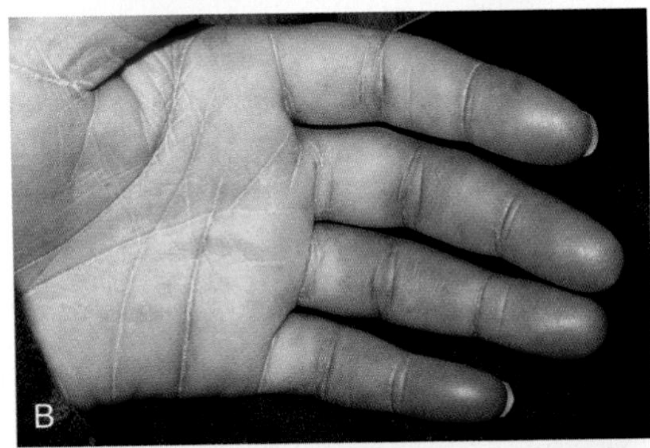

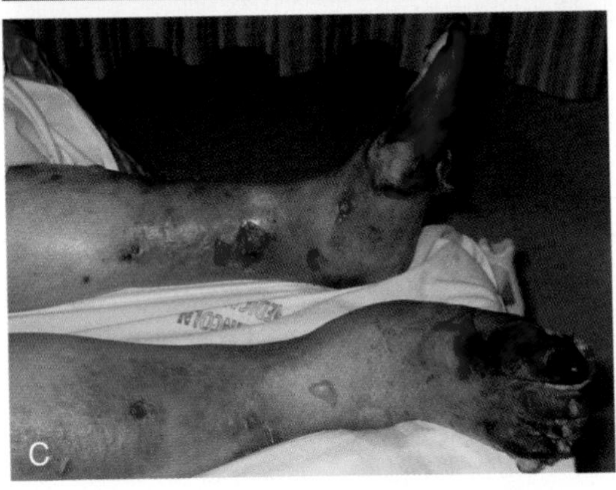

FIGURE 25–27 **A:** Mild frostbite caused by excessive use of therapeutic ice packs. (Courtesy of Jim Roberts, MD.) **B:** Moderately severe frostbite. (Courtesy of Claritza Rios, MD.) **C:** Severe frostbite. (Courtesy of Kabir Yadev, MD.)

REFERENCES

1. Murphy JV, Banwell PE, Roberts AH, McGrouther DA. Frostbite: pathogenesis and treatment. *J Trauma* 2000;48:171–178.
2. Biem J, Koehncke N, Classen D, Dosman J. Out of the cold: management of hypothermia and frostbite. *CMAJ* 2003;168:305–311.

Chilblains

Anthony Morocco

Clinical Presentation

Skin lesions develop 12 to 24 hours after cold exposure.[1] Erythematous, papular, bilateral, symmetric lesions develop most commonly on the toes and dorsal proximal phalanges but may also occur on the face and ears. Patients may complain of burning pain and pruritus. Initial papules and plaques may progress to painful, purple, indurated lesions.[2]

Pathophysiology

Chilblains, also known as pernio or perniosis, are inflammatory skin lesions that occur in nonfreezing, cold, humid climates. Pernio may also be a presenting symptom of patients with connective tissue diseases such as systemic lupus erythematosus (SLE) or other disorders.

Pernio results in a number of pathologic changes in the skin, including vasculitis with lymphocytic infiltration of dermal blood vessels, edema, and fatty necrosis.

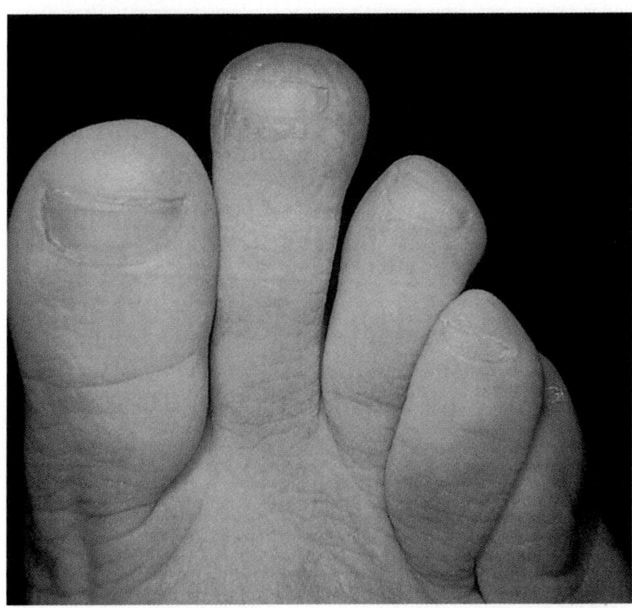

FIGURE 25-28 Inflammatory skin lesions of chilblains caused by severe exposure to cold. (From Dockery, with permission.)

Diagnosis

Pernio should be included in the differential diagnosis for skin lesions in cold climates, particularly in at-risk patients such as young women and those with connective tissue diseases. The differential diagnosis includes atheromatous emboli, erythema nodosum, cold panniculitis, erythromelalgia, nodular vasculitis, and erythema induratum. Workup for associated connective tissue disease should be performed in patients with chronic symptoms. Other causes and associated conditions include Raynaud's disease, macroglobulinemia, chronic myelomonocytic leukemia, anorexia nervosa, and dysproteinemias.[1]

Clinical Complications

Recurrent cold exposure can result in chronic lesions, with scarring and vascular disease. Associated connective tissue disease may result in numerous other complications.

Management

Cold exposure should be avoided by susceptible individuals. Local treatment for pruritus consists of antihistamines. Nifedipine may aid in symptom resolution and healing in severe cases. Uncomplicated pernio lesions usually resolve spontaneously in 1 to 3 weeks.[1]

REFERENCES

1. Giusti R, Tunnessen WW Jr. Picture of the month. Chilblains (pernio). *Arch Pediatr Adolesc Med* 1997;151:1055–1056.
2. Goette DK. Chilblains (perniosis). *J Am Acad Dermatol* 1990;23: 257–262.

Trenchfoot

Anthony Morocco

Clinical Presentation

Patients develop symptoms after hours to days of exposure to cold, wet conditions. During and immediately after exposure, the feet are pulseless, numb, and edematous. A period of hyperemia then occurs, which lasts several days, with severe pain, worsening edema, and formation of bullae. After this period, pain decreases, but cold hypersensitivity and hyperhydrosis may occur.[1]

Pathophysiology

Trenchfoot, also called immersion foot, is a cold injury that occurs after prolonged exposure to water at nonfreezing temperatures. It has been well described in soldiers during several wars over the past century, from the trenches of World War I to the Falklands campaign. Although trenchfoot classically occurs after exposure to very cold water (less than 40° F), warmer water temperatures can cause similar injury, referred to as tropical immersion foot.[2] Tight or wet socks and ill-fitting boots encourage the development of trenchfoot, and even those who wear waterproof footwear may be affected because of the accumulation of sweat. Similar cold injury to the hands also occurs.

Impaired blood flow due to cold and vasoconstriction are probably responsible for the tissue injury. Trenchfoot differs fundamentally from frostbite in that freezing of tissues and ice crystal formation do not occur. Peripheral nerve injury results in the chronic symptoms.

Clinical Complications

Cold sensitivity and hyperhydrosis may persist for months. Though gangrene and tissue loss are rare, permanent nerve injury, reflex sympathetic dystrophy, and disability may occur.[1]

Management

Initial rewarming in water at 104° to 108° F is recommended. Further care is nonspecific and supportive and includes elevation of the affected limbs to limit edema, application of dry bandages, tetanus prophylaxis, and monitoring for secondary infection.[2] Preventative measures to avoid wet feet and early recognition of symptoms are most important.

REFERENCES

1. Ungley CC, Channell GD, Richards RL. The immersion foot syndrome. 1946. *Wilderness Environ Med* 2003;14:135–141.
2. Murphy JV, Banwell PE, Roberts AH, McGrouther DA. Frostbite: pathogenesis and treatment. *J Trauma* 2000;48:171–178.

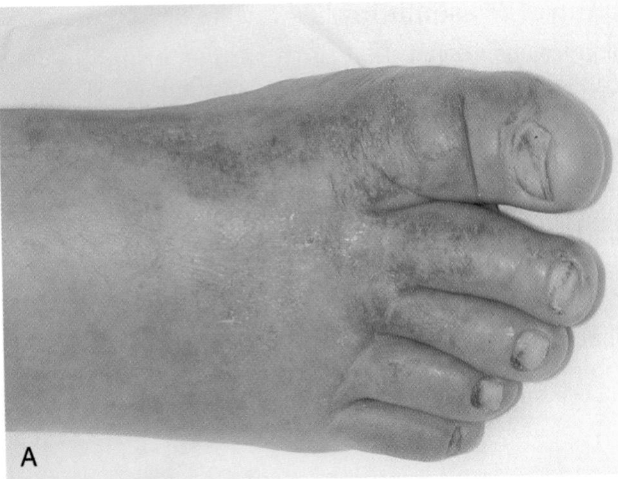

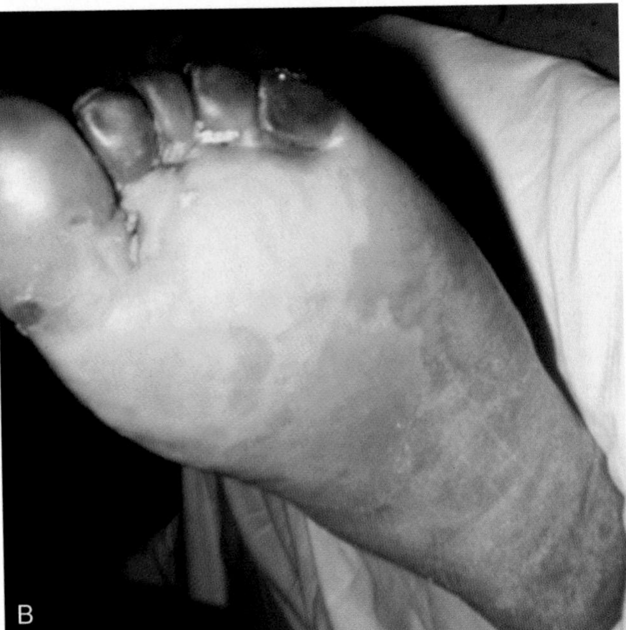

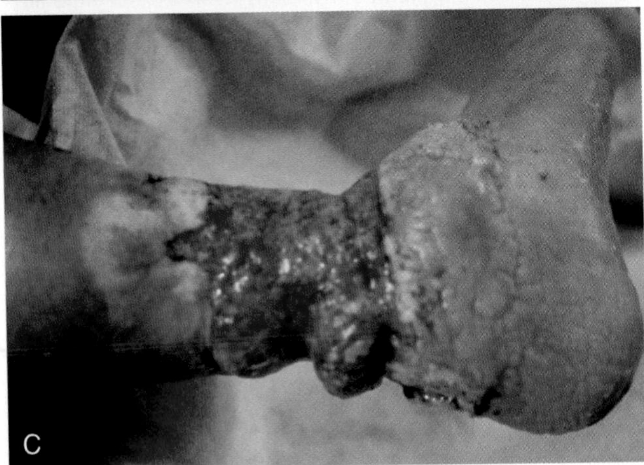

FIGURE 25–29 **A:** Mild trenchfoot. (Courtesy of Robert Hendrickson, MD.) **B:** Moderately severe trenchfoot. (Copyright James R. Roberts, MD.) **C:** Severe trenchfoot. (Courtesy of B. Zane Horowitz, MD.)

Heat-Related Illness and Hyperthermia

Anthony Morocco

Clinical Presentation

Patients with heat exhaustion presents with elevated body temperature (38° to 40° C), vomiting, headache, confusion, tachycardia, and hypotension. In those with heat stroke (body temperature greater than 40° C), the symptoms worsen, with cessation of sweating, arrhythmias, shock, delirium, seizures, and coma.[1] Patients with malignant hyperthermia (MH) present with muscle rigidity and elevated temperature after anesthesia. Neuroleptic malignant syndrome (NMS) causes hyperthermia, "lead-pipe" muscle rigidity, mental status change, and autonomic instability.[2]

Pathophysiology

Hyperthermia has a variety of causes, including environmental exposure, extreme exertion, drug effects, infection, seizures, brain injury, and hyperthyroidism. Heat exhaustion and heat stroke represent progressive degrees of heat illness.

Heat stroke commonly occurs during hot weather, in elderly patients with debilitating medical problems and in younger patients who engage in excessively strenuous physical activity. A large number of medications can cause or predispose patients to hyperthermia. Mechanisms include agitation that results in increased muscle activity and increased heat production (sympathomimetics), impaired sweating and heat loss (anticholinergics), and altered central thermoregulatory control.[2] MH results from abnormal calcium regulation in skeletal muscle and is triggered by inhaled anesthetics and neuromuscular blocking agents. NMS is an idiosyncratic reaction and most likely is related to alterations in dopaminergic activity.

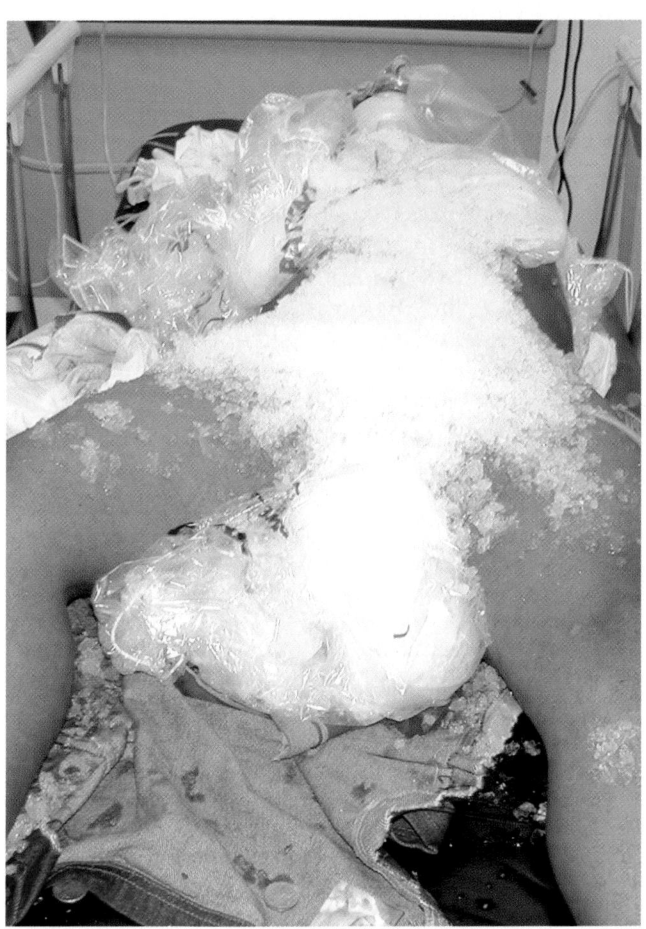

FIGURE 25–30 This patient smoked crack cocaine over several summer days and developed a temperature of 108.8° Fahrenheit. (Courtesy of Robert Hendrickson, MD.)

Diagnosis

Patients at risk for hyperthermia should have their temperature taken with a thermometer capable of measuring very high temperatures, if possible. Laboratory testing should include electrolytes, renal function, urinalysis, liver enzymes, and coagulation studies.

Clinical Complications

Heat stroke may result in multiple complications including rhabdomyolysis, renal failure, hepatic necrosis, disseminated intravascular coagulation (DIC), and death.[1] MH can cause hypotension, hypoxia, hyperkalemia, and dysrhythmias.

Management

Rapid cooling of the patient is essential. Temperatures in excess of 104° F may require that the patient be packed in ice. Wetting and fanning the patient to promote evaporative cooling is no longer considered effective. Cooling maneuvers should cease when temperature falls below 102° F, to prevent iatrogenic hypothermia.[1] MH should be treated with cessation of the causative agent, aggressive cooling, and intravenous dantrolene. NMS may be treated with aggressive supportive care and administration of benzodiazepines, bromocriptine, and dantrolene.

REFERENCES

1. Wexler RK. Evaluation and treatment of heat-related illnesses. *Am Fam Physician* 2002;65:2307–2314.
2. Chan TC, Evans SD, Clark RF. Drug-induced hyperthermia. *Crit Care Clin* 1997;13:785–808.

Lightning Injuries

Anthony Morocco

Clinical Presentation

Lightning strike can cause immediate cardiac and respiratory arrest; 89% of patients present with burns, though only 5% have deep burns. The skin may show erythema, blistering, or linear charring. A feathering pattern called Lichtenberg figures and punctate full-thickness burns are pathognomonic. Substantial injury to muscle and other internal organs may occur with minimal superficial evidence of injury. Tympanic membrane rupture occurs in up to 50% of patients. Transient autonomic instability, with hypertension and peripheral vasospasm, may be evident; it is caused by massive release of catecholamines.[1]

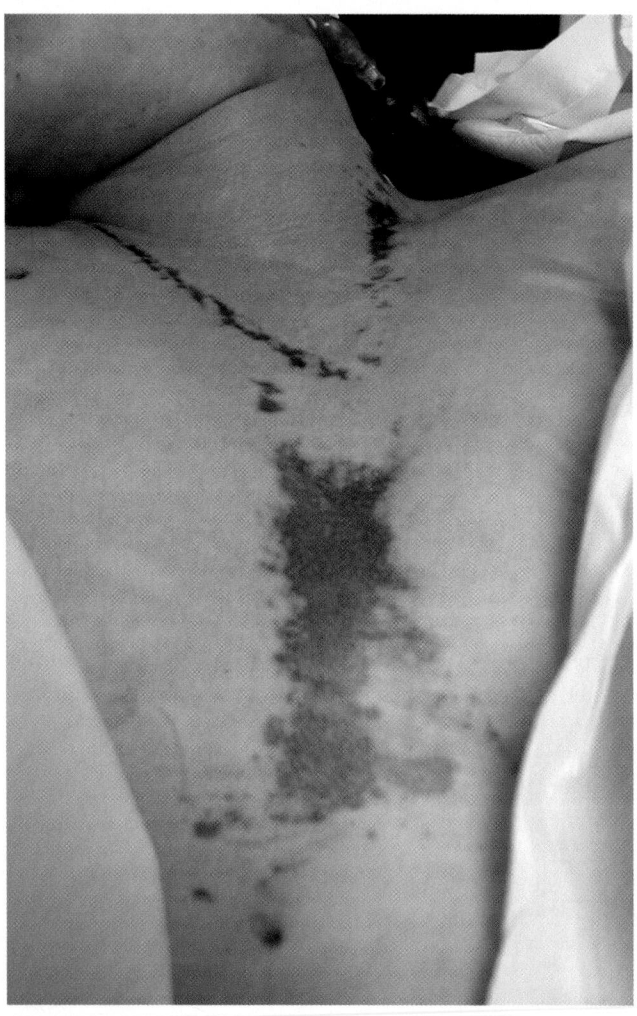

FIGURE 25-31 Fatal lightning injury. Note residual burn outline of patient's necklace. (Courtesy of Anthony Morocco, MD.)

Pathophysiology

Lightning strikes account for about 100 deaths and many more injuries each year in the United States. Victims are typically men between the ages of 15 to 44 years who are engaged in recreational activities.[1,2] Electrical injury is caused by thermal damage, direct effect of current on tissues, and trauma. A lightning strike results in a massive direct current (DC) of 10,000 to 20,000 amperes, lasting just a few microseconds.[1-3] Direct strikes are most damaging. A victim may also be injured by the flow of current after a lightning strike on nearby ground, people, or other objects. Significant burns are less likely with lightning strike than with other electrical injuries, although head and neck burns resulting from current entry and clothing ignition may occur. Trauma to lungs and viscera occurs as the result of shock waves of up to 20 atmospheres that are generated by the sudden superheating of air.[1]

Clinical Complications

Thirty percent of victims die, and 74% develop permanent sequelae.[3] Neurologic sequelae may include reflex sympathetic dystrophy, neuritis, transient paralysis or keraunoparalysis, paraplegia, and amnesia. Eye damage may be both immediate (corneal ulceration, vitreous hemorrhage) and delayed (cataract formation).[1]

Management

Victims may require immediate cardiopulmonary resuscitation (CPR). Survivors of lightning strikes may have minimal injuries and may not require hospital admission. However, patients should remain on cardiac monitoring if there is a history of unconsciousness, abnormal electrocardiogram (ECG), or arrhythmia, or if the history is suspicious for same. Associated traumatic injuries should be ruled out. Aggressive intravenous fluids and alkalinization of the urine are indicated for the few patients with severe burns and rhabdomyolysis. Transfer to a specialized burn unit should be considered for serious cases.[1]

REFERENCES

1. Jain S, Bandi V. Electrical and lightning injuries. *Crit Care Clin* 1999;15:319–331.
2. Zimmermann C, Cooper MA, Holle RL. Lightning safety guidelines. *Ann Emerg Med* 2002;39:660–664.
3. Lightning associated deaths—United States, 1980–1995. *MMWR Morb Mortal Wkly Rep* 47:391-394, 1998.

High-Altitude Illness

Anthony Morocco

Clinical Presentation

Acute mountain sickness (AMS) usually occurs after 12 to 24 hours at altitude, although symptoms may appear after 2 to 96 hours.[1] Patients complain of throbbing bitemporal headache accompanied by gastrointestinal upset, anorexia, fatigue, and dizziness.[1] Disordered sleep is common, as is periodic breathing similar to Cheyne-Stokes breathing.[1] Progression to high-altitude cerebral edema (HACE) is heralded by ataxia, lassitude, and mental status changes. High-altitude pulmonary edema (HAPE) is characterized by dry cough, shortness of breath, and fatigue; symptoms may progress to orthopnea and frothy pink sputum production.

Pathophysiology

The term *high-altitude illness* refers to a spectrum of conditions that occur at altitudes greater than 2500 meters. These include AMS, HAPE, and HACE.[1]

The normal response to high altitude involves the hypoxic ventilatory response (HVR) to decreased ambient oxygen. The HVR causes increased ventilation and is the first step in acclimatization. Patients with decreased HVR are at higher risk for AMS. Increased bicarbonate excretion by the kidneys occurs after 1 to 2 days and corrects the alkalosis caused by increased carbon dioxide exhalation. After several days at altitude, the red cell mass begins to increase, resulting in increased oxygen-carrying capacity.[1]

Clinical Complications

HACE may progress to coma in 12 hours to 9 days; the mortality rate after coma is 60%.[1] HACE may result in permanent cognitive impairment and ataxia. HAPE may progress to respiratory failure.[1] Other conditions related to high altitude include thromboembolism, stroke, syncope, peripheral edema, retinopathy, pharyngitis, cough, immune compromise, and exacerbation of conditions such as chronic obstructive pulmonary disease (COPD) and sickle cell disease.[1]

Management

AMS that does not progress to HACE or HAPE usually resolves in 1 to 3 days without treatment after acclimatization. The most effective treatment is descent, and descent of even 500 to 1000 m may alleviate the condition.[1] Prochlorperazine is effective for nausea and increases HVR. Acetazolamide enhances bicarbonate excretion and increases ventilation, thereby enhancing acclimatization and improving sleep. Severe AMS, HACE, or HAPE requires immediate descent and may be treated with dexamethasone and supplemental oxygen.[1] Portable hyperbaric chambers may be useful for patients who cannot descend.

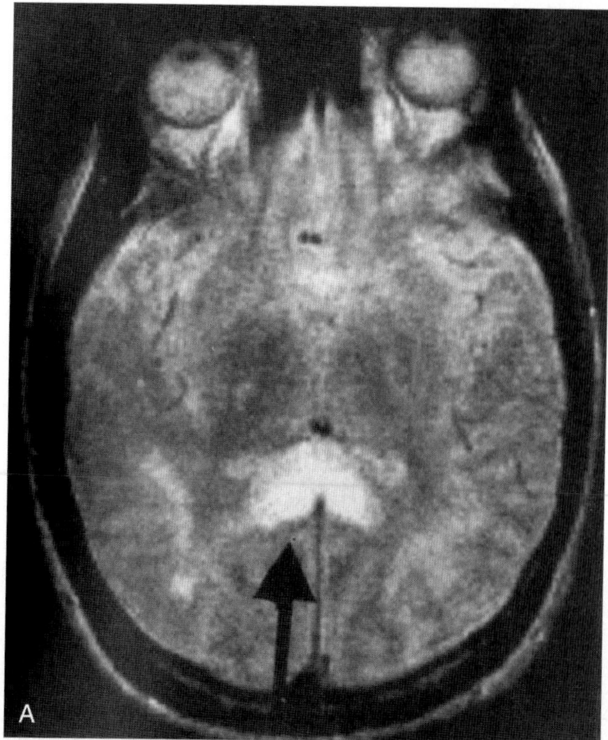

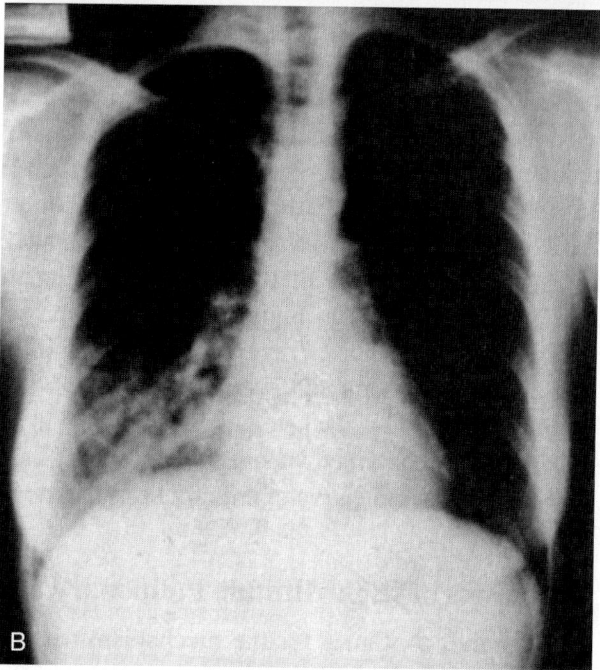

FIGURE 25–32 **A:** High-altitude cerebral edema (HACE) as seen on a magnetic resonance image of brain. **B:** Chest radiograph showing high-altitude pulmonary edema (HAPE). (**A** and **B,** From Auerbach, with permission.)

REFERENCES

1. Zafren K, Honigman B. High altitude medicine. *Emerg Med Clin North Am* 1997;15:191–222.

25-33

Dysbarism

Anthony Morocco

Clinical Presentation

Symptoms of barotrauma depend on the affected area. Ear involvement may cause intense pain, vertigo, hearing deficit, nausea, vomiting, and facial nerve palsy. Pain may also develop in a tooth, a sinus, or the gut. Pulmonary barotrauma manifests as chest pain, shortness of breath, and subcutaneous emphysema, and patients with arterial gas embolism (AGE) may develop significant neurologic deficits, confusion, and seizures immediately after surfacing. Decompression sickness (DCS) manifests with a number of symptoms typically occurring within 1 hour after a dive. These include joint pains and skin rashes (type I DCS), or cardiovascular compromise and neurologic deficits (type II DCS).

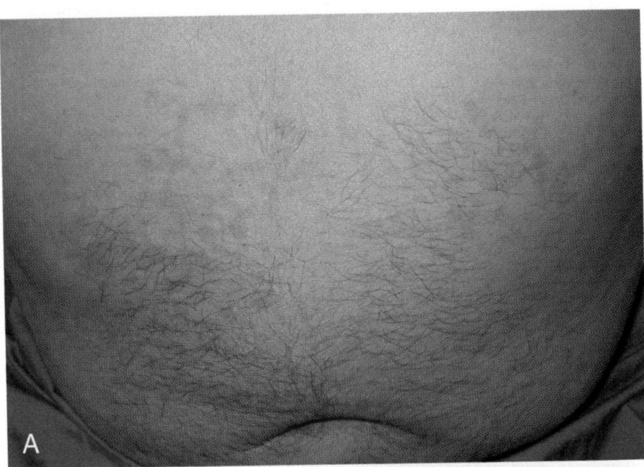

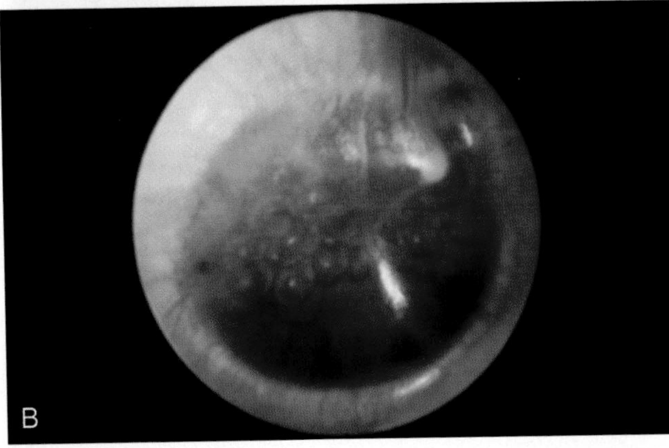

FIGURE 25–33 **A:** Skin lesions from "the bends." (Courtesy of Gregory Juhl, MD.) **B:** Barotrauma of the eardrum. (From Benjamin, with permission.)

Pathophysiology

The term dysbarism refers to the group of disorders that occur as the result of ambient pressure changes and the breathing of compressed gases while scuba diving.[1] A pressure change of 1 atmosphere (760 mg Hg) occurs for every 33 feet of depth change. Barotrauma is related to pressure change in any gas-filled structure in the body. Decompression illness (DCI) is the formation of gas bubbles within the blood and tissue. Types of DCI include decompression sickness, also known as the bends, and arterial gas embolism.

Barotrauma occurs because of a failure to equilibrate pressure in body air spaces with the changing ambient pressure during a dive. Pulmonary barotrauma results from breath-holding during ascension. The decreased ambient pressure causes expansion of lung gases, resulting in gas bubble entry into capillaries (AGE), pneumothorax, and pneumomediastinum. DCS occurs when gas bubbles form in supersaturated tissues, causing pain due to vascular occlusion, pressure, and nerve dysfunction. Bubbles may form in joints, skin, peripheral nerves, or the spinal cord.[1]

Diagnosis

A complete history should be obtained, including timing of symptom onset, time and depth of diving activity, and presence of any predisposing conditions. The diagnosis of dysbarism is clinical, although a chest radiograph should be obtained if pneumothorax is suspected.[1]

Clinical Complications

Recompression and time relieve most symptoms, but some patients have permanent sequelae. AGE can cause rapid death due to respiratory or cardiac arrest, or drowning if symptoms begin while the victim is still in the water.[1]

Management

Patients exhibiting symptoms of DCI should be placed in a supine position and immediately given high-flow oxygen and isotonic intravenous fluids. Patients should be evaluated as soon as possible for recompression therapy. Normobaric or hyperbaric oxygen allows faster resorption of inert gas bubbles in tissues. Multiple treatments may be required.[1]

REFERENCES

1. Moon RE. Treatment of diving emergencies. *Crit Care Clin* 1999;15:429–456.

Near-Drowning

Anthony Morocco

Clinical Presentation

Patients may present with a mental status ranging from alert to comatose. They may be confused, disoriented, seizing, or posturing. Respiratory effort may be diminished, with clinical signs of pulmonary edema and hypoxia. Patients may also be hypothermic.[1]

Pathophysiology

The term *near-drowning* refers to survival after transient asphyxia due to submersion. Young children are at high risk for drowning and near-drowning, with incidents commonly involving home swimming pools and buckets. In adolescents and adults, alcohol is a significant contributing factor in 25% to 50% of drownings. Other risk factors include hypoglycemia, cardiac arrhythmias, seizures, depression, trauma, and hypothermia.[1]

Inspiration of water results in pulmonary edema, alteration of pulmonary surfactant and capillary permeability, and impaired gas exchange. Inspiration against a closed glottis during submersion and neurogenic pulmonary edema contribute to respiratory dysfunction. Hyponatremia or hypernatremia can occur depending on the near-drowning environment: freshwater moves along the osmotic gradient into the circulation, whereas saltwater pulls free water into the alveoli.[1]

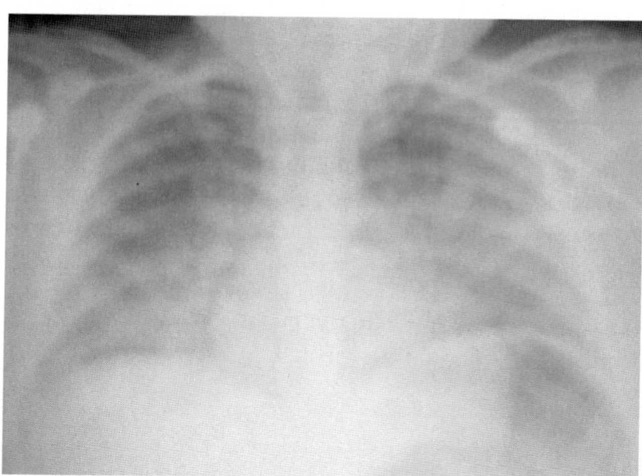

FIGURE 25–34 Bilateral infiltrates in a patient with hypoxemia after near-drowning. (Courtesy of Robert Hendrickson, MD.)

Diagnosis

Laboratory testing reveals respiratory and metabolic acidosis, in addition to hypernatremia or hyponatremia. Chest radiography is almost always abnormal, with bilateral infiltrates and, rarely, pneumomediastinum.[1]

Clinical Complications

Patients may exhibit worsening pulmonary status and chest radiographic appearance in the first hours after admission, with subsequent development of acute respiratory distress syndrome (ARDS). Mechanically ventilated patients have a high risk of bacterial pneumonia. Hypoxic encephalopathy, rhabdomyolysis, and renal insufficiency may occur. Eighty percent of patients who reach the hospital survive.[1]

Management

Patients should receive supplemental oxygen; obtunded patients and those with respiratory distress should be endotracheally intubated. Hypothermic patients should be rapidly rewarmed. However, maintenance of mild hypothermia (32° to 34° C) may be beneficial for unconscious postarrest patients. A careful evaluation should be performed to look for any coexisting trauma or dysbarism. Well-appearing patients should be observed 4 to 6 hours before discharge.[1]

REFERENCES

1. Moon RE, Long RJ. Drowning and near-drowning. *Emerg Med* 2002; 14:377–386.

Electrical Injuries

Anthony Morocco

Clinical Presentation

Patients may present with a range of skin burns, from mild erythema to full-thickness injury with damage to deeper structures. Severe electrical arc burns may be seen on the volar forearm, elbow, and axilla after entry of current at the palm. Children may present with oral burns after biting an electrical cord. Victims may also present with cardiac and respiratory arrest.[1]

Pathophysiology

Electrical injury is caused by thermal damage, direct effect of current on tissues, and trauma related to muscle contraction and falls. Cardiac effects may occur due to thermal damage, vasospasm, or current-induced ventricular fibrillation (low voltage) or asystole (high voltage). Alternating current (AC) is more dangerous than direct current (DC). AC causes tetanic muscle contractions, often resulting in the victim's involuntarily holding on and prolonging contact with the electrical source. Factors affecting the resistance to current flow include moisture, body tissue, size of body part, and magnitude and duration of current. Head-to-feet flow is more dangerous than arm-to-arm flow.[1]

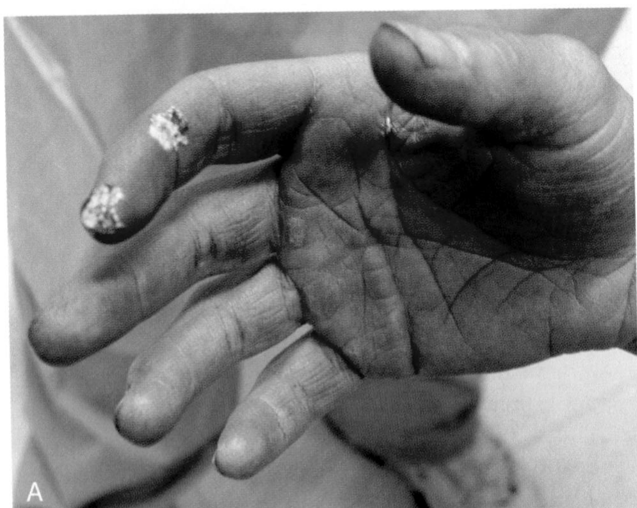

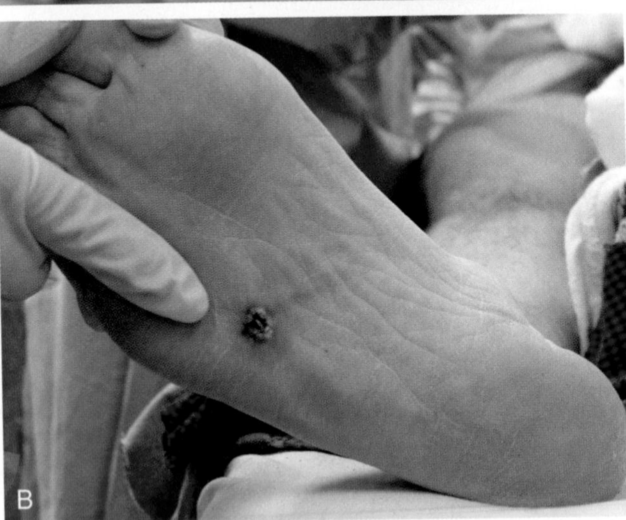

FIGURE 25-35 **A:** Entrance wound from electrical injury. **B:** Exit wound from electrical injury. (**A** and **B**, Courtesy of John Fojtik, MD.)

Clinical Complications

Injury to muscle and internal organs may occur with minimal superficial evidence of injury. Complications include compartment syndrome, vascular injury with later aneurysm formation, spinal cord and peripheral nerve injuries, gastric ulcer, and adynamic ileus.[1]

Management

Victims may require immediate cardiopulmonary resuscitation (CPR)/advanced cardiac life support (ACLS). Associated traumatic injuries should be ruled out. Patients need careful monitoring if there is a history of unconsciousness, abnormal electrocardiogram (ECG), arrhythmia, or evidence of current passage through the thorax. ECG and myocardial-bound creatine kinase (CKMB) measurements are not reliable indicators of myocardial injury. Intravenous fluid requirements are generally higher than with thermal burns because of greater deep tissue damage. Alkalinization of the urine is indicated for rhabdomyolysis. In cases of compartment syndrome, fasciotomy should be considered. Transfer to a burn center should be considered in all cases.[1]

REFERENCES

1. Jain S, Bandi V. Electrical and lightning injuries. *Crit Care Clin* 1999;15:319–331.

Radiation Injury

Anthony Morocco

Clinical Presentation

Radiation injuries may occur from local or whole-body exposure. Localized doses can cause immediate or delayed skin changes. Doses of 3 to 4 Gray (Gy) cause epilation; 10 to 15 Gy causes erythema. Ulceration (25 Gy), blistering (100 Gy), and necrosis can occur in 1 to 2 weeks. Necrosis can occur several months or years later due to vascular injury. Whole-body doses may lead to gastrointestinal, bone marrow, or central nervous system damage. Whole-body exposure to 1 Gy causes nausea and vomiting after 48 hours in 10% of patients; 4 Gy results in vomiting in 90% of victims within 12 hours, with a 50% mortality rate in the absence of treatment. Exposures greater than 30 Gy cause rapid central nervous system and cardiovascular collapse, with death occurring in 24 to 72 hours.[1]

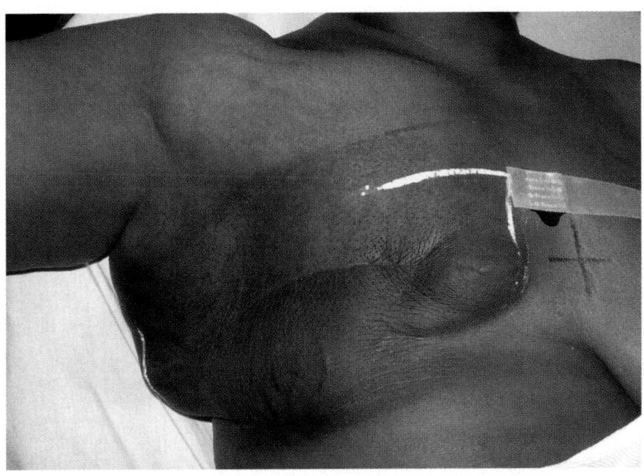

FIGURE 25–36 Radiation burn secondary to radiation therapy after mastectomy for breast cancer. (Courtesy of Mark Silverberg, MD.)

Pathophysiology

Ionizing radiation exists in several forms, which differ in their ability to penetrate and damage the human body. Gamma rays and x-rays penetrate completely, beta particles penetrate a few centimeters, and alpha particles penetrate less than 0.1 mm. The measurement of radioactivity is expressed in several ways. The gray measures dose absorbed by specific tissues (1 Gy = 100 radiation absorbed dose). The Sievert is the effective dose (1 Sv = 100 radiation equivalent, man) and takes into account the differences among types of radiation. Important variables are duration of exposure and distance from the source, because dose is inversely proportional to the square of the distance. Ionizing radiation causes damage to body tissues via free radical formation and direct injury to DNA and other cellular structures. Rapidly dividing cells are preferentially affected.[1]

Clinical Complications

Exposure to greater than 6 Gy causes bone marrow failure and death without treatment; 10 Gy is the maximum survivable dose with optimal medical care.[1] Malignancy is a potential long-term complication. Tumors may develop 5 to 10 years or longer after exposure, whereas leukemia may occur within 2 years.[1]

Management

Potassium iodide should be administered within several hours after nuclear detonation or nuclear reactor discharge to prevent thyroid uptake of radioactive iodine. Intensive supportive care and long-term wound care may be necessary.[1]

REFERENCES

1. Mettler FA Jr, Voelz GL. Current concepts: major radiation exposure—what to expect and how to respond. *N Engl J Med* 2002;346:1554–1561.

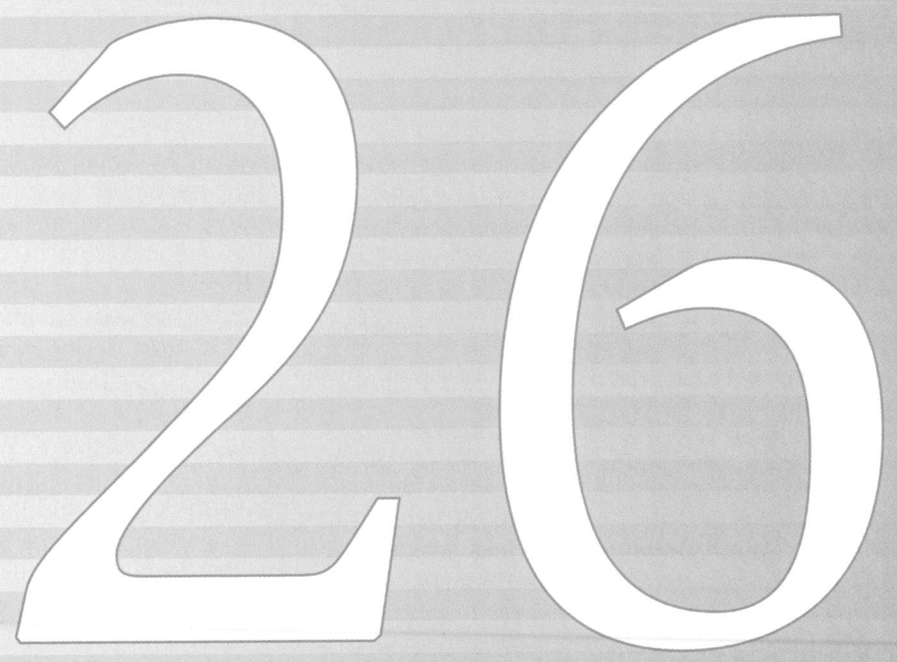

Occupational

Welder's Flash

Michael Greenberg

Clinical Presentation

Patients with Welder's flash (WF) present in a delayed fashion (usually 6 to 12 hours) after welding or observing welding activities. Presenting complaints typically include intensely severe bilateral eye pain, photophobia, lacrimation, blepharospasm, and a gritty or "sandy" feeling or foreign-body sensation of the eyes.[1,2]

Pathophysiology

Exposure to UV-B and UV-C radiation may cause a superficial punctate keratopathy that appears several hours after exposure. Welder's flash is a superficial punctate keratopathy caused by exposure to ultraviolet (UV) radiation related to arc welding. This may be thought of as an ocular analogue of acute blistering sunburn.[1,2] WF may be caused by even momentary or peripheral exposure to UV-C during arc welding.[1,2]

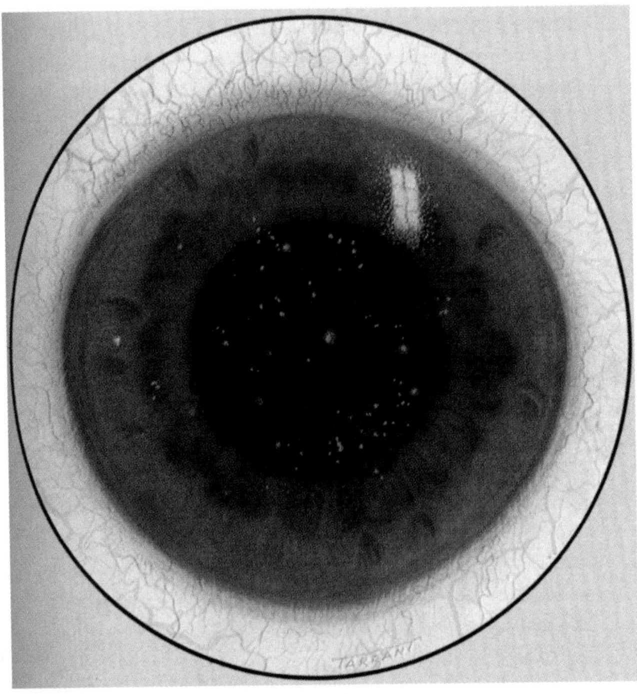

FIGURE 26–1 Superficial punctate keratitis consistent with welder's flash. (From Perkins ES, Hansell P. *An atlas of diseases of the eye,* 2nd ed. Baltimore, Williams & Wilkins, 1971, with permission.)

Diagnosis

The diagnosis rests on obtaining a history of exposure to UV-C radiation during welding without appropriate eye protection. Diagnostic confirmation should be obtained by performing slit-lamp microscopy after applying topical anesthetic drops.[1,2] Without anesthesia, these patients may not tolerate the slit-lamp examination. The skin of the eyelids and face may be erythematous. The cornea should be stained with fluorescein, which reveals focal loss of epithelial cells in a diffuse, punctate pattern. Symptoms usually disappear within 48 hours, and permanent damage, although possible, is uncommon.

Clinical Complications

Complications are very rare and may include infection or corneal ulcers.[1,2]

Management

Treatment requires control of blepharospasm with cycloplegic medications. After slit-lamp microscopy under topical anesthesia, the patient's pain may re-occur. The physician should resist the urge to discharge the patient with a bottle of topical anesthetic, because patients may use this source of temporary relief instead of attending follow-up visits. Some authorities recommend eye patching, but this can be problematic in the bilaterally affected individual.[1,2]

REFERENCES

1. Wilkenfeld M, Crowley KA, Dawodu O. Occupational eye injury due to phototoxicity. *J Occup Environ Med* 2002;44:488–489.
2. Tenkate TD. Ultraviolet radiation: human exposure and health risks. *J Environ Health* 1998;61:9–15.

Tar and Asphalt Burns

Michael Greenberg

Clinical Presentation

The majority of tar and asphalt burns occur in workers who use hot tar or asphalt in the course of their work. Patients present after skin exposure and usually come to the emergency department directly from their worksite.

Pathophysiology

Tar and asphalt are used as protective coatings in various industrial settings, including roofing and road paving. These materials are petroleum distillates with very high boiling points. Because these materials do not cool quickly after being heated, the opportunity exists for prolonged heat transfer to underlying tissues. Because the skin flora is trapped beneath the burn, these injuries are prone to infection. Frequently these burns are associated with vehicular accidents, falls from heights, and explosions, indicating that serious associated multisystem trauma may coexist.[1]

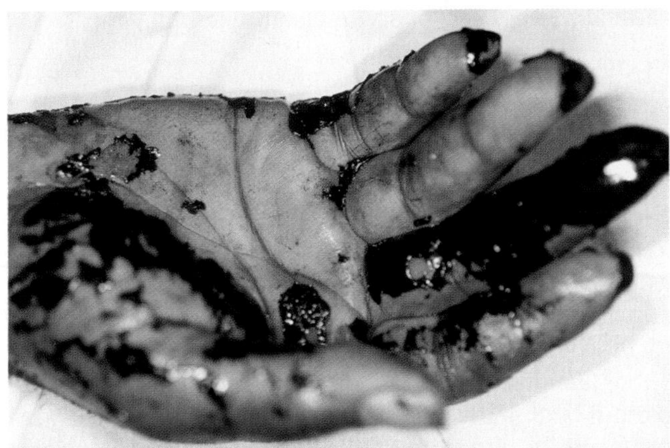

FIGURE 26–2 Tar burns of the hand. (From Roberts, JR. Minor Burns: Tar, cement, and chemicals. *Emerg Med News* 2003; XXV(5):20–23, with permission.)

Diagnosis

The diagnosis is usually obvious and is based on history and physical examination.

Clinical Complications

Complications include superinfection, associated trauma, and other issues depending on burn location (e.g., hands, eyes, perineum).

Management

Various approaches have been taken, including leaving the tar or asphalt in place to solidify and applying various materials to aid in removal. Proposed removal agents include butter, sunflower oil, De-Solv-it,® neomycin, baby oil, gasoline, mayonnaise, ice, acetone, alcohol, and kerosene.[1,2] In any case, removal may be problematic and may take several hours to complete. Sharp débridement for removal is not encouraged because it is painful and may result in the removal of viable underlying skin and skin appendages. Cold water is recommended as a first-aid measure to eliminate the burning process.[1,2]

REFERENCES

1. Baruchin AM, Schraf S, Rosenberg L, et al. Hot bitumen burns: 92 hospitalized patients. *Burns* 1997;23:438–441.
2. Turegun M, Ozturk S, Selmanpakoglu N. Sunflower oil in the treatment of hot tar burns. *Burns* 1997;23:442–445.

Hydrofluoric Acid Injury

James M. Madsen

Clinical Presentation

Exposure to concentrated hydrofluoric (HF) acid (15% to 20% or greater) can be extremely painful, with vesication and necrosis. More dilute solutions may not cause immediate pain nor become visible for several hours, but they may penetrate deeply and cause subcutaneous blanching, gangrene, and systemic and sometimes fatal electrolyte disturbances, including hypocalcemia and hypomagnesemia.[1,2]

Pathophysiology

Hydrofluoric acid "burns" are more correctly designated as chemical injuries rather than thermal burns. This form of chemical injury is often occupationally related (in those who work with glass, brick, metal, electronics, and reformulated fuels), but may also be related to household rust removers or exposure to HF solutions or vapors. These injuries have special clinical features.

Release of hydronium ions may cause local tissue damage, liquefactive necrosis, severe pain due to potassium release from nerve endings, and hyperkalemia. Systemic effects arise from deep penetration of dilute acid and subsequent release of fluoride ions, which can precipitate calcium and magnesium from soft tissues and bone.[1]

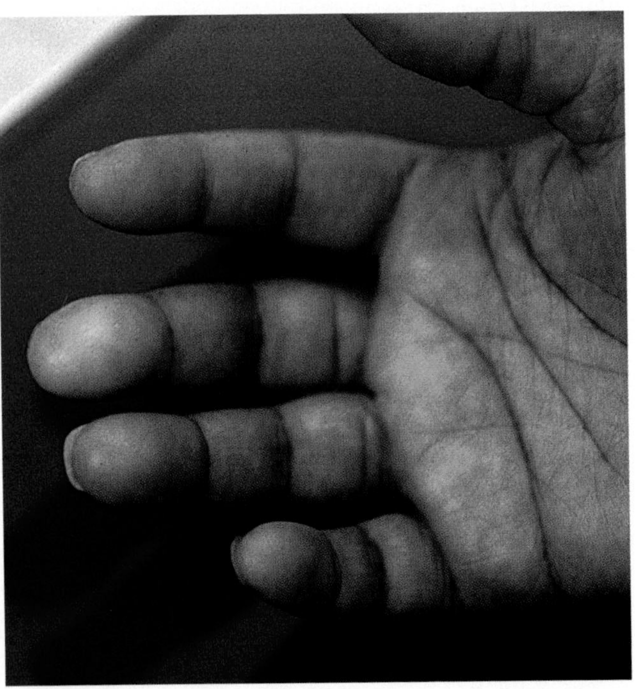

FIGURE 26–3 Burns of the digital pads caused by 3% hydrofluoric acid. (Courtesy of Richard Hamilton, MD.)

Diagnosis

A high index of suspicion and a thorough history are important, especially with exposure to more dilute and more penetrating solutions. Identification of HF, its concentration, and other substances in the solution is important, as are clinical and laboratory investigations of serum electrolytes and electrocardiographic monitoring.[1,2]

Clinical Complications

Gangrenous necrosis of skin, subcutaneous tissue, and even bone may occur, as may secondary infections. Death in fatal cases usually results from disturbances of cardiac rhythm secondary to electrolyte imbalances.[1]

Management

Prompt skin decontamination should be followed by intermittent application of iced benzalkonium chloride or iced tetracaine benzethonium chloride, which may help alleviate pain. Monitoring of electrocardiographic values and serum electrolytes is mandatory. Calcium gluconate as a topical gel or bath is considered to be only marginally helpful, because these preparations do not penetrate to the deeply involved tissues in an efficient fashion. Subcutaneous injections of calcium preparations are painful and may not penetrate deeply enough. Intravenously or intraarterially administered calcium gluconate is preferred in cases of extensive injury. Topical antibiotic creams may be used prophylactically.[1,3]

REFERENCES

1. DiLuigi KJ. Hydrofluoric acid burns. *Am J Nursing* 2001;101: 24AAA–24DDD.
2. Elder DS. An accidental acid burn: providing emergency care. *Aust Fam Physician* 2002;31:37–38.
3. Lin TM, Tsai CC, Lin SD, Lai CS. Continuous intra-arterial infusion therapy in hydrofluoric acid burns. *J Occup Environ Med* 2000; 42:892–897.

High-Pressure Injection Injury

James M. Madsen

Clinical Presentation

The index finger of the nondominant hand is most frequently affected and displays a deceptively innocuous-appearing puncture wound. The worker often underestimates the severity of the injury and continues to work until the later development of excruciating pain and swelling. Injected material may extrude from the injection site or track along the hand and forearm.[1,2]

Pathophysiology

High-pressure injection injuries typically occur in an industrial setting and may involve grease, paint, hydraulic fluid, diesel fluid, paint thinner, molding plastic, paraffin, cement, dry-cleaning solvents, water, or other substances under high pressure.[1]

Normally operating high-pressure nozzles deliver pressures of 3,000 to 7,000 pounds per square inch (psi); partial blockage of jets may increase the pressure to 12,000 psi.[1] Injected material can cause direct tissue necrosis, and the high pressures may produce ischemia from tissue distention. Secondary bacterial infection may occur in devitalized tissue.[2]

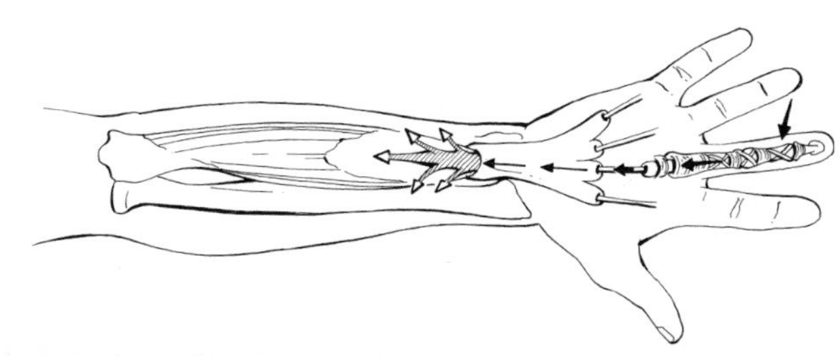

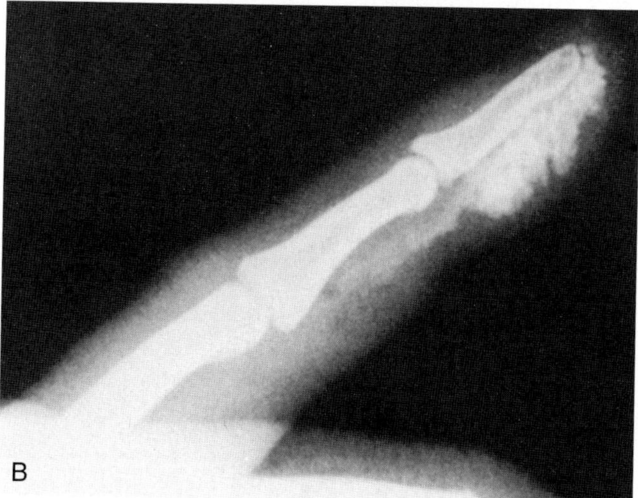

FIGURE 26–4 **A:** Palmar wounds at high pressure may spread into the proximal forearm. (From Seiler, with permission.) **B:** Radiographic appearance of high-pressure injection injury of the digit. (From Proust, with permission.)

Diagnosis

The affected area may be swollen, pale, and anesthetic, although severe pain and tenderness eventually supervene.[1] Subcutaneous emphysema may be felt at the site of the injection and also in the hand and forearm.[1] Radiographs may show air in subcutaneous tissue and in muscle.[1,2]

Clinical Complications

Secondary bacterial infection may be seen. Limb gangrene may necessitate amputation.[1,3] Pigmented material may remain in the anatomic area.[2] Significant reduction of static and dynamic muscle testing may also persist.

Management

Prompt presentation and early clinical recognition are vital.[1] Tetanus immunization should be given as indicated, and broad-spectrum antibiotics should be given prophylactically via the intravenous route while the patient is still in the emergency department.[1] Emergency department management with local incision and drainage is not appropriate, because these injuries require wide surgical exploration (including tendon sheaths and other deep structures) in the operating theater, with aggressive irrigation and débridement. The examining physician may be tempted to simply express whatever fluid was injected, by the application of lateral pressure to the wound margins. This practice is mentioned only so that it may be completely condemned as being inappropriate.[2] In some cases, amputation of the affected part and/or extensive physical rehabilitation are necessary.

REFERENCES

1. Schnall SB, Mirzayan R. High-pressure injection injuries to the hand. *Hand Clin* 1999;15:245–248.
2. Gutowski KA, Chu J, Choi M, et al. High-pressure hand injection injuries caused by dry cleaning solvents: case reports, review of the literature, and treatment guidelines. *Plast Reconstr Surg* 2003;111:174–177.

26–5

Hypothenar Hammer Syndrome

Michael Greenberg

Clinical Presentation

Patients present with days to weeks of acute hand (palmar) pain and swelling in the hypothenar region of the dominant hand. Some present with symptoms in the nondominant hand.[1-3]

Pathophysiology

Hypothenar hammer syndrome (HHS) is a syndrome involving unilateral digital ischemia caused by digital artery occlusions. This is a result of embolization from the palmar artery, caused by the repeated use of the palmar surface of the hand as a blunt force "tool."[1-3]

The pathophysiology of this injury requires direct, forceful, and repeated trauma to the palm of the hand. It is theorized that embolic occlusion of the digital and other small arteries in the hand may originate from a damaged or thrombosed palmar ulnar artery, resulting from this mechanism of injury. Fibromuscular dysplasia is evident in the affected ulnar arteries.[2]

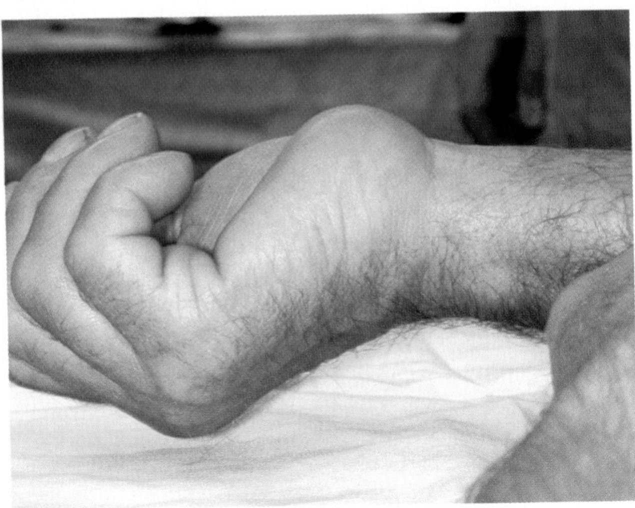

FIGURE 26–5 Note swelling of hypothenar eminence. (Courtesy of Don Fortin, MD.)

Diagnosis

The diagnosis is based on a history of repeated direct trauma to the palmar surface of the hand. This usually occurs in an occupational setting with the use of the hand to align lumber, hammer, or drive materials together. However, this mechanism of injury may also occur in hobbyists and in people who engage in carpentry or similar work as an avocation.[1-3] HHS also occurs in baseball catchers, when the hand is repeatedly subjected to impact from catching a hard-thrown ball. A unilateral Raynaud's phenomenon that spares the thumb and feet may be manifest, and in some cases a palmar mass is evident.[1,2] The diagnosis is verified by angiography. Recently, ultrasound has been used to demonstrate ulnar artery thrombosis in HHS.[3]

Clinical Complications

Complications include the development of aneurysmal dilatation of the ulnar artery, as well as embolic damage to the distal digits that is part and parcel of the HHS itself.

Management

Therapeutic interventions may include oral sympatholytic drugs (phenoxybenzamine, reserpine, calcium-channel blockers), stellate ganglion blockade, local thrombolysis, microvascular surgical reconstruction, and sympathectomy. In addition, patients should be counseled to cease using the hand as a hammering tool and to reduce vascular effects by smoking cessation. Patients identified in the emergency department should be appropriately counseled and referred to an orthopedic or plastic surgeon who specializes in hand surgery.

REFERENCES

1. Wong GB, Whetzel TP. Hypothenar hammer syndrome: review and case report. *Vasc Surg* 2001;35:163–166.
2. Ferris BL, Taylor LM Jr, Oyama K, et al. Hypothenar hammer syndrome: proposed etiology. *J Vasc Surg* 2000;31:104–113.
3. Dean Okereke C, Knight S, McGowan A, Coral A. Hypothenar hammer syndrome diagnosed by ultrasound. *Injury* 1999;30:448–449.

Vibration-Related Disorders

James M. Madsen

Clinical Presentation

Whole-body vibration, usually between 5 to 30 frequency, occurs in commercial-vehicle drivers and others and may manifest as vision problems and low-back pain.[2] Segmental vibration of 200 to 500 Hz affects the upper extremities, resulting in attacks of Raynaud's-like sensorineural (neurologic) and vascular impairment lasting from 15 minutes to 2 hours.[1]

Pathophysiology

Vibration-related disorders include adverse health effects from whole-body or segmental vibration. The most well-defined clinical entity associated with vibration is hand-arm vibration syndrome (HAVS), which is also known as Raynaud's phenomenon of occupational origin.[1] It was previously called vibration white fingers.

Segmental vibration is postulated to induce overactivity of the sympathetic nervous system or a local digital vascular fault. Either way, vasoconstriction of digital arteries leads to an altered "hunting reaction" characterized by hypoperfusion of the fingers followed by vasodilatation, although the vasodilatation may be minimal in HAVS.[1]

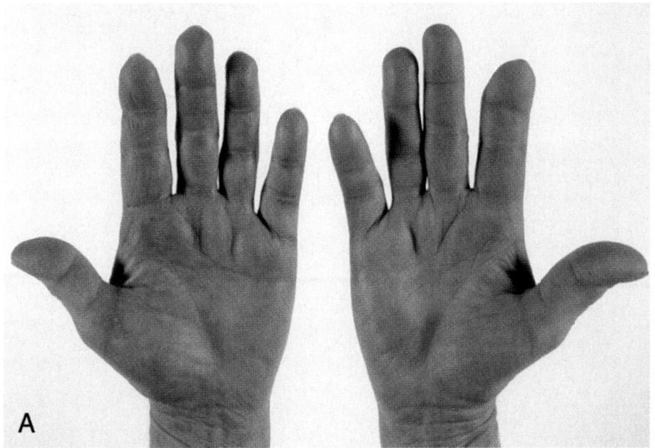

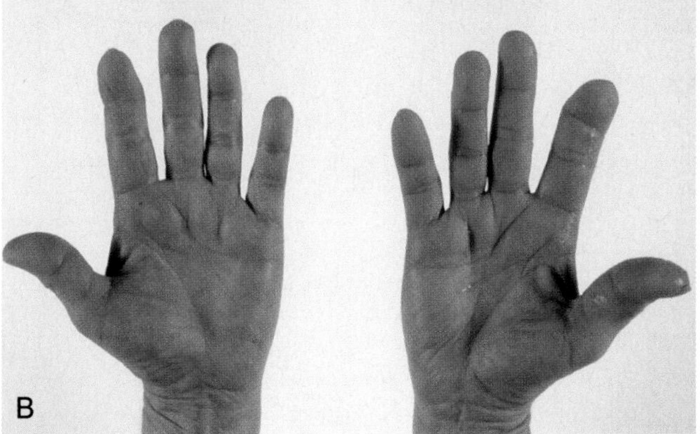

FIGURE 26–6 CREST syndrome: **C**alcinosis, **R**aynaud's phenomenon, **e**sophageal dysmotility, **s**clerodactyly, and **t**elangiectasias. **A:** The patient's fingertips are cyanotic at room temperature. **B:** After the patient has soaked her hands in warm water, the bluish color disappears. (**A** and **B,** From Yamada, with permission.)

Diagnosis

Aids in the diagnosis of HAVS include history (onset may be as rapid as 3 months), cold-provocation testing involving observation of finger color and measurement of finger systolic blood pressure, nerve-conduction studies, and vibrometry testing. The Stockholm scale establishes separate grading criteria for the vascular and neurologic manifestations of the disease.[1,2]

Clinical Complications

HAVS may occur concurrently with carpal tunnel syndrome (CTS) and can mimic it; whether CTS may develop as a complication of HAVS is still unclear.[3] There also appears to be an association between HAVS and hearing loss.

Management

Avoidance or minimization of vibration, including work transfer as needed, is the mainstay of treatment for HAVS. Maintenance of core and hand temperature is helpful, as is night splinting. Medications include calcium-channel blockers and, to reduce platelet deposition, pentoxifylline. Surgical release of the flexor retinaculum may help associated CTS but does not alleviate vascular symptoms.[3]

REFERENCES

1. Issever H, Aksoy C, Sabuncu H, et al. Vibration and its effects on the body. *Med Princ Pract* 2003;12:34–38.
2. Olsen N. Diagnostic aspects of vibration-induced white finger. *Int Arch Occup Environ Health* 2002;75:6–13.
3. Falkiner S. Diagnosis and treatment of hand-arm vibration syndrome and its relationship to carpal tunnel syndrome. *Aust Fam Physician* 2003;32:530–534.

Carpal Tunnel Syndrome

James M. Madsen

Clinical Presentation

Pain, numbness, and tingling in the distribution of the median nerve are classic symptoms, but numbness involving all of the fingers may be more common. Symptoms are usually worse at night and may awaken patients from sleep.[1] Pain and paresthesias may radiate up to the shoulder, and decreased grip strength may progress to atrophy of the thenar musculature.[1]

Pathophysiology

Carpal tunnel syndrome (CTS) is a focal peripheral neuropathy that involves compression of the carpal tunnel in the wrists and resulting compression of the median nerve.

Compression of the carpal tunnel probably causes pain by neural ischemia rather than physical damage to the nerve. The compression may result from edema, which is associated with repetitive motion or with a number of concurrent conditions, including diabetes mellitus, hypothyroidism, various rheumatologic and inflammatory diseases, obesity, and acute trauma.[3]

Diagnosis

History is important. Phalen's test and Tinel's sign are positive in many hand conditions. Magnetic resonance imaging is reasonably discriminatory, unlike plain radiography. Electromyography and nerve-conduction studies are plagued by false-positive and false-negative findings; they are most useful for confirming the diagnosis in suspected cases and for excluding neuropathy and other nerve entrapments.[2]

Clinical Complications

Chronic hand pain, paresthesias, and weakness may lead to long-term disability, especially in workers with severe symptoms. Iatrogenic injury to the median nerve may occur during attempts to inject corticosteroids into the carpal tunnel.

Management

Ergonomic counseling and modifications of work practices may minimize precipitating factors, as may treatment of coexisting related disorders. Nonsteroidal antiinflammatory medications (NSAIDs) and pyridoxine have not been demonstrated to be helpful, but splinting, corticosteroid injections into the carpal tunnel, and, in refractory cases, surgical carpal-tunnel release are beneficial.[2]

REFERENCES

1. Viera AJ. Management of carpal tunnel syndrome. *Am Fam Physician* 2003;68:265–272.
2. Katz JN, Simmons BP. Clinical practice: carpal tunnel syndrome. *N Engl J Med* 2002;346:1807–1812.
3. Atcheson SG, Ward JR, Lowe W. Concurrent medical disease in work-related carpal tunnel syndrome. *Arch Intern Med* 1998;158: 1506–1512.

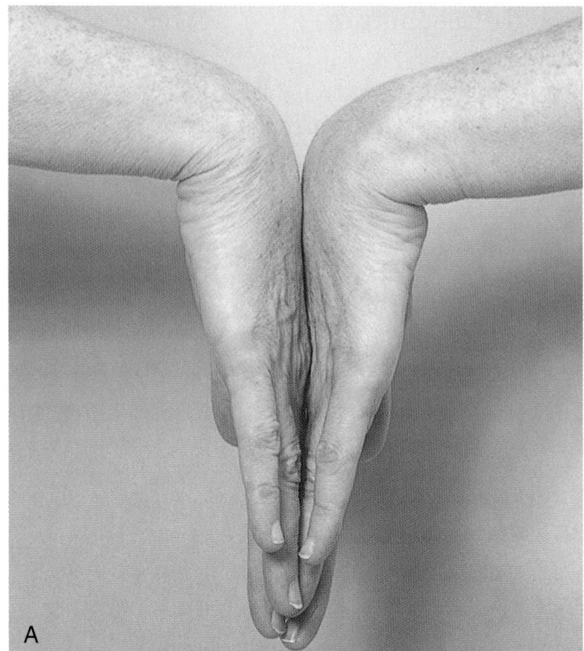

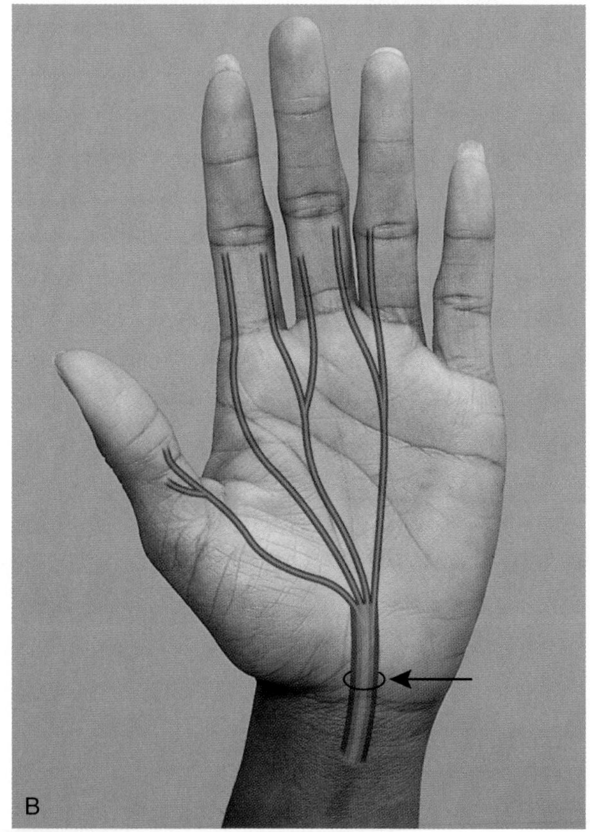

FIGURE 26–7 **A:** Phalen's test is positive if numbness and tingling develop on the palmar surface of the first four digits on flexion of both wrists for 60 seconds. **B:** Tinel's sign is positive if tingling develops on the palmar surface of the first four digits with percussion over the wrist *(arrow)*. (**A** and **B,** From Bickley, with permission.)

Occupational Irritant Contact Dermatitis

James M. Madsen

Clinical Presentation

Typically, occupational irritant contact dermatitis (ICD) is localized, affects workers who have a predisposition to atopy, has a latent period ranging from minutes or hours (with strong irritants) to months (with weak irritants), is characterized by red and scaling fissures, is photopatch negative, and may be chronic.[1] Workers with prolonged exposure to water or to chemicals in solution are particularly at risk.[1–3]

Pathophysiology

Occupational irritant contact dermatitis is usually considered to be a nonimmunologic cutaneous inflammatory response resulting from exposure to one or more exogenous chemical or physical agents found in a workplace setting.[2]

Although immunologic responses may be involved in ICD, the process usually begins without previous sensitization. Direct cytotoxicity or disruption of keratins or lipids in the stratum corneum induces the release of inflammatory cytokines, of which tumor necrosis factor-α is probably the most important for ICD. However, cytokines associated with allergic contact dermatitis may also play a role.[1]

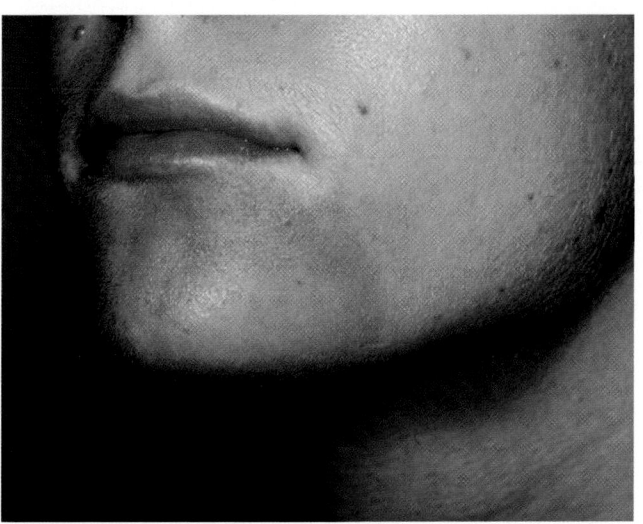

FIGURE 26–8 Irritant contact dermatitis. The localized erythema on this boy's face was caused by irritation from benzoyl peroxide. (From Goodheart, with permission.)

Diagnosis

The history, correlation of anatomic site with potential exposure, a negative patch test, and serum immunoglobulin E (for atopy) help make the diagnosis of ICD. Skin biopsy may show parakeratosis or spongiosis. Nonoccupational causes must be excluded, and putative workplace irritants must be investigated.[1]

Clinical Complications

Rubbing of pruritic lesions of occupational ICD may result in increased absorption of workplace chemicals, chronic lichenification, or secondary infections by bacteria or fungi.

Management

Barrier creams may be more effective than moisturizers, but no barrier cream offers universal protection. Topical corticosteroids such as amcinonide may be helpful, as may phototherapy. Antibiotics are used for secondary bacterial infections. Further exposure must be reduced by engineering or administrative controls and by the use of personal protective equipment such as gloves.[2]

REFERENCES

1. Antezana M, Parker F. Occupational contact dermatitis. *Immunol Allergy Clin North Am* 2003;23:269–290.
2. Chew AL, Maibach HI. Occupational issues of irritant contact dermatitis. *Int Arch Occup Environ Health* 2003;76:339–346.
3. Gould D. Occupational irritant contact dermatitis. *Nurs Stand* 2003;17:53–56, 58, 60.

Occupational Allergic Contact Dermatitis

James M. Madsen

Clinical Presentation

Typically, occupational allergic contact dermatitis (ACD) spreads, has a latent period of 24 to 72 hours, involves vesicles acutely, is photopatch positive, and may clear if diagnosed early. However, it may also become persistent.[1] Workers in almost any occupation can be affected.

Pathophysiology

Occupational allergic contact dermatitis is an immunologically mediated cutaneous inflammatory response resulting from exposure to one or more exogenous chemical or physical agents found in a workplace setting.

ACD requires a sensitization phase in which haptens interact with Langerhans cells in the epidermis. Antigen is then presented to CD45RA+ cells in regional lymph nodes, activating T cells to become memory and effector cells. Rechallenge with antigen begins the elicitation phase, in which activated T cells release inflammatory cytokines and other inflammatory mediators.[1]

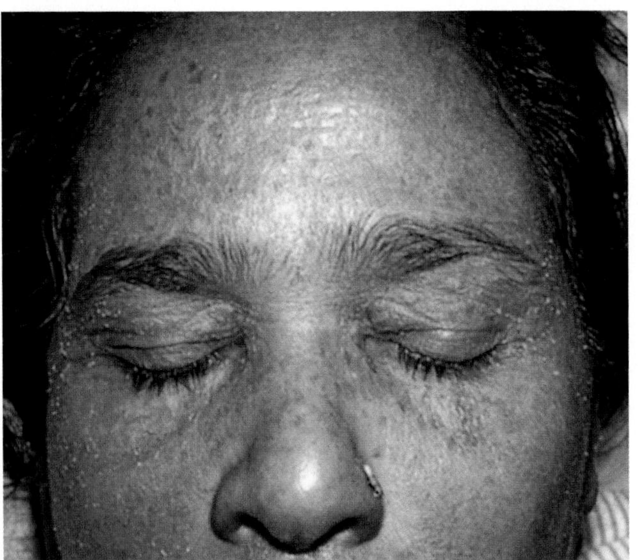

FIGURE 26–9 Acute allergic contact dermatitis from exposure to hair dye. (From Ostler, with permission.)

Diagnosis

Diagnosis of ACD depends on patient history (including exposure history), the pattern of dermatitis, and proper diagnostic patch testing. Patch testing may need to be specific to the putative allergen and should be interpreted by trained and experienced clinicians.[1–3] Exclusion of nonoccupational exposures and identification of specific workplace allergens then define occupational ACD.

Clinical Complications

Occupational ACD may become chronic and may persist or recur even after removal from the work environment. Secondary bacterial or fungal infection may ensue. Iatrogenic ACD may appear after treatment with topical antihistamines.

Management

Oral antihistamines such as hydroxyzine, cool compresses, and topical steroids such as clobetasol, prednisone, and triamcinolone are useful. Systemic corticosteroids may be required in severe cases. Psoralen plus ultraviolet-A (PUVA) therapy and immunosuppressive agents such as azathioprine or cyclosporine are used in refractory cases. Nickel ACD may require treatment with disulfuram.[1–3]

REFERENCES

1. Antezana M, Parker F. Occupational contact dermatitis. *Immunol Allergy Clin North Am* 2003;23:269–290.
2. Andersen KE. Occupational issues of allergic contact dermatitis. *Int Arch Occup Environ Health* 2003;76:347–350.
3. Gawkrodger DJ. Patch testing in occupational dermatology. *Occup Environ Med* 2001;58:823–828.

Occupational Infectious Dermatoses

James M. Madsen

Clinical Presentation

Occupational skin infections usually manifest as one or more skin lesions with the cardinal sign of inflammation, but they can be painless, such as the skin lesion in anthrax. There are scores of infectious dermatoses that can be acquired occupationally—usually, but not always, in outdoor occupations—and the clinical appearance of the lesions is usually disease specific.[1,2]

Pathophysiology

Occupational infectious dermatoses are skin infections that result from exposure to infectious agents in the workplace. They may be acquired by skin contact, or they may arise as cutaneous manifestations of infection acquired via other routes.

The pathophysiology of skin infections depends on the specific agent or agents but usually involves either penetration of microorganisms into the skin from the environment or dissemination of organisms in the blood to the skin.[1,2]

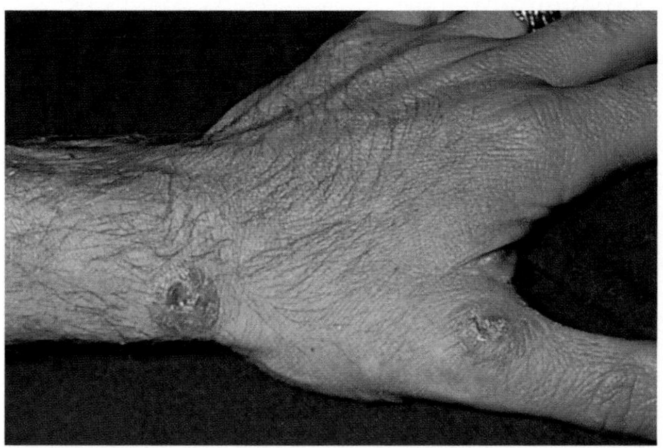

FIGURE 26–10 Sporotrichosis in a gardener. (From Ostler, with permission.)

Diagnosis

Clinical suspicion of any cutaneous infection should prompt a detailed history, including occupational exposure history. Secondary bacterial or fungal infection in a patient with contact dermatitis may be related to the workplace. Fungal or bacterial cultures, biopsies, and worksite visits may be needed.

Clinical Complications

Many occupationally acquired skin infections are self-limited, but many are either the cutaneous manifestations of systemic disease or reach the circulation to cause systemic disease, including sepsis.

Management

After clinical or laboratory identification of the causative organism or organisms, treatment with the appropriate antibiotic, antifungal, or antiviral agent is indicated. Infection-control precautions appropriate to the infection must be observed, and an investigation into patient contacts and potentially affected coworkers is vital to address the source of the infection.[1,2]

REFERENCES

1. Bhumbra NA, McCullough SG. Skin and subcutaneous infections. *Prim Care* 2003;30:1–24.
2. Pittet D, Dharan S, Touveneau S, et al. Bacterial contamination of the hands of hospital staff during routine patient care. *Arch Intern Med* 1999;159:821–826.

Erysipeloid

Michael Greenberg

Clinical Presentation

Erysipeloid is an occupational infectious disease seen in fishermen, butchers, and poultry dressers. Patients present with painful skin lesions several days to 1 week after exposure.[1]

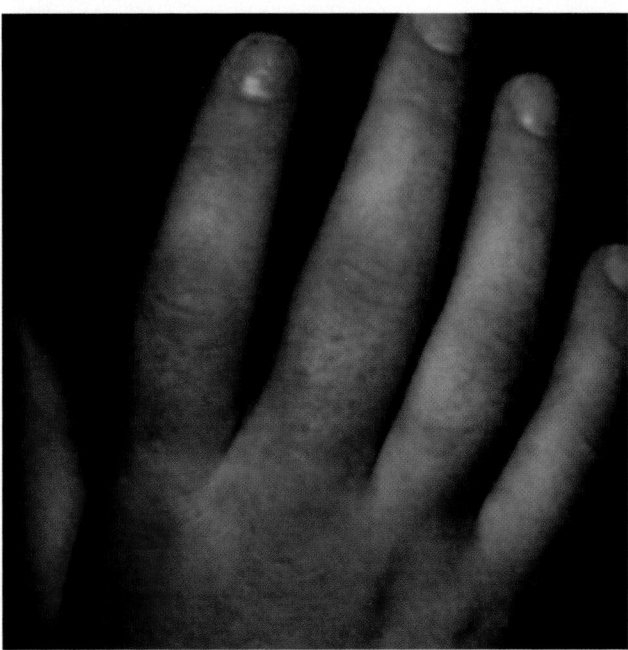

FIGURE 26–11 Erysipeloid. Approximately 3 days after animal or fish contact, a dull red erythema appears at the inoculation site and extends centrifugally. (From Habif, with permission.)

Pathophysiology

The causative organism for erysipeloid, *Erysipelothrix rhusiopathiae,* is a gram-positive, rod-shaped bacteria that infects freshwater and saltwater fish and shellfish as well as poultry. The mode of spread for the infection to human workers is through minor breaks in the skin.[1]

Diagnosis

The diagnosis is based on a carefully obtained work history in conjunction with the identification of painful, raised, purplish papules, usually on the hands. Papules may increase in size and take the form of demarcated, painful, purple-red plaques. At this stage, patients may have lymphangitis as well as lymphadenopathy, fever, and diffuse joint pain.[1]

Clinical Complications

Complications may include septicemia, endocarditis, and secondary local infection.

Management

Skin lesions tend to resolve spontaneously over the course of several weeks, and local care of lesions is essential. Penicillin is effective in curing the disease and eradicating the organism.[1]

REFERENCES

1. Grieco MH, Sheldon C. Erysipelothrix rhusiopathiae. *Ann N Y Acad Sci* 1970;174:523–532.

Silicosis

James M. Madsen

Clinical Presentation

Acute silicosis occurs within 2 years after exposure and manifests with severe dyspnea, cough, fever, and weight loss. Both accelerated silicosis (developing within 5 to 15 years) and chronic silicosis (with a latent period of 2 decades or more) involve the formation of silicotic nodules in the lung. Symptoms may be absent but may include dyspnea, cough, and constitutional symptoms.

Pathophysiology

Silicosis is a pneumoconiosis that is caused by inhalation of dust containing crystalline silica (silicon dioxide) or its less widely distributed polymorphic forms, tridymite or cristobalite.[1]

Alveolar macrophages that have phagocytosed inhaled silica crystals die and release cytotoxic enzymes that lead to accumulation of lipid- and protein-rich fluid (in acute and accelerated silicosis) and the development of fibrotic nodules (in chronic silicosis).[1,2]

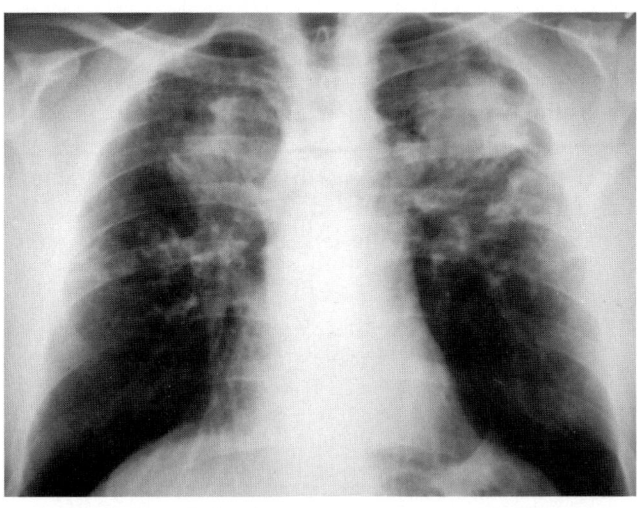

FIGURE 26–12 Chest radiograph shows progressive massive fibrosis in a patient with silicosis. Large, mass-like opacities are present in both upper lobes. There is bilateral hilar retraction and basilar hyperlucency. (From Rom, with permission.)

Diagnosis

The occupational history is crucial. Chest radiography demonstrates pulmonary infiltrates in acute silicosis and nodular densities in chronic silicosis. The nodules are smaller than 1 cm in diameter in simple silicosis and larger in complicated silicosis (progressive massive fibrosis, or PMF). Nodules are primarily in the upper lobes. "Eggshell" calcification of mediastinal lymph nodes may be apparent.

Clinical Complications

Acute silicosis may cause death from silicolipoproteinosis. Silicosis may lead to impaired cell-mediated immunity and increases the risk for development of tuberculosis (with cavitation of silicotic nodules), autoimmune diseases (including rheumatoid arthritis), and chronic obstructive pulmonary disease. Bronchogenic carcinoma may occur after large exposures to silica.[1–3]

Management

Bronchoalveolar lavage has been advocated for acute silicosis. Removal from exposure and cessation of smoking is important, as is oxygen administration and treatment of cor pulmonale in advanced cases. The worker must be medically monitored to detect deteriorating lung function and other complications of silicosis.

REFERENCES

1. Ding M, Chen F, Shi X, et al. Diseases caused by silica: mechanisms of injury and disease development. *Int Immunopharmacol* 2002;2: 173–182.
2. Hnizdo E, Vallyathan V. Chronic obstructive pulmonary disease due to occupational exposure to silica dust: a review of epidemiological and pathological evidence. *Occup Environ Med* 2003;60:237–243.
3. Calvert GM, Rice FL, Boiano JM, et al. Occupational silica exposure and risk of various diseases: an analysis using death certificates from 27 states of the United States. *Occup Envron Med* 2003;60: 122–129.

Asbestosis

James M. Madsen

Clinical Presentation

After a latent period (usually 20 to 40 years), bilateral interstitial fibrosis of pulmonary parenchyma occurs. Related symptoms may include progressive dyspnea on exertion and a dry cough.

Pathophysiology

Asbestosis refers to pneumoconiotic pulmonary fibrosis caused by inhalation of asbestos.[1]

By reason of shape, size, friability, and prolonged biopersistence, amphibole asbestos fibers are the most pathogenic type of asbestos fibers. Fiber injury to epithelial mesothelial cells appears to be related to the production of oxidants and reactive oxygen intermediates, interactions among damaged cells, and release of cytokines.[2]

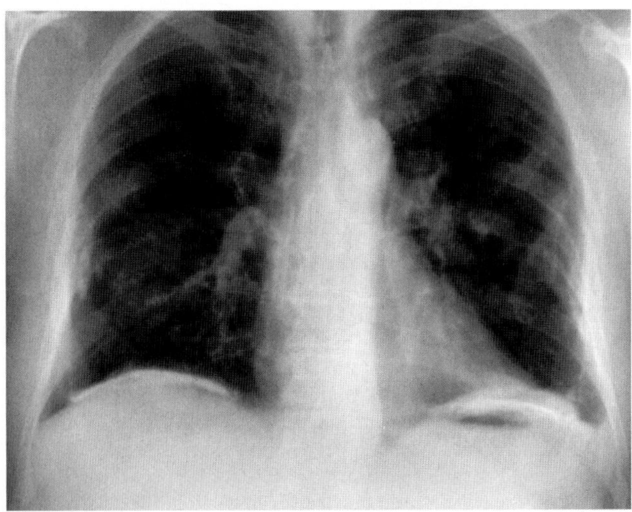

FIGURE 26–13 Discrete, circumscribed pleural plaques with calcification along both chest walls and on top of the diaphragm in a worker who was exposed to asbestos for 2 years in a World War II shipyard. (From Rom, with permission.)

Diagnosis

Asbestosis is diagnosed by a history of exposure combined with radiologic demonstration of interstitial fibrosis (graded according to the International Labour Office [ILO] B-reader classification). High-resolution computed tomography may be particularly useful. Other associated asbestos-related findings, such as pleural plaques, do not define asbestosis. Histologic analysis may show iron- and protein-coated asbestos fibers, but biopsy is not mandatory.[1]

Clinical Complications

Asbestos exposure may lead to a variety of conditions depending on fiber type, fiber size, and the nature, character, and degree of the exposure. These conditions include asbestosis (with progressively decreasing pulmonary function), proliferation of pleural tissue (pleural thickening and plaques, rounded atelectasis, pleural effusions, and mesothelioma), and bronchogenic carcinoma, which, unlike mesothelioma, is synergistic with smoking.[1,3]

Management

Neither steroids nor immunosuppressive agents have demonstrated utility in treating asbestosis. Removal from exposure is usually a moot point, given that the clinically relevant exposures may have occurred decades earlier. Patients with advanced disease may require supplemental oxygen and treatment for cor pulmonale. Immunizations, smoking cessation, and medical monitoring are essential.

REFERENCES

1. Roach HD, Davies GJ, Attanoos R, et al. Asbestos—when the dust settles: an imaging review of asbestos-related disease. *Radiographics* 2002;22(Spec No):S167–S184.
2. Manning CB, Vallyathan V, Mossman BT. Diseases caused by asbestos: mechanisms of injury and disease development. *Int Immunopharmacol* 2002;2:191–200.
3. Weiss W. Asbestosis: a marker for the increased risk of lung cancer among workers exposed to asbestos. *Chest* 1999;115:536–549.

Berylliosis

James M. Madsen

Clinical Presentation

Beryllium exposure can lead to an acute chemical pneumonitis (mostly of historical interest) and to berylliosis, which is characterized symptomatically by progressive dyspnea with or without cough, chest pain, arthralgia, and fatigue. There may be weight loss, and the physical examination may reveal inspiratory crackles, lymphadenopathy, an exanthem, and hepatosplenomegaly.[1]

Pathophysiology

Berylliosis, or chronic beryllium disease (CBD), is a sarcoidosis-like, granulomatous lung disease caused by exposure to beryllium.

Berylliosis occurs in association with human leukocyte antigen HLA-DPB1 alleles that contain glutamine at position 69 in up to 97% of patients (but also 30% to 40% of controls). It is a hypersensitivity disorder maintained by beryllium-specific CD4+ T-helper lymphocytes, which respond to a beryllium-associated peptide by producing interleukin-2 and interferon-γ, leading to granuloma formation.[2,3]

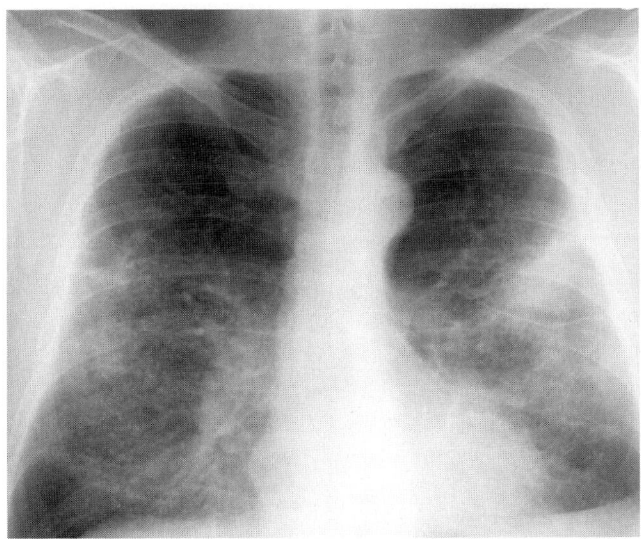

FIGURE 26–14 Posteroanterior chest radiograph of a patient with advanced chronic beryllium disease, caused by past exposure to beryllium oxide ceramic dust. The radiograph illustrates diffuse nodular opacities, formation of conglomerate masses with adjacent areas of emphysema, subpleural thickening, reticular lines and honeycombing, and bilateral hilar adenopathy. (From Rom, with permission.)

Diagnosis

Diagnosis of berylliosis depends on the demonstration of beryllium exposure, bronchoscopy, and bronchoalveolar lavage with a positive beryllium lymphocyte proliferation test (BeLPT). Biopsy may show noncaseating granulomatous lung disease. Symptoms need not be present for the diagnosis.[1]

Clinical Complications

Granulomata may develop in extrapulmonary locations. In the lung, granulomata may enlarge and lead to progressive fibrosis, restrictive findings on pulmonary function tests, and death. Clinical progression is currently unpredictable.[1]

Management

Pulmonary parenchymal involvement can be characterized according to the International Labour Office [ILO] B-reading classification. Removal from workplace exposure may or may not halt disease progression but is recommended. Pharmacologic treatment, which may need to be maintained for life, includes systemic corticosteroids (e.g., prednisone) and methotrexate.[1]

REFERENCES

1. Maier LA. Clinical approach to chronic beryllium disease and other nonpneumoconiotic interstitial lung diseases. *J Thorac Imaging* 2002;17:273–284.
2. Rossman MD. Chronic beryllium disease: a hypersensitivity disorder. *Appl Occup Environ Hyg* 2001;16:615–618.
3. Saltini C, Amicosante M. Beryllium disease. *Am J Med Sci* 2001;321: 89–98.

Pneumoconioses

James M. Madsen

Clinical Presentation

The clinical and radiologic findings vary somewhat, according to the specific type of pneumoconiosis, but typical clinical features range from lack of symptoms in early stages to inspiratory crackles, dyspnea, and a restrictive ventilatory defect.[2]

Pathophysiology

Pneumoconioses are "non-neoplastic reactions of the lungs to inhaled mineral or organic dusts, and the resultant alteration in their structure, excluding asthma, bronchitis and emphysema."[1] They include not only the so-called benign pneumoconioses, such as siderosis, baritosis, and stannosis, but also silicosis, coal-worker's pneumoconiosis, asbestosis, and hard-metal pneumoconioses.

Macrophages that have phagocytosed inhaled dust particles release lysosomal enzymes and inflammatory cytokines that recruit inflammatory cells and induce an alveolitis that damages the pulmonary architecture. This leads to a reparative process characterized by the release of growth factors that induce fibrosis.[3]

Diagnosis

The diagnosis is made based on a history of probable exposure to a specific dust, an appropriate latent period, and radiologic evidence of diffuse parenchymal pulmonary disease with features of pneumoconioses (ranked according to the International Labour Office [ILO] B-reading classification). Inspiratory crackles are often present, and pulmonary function tests may demonstrate a restrictive pattern.[2]

Clinical Complications

Pneumoconiosis may be complicated by secondary infections and may lead to severely impaired pulmonary function. Cancer (including bronchogenic carcinoma) is a known complication of asbestosis and even silicosis.

Management

No specific treatment exists for pneumoconioses. Removal from exposure to the causative dust is the mainstay of management.[2] Monitoring of disease progression and monitoring for associated diseases (e.g., rheumatoid arthritis, lung cancer, mesothelioma) is also important.[1-3]

REFERENCES

1. De Vuyst P, Camus P. The past and present of pneumoconioses. *Curr Opin Pulm Med* 2000;6:151–156.
2. Kuschner WG, Stark P. Occupational lung disease: part 2. Discovering the cause of diffuse parenchymal lung disease. *Postgrad Med* 2003;113:81–88.
3. Fujimura N. Pathology and pathophysiology of pneumoconiosis. *Curr Opin Pulm Med* 2000;6:140–144.

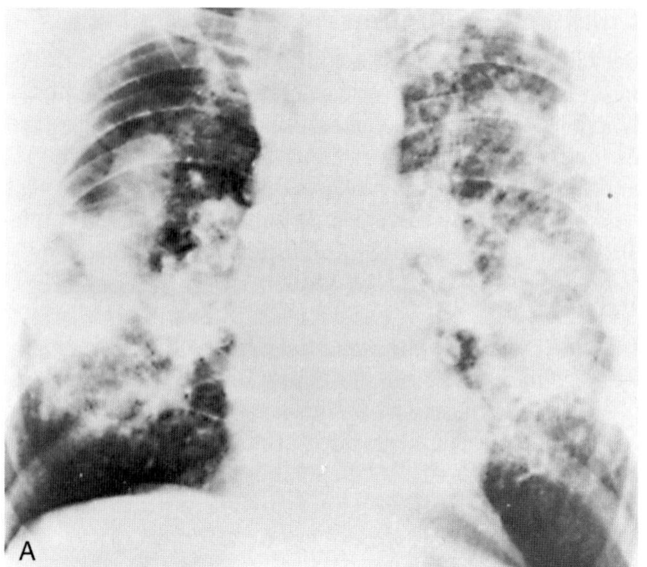

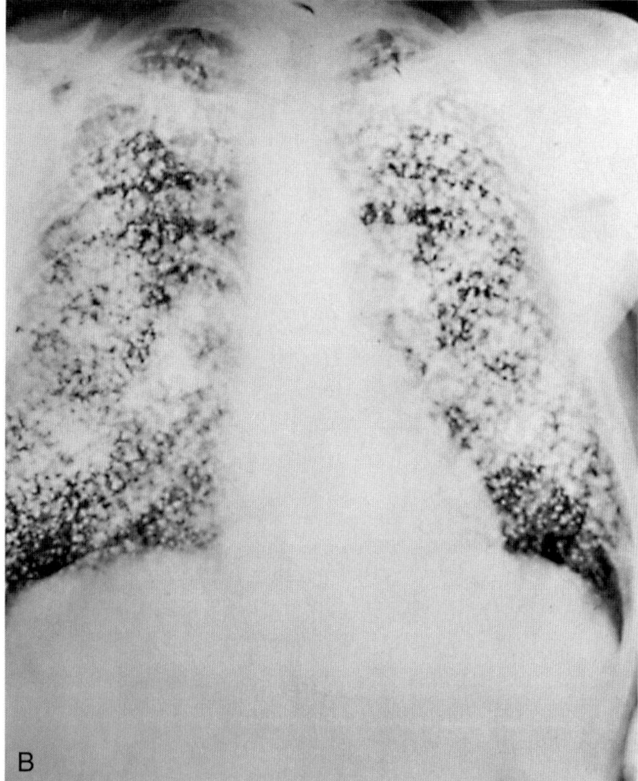

FIGURE 26–15 **A:** Progressive massive fibrosis, category C, of coal worker's pneumoconiosis. **B:** Chest radiography of an asymptomatic 46-year-old man who packaged lithopone (which contains barium sulfate and zinc sulfide) for 10 years. (**A** and **B,** From Rom, with permission.)

Hypersensitivity Pneumonitis

James M. Madsen

Clinical Presentation

Classically, acute, subacute, and chronic syndromes are described, but there is significant clinical overlap, and symptoms are often nonspecific. Patients usually are nonsmokers and report cough, dyspnea, chest tightness, wheezing, chills, and fever.[1]

Pathophysiology

Hypersensitivity pneumonitis (HP), also termed extrinsic allergic alveolitis, is the name given to a group of immune-mediated inflammatory lung diseases caused by inhalation of any of hundreds of environmental agents, usually airborne organic particulate matter such as bacteria, fungi, avian proteins, and wood dusts.[1] Most exposures in the United States are occupational.

Type III and especially type IV hypersensitivity reactions are involved, and alveolar macrophages and Th1 helper T lymphocytes react to inhaled antigens by secreting regulator mediators. This leads to a mononuclear alveolitis, noncaseating granulomata, bronchiolitis with or without organization, interstitial fibrosis, and, in advanced cases, dense fibrosis with honeycombing.[2]

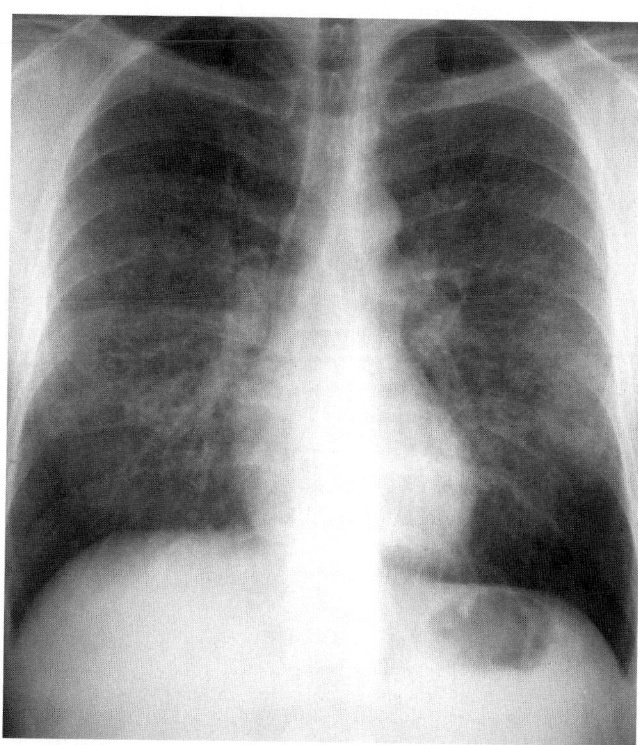

FIGURE 26–16 Posteroanterior chest radiograph showing the typical diffuse, fine, and poorly defined interstitial infiltrates in a case of recent-onset hypersensitivity pneumonitis. (From Rom, with permission.)

Diagnosis

Diagnosis may be difficult and is supported by an appropriate history (including dyspnea on exertion), inspiratory crackles, demonstration of centrilobular ground-glass or nodular opacities by high-resolution computed tomography (plain radiographic films are often normal), and the classic histologic triad (not always present) of bronchiolitis, interstitial lymphocytic infiltration, and granulomata.[2,3]

Clinical Complications

Although most patients recover after exposure termination, disease may progress to end-stage interstitial fibrosis with alveolar destruction in a honeycombing pattern, especially in bird fancier's disease.

Management

The pillar of management is protection from the inciting antigen by use of personal protective equipment (respirators) or removal from the offending work environment. Systemic steroids such as prednisone may be useful for symptomatic relief in severe or chronic disease.[2]

REFERENCES

1. Matar LD, McAdams HP, Sporn TA. Hypersensitivity pneumonitis. *AJR Am J Roentgenol* 2000;174:1061–1066.
2. Yi ES. Hypersensitivity pneumonitis. *Crit Rev Clin Lab Sci* 2002;39: 581–629.
3. Glazer CS, Rose CS, Lynch DA. Clinical and radiologic manifestations of hypersensitivity pneumonitis. *J Thorac Imaging* 2002;17: 261–272.

26-17

Metal Fume Fever

Michael Greenberg

Clinical Presentation

Patients present with malaise, fatigue, chills, muscle aches, sore throat, hoarseness, metallic taste, cough, nausea, dyspnea, and fever approximately 2 to 10 hours after inhalation of metal oxide fumes.[1-3]

Pathophysiology

Metal fume fever (MFF), also called Monday morning fever, brass chills, zinc shakes, or welders' ague, is a syndrome resulting from the unprotected inhalation of metal oxide fumes. MFF is usually an occupational illness, but it may develop in anyone not wearing respiratory protection who inhales heated metal oxide fumes.[1-3]

Several thousand cases of MFF occur in the United States annually.[1] MFF is specifically associated with zinc oxide exposure from welding of galvanized steel or brass. However, some authorities indicate that MFF may also result from exposure to the metal fumes of cadmium, tin, copper, manganese, mercury, or nickel. The latter fumes are usually associated with the development of a true chemical pneumonitis. The pathophysiology is unclear but probably reflects a direct toxic effect of fumes on pulmonary tissue. An exposure-dependent neutrophil alveolitis occurs, in association with release of tumor necrosis factor-α, interleukin-6, and interleukin-8 from pulmonary cells.[1-3]

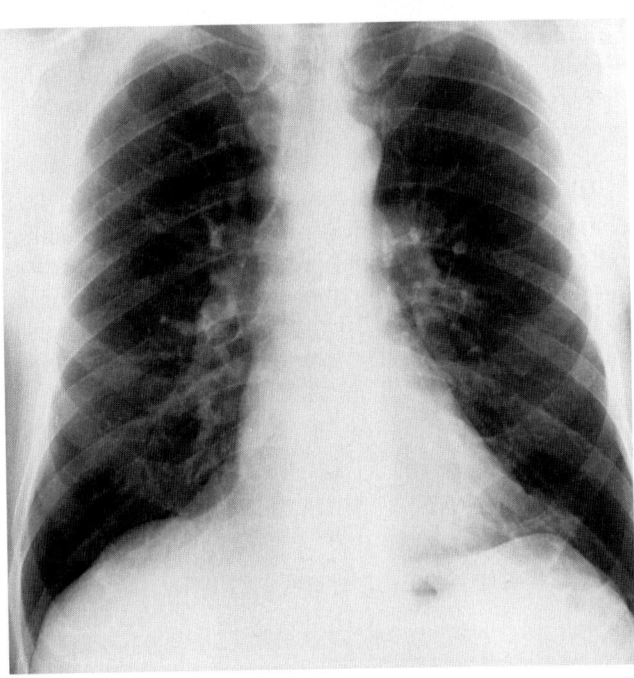

FIGURE 26–17 The chest radiographs of patients with metal fume fever are typically normal, as shown here, despite the presence of significant symptoms. (From Harris and Harris, with permission.)

Diagnosis

Diagnosis is based on history of exposure and clinical findings. MFF tends to resolve spontaneously within 24 hours. The chest radiograph is typically normal in MFF and provides an important differential point in cases with a questionable cause. Most patients exhibit a leukocytosis. A noteworthy feature of MFF is short-term tolerance, in which workers are asymptomatic with repeated exposure.[3]

Clinical Complications

Most sources indicate that there are no significant sequelae after recovery from MFF. However, some consider that occupational asthma or reactive airways dysfunction syndrome may develop after recovery from acute MFF.[1-3]

Management

Therapy requires removal from exposure, fluid hydration, moist oxygen, and bronchodilators as needed. Fever may be treated with acetaminophen or salicylates. Systemic corticosteroids may be considered in severe cases. Patients with hypoxemia or symptoms that do not abate quickly require hospitalization. Traditional chelation therapy has no role in the management of MFF.[2]

REFERENCES

1. El-Zein M, Malo JL, Infante-Rivard C, et al. Prevalence and association of welding related systemic and respiratory symptoms in welders. *Occup Environ Med* 2003;60:655–661.
2. Graeme K, Pollack CV Jr. Heavy metal toxicity: part II: Lead and metal fume fever. *J Emerg Med* 1998;16:171–177.
3. Antonini J, Lewis AB, Roberts JR, et al. Pulmonary effects of welding fumes: review of worker and experimental animal studies. *Am J Ind Med* 2003;43:350–360.

Nail Gun Injuries

Michael Greenberg

Clinical Presentation

Patients with nail gun injuries present after accidental or, in some cases, intentional injury inflicted by penetration of an industrial nail or bolt fired from a pneumatic gun device.[1-5]

Pathophysiology

Pneumatic nail gun devices are commonly used on construction sites and in residences. A standard pneumatic device fires a 3-inch nail, weighing 66.7 g, that can achieve an average velocity of 105.5 feet per second, qualifying it as a low-velocity missile.[1] The degree of penetration and tissue damage depends on the distance of the victim from the gun when fired, the surfaces through which the nail passes before striking the victim, and the specific anatomic site injured.[1-5]

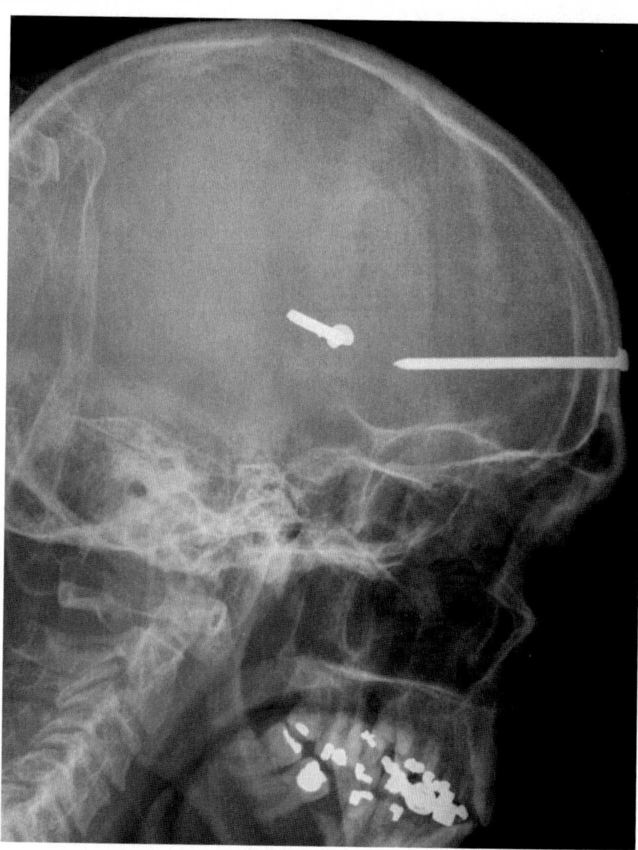

FIGURE 26–18 Pneumatic nail gun injury to the brain. (Courtesy of Robert Hendrickson, MD.)

Diagnosis

The diagnosis usually is evident from the history and physical examination. Confirmation usually is obtained with plain radiographs, although computed tomography and angiography may be required to rule in or out specific organ and vascular injuries. Magnetic resonance imaging is contraindicated while the nail is still retained in the patient.

Clinical Complications

Complications depend largely on the location of the injection injury and the anatomic structures involved. Disability and death have been reported after various nail gun injuries.[1-5]

Management

Advanced trauma life support (ATLS) protocols should be followed, because these injuries represent potentially serious penetrating trauma. Antibiotics need to be considered based on the circumstances of the injury and the patient's underlying medical condition. If removal of an imbedded nail is considered in the emergency department, it should be remembered that many of the nails used with pneumatic firing devices are barbed, making removal a challenge. Removal of nails in extremities is reasonable in the emergency department; however, injuries to the eyes, face, abdomen, or chest usually require admission and surgical removal in the operating theater.

REFERENCES

1. Buchalter GM, Johnson LP, Reichman MV, et al. Penetrating trauma to the head and neck from a nail gun: a unique mechanism of injury. *Ear Nose Throat J* 2002;81:779–783.
2. Nizam I, Choong PF. The nail gun: injuries to the knee and chest. *Injury* 2003;34:240–241.
3. Lipscomb HJ, Dement JM, Nolan J, et al. Nail gun injuries in residential carpentry: lessons from active injury surveillance. *Inj Prev* 2003;9:20–24.
4. Beaver AC, Cheatham ML. Life-threatening nail gun injuries. *Am Surg* 1999;65:1113–1116.
5. Dement JM, Lipscomb H, Li L, et al. Nail gun injuries among construction workers. *Appl Occup Environ Hyg* 2003;18:374–383.

Prepatellar Bursitis

James M. Madsen

Clinical Presentation

Patients presenting with prepatellar bursitis after acute trauma or chronic kneeling may have redness, tenderness, and swelling anterior to the patella. Mild fever may be present, but joint movement is preserved and relatively painless.[1]

Pathophysiology

Prepatellar bursitis, also called housemaid's knee, coal miner's knee, or carpet layer's knee, is an inflammation of the prepatellar bursa.[2] It is common in workers, including roofers, plumbers, and carpenters, who spend significant time kneeling during the course of their work.[3]

Either acute trauma or chronic repetitive trauma to the knee can result in local vasodilation and increased vascular permeability, extravasation of fluid and proteins into the bursa, and consequent stimulation of the inflammatory cascade and activation of leukocytes.[2]

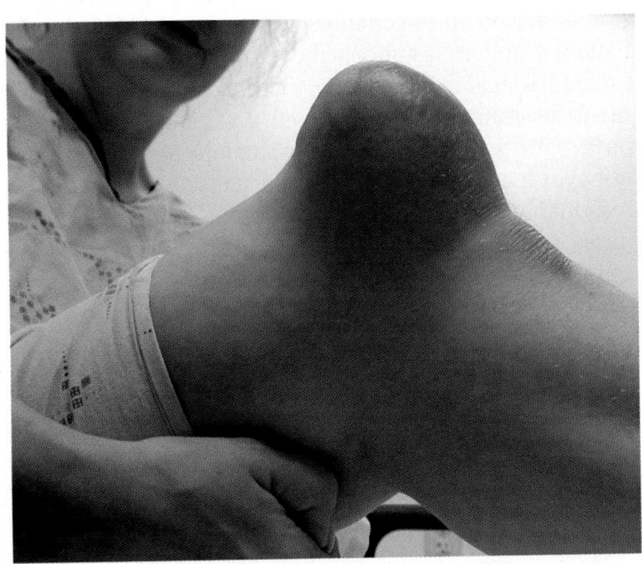

FIGURE 26–19 Prepatellar bursitis. (Courtesy of Ralph Weiche, MD.)

Diagnosis

A history of acute trauma or an occupational history of repeated kneeling, in conjunction with the clinical findings, suggests prepatellar bursitis. Joint aspiration should always be performed if septic bursitis is suspected.[2]

Clinical Complications

Disability may result from the localized pain. The most important complication is septic arthritis, which may arise especially in connection with any breaks in the skin.

Management

Protection by padding or postural adjustment is the definitive treatment. Symptomatic treatment includes relative (active) rest (alternative exercise), ice, compression, elevation, medication (nonsteroidal antiinflammatory drugs and judicious intrabursal injection of a corticosteroid such as betamethasone or triamcinolone), and physical modalities such as ultrasound and high-voltage electrical stimulation.[2]

REFERENCES

1. Golledge C. Carpet layer's knee. *Aust Fam Physician* 1998;27:415.
2. Butcher JD, Salzman KL, Lillegard WA. Lower extremity bursitis. *Am Fam Physician* 1996;53:2317–2324.
3. Jensen LK, Mikkelsen S, Loft IP, et al. Work-related knee disorders in floor layers and carpenters. *J Occup Environ Med* 2000;42:835–842.

Needlestick Injuries

James M. Madsen

Clinical Presentation

The presentation of patients with various blood-borne infections differs according to specific infection, but affected health care workers (HCWs) usually are asymptomatic at the time of presentation (most often within hours after the needlestick injury). A small puncture wound may be evident, with little bleeding or surrounding inflammation. A strong psychological component may be present, even if clinically inapparent.

Pathophysiology

Needlestick injuries are events, usually occurring in a hospital setting, that involve risk of harm from injection (usually inadvertent) by a needle previously used to penetrate the skin of a potentially infectious patient. The potential harm is that of transmission of infection by blood-borne pathogens, mainly hepatitis C virus (HCV), hepatitis B virus (HBV), and human immunodeficiency virus (HIV).[1]

The risks of developing HCV, HBV, or HIV from a single needlestick exposure to blood from an infected source are approximately 30%, 3%, and 0.3%, respectively.[1] The specific pathophysiology and incubation period vary by specific agent. The risks of other diseases also vary by specific disease.

Diagnosis

Diagnosis is made by history and includes an assessment of potential risk based on the circumstances of exposure (volume of blood involved, severity of exposure, pathogen involved, degree of viremia, and immune status of the HCW).[1] Blood (and, as applicable, urine for pregnancy testing) from the HCW should be submitted for analysis, as should blood from the source, if known.[2,3]

Clinical Complications

Depending on the agent, liver dysfunction, acquired immunodeficiency syndrome (AIDS), cancer, and other complications are potential risks. Secondary bacterial infection is rare but may occur.[1–3]

Management

Exposure reporting is mandated by the Occupational Safety and Health Administration (OSHA) for most emergency-department settings. Exposure assessment and postexposure prophylaxis should be guided by standard hospital protocols based on national guidelines (see Table 26–20).[3] Tetanus immunization should be provided as indicated, and HCW counseling should be arranged.[1–3]

REFERENCES

1. Twitchell KT. Bloodborne pathogens: what you need to know. Parts I and II. *AAOHN J* 2003;51:38–45, quiz 46–47; and *AAOHN J* 2003;51:89–97, quiz 98-99.
2. Moran GJ. Emergency department management of blood and body fluid exposures. *Ann Emerg Med* 2000;35:47–62.
3. Beltrami EM, Williams IT, Shapiro CN, et al. Risk and management of blood-borne infections in health care workers. *Clin Microbiol Rev* 2000;13:385–407.

TABLE 26–20 Provisional Public Health Service Recommendations for Chemoprophylaxis after Occupational Exposure to Human Immunodeficiency Virus

Exposure	Antiviral source material	Prophylaxis	Drug regimen
Percutaneous	Blood		
	Highest risk	Recommend	ZDV + 3TC + IDD
	Increased risk	Recommend	ZDV + 3TC ± IDV
	No increased risk	Offer	ZDV + 3TC
	Fluid with visible blood or other potential infectious fluid	Offer	ZDV + 3TC
	Other fluid (e.g., urine)	Do not offer	—
Mucous membrane	Blood	Offer	ZDV + 3TC ± ICV
	Fluid with visible blood or other potential infectious fluid	Offer	ZDV ±3TC
	Other fluid (e.g., urine)	Do not offer	—
Skin with increased risk	Blood	Offer	ZEV + 3TC ± IDV
	Fluid with visible blood or other potential infectious fluid	Offer	ZDV ± 3TC
	Other fluid (e.g., urine)	Do not offer	—

From Schwartz, with permission.
IDV, indinavir; ZDV, zidovudire; 3TC, lamivudire.

Latex Allergy

James M. Madsen

Clinical Presentation

Type IV hypersensitivity produces typical signs and symptoms of allergic contact dermatitis, hours to days after exposure. Type I hypersensitivity may manifest as contact urticaria, systemic urticaria, angioedema, rhinitis, conjunctivitis, bronchospasm, and anaphylaxis.[1] Health care workers and manufacturers of latex products have particularly high rates of occupational sensitization.[1,2]

Pathophysiology

Latex allergy refers to a type IV delayed-hypersensitivity reaction (producing an allergic contact dermatitis) or to a less common but more serious type I immediate-hypersensitivity reaction (ranging from urticaria through anaphylaxis) to proteins, peptides, or other materials associated with the processing of natural rubber latex (NRL).[3] Irritant contact dermatitis may also result from latex exposure.

Exposure to latex elicits hypersensitivity reactions after sensitization. Several NRL proteins (Hev-b1 through Hev-b11) are allergenic; health care workers tend to be particularly sensitive to Hev-b5 and Hev-b6.[3]

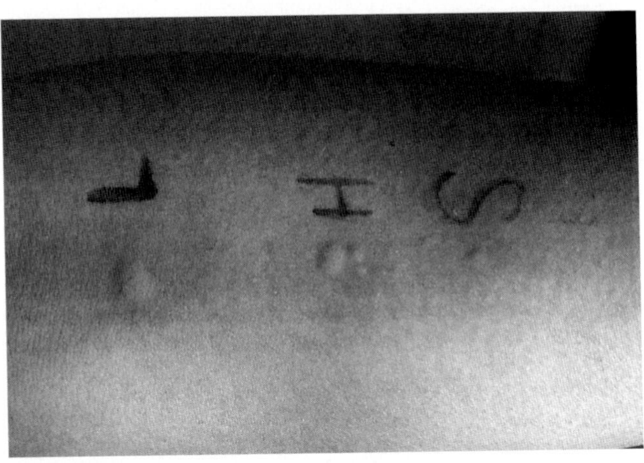

FIGURE 26–21 Positive prick text to eluted latex protein from rubber gloves (L). H, a positive prick test control (histamine); S, a negative control (saline). (From Rom, with permission.)

Diagnosis

The history and physical examination are usually sufficient to make a presumptive diagnosis in the emergency department. Allergic contact dermatitis from latex can be diagnosed by patch testing. Type I hypersensitivity can be evaluated by skin prick testing, by testing of sera via radioallergosorbent test (RAST) or enzyme-linked immunosorbent assay (ELISA) for latex-specific antigens, or by challenge testing.[2] Cross-reactivity to certain fruits is common.[3]

Clinical Complications

Anaphylactic reactions may lead to circulatory collapse and death; allergic contact dermatitis may lead to secondary infections. Either type of reaction may cause long-term disability or necessitate job replacement.[1,3]

Management

Substitution of other materials for latex gloves and other latex products, together with administrative (workplace) controls, allows many latex-sensitive patients to maintain their jobs. Avoidance of exposure decreases latex-specific immunoglobulin E levels.[3] Standard treatment for latex anaphylaxis includes oxygen, fluids, epinephrine, antihistamines, bronchodilators, and corticosteroids.[1]

REFERENCES

1. Toraason M, Sussman G, Biagini R, et al. Latex allergy in the workplace. *Toxicol Sci* 2000;58:5–14.
2. Ahmed DD, Sobczak SC, Yunginger JW. Occupational allergies caused by latex. *Immunol Allergy Clin North Am* 2003;23:205–219.
3. Hepner DL, Castells MC. Latex allergy: an update. *Anesth Analg* 2003;96:1219–1229.

Work-Related Low Back Pain

James M. Madsen

Clinical Presentation

Pain affecting the lower back may include radiation along the sciatic nerve, which suggests compromise of lumbosacral nerve roots; it may be associated with other so-called red flags, such as saddle anesthesia or loss of bowel or bladder function (see Table 26–22); or it may occur as simple back pain (i.e., nonspecific regional low back pain (LBP) without indication of a more serious condition).[1]

Pathophysiology

Work-related low back pain (LBP) is the most common form of occupational back injury. LBP refers to acute or chronic pain, caused or exacerbated by employment, of the lumbosacral region, the buttocks, or the upper legs.[1]

Simple LBP is partly related to psychosocial factors such as job control and job satisfaction and partly related to physical forces (i.e., lifting and forceful movements) and work postures, as well as disease of apophyseal joints in the back.[2] Whole-body vibration may also play a role.[3]

TABLE 26–22 Red Flags in the History and Physical Examination of Patients with Low Back Pain

History
Pain duration greater than 6 wk
Age younger than 18 or older than 50 yr
History of trauma
Sciatica
Neurologic complaints (paresthesias, anesthesia, weakness)
Incontinence of bowel or bladder
Night pain
Unrelenting pain despite rest and analgesics
Fever, chills, and night sweats
History of injection drug use
History of cancer
Physical Examination
Fever
Patient writhing in pain
Point vertebral tenderness
Neurologic deficits
Positive straight-leg raise test

From Harwood-Nuss, with permission.

Diagnosis

The history, especially a detailed occupational history, is important for revealing "red flags" that would signal the possibility of a more serious disorder (see Table 26–22). The physical examination can help to detect malingering; more importantly, it can evaluate sensorimotor deficits and changes in reflexes. Magnetic resonance imaging is sensitive but not specific in detecting disc herniation and should be interpreted with care.[1]

Clinical Complications

Failure to detect serious underlying causes of LBP (e.g., cancer, infection, spinal stenosis) may result in more advanced disease at the time of eventual diagnosis. Simple back pain may lead to disability that becomes more refractory to management the longer the patient is off work.

Management

Once more serious conditions have been excluded, analgesics, muscle relaxants (e.g., cyclobenzaprine) and diazepam may be of short-term benefit, as may epidural steroid injections for sciatica. Bed rest normally should not exceed 4 days. Activity modification, workplace modification, and psychosocial support with early return to work are key elements in the therapeutic plan.[3]

REFERENCES

1. Gerr F, Mani L. Work-related low back pain. *Prim Care* 2000;27: 865–876.
2. Borenstein DG. Epidemiology, etiology, diagnostic evaluation, and treatment of low back pain. *Curr Opin Rheumatol* 2000;12:143–149.
3. Johanning E. Evaluation and management of occupational low back disorders. *Am J Ind Med* 2000;37:94–111.

SECTION V

SPECIAL ISSUES

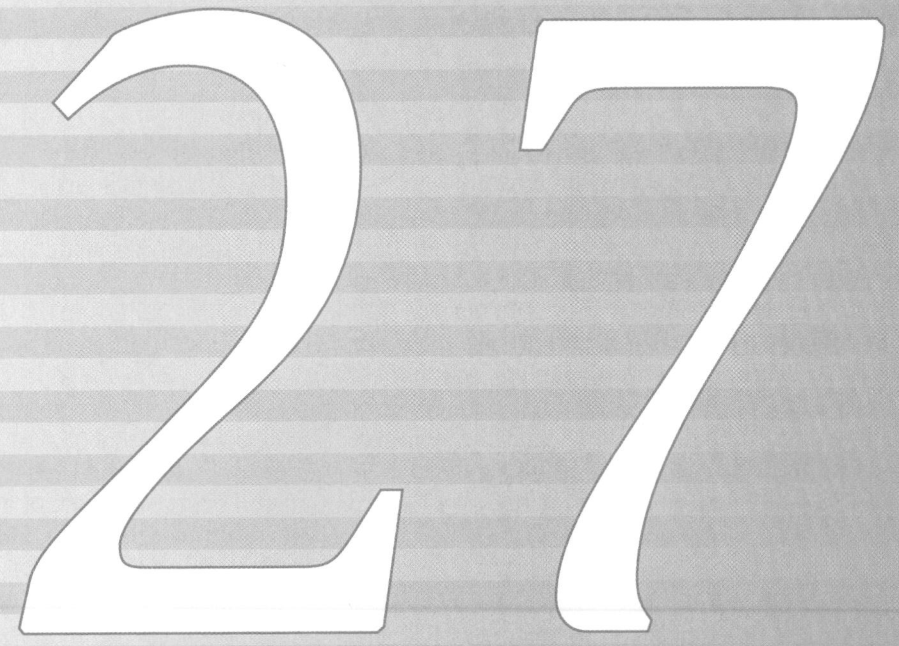

Psychosocial

27–1

Munchausen's Syndrome

Michael Greenberg

Clinical Presentation

Patients with Munchausen's syndrome (MS), who usually are men, can present with any of a myriad of symptoms and complaints referable to one or more body systems.[1] However, all signs and symptoms in these patients are factitious and fabricated.[1–3] Patients may present with complaints of chest pain, shortness of breath, or seizures, or with problems related to self-induced fevers, infections, or bleeding. Feigned memory loss, suicidal thoughts, or hallucinations may be manifest. Patients typically present to many hospitals in different locations, using different names and aliases.

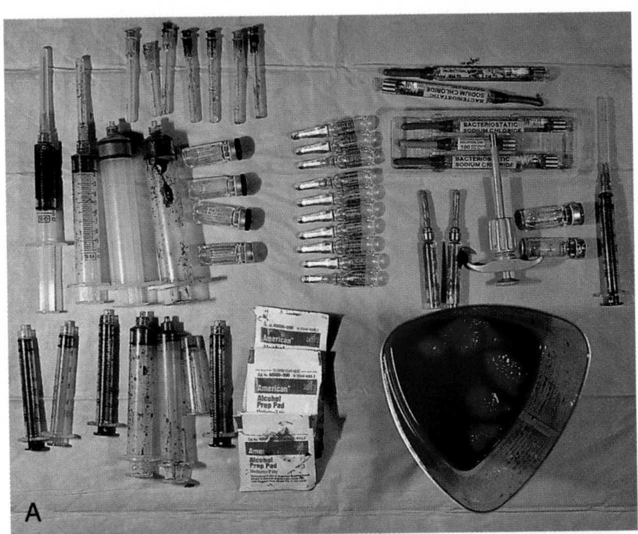

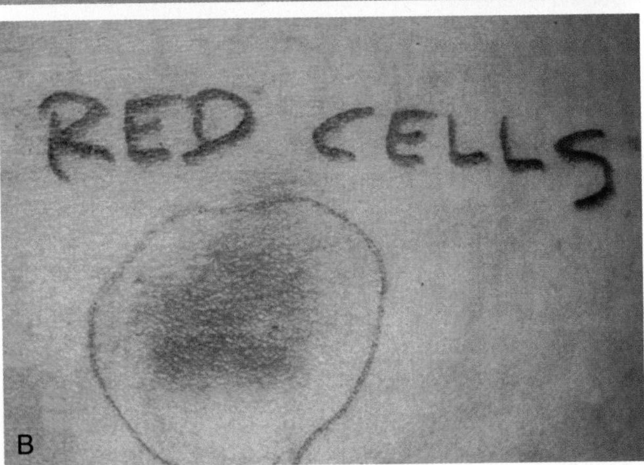

FIGURE 27–1 **A:** View of needle and syringes used by a patient with Munchausen's syndrome to produce the factitious presentation of colonic bleeding. (From Yamada, with permission.) **B:** Skin lesion of psychogenic purpura (autoerythrocyte sensitization) induced by administration of intradermal autologous blood. A saline control elicited no response. (From Greer, with permission.)

Pathophysiology

MS is a form of so-called factitious disorder and is characterized by feigned or simulated illness, "pseudologia fantastica" (persistent and pathologic lying), and "peregrinations," or moving frequently from place to place (or hospital to hospital).[1] Individuals with MS appear to be distinctly different from malingerers, whose goal is to attain some tangible benefit (e.g., occupational- or insurance-derived compensation) from feigned disease. The only apparent goal of an individual with MS is to become a patient and receive unnecessary medical treatment. Most MS patients are men with work experience in health care settings. They are often noted to be "socially conforming" as well as "pleasant and compliant in their relationships with hospital staff".[1]

Diagnosis

The diagnosis of MS is very difficult, especially in the setting of the emergency department. The key to correct diagnosis is to maintain an increased index of suspicion. Valuable clues to this syndrome may be obtained by contacting previous caregivers and institutions who provided care to the patient in the past. MS patients usually allow a wide variety of invasive and even operative procedures to be performed.

Clinical Complications

Complications include unnecessary medication use, unnecessary hospitalizations with the potential for iatrogenic illness, and unnecessary surgical procedures, as well as malpractice lawsuits that may derive from any of these.

Management

Patients with MS are often deemed to be untreatable and virtually impossible to manage. Although the prognosis for these patients is generally poor, attempts should be made to have psychiatric evaluation undertaken at the earliest possible moment.

REFERENCES

1. Turner J, Reid S. Munchausen's syndrome. *Lancet* 2002;359:346–349.
2. Mehta NJ, Khan IA. Cardiac Munchausen's syndrome. *Chest* 2002;122:1649–1653.
3. Chew BH, Pace KT, Honey RJ. Munchausen syndrome presenting as gross hematuria in two women. *Urology* 2002;59:601.

Anorexia Nervosa and Bulimia Nervosa

Judith Eisenberg

Clinical Presentation

Although anorexic patients are more likely to appear cachectic, both anorexic and bulimic patients may present with sequelae of malnutrition.

Pathophysiology

These disorders are characterized by substantial eating disturbances that arise from a distorted body image.[1] Eating disorders are thought to be multifactorial, with neurochemical, genetic, cultural, and psychodevelopmental components. Although there is female gender predominance, there is no difference in incidence related to socioeconomic class or ethnic background. It is estimated that 3% of all young women in the United States suffer from a form of eating disorder.[1,2]

Diagnosis

The diagnostic criteria for anorexia nervosa and bulimia nervosa were set out in the *Diagnostic and Statistical Manual of Mental Disorders,* fourth edition (DSM-IV).[1,2]

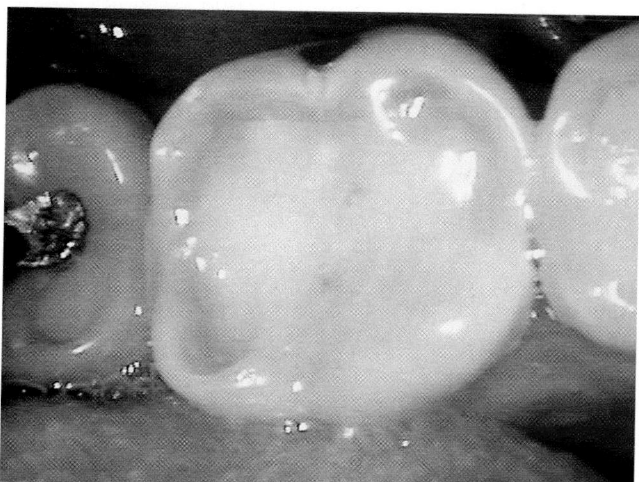

FIGURE 27–2 Dental erosion. Circumscribed, yellowish regions correspond to exposed dentin in areas of enamel loss caused by repeated exposure to gastric contents secondary to chronic gastroesophageal reflux. Similar lesions may be expected in patients with chronic vomiting syndromes. (From Yamada, with permission.)

Criteria for Diagnosis of Anorexia Nervosa

1. Body weight less than 85% of expected weight, or body mass index less than 17.5
2. Intense fear of weight gain
3. Inaccurate perception of own body weight, size, or shape
4. Amenorrhea in girls after menarche

Criteria for Diagnosis of Bulimia Nervosa

1. Recurrent binge eating at least twice a week for 6 months
2. Recurrent purging, excessive exercise, or fasting at least twice a week for 3 months
3. Excessive concern about body weight or shape
4. Absence of anorexia nervosa

Clinical Complications

Potential complications include cardiac dysrhythmias, electrolyte abnormalities, decreased gastrointestinal motility with increased risk of perforation, hypotension, depression, and increased risk for suicide. Inadequate caloric intake may be severe enough to result in hair loss, amenorrhea, and growth arrest. Electrolyte and fluid losses may be exacerbated by laxative abuse. Bulimic patients may have dental caries, loss of dentin, and dorsal hand abrasions from forced emesis. These patients are also at increased risk for Mallory-Weiss tears from repetitive purging.[1,2]

Management

Treatment involves a multidisciplinary approach, with medical therapy aimed at correcting the sequelae of nutritional derangements from severe weight loss, and psychiatric treatment to correct the skewed body image and resultant depression. Psychopharmacology has not been very useful in anorexic patients, but selective serotonin reuptake inhibitors (SSRIs) have some reported benefit in bulimic patients.[2]

REFERENCES

1. Vitousek K, Manke F. Personality variables and disorders in anorexia nervosa and bulimia nervosa. *J Abnorm Psychol* 1994;103: 137–147.
2. Becker AE, Grinspoon SK, Klibanski A, Herzog DB. Current concepts: eating disorders. *N Engl J Med* 1999;340:1092–1098.

Trichotillomania

Michael Greenberg

Clinical Presentation

Patients with trichotillomania present with patchy alopecia.

Pathophysiology

Trichotillomania is a disorder involving the compulsive and repetitive pulling and extraction of body hair.[1,2] The cause for trichotillomania is not known; however, some have characterized this psychiatric disorder as a form of castration surrogate, because hair often is portrayed as a symbol of sexuality and virility.

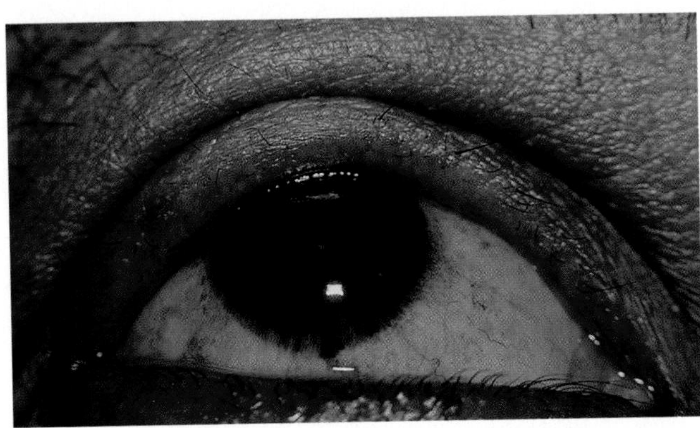

FIGURE 27–3 Trichotillomania. This patient was asymptomatic and admitted to intentionally plucking her eyelashes. (From Tasman, with permission.)

Diagnosis

Trichotillomania is diagnosed based on clinical findings. However, many patients hide the disorder under wigs, hats, or other coverings and avoid situations in which the disorder would become obvious (e.g., water sports). Scalp biopsy may be necessary in some cases if the cause is unclear. Trichotillomania may involve other than head hair; trichotillomaniacs may also pull eyebrows, pubic hair, chest hair, and axillary hair.[1,2]

Clinical Complications

Complications include various psychiatric comorbidities as well as obvious cosmetic issues.

Management

Maximally effective treatment involves the coadministration of pharmacotherapy with behavioral modification therapy. Selective serotonin reuptake inhibitors (SSRIs) are the most popular medications used for this disorder, but virtually every known psychotropic medication has been tried in the treatment of trichotillomania.[1,2]

REFERENCES

1. Papadopoulos AJ, Janniger CK, Chodynicki MP, Schwartz RA. Trichotillomania. *Int J Dermatol* 2003;42:330–334.
2. Diefenbach GJ, Reitman D, Williamson DA. Trichotillomania: a challenge to research and practice. *Clin Psychol Rev* 2000;20: 289–309.

Self-Inflicted Wounds

Michael Greenberg

Clinical Presentation

Patients present with a variety of wounds that appear to have been self-inflicted. These may include puncture wounds, lacerations, abrasions, and thermal or chemical burns. In many cases, if closely questioned, patients admit causing the wounds.[1–3]

Pathophysiology

Deliberate self-harm by self-inflicted wounds has a prevalence in the range of 750 per 100,000 patients and is increasing.[4] Most self-inflicted wounds represent early stages of suicidal gestures that may have been interrupted by others or terminated by the self-inflicting individual. The underlying psychopathology associated with self-harm is often associated with early childhood abuse or important (often parental) losses.[1,2] Specific wounds are identified with suicidal attempts. Common wounds are so-called "hesitation marks" on the volar wrists or forearms; these are produced by lateral cutting of the skin, just into the dermis, by a knife, glass edge, or other sharpened object.[1–3]

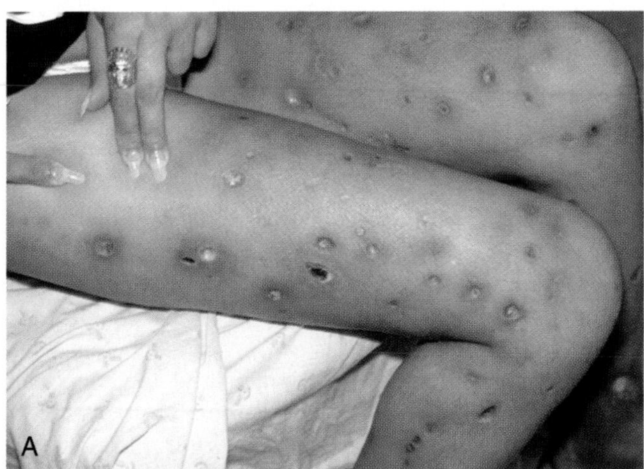

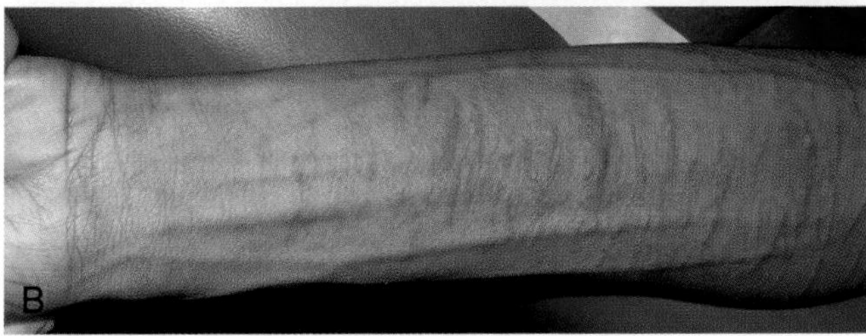

FIGURE 27–4 **A:** Neurotic excoriations (factitia). The self-induced ulcers are seen in a patient who was convinced that she was infested with lice. (From Goodheart, with permission.) **B:** Multiple "hesitation marks" of the volar forearm. (Courtesy of Olufunmilayo Ogudele, MD.)

Diagnosis

The diagnosis is based on history and physical findings and is usually obvious. However, some means of occult self-harm are extremely difficult to ascertain.

Clinical Complications

Complications include infection, disability, and death. After self-inflicted injury, there is "a significant and persistent risk of suicide which varies markedly between genders and age groups."[3] This increased risk may last for a period of years.[3]

Management

Immediate attention to life-threatening problems is essential, as is meticulous wound care. Early, on-site psychiatric intervention is critical for patients who engage in self-harming behaviors, because earlier intervention is associated with better prognosis.[1–4]

REFERENCES

1. Brickman AL, Mintz DC. Datapoints: U.S. rates of self-inflicted injuries and suicide, 1992–1999. *Psychiatr Serv* 2003;54:168.
2. Horrocks J, House A. Self-poisoning and self-injury in adults. *Clin Med* 2002;2:509–512.
3. Hawton K, Zahl D, Weatherall R. Suicide following deliberate self-harm: long-term follow-up of patients who presented to a general hospital. *Br J Psychiatry* 2003;182:537–542.
4. Hafeez U, Goodyear HM. Self-mutilation: do not overlook the obvious. *Eur Acad Dermatol Venereol* 2003;17:369–370.

27–5

Post-Traumatic Stress Disorder

Judith Eisenberg

Clinical Presentation

Patients with post-traumatic stress disorder (PTSD) may present with complaints of fatigue from attempting to stay awake for prolonged periods to avoid nightmares. This sleep deprivation may also manifest as irritability or difficulty concentrating. Somatic symptoms such as asthma, hypertension, or chronic pain are not uncommon. Some patients report that they cannot cope with the nightmares or flashbacks and feel suicidal as a result[1,2] (see Tables 27–5A and 27–5B).

TABLE 27–5A **Predisposing Vulnerability Factors in Post-traumatic Stress Disorder**

Presence of childhood trauma
Borderline, paranoid, dependent, or antisocial personality disorder traits
Inadequate family or peer support system
Being female
Genetic vulnerability to psychiatric illness
Recent stressful life changes
Perception of an external locus of control (natural cause) rather than an internal one (human cause)
Recent excessive alcohol intake

From Kaplan and Sadock, with permission.

TABLE 27–5B **Psychodynamic Themes in Post-traumatic Stress Disorder**

The subjective meaning of a stressor may determine its traumatogenicity.
Traumatic events may resonate with childhood traumas.
Inability to regulate affect may result from trauma.
Somatization and alexithymia may be among the aftereffects of trauma.
Common defenses used include denial, minimization, splitting, projective disavowal, dissociation, and guilt (as a defense against underlying helplessness).
Mode of object relatedness involves projection and introjection of the following roles: omnipotent rescuer, abuser, and victim.

From Kaplan and Sadock, with permission.

Pathophysiology

According to the *Diagnostic and Statistical Manual of Mental Disorders,* fourth edition (DSM-IV), this disorder is an abnormal response to a perceived traumatic event that is characterized by reliving the event, avoiding reminders of the event, and maintaining a persistent state of hypervigilance for at least 1 month.[1,2] Those who have experienced interpersonal violence are more likely to develop PTSD than those who have been involved in natural disasters or motor vehicle accidents.[1,2] Studies have shown that patients with PTSD have increased circulating levels of norepinephrine, more sensitive α-adrenergic receptors, and increased levels of thyroid hormones.[1]

Clinical Complications

Persistent untreated hypertension may result in cardiovascular insults. Patients may be misdiagnosed for years and may receive unnecessary steroid and β-agonist treatment for perceived asthma. Narcotic addiction is a potential problem with any chronic pain complaint.[1,2]

Management

Nonpharmacologic treatment includes exposure and cognitive therapy, as well as anxiety management techniques. Group therapy has been helpful to reduce the isolation that patients commonly promote to feel safe. Initial pharmacologic treatment is with the selective serotonin reuptake inhibitor (SSRI) class; of these, sertraline was the first to be approved by the U.S. Food and Drug Administration (FDA) with the treatment of PTSD as a specific indication for use.[2] Other SSRIs were subsequently approved for this purpose. If there is no response, then either nefazodone or venlafaxine should be prescribed. Benzodiazepines have not been shown to be helpful in chronic PTSD.[1,2]

REFERENCES

1. Yehuda R. Current concepts: post-traumatic stress disorder. *N Engl J Med* 2002;346:108–114.
2. Bryant RA, Friedman M. Medication and non-medication treatments of post-traumatic stress disorder. *Curr Opin Psychiatry* 2001; 14:119–123.

Critical Incident Stress Debriefing

Judith Eisenberg

A common schema for critical incident stress debriefing (CISD) is the Mitchell method—a multi-step, "group psychological process developed to help mitigate the effects of severe stress and post-traumatic stress disorder (PTSD)"[1] (see Table 27–6). This method involves a single session and allows the participant to reach a sense of closure regarding the event. CISD usually takes place within 2 to 7 days after the crisis event.[1–3]

Background

CISD techniques were developed in the 1980s to address the needs of emergency medical services personnel who were traumatized after mass casualty incidents. CISD has progressed to become an integral part of many fire, police, and Emergency Medical Services postincident protocols. These methods have also been used in the civilian arena, most recently in the wake of the terrorist attacks of September 11, 2001.[2]

TABLE 27–6 The Six Phases of a Critical Incident Stress Debriefing (CISD)*

1. Introductory phase
2. Fact phase
3. Feeling phase
4. Symptom phase
5. Teaching phase
6. Reentry phase

*The CISD optimally should be implemented within 3 hours after the incident.

Adapted from Oster N, Doyle C. Critical incident stress and challenges for the emergency workplace. *Emerg Med Clin North Am* 2000;18:339–353.

Components of CISD

The important components of CISD are as follows[1–3]:

1. Immediate intervention after a traumatic event is provided to prevent the formation of maladaptive behaviors that may worsen over time.
2. Symptomatic relief is provided using short-term psychotropic medications along with strategies to reduce the stress in the worker's environment.
3. The Mitchell model provides a framework for debriefing over 1 to 3 hours. First, the participants are allowed to establish the facts of the incident in a purely intellectual manner. The group leader then encourages the participants to express their feelings regarding the event, by asking questions such as, "How did you feel when you first came on scene?" In the last step of the debriefing, the leader helps the group identify possible symptoms of PTSD, teaches techniques for dealing with stress, and guides the participants in discussing coping mechanisms they can use on their return to work.[3]

REFERENCES

1. Hokanson M, Wirth B. The critical incident stress debriefing process for the Los Angeles County Fire Department: automatic and effective. *Int J Emerg Ment Health* 2000;2:249–257.
2. van Emmerick AAP, Kamphuis JH, Hulsbosch AM, Emmelkamp PMG. Single session debriefing after psychological trauma: a meta-analysis. *Lancet* 2002;360:766–771.
3. Everly GS, Flannery RB, Mitchell JT. Critical incident stress debriefing: a review of the literature. *Aggression and Violent Behavior* 2000;5:23–40.

The CAGE Screening Test for Alcoholism

Judith Eisenberg

CAGE is a mnemonic for four questions developed to quickly assess a patient's risk for current alcohol dependence in the primary care setting[1,2] (see Table 27–7).

Utility

Many large-scale studies have been done using this questionnaire. The *Diagnostic and Statistical Manual of Mental Disorders,* third edition, revised (DSM-III-R), applied this questionnaire to the surveys done in the year before its release in 1987 and found that two positive responses to the CAGE questions yielded a sensitivity of 74.6% and a specificity of 91.6% for alcohol dependence.[1] Subsequent studies have shown there is no difference in the results of these screening questions when they are given orally and when they are administered as a written questionnaire. A positive response to all four questions was shown to have a positive predictive value of 100% in a study done by the National Institute of Alcohol Abuse and Alcoholism.[2]

TABLE 27–7 CAGE Questions: A Validated Alcoholism Screening Instrument

C	Have you ever felt that you needed to Cut down on your alcohol use?
A	Have people Annoyed you or criticized you about your alcohol use?
G	Have you ever felt bad or Guilty about your alcohol use?
E	Have you ever used alcohol first thing in the morning to steady your nerves or get rid of a hangover? (an Eye-opener)

Adapted from Ewing JA. Detecting alcoholism: the CAGE questionnaire. *JAMA* 1984;252:1905–1907.

Purpose

When performed in a nonjudgmental manner, the CAGE screening questions are a quick and easy tool that can be administered in the primary care office or in the emergency department. The first step in obtaining assistance for alcohol dependence is allowing the patient to hear from a physician that a problem exists. The economic cost of alcoholism certainly justifies an attempt by any physician who encounters a patient with signs and symptoms of alcohol abuse to identify a problem and refer the patient to appropriate resources.[1,2]

REFERENCES

1. Poulin C, Webster I, Single E. Alcohol disorders in Canada as indicated by the CAGE questionnaire. *CMAJ* 1997;157:1529–1535.
2. Samet JH, O'Connor PG. Alcohol abusers in primary care: readiness to change behavior. *Am J Med* 1998;105:302–306.

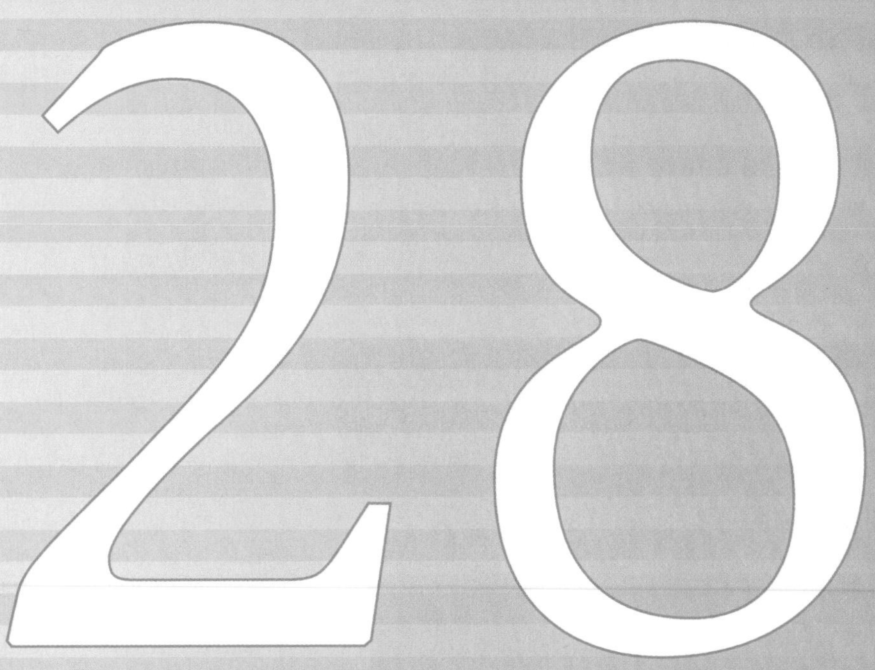

Alternative Medicine

Coining/Spooning

Michael Greenberg

Clinical Presentation

Patients who have undergone coining or spooning present with multiple erythematous linear marks on the back and/or chest.[1,2]

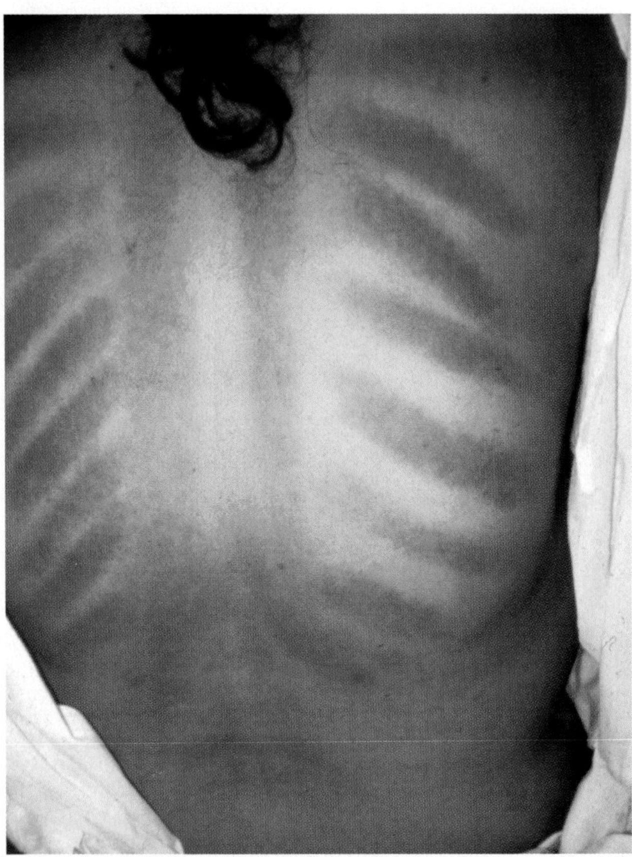

FIGURE 28–1 Characteristic skin lesions of coining. (Copyright James R. Roberts, MD.)

Pathophysiology

"Coining" (*cao gio* in Vietnamese) is an ancient medical technique that originated in the Far East. The practice survives today and may be seen in members of various Asian communities. Coining is used to treat ailments including asthma, viral illnesses, cough, nausea, and vomiting. This practice is seen most frequently among members of the Vietnamese, Chinese, and Laotian immigrant communities.

One popular method of coining involves massaging the skin first with a mentholated oil or ointment, then forcefully stroking the skin with the edge of a coin, a spoon, or a comb. This produces the eccymotic/petechial streaking that is pathognomonic of this technique.

Diagnosis

The diagnosis is based on identification of the typical skin markings. It is important to obtain an adequate history, because the marks associated with these techniques may be mistakenly identified as indicative of child, elder, or spousal abuse.

Clinical Complications

Complications are rare but may include infection and scarring.

Management

In most cases, no treatment is indicated, and evidence of coining is simply an incidental finding.

REFERENCES

1. Crutchfield CE 3rd, Bisig TJ. Images in clinical medicine: coining. *N Engl J Med* 1995;332:1552.
2. Amshel CE, Caruso DM. Vietnamese "coining": a burn case report and literature review. *J Burn Care Rehabil* 2000;21:112–114.

Cupping

Michael Greenberg

Clinical Presentation

Patients who have undergone cupping present with single or multiple erythematous, circular marks on the back, chest, abdomen, or forehead.[1,2]

Pathophysiology

"Cupping" is an ancient medical technique that originated in the Middle East or Far East. The practice survives today and may be seen in members of various Asian and Middle Eastern cultures, among others. Cupping is used in ethnic medicinal practice to treat pain associated with gastrointestinal disorders and lung disease. The technique involves the application of glass or bamboo cups to the skin after pressure within the cup is reduced, which is accomplished by applying heat to the cup or otherwise evacuating air from the cup just before its application to the skin. Because of the reduced pressure, the patient's skin and superficial subcutaneous tissue are drawn into and held in the cup. Some practitioners of this technique move the adhered cup across the skin, creating a pulling of the skin and subcutaneous tissues. These maneuvers create ecchymotic and erythematous cutaneous markings.

Diagnosis

The diagnosis is based on identification of the typical skin markings. It is important to obtain an adequate history, because the marks from these techniques may be mistakenly identified as indicative of child, elder, or spousal abuse.

Clinical Complications

Complications are rare but may include infection and scarring.

Management

In most cases, no treatment is indicated, and evidence of cupping is simply an incidental finding.

REFERENCES

1. Seicol NH. Consequences of cupping. *N Engl J Med* 1997;336:1109.
2. Manber H, Kanzler M. Images in clinical medicine: consequences of cupping. *N Engl J Med* 1996;335:1281.

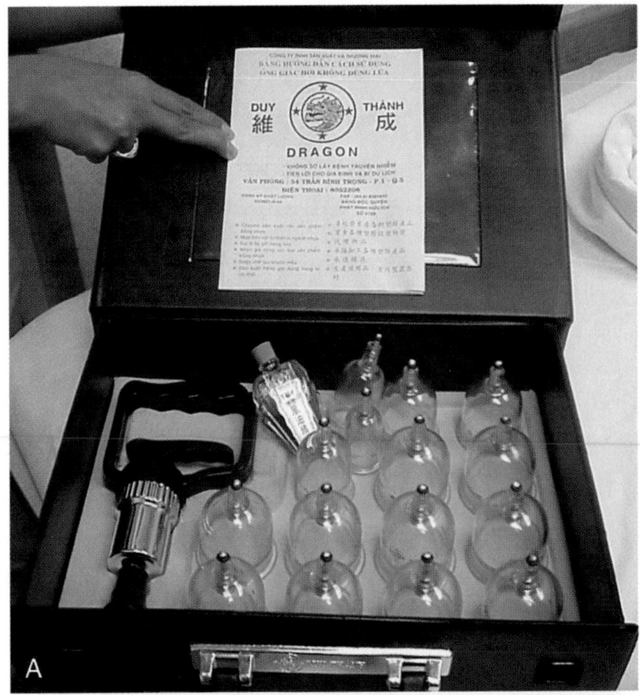

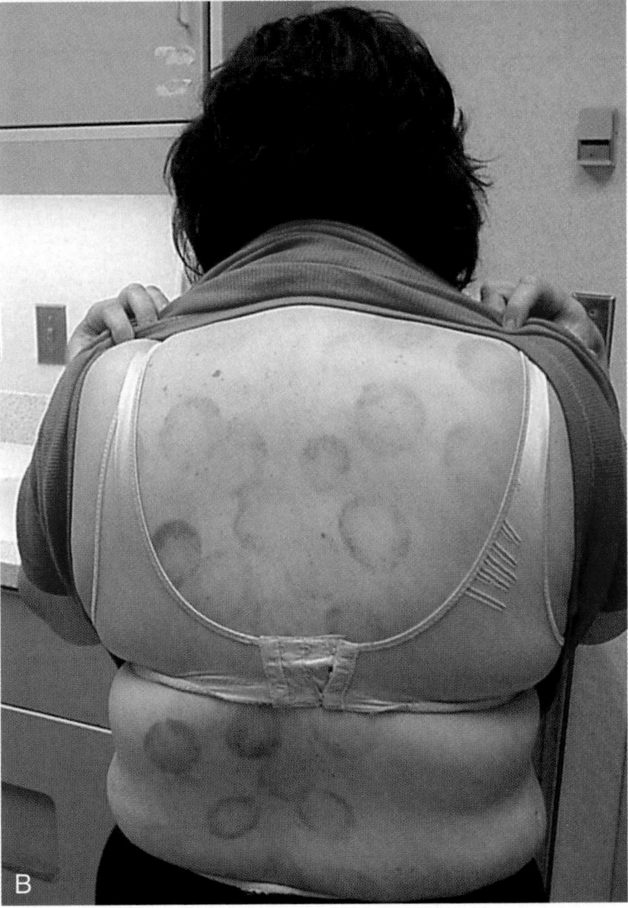

FIGURE 28–2 **A:** Commercially available apparatus for cupping procedures. (Courtesy of Christy Salvaggio, MD) **B:** Skin lesions resulting from cupping. (Courtesy of Christy Salvaggio, MD.)

Acupuncture

Sharad Pandit

Until recently, acupuncture as practiced in China has been poorly understood in the Western world. Chinese medicine holds that the body's vital energy (*chi* or *qi*) circulates through channels, called *meridians,* that have branches connected to bodily organs and functions. Illness is attributed to imbalance or interruption of *chi.*[1]

Traditional acupuncture involves the insertion of stainless steel needles into various body areas. Treatment is applied to "acupuncture points," which are said to be located throughout the body. Originally there were 365 such points. In traditional acupuncture, a combination of points is usually used.

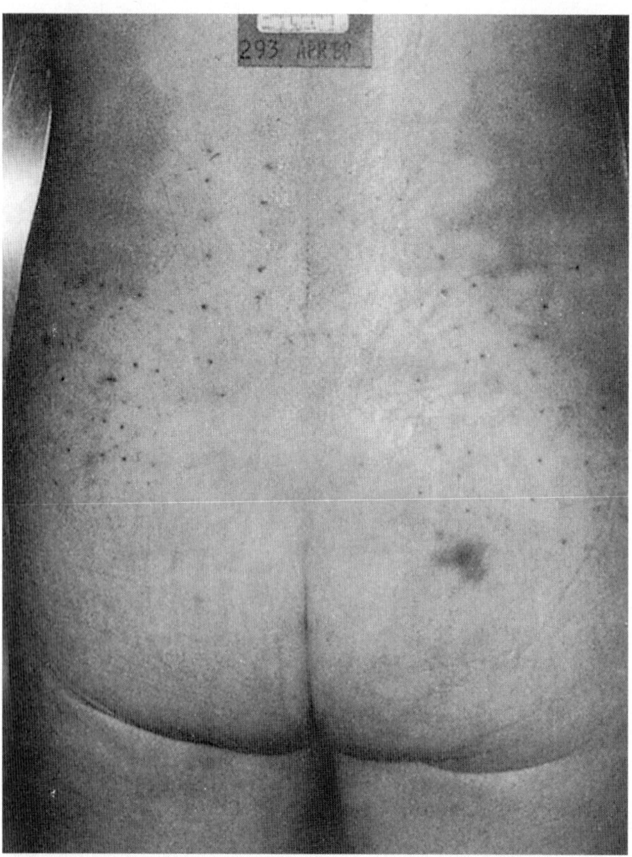

FIGURE 28–3 Acupuncture marks seen postmortem. (From Jones, with permission.)

How acupuncture may relieve pain is unclear. One theory suggests that pain impulses are blocked from reaching the spinal cord or brain at various "gates" to these areas. Another theory suggests that acupuncture stimulates the body to produce narcotic-like substances called endorphins, which reduce pain. Other theories suggest that the placebo effect, external suggestion (hypnosis), and cultural conditioning are important factors. Many studies in animals and humans have demonstrated that acupuncture can cause multiple biologic responses. Considerable evidence supports the claim that opioid peptides are released during acupuncture and that the analgesic effects of acupuncture are at least partially explained by their actions.[1]

Improperly performed acupuncture can cause fainting, local hematoma, pneumothorax (punctured lung), convulsions, local infections, hepatitis B (from use of unsterile needles), bacterial endocarditis, contact dermatitis, and nerve damage.[1]

Acupuncture may be useful for postoperative and chemotherapy-related nausea and vomiting, nausea of pregnancy, and in postoperative dental pain. Acupuncture may be useful as an adjunct treatment in other situations, including addiction, stroke rehabilitation, headache, menstrual cramps, tennis elbow, myofacial pain, osteoarthritis, low back pain, carpal tunnel syndrome, and asthma.[1]

REFERENCES

1. Acupuncture. *NIH Consensus Statement* 1997;15:1–34.

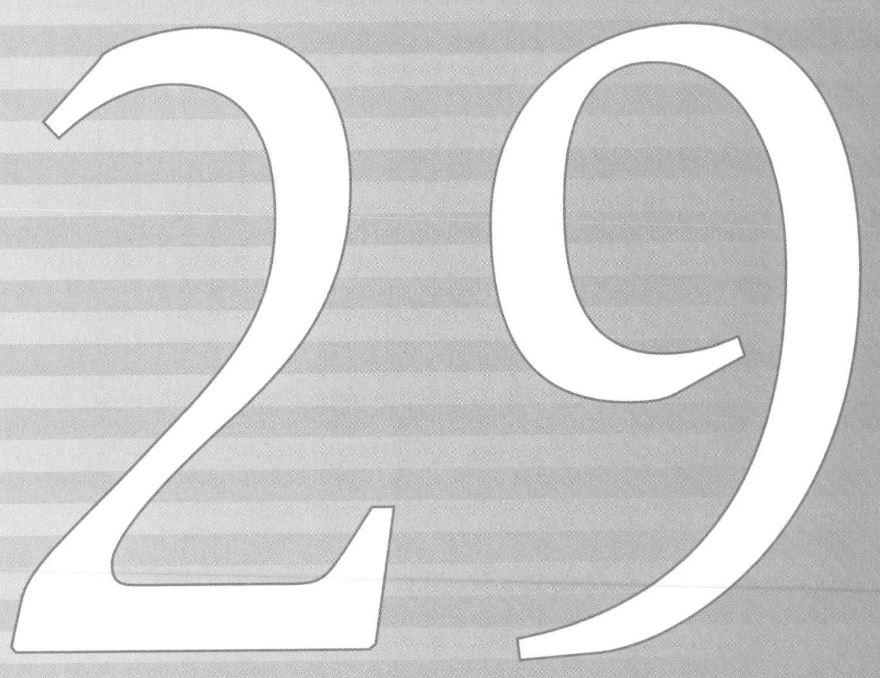

Forensic Emergency Medicine

Identification of Wounds: Shotgun Wounds

Robert Hendrickson

Clinical Presentation

Shotguns are capable of producing a variety of wounds, depending on the ammunition used. Ammunition may be "buckshot," or lead shot, which are multiple, small lead pellets. Lead shot produces entrance wounds that vary in appearance depending on the distance between the gun and the target.[1] Close-range wounds produce a single, large defect and may have a rectangular contusion from the plastic cup that holds the shot.[2] Intermediate-range wounds have a central defect with surrounding lead shot wounds. Long-range wounds produce multiple smaller wounds from individual shot as the shot separates in the air. Shotguns may also be fired with a single slug, or "wad." Wounds from single slugs may appear similar to other gunshot wounds, but with a potentially greater diameter.[2]

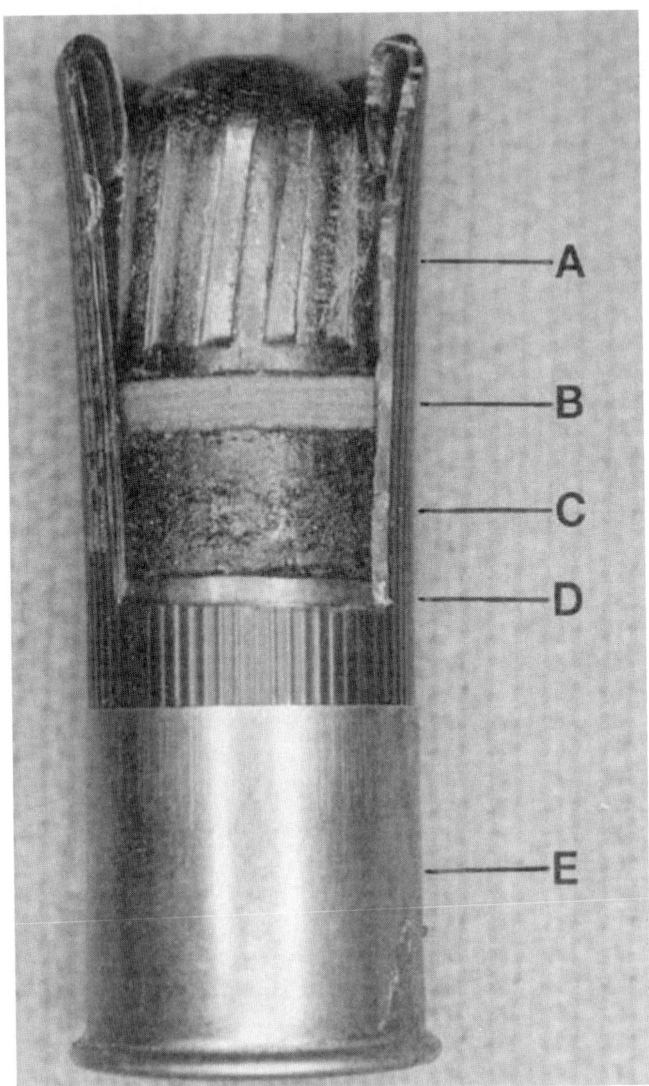

FIGURE 29–1 Cross-sectional representation of conventional 12-gauge shotgun shell loaded with a Foster slug, showing slug **(A)**, hard wadding **(B)**, soft wadding **(C)**, plastic wad **(D)**, and brass head containing powder and primer **(E)**. (From Gestring ML, Geller ER, Akkad N, Bongiovanni PJ. Shotgun slug injuries: case report and literature review. *J Trauma* 1996;40: 650–653, with permission.)

Pathophysiology

As lead shot leaves the barrel of a shotgun, it begins to separate secondary to resistance and gravity. At close range, the shot projectiles travel as a tightly packed group and may produce tissue injury that is similar to that caused by a single, large projectile. As distance from the target increases, the shot separates and produces tissue injury that is more similar to the impact of smaller, individual projectiles. Lead shot injuries rarely cause exit wounds, because the original muzzle energy is divided many times and is essentially dissipated among the individual shot projectiles.

Diagnosis

Diagnosis is by clinical recognition of the typical injury pattern.

Management

Treatment of shotgun injuries is similar to that of other penetrating trauma; however, lead shot may produce injury over a larger surface area than individual projectiles do.[1,2]

REFERENCES

1. DeMuth WE Jr. The mechanism of shotgun wounds. *J Trauma* 1971;11:219–229.
2. Gestring ML, Geller ER, Addak N, Bongiovanni PJ. Shotgun slug injuries: case report and literature review. *J Trauma Infect* 1996;40:650–653.

Identification of Wounds: Blunt Weapon

Robert Hendrickson

Blunt traumatic injuries may produce pattern abrasions, contusions, or lacerations that mimic the striking object.[1] Examples of a pattern abrasion are marks left by a fingernail, carpet, or teeth. Lacerations are produced by blunt force and may reflect the shape of the object. Pattern contusions are the most common pattern injury. Blunt injury from a cylindrical weapon typically leaves a linear, central clearing flanked by parallel contusions. Finger impressions typically appear as circular or oval contusions and may be grouped linearly in the shape of a hand. In addition, contusions may resemble the shape of the offending weapon (e.g., belt, electric cord, hand). Contusion formation and resolution are highly variable. Numerous factors influence the dating of contusions, including the amount of blunt force and tissue characteristics, vascularity, and density.[2] Bite marks typically appear as two curvilinear contusions or abrasions, or both. Bite marks should be treated with great care, because they may contain evidence as to the identity of the assailant. Bite marks should be swabbed with a sterile cotton applicator that has been moistened in sterile saline or water.[1] The sample should be sent to a crime laboratory for identification of DNA and blood group antigen.[1]

REFERENCES

1. Smock WS. Forensic emergency medicine. In: Olshaker JS, Jackson MC, Smock WS, eds. *Forensic emergency medicine.* Philadelphia: Lippincott Williams & Wilkins, 2001.
2. Wilson EF. Estimation of the age of cutaneous contusions in child abuse. *Pediatrics* 1977;60:750–752.

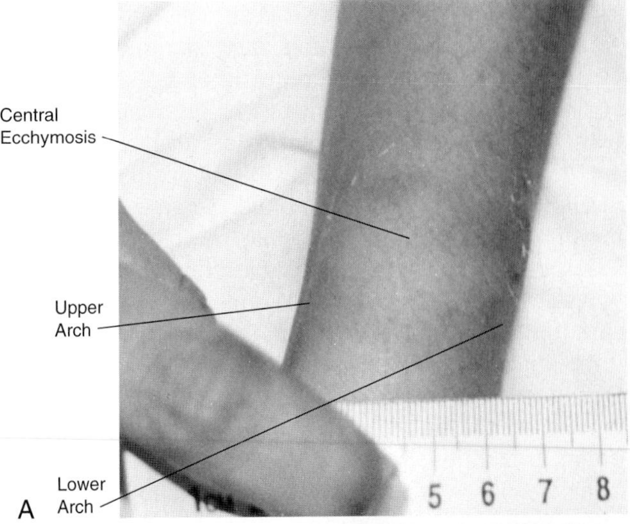

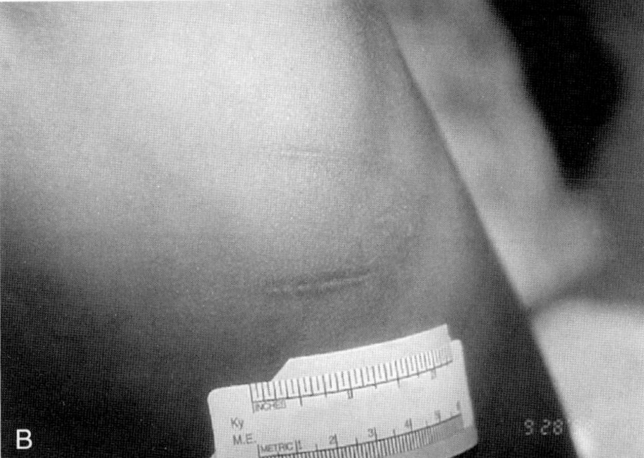

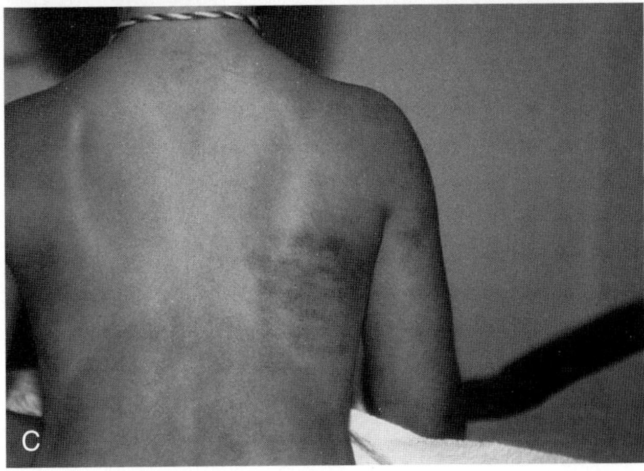

FIGURE 29–2 **A:** Bite mark on the wrist. (From Olshaker, with permission.) **B:** A looped belt injury. **C:** Hand-slap mark. Note parallel linear contusions with central sparing that highlight the imprint of fingers. (**B** and **C,** Courtesy of William Smock, MD, University of Louisville School of Medicine, Louisville, Kentucky. Reprinted from Olshaker, with permission.)

Identification of Wounds: Sharp Weapon

Robert Hendrickson

Injuries caused by sharp weapons fall into two categories: incised wounds and stab wounds.[1] Incised wounds are caused by the drawing of a sharp weapon across the skin, which results in a broad, shallow wound with regular edges. Stab wounds are deeper than they are wide. Stabs wounds may or may not reflect the weapon that produced the wound. Single-edged knives may produce a wound with one sharp edge and one blunt edge, whereas double-edged knives may produce two sharp edges. However, these rules are not always accurate. A single-edged knife can produce two dull edges if the knife was "hilted," with the base of the knife contacting the skin. "Hilted" knives can also produce bruising around the stab wound from the hand of the perpetrator. In addition, wounds may be "V"- or "C"- shaped if the weapon was twisted while in the body.

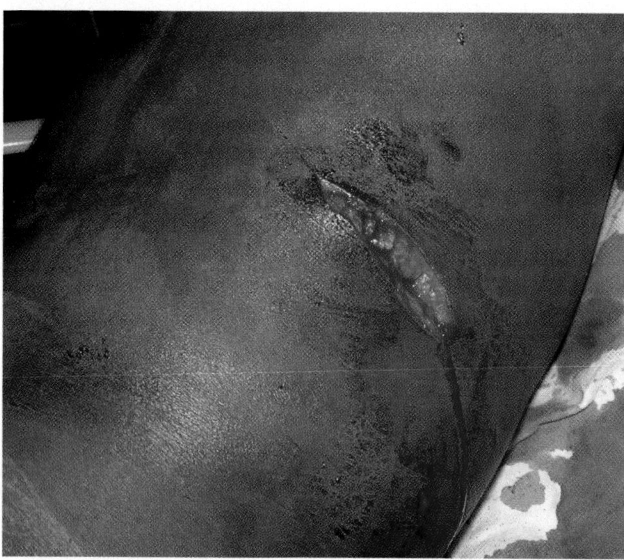

FIGURE 29–3 This stab wound to the left flank violated the peritoneal cavity. (Courtesy of Mark Silverberg, MD.)

The size of a weapon is difficult to assess from a wound, because the tissues are malleable and the angle of the stab affects the width and depth of the wound. Of note, the term "laceration" should not be used to describe injuries that are caused by sharp weapons. Lacerations may be produced only by blunt force or by a tearing motion on the skin.[1]

REFERENCES

1. Smock WS. Forensic emergency medicine. In: Olshaker JS, Jackson MC, Smock WS, eds. *Forensic emergency medicine.* Philadelphia: Lippincott Williams & Wilkins, 2001.

Signs of Death

Robert Hendrickson

In both the prehospital and hospital setting, patients may present in asystolic arrest of unknown duration. The decision to terminate or to not initiate resuscitative efforts may be made if there are signs of irreversible tissue damage or signs of death. Signs of death include decapitation, incineration, fetal maceration, massive cranial destruction, decomposition, rigor mortis, and livor mortis.[1,2]

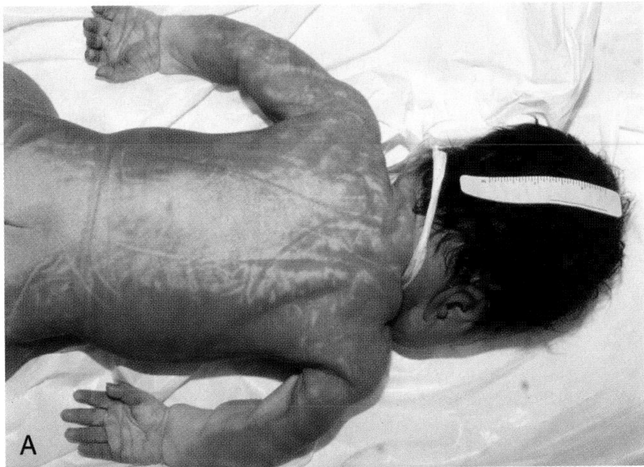

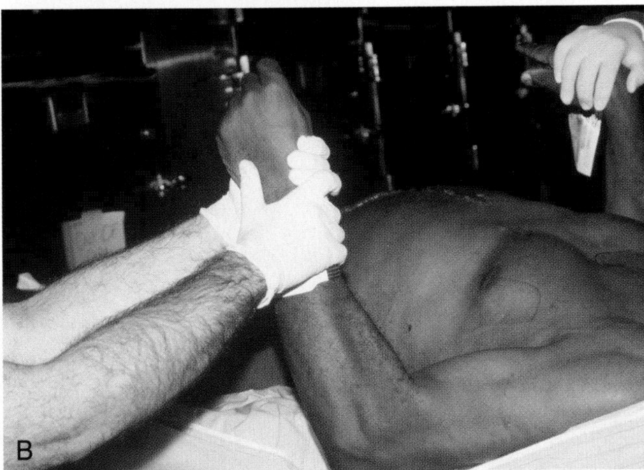

FIGURE 29–4 **A:** Dependent lividity. **B:** Rigor mortis. (**A** and **B,** Courtesy of Charles Catanese, MD.)

The term *rigor mortis* refers to a stiffening of the muscles of the body caused by postmortem reduction of adenosine triphosphate (ATP), which is required in muscle relaxation.[1] Rigor mortis begins to develop shortly after death, increases to full rigidity, and then lessens as the muscle cells decompose. Maximal rigidity typically occurs by 12 hours and resolves by 24 hours; however, the time course is highly variable and changes with air temperature and body habitus. Rigor mortis classically starts in the face and jaw and progresses to the shoulders and upper extremities, then to the trunk and legs. The postmortem interval, or time since death, cannot be calculated in any way based on rigor mortis. Ambient heat increases the rate of development of rigor, and rigor mortis starts and ends relatively rapidly in hot environments and in children. Refrigeration delays the onset of rigor, which then appears in the usual sequence once the body is rewarmed.[1,2]

Livor mortis, or dependent lividity, refers to the pooling of blood in gravitationally dependent areas, typically the sacrum in a supine or seated patient.[1,2]

The rate of decomposition of human tissue is determined primarily by the ambient environmental temperature. Bodies in ice or subzero temperatures do not decompose and thus may be preserved indefinitely. Body decomposition occurs rapidly in the tropics and may be accelerated for bodies in full sunlight.[1,2]

REFERENCES

1. Lockey AS. Recognition of death and termination of cardiac resuscitation attempts by UK ambulance personnel. *Emerg Med J* 2002; 19:345–347.
2. Pepe PE, Swor RA, Ornato JP, et al. Resuscitation in the out-of-hospital setting: medical futility criteria for on-scene pronouncement of death. *Prehosp Emerg Care* 2001;5:79–87.

Smothering and Strangulation

Robert Hendrickson

Smothering refers to asphyxiation caused by external blockage of the airway, typically with a hand or pillow. The typical signs of smothering are the result of trauma to the perioral area, including abrasions and contusions of the mouth, avulsion of teeth, and bite marks on the tongue. Less specific findings include facial petechiae and subconjunctival hemorrhages.[1]

Strangulation refers to asphyxiation caused by external pressure applied to the neck, typically by a hand or ligature. The cause of death varies by type of strangulation. Hangings with significant drops (e.g., judicial hanging) may cause fracture of the upper cervical vertebrae, with medullary disruption leading to unconsciousness and cessation of respiratory effort. Less-traumatic ligature strangulation may cause obstruction of venous and/or arterial flow in the neck or, less commonly, obstruction of the airway. Typical signs include facial plethora, petechiae, and subconjunctival hemorrhages.

Patients who survive smothering or strangulation may develop pulmonary or cerebral edema that can be delayed.[2] Asymptomatic patients should be observed for the onset of symptoms. Symptomatic patients may be treated with supportive care.

REFERENCES

1. Banaschak S, Schmidt P, Madea B. Smothering of children older than 1 year of age: diagnostic significance of morphological findings. *Forensic Sci Int* 2003;134:163–168.
2. Iserson KV. Strangulation: a review of ligature, manual, and postural neck compression injuries. *Ann Emerg Med* 1984;13:179–185.

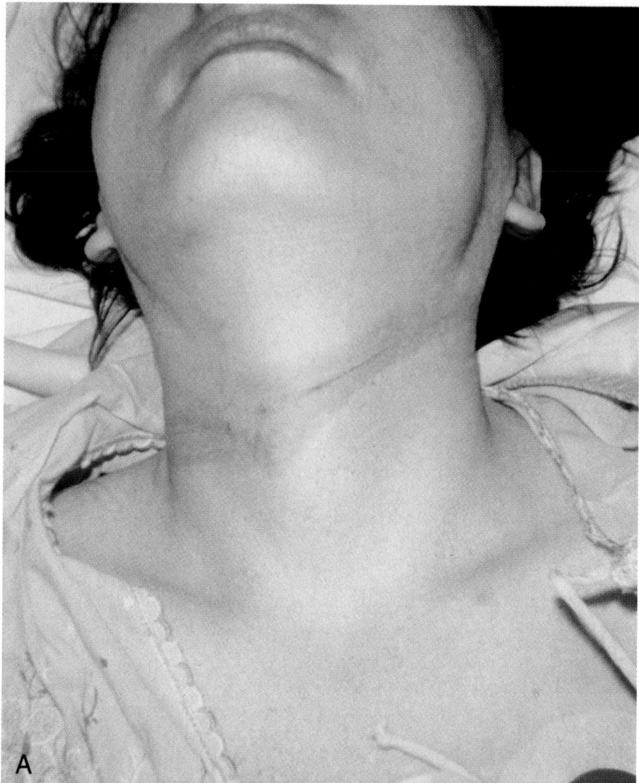

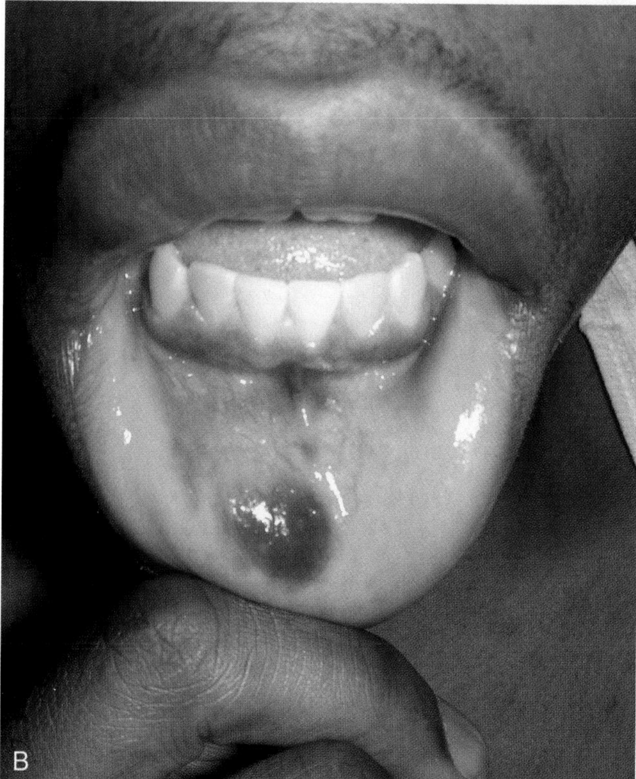

FIGURE 29–5 **A:** Neck marks from rope hanging. (Courtesy of Michael Greenberg, MD.) **B:** Lip ecchymoses due to compression against the teeth during smothering. (Courtesy of Mark Silverberg, MD.)

Estimating Range of Gunshot Wounds

Robert Hendrickson

Entrance wounds are classified as long-range, intermediate-range, close-range, and contact wounds. The approximate range of fire may be estimated by examining the entrance wound characteristics.

A contact wound is generated when the muzzle of the gun is pressed against the skin. On discharge, soot and hot gases are injected into the subcutaneous space, producing soot within the wound. Increased subcutaneous pressure associated with discharge of the gun may press the skin against the muzzle of the gun, producing a contusion ("muzzle marks") and stellate lacerations of the skin.[1]

Close-range wounds are produced by shots fired no more than 6 to 12 inches from the skin.[1] These wounds are identified by the appearance of soot on the skin or clothing around the entrance wound.

Intermediate-range wounds may be identified by the appearance of "tattooing" or "stippling"; these signs occur with shots that are fired within 1 meter.[1] Tattooing and stippling are produced by partially burned gunpowder that is released when the gun is discharged.

Long-range wounds have no identifiable tattooing, muzzle marks, stellate lacerations, or soot. However, long-range wounds may have an "abrasion collar," which is a contused ring of tissue surrounding the entrance wound resulting from friction between the bullet and the skin. These wounds are inflicted by shots from greater than 1 meter.[1]

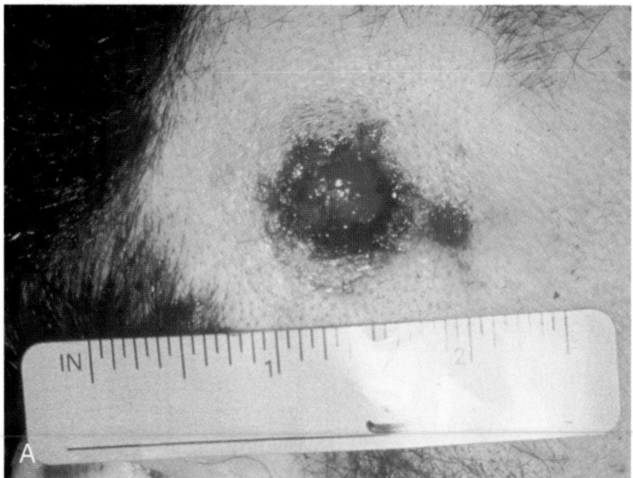

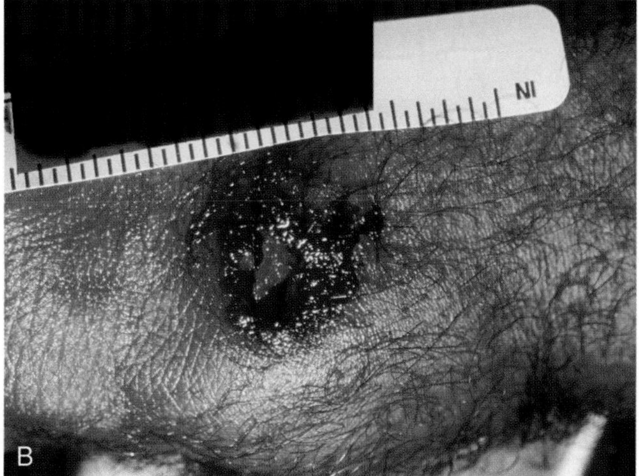

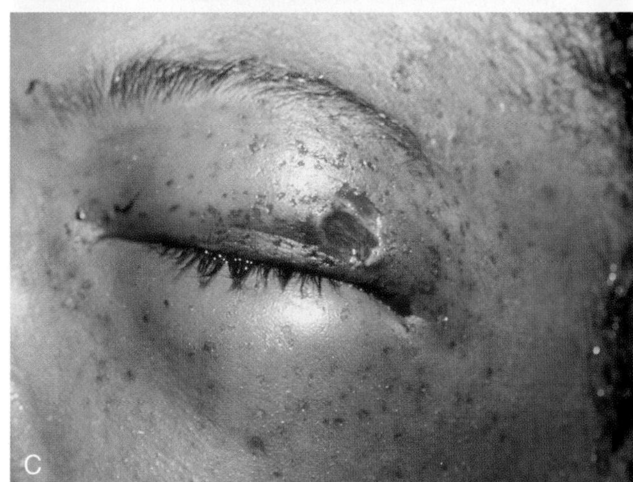

FIGURE 29–6 **A:** Loose-contact entrance wound. Note muzzle mark and seared wound margins. **B:** Close-range entrance wound. Note significant soot around wound. **C:** Intermediate entrance wound. Note tattooing around wound. (**A–C,** Courtesy of Charles Catanese, MD.)

REFERENCES

1. Smock WS. Forensic emergency medicine. In: Olshaker JS, Jackson MC, Smock WS, eds. *Forensic emergency medicine.* Philadelphia: Lippincott Williams & Wilkins, 2001.

29–7

Entrance and Exit Wounds

Robert Hendrickson

Emergency physicians should not document an interpretation of a wound as "entrance" or "exit." The wound should be described in detail and, if possible, photographed. Although entrance and exit wounds can have typical appearances, this determination is not always clear in the acute setting, and misinterpretation may hinder criminal and legal investigations.[1,2]

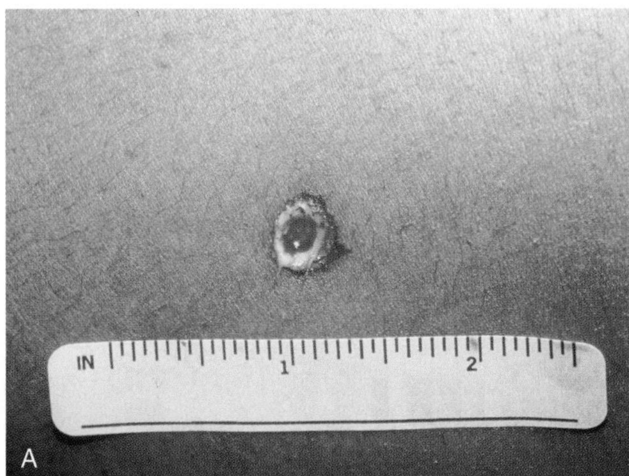

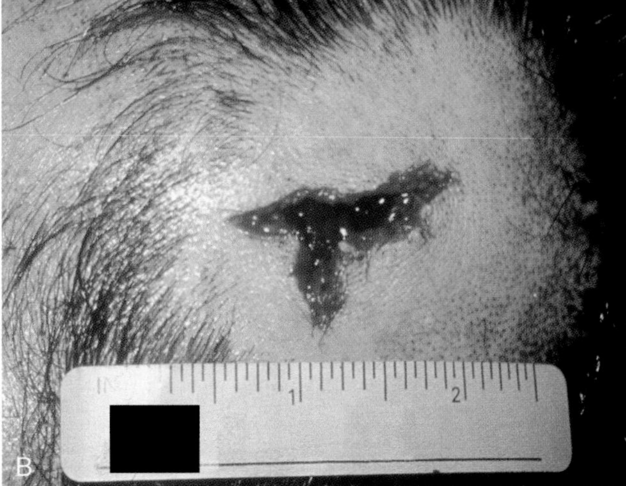

FIGURE 29–7 **A:** Entrance wound. **B:** Exit wound. (**A** and **B**, Courtesy of Charles Catanese, MD.)

Wounds may contain signs that are typical of entrance wounds, including muzzle marks, tattooing, and soot (see "Estimating Range of Gunshot Wounds"). Exit wounds generally have everted, irregular edges and usually lack evidence of soot and tattooing. Exit wounds are not necessarily larger than entrance wounds. In addition, entrance wounds may have everted, irregular edges with stellate lacerations caused by the injection of gases into the subcutaneous tissue.[2]

In Fig. 29–7, the superior wound is an exit wound. The inferior wound is a close-range entrance wound.

REFERENCES

1. Randall T. Clinicians' forensic interpretations of fatal gunshot wounds often miss the mark. *JAMA* 1993;269:2058, 2061.
2. Smock WS. Forensic emergency medicine. In: Olshaker JS, Jackson MC, Smock WS, eds. *Forensic emergency medicine.* Philadelphia: Lippincott Williams & Wilkins, 2001.

Evidence Gathering and Preservation

Robert Hendrickson

Collection of evidence after a crime is generally the role of law enforcement personnel and not the health care worker. However, actions taken in the initial patient encounter can either enhance the ability of law enforcement officials to obtain accurate facts or destroy evidence. Simple steps may be taken to preserve accurate evidence in the emergency department.

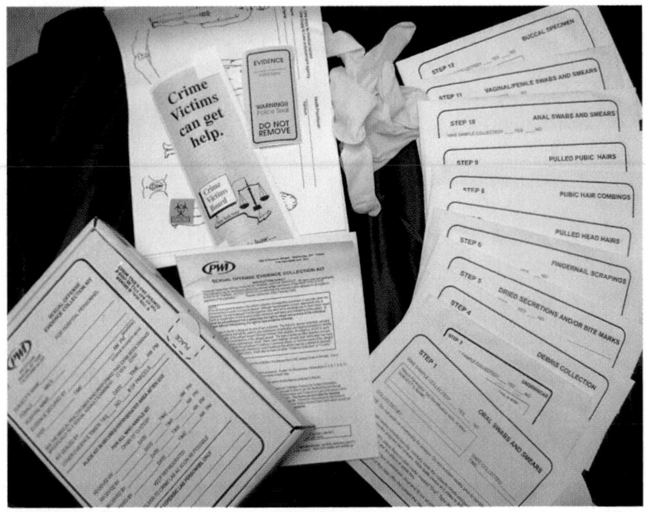

FIGURE 29–8 Clothing may contain important evidence. The emergency physician should avoid cutting clothing in the area of the wound, and ensure proper handling of clothing as evidence. (Courtesy of Mark Silverberg, MD.)

When any victim of trauma is evaluated, an accurate description of all injuries should be recorded. If the injury is caused by penetrating trauma, the clothing should be cut in an area that is distant to the wounds and packaged in paper bags.[1] If the patient fired a gun, the firing hand should be wrapped in a paper bag to prevent removal of gun residue from the hand. Wounds should be adequately described, and potentially photographed, before wound exploration, if possible. When describing wounds, terms such as "entrance wound," "close range," and "exit wound" should be avoided.[1] Instead, a thorough description of the appearance of the wound is more appropriate. When handling bullets, the emergency physician should avoid the use of forceps, because they can scratch the bullet and destroy important evidence.[1] If forceps must be used, their edges should be wrapped in gauze.

REFERENCES

1. Ryan MT, Houry DE. Clinical forensic medicine. *Ann Emerg Med* 2000;36:271–273.

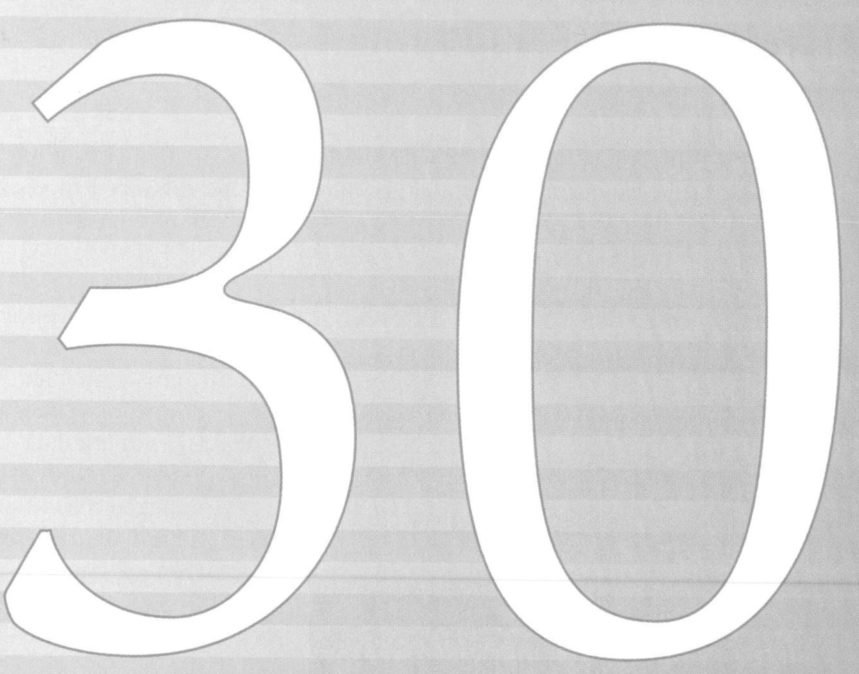

Weapons of Mass Destruction

30-1

Personal Protective Equipment

Anthony Morocco

Personal protective equipment (PPE) is usually classified into four levels based on respiratory and contact protection.[1]

- Level A: Self-contained breathing apparatus and completely sealed chemical-resistant suit. This gives the highest level of protection against inhalation or contact with chemical or biologic agents and should be reserved for on-scene rescuers with exposure to vapor respiratory and contact threats.
- Level B: Self-contained or supplied-air positive-pressure respirator and chemical-resistant suit with gloves and boots. The respiratory protection is equivalent to that of level A, but contact protection is reduced to resist splashes but not vapors. Level B is useful for on-scene rescuers with potential splash and respiratory exposure or oxygen-depleted environments.
- Level C: Air-purifying respirator and chemical resistant suit with gloves and boots. Contact protection is equivalent to that of level B, but respiratory protection is decreased. Respirators filter ambient air through cartridges and may be powered to provide positive pressure (greater protection than nonpowered respirators). Different cartridges or combination of cartridges are used, depending on the type of agent to be filtered (e.g., high-efficiency particulate air [HEPA] filters). Level C is probably the highest level of protection needed for health care facility workers. It is useful when dealing with patients who are contaminated with chemical or biologic agents.
- Level D: Standard work clothing and protection, such as hospital scrubs with gown, mask, and gloves (standard universal hospital precautions).

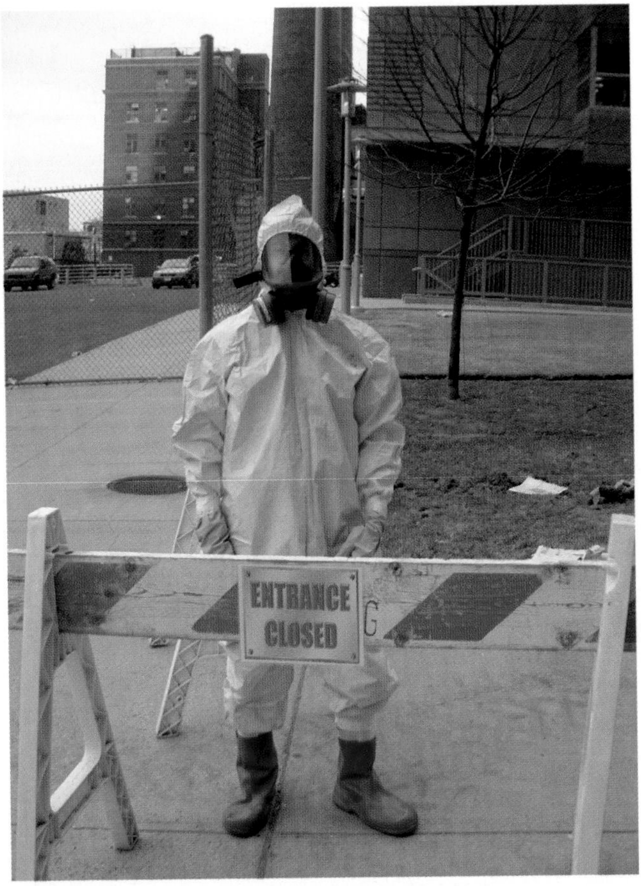

FIGURE 30–1 Level C personal protective equipment with exposure suit, gloves, boots, and mask. (Courtesy of Mark Silverberg, MD.)

The choice of appropriate PPE depends on a number of factors. Higher levels of protection necessitate bulky, heavy, and cumbersome equipment; extensive training and fit-testing for proper use; large expense for equipment and training; lower usable work time due to limited air supply, heat, and exhaustion; difficulty with vision and communication while wearing masks and hoods; and time delays in donning complex suits. For these reasons, the lowest level of protection that is adequate for the potential risk should be employed. In addition, when dealing with patients who are contaminated with radioactive material, health care workers should wear dosimeters.[1]

REFERENCES

1. Hick JL, Hanfling D, Burstein JL, et al. Protective equipment for health care facility decontamination personnel: regulations, risks, and recommendations. *Ann Emerg Med* 2003;42:370–380.

Decontamination

Anthony Morocco

Victims of chemical or biologic weapons may, in some circumstances, require decontamination. Ideally, decontaminations should take place at a site removed from the hospital; however, disaster-level events may result in large numbers of nondecontaminated patients presenting to hospital emergency departments. Therefore, it is vital for hospitals to have adequately trained personnel, appropriate and fit-tested equipment, and a plan for decontamination.

Victims of chemical agents are likely to require more extensive decontamination than those exposed to biologic agents, because chemical agents can be volatile and dermally active. Reaerosolization of biologic particles on victims is possible but is a less immediate risk than chemical exposure.[1]

The first step in decontamination at a health care facility is primary triage, which should be performed outside the hospital proper, by personnel wearing appropriate personal protective equipment (PPE). The level of PPE should be tailored to the exposure, if known. For chemical agents, those performing triage and decontamination should wear level C PPE. For biologic contamination, level D is appropriate, with latex gloves, eye protection, and N-95 masks or high-efficiency particulate air (HEPA) filter masks. For unknown events, level C PPE should be used, with a respirator equipped with a combination organic vapor and HEPA cartridge. Patients with no symptoms are triaged to a self-decontamination or waiting area. Ill patients enter the medical decontamination and emergency treatment area. Actual decontamination starts with removal of all clothing, which may actually remove 75% to 90% of the hazardous agent. Attention should be paid to privacy and appropriate packaging of contaminated items and valuables. This is followed by copious rinsing with warm water and, possibly, washing with soap for 1 to 2 minutes. Excessively hot water and harsh scrubbing may enhance chemical absorption and should be avoided.

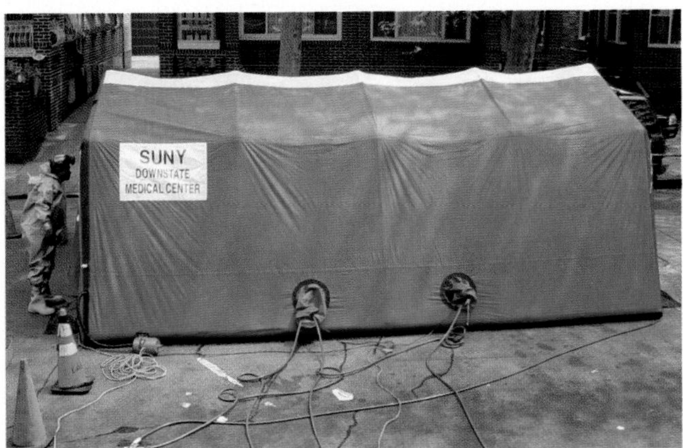

FIGURE 30–2 Decontamination tent. (Courtesy of Mark Silverberg, MD.)

Hypochlorite solution (0.5%) has been recommended to inactivate both biologic and chemical agents. However, because a contact time of 15 to 20 minutes is necessary to deactivate the chemical agents, damage to injured tissues and eyes may occur, and no evidence of superior efficacy versus soap and water exists. For these reasons, hypochlorite solutions are not recommended as part of routine decontamination procedures. The final steps after washing are to dry the patients, place them in gowns, and place ill patients in the emergency department and others in a predetermined holding area.[1]

REFERENCES

1. Macintyre AG, Christopher GW, Eitzen E Jr, et al. Weapons of mass destruction events with contaminated casualties: effective planning for health care facilities. *JAMA* 2000;283:242–249.

Blast Injury

Michael Greenberg

Clinical Presentation

Explosive and incendiary devices are the weapons of choice for terrorists worldwide. Patients who survive the initial event present for care with a wide variety of injuries affecting multiple organ systems.[1–3]

Pathophysiology

Blast injury (BI) is classified as follows (see Table 30–3). Primary BI is caused by an acute change in ambient pressure emanating from the so-called "blast wave" or "overpressure" wave. Primary BI usually affects the respiratory, gastrointestinal, central nervous, and cardiovascular systems and is rarely seen in survivors, because most people who die from BI die from primary BI. Secondary BI results from objects launched as projectiles secondary to the explosive forces. Tertiary BI is caused when an individual is thrown against a fixed object or the ground, or is injured by crushing forces from a structural collapse. Miscellaneous BI involves burns, chemical exposures, and smoke inhalation resulting from the primary explosion.[1–3]

Diagnosis

Diagnosis is based on standard advanced trauma life support (ATLS) protocols and the judicious use of imaging and laboratory studies, as dictated by those protocols.

Clinical Complications

Complications include localized and systemic infections (including tetanus), deeply imbedded foreign bodies, limb amputations, post-traumatic stress disorder, and other ill-defined neuropsychiatric sequelae related to BI.

Management

Treatment should comport with standard ATLS protocols, with special emphasis on extensive and meticulous wound débridement as needed.[1,2]

REFERENCES

1. Argyros GJ. Management of primary blast injury. *Toxicology* 1997;121:105–115.
2. Covey DC. Blast and fragment injuries of the musculoskeletal system. *J Bone Joint Surg Am* 2002;84:1221–1234.
3. Mayorga M. The pathology of primary blast overpressure injury. *Toxicology* 1997;121:17–28.

TABLE 30–3 Mechanisms of Blast Injury

Category	Characteristics	Body Part Affected	Types of Injuries
Primary	Unique to high-order explosives, results from the impact of the overpressurization wave with body surfaces	Gas-filled structures are most susceptible—lungs, gastrointestinal tract, and middle ear	Blast lung (pulmonary barotrauma) Tympanic membrane rupture and middle ear damage Abdominal hemorrhage and perforation; globe (eye) rupture; concussion (traumatic brain injury without physical signs of head injury)
Secondary	Results from flying debris and bomb fragments	Any body part may be affected	Penetrating ballistic (fragmentation) or blunt injuries Eye penetration (can be occult)
Tertiary	Results from individuals' being thrown by the blast wind	Any body part may be affected	Fracture and traumatic amputation Closed and open brain injury
Quaternary	All explosion-related injuries, illnesses, or diseases not due to primary, secondary, or tertiary mechanisms Includes exacerbation or complications of existing conditions	Any body part may be affected	Burns (flash, partial, and full-thickness) Crush injuries Closed and open brain injury Asthma, chronic obstructive pulmonary disease, or other breathing problems from dust, smoke, or toxic fumes Angina Hyperglycemia, hypertension

Courtesy of the Centers for Disease Control and Prevention.

Dispersion of Radioactive Materials

Anthony Morocco

Clinical Presentation

Patients may present with traumatic injuries and stress reactions but not acute radiation injury. However, dispersion of radiologic agents may result in internal contamination via inhalation, ingestion, or wound contamination. Direct contact with a radioactive source results in skin burns. The extent and onset of radiologic injury depend on the penetration and dose of radioactivity.[1]

Pathophysiology

Conventional explosives may be used in a "dirty bomb" to inflict trauma and spread radioactive material over a wide area. A number of different radiologic isotopes are used for industrial, medical, and military applications and therefore may be available to terrorists. Cesium 137, cobalt 60, and iridium 192 are sources within industrial radiographic and radiotherapy equipment. Other radionuclides include tritium, iodine 125, iodine 131, cesium 134, strontium 89, strontium 90, americium, and plutonium.[1]

Ionizing radiation causes damage to body tissues via free radical formation and direct injury to DNA and other cellular structures.[1]

TABLE 30–4 Therapy for Specific Isotopes

Radionuclide	Therapy
Tritium	Force fluids
Cesium	Prussian Blue (currently investigational)
Plutonium and transuranics	Chelating agents such as calcium or zinc diethylenetriaminepentaacetate (DTPA) (currently investigational)
Strontium ingestion	Oral aluminum phosphate or barium sulfate

Courtesy of the Department of Homeland Security Working Group on RDD Prep—Medical Preparedness and Response Sub-Group.

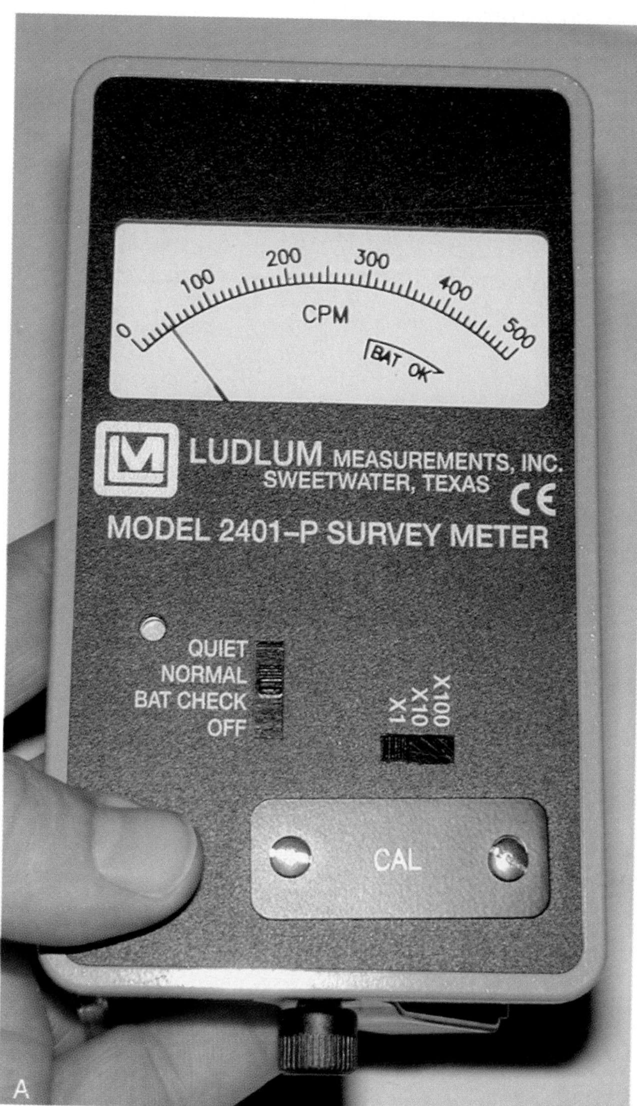

FIGURE 30–4 Radiation survey meter. (Courtesy of Robert Hendrickson, MD.)

Clinical Complications

Radiation doses greater than 6 Gray (Gy) causes bone marrow failure and death without treatment; 10 Gy is the maximum survivable dose with optimal medical care. Malignancy is an important long-term complication. Tumors may develop 5 to 10 years or longer after exposure, whereas leukemia may occur within 2 years.[1]

Management

The hospital radiation safety officer and the Radiation Emergency Assistance Center/Training Site (REAC/TS, telephone 1-865-576-3131) should be contacted. Victims should be undressed and skin decontaminated. Contaminated wounds should be irrigated, and surgical excision may be necessary for retained particles of long-lived isotopes. Hospital workers are at little risk of exposure to any significant radioactivity. Potassium iodide should be administered within several hours after nuclear detonation or nuclear reactor discharge to prevent thyroid uptake of radioactive iodine. Prussian blue binds cesium and decreases gastrointestinal absorption (see Table 30–4). Chelators (calcium diethylenetriaminepentaacetic acid [DTPA] or zinc DTPA) enhance elimination of americium and plutonium. Strontium absorption is decreased by phosphate administration.[1]

REFERENCES

1. Mettler FA Jr, Voelz GL. Current concepts: major radiation exposure—what to expect and how to respond. *N Engl J Med* 2002;346: 1554–1561.

30-5

Acute Radiation Syndrome

Michael Greenberg

Clinical Presentation

Patients with acute radiation syndrome (ARS) may be expected to present minutes to hours after exposure to high energy x-irradiation or gamma irradiation. Specific presenting symptoms depend on the total dose of radiation received. Initial symptoms usually include nausea, vomiting, and anorexia.[1,2]

Pathophysiology

Four clinical phases for ARS have been identified (see Table 30–5B): (1) the prodromal phase, which may range from no symptoms to mild or moderate nausea, vomiting, and diarrhea, depending on degree of exposure, and lasts up to 5 days; (2) the latency phase, which lasts up to 3 weeks and includes dose-dependent hair loss and lymphocytopenia; (3) the phase of overt illness, which includes fatigue, infection, bleeding, thrombocytopenia, hemodynamic instability, coma, and death; and (4) the recovery or demise phase, which occurs after the phase of overt illness.[1,2] See Table 30–5A for dermal manifestations.

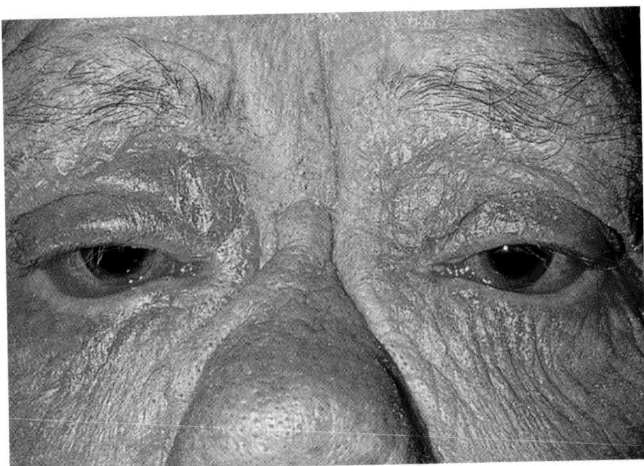

FIGURE 30–5 Erythema, dry scaly skin, and lower ectropion in a patient exposed to local radiation. (From Tasman, with permission.)

Diagnosis

Diagnosis is based on history, clinical findings, and results of the complete blood count.

Clinical Complications

Complications are dose-dependent and may include central nervous system dysfunction, cataracts, sepsis, seizures, coma, and death.[1,2]

Management

Initial treatment may require decontamination efforts followed by meticulous supportive medical care. Because clinical effects are dose-dependent, treatment planning must be individualized, especially if multiple casualties are involved. Cytokine therapy may be helpful in stimulating various bone marrow cell lines that were destroyed or suppressed by radiation exposure.[1,2] Bone marrow transplantation may be an option for treatment in some cases.

REFERENCES

1. Leikin JB, McFee RB, Walter FG, Edsall K. A primer for nuclear terrorism. *Dis Mon* 2003;49:485–516.
2. Allen J, Matthews L. Radiation as a weapon of mass destruction. *Clin Pediatr Emerg Med* 2002;3:248–255.

TABLE 30–5A Dermal Manifestations of Radiation Dose

Dose (Gy)	Clinical Findings	Time Since Exposure
3	Epilation beginning	14–21 days
6	Erythema	(Transient initially; primary erythema occurs at 14–21 days after exposure)
1–15	Dry desquamation	2–3 wk
20–50	Wet desquamation	2–3 wk
>50	Overt radionecrosis and ulceration	4 wk

From the Department of Homeland Security Working Group on RDD Prep—Medical Preparedness and Response Sub-Group.
Gy, Gray.

Acute Radiation Syndrome

Michael Greenberg

TABLE 30–5B Acute Radiation Syndromes

Syndrome	Dose	Prodromal Stage	Latent Stage	Manifest Illness Stage	Recovery Stage
Bone marrow (hematopoietic)	0.7–10 Gy (70–1,000 rads) Mild symptoms may occur as low as 0.3 Gy (30 rads)	Anorexia, nausea and vomiting Occurs 1 hour to 2 days after exposure Lasts for minutes to days	Stem cells in bone marrow are dying, although patient may appear and feel well Lasts 1 to 6 wk	Drop in all blood cell counts for several weeks Anorexia, fever, malaise Primary cause of death is infection and hemorrhage Survival decreases with increasing dose Most deaths occur within a few months after exposure	In most cases, bone marrow cells begin to repopulate the marrow There should be full recovery for a large percentage of individuals from a few weeks up to 2 yr after exposure Death may occur in some individuals at 1.2 Gy (120 rads) The LD50/60 is about 2.5 to 5 Gy (250 to 500 rads)
Gastrointestinal (GI)	10–100 Gy (1,000–10,000 rads) Some symptoms may occur as low as 6 Gy (600 rads)	Anorexia, severe nausea, vomiting, cramps and diarrhea Occurs within a few hours after exposure Lasts about 2 days	Stem cells in bone marrow and cells lining GI tract are dying, although patient may appear and feel well Lasts less than 1 wk	Malaise, anorexia, severe diarrhea, fever, dehydration, electrolyte imbalance Death is caused by infection, dehydration, and electrolyte imbalance Death occurs within 2 wk after exposure	The LD100 is about 10 Gy (1,000 rads)
Cardiovascular (CV) and central nervous system (CNS)	>50 Gy (5,000 rads) Some symptoms may occur as low as 20 Gy (2,000 rads)	Extreme nervousness; confusion; severe nausea, vomiting, and watery diarrhea; loss of consciousness; burning sensations of the skin Occurs within minutes after exposure Lasts for minutes to hours	Patient may return to partial functionality May last for hours but often is less	Return of watery diarrhea, convulsions, coma Begins 5 to 6 hr after exposure Death within 3 days after exposure	No recovery

LD50/60, dose lethal to 50% to 60% of individuals; LD100, dose lethal to 100% of individuals.
Courtesy of the Centers for Disease Control and Prevention.
Gy, Gray; rads, radiation absorbed dose.

30-6

Anthrax

Anthony Morocco

Clinical Presentation

Patients with the most serious form of the disease, inhalational anthrax, initially develop nonspecific symptoms such as headache, fever, cough, and chest pain, with progression to dyspnea, hypotension, obtundation, and other signs of severe systemic illness. Cutaneous anthrax begins as a pruritic papule or macule that enlarges, ulcerates, and forms an eschar. Patients with gastrointestinal anthrax may present with ulceration and edema of the mouth and esophagus or with nausea, vomiting, malaise, and bloody diarrhea associated with bowel involvement.[1]

Pathophysiology

Anthrax is the name for any of the three clinical syndromes caused by *Bacillus anthracis*, a gram-positive, spore-forming bacterium.[1]

The bacterium releases three toxins that cause edema, release of inflammatory mediators, hemorrhage, and cell death. Inhalational anthrax occurs after germination of inhaled *B. anthracis* spores in mediastinal lymph nodes, which may occur up to several weeks after exposure. This form occurs rarely in nature but is likely to develop after exposure to weaponized *B. anthracis.* Cutaneous anthrax may be transmitted to humans by contact with animals (i.e., "woolsorter's disease"). The gastrointestinal form occurs after ingestion of improperly cooked, contaminated meat.[1]

Clinical Complications

Patients with inhalational anthrax rapidly develop mediastinal lymphadenopathy, hemorrhagic mediastinitis, sepsis, and hemorrhagic meningitis. The mortality rate may be as high as 90%. The cutaneous and gastrointestinal forms may also progress to severe systemic illness. Untreated cutaneous anthrax may result in a 20% mortality rate.[1]

Management

Although naturally occurring anthrax is usually susceptible to treatment with penicillin, some strains used for biowarfare have been endowed with resistance to several classes of antibiotics. Culture and susceptibility testing should ultimately be used to guide antibiotic therapy. However, aggressive initial treatment of inhalational anthrax should include early use of intravenous ciprofloxacin or doxycycline, with the addition of one or two other agents such as penicillin, rifampin, or chloramphenicol. Postexposure prophylaxis and treatment of cutaneous anthrax related to bioterrorism consists of oral ciprofloxacin or doxycycline given for at least 60 days.[1]

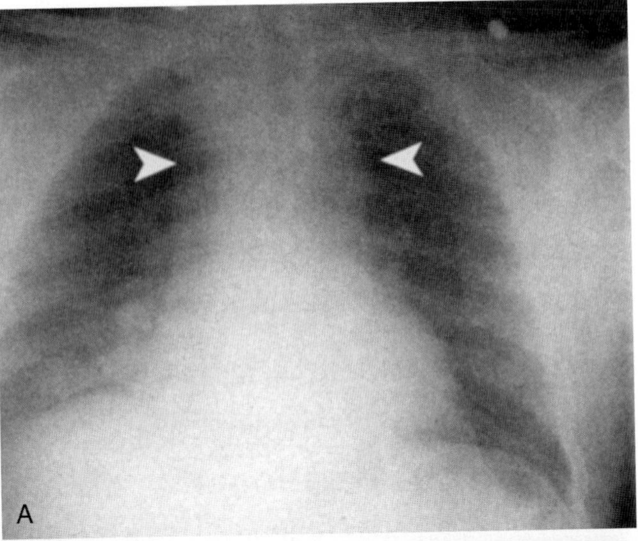

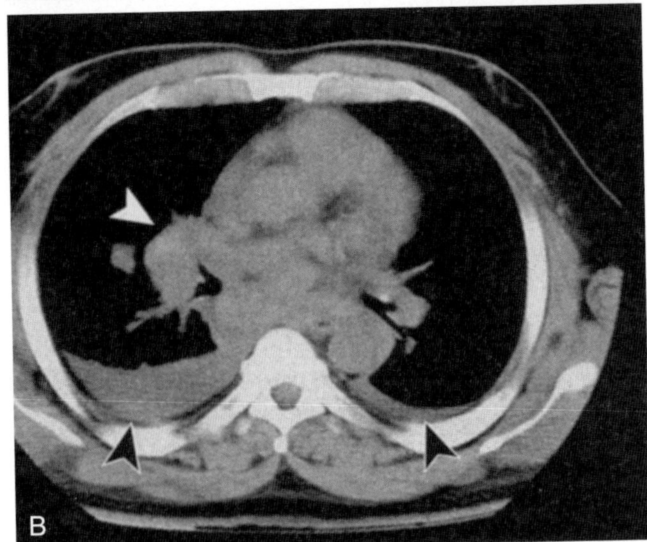

FIGURE 30–6 **A:** Chest radiograph of a 56-year-old man with inhalational anthrax depicts a widened mediastinum, bilateral hilar fullness, right pleural effusion, and bilateral perihilar air-space disease. **B:** Noncontrast spiral computed tomographic scan depicts an enlarged and hyperdense right hilar lymph node *(white arrowhead)*, bilateral pleural effusions *(black arrowheads)*, and edema of the mediastinal fat. (Reprinted with permission from Mayer TA, Bersoff-Matcha S, Murphy C, et al. Clinical presentation of inhalation anthrax following bioterrorism exposure. *JAMA* 2001;286:2549–2553. © 2001 American Medical Association. All rights reserved.)

REFERENCES

1. Inglesby TV, O'Toole T, Henderson DA, Russell PK, Tonat K. Working Group on Civilian Biodefense. Anthrax as a biological weapon, 2002: updated recommendations for management. *JAMA* 2002;287:2236–2252.

Smallpox

Anthony Morocco

Clinical Presentation

The most common form of smallpox (90% of cases) is variola major. The prodromal phase lasts 2 to 3 days and consists of fever, malaise, headache, backache, vomiting, and high fever. A maculopapular rash develops, starting with the mouth and spreading to the hands, forearms, legs, and trunk. Over several days, the rash progresses to enlarging vesicles and finally to deep, 4- to 6-mm diameter pustules. In the malignant or flat form, lesions are flattened and confluent, whereas the hemorrhagic form results in petechiae and larger hemorrhages of the skin and mucous membranes. Variola minor results in smaller, fewer, and more superficial lesions; patients with variola sine eruptione (which occurs in previously vaccinated individuals) may be asymptomatic or develop mild, flu-like symptoms.[1-3]

Pathophysiology

Transmission occurs from person to person via aerosolized respiratory droplets or fomites. Only a few virions are likely needed to initiate infection. The virus enters the mucosa of the respiratory tract and multiplies in local lymph nodes and in the reticuloendothelial system during the 7- to 17-day incubation period.[1,2]

Clinical Complications

Death occurs in 30% of cases of variola major caused by viremia, circulating immune complexes, and hypotension. Pockmarks, most commonly on the face, occur in most survivors. Other complications include encephalitis (1%), arthritis (2% of affected children), viral keratitis, and pneumonia. The hemorrhagic and malignant forms are almost universally fatal, whereas variola minor is fatal in fewer than 1% of cases.[1]

Management

There is currently no specific treatment for smallpox. Strict isolation, aggressive supportive care, and antibiotics for secondary infections are indicated. The vaccinia vaccine is effective in preventing the disease, and immediate postexposure vaccination may attenuate or prevent subsequent illness.[1-3]

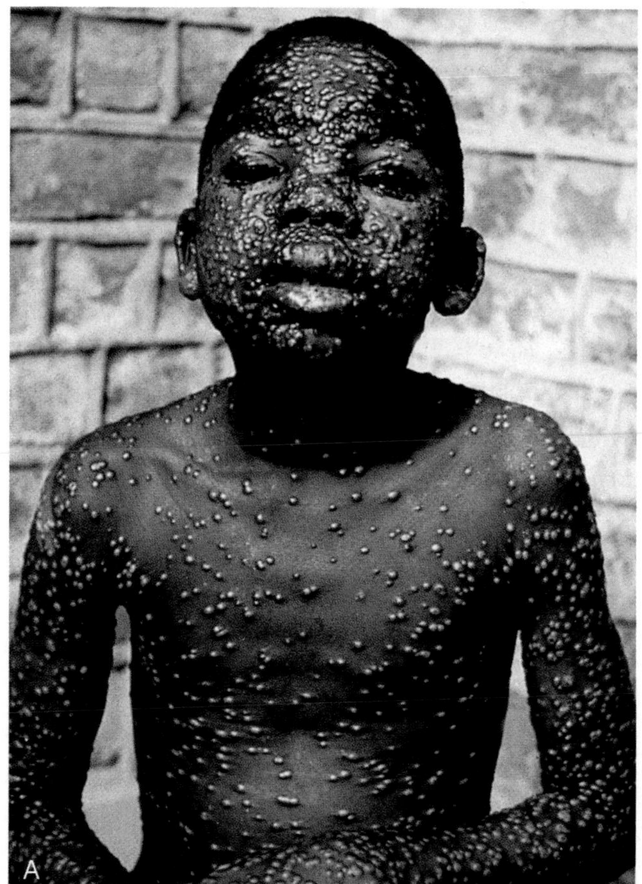

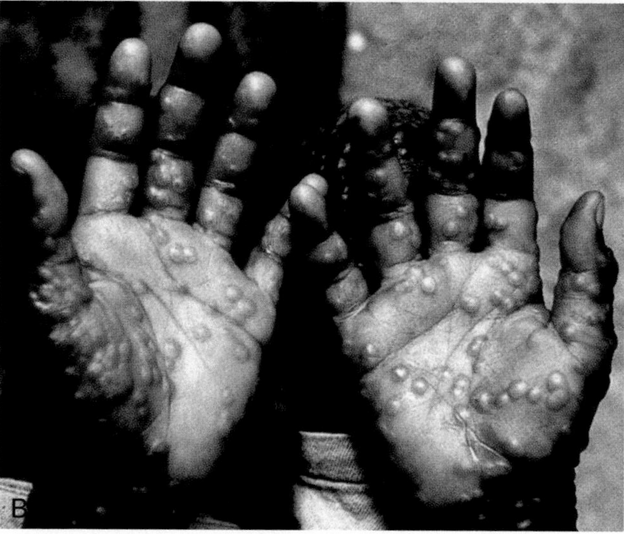

FIGURE 30-7 **A:** Smallpox vesicles are umbilicated and all at similar stages of development. Also note the peripheral and facial predisposition. **B:** Smallpox vesicles. (**A** and **B,** From Ostler, with permission.)

REFERENCES

1. Breman JG, Henderson DA. Current concepts: diagnosis and management of smallpox. *N Engl J Med* 2002;346:1300–1308.
2. Henderson DA, Inglesby TV, Bartlett JG, et al. Working Group on Civilian Biodefense. Smallpox as a biological weapon: medical and public health management. *JAMA* 1999;281:2127–2137.
3. Fenner F, Henderson DA, Arita I, Jezek Z, Ladnyi ID. Smallpox and its eradication. Geneva, Switzerland: World Health Organization; 1988:1460.

Smallpox Vaccination

Anthony Morocco

Clinical Presentation

The vaccine consists of live vaccinia virus injected under the skin over the deltoid or lateral lower leg through multiple punctures made with a bifurcated needle dipped into the vaccination solution.[1]

Patients develop pruritus, pain, and a papule at the immunization site. Regional lymphadenopathy and systemic symptoms of fever, headache, nausea, myalgias, and malaise may develop after 1 week. The papule becomes a pustule and then a scab that detaches within 14 to 21 days. A large reaction (greater than 10 cm) with edema occurs in 10% of vaccinees. A pitted scar usually remains at the site. If a lesser local reaction occurs, the patient is considered to have an inadequate immunization and should undergo another attempt.[1]

Clinical Complications

Secondary bacterial infection may occur at the immunization site. Anaphylaxis, nonspecific rashes, or erythema multiforme may also occur. The vaccinia virus may be transmitted to susceptible contacts. For this reason, health care workers should cover their immunization sites, and vaccination should not be performed on those who have close contact with susceptible individuals. Inadvertent inoculation results in vaccinia lesions in areas such as the eyelid, nose, lips, mouth, genitalia, or anus. Ocular involvement results in conjunctivitis, keratitis, iritis, and corneal scarring.

Generalized vaccinia is a maculopapular or vesicular rash that occurs 6 to 9 days after immunization. The course is generally self-limited except in immunosuppressed patients. Eczema vaccinatum is a severe systemic reaction that occurs most commonly in patients with atopic dermatitis or other chronic skin conditions. Patients develop fever, lymphadenopathy, and extensive skin lesions, with a high risk of secondary infection. Progressive vaccinia occurs in immunosuppressed patients. The inoculation site develops an enlarging, nonhealing, ulcerated, necrotic lesion; severe systemic illness and viremia occur. Postvaccinial encephalitis occurs in infants younger than 12 months of age and may result in permanent cerebral impairment and hemiplegia. Postvaccinial encephalomyelitis occurs in patients older than 2 years of age. Immunization during pregnancy can result in fetal vaccinia and fetal death.[1]

Management

Topical antivirals such as trifluridine may be helpful for ocular vaccinia infection. Vaccinia immunoglobulin (VIG) should be administered for severe ocular disease, eczema vaccinia (to reduce the mortality rate to 7% from 30 to 40%), and progressive vaccinia (100% mortality without treatment).[1]

REFERENCES

1. Cono J, Casey CG, Bell DM. Smallpox vaccination and adverse effects. *MMWR Recomm Rep* 2003;52(RR-4):1–28.

Smallpox Vaccination

Anthony Morocco

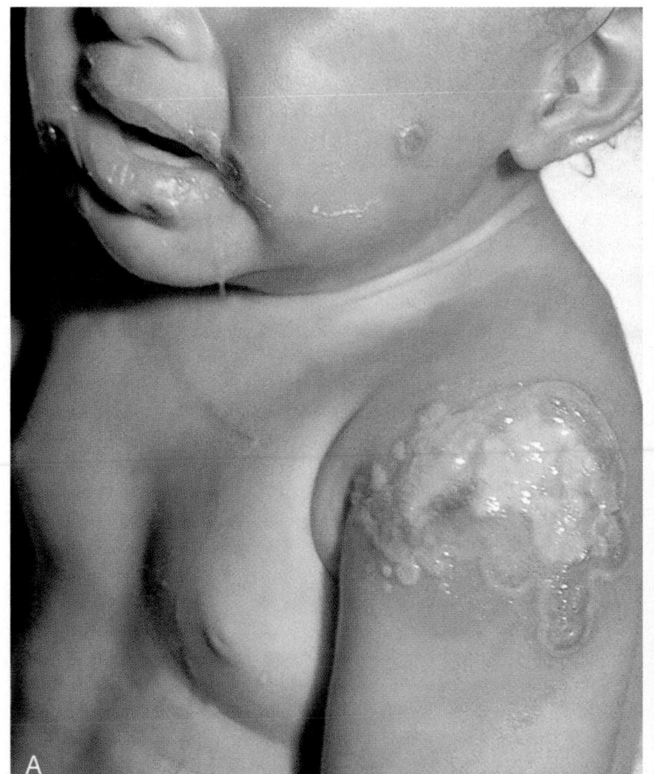

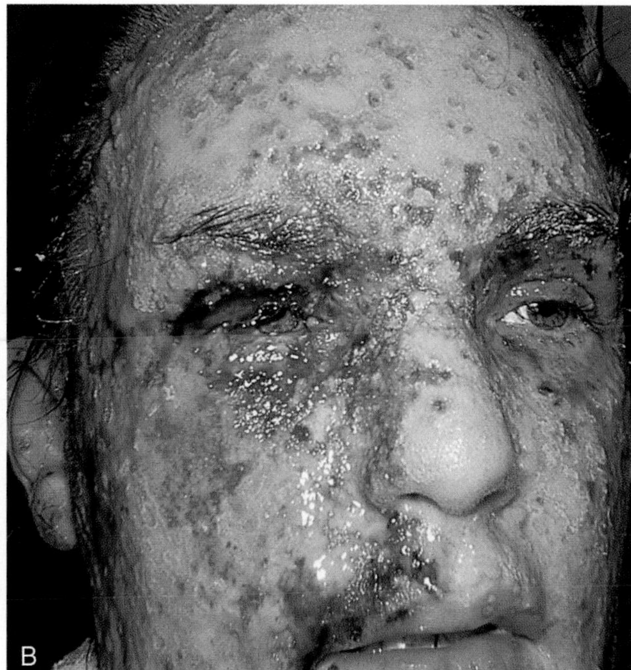

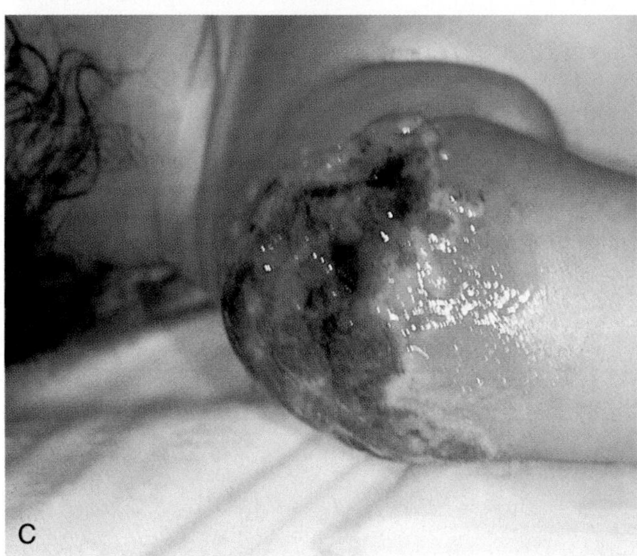

FIGURE 30–8 **A:** Vaccinia, showing severe local reaction with confluent pustules, edema, and erythema. **B:** Eczema vaccinatum (Kaposi varicelliform eruption) in a man with a history of atopic eczema. **C:** Vaccinia necrosum. Necrotizing cellulitis in an immunocompromised infant. (**A–C** From Ostler, with permission.)

Plague

Anthony Morocco

Clinical Presentation

Naturally occurring plague most often occurs in the bubonic form. Patients develop sudden onset of fever, chills, and malaise, followed within 1 day by one or more buboes, which are swollen, painful, nonfluctuant lymph nodes, most commonly in the groin, axilla, or cervical areas. Patients may also present with septicemia without bubo formation in primary septicemic plague. Plague due to bioterrorism would result in primary pulmonary pneumonic plague, in which patients present with fever, cough productive of bloody sputum, and possibly gastroenteritis. Pharyngeal plague with cervical lymphadenopathy may also occur in this setting.[1]

Pathophysiology

Plague, a term often used to refer to any widespread illness or disaster, more specifically refers to the clinical syndromes caused by the gram-negative bacillus, *Yersinia pestis*.

Plague is transmitted from its natural reservoir in rats and other rodents to humans via fleabites. The organism is phagocytized and travels to local lymph nodes, where multiplication and tissue destruction occur, as well as hematogenous spread. The incubation period is 2 to 8 days. Person-to-person transmission occurs only via respiratory droplets in primary and secondary pneumonic plague. Aerosolized *Y. pestis*, as used in a bioterrorist attack, would cause respiratory symptoms in 1 to 6 days.[1]

Diagnosis

The diagnosis may be strongly suspected based on clinical presentation alone. Naturally occurring plague should be considered in areas where it is endemic. Pneumonic plague secondary to bioterrorism would be expected to result in concurrent development of a fulminant pulmonary illness in numerous previously healthy individuals. Gram staining and culture may aid the diagnosis, but hospital laboratories may have difficulty accurately identifying the organism. Special techniques such as polymerase chain reaction (PCR) and immunoassay are available through state health laboratories, the Centers for Disease Control and Prevention (CDC), and military laboratories.

Clinical Complications

Septicemia commonly results from all forms of plague and may lead to shock, disseminated intravascular coagulation (DIC), and death. Skin involvement secondary to small-vessel necrosis may cause purpura and even gangrene of the extremities—hence, the historical name, "black death." Hematogenous spread of the organism may also result in secondary pneumonic plague (12% of cases) and meningeal plague.[1]

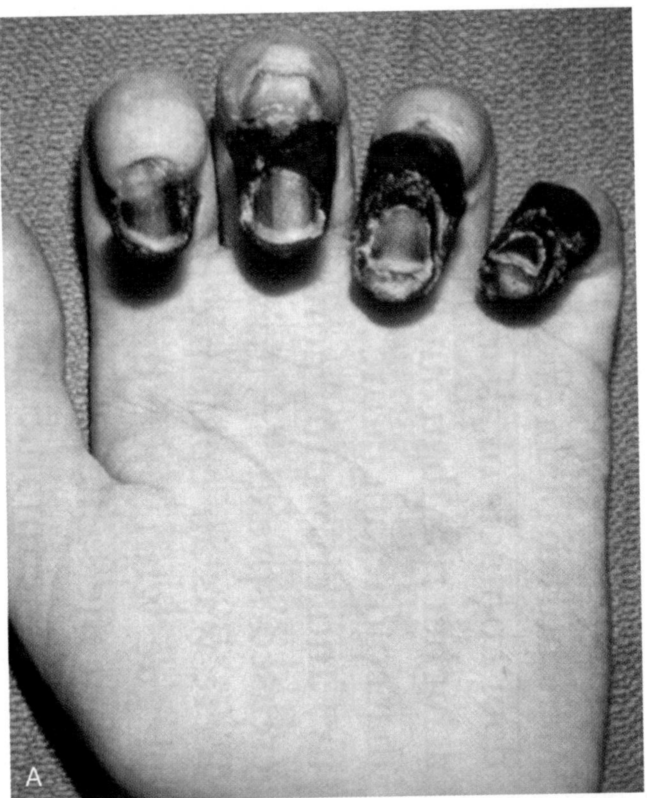

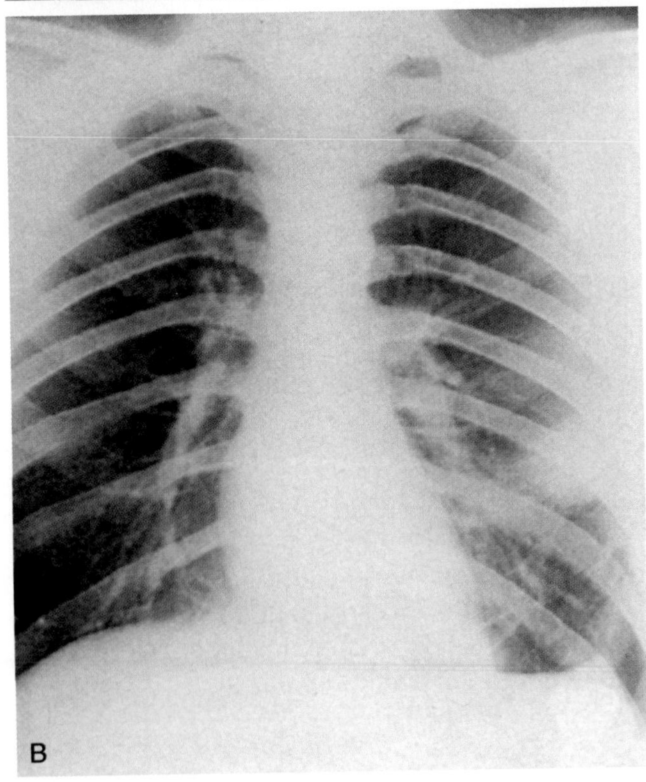

FIGURE 30–9 **A:** Acral gangrene in a patient during the recovery phase of naturally occurring bubonic plague. **B:** Chest radiograph showing extensive lobal consolidation in left lower and left middle lung fields. (Courtesy of Centers for Disease Control and Prevention, Atlanta, Georgia.)

Plague

Anthony Morocco

Management

Early antibiotic treatment is vital to reduce the high mortality rate. However, multidrug-resistant strains of *Y. pestis* that may have been created in the former Soviet Union might be used by terrorists. Parenteral therapy with streptomycin or gentamicin should be initiated in symptomatic patients. Doxycycline, ciprofloxacin, and chloramphenicol are second-line agents. Oral therapy with doxycycline or ciprofloxacin may be used for post-exposure prophylaxis and in cases of mass casualties.[2] Strict respiratory isolation is clearly indicated for any case of suspected plague. A vaccine was previously available, but it does not prevent primary pneumonic plague.

REFERENCES

1. Inglesby TV, Dennis DT, Henderson DA, et al. Working Group on Civilian Biodefense. Plague as a biological weapon: medical and public health management. *JAMA* 2000;283:2281–2290.
2. Gilligan PH. Therapeutic challenges posed by bacterial bioterrorism threats. *Curr Opin Microbiol* 2002;5:489–495.

Hemorrhagic Fever Viruses

Anthony Morocco

Clinical Presentation

Hemorrhagic fever viruses (HFVs) are members of several families and include a number of potential bioweapons such as Ebola, Marburg, Lassa, New World arenaviruses (NWA), Rift Valley fever (RVF), yellow fever (YF), Omsk hemorrhagic fever (OHF), Kyasanur Forest disease (KFD), Crimean-Congo hemorrhagic fever (CCHF), and hantavirus species (HV).[1,2]

Although the viruses vary somewhat in clinical effects, a common HFV syndrome can be described. Patients develop fever, myalgias, prostration, hypotension, variable rash or cutaneous flushing, conjunctivitis, pharyngitis, petechiae, and bleeding from mucous membranes. Unique features include peripheral edema, less prominent hemorrhage, and hearing loss (Lassa); retinitis (RVF); renal syndrome (HV); and pulmonary and central nervous system involvement (OHF, KFD).

Pathophysiology

Natural transmission of most HFVs occurs from animal reservoirs or arthropod vectors. Human-to-human transmission via contact with blood and body fluids, as well as possibly via airborne virus, occurs with Ebola, Marburg, Lassa, and NWA. All the HFVs could be used to infect humans by inhalation of aerosols during a bioterrorist attack. Incubation periods range from 2 to 21 days.[1] The HFVs are RNA viruses and exhibit generalized cytotoxicity. Several mechanisms may be responsible for the hemorrhage and thrombocytopenia, including consumptive coagulopathy, bone marrow failure, vascular endothelial injury, and platelet dysfunction.

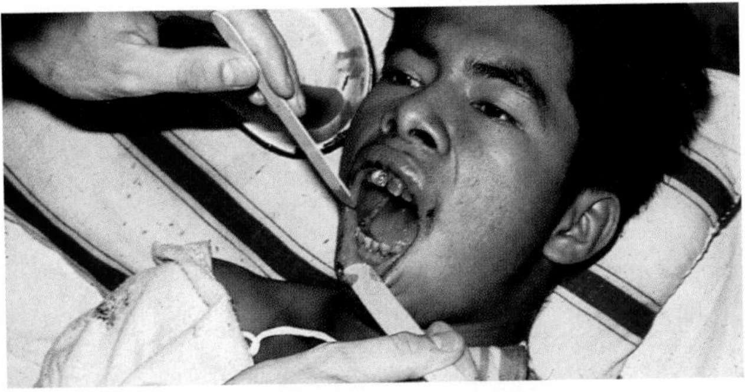

FIGURE 30–10 Gingival hemorrhages occur commonly in hemorrhagic fever. (From Mandell, *Essential Atlas of Infectious Diseases*, with permission.)

Diagnosis

HFV should be suspected in any patient with fever and hemorrhagic complications, particularly if a relevant travel history exists. The presence of multiple concurrent cases in previously healthy individuals away from endemic areas suggests bioterrorism. Basic laboratory studies may reveal thrombocytopenia, leucopenia, and hematuria. Polymerase chain reaction (PCR) tests, antigen detection by enzyme-linked immunosorbent assay (ELISA), and viral culture to confirm the presence of an HFV are available through the Centers for Disease Control and Prevention (CDC).

Clinical Complications

In addition to hemorrhagic complications, disseminated intravascular coagulation (DIC), renal failure, jaundice, and central nervous system dysfunction may occur. Mortality rates vary widely among the HFVs. Ebola (50% to 90% mortality) and Marburg (23% to 70%) have highest rates; Lassa (15% to 20%), NWA (15% to 30%), and YF (20%) have intermediate rates; and RVF and OHF have the lowest rates (less than 1%).[1]

Management

Patients with suspected HFV should be placed in strict respiratory and contact isolation, and public health officials should be contacted immediately. Meticulous supportive care is essential. The antiviral drug ribavirin may be useful for Lassa, RVF, HV, CCHF, and NWA. The drug is not recommended for postexposure prophylaxis, but it should be used in symptomatic patients before virus identification. A vaccine is available only for YF but is not useful for postexposure prophylaxis.

REFERENCES

1. Borio L, Inglesby TV, Peters CJ, et al. Working Group on Civilian Biodefense. Hemorrhagic fever viruses as biological weapons: medical and public health management. *JAMA* 2002;287:2391–2405.
2. Kortepeter M, Christopher G, Cieslak T, et al. *USAMRIID's medical management of biological casualties handbook*, 4th ed. February 2001. Available at: http://www.usamriid.army.mil/education/bluebookpdf/Mmbch4AdobePDFVer4-02.pdf

Tularemia

Anthony Morocco

Clinical Presentation

With naturally occurring tularemia, there can be a myriad of presentations and widely varying severity of illness. Ulceroglandular, glandular, oculoglandular, oropharyngeal, pneumonic, and typhoidal forms occur. Suppurative, necrotic lesions and regional lymphadenopathy occur in the cutaneous forms, whereas fever, malaise, body aches, and often gastrointestinal symptoms with no focal signs occur in the typhoidal form. Inhalational illness may initially manifest with systemic signs and symptoms before the development of respiratory difficulties.

Pathophysiology

Tularemia is a zoonosis caused by the gram-negative coccobacillus, *Francisella tularensis.*

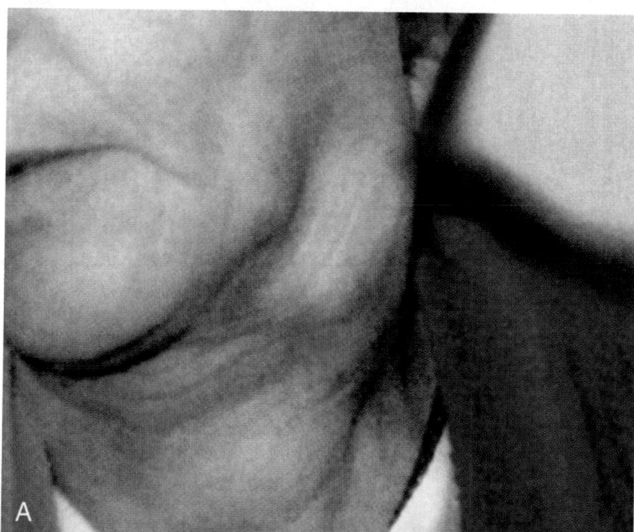

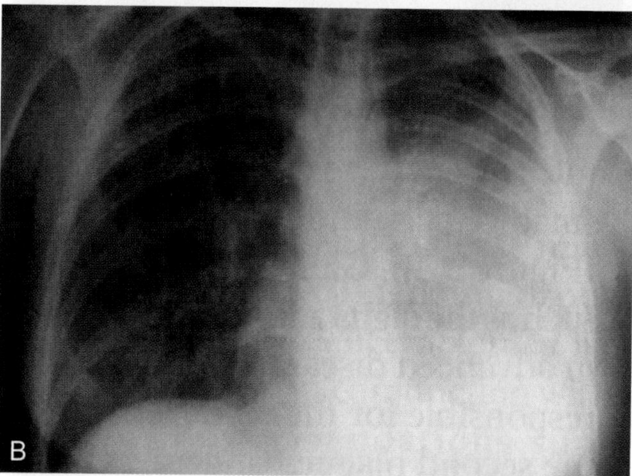

FIGURE 30–11 **A:** Patient with marked swelling and fluctuant suppuration of several anterior cervical lymph nodes after ingestion of food or water contaminated with tularemia. (Courtesy of World Health Organization, Geneva, Switzerland.) **B:** Infiltrates in left lower lung, tenting of diaphragm, and enlargement of left hilum. (Courtesy of Armed Forces Institute of Pathology, Washington, D.C.)

Two major subspecies exist, types A and B, with the former being the much more virulent pathogen. Small mammals such as rabbits are a reservoir, and humans may contract the disease after an arthropod bite or exposure to contaminated animal tissues, water, soil, or food. Bioterrorism-related cases could result from inhalation of aerosolized bacteria, with likely symptoms developing 3 to 5 days after exposure. The organism is taken up by macrophages and migrates to regional lymph nodes, where it further multiplies and may disseminate. Granulomatous lesions occur after suppuration and necrosis.

Diagnosis

The diagnosis may be strongly suspected based on clinical presentation alone. Naturally occurring tularemia should be considered in at-risk populations such as rabbit hunters. Pneumonic tularemia secondary to bioterrorism should be suspected if numerous previously healthy individuals concurrently develop fever and respiratory complaints. Chest radiographic findings such as infiltrates, effusion, and hilar lymphadenopathy may be absent early in the disease. Cultures may aid the diagnosis, but special procedures are necessary. Other techniques, such as direct fluorescent antibody or immunohistochemical stains, polymerase chain reaction (PCR), immunoassays, and antigen detection, may be available through research or reference laboratories.[1]

Clinical Complications

Septicemia may result from any form of tularemia, and death occurs in 1.4% of all naturally infected patients. Hematogenous spread may cause secondary pneumonia and meningitis.

Management

Parenteral therapy with streptomycin or gentamicin should be initiated in symptomatic patients. Doxycycline, ciprofloxacin, and chloramphenicol are second-line agents. Oral therapy with doxycycline or ciprofloxacin may be used for postexposure prophylaxis and in cases of mass casualties.[2] Respiratory isolation is not indicated, because there is no known human-to-human transmission. A live attenuated vaccine has been used in tularemia researchers, but it is not fully protective. Multidrug-resistant and vaccine-resistant strains of *Yersinia pestis* that may have been created in the former Soviet Union might be used by terrorists.

REFERENCES

1. Dennis DT, Inglesby TV, Henderson DA, et al. Working Group on Civilian Biodefense. Tularemia as a biological weapon: medical and public health management. *JAMA* 2001;285:2763–2773.
2. Gilligan PH. Therapeutic challenges posed by bacterial bioterrorism threats. *Curr Opin Microbiol* 2002;5:489–495.

Nerve Agents

Anthony Morocco

Clinical Presentation

Symptoms are consistent with cholinergic excess and vary depending on the dose and route of exposure. With low-dose vapor exposure, patients may complain of blurred vision, headache, rhinorrhea, chest tightness, lacrimation, salivation, and bronchorrhea. Larger vapor doses result in copious secretions, fasciculations, seizures, and apnea. Small doses to the skin cause local sweating and fasciculations, followed by nausea, vomiting, and diarrhea. Low-dose skin exposures may result in an asymptomatic period up to 18 hours before the onset of gastrointestinal symptoms. Larger skin exposures generally cause severe systemic toxicity within 30 minutes. On physical examination, tachycardia or bradycardia may be present, but blood pressure is normal or elevated. Miosis occurs with direct exposure to the eye or with large systemic doses, but not with small skin exposure.[1]

Pathophysiology

The nerve agents are a group of highly neurotoxic compounds used in chemical warfare. They include tabun (GA), sarin (GB), soman (GD), cyclosarin (GF), and VX. Although they often are referred to as "nerve gases," all of the nerve agents are liquids at room temperature and are dispersed in liquid, aerosol, or vapor form.[1]

The nerve agents are organic phosphorous compounds that inhibit the enzyme acetylcholinesterase. This enzyme normally hydrolyzes acetylcholine at the synaptic junction. In the presence of a nerve agent, there is an accumulation of this neurotransmitter, resulting in the symptoms of cholinergic excess. The reaction of nerve agent with the enzyme occurs in two steps: an initial reversible phosphorylation reaction, followed minutes to days later by the loss of a side chain. The second step, called "aging," differs substantially in time course among the nerve agents and is irreversible.[1]

Diagnosis

Identification of a nerve agent release is based on the observation of symptoms of cholinergic excess occurring simultaneously in a large number of patients. Chemical detection equipment may aid in the diagnosis and is becoming more widely available to hospitals and emergency personnel. Laboratory evidence of decreased plasma and red blood cell cholinesterase activity may be helpful but is often not readily available. The diagnosis of organic phosphorous pesticide poisoning should be considered, because this entity is clinically indistinguishable from nerve agent exposure.[1]

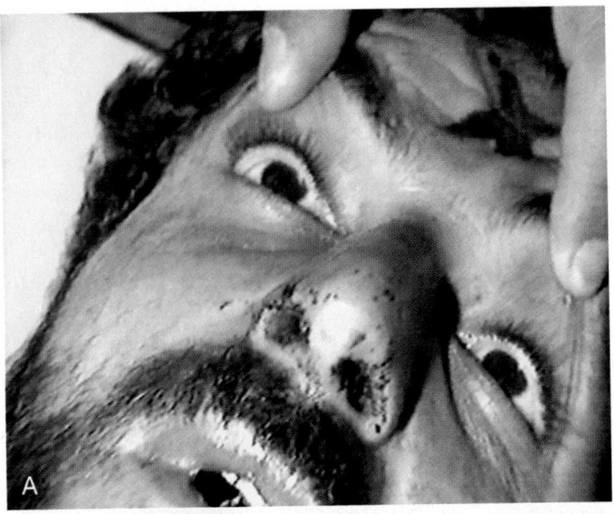

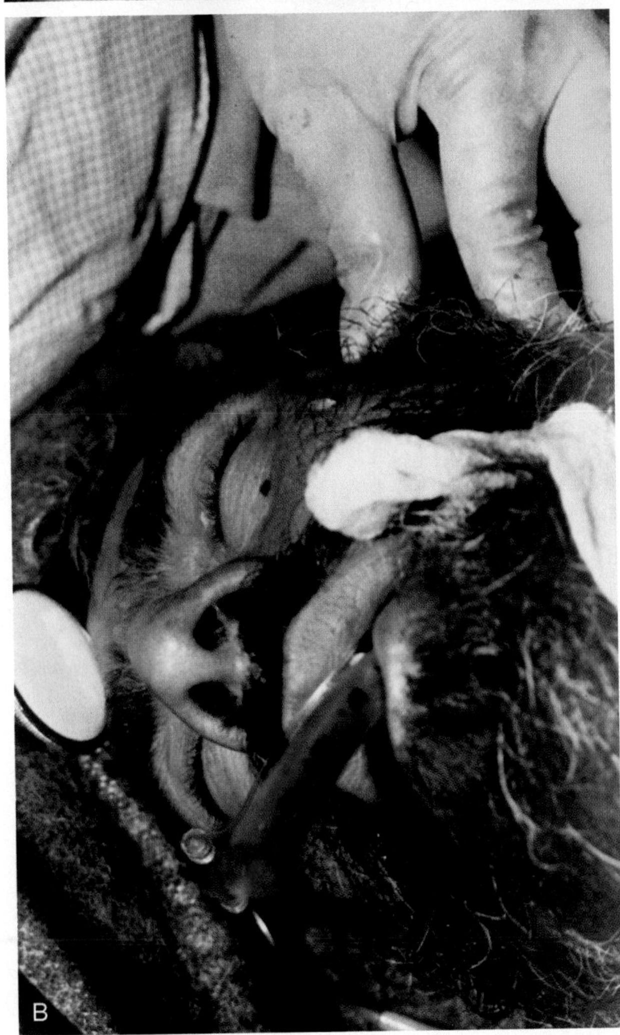

FIGURE 30–12 **A:** Victim of a sarin release in Iran, 1987. Note pinpoint pupils and muscular weakness (ptosis). **B:** Victim of a nerve agent in Iran, 1985. Note the copious secretions and muscular weakness. (**A** and **B,** From Foroutan, with permission.)

Nerve Agents

Anthony Morocco

Clinical Complications

Large doses of nerve agent by any route cause rapid loss of consciousness, seizures, and death. Long-term effects are unclear. Exposures to organic phosphorous pesticides have produced an "intermediate syndrome," long-term neuropsychiatric effects, and polyneuropathy that have not been reported after nerve agent exposure.[1]

Management

The first concern is to decontaminate the patient. After vapor exposure, only removal of clothing is necessary. Liquid exposures require removal of clothing and washing of the skin with water and soap, if available. Health care workers have become symptomatic after treating patients who were not decontaminated. Atropine is a cholinergic antagonist that acts at the muscarinic receptors; the dose is 2 mg initially, repeated every 2 to 5 minutes to effect. Large doses may be required. Parenteral atropine should not be used to reverse miosis, although topical atropine or homatropine may be used.

Pralidoxime (2-PAM) separates the nerve agent from the acetylcholinesterase, thereby regenerating the enzyme. Pralidoxime is not effective after aging has occurred. Unlike atropine, pralidoxime results in improvement of nicotinic receptor–related symptoms (muscle weakness, fasciculations, paralysis, and tachycardia). The dose is 1 g given intravenously over 20 to 30 minutes, or 1 g given intramuscularly. Pralidoxime is not effective against GA, and it is unlikely to be helpful after GD exposure because of its very short aging time (2 to 6 minutes); however, it is not possible to clinically differentiate the nerve agents used. Diazepam is also recommended for severe nerve agent intoxication, to reduce convulsive activity. The Mark I kit is used by military personnel for nerve agent casualties. Each kit contains 2 mg atropine and 600 mg pralidoxime in intramuscular autoinjectors. Treatment for mild toxicity is one kit; moderate toxicity, one to two kits; and severe toxicity, three kits plus 10 mg diazepam.[1]

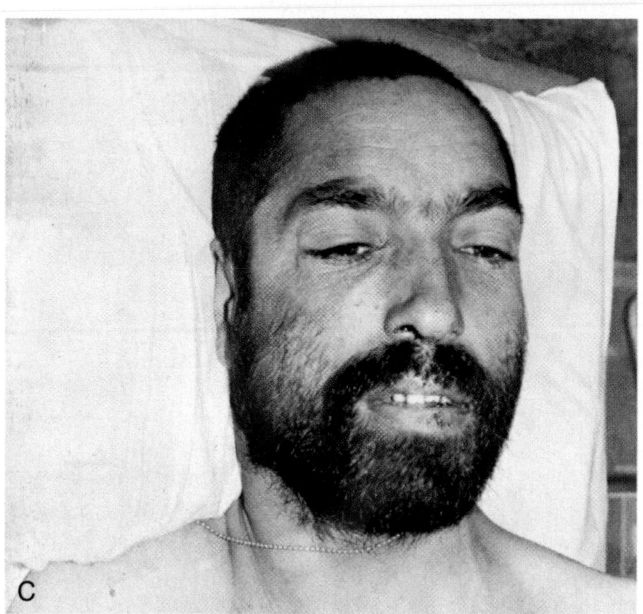

FIGURE 30–12, cont'd. C: Victim of a nerve agent in Iran, 1985. Note the patient's ptosis, miosis, and muscular weakness of the jaw. (From Foroutan, with permission.)

REFERENCES

1. *USAMRICD's medical management of chemical casualties handbook,* 3rd ed. Aug 1999. Available at: www.unh.org/CHEMCASU/titlepg.html.

Vesicants

Anthony Morocco

Clinical Presentation

The vesicants are a class of chemical warfare agents that cause damage to body tissues on contact. These agents include sulfur mustard (H and HD), lewisite (L), and phosgene oxime (CX).

The vesicants L and H differ primarily in time to onset of symptoms. L causes immediate burning of the skin and mucous membranes, whereas H causes delayed symptoms and injury. L may result in less severe injuries, because the immediate symptoms cause exposed patients to flee the scene and decontaminate themselves, thus limiting exposure. Those exposed to H may be unaware until onset of erythema and burning, 2 to 48 hours later. Skin erythema and blisters form, followed by areas of necrosis. Increasing inhaled doses cause mucous membrane burning, cough, laryngospasm, and severe lung injury. Pseudomembrane formation and mucosal necrosis, preferentially affecting the upper respiratory tract, may occur. The scrotum is commonly affected, because H penetration is best in warm, moist areas with thin skin. The eyes are particularly sensitive to H vapor, with injury ranging from conjunctivitis to severe corneal injury. CX is an urticant; it causing immediate mucous membrane and skin irritation, but not blistering.[1,2]

Pathophysiology

The precise mechanisms of action of the vesicants are unknown. L contains the toxic trivalent form of arsenic. H forms reactive cyclic ethylene sulfonium ions that most likely react with and damage numerous cellular proteins to produce DNA alkylation. H also possesses mild cholinergic properties.

Diagnosis

Immediate versus delayed clinical effects differentiate H and L exposure. Patients may report smelling geraniums during exposure to L. Thiodiglycol, a urinary metabolite of H, is detectable.[1,2]

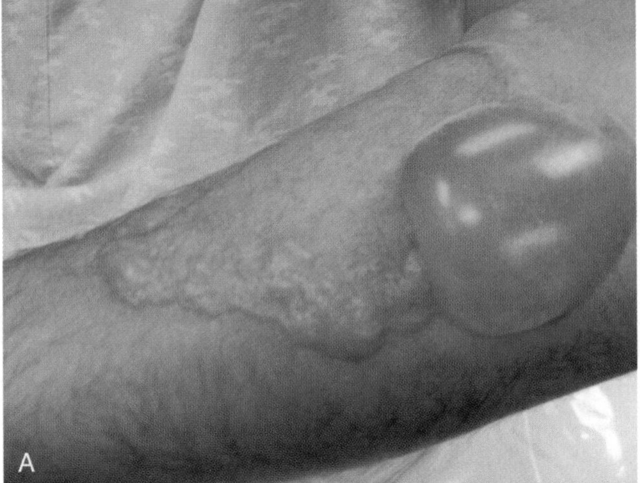

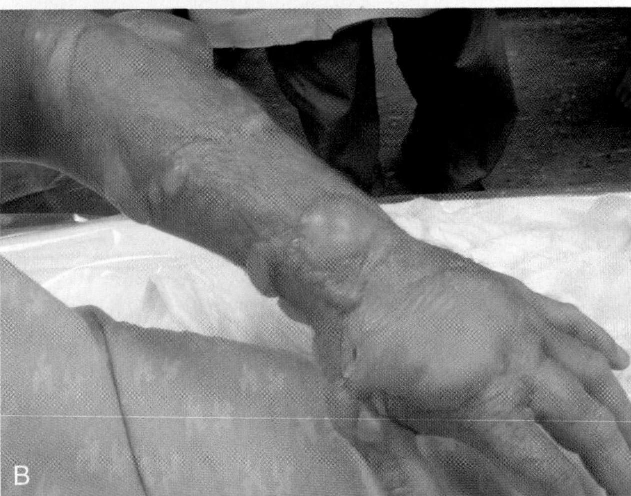

FIGURE 30–13 **A** and **B:** Second degree chemical injury in a military bomb disposal technician who inadvertently came into contact with sulfur mustard. Note extensive blistering with bullae and blisters containing brown-tan fluid. It is anticipated that the blister fluid does not contain sulfur mustard. (Courtesy of Michael Greenberg, MD and Leslie Carroll, MD.)

Clinical Complications

Death most commonly occurs as a result of respiratory injury. Secondary bacterial infection, immunosuppression due to bone marrow damage (H), gastrointestinal mucosal injury, and central nervous system involvement may occur after large exposures. Blindness rarely occurs after corneal injury and panophthalmitis. Long-term effects include skin and respiratory tract cancers, tracheobronchial stenosis, and glaucoma.[1,2]

Management

Immediate decontamination, including eye irrigation, is vital. Skin damage is treated the same as for thermal burns, except that intravenous fluid requirements are not as high after vesicant injury. Respiratory involvement suggests the need for early intubation, because edema and laryngospasm may develop. No specific antidote is available for H or CX. British anti-lewisite (BAL) may be useful after L exposure, but no topical formulation is commercially available.[1,2]

REFERENCES

1. Chemical casualties: vesicants (blister agents). *J R Army Med Corps* 2002;148:358–370.
2. Devereaux A, Amundson DE, Parrish JS, Lazarus AA. Vesicants and nerve agents in chemical warfare: decontamination and treatment strategies for a changed world. *Postgrad Med* 2002;112:90–96.

Ricin

Anthony Morocco

Clinical Presentation

Routes of exposure may be oral, inhalational, ocular, dermal, or parenteral.[1] Person-to-person transmission does not occur. The clinical presentation depends specifically on the route of exposure. Ricin poisoning may resemble routine gastroenteritis or viral respiratory illness and therefore may at first be difficult to diagnose.

Symptom onset occurs 4 to 8 hours after inhalation of the toxin. Patients may complain of cough, chest tightness, dyspnea, fever, nausea, and arthralgias. High doses cause progression to pulmonary edema within 18 to 24 hours. After ingestion, patients may present with severe nausea, vomiting, and diarrhea.[1–3]

Pathophysiology

Ricin is a toxin derived from the beans of the castor plant (*Ricinus communis*). The toxin is easily extracted from the waste mash produced during castor oil production, which is 5% ricin by weight. Ricin has been procured for use as a terrorist weapon on a number of occasions.[1]

Ricin toxin contains a "B" chain, which facilitates entry into cells, and an "A" chain, which exerts toxicity by binding ribosomes and inhibiting protein synthesis. The result is cell death and a systemic inflammatory response syndrome with capillary leak.[1–3]

Diagnosis

Ricin dissemination should be suspected if a large number of patients present with respiratory or gastrointestinal symptoms where a terrorist attack is suspected. Enzyme-linked immunosorbent assay (ELISA) testing of serum and respiratory secretions can confirm the diagnosis but may not be available in time for clinical decision-making. Other diagnostic testing may reveal bilateral infiltrates on chest radiographs and leukocytosis.[1–3]

Clinical Complications

Lung injury may lead to respiratory failure, acute respiratory distress syndrome (ARDS), and death within 36 to 72 hours. Gastrointestinal exposure results in massive fluid losses through diarrhea, vomiting, and hemorrhagic necrosis of the liver, spleen, and kidneys. Intramuscular injection of ricin toxin results in local necrosis and injury to multiple organ systems.[1–3]

Management

Treatment requires aggressive supportive care; there is no specific antidote. Gastrointestinal decontamination with gastric lavage should be considered early after ingestion. Lung injury necessitates respiratory support, and gastrointestinal injury requires replacement of extensive gastrointestinal fluid losses.[1] Suspected or known cases of ricin poisoning should be reported to a regional poison center, local and state health officials, and the Centers for Disease Control and Prevention (CDC) and other federal agencies as soon as possible.[1]

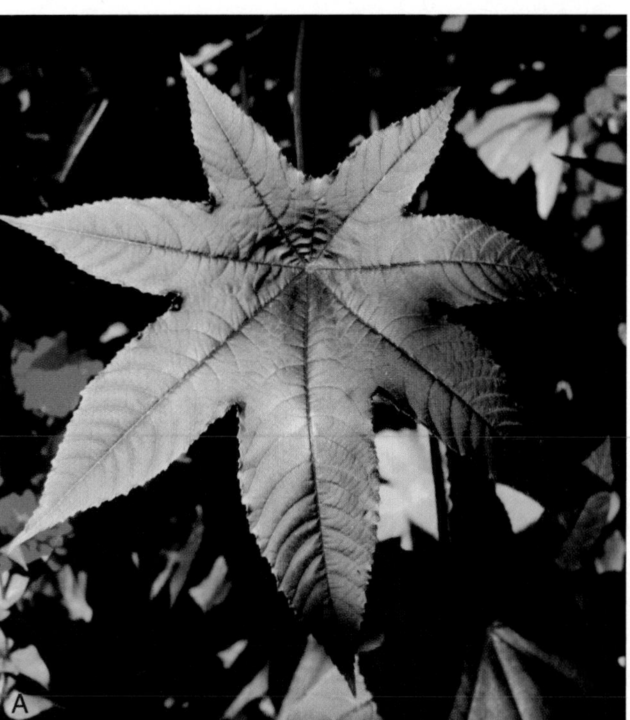

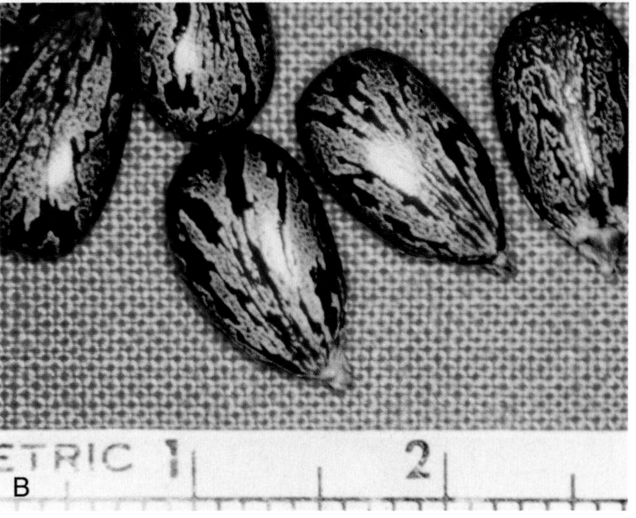

FIGURE 30–14 **A:** The leaf of *Ricinus communis.* **B:** Castor beans. (**A** and **B,** Courtesy of Robert H. Poppenga, DVM, PhD.)

REFERENCES

1. Investigation of a ricin-containing envelope at a postal facility. *MMWR Morb Mortal Wkly Rep* 2003;52:1129–1131.
2. Challoner KR, McCarron MM. Castor bean intoxication. *Ann Emerg Med* 1990;19:1177–1183.
3. Olsnes S, Kozlov JV. Ricin. *Toxicon* 2001;39:1723–1728.

Pulmonary/Choking Agents

Anthony Morocco

Clinical Presentation

Phosgene causes delayed lung injury, with symptom onset occurring 20 minutes to 24 hours after exposure, depending on the dose. Patients develop shortness of breath, chest tightness, hypoxemia, and crackles on lung examination. Very high concentrations may also produce early symptoms of mucous membrane irritation. Exposure to ammonia or chlorine produces immediate burning of mucous membranes, skin, and eyes. Patients may develop cough and stridor.[1]

Pathophysiology

Several agents might be used as weapons because of their potential pulmonary toxicity. Phosgene, chlorine, ammonia, hydrogen fluoride, hydrogen chloride, methyl isocyanate, and phosphine are widely available in industry. Among these, chlorine and phosgene were used as weapons during World War I. Other potential pulmonary agents include the fumigant chloropicrin, diphosgene, sulfur dioxide, and riot control agents such as tear gas (CS). The vesicants and cyanogen chloride

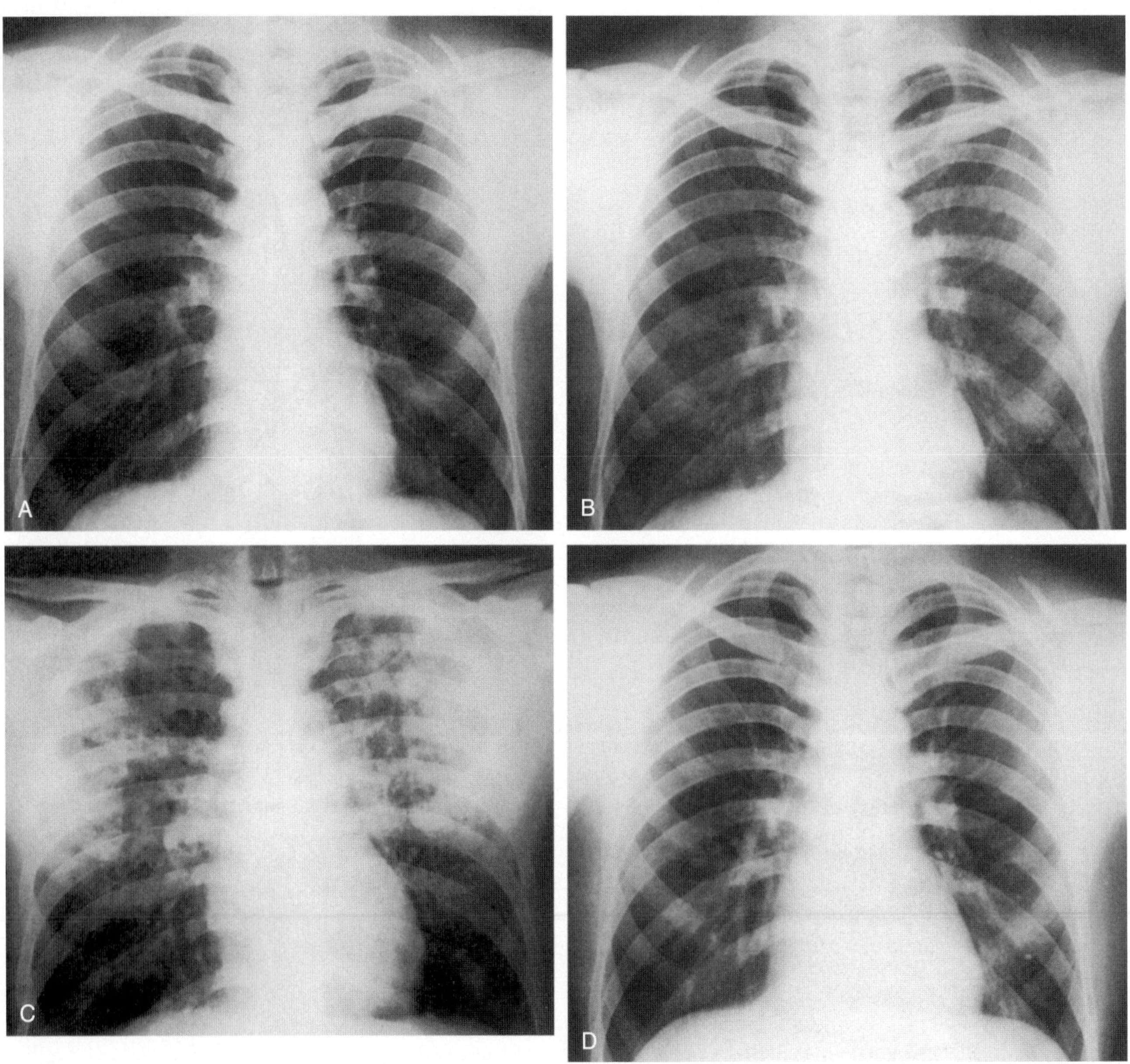

FIGURE 30–15 The development of chest roentgenographic signs in acute phosgene exposure. **A:** One year before exposure. **B:** Six hours after phosgene inhalation. Early pulmonary edema can be seen. **C:** Ten hours after phosgene inhalation: overt pulmonary edema. **D:** Five days after phosgene inhalation: complete regression with clear chest film. (From Borak J, Diller WF. Phosgene exposure: mechanisms of injury and treatment strategies. *J Occup Envir Med* 2001;43:110–119, with permission.)

may also act as lung irritants in addition to their systemic and dermal toxicities.[1]

Agents that are highly water soluble (e.g., ammonia) act primarily in the upper airways, whereas agents that are less water soluble (e.g., phosgene) act in the more distal aspects of the pulmonary tree. At high gas concentrations this distinction does not apply, because these agents are capable of causing damage in both areas. Irritant gases act by producing corrosive solutions on contact with water (e.g., hydrochloric acid from chlorine, ammonium chloride from ammonia). Phosgene reacts with a number of cellular compounds to produce damage and pulmonary capillary leak.

Diagnosis

No specific tests are available for most pulmonary agents. Phosgene may be recognized by the smell of fresh hay during exposure and by the delayed onset of pulmonary edema.

Clinical Complications

Phosgene-induced injury may progress to pulmonary edema, respiratory failure, and death. Prolonged exposure to high concentrations of compounds such as ammonia or chlorine may cause severe lung injury. Chronic lung disease, such as bronchitis, bronchiolitis obliterans, bronchiectasis, or airway hyperreactivity, may develop after recovery from the initial injury.[1]

Management

Supplemental humidified oxygen should be given. Treatment with bronchodilators and corticosteroids may be beneficial for patients with bronchospasm and reactive airway disease. Endotracheal intubation and mechanical ventilation may be required for those with laryngospasm, upper airway edema, lung injury, or pulmonary edema. Asymptomatic patients may require prolonged observation (24 hours) after exposure to an agent with delayed symptoms, such as phosgene.[1]

REFERENCES

1. Harrison RJ. Chemicals and gases. *Prim Care* 2000;27:917–982.

Botulinum Toxin

Anthony Morocco

Clinical Presentation

The severity of symptoms and their time of onset depend on the dose of toxin. Symptoms begin to appear 2 hours to 8 days after exposure. Patients who develop botulism by inhalation or ingestion of the toxin exhibit the same neurologic symptoms, but not the gastrointestinal symptoms that may be present in the naturally occurring disease. Invariably, a descending paralysis occurs, beginning with bulbar signs such as ptosis (73%), gaze paralysis (65%), and dilated or fixed pupils (44%). Patients complain of blurred vision, dysarthria, dysphonia, and dysphagia. Most patients (90%) have an alert mental status. Gradual decrease or loss of reflexes (40%) and respiratory muscle paralysis may occur.[1]

Pathophysiology

Botulism is a syndrome of paralysis caused by a toxin from the bacterium, *Clostridium botulinum.* The botulinum toxin has been called the "most poisonous substance known," because it is potentially lethal at nanogram doses. Botulinum toxin is considered a potential weapon of bioterrorism, through aerosol release or contamination of the food supply.

Botulinum toxin exists in seven serotypes, designated by the letters A through G. Types A, B, E, and, rarely, F are known to cause the natural disease. Toxin is absorbed from the gastrointestinal tract and lungs, but it does not penetrate intact skin. The lethal human oral dose is estimated to be 70 ng. The toxin prevents the release of acetylcholine by blocking the fusion of neurotransmitter-containing vesicles with the presynaptic membrane, primarily at the neuromuscular junction.[1]

Diagnosis

The diagnosis of botulism should be strongly suspected in any patient with descending paralysis and a clear sensorium. Bioterrorism should be suspected in the following circumstances: an outbreak with a common geographic area but no common food source; identification of toxin types C, D, F, G, or E without an aquatic food source; or occurrence of a large number of cases. A mouse bioassay to confirm the diagnosis and toxin type is available through the Centers for Disease Control and Prevention (CDC). Electromyography (EMG) may help confirm the diagnosis and to differentiate botulism from potential misdiagnoses such as Guillain-Barré syndrome and Miller-Fisher syndrome.

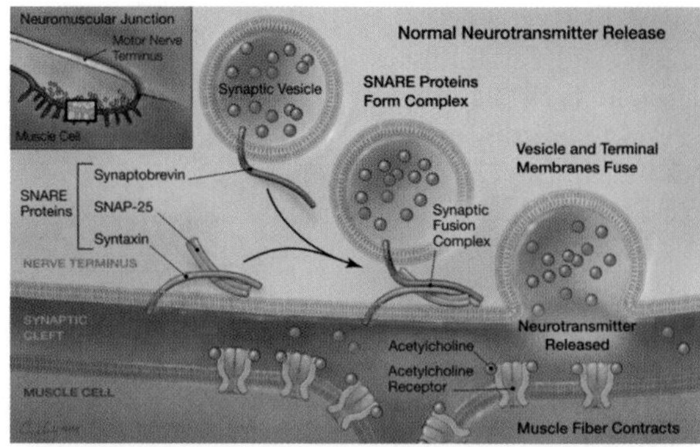

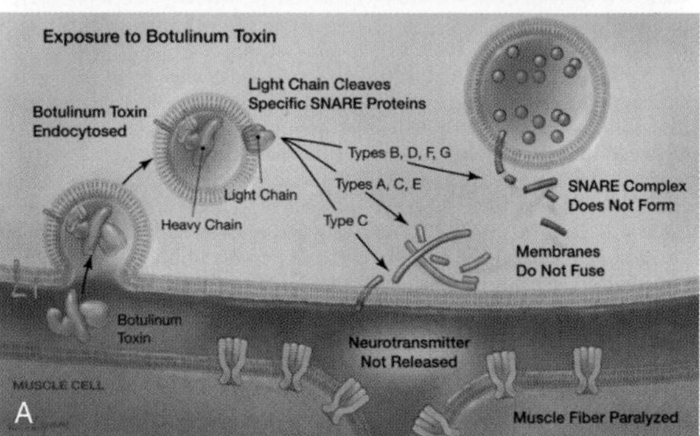

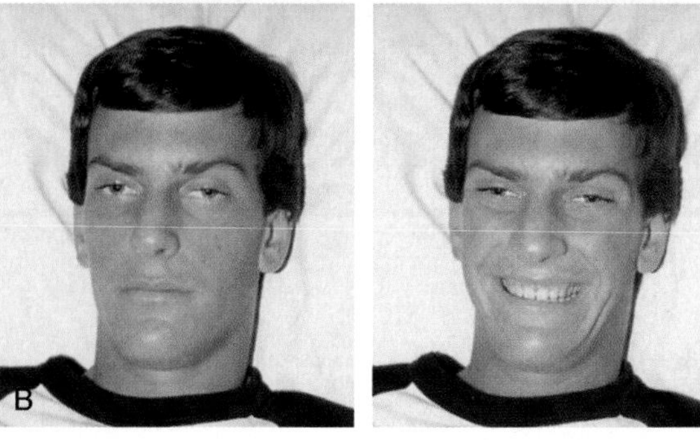

FIGURE 30–16 **A:** SNARE proteins allow vesicle binding, release of acetylcholine, and normal muscle contraction. Botulinum toxin cleaves SNARE proteins and inhibits acetylcholine release, causing muscular weakness. **B:** Patient with mild botulism. When at rest, the patient has bilateral ptosis, disconjugate gaze, and mydriasis. When asked to maximally smile, the patient has no periorbital creases, bilateral ptosis, and an asymmetric smile. (From Arnon SS, Schechter R, Ingelsby TV et al. Working Group on Civilian Biodefense. Botulinum toxin as a biological weapon: medical and public health management. *JAMA* 2001;285:1059–1070, with permission.)

Botulinum Toxin

Anthony Morocco

Clinical Complications

Patients may require prolonged mechanical ventilation, which may result in complications such as nosocomial infections.[1]

Management

Treatment consists primarily of supportive care. Recovery occurs in weeks to months as new axons sprout to create new neuromuscular junctions. An equine antitoxin is available through the CDC. Antitoxin may limit progression of the disease, but it does not improve existing paralysis, so it should be administered as early as possible. This trivalent antitoxin is effective for types A, B, and E only. The U.S. Army has an investigational heptavalent antitoxin that is effective against all seven toxin types. Secondary infections should not be treated with clindamycin or aminoglycosides, because they can worsen the neuromuscular blockade.

REFERENCES

1. Arnon SS, Schecter R, Inglesby TV, et al. Working Group on Civilian Biodefense. Botulinum toxin as a biological weapon: medical and public health management. *JAMA* 2001;285:1059–1070.

Cyanide

Anthony Morocco

Clinical Presentation

Two potential cyanide chemical warfare agents exist: a gas, hydrogen cyanide (HCN), also known by the military designation AC; and a liquid, cyanogen chloride (CNCl), which is designated CK.[1,2]

Exposures to large concentrations of AC or CK cause rapid loss of consciousness, seizures, and death. Lower-level exposures to AC result in symptoms of apprehension, dizziness, headache, nausea, and vomiting. Continued exposure results in gradual loss of consciousness, seizures, and apnea. CK shares the effects of AC but is also a mucous membrane irritant, causing lacrimation, rhinorrhea, and bronchorrhea. A "cherry-red" appearance of the skin has been described in some cyanide victims; it is caused by high venous blood oxygen content due to decreased oxygen utilization.[1,2]

Pathophysiology

Cyanides are rapidly absorbed in the lungs and gastrointestinal tract. Cyanide binds the iron atom in mitochondrial cytochrome a_3; this inhibits the electron transport chain and thus disrupts aerobic metabolism. Only relatively inefficient anaerobic metabolism can take place, and the result is hyperlactemia, acidemia, and cell death.[1,2]

Diagnosis

Cyanides cause a characteristic odor of bitter almonds that may be detectable on the patient. However, 50% of the population cannot detect this odor. Laboratory abnormalities that aid in diagnosis include elevated whole-blood cyanide level, hyperlactemia, acidemia, and elevated venous oxygen saturation.[1,2]

Clinical Complications

Survivors of serious cyanide poisoning may develop long-term neurologic sequelae such as basal ganglia damage and parkinsonian symptoms.[1,2]

Management

Treatment of cyanide poisoning consists of decontamination, aggressive supportive care, and therapy to decrease mitochondrial cyanide and enhance elimination. Pharmacologic treatment is contained in the cyanide antidote kit. Amyl nitrite and sodium nitrite are used to induce methemoglobin formation. The amyl nitrite is used via inhalation and only if no intravenous access exists. The oxidized iron in methemoglobin has a higher affinity for cyanide than does the cytochrome a_3; therefore, it pulls cyanide from the mitochondria to the red blood cells. Nitrites should be used cautiously, because they may cause hypotension and decreased oxygen delivery due to excessive methemoglobin formation. The antidote kit also contains sodium thiosulfate, which acts as a substrate for the hepatic rhodanese enzyme as it catalyzes the conversion of cyanide to thiocyanate. This is the natural metabolic pathway to detoxify cyanide and facilitate urinary excretion. Thiosulfate is benign and should be given in all cases of suspected cyanide exposure; nitrites should be reserved for cases of severe poisoning.[1,2]

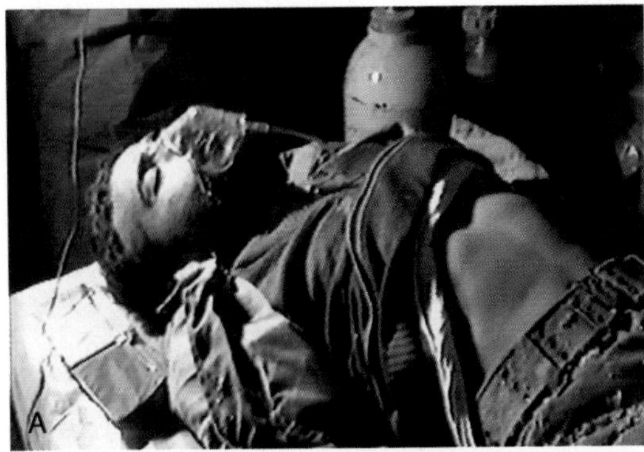

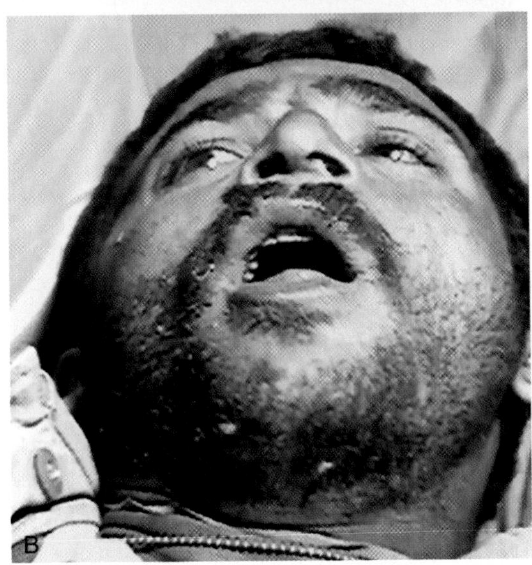

FIGURE 30–17 **A** and **B:** Iranian military victim of cyanide poisoning. Note the respiratory distress. Lack of significant secretions and normal pupil size may help differentiate cyanide from nerve agent use. (**A** and **B,** From Foroutan, with permission.)

REFERENCES

1. *USAMRICD's medical management of chemical casualties handbook,* 3rd ed. Aug 1999. Available at: www.unh.org/CHEMCASU/titlepg.html.
2. Kerns W, Isom G, Kirk MA. Cyanide and hydrogen sulfide. In: Goldfrank LR, Flomenbaum NE, Lewin NA, Howland MA, Hoffman RS, Nelson LS, eds. *Goldfrank's toxicologic emergencies,* 7th ed. New York: McGraw-Hill, 2002:1498–1510.

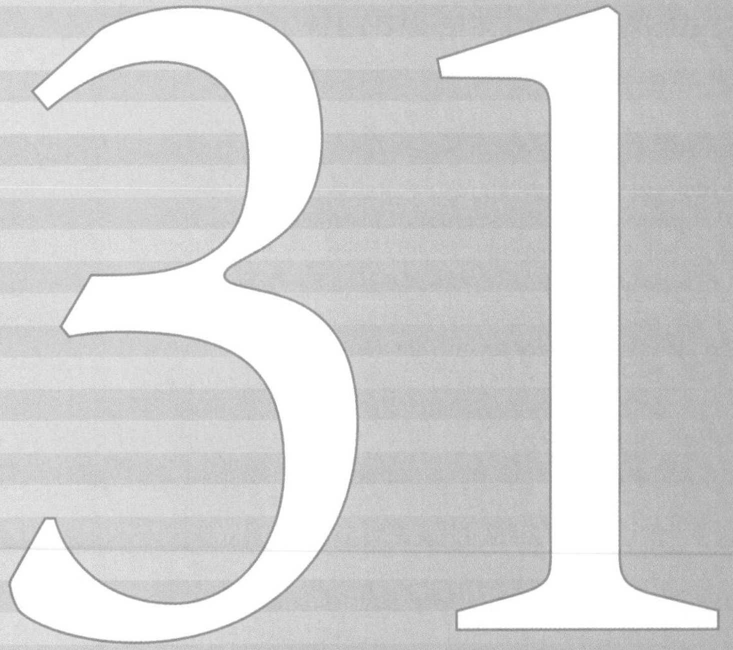

Complications of Procedures

Nasogastric Tube Complications

Mark Silverberg

Indications

Nasogastric tubes (NGTs) can be used to decompress the upper gastrointestinal tract if enteric obstruction exists. In the past, NGTs were used to remove stomach contents after an overdose, but this procedure has fallen into disuse. If a patient cannot tolerate oral intake, NGTs can serve as a route of delivery for medications, oral contrast media, or enteral nutrition.[1]

Predisposing Factors

Older age and the existence of comorbid conditions increase the risk of complications in general.[2] Patients who are anticoagulated are at high risk for bleeding from nasal trauma during tube placement. Altered mental status, prolonged supine position, neuromuscular disease, and structural abnormalities make aspiration and tube malposition more likely.[1,2]

Complications

Complications may be traumatic in nature and include injury to or bleeding from the nasopharyngeal structures and the apparatus of phonation.[1,2] Hemorrhage may be severe enough to critically compromise the airway.[1] Necrosis of nasal cartilage may occur if the tube is not properly secured in place.[1] Malpositioning of the NGT intracranially, into false passages, or into the trachea is common.[1] Inadvertent entry into the respiratory tract can result in pulmonary injury, hydrothorax, pneumothorax, empyema or pulmonary abscess formation, or potentially lethal installation of fluid into the lungs.[2] After the tube is in place, it can become clogged, cracked, kinked, knotted, or dislodged.[2] Sinusitis and esophageal stricture can occur from prolonged NGT use.[2]

Complication Prevention

Nasal trauma can be avoided and NGT passage facilitated by administration of intranasal viscous lidocaine and use of adequate amounts of lubricant for comfort, and/or use of lidocaine with epinephrine for comfort and vasoconstriction.[1] To prevent NGT dislodgement, the proximal end of the tube can be secured with tape or a nasal bridle.[2] However, use of the bridle may be associated with erosion of the nasal septum.[2] Deep placement of the NGT into the small bowel significantly reduces the frequency of aspiration pneumonia compared with intragastric feeding, as does keeping the head of the bed elevated and adding a prokinetic agent.[2] Verification of tube position by plain radiography is always advisable.

Complication Treatment

Procedure-related epistaxis is usually self-limited and rarely requires nasopharyngeal packing.[2] Aspiration pneumonia should be treated in the usual fashion with systemic antibiotics. If the position of an NGT is questionable, the tube should be removed and replaced.

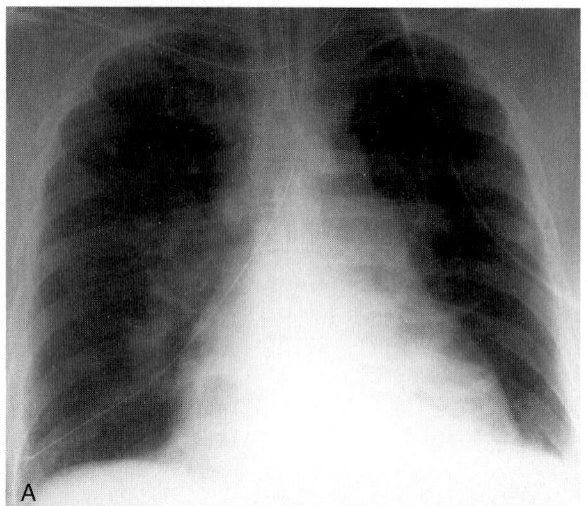

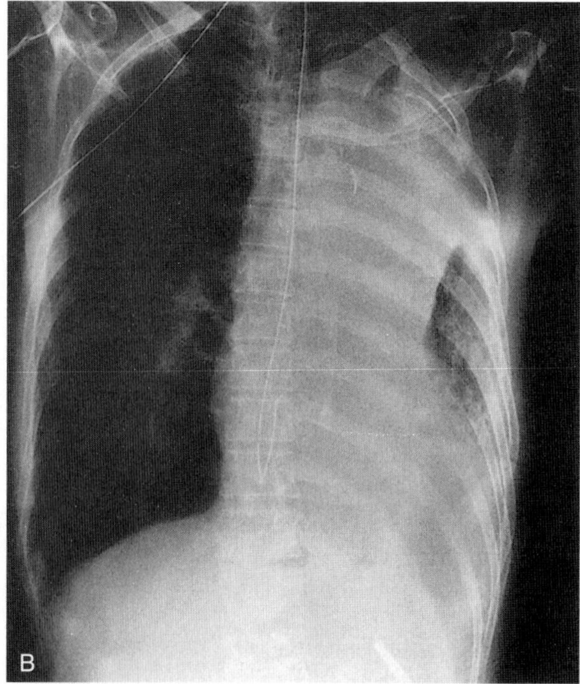

FIGURE 31–1 **A:** A nasogastric tube (NGT) advanced into the main-stem branches. (Courtesy of Mark Silverberg, MD.) **B:** Chest radiograph taken 1 hour after administration of a colonoscopy preparation solution into the left lung. Opacity of the left lung was caused by administration of the solution through the NGT. (From Ovassapian, with permission.)

REFERENCES

1. Gallacher BP. An atraumatic nasogastric tube guide probe. *Am J Emerg Med* 1995;13:252–253.
2. McClave SA, Chang WK. Complications of enteral access. *Gastrointest Endosc* 2003;58:739–751.

Endotracheal Intubation Complications

Mark Silverberg

Indications

Endotracheal intubation (ETI) is indicated for definitive airway control in patients with respiratory failure, hypoxemia, inability to maintain an airway themselves, or high risk of aspiration, in addition to patients undergoing operative procedures. Occasionally, ETI is indicated if the behavior of the patient presents a risk to his or her well-being.

Predisposing Factors

Preexisting poor dentition or a "difficult airway" predisposes the patient to potential laryngoscopic dental trauma.[1] Facial trauma with or without basilar skull fractures increases the risk of misplacement of the endotracheal tube (ETT).[1] Anticoagulation or coagulopathy increases the risk of oropharyngeal bleeding, which may make cord visualization difficult. Preexisting temporomandibular joint disease may predispose to jaw dislocations or decreased mouth aperture, increasing the likelihood of ETT misplacement.[1] Concomitant use of a nasogastric tube may increase the risk for aspiration.[1]

Complications

Acute complications of ETI include local trauma from the laryngoscope, ETT, or cuff that leads to injury to the teeth, tongue, uvula, buccal mucosa, epiglottis, arytenoids, trachea, esophagus, or lingual nerve.[1] The ETT can cause trauma as it is passed, leading to vocal cord injury or paralysis, and it can even be lost into the esophagus or trachea.[1] It can be misplaced into any number of sites, including the esophagus, cranium, and neck soft tissues.[1] Aspiration of vomit or foreign bodies (e.g., teeth, the laryngoscope bulb, other instrumentation) may occur during the intubation procedure.[1] Chronically, subglottic stenosis can develop secondary to granuloma formation if the ETT must remain in place for a long period or as a result of cuff inflation.[1]

Complication Prevention

To prevent blade trauma, the laryngoscopist should pay careful attention to the proximal portion of the blade during the intubation procedure. Proton-pump inhibitors or histamine type 2 (H_2) receptor blockers may be administered before intubation to decrease the risk of damage caused by aspiration, but this remains controversial.[1] A fluid-filled cuff may be used when working with nitrous oxide to prevent diffusion of the gas into an air-filled cuff and to stop overinflation.[1]

Complication Treatment

Oral trauma may be treated in the usual fashion, and the patient's tetanus status should be checked and updated if necessary. Tube placement should be confirmed in the usual manor, and the tube should be adjusted or removed if it is in the wrong place. Vocal cord paralysis usually recovers spontaneously.[1]

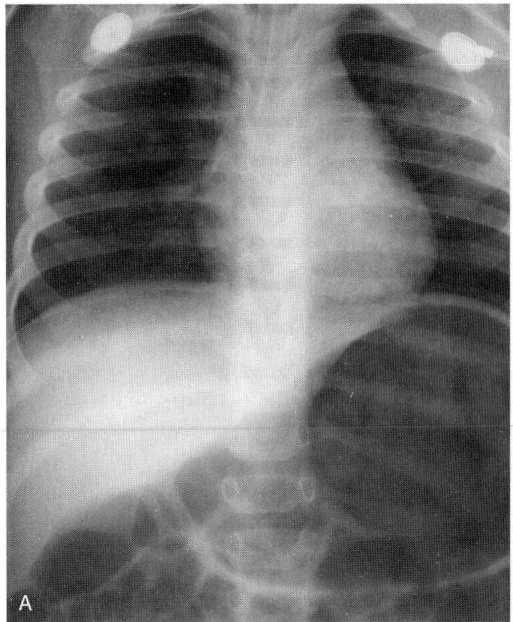

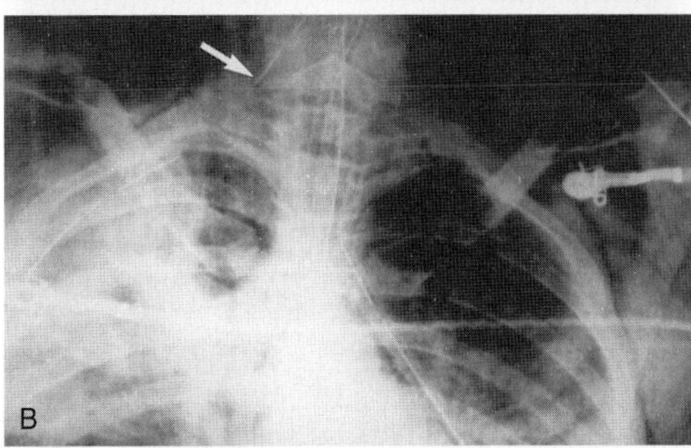

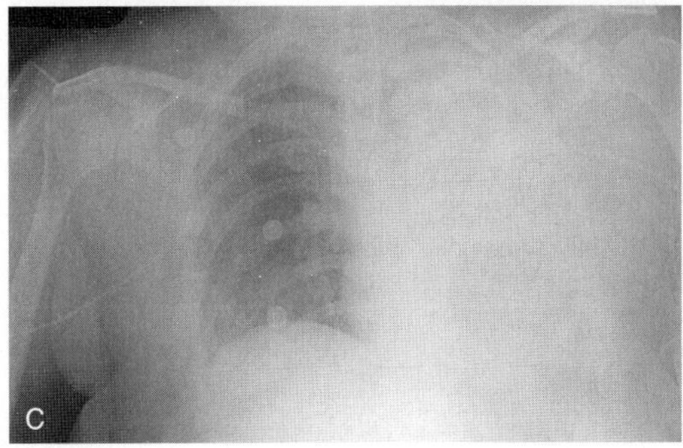

FIGURE 31–2 **A:** Endotracheal tube (ETT) in the esophagus, with distended stomach. Also note the second endotracheal tube in the trachea. (Courtesy of Robert Hendrickson, MD.) **B:** Laryngotracheal separation. The tip of the ETT is visible in the soft tissues of the right neck *(arrow)*. There is massive subcutaneous emphysema. (From Bailey, with permission.) **C:** A right main bronchus intubation with total atelectasis on the left. (Courtesy of Mark Silverberg, MD.)

REFERENCES

1. Weber S. Traumatic complications of airway management. *Anesthesiol Clin North Am* 2002;20:503–512.

Internal Jugular and Subclavian Central Line Complications

Mark Silverberg

Indications

Common indications for central venous catheter (CVC) placement are hemodialysis, hemodynamic monitoring, fluid resuscitation when peripheral access is difficult or inadequate, and centrally administered medications such as catecholamines or parenteral nutrition.[1]

Predisposing Factors

Many factors predispose certain patient populations to complications of CVC placement. Asthmatics and patients with chronic obstructive pulmonary disease have hyperinflated lungs, making pneumothorax more likely. Cancer patients may be hypercoagulable and have been reported to have rates of catheter-related thrombosis greater than 50% in some instances.[1]

Complications

Many complications have been documented in association with CVC placement, with an overall complication rate of 1% to 10%.[1] Complications can be vascular, infectious, or physical in nature. According to the meta-analysis of Ruesch and colleagues,[1] vascular complications such as arterial punctures were most common and were seen more frequently when a line was placed via the internal jugular approach rather than the subclavian route. In contrast, the physical complication of catheter malpositioning (subcutaneous, arterial, or erroneous venous location) was less likely when attaining internal jugular access, compared with subclavian cannulation. No statistical difference was noticed between the two approaches when comparing the incidence of vessel thrombosis/stenosis or hemothorax/pneumothorax.[1] Catheter-related infection remains an important cause of nosocomial infection; bacteremia and insertion-site infections were found to be more common with internal jugular lines, but the data were not statistically significant. Other, less common complications include vessel or cardiac perforation, cardiac tamponade, air or solid emboli (including guidewires), and injuries to the thoracic duct, esophagus, trachea, or nerves.

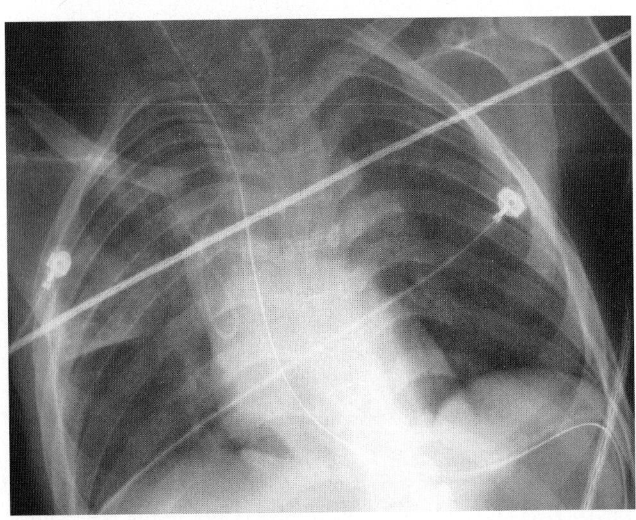

FIGURE 31-3 Left internal jugular venous catheter enters right atrium then loops back into right subclavian vein. (Courtesy of Mark Silverberg, MD.)

Complication Prevention

Ultrasound guidance is an effective method for decreasing the incidence of arterial puncture or pneumothorax formation.[1] Infection rates can be reduced by following strict aseptic techniques and conscientious handwashing protocols.

Complication Treatment

Treatment depends on the nature of the particular complication. Hematoma formation may be treated traditionally with warm packs and direct pressure if the puncture site is accessible. Large vascular injuries may require surgical repair. Pneumothoraces should be treated with chest tube placement. In cases of central-line infection, the catheter should be removed and the tip cultured for pathogen identification and sensitivity. Vessel thrombosis should be treated as any other venous thrombus.[1]

REFERENCES

1. Ruesch S, Walder B, Tramèr M. Complications of central venous catheters: internal jugular versus subclavian access—a systematic review. *Crit Care Med* 2002;30:454–460.

Femoral Line Complications

Mark Silverberg

Indications

Common indications for central venous catheter (CVC) placement include hemodialysis, hemodynamic monitoring, fluid resuscitation when peripheral access is difficult or inadequate, and centrally administered medications or parenteral nutrition.

Predisposing Factors

The inguinal region of the leg should be free of preexisting infection during the insertion process; otherwise, line sepsis is more likely.[1] Patients who are anticoagulated are at increased risk for excessive bleeding and hematoma formation during catheter insertion.[1] In contrast, patients are at increased risk for deep vein thrombosis (DVT) if they are in a hypercoagulable state (e.g., protein C or S deficiency, presence of the lupus anticoagulant).[1] Other risk factors for DVT include recent surgery, pelvic fracture, and lower-extremity ischemia.[1]

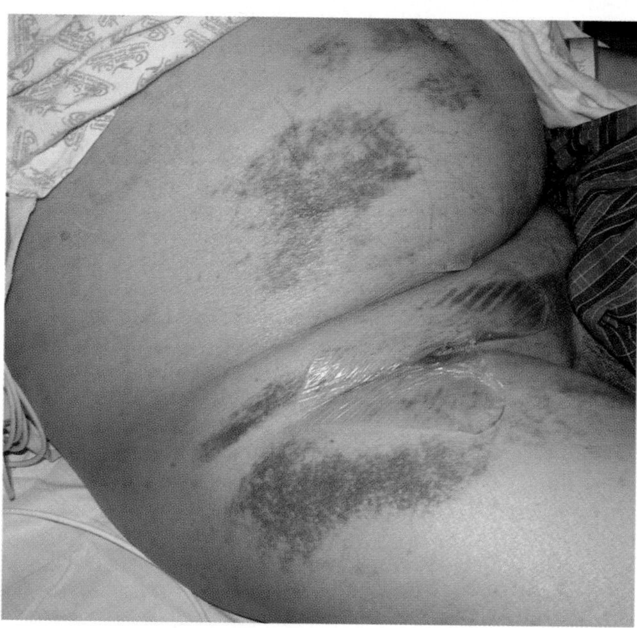

FIGURE 31–4 Hematoma secondary to right femoral venous catheter placement. (Courtesy of Mark Silverberg, MD.)

Complications

The most common complications occur during line insertion and include arterial puncture, hematoma formation, and local bleeding.[1] Malpositioning of the catheter into various abdominal and pelvic vascular sites has also been documented.[1] Other complications seen after line placement include local and systemic infections, extremity ischemia/cyanosis, thrombophlebitis, fibrin sleeve formation, and DVT with or without pulmonary embolization.[1]

Complication Prevention

A clear dressing should be applied to the catheter insertion site so that complications can be identified early. These dressings should be changed regularly to prevent infection.[1] Newer catheters made from silicone or polyurethane have lower rates of thrombosis compared with polyvinyl or polyethylene catheters and should always be used to prevent DVT formation.[1]

Complication Treatment

Insertion-site bleeding can be controlled with direct pressure.[1] The catheter should be repositioned if it is incorrectly located.[1] If a local or systemic infection develops, blood samples for culture should be drawn from a peripheral vein and from the femoral catheter, and empiric antibiotic therapy should be started. The catheter should be removed, and the tip should be cut off and sent to the laboratory for culture.[1] If leg swelling develops or a DVT is suspected, a lower-extremity Doppler ultrasound study or contrast venography may be performed to confirm suspicions.[1] A catheter-induced DVT should be treated in the classic fashion with anticoagulation.[1]

REFERENCES

1. Durbec O, Viviand X, Potie F, Vialet R, Albanese J, Martin C. A prospective evaluation of the use of femoral venous catheters in critically ill adults. *Crit Care Med* 1997;25:1986–1989.

Chest Tube Complications

Mark Silverberg

Indications

Placement of a chest tube (CT) is commonly indicated in the presence of a pneumothorax, hemothorax, chylothorax, or empyema; postoperatively after cardiothoracic surgery; and in severe cases of hypothermia for rewarming.[1]

Predisposing Factors

Positive-pressure ventilation and lung overinflation predispose patients to lung injuries when the pleural space is violated, as do poor lung compliance, adhesions, and gestational age less than 28 weeks in a newborn.[1] CTs placed on the left side have a higher complication rate, for unknown reasons.[1] Placing of multiple tubes has led to a higher chance of empyema, and reexpansion of a pneumothorax that has been present for longer than 24 hours is associated with a greater incidence of pulmonary edema.[1]

Complications

The overall complication rate associated with CT placement is approximately 1% in experienced hands.[1] Common complications include persistent pneumothorax/effusion; nonfunctioning tube or kinking of the tube; empyema; and injuries to intrathoracic organs, the intercostal bundle or diaphragm, or abdominal contents.[1] Inadvertent placement of a CT in an extrathoracic location can also occur.[1] Other, less common complications include Horner's syndrome, winging of the scapula, bronchopleural fistula, and retained tubes or tube fragments.[1,2]

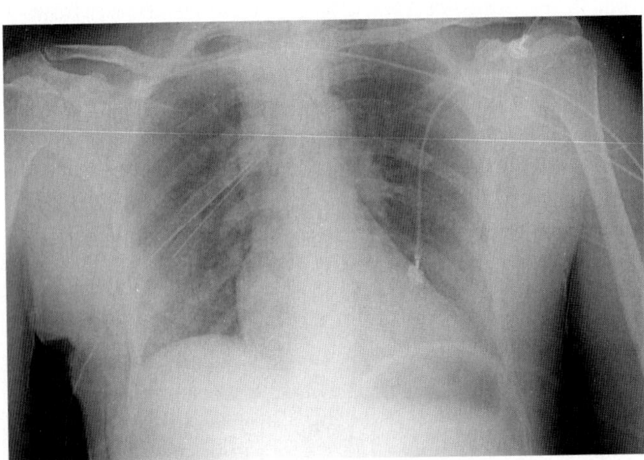

FIGURE 31–5 Right thoracostomy tube kinked against mediastinum. (Courtesy of Jerrica Chen, MD.)

Complication Prevention

To prevent injury to the neurovascular bundle (which courses below the rib margins) during insertion, the CT should be placed through an incision so that the tube enters the thoracic cavity above the rib.[1] It should not be put in below the fourth space, to avoid diaphragm injury or violation.[1] To prevent lung injury, the physician should place a finger within the chest cavity before tube insertion and sweep it in a 360-degree circle to make sure no adhesions exist.[1] The tube should then be guided between the ribs with a clamp or fingers to make sure its final location is within the chest cavity.[1]

Complication Treatment

A persistent pneumothorax or effusion can be treated with additional CTs; pleurodesis with talc, tetracycline, or silver nitrate; or pleurectomy and wedge resection (if less invasive measures fail).[1] Nonfunctioning tubes should be checked for clogs, leaks, or kinks.[1] Empyema may be treated with systemic or intrathoracic antibiotics.[1] Retained CTs or fragments should be removed under fluoroscopic guidance.[1]

REFERENCES

1. Gilbert TB, McGrath BJ, Soberman M. Chest tubes: indications, placement, management, and complications. *J Intensive Care Med* 1993;8:73–86.
2. Hassan WU, Keaney NP. Winging of the scapula: an unusual complication of chest tube placement. *J Accid Emerg Med* 1995;12:156–157.

Diagnostic Peritoneal Lavage Complications

Mark Silverberg

Indications

Diagnostic peritoneal lavage (DPL) may be performed on stable patients with either blunt or penetrating abdominal trauma and no obvious indication for laparotomy, or on unstable patients who cannot be sent for computed tomographic scanning. Stable patients may have DPL performed because of an unreliable or equivocal physical examination or before administration of general anesthesia for a nonabdominal injury.[1]

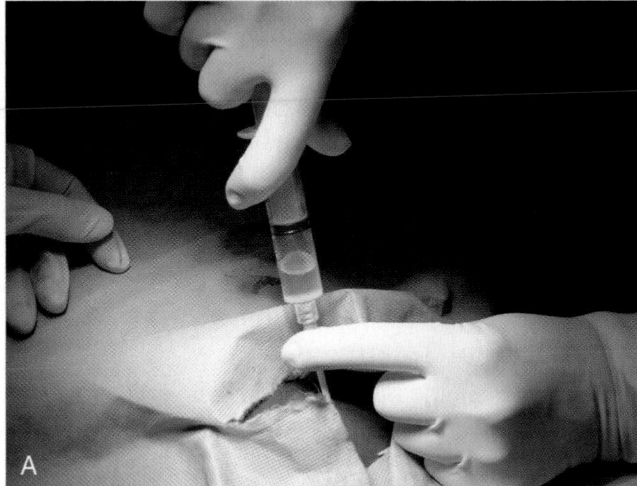

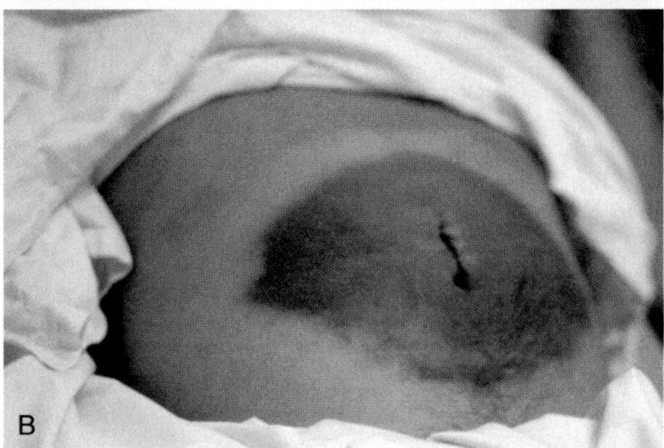

FIGURE 31–6 **A:** Diagnostic peritoneal lavage (DPL) catheter placed into the bladder; note return of urine into syringe. (Courtesy of Mark Silverberg, MD.) **B:** Bleeding or infection may occur at the site of a DPL catheter. (Courtesy of B. Zane Horowitz, MD.)

Predisposing Factors

In the hands of experienced operators, DPL is a relatively safe procedure. The most common risk factors for complications are previous abdominal surgery, an anterior pelvic fracture, and pregnancy.[1]

Complications

Complications include injuries to intraabdominal organs such as bowel, stomach or mesentery, bladder, intraabdominal vessels, or ovaries; abdominal wall injuries or infection; retroperitoneal or abdominal wall fluid infusion; peritonitis; and DPL fluid not returning from the peritoneal cavity.[1] Although laparotomy for a positive DPL result in the absence of actual intraabdominal injury is not a true complication, it is a possibility if a closed DPL procedure is performed in the setting of an anterior pelvic fracture and the catheter tip is placed into an abdominal wall hematoma.[1]

Complication Prevention

Aseptic technique, including sterile gown, gloves, hat, and mask, should always be used to prevent infection.[1] Placement of a Foley catheter and a nasogastric tube before the DPL procedure is started decreases the chance of a bladder or gastric injury.[1] In the patient who is obese or has a pelvic fracture, an open technique for DPL should be employed.[1] If a prior laparotomy scar is present, the DPL should be done away from the previous surgery site.[1] If the patient is pregnant, the procedure should be performed above the uterine fundus.[1] If the DPL fluid does not return out of the abdomen, the physician can either infuse a second liter of fluid and try again or perform the procedure at a second site.[1]

REFERENCES

1. Nagy KK, Roberts RR, Joseph KT, et al. Experience with over 2500 diagnostic peritoneal lavages. *Injury* 2000;31:479–482.

Peripheral Intravenous Catheter Complications

Mark Silverberg

Indications

There are numerous indications for insertion of a peripheral intravenous (IV) catheter, ranging from blood sampling to fluid hydration therapy to administration of parenteral medications.

Predisposing Factors

Multiple factors predispose individuals to complications of IV catheters. The most important element is the length of time the catheter remains in the vessel.[1,2] The longer the catheter remains inserted, the more likely it is that an infection or other complication will occur. Additionally, once a complication is identified, delays in addressing the issue may lead to further complications.[2] Various infusates, including certain antibiotics, potassium, parenteral nutrition, chemotherapeutic agents, and blood products, may predispose to IV catheter–related complications.[2]

Complications

Common complications of IV catheters include localized infections and infiltration.[1–3] Infection is usually caused by a single organism (most commonly staphylococci), but multiple organisms can be isolated from catheter-related infections.[1,2] Cellulitis, superficial thrombophlebitis, and abscess formation are common minor complications. Suppuration of the blood vessel beyond the insertion site, catheter-related bacteremia, and bacterial endocarditis are common major complications.[1,2]

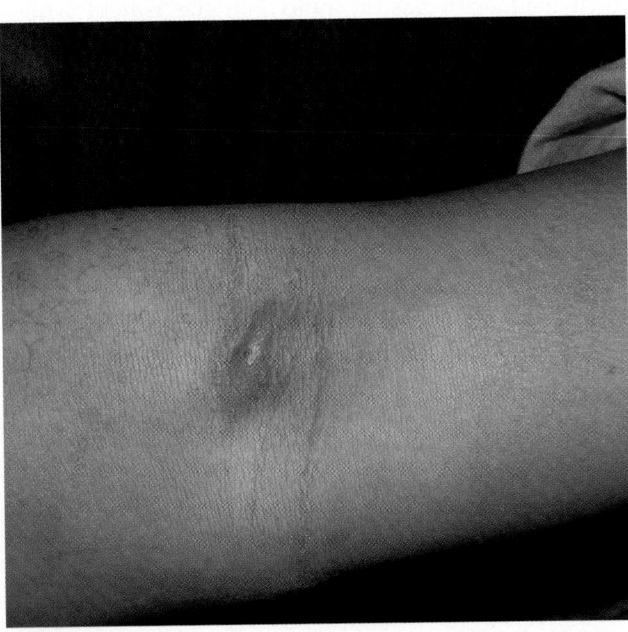

FIGURE 31–7 An intravenous catheter inserted with poor sterile technique has led to thrombophlebitis. (Courtesy of Mark Silverberg, MD.)

Complication Prevention

Many health care companies have attempted to produce IV catheters that are less likely to develop complications. They have marketed antibiotic-bonded catheters and silver-impregnated subcutaneous cuffs, but these innovations add to health care costs.[1] Adherence to the Centers for Disease Control and Prevention (CDC) recommendations for IV catheter placement is the most reliable way to decrease catheter-related complications. The CDC recommends aseptic placement technique, application of povidone-iodine ointment to the insertion site, dressing changes every 24 to 48 hours, and, most importantly, removal of the catheter within 72 hours after insertion.[1–3]

Complication Treatment

The catheter should be removed and either its tip or the surrounding pus should be sent for culture.[1,2] Blood cultures may also prove useful in identifying offending organisms. Empiric antibiotic therapy should be started if a catheter-related infection is suspected. For more serious complications, echocardiography, consultation with an infectious disease specialist, and operative vein stripping may be necessary.[1]

REFERENCES

1. Arnow PM, Quimosing EM, Beach M. Consequences of intravascular catheter sepsis. *Clin Infect Dis* 1993;16:778–784.
2. Soifer NE, Borzak S, Edlin BR, Weinstein RA. Prevention of peripheral venous catheter complications with an intravenous therapy team: a randomized controlled trial. *Arch Intern Med* 1998;158:473–477.
3. CDC Working Group. Guidelines for prevention of intravenous therapy-related infections. *Infect Control* 1981;3:62–79.

Arterial Catheter Complications

Mark Silverberg

Indications

Arterial lines usually are placed for blood-pressure monitoring in the setting of hypotension, hypertension, or trauma.[2] They can also be used to deliver medications into the arterial circulation, such as calcium in the case of hydrofluoric acid injuries.

Predisposing Factors

Raynaud's phenomenon and thromboangiitis obliterans have been implicated as risk factors for development of thrombi and emboli.[1] Risk factors for distal tissue ischemia include hypoxia, prolonged hypotension, sepsis, and use of intravenous vasomodulators such as epinephrine or dopamine.[2]

Complications

The most common complications of arterial line placement are hematoma formation and bleeding due to arterial puncture at the insertion site.[1,2] Vasospasm, thrombus formation, and emboli production may also occur.[1,3]

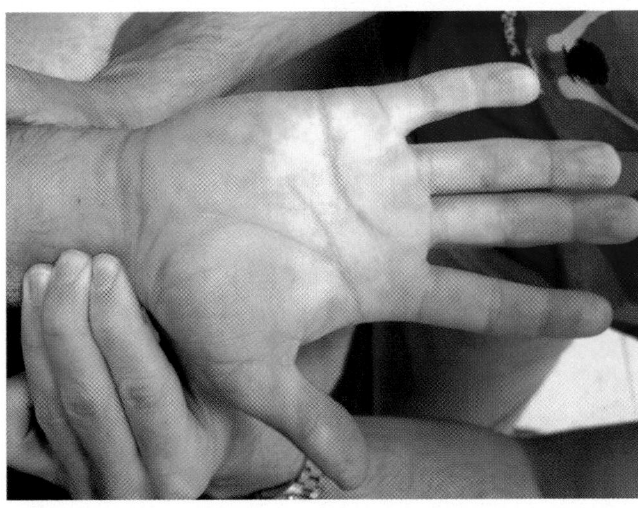

FIGURE 31–8 Ulnar artery insufficiency: a positive Allen test. (Courtesy of Michael Stein, PA.)

Cellulitis around the catheter may occur and is usually caused by skin flora such as *Staphylococcus epidermidis* or *Staphylococcus aureus.*[2] Such localized infections may on rare occasions spread and cause sepsis, which may lead to death if untreated.[1,2] Pseudoaneurysm formation at the site of an infected radial-artery catheter has been reported.[1] Nerve and tendon injuries have also been documented.[2] Less common complications include tissue necrosis and limb shortening and amputation due to ischemia from extravasation of vasoactive substances such as dopamine and norepinephrine.[3]

Complication Prevention

It is recommended that the Allen test be performed before catheter insertion to ensure that the palmar arterial arch is intact.[1–3] However, this practice has never been proven to prevent distal ischemia.[1] Some recommend Doppler ultrasonography in addition to the Allen test to demonstrate two-vessel flow to the hand.[2] To be safe, most advocate catheterizing the radial artery of the nondominant hand in case a complication does arise.[1] Smaller-sized Teflon catheters should be used, if possible, because they are less thrombogenic than those made of polypropylene.[2]

Complication Treatment

Arterial catheters should be removed if ischemia or infection develops. Other measures, such as limb elevation and warming of the opposite limb to evoke a vasodilation reflex, also have been used. Topical nitroglycerin has been advocated in some cases.[3]

REFERENCES

1. Bowdle TA. Complications of invasive monitoring. *Anesthesiol Clin North Am* 2002;20:571–588.
2. Kahler AC, Mirza F. Alternative arterial catheterization site using the ulnar artery in critically ill pediatric patients. *Pediatr Crit Care Med* 2002;3:370–374.
3. Baserga MC, Puri A, Sola A. The use of topical nitroglycerin ointment to treat peripheral tissue ischemia secondary to arterial line complications in neonates. *J Perinatol* 2002;22:416–419.

Foley Catheter Complications

Mark Silverberg

Indications

Placement of a Foley catheter is indicated if the patient is unresponsive, to monitor urine output, to retrieve a sterile sample of urine, or to treat acute retention.

Predisposing Factors

Strictures or prostatic hypertrophy may increase the risk for complications during Foley catheter placement.[1] Additionally, a catheter that remains in place for a prolonged period also carries a higher risk of problems.[1]

Complications

Urethral injury can occur from forceful insertion or from blowing up the balloon before it has reached the bladder; this can lead to hematuria or false passages.[1] The bladder can also be perforated, but this is more likely to occur if the catheter has been in place for a long time and has caused erosions or thinning due to chronic cystitis.[1] Such bladder infections are common and may ascend to become pyelonephritis or urosepsis; they occasionally may result in death.[1] Excessive traction on the catheter can lead to penile lacerations.[1] Lastly, longstanding Foley catheters can be difficult to remove from some patients, either because the catheter has become knotted or, more likely, because of an inability to deflate the balloon due to obstruction of the inflation portal.[1]

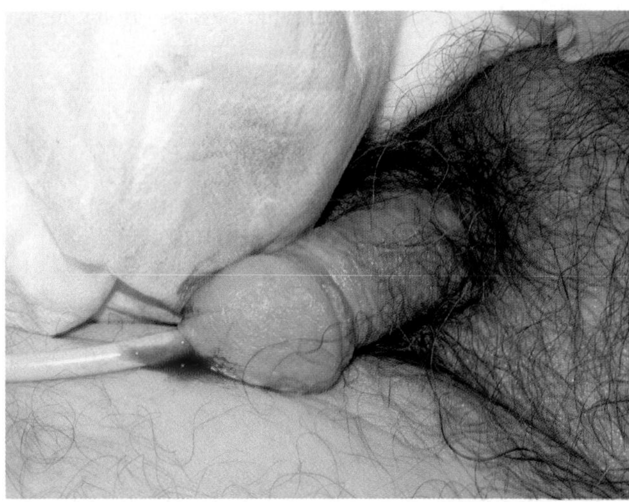

FIGURE 31–9 Traumatic insertion of Foley catheter. (Courtesy of Mark Silverberg, MD.)

Complication Prevention

To prevent infection, sterile technique should always be employed. Many authors have attempted to prevent bacterial overgrowth by putting antibiotics into the Foley bag or giving them systemically; however, only early removal seems to prevent cystitis.[1] To reduce pain and trauma, trained individuals should place Foley catheters, using copious amounts of lubrication and only mild insertion pressure. The balloon should never be blown up until urine is visualized in the collecting tube. If no urine is returned and the catheter is fully inserted, gentle abdominal pressure may clear lubrication from the catheter lumen. Sterile water should be used to inflate the balloon, because air can diffuse out and saline solutions can crystalize, leading to Foley extraction problems.[1] To prevent penile erosions, the catheter should be taped in a comfortable position.[1]

Complication Treatment

Cystitis may be treated with antibiotics in addition to catheter removal, if removal is possible.[1] If a Foley catheter cannot be removed, the inflation port can be cut off in case the valve is malfunctioning, and a guidewire can gently be passed to remove any sediment.

REFERENCES

1. Cancio LC, Sabanegh ES Jr, Thompson IM. Managing the Foley catheter. *Am Fam Physician* 1993;48:829–836.

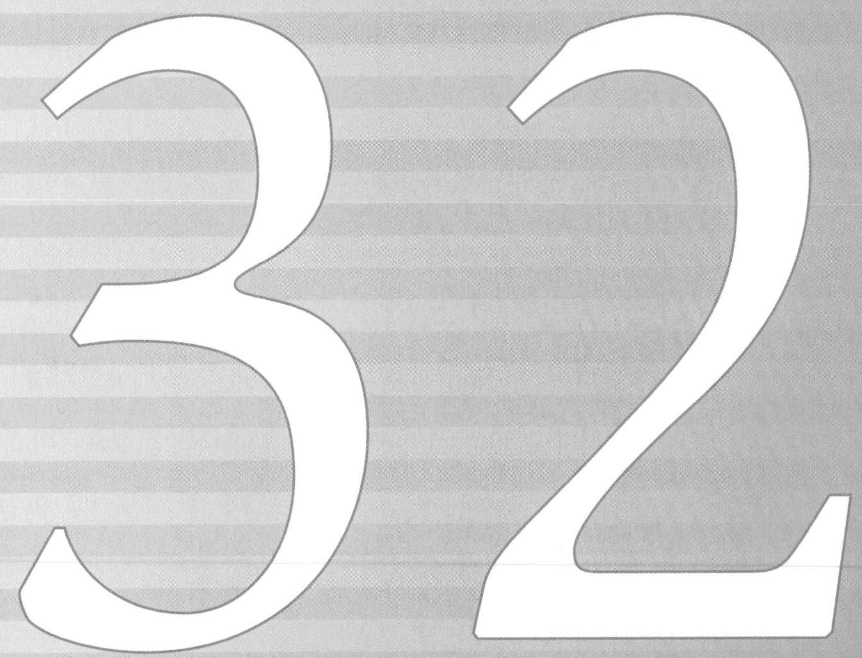

Complications of Drug Abuse

Substance Abuse: Infectious Disease Complications

Anthony Morocco

A variety of infections occur in injection drug users. They are caused by diverse organisms that include bacteria, viruses, and fungi. Injection drug and alcohol abusers are also more likely to develop community-acquired and aspiration pneumonia, as well as tuberculosis.

Soft-Tissue Infections

Soft-tissue infections are usually caused by skin flora, most commonly *Streptococcus* and *Staphylococcus* species. Anaerobic bacteria are also commonly involved and may be introduced if the user licks the needle before injection. (This activity is thought by some drug users to "clean" a previously used needle.) An unusual infection is wound botulism, which is related to the production of toxin by *Clostridium botulinum.* This condition has recently been associated with the use of black tar heroin.[1]

Endocarditis

Endocarditis occurs in injection drug users after progressive valvular damage and fibrin deposition, which allow microorganism adherence. The estimated incidence is 2 cases per 1,000 addicts per year, with the right and left sides of the heart equally affected. The most common pathogen is *Staphylococcus aureus,* followed by *Streptococcus* species. Echogenic vegetations may be visualized on echocardiography even after bacterial eradication, and 20% of patients require surgical intervention. Septic emboli may affect the lungs or any end organ.[1]

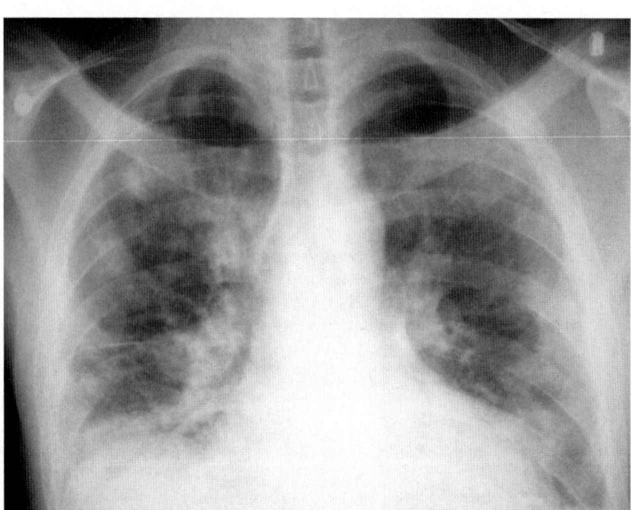

FIGURE 32–1 Multiple, bilateral septic emboli in an intravenous drug abuser. (Courtesy of Michael Greenberg, MD.)

Viral Infections

Injection drug users may develop viral illnesses such as hepatitis B and C and human immunodeficiency virus (HIV) infection. Acquired immunodeficiency syndrome (AIDS) also results in increased susceptibility to a multitude of opportunistic infections. Bacterial pneumonia is four times more common among drug users who are HIV-positive. Tuberculosis is also more common in HIV patients, and it commonly results in extrapulmonary disease in this population. Other HIV-related infections are caused by cytomegalovirus (CMV), toxoplasmosis, *Mycobacterium avium-intracellulare,* and *Cryptococcus* species.

Other Infections

Other potential infections caused by injection drug use include osteomyelitis, septic arthritis, malaria, epidural abscess, and brain abscess.[1] Vertebral osteomyelitis occurs after hematogenous seeding of the bone or facet joints. The infection may spread locally to cause epidural abscess and myelitis.[2] Septic arthritis and costochondritis occur after hematogenous spread of bacterial and occasionally fungal pathogens. Injection drug users may develop unusual locations for these infections, such as sternoclavicular, acromioclavicular, and sacroiliac joints.[2]

A number of ophthalmic infections occur in injection drug users, including endophthalmitis due to *Candida, Aspergillus, Bacillus,* and *Staphylococcus* species.

REFERENCES

1. Stein MD. Medical consequences of substance abuse. *Psychiatr Clin North Am* 1999;22:351–370.
2. Gotway MB, Marder SR, Hanks DK, et al. Thoracic complications of illicit drug use: an organ system approach. *Radiographics* 2002;22(Spec No):S119–S135.

Substance Abuse: Cardiovascular Complications

Anthony Morocco

Injection Drug Use

Use of illicit substances may cause a variety of cardiovascular complications. Injection drug use may result in bacterial endocarditis, leading to permanent valve damage and congestive heart failure, as well as disseminated infection. Talc and other inert substances may be found as adulterants in commonly injected drugs such as cocaine, heroin, and methamphetamine. Pills such as methylphenidate and oxycodone also contain inert ingredients such as talc and cellulose, which are introduced into the vasculature when the pills are crushed, mixed with water, and injected. Deposition of talc or cotton in the pulmonary vasculature may occlude vessels and result in granuloma formation and pulmonary hypertension. Neovascularization of the retina may also occur due to talc. Cotton fibers may be inadvertently injected intravenously when cotton (e.g., cigarette filters) is used to filter the drug solution before use.[1,2] Several vascular complications may result from intravenous drug use, including pseudoaneurysm formation, necrotizing angiitis, needle embolus, and mycotic aneurysm.[1] Subclavian and carotid pseudoaneurysms may result from injection into the supraclavicular fossa (colloquially known as a "pocket shot").[2]

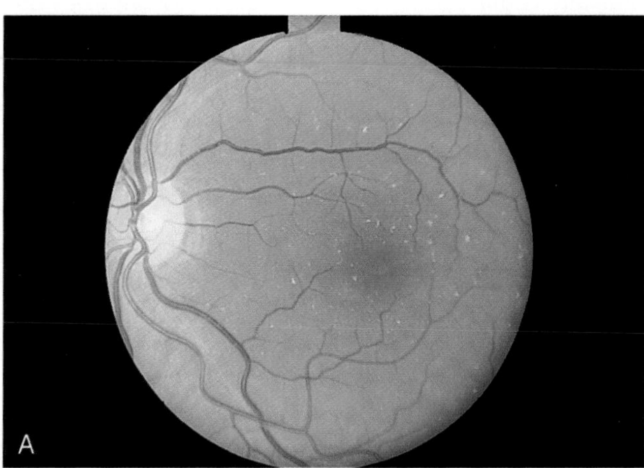

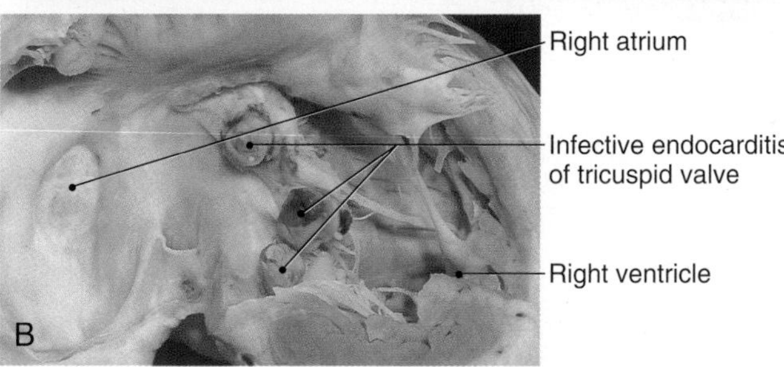

FIGURE 32–2 A: Talc particles are evident in the small retinal vessels of an eye of a chronic intravenous drug abuser with peripheral retinal neovascularization. (From Tasman, with permission.) **B:** Tricuspid endocarditis and vegetations in an intravenous drug user. (From Becker, with permission.)

Cocaine

Cocaine use is associated with serious cardiotoxicity, including myocardial infarction, arrhythmias, and sudden death. Mechanisms may include coronary vasospasm, increased myocardial oxygen demand, premature atherosclerosis, and enhanced platelet aggregation. Cocaine exerts a sodium-channel blocking effect similar to the class I antiarrhythmic drugs.[1] Cocaine may also cause cerebral vasospasm, hemorrhagic or ischemic stroke, cerebral vasculitis, or mesenteric arterial vasoconstriction and ischemia. Cocaine is associated with the development and propagation of aortic dissection due to vasoconstriction, hypertension, and tachycardia.[1,2]

Ethanol

Ethanol abuse may result in cardiomyopathy and atrial fibrillation ("holiday heart"). It is associated with hypertension, stroke, subarachnoid hemorrhage, and sudden cardiac death.[1]

REFERENCES

1. Stein MD. Medical consequences of substance abuse. *Psychiatr Clin North Am* 1999;22:351–370.
2. Gotway MB, Marder SR, Hanks DK, et al. Thoracic complications of illicit drug use: an organ system approach. *Radiographics* 2002; 22(Spec No):S119–S135.

Substance Abuse: Skin Complications

Anthony Morocco

Scarring and Stigmata

Injection drug users develop several varieties of scarring and other cutaneous stigmata. Track marks are hyperpigmented or hypopigmented atrophic scars at injection sites that often trace the path of the vein. Subcutaneous "pockets" may develop in areas of deep-vein injection, such as the groin. Chronic venous ulcers on the feet and legs develop due to trauma, repeated infections, thrombosis, and lymphatic injury. Other changes include varicose veins, hyperpigmentation, venous eczema, and lipodermatosclerosis (skin fibrosis).[1]

Infections of the Skin

Skin infections, such as cellulitis and abscesses, are common among injection drug users. The most common sites of infection are injection sites in the extremities and groin. In addition, users may inject into other areas, including deep central veins such as the subclavian (i.e., "pocket shot" in the supraclavicular fossa). Users who have difficulty accessing veins may also practice "skin popping," which involves subcutaneous or intramuscular drug injection. Sources of infection include dirty needles, contaminated drugs, and unclean injection sites. Tissue trauma, ischemia, and necrosis due to repeated injections increase susceptibility to infection. Skin and oropharyngeal flora, *Streptococcus* and *Staphylococcus* species, are the most common causes of infection, but anaerobic bacteria such as *Fusobacterium* are also commonly involved. Oral bacteria such as *Eikenella* may be introduced when users lick the needle or crush pills in the teeth before dissolving them into solution for injection. Cutaneous abscesses may spread locally or hematogenously to cause tenosynovitis, septic arthritis, arterial pseudoaneurysm, and osteomyelitis. Specific areas of concern are cervical abscesses, which can result in airway compromise, and femoral triangle abscesses, which can spread to the retroperitoneal space. The diagnosis of abscess may not be straightforward in these patients. Many patients may not exhibit fluctuance or fever at presentation. Treatment consists of incision and drainage of abscesses, with intravenous antibiotics for cellulitis.[1]

Less common organisms implicated in outbreaks of skin infections include various *Clostridium* species and *Bacillus anthracis.* Wound botulism occurs due to injection of heroin contaminated by *Clostridium botulinum* spores. This condition has recently been associated with the use of black tar heroin.[1]

Necrotizing Fasciitis

Necrotizing fasciitis may also occur, particularly in users who practice "skin popping." This diagnosis is made by close inspection of the wound and surrounding tissue on incision and drainage. Associated findings may include hemodynamic instability, subcutaneous gas, rapid extension to surrounding tissue, pain out of proportion to local findings, and death.[1]

REFERENCES

1. Ebright JR, Pieper B. Skin and soft tissue infections in injection drug users. *Infect Dis Clin North Am* 2002;16:697–712.

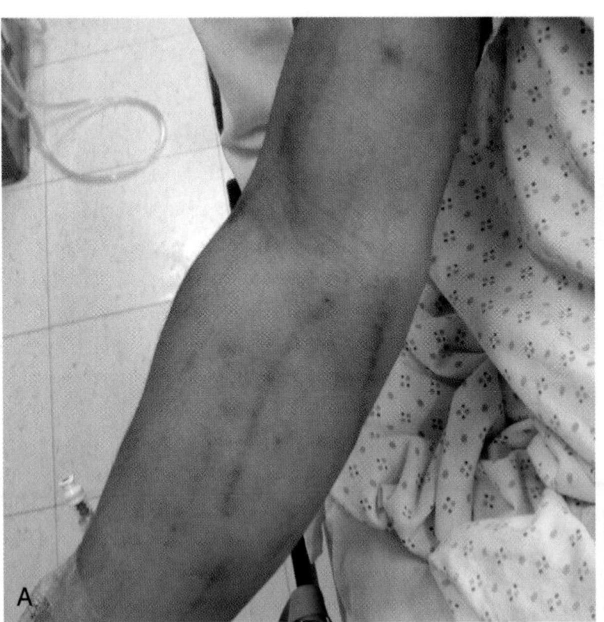

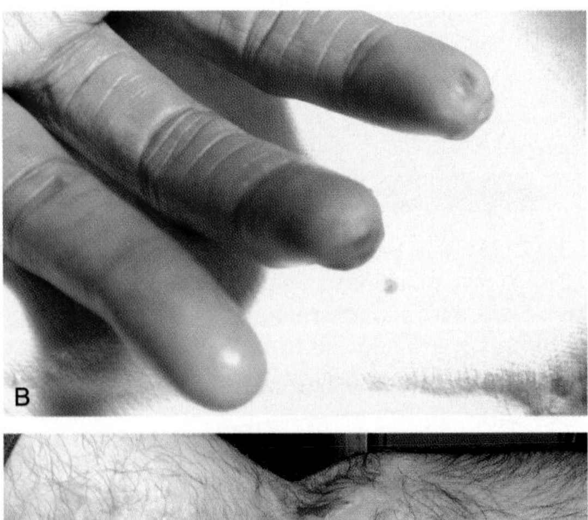

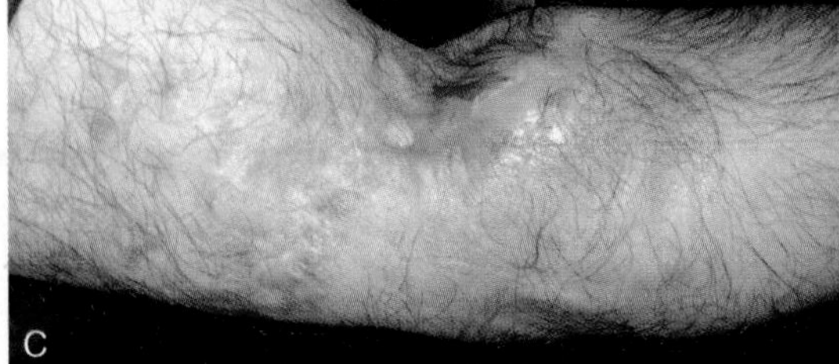

FIGURE 32–3 **A:** Track marks in an intravenous heroin abuser. (Courtesy of Robert Hendrickson, MD.) **B:** "Crack fingers." Pictured are typical finger burns caused by a pipe used to smoke crack or methamphetamines. Typical burn locations are the ulnar surface of the thumb pad and the radial surface of the index finger pad. (Courtesy of Anthony Morocco, MD.) **C:** Antecubital abscess secondary to injection of heroin. (Courtesy of Mitzi Mae Lim, MD.)

Substance Abuse: Pulmonary Complications

Anthony Morocco

Injection Drug Use

Contaminants such as talc (magnesium silicate), cellulose, cotton, and other inert substances are commonly found in injected drug solutions used by drug abusers. Talc and cotton particles may deposit in the pulmonary vasculature, resulting in granulomatous reactions and chronic dyspnea.[1] Talc-induced lung disease, or "talcosis," may appear as diffuse nodular disease and lymphadenopathy on chest radiography, with progression to fibrosis.[2] Emphysema and bullae formation are associated with injection drug use. Methylphenidate injection in particular results in panacinar emphysema. It is unclear whether this condition is caused by talc, by other contaminants, or by direct pulmonary drug toxicity.[2]

Pulmonary infections such as community-acquired pneumonia, aspiration pneumonia, and tuberculosis are more common in drug users, particularly those with human immunodeficiency virus (HIV) infection. Bronchiectasis occurs in chronic injection drug users after recurrent lung infection and injury. Septic emboli occur after tricuspid valve endocarditis and appear as multifocal, cavitating lung lesions.[2]

Heroin overdose is associated with the development of noncardiogenic pulmonary edema. This condition occurs in 1% to 2% of cases and develops within the first few hours after drug use. Patients develop hypoxia and bilateral infiltrates, although unilateral pulmonary edema may be seen. The specific cause is not known, and it generally resolves within 24 hours.[3]

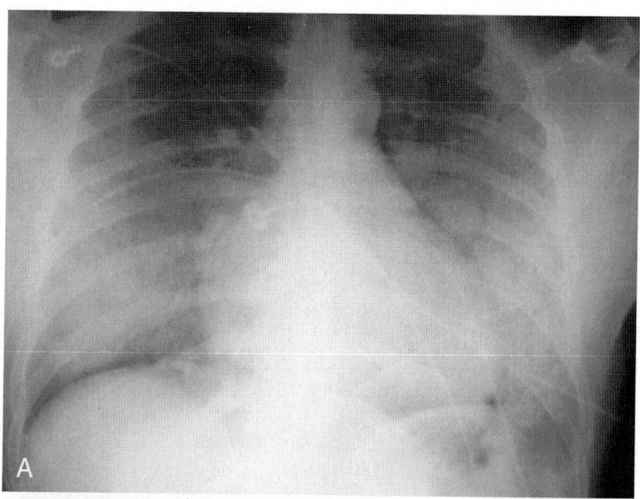

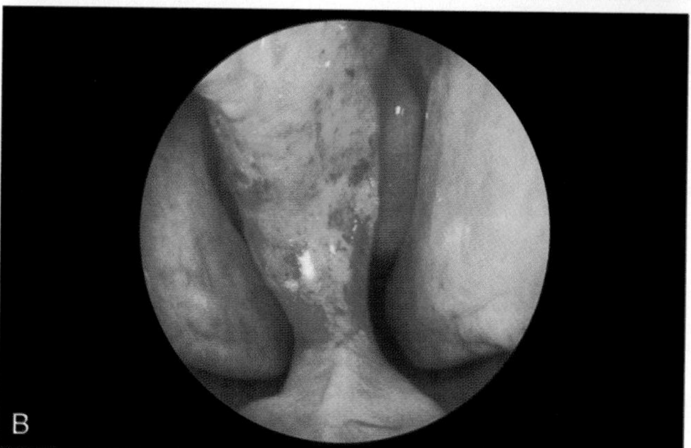

FIGURE 32–4 **A:** Crack-induced pneumonitis. (Courtesy of Robert Hendrickson, MD.) **B:** Large nasal septal perforation caused by chronic cocaine insufflation. (From Benjamin, with permission.)

Crack Cocaine

Crack cocaine smoking may result in pulmonary edema, lung injury, and pulmonary hemorrhage. "Crack lung" is characterized by chest pain, hemoptysis, and diffuse alveolar infiltrates. Crack smoking may also cause barotrauma, resulting in pneumomediastinum and pneumothorax. Pneumothorax also occurs after attempted injection into the subclavian or internal jugular veins ("pocket shot").[1,2] A variety of upper-airway injuries may occur due to cocaine use. Chronic rhinitis, altered olfaction, and nasal septal ischemia with subsequent necrosis and perforation may occur after repeated cocaine insufflation because of the vasoconstrictive effects of the drug.[1] Crack pipes contain a makeshift filter screen that may be inadvertently inhaled, causing upper-airway burns. Severe cutaneous and airway burns may also occur when the free base form of cocaine is produced or smoked.

REFERENCES

1. Stein MD. Medical consequences of substance abuse. *Psychiatr Clin North Am* 1999;22:351–370.
2. Gotway MB, Marder SR, Hanks DK, et al. Thoracic complications of illicit drug use: an organ system approach. *Radiographics* 2002; 22(Spec No):S119–S135.
3. Sporer KA, Dorn E. Heroin-related noncardiogenic pulmonary edema: a case series. *Chest* 2001;120:1628–1632.

32-5

Substance Abuse: Wound Botulism

Michael Greenberg

Clinical Presentation

Patients with wound botulism (WB) related to substance abuse present with findings consistent with botulism, including descending flaccid muscular paralysis, diplopia, blurred vision, ptosis, dysarthria, and muscle weakness (predominantly proximal). They may present initially with lower cranial nerve palsies.[1]

Pathophysiology

WB develops when anaerobic conditions within an abscessed or subcutaneous wound allow for generation of *Clostridium botulinum* spores with multiplication of the organisms and production and absorption of botulinum toxin. WB has been associated specifically with the use of Mexican black tar heroin (BTH), a form of heroin that is contaminated, presumably during the "cutting process," with dirt or shoe polish.[1] Clusters of WB cases have been identified in drug users.[1–5] In this population, the predominant botulinum serotype is type A.[5]

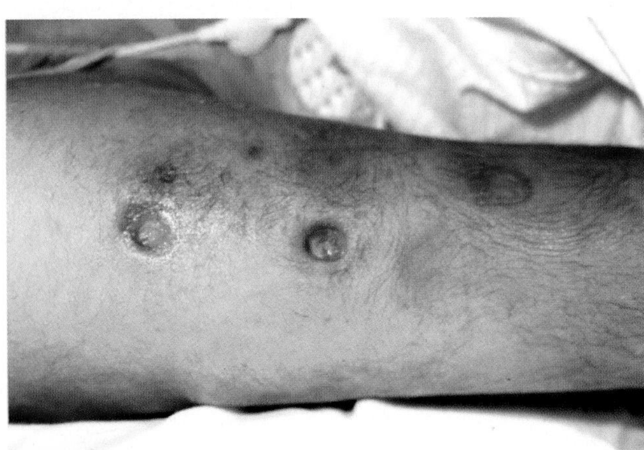

FIGURE 32–5 Indica of "skin popping" in a heroin addict who developed wound botulism. (From Jensenius M. A heroin user with a wobbly head. *Lancet* 2000;356:1160, with permission.)

Diagnosis

The diagnosis is based on clinical findings and confirmed by neurophysiologic and serologic testing and by identification of the organism and/or toxin. WB must be suspected in intravenous and subcutaneous injection drug users, especially those who have used BTH.[1,3–5] In addition, WB has been reported in drug abusers who have snorted BTH.[1]

Clinical Complications

Complications include residual weakness and chronic autonomic dysfunction as well as death (case-fatality rate, 15%).[2]

Management

WB is a potentially life-threatening condition, and all cases must be treated emergently and aggressively. Once the disease is even suspected, the immediate administration of antitoxin and anticlostridial antibiotics, surgical débridement of wounds, and intensive monitoring to identify respiratory failure requiring mechanical ventilation should be performed.

REFERENCES

1. Wound botulism among black tar heroin users—Washington, 2003. *MMWR Morb Mortal Wkly Rep* 2003;52:885–886.
2. Jensenius M, Levstad R, Dhaenens G, Rorvik LM. A heroin user with a wobbly head. *Lancet* 2000;356:1160.
3. Sandrock CE, Murin S. Clinical predictors of respiratory failure and long-term outcome in black tar heroin-associated wound botulism. *Chest* 2001;120:562–566.
4. Jones JA, Salmon JE, Djuretic T, et al. An outbreak of serious illness and death among injecting drug users in England during 2000. *J Med Microbiol* 2002;51:978–984.
5. Merrison AF, Chidley KE, Dunnett J, Sieradzan KA. Wound botulism associated with subcutaneous drug use. *BMJ* 2002;325: 1020–1021.

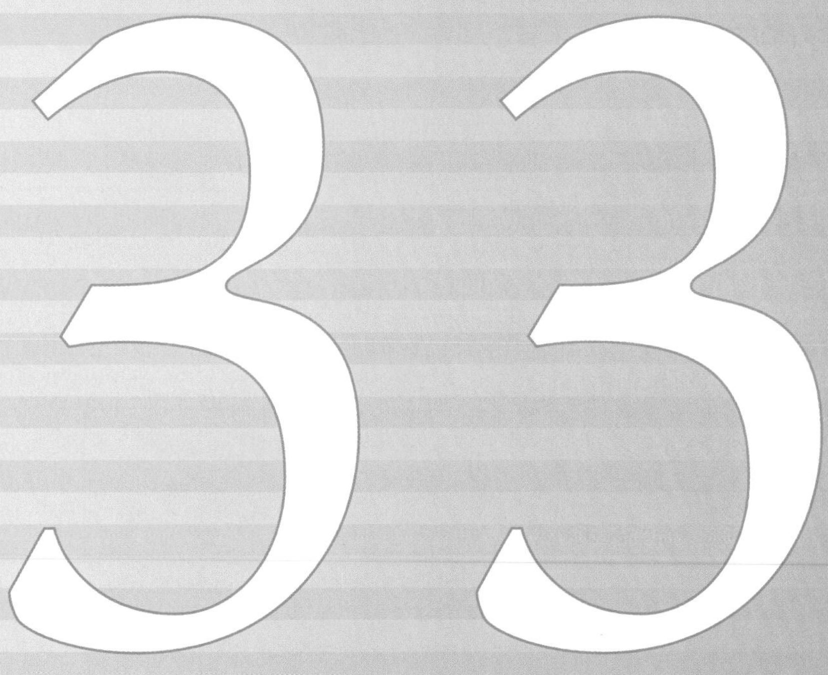

33 Human Immunodeficiency Virus–Related

33–1

AIDS-Defining Opportunistic Illnesses

Michael Greenberg

Acquired immunodeficiency syndrome (AIDS)–defining opportunistic illnesses (OIs) include 26 clinical conditions that affect people with advanced human immunodeficiency virus (HIV) disease.

An HIV-infected person receives a diagnosis of AIDS after developing one of the AIDS indicator illnesses defined by the Centers for Disease Control and Prevention (CDC). AIDS-defining OIs are the major cause of morbidity and mortality among persons infected with HIV. Table 33–1 lists the current CDC-defined OIs.

REFERENCES

www.cdc.gov/hiv/dhap.htm. Last updated 8/9/04.

TABLE 33–1 AIDS-Defining Opportunistic Illnesses

Pneumocystis carinii pneumonia
Esophageal candidiasis
Kaposi's sarcoma
Wasting syndrome
Mycobacterium avium complex
Pulmonary tuberculosis
Extrapulmonary cryptococcosis
HIV encephalopathy
Cytomegalovirus retinitis
Cytomegalovirus disease
Toxoplasmosis of brain
Chronic cryptosporidiosis
Recurrent pneumonia
Extrapulmonary tuberculosis
Chronic herpes simplex
Immunoblastic lymphoma
Progressive multifocal leukoencephalopathy
Invasive cervical cancer
Disseminated histoplasmosis
Burkitt's lymphoma
Other disseminated mycobacterial infections
Primary brain lymphoma
Pulmonary candidiasis
Disseminated coccidioidomycosis
Recurrent *Salmonella* septicemia
Chronic isosporiasis

MMWR 1999;48(SS-2):1–22.
www.cdc.gov/mmwr/preview/mmwrhtm/00056917.htm

Acute HIV Seroconversion Disease

Michael Greenberg

Clinical Presentation

Within 4 weeks after the initial infection with human immunodeficiency virus (HIV)-1, a substantial number of patients develop an acute illness that clinically resembles mononucleosis.[1,2] This illness is characterized by sore throat, low-grade fever, fatigue, headache, and lymphadenopathy. In addition, an evanescent, faintly red, nonpruritic rash may develop.[1,2] This rash usually involves the face and tends to have a more central than peripheral distribution. In conjunction with this rash, oral and pharyngeal ulcerations may occur. Table 33–2 describes some of the clinical and demographic characteristics of one primary HIV cohort.

TABLE 33–2 Clinical and Demographic Characteristics of a Primary HIV Cohort

Clinical Characteristics	Symptoms of PH1 [Median (Range)]
HIV-1 RNA (copies/mL)	377,683 (1,255–>1,600,000)
CD4-positive T-cell count (×10⁶/L)	504 (216–1,104)
Demographic Characteristics	**Symptoms of PH1 [No. Patients (%)]**
Total no. of patients	39
Mode of HIV exposure	
Male-male sexual contact	35 (90%)
Heterosexual contact	2 (5%)
Injection drug use	1 (3%)
Needlestick exposure	1 (3%)
Gender	
Male	36 (96%)
Female	3 (8%)
Race/Ethnicity	
African-American	1 (3%)
Latino	4 (10%)
White	29 (74%)
Other	5 (13%)
Age in years (median [range])	32 (21–62)

PHI, primary HIV infection.
Adapted from Hecht FM, Busch MP, Rawal B, et al. Use of laboratory tests and clinical symptoms for identification of primary HIV infection. *AIDS* 2002;16:1119–1129.

Pathophysiology

This phase of clinical illness usually lasts 1 to 4 weeks and has been associated with seroconversion for HIV-1 in 53% to 95% of cases.[1,2]

Diagnosis

The diagnosis is made on the basis of information obtained from the history and physical examination. Laboratory findings may include thrombocytopenia, leucopenia, and liver transaminase elevations.[1,2]

Management

Unless the patient is acutely ill enough to warrant hospitalization, the workup may be initiated in the emergency department. This workup includes ruling out intercurrent infection and obtaining relevant baseline laboratory tests, including HIV status testing, CD4-positive T-lymphocyte count, HIV viral load testing, and routine tests. Consultation with an infectious disease specialist should be initiated in the emergency department, because antiretroviral therapy should be initiated as soon as possible.[1,2]

REFERENCES

1. Pederson C, Lindhart B, Jensen B, et al. Clinical course of primary HIV infection: consequences for subsequent course of infection. *BMJ* 1989;299:154–157.
2. Tindall B, Barker S, Donovan B, et al. Characterization of the acute clinical illness associated with immunodeficiency virus infection. *Arch Intern Med* 1988;148:945–949.

HIV Wasting Syndrome

Michael Greenberg

Clinical Presentation

HIV wasting syndrome is defined by the Centers for Disease Control and Prevention (CDC) as a weight loss of at least 10% in association with diarrhea or chronic weakness and documented fever for at least 30 days not attributable to conditions other than infection with human immunodeficiency virus (HIV).[1]

Pathophysiology

Multiple factors are thought to contribute to the development and propagation of this syndrome. These factors usually represent sequelae of HIV disease, acquired immunodeficiency syndrome (AIDS), or complications thereof and include anorexia, malabsorption, metabolic abnormalities, and hypogonadism.[1] In addition, excessive cytokine production may be associated with wasting and may be partly responsible for the establishment of a vicious cycle of wasting propagated by increased levels of cytokines, which in turn are generated by wasting.[1]

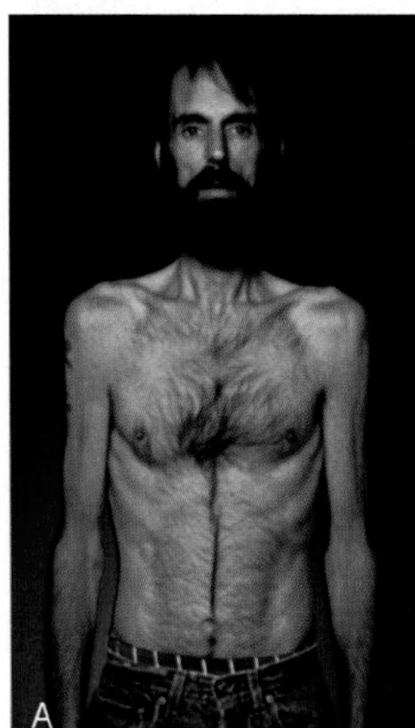

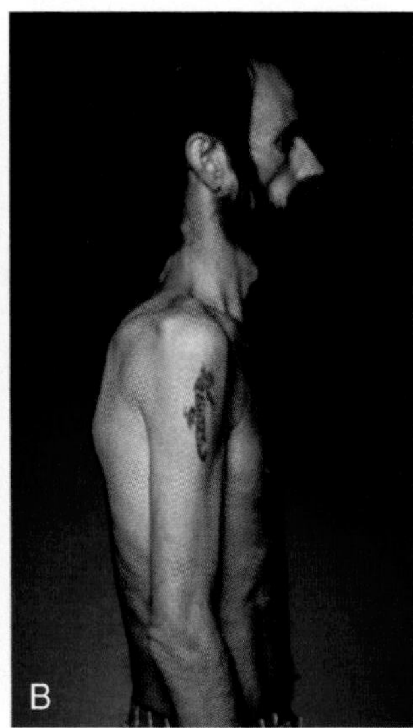

FIGURE 33–3 The wasting syndrome in acquired immunodeficiency syndrome (AIDS) is accompanied by marked muscle wasting with variable loss of body fat. Patients with the wasting syndrome show tissue loss in the extremities and viscera. (From Mandell, *Atlas of AIDS,* with permission.)

Diagnosis

The diagnosis of HIV-related wasting syndrome usually is obvious on observation of the patient, and specific clinical testing usually is not necessary to confirm the diagnosis. However, techniques involving anthropometric measurements, body composition determinations, and nutritional assessments may be helpful for clinicians who care for these patients on a long-term basis. Because treatment of the underlying HIV disease is expected to help control wasting, it is important for emergency physicians to recognize these patients for primary diagnosis, or to facilitate proper treatment and intervention for those who have already been diagnosed.

Clinical Complications

Weight loss related to HIV disease has been associated with the development of acute infections as well as malabsorption.

Management

The emergency physician must determine when and if patients afflicted with wasting syndrome require hospital admission. Clinically important dehydration, weakness, and severe wasting should dictate hospitalization. Physicians who care for these patients over the long term may employ various modalities to correct wasting, including the use of appetite-stimulant drugs, anabolic steroids, growth hormone, and various growth factors. In addition, the drug thalidomide has been shown to increase weight in wasted HIV patients by roughly 4%.[3]

REFERENCES

1. Centers for Disease Control and Prevention. Revision of the CDC surveillance case definition of acquired immunodeficiency syndrome. *MMWR Morb Mortal Wkly Rep* 1987;36:3S–15S.
2. Klausner JD, Makonkawkeyoon S, Akarasewi P, et al. The effect of thalidomide on the pathogenesis of human immunodeficiency virus type I and *M. tuberculosis* infection. *J Acquir Immune Defic Syndr Hum Retrovirol* 1996;11:247–257.
3. Cohen PT, Sande MA, Volberding PA, et al. *The AIDS knowledge base,* 3rd ed. Philadelphia: Lippincott Williams & Wilkins, 1999.

Oropharyngeal Candidiasis

Michael Greenberg

Clinical Presentation

Adult patients with oropharyngeal candidiasis (OPC) present with sore throat, difficulty swallowing, and changes in ability to taste, in conjunction with whitish plaques and deposits on the tongue, oral cavity, and pharynx. Neonates and infants present with excessive crying, poor feeding, and failure to suck properly.[1–3]

Pathophysiology

OPC is found in various patient groups, including those with human immunodeficiency virus (HIV) disease, nutritional deficiencies, or malignancies and those who have undergone organ transplantation, and as a side effect of some medications. Most OPC is caused by overgrowth of *Candida albicans*. However, other *Candida* species may also be causative of OPC.[3]

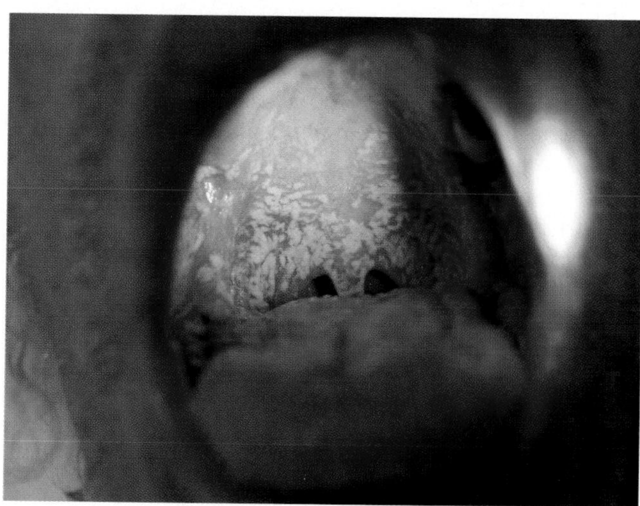

FIGURE 33–4 Oropharyngeal candidiasis. (Courtesy of Colleen Campbell, MD.)

Diagnosis

The diagnosis is a clinical one. It usually is obvious on visualization of the oral cavity and pharynx.

Clinical Complications

Complications include reoccurrence, intractability, drug resistance, extension to esophageal disease, and systemic candidal infection.[1–3]

Management

Topical fluconazole has been highly effective; however, resistant organisms have emerged. Some cases require systemic antifungal therapy. If candidal disease restricts intake of fluid or food or in any way compromises the airway, hospitalization is essential. Therapy should be initiated for all patients identified in the emergency department; those who are not admitted should be referred for follow-up within 24 hours.[1–3]

REFERENCES

1. Hoppe J. Treatment of oropharyngeal candidiasis and candidal diaper dermatitis in neonates and infants: review and reappraisal. *Pediatr Infect Dis* 1997;16:885–894.
2. Penzak SR, Gubbins PO. Preventing and treating azole-resistant oropharyngeal candidiasis in HIV-infected patients. *Am J Health Syst Pharm* 1998;55:279–283.
3. Redding SW. The role of yeasts other than *Candida albicans* in oropharyngeal candidiasis. *Curr Opinion Infect Dis* 2001;14:673–677.

33–5

Oral Hairy Leukoplakia

Jason Kitchen

Clinical Presentation

Patients with oral hairy leukoplakia (OHL) present with white thickening of the tongue at the lateral border, with vertical "hairy" projections.[1–3] Lesions may extend to the tongue's ventral and dorsal surfaces, where it is usually flat and plaque-like. Lesions can be unilateral or bilateral, and they vary in size from a few millimeters to covering almost the entire surface of the tongue.[1]

Pathophysiology

OHL is believed to be an Epstein-Barr virus (EBV)–induced hyperplasia of the upper portions of the epithelial surface of the tongue. No malignant transformation has been identified.[1–3]

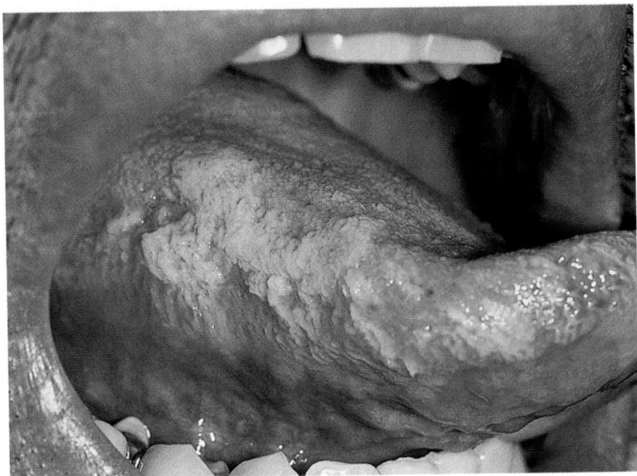

FIGURE 33–5 Oral hairy leukoplakia caused by the Epstein-Barr virus in a patient with acquired immunodeficiency syndrome (AIDS). This is commonly seen before the onset of AIDS. (From Ostler, with permission.)

Diagnosis

In the HIV-infected patient, the diagnosis is made on clinical appearance. Confirmation can be made by biopsy, and EBV can be demonstrated in lesions.[1–3] A rapid method for differentiating OHL from oral candidiasis is to wipe the lesions with gauze. In the case of candidiasis, the white plaques can be removed, leaving a tender red base. OHL lesions cannot be removed.[1–3]

Clinical Complications

OHL can become superinfected with *Candida albicans*, which can cause soreness and burning. HIV-infected patients presenting with the condition are considered to be at an increased risk for progression to acquired immunodeficiency syndrome (AIDS).[2]

Management

Treatment is not needed in most cases. However, OHL regresses in response to acyclovir, ganciclovir, foscarnet, and zidovudine but tends to recur when antiviral drugs are discontinued.[1–3] Topical application of podophyllum resin has also been used.[1,2]

REFERENCES

1. Patton LL, van der Horst C. Oral infections and other manifestations of HIV disease. *Infect Dis Clin North Am* 1999;13:879–900.
2. Greenspan JS. Sentinels and signposts: the epidemiology and significance of the oral manifestations of HIV disease. *Oral Dis* 1997;3[Suppl 1]:S13–S17.
3. Kessler HA, Benson CH, Urbanski P. Regression of oral hairy leukoplakia during zidovudine therapy. *Arch Intern Med* 1988;148: 2496–2497.

Clinical Presentation

Patients with HIV-associated periodontitis (HAP) present with complaints of tooth and gum pain, although some are asymptomatic. Multiple teeth are usually involved, with the anterior, inferior teeth most often affected.[1,2]

HIV-Associated Periodontitis

Grant Wei

Patients with HIV-associated periodontitis (HAP) present with complaints of tooth and gum pain, although some are asymptomatic. Multiple teeth are usually involved, with the anterior, inferior teeth most often affected.[1,2]

Pathophysiology

HAP is also known as necrotizing ulcerative gingivitis, necrotizing ulcerative periodontitis, or necrotizing stomatitis. It is a necrotic disease of the gums, soft tissues, and bone surrounding the teeth.[1] The incidence of HAP is less than 2% per year.[1] The mixed microflora typically found with the disease is similar to that of classic periodontitis (e.g., *Porphyromas gingivalis, Prevotella intermedia, Fusobacterium nucleatum*). However, *Candida* and other anaerobic species (e.g., *Clostridium, Enterococcus*), as well as several viruses, including cytomegalovirus and Ebstein-Barr virus, have also been found in greater numbers of tissue biopsies of HAP, compared with classic periodontitis.[1,2]

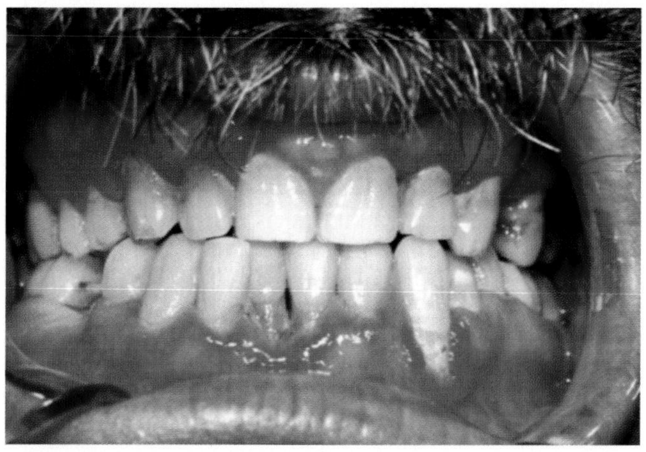

FIGURE 33–6 Necrotizing periodontitis (HIV periodontitis). (From Katz MH, Greenspan D, Westenhouse J, et al. Progression to AIDS in HIV infected homosexual and bisexual men with hairy leukoplakia and oral candidiasis. *AIDS* 1992;6:95-100.)

Diagnosis

The diagnosis of HAP is made clinically, although HAP is associated with HIV infection early in life, younger age, and with the presence of oral candidiasis. Response to the treatment regimen described here is reported to be near-diagnostic, although wound cultures and tissue biopsy may be required for lesions that do not respond to initial treatment.[1-3]

Clinical Complications

Clinical complications of HAP result from extension of the necrosis from the gums and papilla into the bone or contiguous tissues. Loss of tooth attachment may result from uncontrolled or rapidly progressive disease.[1,2]

Management

Treatment requires referral to a dental/oral surgeon for débridement of the lesions, systemic metronidazole, and chlorhexidine mouthwash. Oral hygiene regimens should be encouraged and reinforced.[1-3]

REFERENCES

1. Robinson PG. The significance and management of periodontal lesions in HIV infection. *Oral Dis* 2002;8[Suppl 2]:91–97.
2. Robinson PG, Adegboye A, Rowland RW, Yeung S, Johnson NW. Periodontal diseases and HIV infection. *Oral Dis* 2002;8[Suppl 2]: 144–150.
3. Robinson PG, Sheiham A, Challacombe SJ, Wren MW, Zakrzewska JM. Gingival ulceration in HIV infection: a case series and case control study. *J Clin Periodontol* 1998;25:260–267.

33–7

Kaposi's Sarcoma

Michael Greenberg

Clinical Presentation

Several clinical variants of Kaposi's sarcoma (KS) exist, including classic KS, endemic KS, immunosuppression- and transplantation-related KS, and epidemic or acquired immunodeficiency syndrome (AIDS)-associated KS. Approximately 95% of AIDS-related KS is seen in homosexual or bisexual men.[1–3]

Pathophysiology

KS is an uncommon tumor of vascular origin and was one of the first recognized manifestations of AIDS.[1] KS is the most common tumor in human immunodeficiency virus (HIV)-infected persons and is considered an AIDS-defining illness by the Centers for Disease Control and Prevention (CDC). KS appears to be caused, in part, by a sexually transmissible agent known as human herpesvirus-8 (HHV-8).[1–3] The pathogenesis of HIV-related KS is complex and is thought to involve multiple factors such as altered gene expression with regard to response to cytokines and stimulation of KS tissue growth by an HIV-1–transactivating protein.[3]

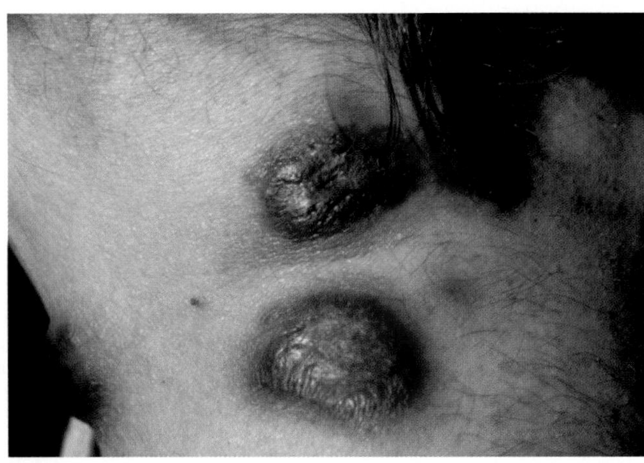

FIGURE 33–7 Epidemic Kaposi's sarcoma. Note the resemblance to the lesions of bacillary angiomatosis. (From Goodheart, with permission.)

Diagnosis

KS is usually recognized as tumors of the skin and mucosa; these are asymptomatic, pink to purple or dark brown, round to oval areas that thicken over time into plaques and nodules. In AIDS patients, KS lesions tend to have a symmetric distribution along skin cleavage lines.[1–3]

Management

Because newly diagnosed KS may be the first manifestation of AIDS, steps need to be taken to enroll the patient into an appropriate treatment regimen under the care of appropriate specialists. Most KS patients are begun on antiretroviral therapy, but radiation therapy, cryotherapy, photodynamic therapy, and surgical excision are often added as adjuncts. However, there is no cure known for KS to date. The goal of all current therapies is to provide palliation and reduce morbidity through shrinking lesions, controlling pain, and slowing the progression of the disease.[3]

REFERENCES

1. Mitsuyasu RT. Update on the pathogenesis and treatment of Kaposi sarcoma. *Curr Opinion Oncol* 2000;12:174–180.
2. Antman K, Chang, Y. Medical progress: Kaposi's sarcoma. *N Engl J Med* 2000;342:1027–1038.
3. Dezube BJ. New therapies for the treatment of AIDS-related Kaposi sarcoma. *Curr Opinion Oncol* 2000;12:445–449.

Toxoplasmosis

Grant Wei

Clinical Presentation

Patients with toxoplasmosis complain of ocular "floaters," blurred vision, pain, and redness. In immunosuppressed patients, the disease may be bilateral and multifocal, with greater severity and more rapid progression.[1] Encephalitis manifests with headache, altered mental status, seizures, and focal neurologic signs.[2,3]

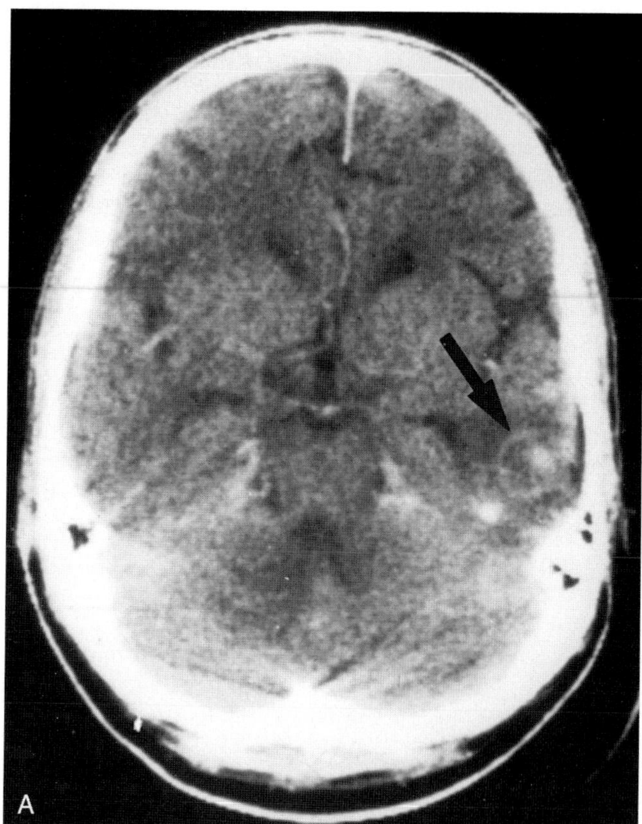

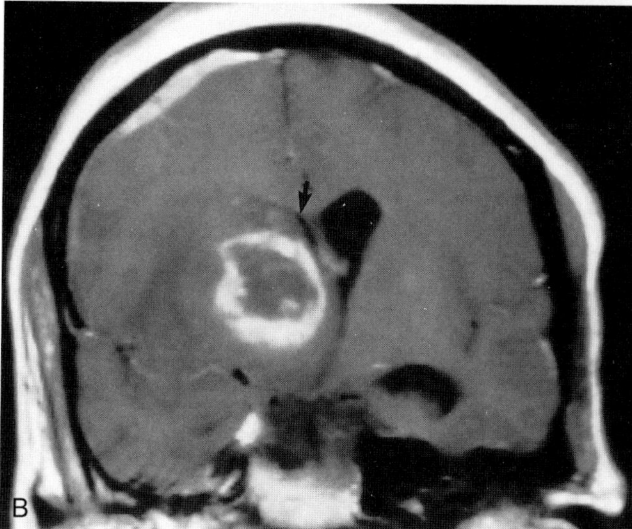

FIGURE 33–8 Toxoplasmosis in patients with AIDS. **A:** Axial postcontrast head computed tomogram shows a ring-enhancing lesion *(arrow)* in the left posterior temporal lobe. **B:** Coronal postcontrast T1-weighted magnetic resonance image shows an enhancing lesion with irregular margins *(arrow)*. (**A** and **B**, From Harris, with permission.)

Pathophysiology

Acute infection usually is self-limited and is associated with fever, lymphadenopathy, myalgias, and headache.[2,3] *Toxoplasma gondii* is a widespread intracellular parasite with a definitive host stage in cats. In the United States, it is estimated that 16% to 40% of the population is infected, and in other parts of the world up to 80%.[2] Ingestion of oocysts from cat litter or soil, ingestion of bradyzoites from undercooked meat, or transplacental spread of tachyzoites may lead to disease.[2,3]

Diagnosis

In patients with suspected encephalitis, computed tomographic scans with contrast (showing ring enhancing lesions with edema) and without contrast (showing multiple subcortical lesions) and magnetic resonance imaging studies are useful. Serologic studies with immunoglobulin M (IgM) and immunoglobulin E (IgE) antibody titers and polymerase chain reaction (PCR) analysis of spinal fluid, biopsy samples, or vitreous fluid can also show infection. Definitive diagnosis is made by finding *T. gondii* on biopsy.[1-3]

Clinical Complications

Ocular toxoplasmosis can result in visual impairment or glaucoma; encephalitis can lead to changed mental status, ataxia, seizures, coma, and death.[1,3] Congenital toxoplasmosis is associated with mental retardation, blindness, and seizure disorders.[2,3]

Management

Patients with suspected toxoplasma encephalitis should be admitted and treated with sulfadiazine, leucovorin, and pyrimethamine. Patients with suspected ocular toxoplasmosis should have urgent follow-up with an ophthalmologist. If the patient is immunosuppressed, pregnant, or newborn, or has experienced visual acuity change or severe disease, treatment with sulfadiazine, pyrimethamine, leucovorin, and corticosteroids should be initiated.[1-3]

REFERENCES

1. Hovakimyan A, Cunningham ET Jr. Ocular toxoplasmosis. *Ophthalmol Clin North Am* 2002;15:327–332.
2. Hill D, Dubey JP. *Toxoplasma gondii:* transmission, diagnosis and prevention. *Clin Microbiol Infect* 2002;8:634–640.
3. Lynfield R, Guerina NG. Toxoplasmosis. *Pediatr Rev* 1997;18:75–83.

HIV-Related Molluscum Contagiosum

Brenda L. Liu

Clinical Presentation

Molluscum contagiosum (MC) appears as pearly, flesh-colored, painless papules, usually between 2 and 5 mm in diameter, with central umbilication.[1-3] The number of lesions averages between 10 and 20.[2,3] In human immunodeficiency virus (HIV)-infected individuals, lesions are often 1 to 6 cm in diameter.[1,3] MC lesions are found in the groin, axilla, antecubital area, and popliteal fossa.[2,3] Lesions that are sexually transmitted are found predominantly on the groin, lower abdomen, and upper thighs.[2,3]

Pathophysiology

MC is caused by a DNA poxvirus adapted to epidermal cells,[1] which causes hypertrophy and hyperplasia of keratinocytes.[2,3] In HIV-infected individuals, the CD4-positive T-lymphocyte count is often less than 100 cells/mm^3.[1] Lesions have a virus-rich core; therefore, MC is highly contagious and is spread by direct contact, by contact with infected material (e.g., clothing, towels), and by autoinoculation.[2,3] Incubation periods range from 1 week to several months.[2,3]

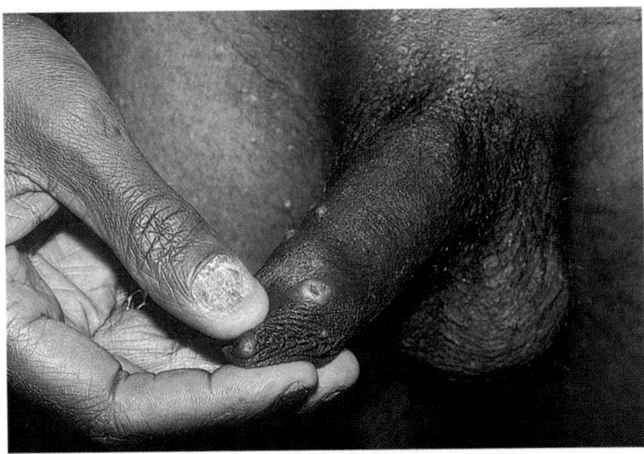

FIGURE 33–9 Molluscum contagiosum. This patient has "giant" molluscum lesions on the shaft of his penis, as well as other scattered smaller lesions. Also note onychomycosis of the thumbnail. (From Goodheart, with permission.)

Diagnosis

The diagnosis is a clinical one, based on physical examination.[1-3] Material expressed from the lesions may be analyzed by light microscopy with Giemsa staining or by electron microscopy to reveal pathognomonic cytoplasmic inclusions, known as "molluscum bodies."[1-3]

Clinical Complications

MC can be a self-limited and benign infection in immunocompetent individuals. Immunocompromise should be suspected in patients with long-standing or widespread lesions.[2,3] MC dermatitis, seen as erythema of the skin surrounding the lesion, can occur and is most likely an immunologic reaction to the papule.[3]

Management

MC requires minimal care in the emergency department; however, patients should be educated regarding the method of transmission. Patients with MC should be referred to their primary care physician, a dermatologist, or an infectious disease specialist for further evaluation and management. Definitive treatment may include removal by curettage, cryotherapy, electrodissection, or treatment with antiviral agents such as cidofovir and imiquimod.[1-3] In HIV-infected individuals, MC may be successfully treated with combination antiretroviral therapy.[1-3]

REFERENCES

1. Garman ME, Tyring SK. The cutaneous manifestations of HIV infection. *Dermatol Clin* 2002;20:193–208.
2. Perna AG, Tyring SK. A review of the dermatologic manifestations of poxvirus infections. *Dermatol Clin* 2002;20:343–346.
3. Diven DG. An overview of poxviruses. *J Am Acad Dermatol* 2001;44:1–16.

Coccidioidomycosis

Grant Wei

Clinical Presentation

Patients with coccidioidomycosis may present with arthralgias, myalgias, self-limited "influenza-like" illness, dry cough, fever, fatigue, pleuritic chest pain, weight loss, night sweats, and rashes (erythema multiforme or erythema nodosum). Signs of dissemination include bony or joint pain, headache, nausea, vomiting, focal neurologic signs, and changed mental status (fewer than 1% of cases).[1,2]

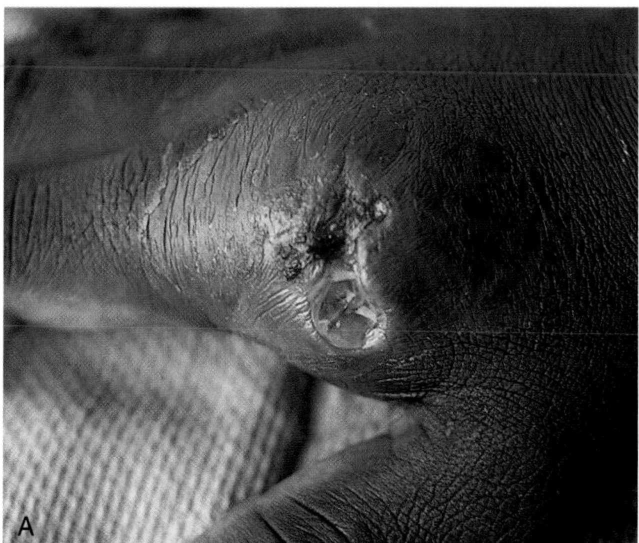

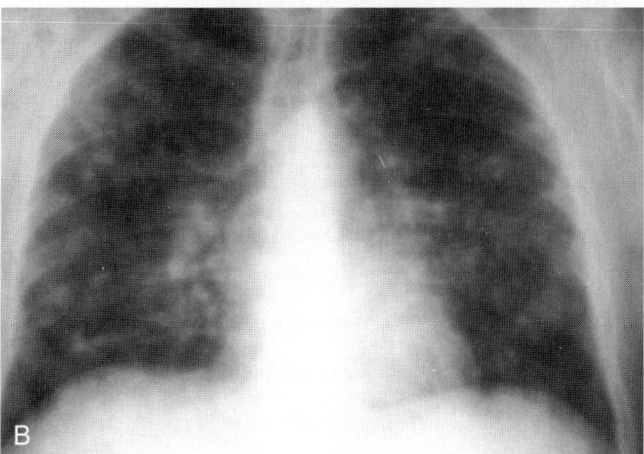

FIGURE 33–10 **A:** Coccidioidomycosis producing deep, painful abscess and local bone invasion. Infection developed after injury to the hand. (Courtesy of Jane Rosensweig, MD.) (From Ostler, with permission.) **B:** Pulmonary coccidioidomycosis. Radiograph shows extensive bilateral nodular infiltrates. (From Mandell, *Essential atlas of infectious diseases,* with permission.)

Pathophysiology

Coccidioidomycosis is endemic in the southwestern United States, primarily in the San Joaquin Valley of California and in Texas, northern Mexico, and Central and South America.[1,2] The disease is caused by inhaled spores that convert to "spherules," which are released as endospores. Endospores cause local inflammatory reactions and pneumonitis. Dissemination occurs by lymphohematogenous spread.[1,2]

Diagnosis

Definitive diagnosis is made by growing the organisms from culture or by seeing spherules in a tissue biopsy specimen. The laboratory should be notified if the disease is suspected, because it is highly infectious. Chest radiography may show infiltrates with ipsilateral hilar adenopathy and pleural effusions.[1,2] Computed tomographic scanning may show dilated ventricles (hydrocephalus), and lumbar puncture may show low glucose, elevated protein, and pleocytosis in the cerebrospinal fluid.[1]

Clinical Complications

Complications include pneumonia and subsequent chronic pulmonary nodules or cavities, as well as skin lesions (plaques, abscesses, and granulomata), meningitis, osteomyelitis, and joint infection (90% in a single joint, most commonly the knee).[1,2]

Management

Immunocompetent patients with newly diagnosed or suspected coccidioidomycosis may be referred to primary care follow-up without treatment if there are no signs or symptoms of extrapulmonary infection or severe complaints. Patients with immunosuppression or with severe or persistent disease should be considered for admission and treatment with amphotericin B and/or oral fluconazole, ketoconazole, or itraconazole. Any patient with suspected meningitis or respiratory compromise should be admitted and started on amphotericin B. The type and urgency of consultation is based on disease manifestation and may involve pulmonary, infectious disease, orthopedic surgery, neurosurgery, and thoracic surgery specialists.[1-3]

REFERENCES

1. Chiller TM, Galgiani JN, Stevens DA. Coccidioidomycosis. *Infect Dis Clin North Am* 2003;17:41–57.
2. Goldman M, Johnson PC, Sarosi GA. Fungal pneumonias: the endemic mycoses. *Clin Chest Med* 1999;20:507–519.
3. Galgiani, JN. Coccidioidomycosis: a regional disease of national importance. Rethinking approaches for control. *Ann Intern Med* 1999;130:293–300.

Cryptosporidiosis

Michael Greenberg

Pathophysiology

Cryptosporidiosis is a parasitic infection caused by organisms of the genus *Cryptosporidium. Cryptosporidium* is a genus of intracellular parasites within which 10 species have been identified. *Cryptosporidium parvum* is the species most often associated with human infection. The intestinal epithelium is the primary site of infection for this organism, and infection results in diarrhea that is usually self-limited in immunocompetent individuals but potentially life-threatening in immunocompromised persons. Infection with *C. parvum* is especially dangerous for persons with acquired immunodeficiency syndrome (AIDS).[1]

Diagnosis

Cryptosporidiosis must be considered in any patient with persistent diarrhea, especially in patients who may be immunocompromised from various causes, including AIDS. The diagnosis is made by identification of the organism using microscopic techniques applied to tissues or body fluids.

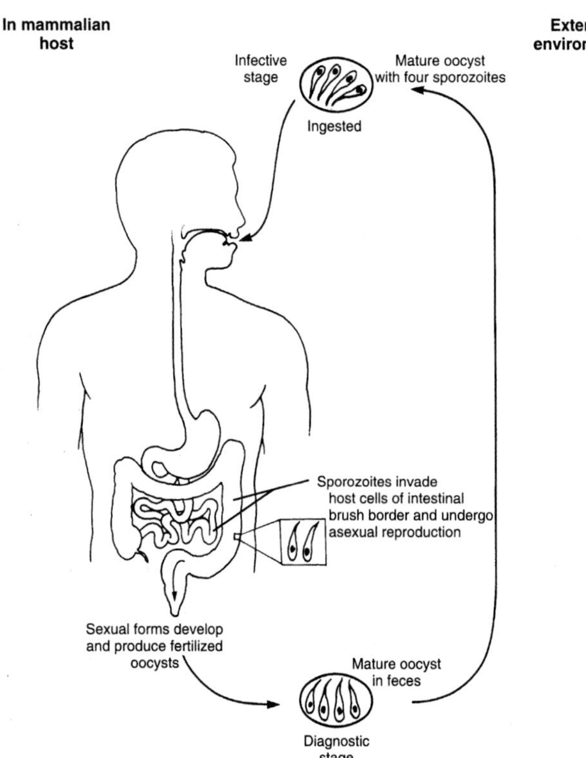

FIGURE 33–11 Life cycle of *Cryptosporidium*. (From McClatchey, with permission.)

Clinical Complications

Cryptosporidial infections in extraintestinal sites (pulmonary, middle ear, biliary tract, pancreas, and stomach) may occur in AIDS patients and are problematic. The biliary tract is reportedly the most common extraintestinal site for this infection, and it may actually serve as a reservoir for cryptosporidia, influencing the chronicity of the infection. Although biliary cryptosporidiosis increases morbidity, it may not change survival statistics.[1–3] In 1993, major outbreaks of cryptosporidiosis transmitted via public drinking water occurred in Milwaukee, Wisconsin, and Las Vegas, Nevada. More than 400,000 people were afflicted in the Milwaukee outbreak, and several thousand were afflicted in the Las Vegas episode.[4]

Management

The treatment of cryptosporidiosis is difficult because currently there are no antimicrobial agents that are capable of totally eradicating the organism.[3] Patients require excellent supportive care to treat and prevent dehydration. The best course of therapy for AIDS patients involves augmentation of the immune function by the use of standard antiretroviral drugs.[1–3] In addition, the combination of drugs such as paromomycin, azithromycin, and nitazoxanide with antidiarrheal agents is a mainstay of therapy.[1–3]

REFERENCES

1. Manabe YC, Clark DP, Moore RD, et al. Cryptosporidiosis in patients with AIDS: correlates of disease and survival. *Clin Infect Dis* 1998;27:536–542.
2. Chappell CL, Okhuysen PC. Cryptosporidiosis. *Curr Opin Infect Dis* 2002;15:523–527.
3. Chen XM, Keithly JS, Paya CV, LaRusso NF. Current concepts: cryptosporidiosis. *N Engl J Med* 2002;346:1723–1731.
4. Gostin LO, Lazzarini Z, Neslund VS, Osterholm MT. Water quality laws and waterborne diseases: *Cryptosporidium* and other emerging pathogens. *Am J Pubic Health* 2000;90:847–853.

HIV Colitis

Jennifer Wiler

Clinical Presentation

Patients with human immunodeficiency virus (HIV) colitis present with a myriad of gastrointestinal complaints, including watery or bloody diarrhea, fever, anorexia, weight loss, periumbilical cramps, bloating, nausea, vomiting, urgency, or tenesmus. In severe cases, patients may present with dehydration and hemodynamic instability secondary to significant fluid and electrolyte loss, or with severe acute abdominal pain.[1-3]

Pathophysiology

The most common cause of colitis in HIV is bacterial, but as the degree of immunodeficiency worsens, infection with opportunistic pathogens and neoplasms becomes more frequent.[2] Enterocolitis may be caused by HIV itself or it may be the result of extended antibiotic therapy.[3]

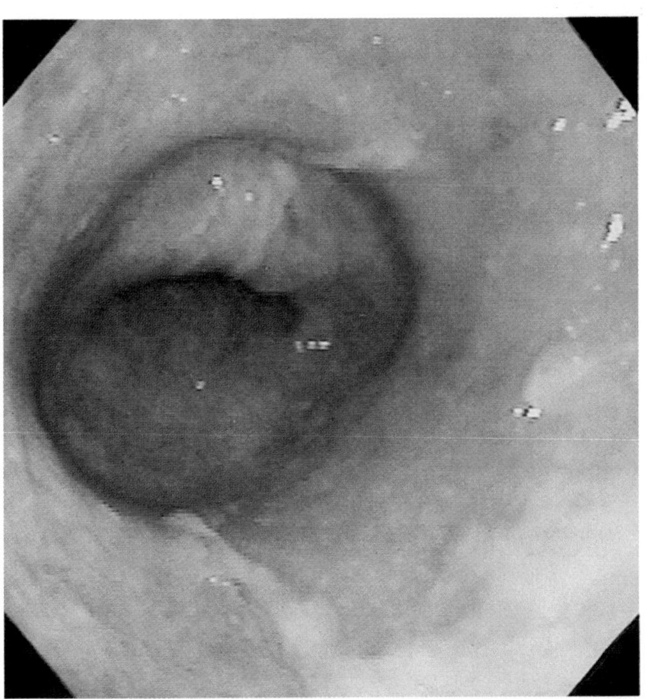

FIGURE 33–12 Bacterial infections with *Salmonella* species, *Shigella flexneri,* and *Campylobacter jejuni* cause similar clinical illnesses in persons infected with human immunodeficiency virus (HIV)-1. (From Yamada, with permission.)

Diagnosis

The diagnosis is based on clinical suspicion and a known diagnosis of HIV/acquired immunodeficiency syndrome (AIDS). Laboratory evaluation of the stool for occult blood, leukocytes, ova, parasites, acid-fast bacilli, *Clostridium difficile* toxin, and bacterial culture may aid in diagnosis of the offending pathogen.[1-3]

Clinical Complications

Clinical complications include dehydration, electrolyte abnormalities (including hypokalemic metabolic alkalosis), bacteremia, severe gastrointestinal hemorrhage, and perforated viscera.[3]

Management

Evaluation in the emergency department should focus on the severity of the symptoms. Stool should be collected for laboratory evaluation. Rehydration, administration of antidiarrheal agents, electrolyte replacement, and empiric antibiotic treatment may be necessary. Samples for appropriate cultures should be taken. Hospitalization is required for patients with severe dehydration, intractable diarrhea, toxicity, or marked abdominal pain.[1]

REFERENCES

1. Du Pont HL. Guidelines on acute infectious diarrhea in adults. The Practice Parameters Committee of the American College of Gastroenterology. *Am J Gastroenterol* 1997;92:1962–1975.
2. Monkemuller KE, Wilcox CM. Diagnosis and treatment of colonic disease in AIDS. *Gastrointest Endosc Clin North Am* 1998;8:889–911.
3. Smith PD, Quinn TC, Strober W, Janoff EN, Masur H. NIH conference: Gastrointestinal infections in AIDS. *Ann Intern Med* 1992;116:63–77.

HIV-Related Vasculitis

Jennifer Wiler

Clinical Presentation

Clinical presentation depends on the organ systems affected. Constitutional symptoms can include weakness and malaise, or fever and weight loss.[1-4]

Pathophysiology

A wide range of inflammatory vascular diseases may develop in human immunodeficiency virus (HIV)-infected patients, including systemic necrotizing vasculitis, polyarteritis nodosa, bacteria-induced vasculitis, hypersensitivity vasculitis, Henoch-Schönlein purpura, angiocentric immunoproliferative vasculitis, benign lymphocytic angiitis, large-vessel vasculitis, and primary angiitis (a rare central nervous system vasculitis associated with high mortality).[1-4] Functional and morphologic endothelial damage is caused by HIV-1.[4] However, extensive studies have demonstrated no evidence of viral antigens in the inflammatory infiltrates associated with HIV-related vasculitic lesions. It is T lymphocytes, particularly CD3-, CD8-, and CD4-positive T cells, that are thought to be important immunologic mediators in the development of this condition.[1,2] Among the infective causes of HIV vasculitis, cytomegalovirus and tuberculosis are the most common.[2]

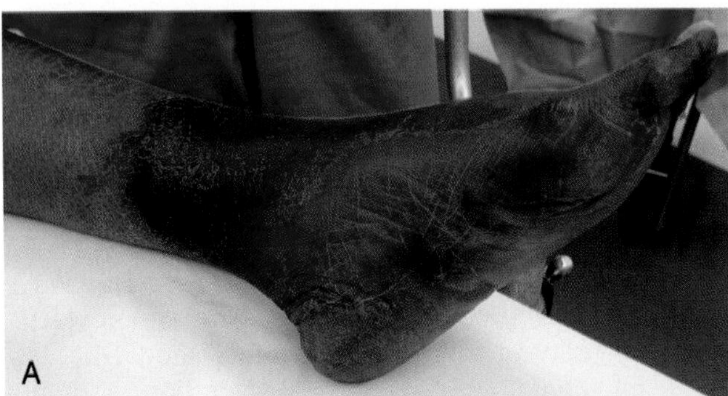

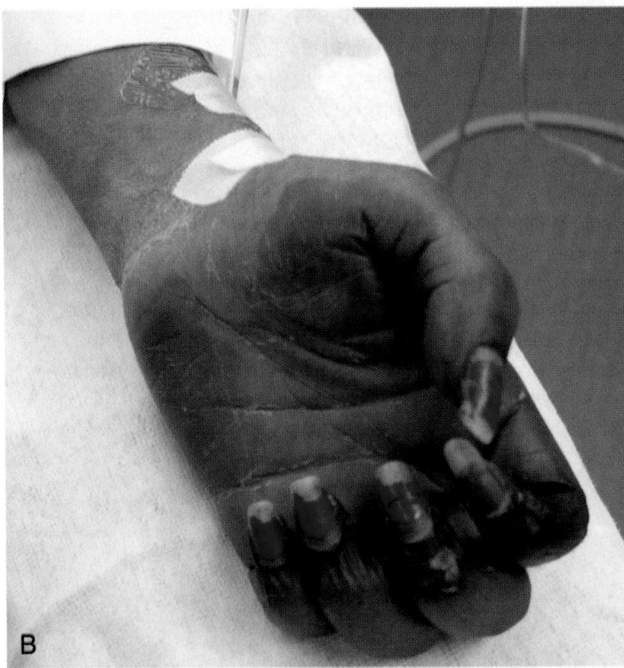

FIGURE 33–13 **A** and **B:** HIV-related vasculitis. (Courtesy of Michael Weingarten, MD.)

Diagnosis

The diagnosis of vasculitis is based on clinical suspicion and is confirmed by immunohistochemistry and, occasionally, by lesion biopsy.

Clinical Complications

Clinical complications of HIV-induced vasculitis depend on the involved organ systems and the extent of vasculitic infiltration. Serious complications can include organism superinfection, sepsis, vascular compromise, malignancy, ischemia, renal failure, stroke, aneurysm formation, and death.[1-4]

Management

Treatment for each of the HIV-related vasculitic conditions is varied and often depends on the underlying cause. Patients with some forms of vasculitis require pharmacologic suppression of immunologic mediators or plasma apheresis, whereas others require only supportive care.[1-4]

REFERENCES

1. Calabresi LH, Estes M, Yen-Lieberman B, et al. Systemic vasculitis in association with human immunodeficiency virus infection. *Arthritis Rheum* 1989;32:569–576.
2. Chetty R. Vasculitides associated with HIV infection. *J Clin Pathol* 2001;54:275–278.
3. Barbaro G. Cardiovascular manifestations of HIV infection. *Circulation* 2002;106:1420–1425.
4. Terada LS, Gu Y, Flores SC. AIDS vasculopathy. *Am J Med Sci* 2000;320:379–387.

Mycobacterium avium Complex

Jennifer Wiler

Clinical Presentation

Disseminated *Mycobacterium avium* complex (MAC) disease typically manifests in immunocompromised patients with weakness, chills, night sweats, diarrhea, weight loss, abdominal pain, anemia, and thrombocytopenia.[2] Of the acquired immunodeficiency syndrome (AIDS) cases reported to the Centers for Disease Control and Prevention (CDC) between 1981 and 1987, disseminated nontuberculous mycobacteria occurred in 5.5%, with 95% being MAC.[1–3]

Pathophysiology

MAC refers to infections caused by either *Mycobacterium avium* or *Mycobacterium intracellulare,* which can result in pneumonia, superficial lymphadenitis, soft tissue infection, and disseminated disease. MAC is an AIDS-defining illness.[1–3] MAC organisms are commonly found in soil, food, and water. They enter the respiratory and gastrointestinal tracts and are disseminated into the bloodstream. Most signs and symptoms of MAC disease are the result of elaboration of cytokines.[3]

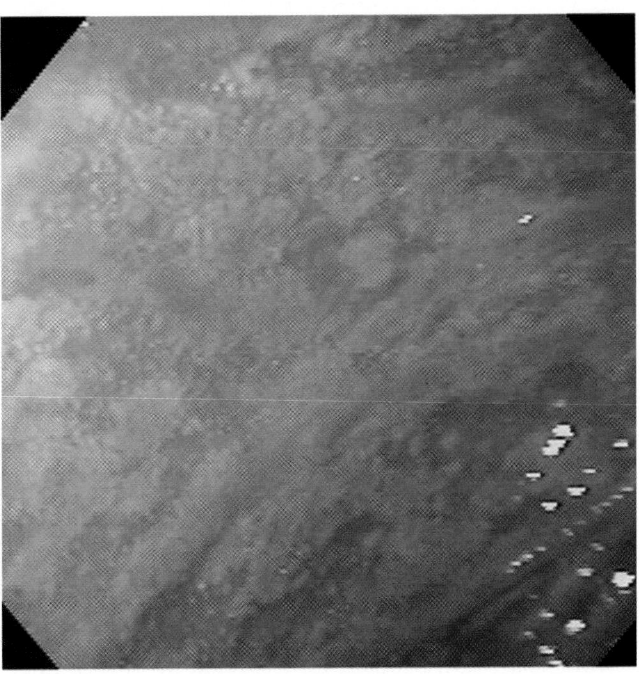

FIGURE 33–14 Endoscopic image of the duodenum in an acquired immunodeficiency syndrome (AIDS) patient with disseminated *Mycobacterium avium* complex infection. (From Yamada, with permission.)

Diagnosis

An acute pulmonary infiltrate, nodule, or cavitation on the chest radiograph in a patient with cough, sputum production, or dyspnea is suspicious for pneumonia. Laboratory identification of MAC is achieved by sputum culture and acid-fast bacteria stain and smear. Lesion biopsy may be required to confirm the diagnosis.[1] Disseminated infection is identified with positive blood cultures and DNA species probes.[2]

Clinical Complications

MAC is rarely the direct cause of death but increases the risk for superinfection. Death may result from malnutrition or other infections.[3]

Management

Patients with suspected MAC infection should be referred to a clinician who specializes in HIV-related infections. Suspected opportunistic infection should be treated initially with broad-spectrum empiric antibiotics until the pathogen is identified. Treatment of the disease is with multiple antituberculosis mediations.[2]

REFERENCES

1. Diagnosis and treatment of disease caused by non-tuberculous mycobacteria. Official Statement of the American Thoracic Society. *Am J Respir Crit Care* 1997;156:S1–S25.
2. Hewitt RG, Papandonatos GD, Shelton MJ, Hsiao CB, Harmon BJ, Kaczmarek SR, Amsterdam D. Prevention of disseminated *Mycobacterium avium* complex infection with reduced dose clarithromycin in patients with advanced HIV disease. AIDS 1999;13:1367–1372.
3. Horsburgh CR Jr. *Mycobacterium avium* complex infection in the acquired immunodeficiency syndrome. *N Engl J Med* 1991;324: 1332–1338.

Pneumocystis carinii Pneumonia

Polly Dole

Clinical Presentation

The classic presentation of *Pneumocystis carinii* pneumonia (PCP) includes exertional dyspnea, fever, and nonproductive cough.

Pathophysiology

The organism *P. carinii* enters the lungs via respiration and attaches to alveolar cells. Proliferation produces a foamy, eosinophilic exudate that fills the alveolar spaces, leading to decreased oxygenation, a thickened interstitium, and eventual fibrosis.[1] A key risk factor for PCP infection is seropositive human immunodeficiency syndrome (HIV) status. Among HIV-positive patients, risk factors include a CD4-positive T-lymphocyte count lower than 200 cells/mm^3, unexplained fever greater than 37.7° C (100° F) for longer than 2 weeks, a history of oropharyngeal candidiasis, and one or more previous episodes of PCP.[1]

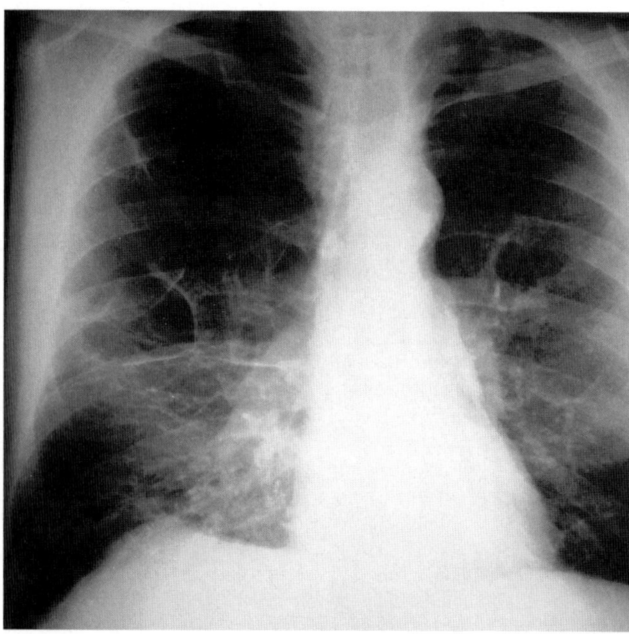

FIGURE 33–15 *Pneumocystis carinii* pneumonia. (Courtesy of Mark Silverberg, MD.)

Diagnosis

Patients are often noted to be hypoxemic. Lung auscultation may reveal fine rales, or it may be normal.[1] Chest radiography may show diffuse bilateral interstitial or perihilar infiltrates, or it may be normal. An elevated lactate dehydrogenase level can indicate disease severity. Diagnosis of PCP is made with the use of stains to identify the organism cyst wall and trophozoite. If clinical suspicion is high and bronchial alveolar lavage is negative, transbronchial biopsy may be needed.[1]

Clinical Complications

Pneumothorax and ventilator-dependent respiratory failure may occur. Medications used for treatment have distinct side-effect profiles that limit their use.[1]

Management

The best prognostic indicator is the alveolar-to-arterial oxygen difference ($[A–a]DO_2 = 150 - 1.2(PaCO_2) - PaO_2$).[1] Mild infection is defined by an $[A–a]DO_2$ less than 35 mm Hg, with a PaO_2 greater than 70 mm Hg; moderate infection by an $[A–a]DO_2$ of 35 to 45 mm Hg with a PaO_2 greater than 70 mm Hg; and severe infection by a $[A–a]DO_2$ greater than 45 mm Hg with PaO_2 greater than 50 mm Hg. Mild to moderate PCP can be treated with oral medications. The first choice is trimethoprim-sulfamethoxazole (TMP-SMX), followed by trimethoprim and dapsone or clindamycin and primaquine, with atovaquone as a last choice. Moderate to severe PCP necessitates intravenous therapy. The first choice is again TMP-SMX, followed by trimetrexate, leucovorin and oral dapsone, or clindamycin and oral primaquine, with pentamidine as a last choice.[1] A 3-week course of prednisone, or methylprednisolone if intravenous medication is indicated, is warranted for moderate to severe infections and for all infections in acquired immunodeficiency syndrome patients.[1]

REFERENCES

1. Wilkin A, Feinberg J. *Pneumocystis carinii* pneumonia: a clinical review. *Am Fam Physician* 1999;60:1699–1714.

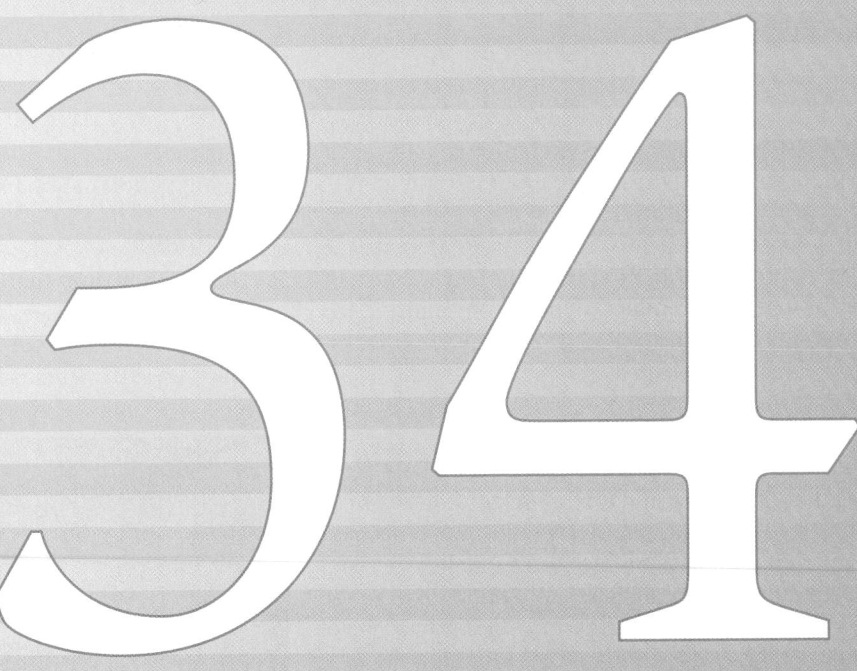

34 Abuse

Child Abuse

Charles Felzen Johnson

Child abuse (CA) is defined as intentional injuries to children that are significant or threatening to the child's physical or psychological welfare. From a medical standpoint, an impact that results in a bruise, fracture, or damage to an internal organ should be considered significant. The failure to protect a child from injury is reportable as safety neglect. Physicians are among the mandated reporters of suspected CA.

Clinical Presentation

Intentional injuries may include such things as inflicted caustic or thermal burns, fractures, impact injuries from various objects (most commonly the hand), and acceleration-deceleration injuries to the head.[1] In addition, children may be pinched, strangled, punctured, smothered, or shaken by caretakers. Children may be burned in hot water in the process of bathing, either intentionally or if the water temperature is not checked (safety neglect). Caretakers who intentionally injure a child rarely indicate this fact when they bring the child to the emergency department, and a variety of plausible, implausible, and changing explanations may be offered.[1]

Diagnosis

A thorough history that includes the cause, timing, treatment of, and witnesses to the injury should be obtained. Potential victims of CA should be examined thoroughly, including skin, mucosa, and the fundus. Bruises, the

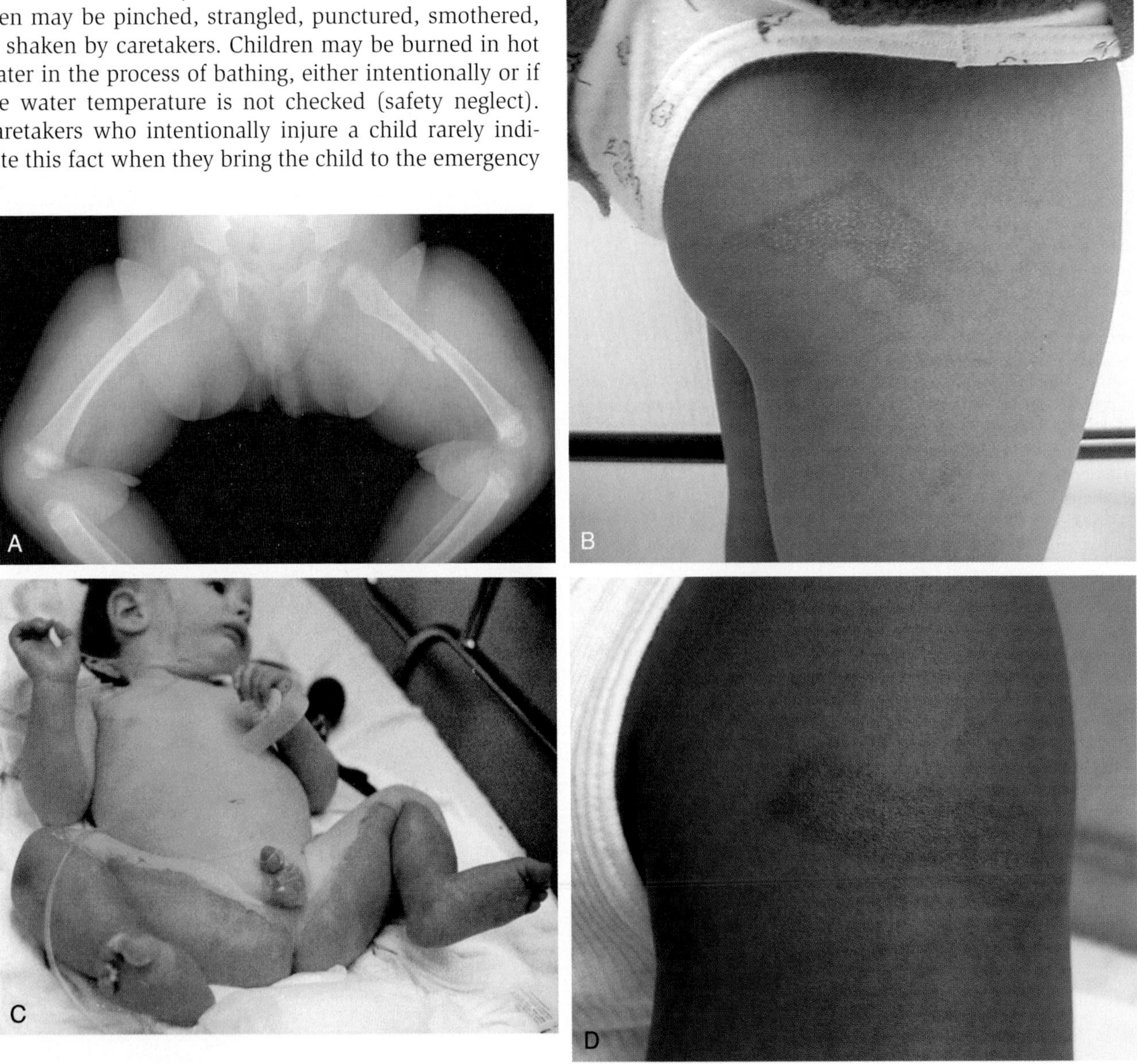

FIGURE 34–1 Child abuse. **A:** Abusive femur fracture. (Courtesy of Mark Silverberg, MD.) **B:** Iron imprint. (Courtesy of Christy Salvaggio, MD.) **C:** Thermal burns. (Courtesy of B. Zane Horowitz, MD.) **D:** Red mark with three clear dots across, matching the belt with which this child was hit. (Courtesy of Mark Silverberg, MD.)

Child Abuse

Charles Felzen Johnson

most common consequence of intentional injury, change color over time, but the time course is unreliable. Familiarity with the patterns made on the skin by various common materials aids the physician in recognizing CA. Hand prints or instruments may be outlined or silhouetted on the skin.[1]

The shaken infant may present in various stages of central nervous system dysfunction, and meningitis may be suspected. Investigation may reveal subdural hematomas, bloody spinal fluid (often misinterpreted as iatrogenic), or retinal hemorrhages (85% of shaken infants).[1] Because there may be a combination of shaking and impact, the term "intentional head injury" is preferred.

Clinical Complications

Complications relate to the individual injury and the delay before seeking medical attention.

Management

If the injury and the cause are not compatible, then a suspected CA report should be made to local children's protective services or law enforcement agencies or both. This is best accomplished through the use of standardized forms. Children younger than 2 years of age with intentional trauma should have a skeletal survey and possibly a computed tomogram of the head. The accident scene and home should be investigated. All witnesses should be interviewed. Other children in the home of the injured child should be examined.[1]

REFERENCES

1. Johnson CF. Inflicted injury versus accidental injury. *Pediatr Clin North Am* 1990;37:791–814.

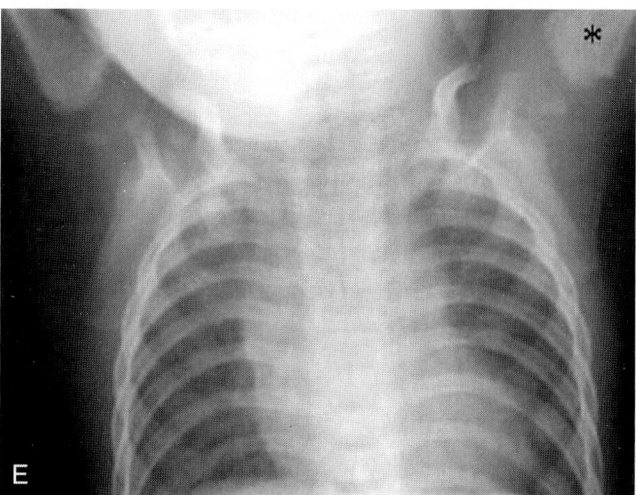

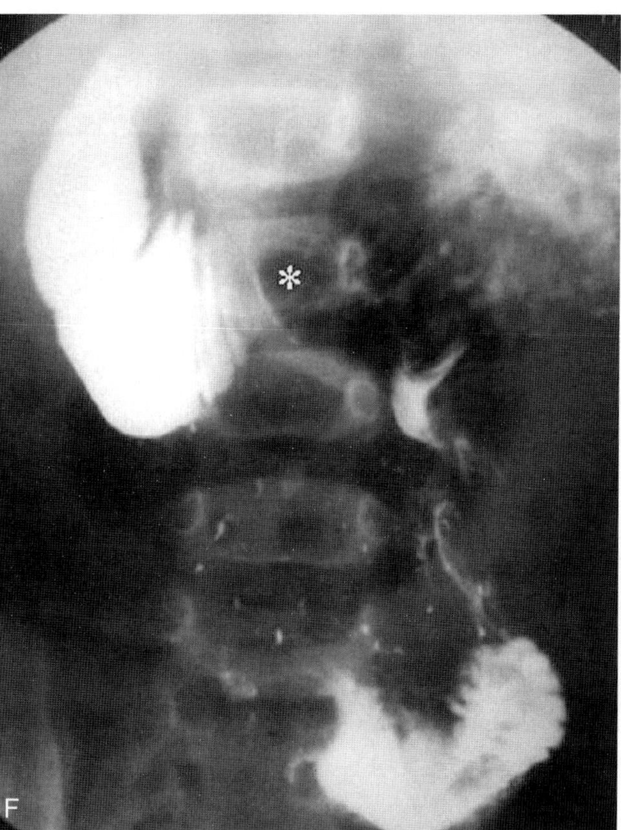

FIGURE 34–1, cont'd. Child abuse. **E:** Anteroposterior chest radiograph in a 7-month-old infant obtained for "rule-out pneumonia." Note the healing fracture of the proximal left humerus in this victim of physical abuse. (Courtesy of Evan Geller, MD.) **F:** Anteroposterior radiograph of the abdomen from an upper gastrointestinal study in an abused child with blunt abdominal trauma and bowel wall hematoma. (Courtesy of Evan Geller, MD.)

34–2

Shaken Baby Syndrome

Michael Greenberg

Clinical Presentation

Patients with shaken baby syndrome (SBS) present with a spectrum of problems, which depend on the time since shaking as well as the degree and severity of the shaking event. After minimal shaking, some patients have no clinically evident problems. Others present with lethargy, feeding problems, vomiting, and irritability. Severely shaken patients may present with seizures, coma, or death, sometimes with opisthotonos and distended fontanelles.[1–4]

Pathophysiology

The primary injury-inducing forces involve rotational (as opposed to translational) forces transmitted to the head and brain.[4] These rotational forces are generated by shaking the child and result in the brain's moving about its central axis and at the brainstem. This causes stretching and tearing of the bridging veins between the dural venous sinuses and the cortex.[4] As a result, small amounts of blood may seep into the subdural space, thus providing definite evidence of injury induced by shaking. Forceful shaking also induces diffuse axonal injury. In addition, forceful shaking results in brain tissue hypoxia, cerebral edema, and elevations in intracranial pressure.[1–4]

Shaken infants often manifest ocular as well as bony injuries. As many as 95% of babies with intracranial injury not associated with high-speed trauma are victims of shaking.[4]

Diagnosis

The key to diagnosis is the maintenance of a high index of suspicion. Physicians must never accept illogical explanations for intracranial or other injuries. Retinal hemorrhages confirm the diagnosis of SBS. Plain skull radiographs may be necessary but in general do not confirm the diagnosis of SBS. Computed tomography without contrast is often the first study done in these cases. However, magnetic resonance imaging with diffusion-weighted sequences is currently considered to be the most sensitive imaging study for SBS diagnosis.[1–4]

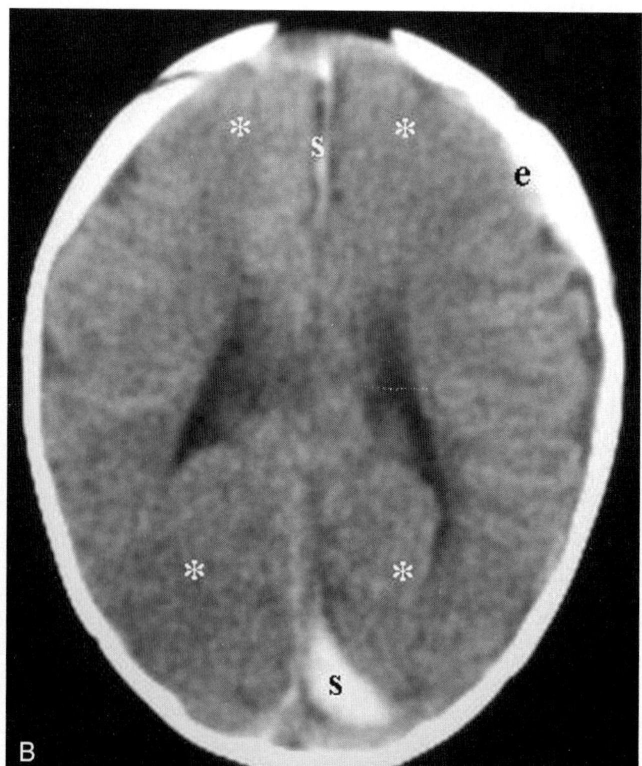

FIGURE 34–2 Shaken baby syndrome. **A:** Axial image from an abdominal computed tomography (CT) study with oral and intravenous contrast. Note the bowel wall (b) and hematoma (H) with mass effect. **B:** Nonenhanced axial head CT demonstrating bifrontal and occipital hypodensities (*), subdural hemorrhage (s), a small left parietal epidural hematoma (e), and effacement of the normal sulci consistent with cerebral edema. (**A–C,** Courtesy of Evan Geller, MD.)

Shaken Baby Syndrome

Michael Greenberg

Clinical Complications

Complications include bilateral or unilateral retinal hemorrhages, coagulopathies, metaphyseal fractures caused by flailing of the limbs during shaking, posterior rib fractures caused by pressure from holding the child during shaking, subdural hematomas, blindness, microcephaly, permanent brain damage, and death.[1-4]

Management

Emergency treatment first addresses the standard ABCs of resuscitation (airway, breathing, and circulation), monitoring, and control of intracranial pressure. If there is a suspicion of shaking, the child should be admitted to a pediatric facility. Social and law enforcement officials should be involved in the case at the earliest appropriate time.

REFERENCES

1. Morad Y, Kim Y, Mian M, et al. Nonophthalmologist accuracy in diagnosing retinal hemorrhages in the shaken baby syndrome. *J Pediatr* 2003;142:431–434.
2. Tsao K, Kazlas M, Weiter JJ. Ocular injuries in shaken baby syndrome. *Int Ophthalmol Clin* 2002;42:145–155.
3. King WJ, MacKay M, Sirnick A, Canadian Shaken Baby Syndrome Group. Shaken baby syndrome in Canada: clinical characteristics and outcomes of hospital cases. *CMAJ* 2003;168:155–159.
4. Blumenthal I. Shaken baby syndrome. *Postgrad Med J* 2002;78: 732–735.

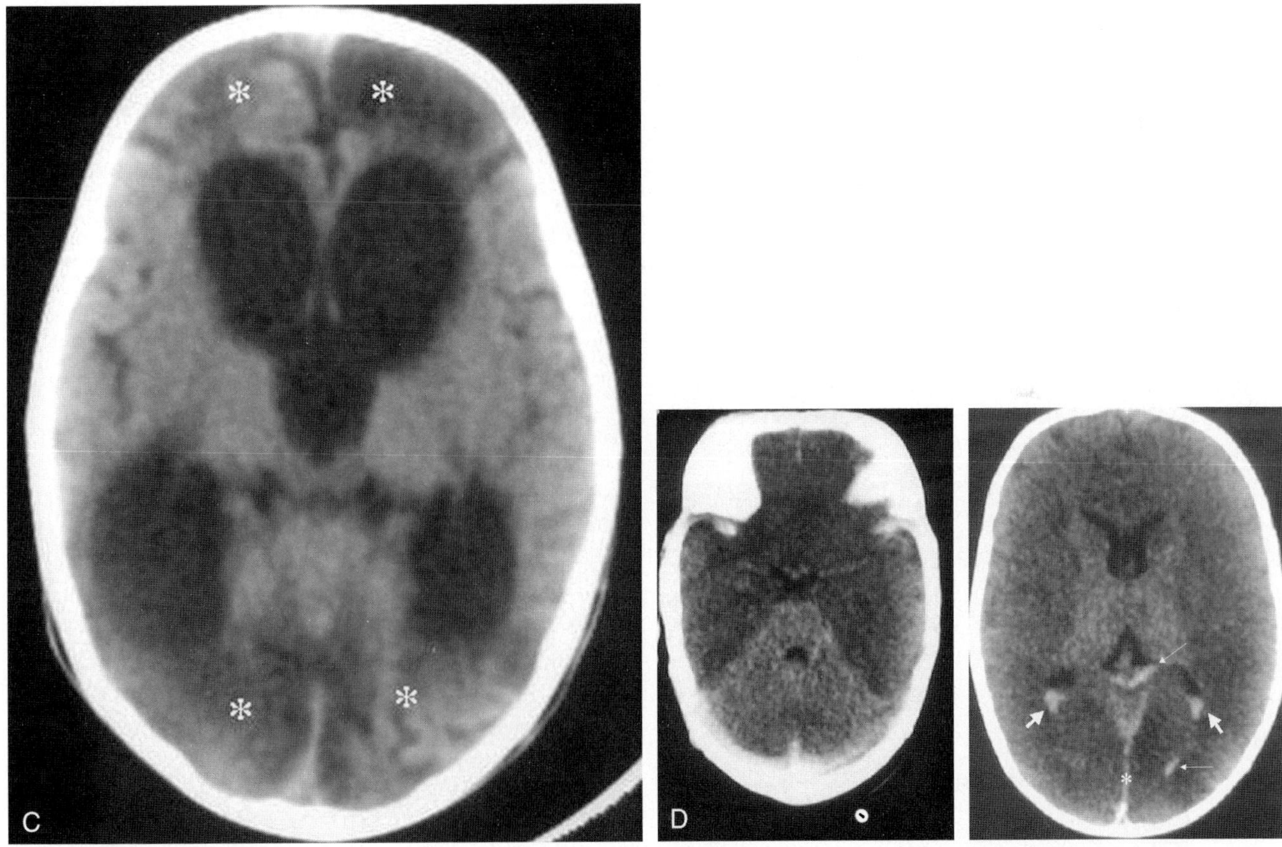

FIGURE 34–2, cont'd. Shaken baby syndrome. **C:** Same patient as in **B,** 1 year later. Note infarctions in the anterior and posterior cerebral artery distributions (*) and *"ex-vacuo"* dilation of the ventricular system. **D:** Nonenhanced head computed tomography (CT) in a victim of child abuse, demonstrating the "reversal sign" of diffuse cerebral injury after anoxic insult. Note the higher attenuation of the thalami and basal ganglia. Also note blood within the occipital horns of the lateral ventricles *(short arrows)*, blood within the posterior interhemispheric fissure (*), and shear injury of the splenium of the corpus callosum *(long arrows)*. (**C** and **D,** Courtesy of Evan Geller, MD.)

Skeletal Survey in Physical Abuse

Evan Geller

The skeletal survey should be the initial imaging study in children younger than 2 years of age who are suspected victims of nonaccidental injury.[1] The skeletal survey should include the following projections:

- Humerus, radius/ulna, wrist, and hand (anteroposterior [AP])
- Femur, tibia/fibula, ankle, and foot (AP)
- Chest, including thoracic spine and ribs (AP and lateral [LAT])
- Abdomen to include lumbosacral spine and bony pelvis (AP)
- Lumbosacral spine (LAT)
- Cervical spine (AP and LAT)
- Skull (AP and LAT)

The goal of the survey is to identify fractures that are not clinically evident as a sign of past abuse. The value of the skeletal survey as a screening study for physical abuse diminishes beyond 2 years of age and is of little utility in children older than 5 years of age.[1]

Diagnosis

Findings on the skeletal survey may be classified according to their specificity for physical abuse. High-specificity lesions include the following: (1) rib fractures, especially of the posterior ribs; (2) metaphyseal "corner" or "bucket-handle" fractures of the long bones; and (3) fractures of the sternum, scapulae, or spinous processes (the 3 S's); these bones require a great force to fracture. Examples of high specificity lesions are given in Figure 34–3D,E.

Lesions of moderate specificity include (1) fractures in different stages of healing; (2) fracture of the femur/tibia in a nonambulating child; (3) complex skull fractures (e.g., depressed, stellate); and (4) digital fractures. Lesions of low specificity include (1) fracture of the femur/tibia in an ambulating child and (2) nondisplaced, linear skull fracture.

Management

If a fracture of a long bone is suspected on a single view, it is important to obtain an additional view of the injured segment. A "babygram" (Fig. 34–3C) is not an acceptable alternative to a properly performed skeletal survey, because geometric distortion and underexposure or overexposure may obscure subtle injuries. If multiple fractures are discovered on a skeletal survey, it is important to exclude an underlying bone dysplasia (e.g., osteogenesis imperfecta) or metabolic disorder (e.g., rickets) as a potential cause. If an initial skeletal survey is normal or is inconclusive relative to the degree of clinical concern, a bone scan or follow-up skeletal survey in 2 weeks may be indicated.[2] Magnetic resonance imaging

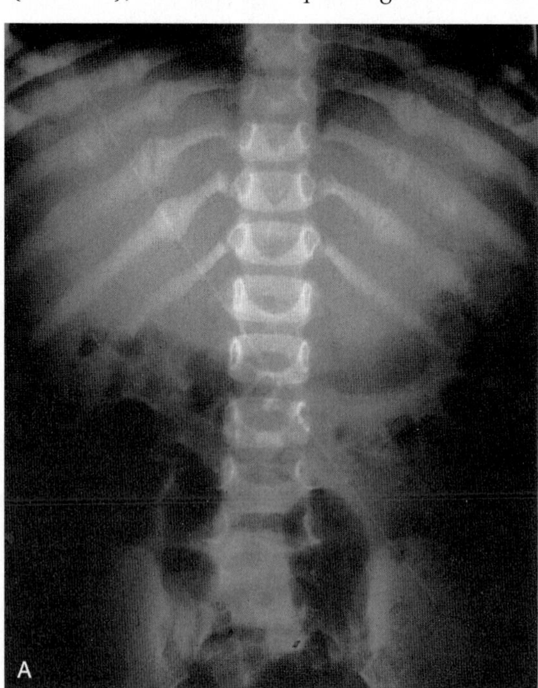

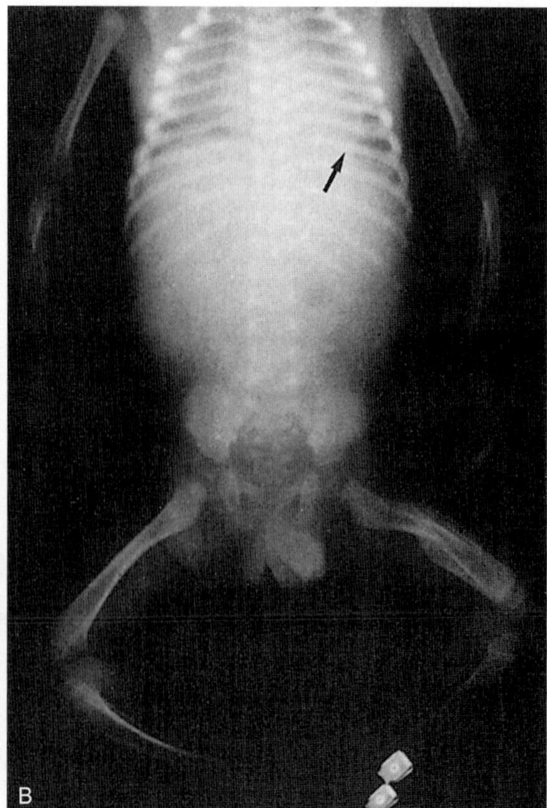

FIGURE 34–3 Skeletal survey in physical abuse. **A:** Infant with multiple old rib injuries and gastric distention. (From Reece, with permission.) **B:** Radiograph of the trunk and extremities of a victim of child abuse, showing healed misaligned fracture of the left femur and healing rib fractures *(arrow)* on the left. (From Jones, with permission.)

Skeletal Survey in Physical Abuse

Evan Geller

or sonography or both may be indicated in the evaluation of epiphyseal separations if these are suspected on plain films. Consultation with a pediatric radiologist should be considered.

REFERENCES

1. Diagnostic imaging of child abuse. *Pediatrics* 2000;105:1345–1348.
2. Kleinman PK, Nimkin K, Spevak MR, et al. Follow-up skeletal surveys in suspected child abuse. *AJR Am J Roentgenol* 1996;167: 893–896.

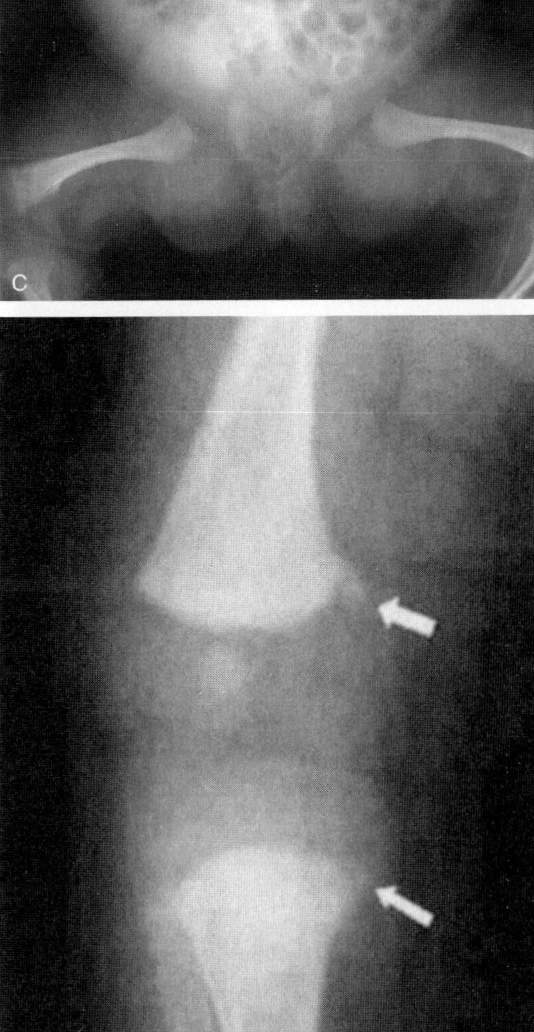

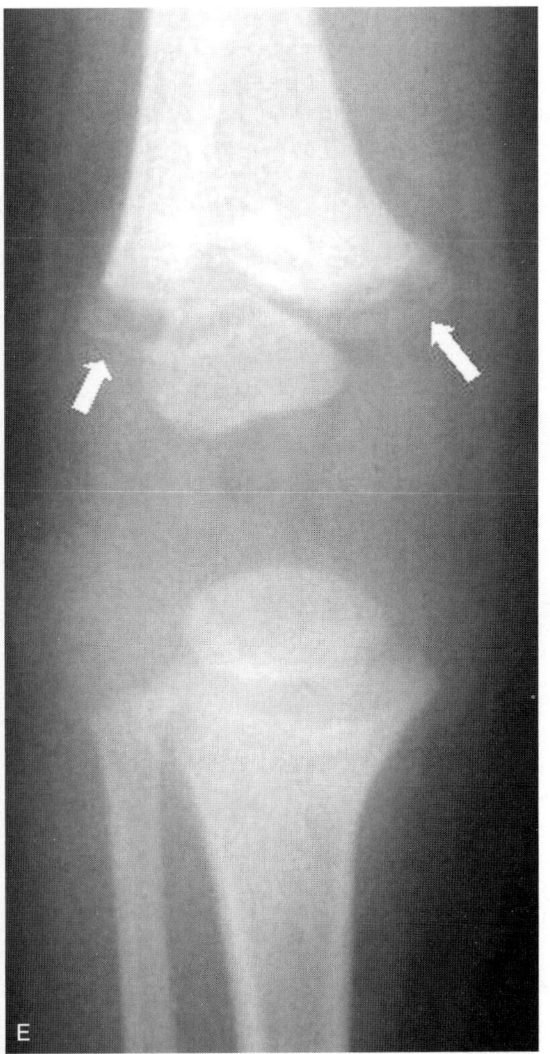

FIGURE 34–3, cont'd. Skeletal survey in physical abuse. **C:** "Babygram": a single frontal radiograph of the long bones and axial skeleton may mask subtle injuries due to geometric distortion and exposure variation. **D:** Frontal radiograph of the knee showing a characteristic metaphyseal "corner" fracture of the distal femur *(arrows)*. **E:** Another infant's knee demonstrating the typical and highly specific "bucket-handle" fracture of the distal femur *(arrows)*. (**C–E,** Courtesy of Evan Geller, MD.)

Abuse-Related Head Trauma

Stephen Boos

Clinical Presentation

Patients with abusive head trauma may present with obvious signs of traumatic injury, including bruising, lacerations, or slap marks. However, head injuries may be occult, revealing few or no external signs of trauma.

Pathophysiology

A wide variety of head injuries may be inflicted during child abuse, and these injuries account for 80% of pediatric deaths due to abuse.[1]

Shaken baby syndrome (SBS) is an abusive head injury that occurs during vigorous shaking or by direct trauma.[1] Clinical signs of brain injury may be present, including decreased mental status, neurologic deficits, seizures, and retinal hemorrhage. Other signs associated with vigorous shaking include finger-shaped bruises on the thorax and fractures of the lower-extremity long bones.[1] External signs of head trauma may not be evident (50% to 75%) on visual examination.[1,2] SBS is produced by acceleration/deceleration of the head that is typical during shaking in addition to blunt trauma. Shear forces and blunt injury may produce diffuse axonal injury, subarachnoid hemorrhage, and subdural hematoma.[1]

Diagnosis

All children with head injuries require an assessment for child abuse, including a thorough history, examination for other injuries, and evaluation of the family and social interactions. Examination of the retina is essential, because 70% to 85% of patients with SBS have retinal hemorrhage.[1] If there is suspicion for abuse or evidence of SBS, a skeletal survey and/or additional radiologic/laboratory evaluation may be performed, and social services should be contacted.

An attempt should be made to match the mechanism of the injury with the physical findings. For example, in accidental falls (less than 8 feet), external signs of trauma are common, only 1% to 2% of children develop skull fractures, and few patients develop epidural hematomas.[1] In contrast, victims of abuse may have no signs of external trauma, but they have a high incidence

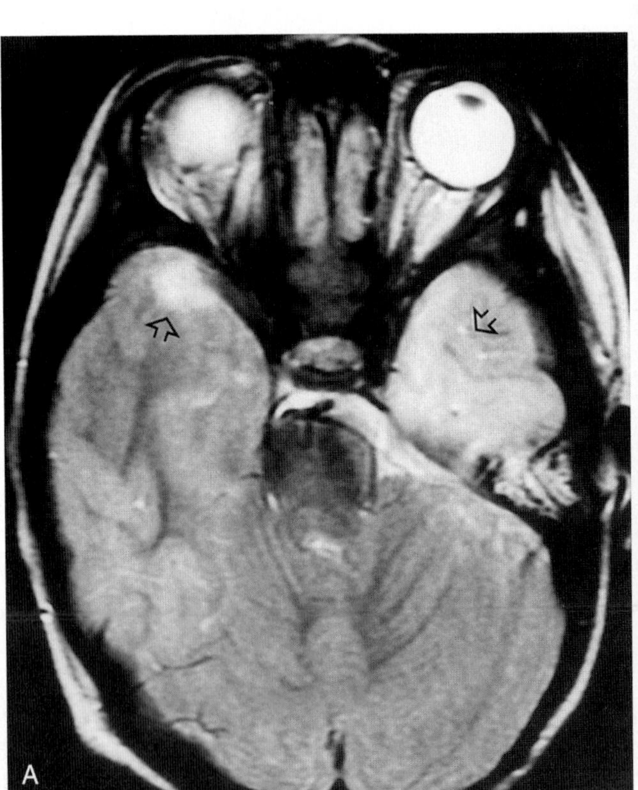

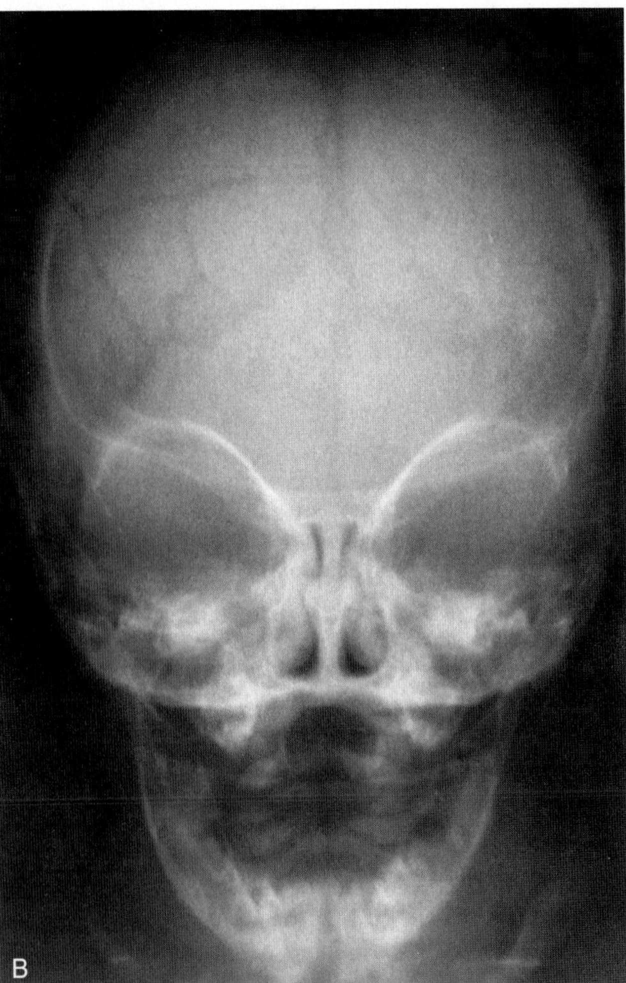

FIGURE 34–4 Abusive head trauma. **A:** Axial T2-weighted magnetic resonance image of the brain in a 20-month-old shaken-impact victim shows high signal (white) in the anterior portions of both temporal lobes *(arrows)*. **B:** Complex right posterior parietal "eggshell" fracture. (**A** and **B,** From Reece, with permission.)

Abuse-Related Head Trauma

Stephen Boos

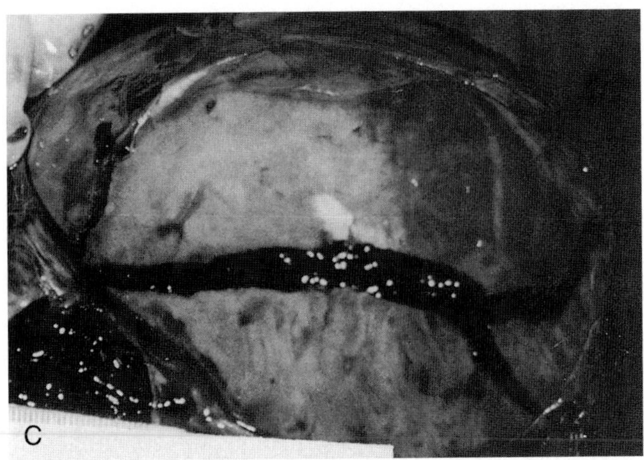

FIGURE 34–4, cont'd. Abusive head trauma. **C:** Complex skull fracture found in a child abuse victim. (From Jones, with permission.)

of subdural and subarachnoid bleeding (90% to 98%).[1] An exception is children younger than 2 years of age, who may develop skull fractures with smaller falls (approximately 3 feet).[2]

Clinical Complications

Between 7% and 30% of victims of abusive head injury die, and between 30% and 50% have significant long-term cognitive/neurologic deficits.[1]

Management

Patients with obtundation or focal neurologic deficits require an emergency computed tomographic scan and may require airway control as well as neurosurgical consultation. An evaluation for additional acute trauma (e.g., splenic laceration) and chronic trauma (e.g., long bone or rib fractures) should be initiated.

REFERENCES

1. Case ME, Graham MA, Handy TC, et al. Position paper on fatal abusive head injuries in infants and young children. *Am J Forensic Med Pathol* 2001;22:112–122.
2. Schutzman SA, Greenes DS. Pediatric minor head trauma. *Ann Emerg Med* 2001;37:65–74.

Child Abuse: Bruising

Michael Greenberg

Clinical Presentation

Bruising is probably the most common presenting complaint raising the suspicion for child abuse. The probability of abuse as indexed by bruising depends on multiple factors, including the child's age, the site of the bruises, and the pattern of the bruises.[1,2]

Pathophysiology

Bruising develops when capillaries are damaged, causing blood to leave the vascular space and enter the interstitial tissue spaces.[1] The stage of hemoglobin degradation within the interstitium determines the color of the bruise at any given time.[1,2] The apparent color of the bruise may be altered by the skin color and tone and by the lighting under which the bruise is observed.[1,2] The object used to strike the skin often creates a "negative image" of the object "surrounded by a rim of petechiae where capillaries have been stretched and torn."[1] However, injuries that are of higher impact create a "positive image" of the object due to direct vessel rupture. Common patterned bruises in abuse include those produced by hairbrushes, slap marks, belts, cords, shoes, and sticks.[1]

Bruising on the extremities is more expected in accidental incidents. Bruising of the face, ears, buttocks, thighs, abdomen, and chest are much more suspicious of abuse than accident. Physicians are often called upon to determine the age of bruises in an attempt to determine the perpetrator of abuse. The ability to visually determine the age of bruises "remains an inexact science despite recent composite charts that suggest otherwise."[2] In some cases, valid medical explanations for bruises exist. Such disorders as leukemia, thrombocytopenia, Ehlers-Danlos syndrome, and various bone marrow failure disorders may predispose patients to easy bruisability and should not be mistaken for bruising associated with child abuse.

Diagnosis

Diagnosis is based on clinical observation with special attention to the age of the child, the pattern of bruising, and the site of bruising.

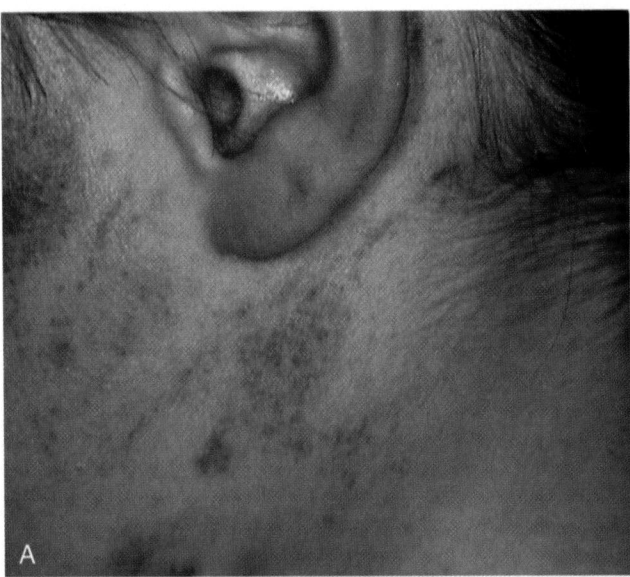

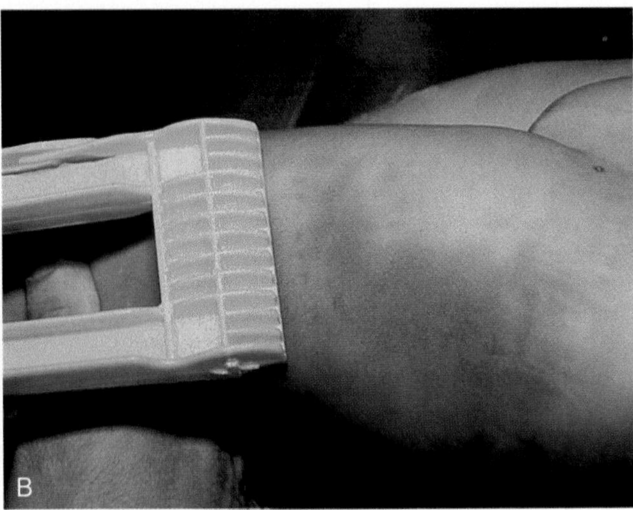

FIGURE 34–5 Child abuse: bruising. **A:** A three-year-old boy with classic hand imprint pattern injury to the face. **B:** A plastic wagon handle used to beat the child is compared with the patterned bruising of the left thigh. Note that the wagon handle was partially broken by the force of the beating. (**A** and **B,** From Reece, with permission.)

Child Abuse: Bruising

Michael Greenberg

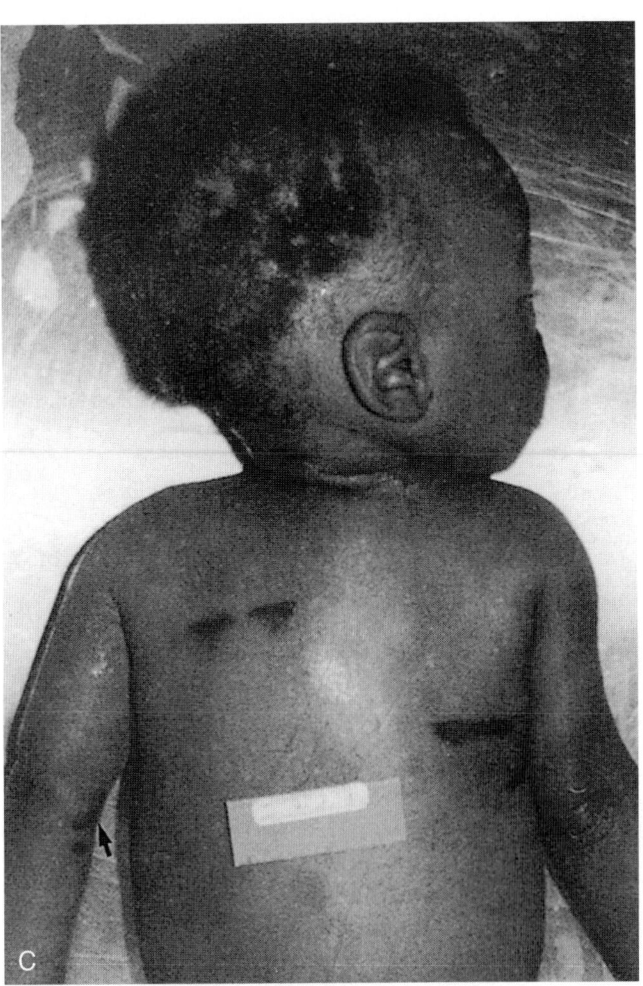

FIGURE 34–5, cont'd. Child abuse: bruising. **C:** Abrasions and bruises on the back of a victim of abuse. (From Jones, with permission.)

Clinical Complications

Complications include failure to recognize bruises indicative of abuse.

Management

Prompt attention to associated acute injuries is essential. Because the most sensitive indicator of child abuse is the care provider's index of suspicion, children must be taken into protective custody or otherwise shielded from abusers if abuse is even suspected.

REFERENCES

1. Barber MA, Sibert JR. Diagnosing physical child abuse: the way forward. *Postgrad Med J* 2000;76:743–749.
2. Schwartz AJ, Ricci LR. How accurately can bruises be aged in abused children? Literature review and synthesis. *Pediatrics* 1996; 97:254–257.

Child Abuse: Burns

Michael Greenberg

Clinical Presentation

Patients present with a history of burn injury that does not match the pattern of the burn injury.[1–3]

Pathophysiology

Approximately 10% of child abuse cases involve intentional burning.[3] Intentionally inflicted burns may be categorized as immersion burns, splash burns, flexion burns, and contact burns.[1] Certain specific burn injury patterns are characteristic (but not necessarily diagnostic) of abuse. These include deep partial- or full-thickness (formerly referred to as second- and third-degree) burns in symmetric and circumferential distribution. Other patterns that may be indicative of abuse by burning are isolated burns of the buttocks or lower extremities and burns that produce characteristic patterns (e.g., hot iron, hot plate, hot utensils).

Diagnosis

Immersion burns tend to be of equal depth, with sharp and straight lines of demarcation bordering unburned areas. In contrast, accidental immersion burns involving a foot or hand result in peripheral splash marks with poor margin demarcation. Splash burns result when hot fluid is thrown or poured on the patient.[1] These injuries do not show sharp lines of demarcation, and the differentiation between accidental and intentional splash injuries may be difficult.[1] Flexion burns result when the victim is cowering in fear and holding upper and lower extremity joints in flexion as a protective measure.[1] Contact burns are defined by the physical configuration of the hot object as it contacts the skin.[1] Other intentional burning incidents may involve hot hair dryers, microwave ovens,

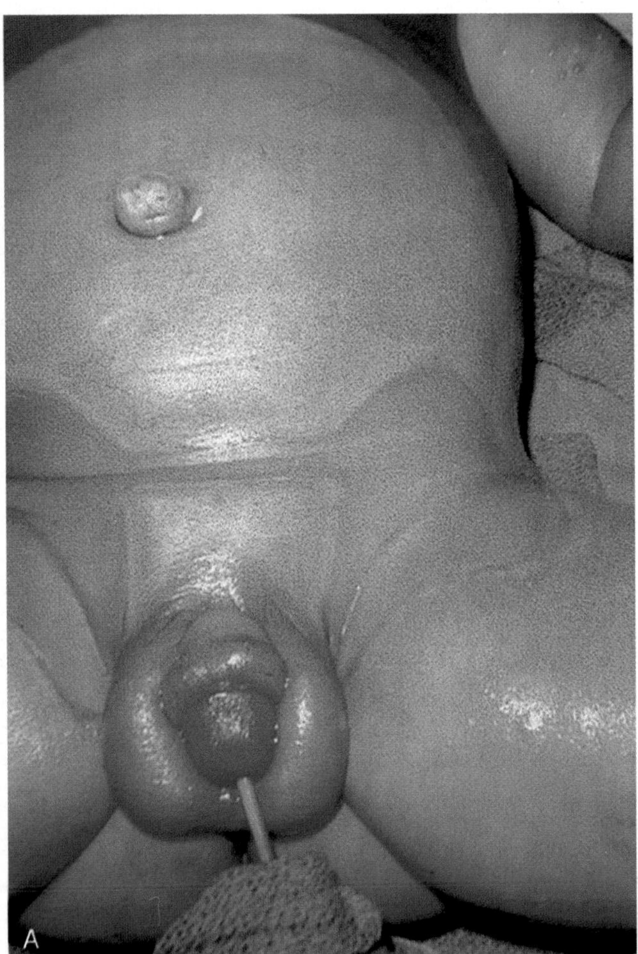

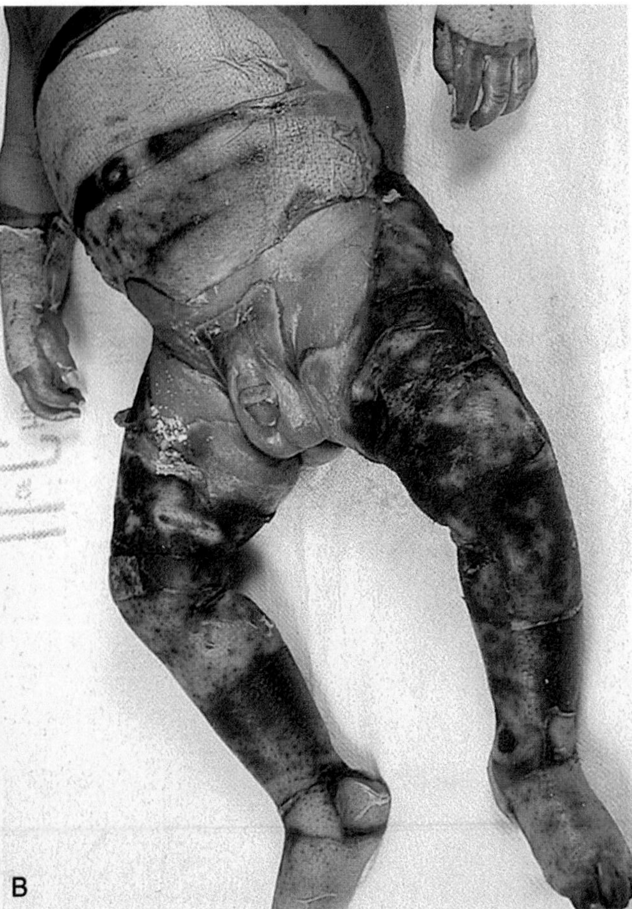

FIGURE 34–6 Child abuse: burns. **A:** Photograph taken at time of admission shows the sharp margins of the burn with sparing of the groin region. **B:** At autopsy, the appearance of the burn is much different, but the sharply demarcated burn patterns remain obvious. (**A** and **B,** From Reece, with permission.)

and various heated tools. A high index of suspicion is essential to avoid missing abuse-related burns.

Clinical Complications

Complications include infection, other concomitant abuse-related physical trauma, and the long-term psychological impact of having been abused by burning.

Management

Treatment should follow accepted burn wound protocols and is based in part on the extent and degree of the burn injuries. Immediate separation of the child from the abuser is required, and legally based protective custody proceedings should be initiated at the earliest reasonable time in the emergency department according to applicable local and state laws. It is incumbent upon emergency physicians to have knowledge of the laws that govern child abuse in the locale where they practice. Photographs of the burns may be helpful both clinically and in subsequent legal proceedings and should be taken at the earliest appropriate time.

REFERENCES

1. Peck MD, Priolo-Kapel D. Child abuse by burning: a review of the literature and an algorithm for medical investigations. *J Trauma* 2002;53:1013–1022.
2. Mukadam S, Gilles EE. Unusual inflicted hot oil burns in a 7-year-old. *Burns* 2003;29:83–86.
3. Feldman KW, Schaller RT, Feldman JA, McMillon M. Tap water scald burns in children 1997. *Injury Prev* 1998;4:238–242.

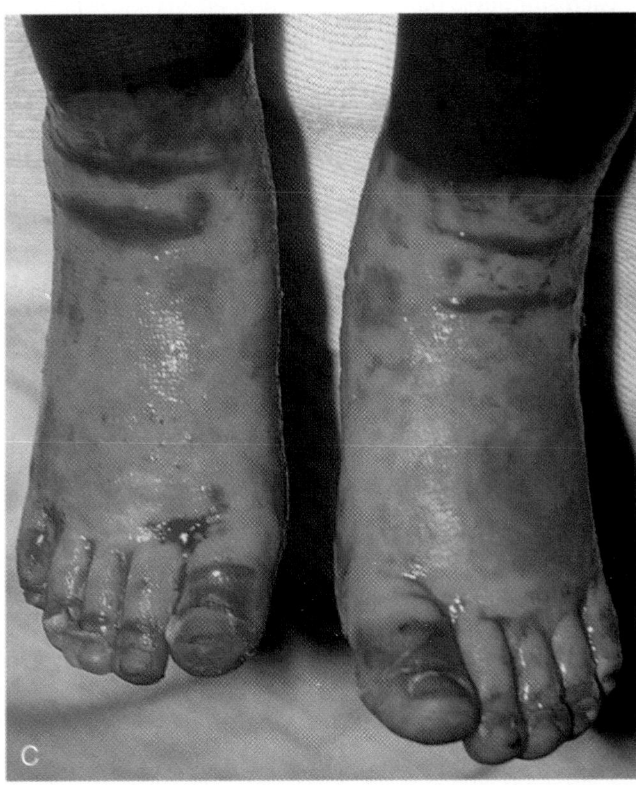

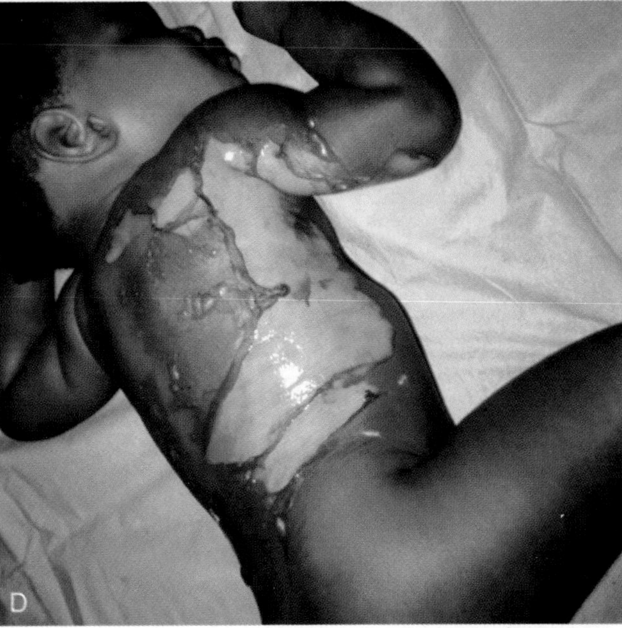

FIGURE 34–6, cont'd. Child abuse: burns. **C:** Immersion burn of the extremities. (From Reece, with permission.) **D:** Abusive thermal burn of the back. (Courtesy of David Wagner, MD.)

Abuse: Bite Marks

Angelo P. Giardino

Clinical Presentation

Human bite marks may be oval, arched, or rounded. The pattern depends on where the bite is and whether one or both dental arches leave a mark. The typical size of an adult dental arch (measured canine to canine) is approximately 2.5 to 4 cm. There may be an area of central ecchymosis if the blood vessels of the victim's skin become trapped between the jaws of the biting individual and a suction force is created. Animal bites from cats and dogs tend to puncture the skin; the cross-sectional size of the teeth tends to be smaller, the teeth marks tend to be circular, and the number of incisors may be greater than with human bite marks.

Aging of bite marks is far from an exact science. Those that do not break the skin may act similar to either a superficial or a deep bruise, and last from minutes to days or weeks. Those that break the skin can be expected to be visible for several days to weeks, depending on the depth of the injury, the care the bite receives, and any complications that occur.[1–3]

Pathophysiology

Human bites involve a complex injury pattern that combines crushing pressure, cutting, and dragging of teeth across the skin surface.

Diagnosis

Recognition, thorough evaluation, and accurate documentation are essential. Before the bite mark is cleansed, samples may be taken using sterile cotton swabs moistened with sterile saline to preserve forensic evidence. Control swabs should be taken from nonbitten areas; each sample should be allowed to air dry and should be submitted separately. Photographs should be taken from many different angles, with a reference scale included in the photographic field. If a forensic odontologist is available, impressions may be made of the wound.[1–3]

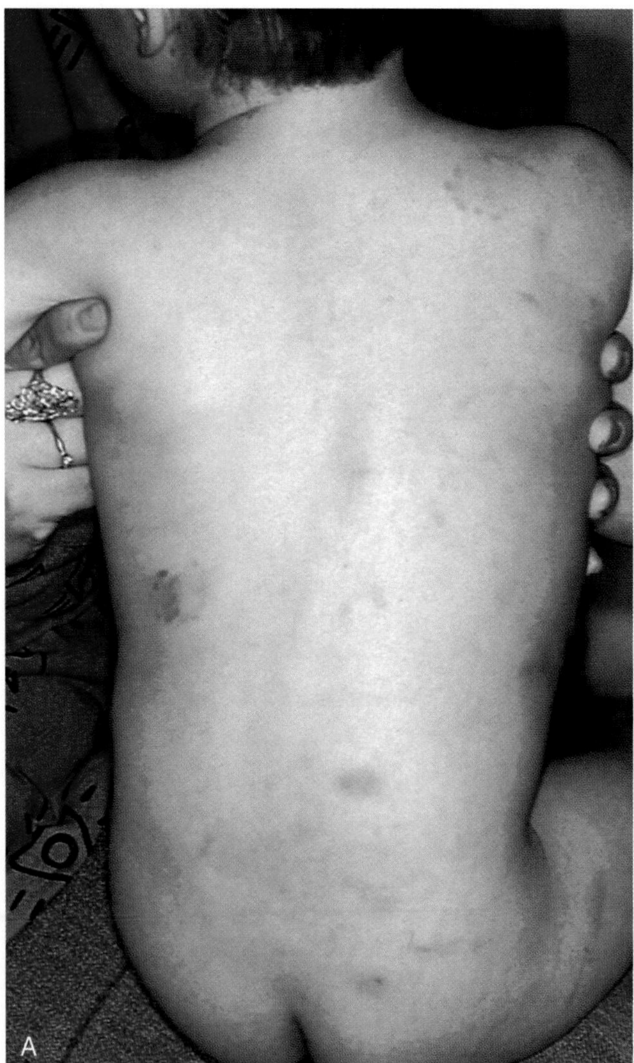

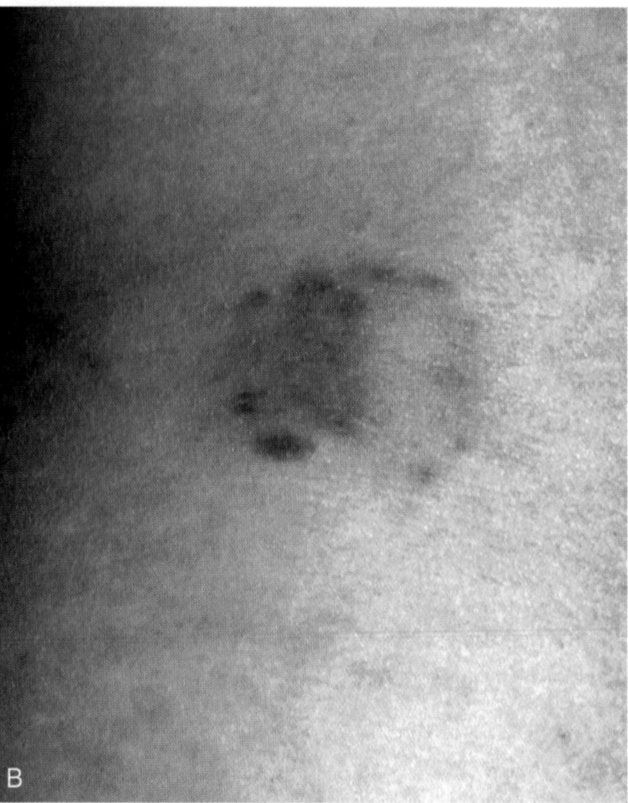

FIGURE 34–7 Child abuse: bite marks. **A:** Full back view demonstrates two bites (right shoulder and left flank) in relation to neighboring anatomy. **B:** Close-up view of the flank bite demonstrates detail of teeth imprint. Size of teeth and arch suggest that the bite came from another child. (**A** and **B,** From Reece, with permission.)

Abuse: Bite Marks

Angelo P. Giardino

Clinical Complications

Complications include infection, underlying associated injuries, and psychological damage.

Management

The wound needs to be adequately evaluated, forensic evidence collected, and photographs taken. The extent of the injury should be determined, the wound cleansed, and appropriate antibiotic therapy considered. If extensive tissue damage is present, consultation with a general or plastic surgeon may be necessary. Reporting of the suspected child abuse is mandatory.[1–3]

REFERENCES

1. Guidelines for bite mark analysis. American Board of Forensic Odontology, Inc. *J Am Dent Assoc* 1986;112:383–386.
2. Baker MD, Moore SE. Human bites in children: a six-year experience. *Am J Dis Child* 1987;141:1285–1290.
3. Barsley RE. Forensic and legal issue oral diagnosis. *Dent Clin North Am* 1993;37133–156.

Child Abuse: Abdominal Injuries

Michael Greenberg

Clinical Presentation

Patients with abusive abdominal injuries may present with a wide variety of signs and symptoms that generally are not specific indicators for child abuse. An elevated index of suspicion is the most important factor to accurately determine child abuse of any sort.[1–4]

Pathophysiology

Abdominal injuries are uncommonly associated with child abuse. However, if abdominal injury occurs as part of child abuse, mortality is a serious risk. One study reported a mortality rate of 45% when blunt abdominal trauma was inflicted in the setting of child abuse.[2] The clinical aspects of abdominal trauma that differentiate abuse-related injuries from accidental injuries have not been completely defined. Some reports indicate that the liver is the most commonly injured intraabdominal organ in abuse.[3] Others have reported that small-bowel injury may be more common in abuse as opposed to unintentional accidents.[1] A common excuse for injury offered by parents is that the child "fell on stairs." However, recent work has demonstrated that there is "no evidence to support the contention that an unobstructed fall on stairs could be consistent with perforation of the small intestine."[4]

Diagnosis

Abuse must be considered in any case of pediatric abdominal injuries without a clear or logical explanation. Abdominal bruising in children may be a clue to abdominal injury related to abuse.

Clinical Complications

Complications include failure to recognize injuries indicative of abuse.

Management

Prompt attention to associated acute injuries is essential. Because the most sensitive indicator of child abuse is the care provider's index of suspicion, children must be taken into protective custody or otherwise shielded from abusers if abuse is even suspected.

REFERENCES

1. Barber MA, Sibert JR. Diagnosing physical child abuse: the way forward. *Postgrad Med J* 2000;76:743–749.
2. Cooper A, Floyd T, Barlow B, et al. Major blunt abdominal trauma due to child abuse. *J Trauma* 1988;28:1483–1487.
3. DiGiacomo JC, Frankel H, Haskell RM, et al. Unsuspected child abuse revealed by delayed presentation of periportal tracking and myoglobinuria. *J Trauma* 2000;49:348–350.
4. Huntimer CM, Muret-Wagstaff S, Leland NL. Can falls on stairs result in small intestine perforations? *Pediatrics* 2000;106:301–305.

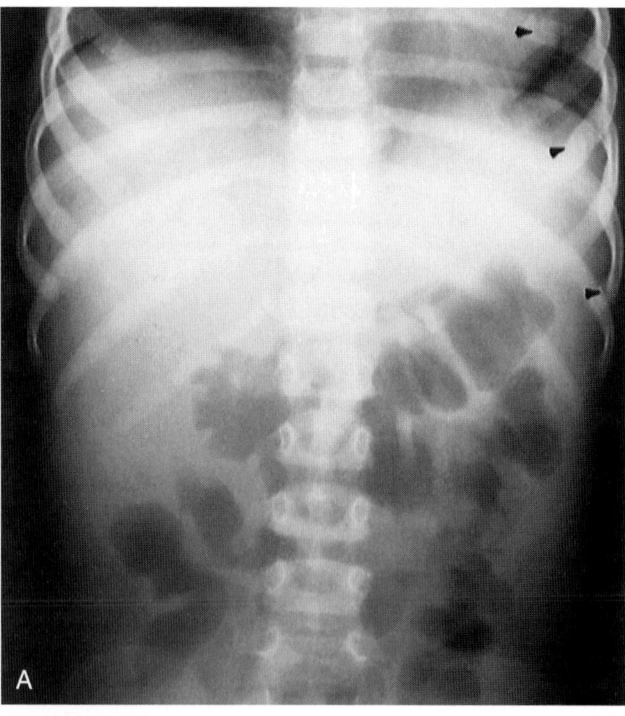

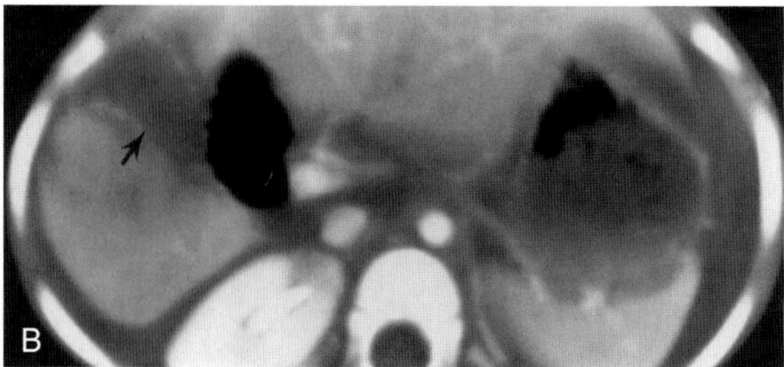

FIGURE 34–8 Child abuse: abdominal injuries. **A:** Abdominal radiograph shows peritoneal fluid with bowel loops "floating" in the midabdomen, as well as multiple rib fractures *(arrows)*. **B:** Computed tomographic scan shows a liver laceration *(arrow)* with a large hemoperitoneum. (**A** and **B,** From Reece, with permission.)

Child Abuse: Abdominal Injuries

Michael Greenberg

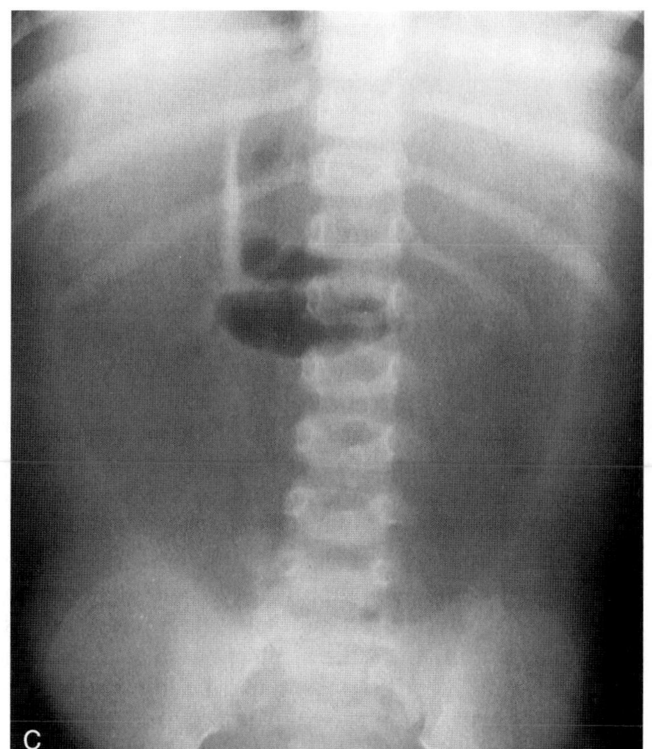

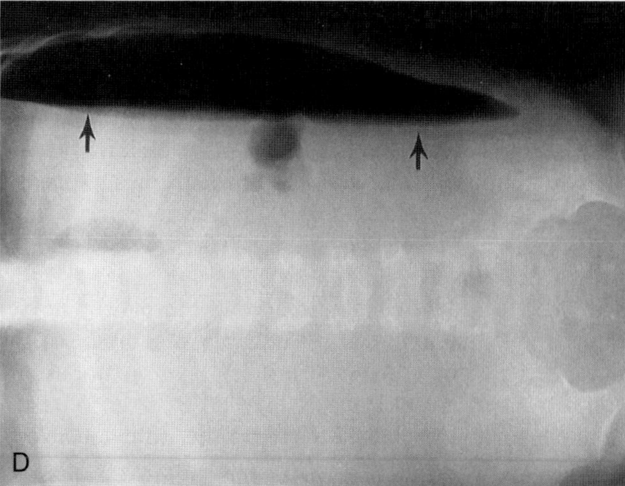

FIGURE 34–8, cont'd. Child abuse: abdominal injuries. **C:** Abdominal radiograph reveals massive pneumoperitoneum. **D:** A lateral decubitus view shows an air–fluid level *(arrows)* with free peritoneal fluid. (**C** and **D,** From Reece, with permission.)

Child Abuse: Sexual Abuse

Michael Greenberg

Clinical Presentation

Children who have been sexually abused may present after violent assaults, kidnappings, or similar crimes. Others may be brought to the emergency department by parents, relatives, or friends because of suspicion of possible sexual abuse. Older children may, at times, present unaccompanied by adults.[1–3]

Pathophysiology

Up to 12% of adolescent girls and 4% to 5% of boys have been victims of sexual assault.[1,3] Sexual abuse may reflect a single acute event or a long-standing situation of abuse. A variety of injuries may be inflicted during sexual abuse, and these injuries may reflect the nature of the abuse.

Diagnosis

A high index of suspicion for sexual abuse of any child must be maintained. However, special care must be exercised to avoid mistaking various nonabuse injury patterns for abuse. Similarly, physicians must be vigilant to avoid missing the diagnosis of child sexual abuse. Specifically, physicians must never accept illogical explanations for suspicious injuries, illnesses, or social situations. The maintenance of a high index of suspicion is essential to diagnosing sexual child abuse.

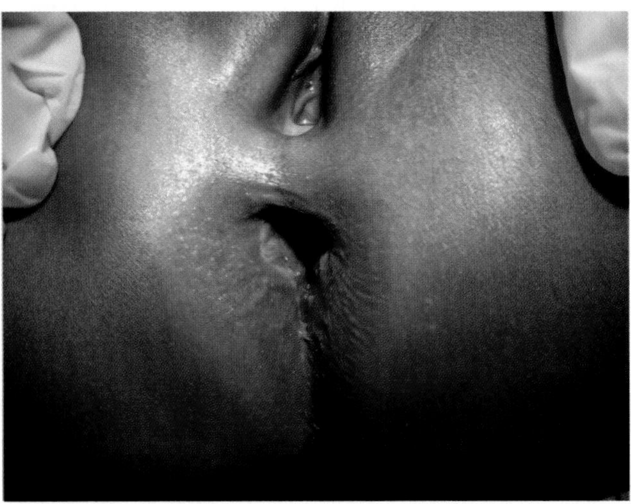

FIGURE 34–9 Child abuse: sexual abuse. Relaxation of the rectal sphincter and gaping of the anus may occur after death. Evidence of abuse includes perianal scarring and lacerations. (Courtesy of Mark Silverberg, MD.)

Clinical Complications

Complications include various traumatic injuries, sexually transmitted diseases, unwanted pregnancy, and long-term, severe psychological effects.

Management

Written protocols should be in place addressing the means and modalities for assessment of the sexually abused child, as well as the procedures for incorporating social and law enforcement officials into the process of evaluation and treatment of these children. This may require specialized teams that include pediatric gynecologists, social workers, rape counselors, and others. Attention to the immediate medical needs of the patient is paramount. Identification of specific injuries, screening for sexually transmitted diseases, and pregnancy screening are essential. Protocols should be in place to provide guidance with regard to the administration of contraception to rape victims. Special techniques may be needed to assess the sexually abused child, including colposcopy to identify genital and perianal abnormalities and Wood's lamp illumination to identify seminal fluid on the skin.

REFERENCES

1. Fleming J. Childhood sexual abuse: an update. *Curr Opin Obstet Gynecol* 1998;10:383–386.
2. Atabaki S, Paradise JE. The medical evaluation of the sexually abused child: lessons from a decade of research. *Pediatrics* 1999; 104:178–186.
3. Santucci KA, Hsiao AL. Advances in clinical forensic medicine. *Curr Opin Pediatr* 2003;15:304–308.

Conditions That Mimic Sexual Abuse

Lori D. Frasier

Presentation of a child to the emergency department (ED) with anogenital complaints must always raise concerns of possible sexual abuse. There are many conditions that affect the genital area that are frequently confused with sequelae of abuse. These conditions typically mimic trauma or sexually transmitted diseases. However, on careful evaluation by experienced clinicians, an alternative explanation exists.[1,2]

Clinical Presentation

Perhaps the most frequent "mimic" of sexual abuse diagnosed in the ED is the misinterpretation of normal examination findings.[1] These findings include hymenal notches, partial clefts, and asymmetry, as well as the size of the hymenal orifice. Physicians without specialized training in the evaluation of child sexual abuse have difficulty recognizing normal anatomy in the prepubertal child. Also, more than 90% of prepubertal girls who allege vaginal penetration have a normal examination when seen in a sexual-abuse referral clinic. Anal findings are even more rare, with more than 98% of children who present with a history of anal penetration having normal findings.[1,2]

Diagnosis

Most suspicious conditions fall into the following categories: those resembling sexual trauma, those resembling sexually transmitted diseases, and minor congenital malformations. The conditions that are most commonly confused with the sequelae of sexual abuse are listed in Table 34–10.[1,2]

Clinical Complications

Accurate diagnosis of trauma related to sexual abuse is critically important in the protection of children. However, overdiagnosis of abuse due to failure to recognize alternative conditions may result in false allegations and unnecessary trauma to the family and the child.[1,2]

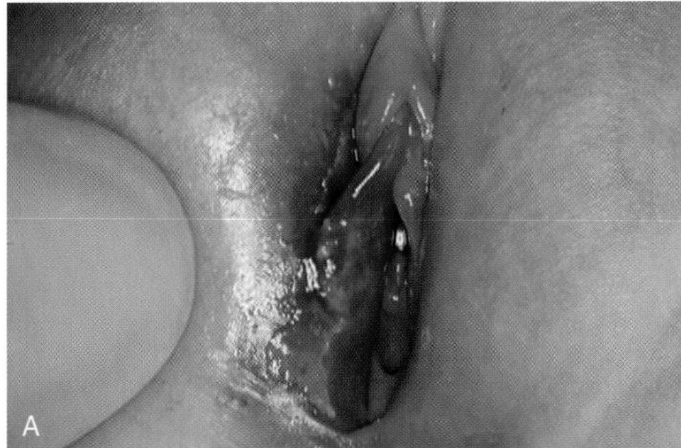

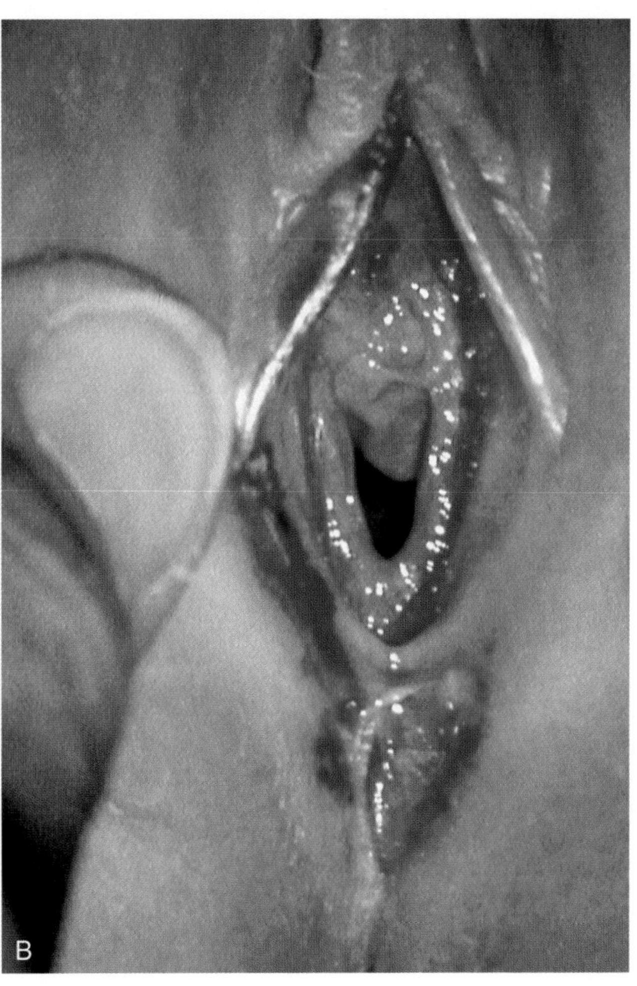

FIGURE 34–10 Conditions that mimic sexual abuse. **A:** A 6-year-old girl with an acute crush injury to the labia minora and majora after falling on a metal bar of a jungle gym. Note that the injury does not involve the hymenal membrane recessed in the vaginal canal. **B:** Lichen sclerosus in an 8-year-old girl evaluated for sexual abuse after she had vaginal bleeding on returning from a 2-week visit with her divorced father. The subepidermal hemorrhages are characteristic. (**A** and **B,** From Reece, with permission.)

Conditions That Mimic Sexual Abuse

Lori D. Frasier

Management

In the absence of obvious trauma, the ED physician should defer the determination of whether a nonacute finding is the result of sexual abuse to a specialized sexual abuse evaluation program.

REFERENCES

1. Bays J, Jenny C. Genital and anal conditions confused with child sexual abuse trauma. *Am J Dis Child* 1990;144:1319–1322.
2. Siegfried EC, Frasier LD. Anogenital skin diseases of childhood. *Pediatr Ann* 1997;26:321–331.

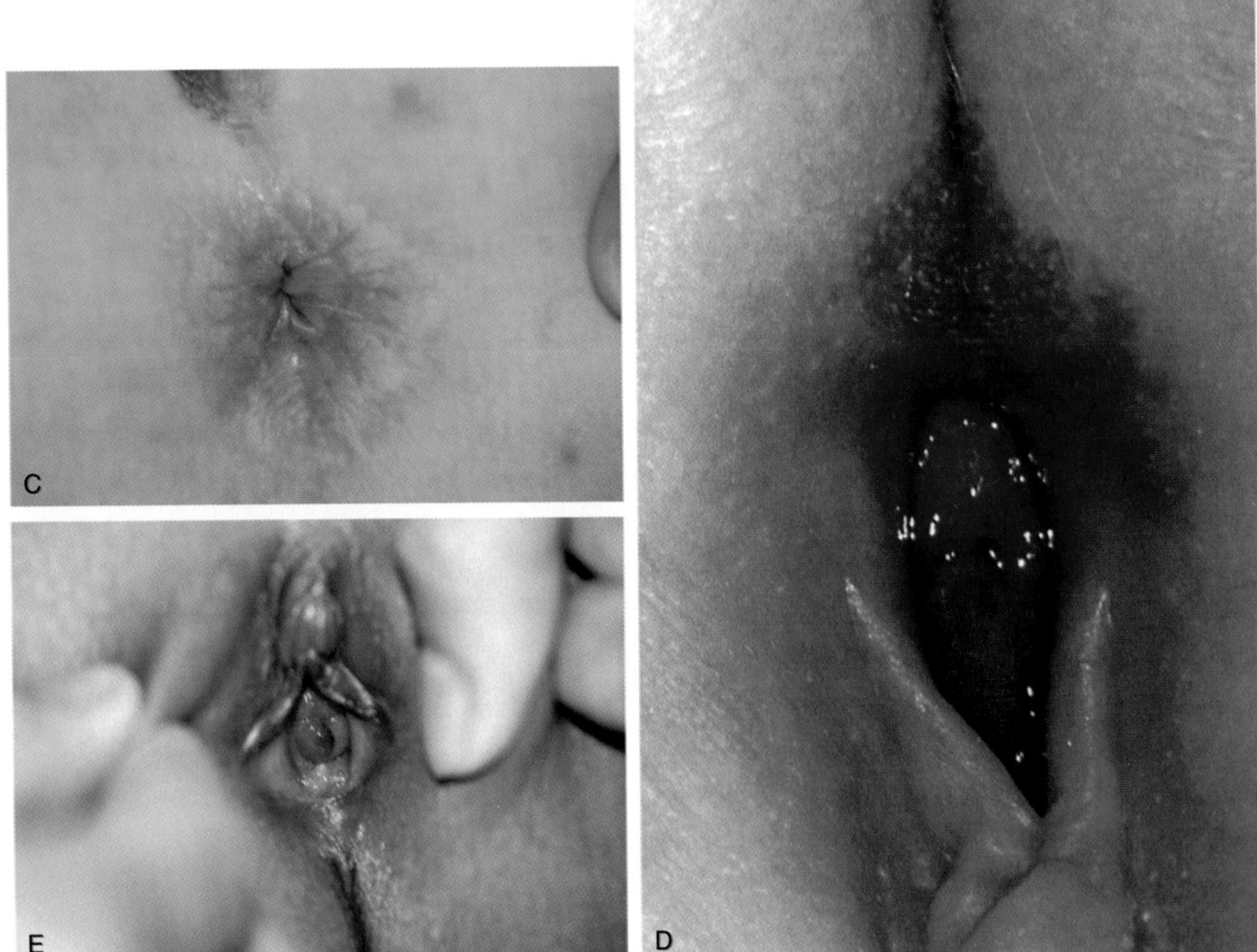

FIGURE 34–10, cont'd. Conditions that mimic sexual abuse. **C:** Lichen sclerosus with hypopigmentation and fissuring of the perianal area. **D:** Hemangioma of the posterior fourchette and perineal body, mistaken for trauma due to abuse. The lesion blanched with pressure. **E:** Urethral caruncle or partial urethral prolapse in a 3-year-old African-American girl, which caused bleeding and concerns about sexual abuse. (**C–E,** From Reece, with permission.)

Conditions That Mimic Sexual Abuse

Lori D. Frasier

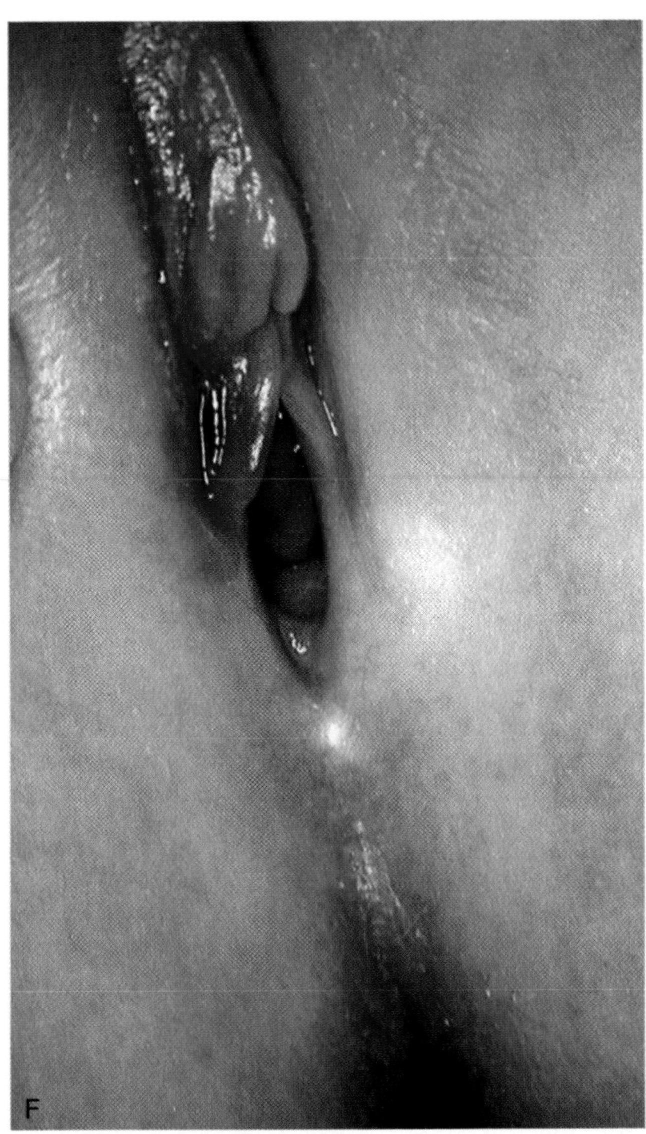

FIGURE 34–10, cont'd. Conditions that mimic sexual abuse. **F:** Straddle injury to the right labium. The hymen was undamaged. (From Reece, with permission.)

TABLE 34–10 Conditions Most Commonly Confused with Sequelae of Sexual Abuse

Conditions resembling sexual trauma

- Lichen sclerosis et atrophicus
- Vaginal bleeding: hematuria, precocious puberty, vaginal tumors, ovarian tumors, infections, withdrawal bleeding (newborn), extravaginal source (irritation of mucosa or skin)
- Urethral prolapse
- Straddle injuries (accidental) involving genitals or anal area
- Henoch-Schönlein purpura (primary genital presentation)
- Disorders of clotting or coagulation with primary genital presentation
- Vascular malformations, hemangiomas with isolated anogenital presentation
- Prominent hemorrhoidal veins in the perianal area resembling bruising
- Perianal group A streptococcal dermatitis
- Rectal fissures
- Rectal bleeding from primary gastrointestinal source
- Erythema from irritant contacts (e.g., poor hygiene, bubble baths, perfumed soaps, lotions, nickel)

Conditions resembling sexually transmitted diseases *(usually manifested as vaginal discharge)*

- Group A streptococcal vaginitis or perianal dermatitis (may also appear as perianal trauma with bleeding)
- Nonvenereal bacterial infections: *Haemophilus influenzae, Staphylococcus, Pneumococcus, Neisseria meningitidis, Shigella* species
- Nonvenereal viral infections: molluscum contagiosum
- Other: vaginal foreign body (serosanguineous discharge)

Congenital anogenital abnormalities

- Failure of midline fusion
- Rectus diastasis (external rectal sphincter)
- Hymenal abnormalities (septate, cribriform, imperforate)

Normal Prepubertal and Pubertal Anatomic Variants in the Female External Genital Anatomy

Angelo P. Giardino

The external genital structures in the female are referred to as the vulva and consist of the following: mons pubis, labia majora, labia minora, clitoris, urethral meatus, hymen, fossa navicularis (concave area between posterior attachment of the hymen and posterior fourchette), and posterior fourchette (area where labia minora join posteriorly). Normal variations in these structures occur congenitally, and their appearance changes under the influence of estrogen. The shape, size, and contour of the hymenal opening is an area of particular clinical interest because of its relevance to inflicted trauma and sexual abuse.[1–3]

Clinical Presentation

Huffman described four stages of estrogen effects on the appearance of the female external genitalia. Stage 1 (postneonatal regression, approximately 0 to 2 months) shows evidence of profound estrogen effect (thickened, pink, lubricated mucous membranes) secondary to the presence of maternal hormones. Stage 2 (early childhood, approximately 2 months to 7 years) shows a typical immature appearance because of a relative paucity of endogenous estrogen (thin, red, translucent membranes with lacy vascular pattern visible). Stage 3 (late childhood, beginning sometime after age 7 years) shows the steadily increasing effects of endogenous estrogen (thickening, pinkish, opaque mucous membranes). Stage 4 (premenarche, seen at the onset of pubertal development) shows evidence of estrogen effect (thickened, pink, lubricated mucous membranes).[1–3]

An opening in the hymenal membrane is expected. An imperforate hymen that describes no opening would be abnormal and would require further evaluation.

The shape of the hymenal orifice may vary. The most common shapes are annular (40% to 50% of girls), in which a circular opening is surrounded by hymenal tissue; crescentic (30% to 40%), in which a half-moon opening has the majority of the tissue between the

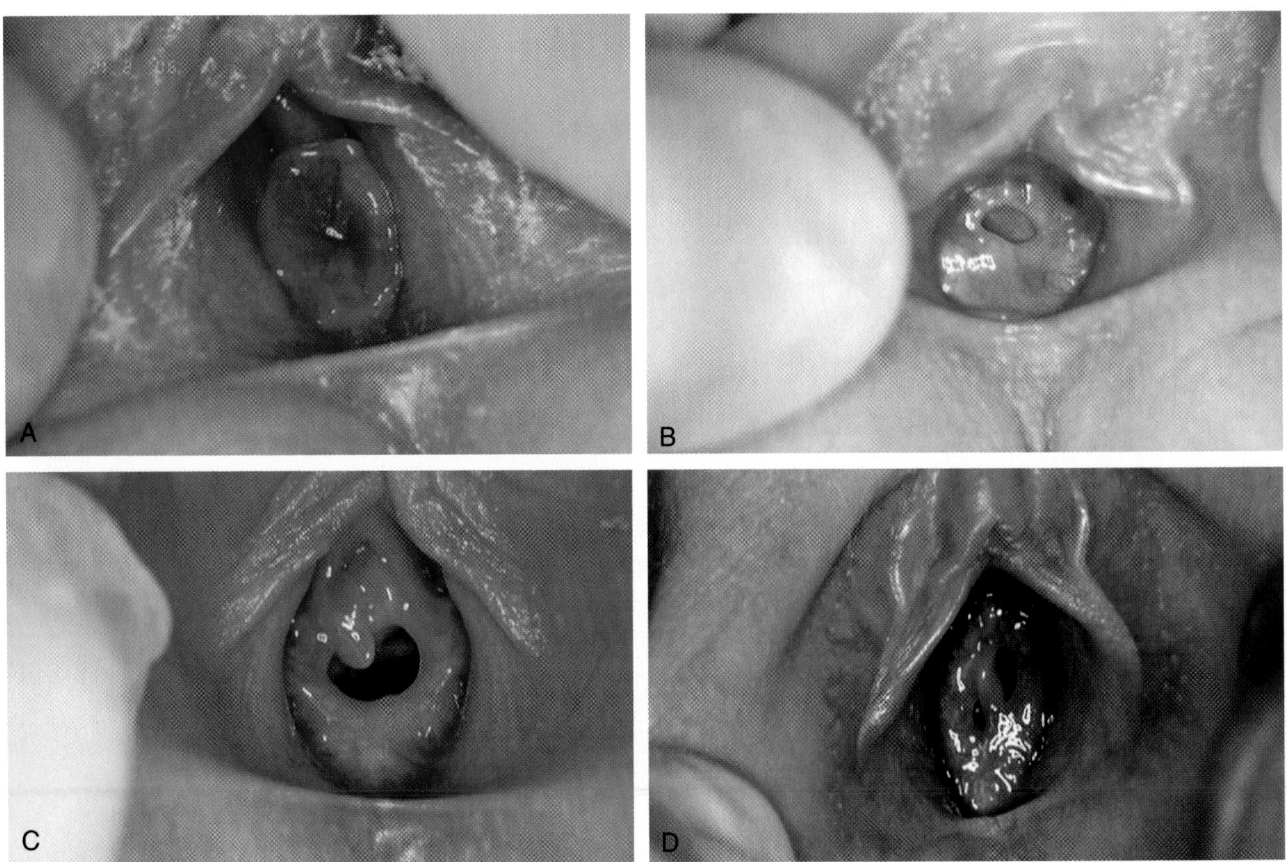

FIGURE 34–11 Normal prepubertal and pubertal anatomic variants in the female external genital anatomy. **A:** This 15-month-old girl has a flared configuration of the annular orifice. Note thickened normal variation of the membrane. **B:** A girl aged 2 years 3 months has a superior and eccentrically oriented annular orifice. The external surface of the membrane is translucent. **C:** A girl aged 9 years 8 months has a prominent hymenal membrane projection of tissue at the 11 o'clock position, with a small bump at the 5 o'clock position that may have been previously attached, forming a septum. **D:** A girl aged 5 years 7 months has a septum of the hymen, resulting in two orifices. (**A–D,** From Reece, with permission.)

Normal Prepubertal and Pubertal Anatomic Variants in the Female External Genital Anatomy

Angelo P. Giardino

2 o'clock and 10 o'clock positions; fimbriated (10% to 20%), in which the hymenal tissue bunches up around the opening, with multiple folds visible; septate (less than 5% of girls) in which a band of tissue bisects the opening; and cribriform (less than 1% of girls), in which multiple bands of tissue create several smaller openings in the orifice.[1–3]

The size of the hymenal orifice is quite variable and may vary even during a given physical examination, based on the child's age, positioning, comfort, and relaxation during the examination, as well as examiner technique and method used for measurement. Experts have urged caution with regard to use of hymenal orifice size in sexual abuse evaluations.

The contour of the hymen may also vary from the expected smooth edge. Outgrowths or prominences, called bumps, are seen in almost half of girls who have not been abused. Notches or superficial areas of decreased tissue or irregularity are seen much less frequently than bumps and may be found in approximately 5% of nonabused girls; the incidence of hymenal tags on examination is similar.

Diagnosis

The differentiation of normal and abnormal external genital appearance is particularly important in the context of the suspected sexual abuse examination. Adams developed a two-part classification system that assesses genital and anal findings on examination and also provides an overall assessment.[2] In Part One, the Adams comprehensive classification categorizes genital and anal findings into one of four categories: (1) normal/not related to abuse; (2) nonspecific for abuse; (3) concerning for abuse; and (4) clear evidence for abuse. In Part Two, the overall assessment draws on information beyond the physical examination and considers history and laboratory findings, categorizing the overall assessment into one of four categorizes: (1) no evidence; (2) possible abuse; (3) probable; and (4) definite evidence.

Management

A growing body of literature confirms the reality of variation in the appearance of the external genitalia of both prepubertal and pubertal girls. These variations are most prominent with regard to the shape, size, and contour of the hymenal orifice. The majority of children who have been sexually abused present with no genital abnormality, so understanding of the range of normal vulvar findings remains essential.

REFERENCES

1. Adams JA, Harper K, Knudson S, Revilla J. Examination findings in legally confirmed child sexual abuse: it's normal to be normal. *Pediatrics* 1994;94:310–317.
2. Adams JA. Evolution of a classification scale: medical evaluation of suspected child sexual abuse. *Child Maltreat* 2001;6:31–36.
3. Atabaki S, Paradise JE. The medical evaluation of the sexually abused child: lessons from a decade of research. *Pediatrics* 1999; 104:178–186.

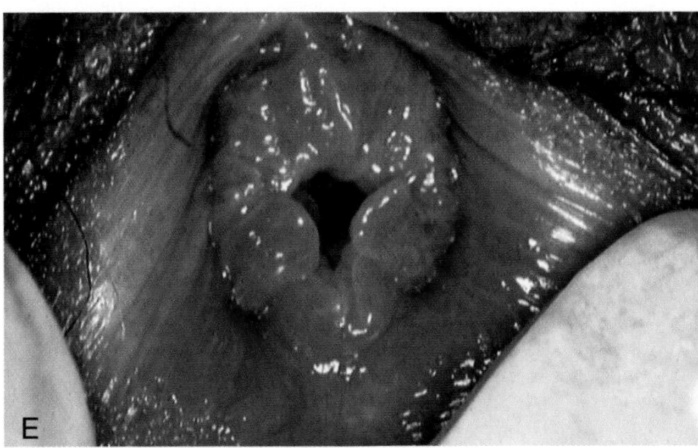

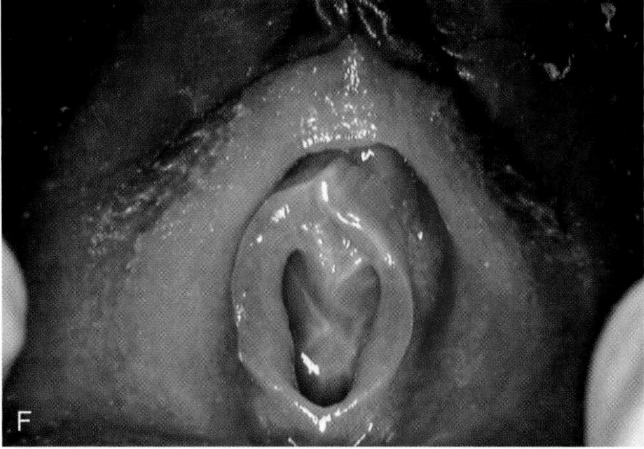

FIGURE 34–11, cont'd. Normal prepubertal and pubertal anatomic variants in the female external genital anatomy. **E:** A 12-year-old girl with Tanner stage III anatomy. Multiple congenital clefts circumferentially lead to a fimbriated or "frilly" appearance of hymen. Note that the clefts do not extend to the vaginal wall. **F:** A girl aged 11 years 4 months with Tanner stage III anatomy. Note that the annular orifice has a flared appearance but there are no interruptions in the edge circumferentially. (**E** and **F,** From Reece, with permission.)

Domestic Abuse

Michael Greenberg

Clinical Presentation

The various potential clinical presentations of domestic abuse (DA) are reflected by the following definition of DA: "a pattern of coercive control consisting of physical, sexual, and/or psychological assault against former or current intimate partners."[1] Specific presentations may be reflected by the following definition: "physical violence varying in severity and including pushing, shoving, punching, kicking, restraining, tying down, assaulting with a weapon, refusing to help during injury or illness, and placing a family member in a dangerous situation."[2]

Pathophysiology

DA is a critical public health issue. As many as 2 million women are injured by domestic partners each year, and up to 50% of homicides committed against women are perpetrated by their current or previous domestic partners. The vast majority of DA incidents involve men harming women. As many as 30% of all emergency department visits may result from DA, and substantial numbers of patients admitted to trauma services have been identified as victims of DA. DA is noted to be frequently unrecognized and often underreported by health care providers.[3,4]

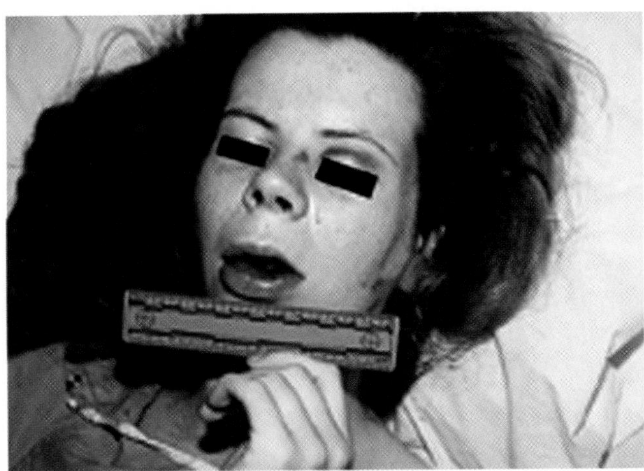

FIGURE 34–12 Domestic abuse. A victim of intimate partner abuse exhibits swelling and contusion of the left side of the nose and the upper and lower lips, with lip lacerations, caused by multiple blows with a closed fist. (From Olshaker, with permission.)

Diagnosis

The diagnosis of DA requires a high index of suspicion as well as a patterned practice of inquiry regarding DA. Specifically, all patients in whom DA is suspected should be asked if they have been struck or hurt by anyone in the past year. Also, they should be asked if they "feel safe" in their current relationship. Finally, they should be asked if there is any one from a prior relationship who is making them feel unsafe at the present time. An affirmative answer to any of these queries requires intervention.

Clinical Complications

DA may result in disabling injuries, acute and chronic psychological damage and impairment, or death.[1–4]

Management

The first priority is a complete history and physical examination and treatment of any injuries. The primary intervention for DA involves removal of the victim from the environment in which the DA is occurring to a safe environment.

REFERENCES

1. Eisenstat SA, Bancroft L. Domestic violence. *N Engl J Med* 1999;341:886–892.
2. Heinzer MM, Krimm JR. Barriers to screening for domestic violence in an emergency department. *Holistic Nurs Pract* 2002;16:24–33.
3. Davis JW, Parks SN, Kaups KL, et al. Victims of domestic violence on the trauma service: unrecognized and underreported. *J Trauma* 2003;54:352-355.
4. Melnick DM, Maio RF, Blow FC, et al. Prevalence of domestic violence and associated factors among women on a trauma service. *J Trauma* 2002;53:33–37.

Elder Abuse and Neglect

Michael Greenberg

Clinical Presentation

Elder abuse and neglect (EAN) can take various forms, and no single presenting scenario is applicable to all situations. However, EAN commonly takes the form of one or more of the following: withholding food, water, or other necessities; physical abuse; psychological or emotional abuse; sexual abuse; withholding essential medical or dental services; financial abuse; self-neglect; or other violations of civil rights.[1–3]

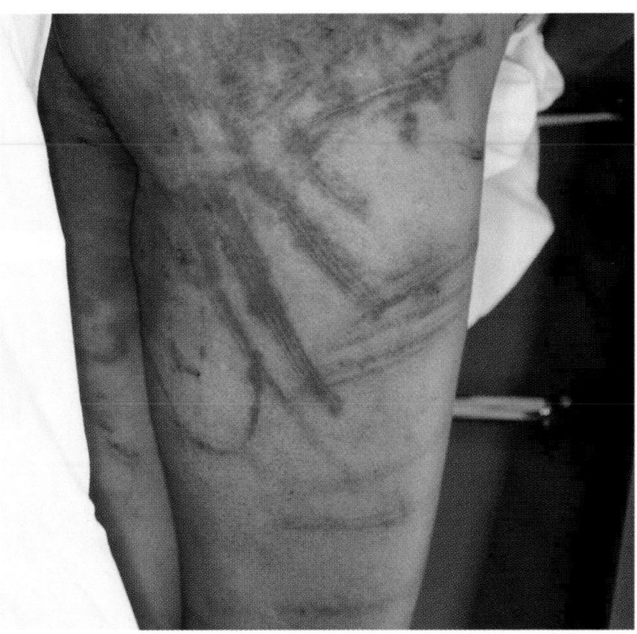

FIGURE 34–13 Elder abuse and neglect. Multiple bruises. (Courtesy of Michael Greenberg, MD.)

TABLE 34–13 **Screening Questions for Elder Abuse**

Has anyone at home ever hurt you?
Has anyone ever touched you without your consent?
Has anyone ever made you do things you didn't want to do?
Has anyone taken anything that was yours without asking?
Has anyone ever scolded or threatened you?
Have you ever signed any documents that you didn't understand?
Are you afraid of anyone at home?
Are you alone a lot?
Has anyone ever failed to help you take care of yourself when you needed help?

From the American Medical Association. Diagnostic and Treatment Guidelines on Elder Abuse and Neglect. www.ama-assn.org/amal/pub/upload/mm/386/elderabuse.pdf

Pathophysiology

Self-neglect constitutes the majority of all EAN situations. Risk factors for self-neglect include alcoholism, drug abuse, dementia, living alone, depression, bereavement, poverty, physical impairments, and psychiatric disorders.[1–3]

Diagnosis

Physical abuse may be uncovered on physical examination. Findings consistent with EAN include bruising, skin tears, trauma, degraded personal hygiene, malnutrition, dehydration, pressure ulcers, contractures, lice, scabies, and patients who seem fearful of examination. Self-neglect may be diagnosed by identification of the noted risk factors.[1–3]

Clinical Complications

Complications include untreated injuries, untreated or undertreated medical conditions, worsening of mental problems, localized and systemic infections, and premature death.

Management

Untreated or undertreated medical conditions must be attended to promptly. In most jurisdictions, EAN is reportable to social and law enforcement authorities. Failure to report could have negative consequences for the patient as well as substantial negative legal consequences for the care provider.

REFERENCES

1. Harrell R, Toronjo C, McLaughlin J, et al. How geriatricians identify elder abuse and neglect. *Am J Med Sci* 2002;323:34–38.
2. Levine J. Elder neglect and abuse: a primer for primary care physicians. *Geriatrics* 2003;58:37–44.
3. Shugarman L, Fries B, Wolf R, et al. Identifying older people at risk of abuse during routine screening practices. *J Am Geriatric Soc* 2003;51:24–31.

FIGURE CREDITS

FIG. 23-3 from American College of Radiology teaching collection.

FIGS. 10-25A, 16-19, 20-31B, 21-2B, 21-4B, 21-6B, 21-9, and **24-55** from Anderson SC, Poulsen KB. Anderson's Atlas of Hematology. Philadelphia: Lippincott Williams & Wilkins, 2003.

FIG. 30-11B from Armed Forces Institute of Pathology, Washington, D.C.

FIG. 30-16 from Arnon SS, Schechter R, Ingelsby TV et al. Working Group on Civilian Biodefense. Botulinum toxin as a biological weapon: medical and public health management. JAMA 2001;285:1059–1070. Copyright © 2001 American Medical Association. All rights reserved.

FIGS. 25-32A&B from Auerbach PS, ed. Wilderness Medicine: Management of Wilderness and Environmental Emergencies, Third Edition. St. Louis: Mosby-Year Book, Inc., 1995.

FIG. 16-26 from Avery GB, Fletcher MA, MacDonald MG. Neonatology: Pathophysiology and Management of the Newborn, 5th Ed. Philadelphia: Lippincott Williams & Wilkins, 1999:1326.

FIGS. 17-7, 19-15, 31-2B from Bailey BJ, Karen H. Calhoun et al, eds. Head & Neck Surgery, Third Edition. Philadelphia: Lippincott Williams & Wilkins, 2001.

FIG. 20-3A from Barat LM, Bloland PB. Drug resistance among malaria and other parasites. Infect Dis Clin North Am 1997;11:969–987.

FIG. 24-17 from Bartolomé B, Córdoba S, Nieto S, et al. Acute arsenic poisoning: clinical and histopathologic features. British Journal of Dermatology 1999; 141:1106-1109.

FIGS. 15-35A, 15-37, 15-57, 15-73A&B from Beaty JH, Kasser JR, eds. Rockwood and Wilkins' Fractures in Children, Fifth Edition. Philadelphia: Lippincott Williams & Wilkins, 2001.

FIGS. 7-8, 7-16B, 7-23B, 7-29, 32-2B from Becker AE, Anderson RH: Cardiac Pathology. New York: Raven Press, 1983.

FIGS. 1-1A-D, 1-5B, 1-7, 1-8, 1-9, 1-15, 5-1, 5-2, 5-3, 5-4A, 5-5, 5-8, 5-9, 5-10 (Courtesy of Dr. Allen W. Tarro), **5-12, 5-14B, 5-15, 5-16, 5-17, 5-18, 5-19B, 5-20, 5-21, 5-22, 5-25, 5-36, 5-37** (Courtesy of Dr. Jeremy Freeman), **5-41, 6-3, 6-11, 11-9, 16-6, 16-9B, 17-1B-D, 20-19A, 21-6A** (Courtesy of Dr. Sandy Sharp), **22-5D, 25-33B, 32-4B** from Benjamin B, Bingham B, Hawke M, Stammberger H. A Color Atlas of Otorhinolaryngology. Philadelphia: J.B. Lippincott Company, 1995. Artwork © Bruce Benjamin, Brian Bingham, Michael Hawke, and Heinz Stammberger.

FIGS. 4-4B, 4-29 from Benson WE, Jeffers JB. Blunt Trauma. In: Tasman W, Jaeger EA, eds. Duane's Clinical Ophthalmology. Philadelphia: Lippincott Williams & Wilkins, 1997.

FIG. 15-25 from Berger RA, Doyle JR, Botte MJ. Wrist. In: Doyle JR, Botte MJ, eds. Surgical Anatomy of the Hand and Upper Extremity. Philadelphia: Lippincott Williams & Wilkins, 2003.

FIGS. 26-7A&B from Bickley LS, Hoekelman, eds. Bates' Guide to Physical Examination and History Taking, Seventh Edition. Philadelphia: Lippincott, Williams & Wilkins, 1999.

FIG. 20-6 from Binotto MA, Guilherme L, Tanaka AC, Rheumatic Fever. Images Paediatr Cardiol 2002;11:12-25.

FIG. 24-32 from H.C. "Skip" Bittenbender, PhD, and the Farmer's Bookshelf, College of Tropical Agriculture and Human Resources, University of Hawaii at Manoa [http://www.CTAHR.Hawaii.edu/fb/]

FIG. 3-13 from Blume WT, Kaibara M, Young GB. Atlas of Adult Electroencephalography. Philadelphia: Lippincott Williams & Wilkins, 2002.

FIG. 30-15 from Borak J, Diller WF. Phosgene exposure: mechanisms of injury and treatment strategies. J Occup Envir Med 2001;43:110–119.

FIG. 3-14A from Britt RH, Enzmann DR. Clinical stages of human brain abscesses on serial CT scans after contrast infusion. Computerized tomographic, neuropathological, and clinical correlations. J Neurosurg 1983; 59(6):972-89.

FIGS. 3-29, 3-30, 15-20, 15-22A&B, 15-23A&B, 15-39, 15-50A&B, 15-56A-C, 17-21A&B from Bucholz RW, Heckman JD, eds. Rockwood and Green's Fractures in Adults, Fifth Edition. Philadelphia: Lippincott Williams & Wilkins, 2002.

FIG. 24-53 from Burneo JG, Anandan JV, Barkley GL. A prospective study of the incidence of the purple glove syndrome. Epilepsia 2001;42:1156–1159.

FIG. 3-6 from Cannon ML, Antonio BL, McCloskey JJ, Hines MH, Tobin JR, Shetty AK. Pediatr Cavernous sinus thrombosis complicating sinusitis. Crit Care Med 2004;5(1):86–8.

FIGS. 19-8B, 20-7C, 30-9B Courtesy of the Centers for Disease Control.

FIGS. 20-14, 20-16 Courtesy of the Centers for Disease Control's Division of Vector-Borne Infectious Diseases.

FIG. 7-27 from Chatterjee K, et al. Cardiology: An Illustrated Text-Reference. New York: Gower, 1992.

FIG. 13-12 from Richard Fischer, MD, and eMedicine.com, Inc., 2003.

FIG. 9-1 from Cohen ME, Kegel JG. Candy cocaine esophagus. Chest 2002;121:1701–1703.

FIG. 5-4B from Cotton RT, Myer CM III. Practical Pediatric Otolaryngology. Lippincott Williams & Wilkins, 1998.

FIGS. 2-3, 25-1B from Dart RC, ed. Medical Toxicology, Third Edition. Philadelphia: Lippincott Williams & Wilkins, 2004.

FIGS. 7-1B&C, 7-2B from Davies MJ. Atlas of Coronary Artery Disease. Philadelphia: Lippincott-Raven, 1998.

FIGS. 14-10, 14-21, 15-51, 25-17, and **25-28** from Dockery GL, Crawford ME. Color Atlas of Foot & Ankle Dermatology. Philadelphia: Lippincott-Raven, 1999.

FIG. 24-20 from Donnelly R. Methemoglobinemia. NEJM 2000;343:337. Copyright © 2000 Massachusetts Medical Society. All rights reserved.

FIGS. 11-7A, 12-3B, 13-1B-D, 13-8A&B, 13-9, 13-10, 13-14A from Doubilet PM, Benson CB. Atlas of Ultrasound in Obstetrics and Gynecology: A Multimedia Reference. Philadelphia: Lippincott Williams & Wilkins, 2003.

FIG. 18-2 from Dudgeon DL, Kellogg DR, Gilchrist GS, et al. Purpura fulminans. Arch Surg 1971;103:351–358. © 1971, AMA.

FIG. 24-33 from Glenn Everett. Khat wrapped in banana leaves and smuggled in a suitcase. Microgram Bulletin 2002;35:237.

FIGS. 1-5C&D, 10-9A&B, 10-14, 14-12, 16-22, 16-28A&B, 16-47, 16-48, 17-45A&B, 25-10, 25-23, 30-17 from Fleisher GR, Ludwig S, Baskin MN, eds. Atlas of Pediatric Emergency Medicine. Philadelphia: Lippincott Williams & Wilkins, 2004.

FIGS. 8-11, 10-5A&B, 10-15, 16-34, 16-36A, 16-39A&B, 20-13A&B, 20-30 from Fleisher GR, Ludwig S, Henretig FM, Ruddy RM, Silverman BK, eds. Textbook of Pediatric Emergency Medicine, Fourth Edition. Philadelphia: Lippincott Williams & Wilkins, 2000.

FIGS. 30-12, 30-17 from Foroutan A. Medical Review of Iraqi Chemical Warfare. Teheran: Baqiyatallah University of Medical Sciences (In Persian), 2003.

FIGS. 7-2A, 7-3A, 7-32, 7-33A&B, 7-35, 7-37, 7-38A-D, 7-40, 8-2B, 22-8, 22-17B, 24-23A-C from Fowler NO. Clinical Electrocardiographic Diagnosis: A Problem-Based Approach. Philadelphia: Lippincott Williams & Wilkins, 2000.

FIG. 29-1 from Gestring ML, Geller ER, Akkad N, Bongiovanni PJ. Shotgun slug injuries: case report and literature review. J Trauma 1996;40:650–653.

FIG. 8-17 from George RB, Light RW, Matthay MA, Matthay RA, eds. Chest Medicine: Essentials of Pulmonary and Critical Care Medicine, Fourth Edition. Philadelphia: Lippincott Williams & Wilkins, 2000.

FIGS. 10-11, 12-4, 12-6, 12-8, 12-10, 13-3, 14-1, 14-17, 14-27, 14-29, 14-30, 14-37A, 14-43, 14-44, 14-47, 14-53, 16-5B, 16-7, 16-8B, 16-12A-C, 16-13B, 16-14, 16-17B, 20-2A&D, 20-33, 22-4, 24-51A, 24-52, 25-9B, 26-8, 27-4A, 33-7, 33-9 from Goodheart HP. Goodheart's Photoguide to Common Skin Disorders, Diagnosis and Management, Second Edition. Philadelphia: Lippincott Williams & Wilkins, 2003.

FIG. 10-12B from Graham SD Jr, Glenn JF, eds. Glenn's Urologic Surgery, Fifth Edition. Philadelphia: Lippincott Williams & Wilkins, 1998.

FIG. 9-46 from Greenfield LJ, Mulholland MW, Oldham KT, Zelenock GB, Lillemoe KD, eds. Surgery: Scientific Principles and Practice, Third Edition. Philadelphia: Lippincott Williams & Wilkins, 2001.

FIGS. 18-2A, 21-3, 21-5, 24-57, 27-1B from Greer JP, Foerster J, Lukens JN, Rodgers GM, Paraskevas F, Glader BE, eds. Wintrobe's Clinical Hematology, Eleventh Edition. Philadelphia: Lippincott Williams & Wilkins, 2003.

FIGS. 3-14B (Courtesy of Joo Ho Sung), **3-22B** from Griggs RC, Joynt RJ, eds. Baker and Joynt's Clinical Neurology, 2003 Edition. Philadelphia: Lippincott Williams & Wilkins, 2003.

FIGS. 8-3D, 20-1, 25-21, 26-11 from Habif TP. Clinical Dermatology: A Color Guide to Diagnosis and Therapy. Philadelphia: Mosby, 2004.

FIGS. 14-40, 21-4A and **21-7A** from Handin RI, Lux SE, Stossel TP, eds. Blood: Principles and Practice of Hematology, Second Edition. Philadelphia: Lippincott Williams & Wilkins, 2003.

FIGS. 3-28, 16-10, 17-8, 17-16, 26-17, 33-8A&B from Harris JH Jr., Harris WH. The Radiology of Emergency Medicine, Fourth Edition. Philadelphia: Lippincott Williams & Wilkins, 2000.

FIG. 17-18A from Harwood-Nuss A, Wolfson AB, Linden CH, Shepherd SM, Stenklyft PH, eds. The Clinical Practice of Emergency Medicine, Third Edition. Philadelphia: Lippincott Williams & Wilkins, 2001.

FIG. 20-35B from Hendrickson RG, Olshaker J, Duckett O. Rhinocerebral mucormycosis: a case of a rare but deadly disease. Journal of Emergency Medicine, V17: 641-645, 1999, with permission from Elsevier.

FIG. 25-20B from © Hogle Zoo, Salt Lake City, UT. http://www.hoglezoo.org.

FIGS. 23-4, 23-9, 23-10, 23-11 from Hunder GG. Atlas of Rheumatology, 3rd Ed. Philadelphia: Current Medicine, Inc., 2001.

FIGS. 7-5B (Courtesy of Joel M. Felner, MD, Atlanta, GA), **7-6C, 7-7B** (Courtesy of Stephen D. Clements, Jr., MD, Atlanta, GA), **7-9A** (Courtesy of Michael Van Aman, MD, Columbus, OH), **7-9B, 7-21, 7-25B** (Courtesy of the X-ray Department, Henrietta Egleston Hospital for Children, Atlanta, GA), **7-26A, 7-28A, 7-30, 9-32, 17-28, 22-4C, 22-5C** from Hurst JW, Alpert JS. Diagnostic Atlas of the Heart. New York: Raven Press, 1994.

FIGS. 3-5, 7-4B&C, 7-10B, 7-13, 7-14, 7-15, 7-16A (Courtesy of Robert G. Sybers, MD and Wade H. Shuford, MD, Atlanta, GA), **7-23A** (Courtesy of Robert G. Sybers, MD and Wade H. Shuford, MD, Atlanta, GA), **7-24A, 7-25A, 7-26B, 8-2C, 8-3C, 16-50B** from Hurst JW. Atlas of the Heart. New York: Gower, 1988.

FIGS. 8-1C, 8-2A from Hurst JW, ed. The Heart, 6th Edition. New York: McGraw-Hill, 1986.

FIG. 20-10B from Isaacs L. Necrotizing Fasciitis: Diagnosis and Treatment. Emergency Medicine News 2002;XXIV(8):4.

FIG. 32-5 from Jensenius M. A heroin user with a wobbly head. Lancet 2000;356:1160.

FIGS. 16-30B, 17-4, 18-3, 18-4, 28-3, 34-3B, 34-4C, 34-5C from Jones NL. Atlas of Forensic Pathology. Philadelphia: Lippincott Williams & Wilkins, 1996

FIGS. 1-19, 7-3B, 7-7A, 23-20B from Kassner EG. Atlas of Radiologic Imaging. New York: Gower, 1989.

FIG. 33-6 from Katz MH, Greenspan D, Westenhouse J, et al: Progression to AIDS in HIV infected homosexual and bisexual men with hairy leukoplakia and oral candidiasis. AIDS 1992;6:95–100.

FIG. 5-13 from Khalak R. Images in clinical medicine: cauliflower ear. N Engl J Med 1996;335:339. Copyright 1996 Massachusetts Medical Society. All rights reserved.

FIGS. 23-2B, 23-15, 23-16 from Koopman WJ, ed. Arthritis and Allied Conditions: A Textbook of Rheumatology, 14th Ed. Philadelphia: Lippincott Williams & Wilkins, 2001.

FIG. 17-46 adapted from Koraitim MM. Pelvic fracture urethral injuries: the unresolved controversy. J Urol 1999; 16:1443–1441.

FIGS. 4-13B&C from Kostick DA, Linberg JV. Lacrimal Gland Tumors. In: Tasman W, Jaeger EA, eds. Duane's Clinical Ophthalmology. Philadelphia: Lippincott Williams & Wilkins, 1995.

FIG. 15-35B from Koval KJ, Zuckerman JD, eds. Atlas of Orthopaedic Surgery: A Multimedia Reference. Philadelphia: Lippincott Williams & Wilkins, 2004.

FIG. 16-3 from CW Leung, Department of Pediatrics and Adolescent Medicine, Princess Margaret Hospital, Lai Chi Kok, Kowloon, Hong Kong.

FIGS. 33-3A&B from Mandell GL, Mildvan D, eds. Atlas of AIDS, Third Edition. Philadelphia: Current Medicine, Inc., 2001.

FIGS. 6-1, 11-2B, 11-3B, 11-4, 12-12, 20-5, 20-31A, 30-10 (Courtesy of K. Johnson, MD), **33-10B** from Mandell GL, ed. Essential Atlas of Infectious Diseases, Second Edition. Philadelphia: Current Medicine, Inc., 2001.

FIG. 10-24 from Massry SG, Glassock RJ, eds. Massry & Glassock's Textbook of Nephrology, Fourth Edition. Philadelphia: Lippincott Williams & Wilkins, 2000.

FIG. 30-6 from Mayer TA, Bersoff-Matcha S, Murphy C, et al. Clinical presentation of inhalational anthrax following bioterrorism exposure. JAMA 2001;286:2549–2553. Copyright 2001 American Medical Association. All rights reserved.

FIG. 33-11 from McClatchey KD, ed. Clinical Laboratory Medicine, Second Edition. Philadelphia: Lippincott Williams & Wilkins, 2002.

FIG. 15-83 MediClip image. Copyright 2003 Lippincott Williams & Wilkins. All rights reserved.

FIG. 16-21 from O'Doherty N. Atlas of the Newborn. Philadelphia: JB Lippincott, 1979:32

FIG. 15-70A from Ogden JA. Skeletal Injury in the Child, 2nd Edition. Philadelphia: WB Saunders, 1990.

FIGS. 29-2A-C and **34-12** from Olshaker JS, Jackson MC, Smock WS, eds. Forensic Emergency Medicine. Philadelphia: Lippincott Williams & Wilkins, 2001.

FIGS. 5-31, 7-24C-E, 8-13B, 12-1, 12-7 (Courtesy of Dr. William Henessy), **14-33, 16-5A, 16-23, 16-25, 19-1, 20-7A, 20-11, 20-12, 20-17A, 20-19B&C, 20-26, 20-28** (Courtesy of Dr. Mitchell Friedlaender), **20-32** (Courtesy of Alson E. Braley), **20-35A, 20-36, 23-7, 23-14A, 23-17, 23-19, 26-9, 26-10, 30-7A&B, 30-8A-C** (A&C, Courtesy of Dr. Paul Fasal), **33-5, 33-10A** (Courtesy of Dr. Jane Rosensweig) from Ostler HB, Maibach HI, Hoke AW, Schwab IR. Diseases of the Eye and Skin: A Color Atlas. Philadelphia: Lippincott Williams & Wilkins, 2004.

FIGS. 1-13A-E, 16-1B, 22-6C, 31-1B from Ovassapian A. Fiberoptic Endoscopy and the Difficult Airway, Second Edition. Philadelphia: Lippincott-Raven, 1996.

FIG. 17-30 from Peitzman AB, Rhodes M, Schwab CW, Yealy DM, Fabian T. The Trauma Manual, Second Edition. Philadelphia: Lippincott Williams & Wilkins, 2002.

FIGS. 7-28B, 7-41 from Perkin GD, Blackwood W, Rose FC, Shawdon HH. Atlas of Clinical Neurology. New York: Gower, 1986.

FIG. 26-1 from Perkins ES, Hansell P. An Atlas of Diseases of the Eye, 2nd Ed. Baltimore: Williams & Wilkins, 1971.

FIG. 3-10 from Plum F, Posner JB. The Diagnosis of Stupor and Coma, Third Edition. New York: Oxford University Press, 1982.

FIG. 26-4B from Proust AF. Special injuries of the hand. Emerg Med Clin North Am 1993;11:770.

FIG. 24-18 from Putnam JJ. Quicksilver and slow death. National Geographic 1972;142:507.

FIG. 8-5 from Rainer TH, Cameron PA, Smit D, et al. Evaluation of WHO criteria for identifying patients with severe acute respiratory syndrome out of the hospital: prospective observational study. BMJ 2003;326:1354–1358.

FIGS. 3-2B, 16-12D, 34-3A, 34-4A&B, 34-5A&B, 34-6A-C, 34-7A&B, 34-8A-D, 34-10A-F, and **34-11A-G** from Reece RM, Ludwig S, eds. Child Abuse: Medical Diagnosis and Management, Second Edition. Philadelphia: Lippincott Williams & Wilkins, 2001.

FIG. 12-11B from Rein MF. In: Holmes KK et al, eds. Sexually Transmitted Diseases. New York: McGraw-Hill, 1984.

FIG. 26-2 from Roberts James R. Minor Burns: Tar, Cement, and Chemicals. Emergency Medicine News 2003;XXV(5):20–23.

FIG.15-38 from Roberts JR. Olecranon Bursitis: The Technique of Bursal Aspiration. Emergency Medicine News 2002;24(12):20-21

FIGS. 15-6A&B, 15-26A&B, 15-38A&B, 15-78, 17-56, 26-2 from Roberts JR. Robert's Practical Guide to Common Medical Emergencies. Philadelphia: Lippincott-Raven, 1996.

FIGS. 26-12, 26-13, 26-14, 26-15 (B, Courtesy of Ben Felson, M.D., University of Cincinnati), **26-16, 26-21** from Rom WN, ed. Environmental & Occupational Medicine, 3rd Ed. Philadelphia: Lippincott-Raven, 1998.

FIG. 25-1A Copyright Rocky Mountain Poison Center, Dean Olsen.

FIG. 13-2 from Rubin E, Farber JL. Pathology, 3rd Edition. Philadelphia: Lippincott Williams & Wilkins, 1999.

FIG. 24-8A from Rumack BH, Matthew H. Acetaminophen poisoning and toxicity. Pediatrics 1975;55:871.

FIG. 24-19 from Rusyniak DE, Furbee RB, Kirk MA. Thallium and arsenic poisoning in a small midwestern town. Ann Emerg Med. 2002 Mar;39(3):307–11. Copyright 2002 The American College of Emergency Physicians.

FIGS. 11-5B&C, 11-8, 13-1A from Sauerbrei EE, Nguyen KT, Nolan RL. A Practical Guide to Ultrasound in Obstetrics and Gynecology, Second Edition. Philadelphia: Lippincott-Raven, 1998.

FIG. 7-12 from Safi JH, Winnerkvist A, Miller CC 3rd, et al. Effect of extended cross-clamp time during thoracoabdominal aneurysm repair. Ann Thorac Sur 1998;66:1204–1209.

FIG. 3-15 from Scheld WM, Whitley RJ, Marra CM, eds. Infections of the Central Nervous System, Third Edition. Philadelphia: Lippincott Williams & Wilkins, 2004.

FIG. 1-16, 13-14B from Schwartz GR, ed. Principles and Practice of Emergency Medicine, Fourth Edition. Philadelphia: Lippincott Williams & Wilkins, 1999.

FIG. 9-12C from Schwartz MD, Morgan BW. Massive Verapamil Pharmacobezoar Resulting In Esophageal Perforation. Int J Med Toxicol 2004;7(1):4.

FIG. 26-4A from Seiler JG III. Essentials of Hand Surgery. Philadelphia: Lippincott Williams & Wilkins, 2001.

FIG. 16-40 from Shah B, Laude T. Atlas of Pediatric Clinical Diagnosis. Philadelphia: WB Saunders, 2000.

FIG. 14-37B from Skarin AT. Atlas of Diagnostic Oncology. New York: Gower, 1991.

FIG. 14-39 from The Skin Cancer Foundation, New York, NY. Basal Bell Carcinoma. The Most Common Skin Cancer. Copyright © 1986, Revised 1999.

FIG. 20-3B from Smith JW et al. Diagnostic Medical Parasitology: Blood and Tissue Parasites. Chicago: American Society of Clinical Pathologists, 1976.

FIGS. 20-15, 20-22, 20-23, 20-25 from Smith JW, Ash LR, Thompson JH Jr. et al: Intestinal helminths. In: Atlas of Diagnostic Medical Parasitology Series. Chicago: American Society of Clinical Pathologists, 1984.

FIGS. 7-24B, 23-1, 23-6, 23-13A, 23-14B, 23-18, from Sontheimer RD, Provost TT, eds. Cutaneous Manifestations of Rheumatic Diseases, Second Edition. Philadelphia: Lippincott Williams & Wilkins, 2004.

FIGS. 15-12, 16-16, 16-36B, 16-51 from Staheli. The Practice of Pediatric Orthopedics. Philadelphia: Lippincott Williams & Wilkins, 2001.

FIG. 17-13 from Sumchai A, Sternback G. Hangman's fracture in a 7-week-old infant. Ann Emerg Med 1991;20:87

FIGS. 6-12, 11-2A, 11-3A, 12-9C from Sweet RL, Gibbs, RS. Atlas of Infectious Diseases of the Female Genital Tract. Philadelphia: Lippincott Williams & Wilkins, 2004.

FIGS. 1-14, 15-1A, 16-9A, 16-20, 17-34, 24-7A&B, from Swischuk LE. Emergency Imaging of the Acutely Ill or Injured Child. Philadelphia: Lippincott Williams & Wilkins, 2000.

FIGS. 3-19, 3-20, 3-23, 3-24, 3-25, 3-26, 4-2, 4-3, 4-5, 4-6, 4-7 (Courtesy of William C. Benson, MD, Philadelphia, PA), **4-8, 4-11, 4-13A, 4-14, 4-15, 4-16, 4-17B, 4-18, 4-19, 4-20, 4-21, 4-23, 4-25A, 4-27, 4-28, 4-30, 4-31, 4-32, 4-33, 4-34, 4-35, 4-36, 4-38, 4-39, 4-41, 4-43, 4-45, 4-46, 4-47, 5-7, 14-52, 17-9B, 19-13B, 22-5A&B, 22-6A, 23-8A, 24-12, 27-3, 30-5, 32-2A** from Tasman W, Jaeger EA, eds. The Wills Eye Hospital Atlas of Clinical Ophthalmology, Second Edition. Philadelphia: Lippincott Williams & Wilkins, 2001.

FIGS. 24-34A&B, 24-35, 24-36, 24-37, 24-38, 24-40, 24-41A from U.S. Drug Enforcement Agency.

FIG. 1-10 Copyright 2004, Ron M. Walls, MD, used with permission.

FIGS. 1-11, 1-12A&B Copyright 2004, Ron M. Walls, MD and STRATUS Center for Medical Simulation, Bringham and Women's Hospital, used with permission.

FIGS. 25-2, 25-4 Copyright Dr. Julian White.

FIGS. 20-7B, 30-11A Courtesy of the World Health Organization.

FIGS. 5-33, 5-35, 9-2A&B, 9-3D (Courtesy of Drs. Anna Sasaki and Daniel Zovich), **9-3E, 9-4, 9-5, 9-6A&B, 9-7B, 9-8, 9-9, 9-12B, 9-13** (Courtesy of Dr. James DiSario), **9-14A&B, 9-18, 9-19, 9-20B, 9-23B, 9-24A&B, 9-25A&B, 9-26, 9-27, 9-30A&B, 9-31, 9-33A&B** (A, Courtesy of Jeffrey P. Callen), **9-35B&C, 9-36C, 9-37A-D** (C, Courtesy of Harold Schwartz, MD; D, Courtesy of Caroline Taylor, MD), **9-38** (Courtesy of Dr. Randall Radin, University of Southern California), **9-39** (Courtesy of Dr. Sue Ellen Hanks, University of Southern California), **9-40B-F, 9-43, 9-44, 9-45A&B, 9-47, 9-48, 12-5, 12-9B, 16-11, 16-41, 20-9B&C, 20-20** (Courtesy of Patrick Murray, Ph.D.), **20-21, 20-24** (Courtesy of Richard L. Guerrant, MD, Charlottesville, VA), **20-27A-C** (A, Courtesy of Patrick Murray, Ph.D.), **21-1A-C, 22-18, 23-12A, 24-8B, 24-9B, 26-6A&B, 27-1A, 27-2, 33-12, 33-14** from Yamada T, Alpers DH, Kaplowitz N, Laine L, Owyang C, Powell DW, eds. Atlas of Gastroenterology, Third Edition. Philadelphia: Lippincott Williams & Wilkins, 2003.

FIGS. 25-5, 25-11, 25-13, 25-14, 25-15, 25-19B © Robert Yin 2004.

INDEX

Page numbers followed by *f* refer to figures.

B

C

D

E

F

G

H

I

J

K

L

M

O

P

Q

R

S

T

U

V

W

X

Y

Z